AF785260

Salmonella in Domestic Animals

2nd Edition

FSC
www.fsc.org
MIX
Paper from responsible sources
FSC® C013604

Salmonella in Domestic Animals

2nd Edition

Edited by

Paul A. Barrow

School of Veterinary Medicine and Science, University of Nottingham, UK

and

U. Methner

Friedrich-Loeffler-Institute, Institute of Bacterial Infections and Zoonoses, Germany

www.cabi.org

Front cover photo courtesy of Elisabeth Liebler-Tenorio and Ulrich Methner.

Cover design by Wolfram Maginot, Friedrich-Loeffler-Institute, Jena, Germany.

CABI is a trading name of CAB International

CABI Head Office
Nosworthy Way
Wallingford
Oxfordshire OX10 8DE
UK

Tel: +44 (0)1491 832111
Fax: +44 (0)1491 833508
E-mail: info@cabi.org
Website: www.cabi.org

CABI North American Office
38 Chauncey Street
Suite 1002
Boston, MA 02111
USA

Tel: +1 800 552 3083 (toll free)
Fax: +1 (0)617 395 4051
E-mail: cabi-nao@cabi.org

© CAB International 2013 (Chapters 1–11 and 13–25) © Crown copyright 2013 (Chapter 12). Reproduced with the permission of the Controller of Her Majesty's Stationery Office/Queen's Printer for Scotland and Animal Health and Veterinary Laboratories Agency. All rights reserved. No part of this publication may be reproduced in any form or by any means, electronically, mechanically, by photocopying, recording or otherwise, without the prior permission of the copyright owners.

A catalogue record for this book is available from the British Library, London, UK.

Library of Congress Cataloging-in-Publication Data

Salmonella in domestic animals. -- 2nd edition / edited by P.A. Barrow and U. Methner.
p. ; cm.
Includes bibliographical references and index.
ISBN 978-1-84593-902-1 (alk. paper)
1. Salmonella infections in animals. 2. Domestic animals. I. Barrow, P. A., editor of compilation. II. Methner, U. (Ulrich), editor of compilation.
[DNLM: 1. Salmonella Infections, Animal. 2. Animals, Domestic.
3. Salmonella--pathogenicity. SF 809.S24]

SF809.S24S25 2013
636.089'6927--dc23

2012049903

ISBN-13: 978 1 84593 902 1

Commissioning editor: Rachel Cutts
Editorial assistant: Alexandra Lainsbury
Production editor: Shankari Wilford

Typeset by AMA DataSet Ltd, Preston
Printed and bound in the UK by CPi Group (UK) Ltd, Croydon, CR0 4YY

Contents

The colour plate section can be found following p. 68

Contributors

Muna F. Anjum, Animal Health Veterinary Laboratories Agency, Weybridge Laboratory, Woodham Lane, New Haw, Addlestone, Surrey KT15 3NB, UK. E-mail: muna.anjum@ahvla.gsi.gov.uk

Robert J. Atterbury, School of Veterinary Medicine and Science, University of Nottingham, Sutton Bonington, Loughborough, LE12 5RD, Leicestershire, UK. E-mail: robert.atterbury@nottingham.ac.uk

Paul A. Barrow, School of Veterinary Medicine and Science, University of Nottingham, Sutton Bonington Campus, Sutton Bonington, Loughborough, Leicestershire LE12 5RD, UK. E-mail: paul.barrow@nottingham.ac.uk

Andreas J. Bäumler, Department of Medical Microbiology and Immunology, School of Medicine, University of California at Davis, One Shields Ave., Davis, CA 95616, USA. E-mail: ajbaumler@ucdavis.edu

Angela Berndt, Institute of Molecular Pathogenesis at the Friedrich-Loeffler-Institute, Federal Research Institute for Animal Health, Naumburger Str. 96a, D-07743 Jena, Germany. E-mail: angela.berndt@fli.bund.de

Filip Boyen, Laboratory of Veterinary Bacteriology and Mycology, Department of Pathology, Bacteriology and Avian Diseases, Faculty of Veterinary Medicine, Ghent University, Salisburylaan 133, B9820 Merelbeke, Belgium. E-mail: Filip.boyen@UGent.be

Malcolm A. Cobb, School of Veterinary Medicine and Science, University of Nottingham, Sutton Bonington Campus, Loughborough, Leicestershire LE12 5RD, UK. E-mail: malcom.cobb@nottingham.ac.uk

Robert W. Crawford, Department of Medical Microbiology and Immunology, School of Medicine, University of California at Davis, One Shields Ave., Davis, CA 95616, USA. E-mail: rwcrawford@ucdavis.edu

Robert H. Davies, Animal Health Veterinary Laboratories Agency, Weybridge Laboratory, Woodham Lane, New Haw, Addlestone, Surrey KT15 3NB, UK. E-mail: rob.davies@ahvla.gsi.gov.uk

Kris De Smet, SANCO, European Commission, Rue Belliard 232, 1049 Brussels, Belgium. E-mail: Kris.De-Smet@ec.europa.eu

Séamus Fanning, UCD Centre for Food Safety, School of Public Health, Physiotherapy & Population Science, UCD Veterinary Sciences Centre, University College Dublin, Belfield, Dublin 4, Ireland. E-mail: sfanning@ucd.ie

Neil Foster, School of Veterinary Medicine and Science, University of Nottingham, Sutton Bonington Campus, Loughborough, Leicestershire LR12 5RD, UK. E-mail: n.foster@nottingham.ac.uk
Jeffrey T. Gray, Office of the Vice President for Research, Des Moines University, Des Moines, Iowa 50312, USA. E-mail: Jeffrey.GrayPhD@dmu.edu
Freddy Haesebrouck, Laboratory of Veterinary Bacteriology and Mycology, Department of Pathology, Bacteriology and Avian Diseases, Faculty of Veterinary Medicine, Ghent University, Salisburylaan 133, B9820 Merelbeke, Belgium. E-mail: Freddy.Haesebrouck@UGent.be
Hafez Mohamed Hafez, Free University of Berlin, Department of Veterinary Medicine, Institute of Poultry Diseases, Königsweg 63, 14163 Berlin, Germany. E-mail: hafez@zedat.fu-berlin.de
Ruth Hall, School of Molecular Bioscience, The University of Sydney, NSW 2006, Australia. E-mail: Ruth.hall@sydney.edu.au
Tom Humphrey, National Centre for Zoonosis Research, University of Liverpool, Leahurst Campus Neston, Wirral, CH64 7TE, UK. E-mail: tom.humphrey@liverpool.ac.uk
Fillip van Immerseel, Department of Pathology, Bacteriology and Avian Diseases, Ghent University, Merelbeke, Belgium. E-mail: filip.vanimmerseel@UGent.be
Michael A. Jones, School of Veterinary Medicine and Science, University of Nottingham, Sutton Bonington Campus, Sutton Bonington, Loughborough, Leicestershire LE12 5RD, UK. E-mail: michael.a.jones@nottingham.ac.uk
Pete Kaiser, The Roslin Institute and Royal (Dick) School of Veterinary Studies, University of Edinburgh, Easter Bush, Midlothian EH25 9RG, UK. E-mail: pete.kaiser@roslin.ed.ac.uk
Roberto La Ragione, Department of Microbial and Cellular Sciences, Faculty of Health and Medical Sciences, University of Surrey, Guildford, Surrey GU2 7XH, UK. E-mail: r.laragione@ahvla.defra.gsi.gov.uk; r.laragione@surrey.ac.uk
Pia Mäkelä, European Food Safety Authority, Biological Monitoring Unit, Via Carlo Magno 1/A, 1-43126 Parma, Italy. E-mail: pia.makela@efsa.europa.eu
Geoffrey Mead, Consultant, 17 Harbutts, Bathampton, Bath, Somerset BA2 6TA, UK. E-mail: mead.val@gmail.com
Hannah J. Metcalfe, Department of Pathology and Infectious Diseases, Royal Veterinary College, Hatfield, Hertfordshire, AL9 7TA, UK. E-mail: hjmetcalfe@gmail.com
Ulrich Methner, Institute of Bacterial Infections and Zoonoses at the Friedrich-Loeffler-Institute, Federal Research Institute for Animal Health, Naumburger Str. 96a, D-07743 Jena, Germany. E-mail: Ulrich.methner@fli.bund.de
Geovana Brenner Michael, Institute of Farm Animal Genetics at the Friedrich-Loeffler-Institute, Federal Research Institute for Animal Health, Höltystr. 10, D-31535 Neustadt, Germany. E-mail: geovana.michaelbrenner@fli.bund.de
Satheesh Nair, Health Protection Agency, Centre for Infections, Colindale, London, NW9 5EQ, UK. E-mail: Satheesh.Nair@hpa.org.uk
John E. Olsen, Department of Veterinary Disease Biology, University of Copenhagen, Stigbøjlen 4, DK-1870 Frederiksberg C. Denmark. E-mail: jeo@life.ku.dk
Frank Pasmans, Laboratory of Veterinary Bacteriology and Mycology, Department of Pathology, Bacteriology and Avian Diseases, Faculty of Veterinary Medicine, Ghent University, Salisburylaan 133, B9820 Merelbeke, Belgium. E-mail: frank.pasmans@UGent.be
Wolfgang Rabsch, National Reference Centre for Salmonella and other Enteric Pathogens at the Robert Koch Institute, Burgstrasse 37, D-38855 Wernigerode, Germany. E-mail: rabsch@rki.de
Andrew N. Rycroft, Royal Veterinary College, Hawkshead Lane, North Mymms, Hertfordshire, AL9 7TA, UK. E-mail: arycroft@rvc.ac.uk
Kenneth E. Sanderson, Department of Biological Sciences, University of Calgary, Calgary, Alberta T2N1N4, Canada. E-mail: kesander@ucalgary.ca

Stefan Schwarz, Institute of Farm Animal Genetics at the Friedrich-Loeffler-Institute, Federal Research Institute for Animal Health, Höltystr. 10, D-31535 Neustadt, Germany. E-mail: Stefan.schwarz@fli.bund.de

H.L. Shivaprasad, California Animal Health and Food Safety Laboratory System, Tulare Branch, University of California, Davis, 18830 Road 112, Tulare, CA 93274, USA. E-mail: hlshivaprasad@ucdavid.edu

Sandra Simon, National Reference Centre for Salmonella and other Enteric Pathogens at the Robert Koch Institute, Burgstrasse 37, D-38855 Wernigerode, Germany. E-mail: SimonS@rki.de

Jenny Stavisky, School of Veterinary Medicine and Science, University of Nottingham, Sutton Bonington Campus, Loughborough, Leicestershire LE12 5RD, UK. E-mail: jenny.stavisky@nottingham.ac.uk

Torsten Sterzenbach, Department of Medical Microbiology and Immunology, School of Medicine, University of California at Davis, One Shields Ave., Davis, CA 95616, USA. E-mail: tsterzenbach@ucdavis.edu

Mark Stevens, The Roslin Institute and Royal (Dick) School of Veterinary Studies, University of Edinburgh, Easter Bush, Midlothian EH25 9RG, UK. E-mail: mstevens3@exseed.ed.ac.uk

Nicholas R. Thomson, Wellcome Trust Sanger Laboratory, Hinxton Wellcome Trust Sanger Institute, Wellcome Trust Genome Campus, Hinxton, Cambridge CB10 1SA, UK. E-mail: nrt@sanger.ac.uk

John Timoney, Gluck Equine Research Centre, Department of Veterinary Science, University of Kentucky, Lexington, KY 40546-0099, USA. E-mail: jtimoney@uky.edu

Sergio Uzzau, Dipartimento di Scienze Biomediche, Centre for Biotechnology Development and Biodiversity Research, Università di Sassari, Italy. E-mail: uzzau@uniss.it

Bernardo Villarreal-Ramos, Animal Health and Veterinary Laboratories Agency (Weybridge), New Haw, Addlestone, Surrey KT15 3NB, UK. E-mail: bernardo.villarreal@ahvla.gsi.gov.uk

John Wain, The Norwich Medical School, University of East Anglia and The Laboratory of Gastrointestinal pathogens, HPA, Colindale London, UK. E-mail: john.wain@uea.ac.uk

Andrew Wales, Animal Health Veterinary Laboratories Agency, Weybridge Laboratory, Woodham Lane, New Haw, Addlestone, Surrey KT15 3NB, UK. E-mail: andywales@fastmail.fm

Dirk Werling, Department of Pathology and Infectious Diseases, Royal Veterinary College, Hatfield, Hertfordshire, AL9 7TA, UK. E-mail: dwerling@rvc.ac.uk

Martin Wierup, Department of Biomedical Sciences and Veterinary Public Health, Swedish University of Agricultural Sciences, P.O. Box 7028, 750 07 Uppsala, Sweden. E-mail: martin.wierup@bvf.slu.se

Sebastian E. Winter, Department of Medical Microbiology and Immunology, School of Medicine, University of California at Davis, One Shields Ave., Davis, CA 95616, USA. E-mail: sewinter@ucdavis.edu

Preface

Salmonella enterica subsp. *enterica* remains a major cause of infection and disease in man and animals worldwide. Much of the economic and public health problems arise from diseases of animals or disease-free carriage. In Europe animal salmonellosis as a cause of human infection became increasingly significant as agricultural production began to intensify after World War II. In the 1950s the rapid intensification of the poultry industry in many countries was supported by importation of dried fish meal from South America which contained many *Salmonella* serovars. Much more recently the pandemic involving several phage types of *S.* Enteritidis concentrated the minds of governments which introduced increased surveillance and control measures that have been successful in many countries.

The first edition of this book arose at a time when our understanding of the biology, genetics and immunology was expanding almost exponentially. These changes are continuing and it is a good time 13 years after the appearance of the first edition to stand back and review our knowledge of the organism together with current and new approaches to infection control.

Patterns of livestock production and movement are changing as the world is changing. Elevated wages in the West result in increased production in and importation of poultry meat and processed products from countries in South America and Asia. An improved standard of living in many countries is accompanied by increased meat consumption, mainly pork and poultry but also beef and dairy products. Regulation of meat production in many countries is improving but there are currently huge problems of antibiotic resistance which is becoming a global problem. Poor management and hygiene results in the transmission of many viral and bacterial pathogens of which *Salmonella* is just one. Other changes associated with increasing living standards in South America and Asia include the increasing importance of companion animals in people's lives which are well recognized as sources of infection.

In parallel with global changes in trade and human populations, improvements in technology have enabled us to gain an unprecedented understanding of the biology of *Salmonella*. *S.* Typhimurium has always been one of the key bacterial tools for geneticists with the additional targets of understanding the molecular basis of its physiology and virulence. Variations of random transposon and site-directed mutagenesis have been used extensively and during the last 10 years whole-genome expression studies have followed the increasing availability of the gold mines of whole genome sequences. However, many aspects of *Salmonella* biology and infection biology remain tantalizingly unresolved after the last 10 years of research, and more than 50 years after Professor Buxton's book (*Salmonellosis in Animals: A Review* (1957), CAB International) appeared, such that the organism should remain the focus of worldwide research activity for many more years. In many respects the study of this organism is now a global enterprise. Shrinking research budgets in the West have been replaced with increasing interest in those countries with increasing budgets and where an appreciation of the animal and public health *Salmonella* problem is increasing.

As with the first edition the second maintains its emphasis on the role of *Salmonella* in animal disease. The pattern follows that of the first edition with an initial section on the bacteriology of *Salmonella* to which we have added a chapter on genomes. The section on virulence is an area where the range of knowledge has exploded and we have also added a chapter on immunity. To the section on *Salmonella* infections in animals we have added a chapter on infection of exotic animals as some of these are playing an increasing significance as companion animals. The section on epidemiology and prevention additionally contains a chapter on the environment as a source of infection. We have also included a chapter on legislation because many countries for which *Salmonella* in animals is a relatively new problem may wish to study existing frameworks on which *Salmonella* control has been successfully based. We do not regard a book of this sort as the rightful place for chapters on developments in techniques for isolation, identification and other laboratory tests. These change by the year and are more appropriate for a technical manual and we have thus omitted them from this edition.

The contributing authors either have long experience of research in their own topic or have a particular insight into their subject. We hope that the non-lay public with scientific and/or professional interests in this organism will find the new edition a valuable addition to the *Salmonella* canon.

Paul A. Barrow
Ulrich Methner

1 Taxonomy and Species Concepts in the Genus *Salmonella*

Kenneth E. Sanderson[1]* and Satheesh Nair[2]

[1]*Department of Biological Sciences, University of Calgary, Canada;* [2]*Health Protection Agency, Centre for Infections, London, UK*

'When **I** use a word,' Humpty Dumpty said, in rather a scornful tone, 'it means just what I choose it to mean – neither more nor less.'

'The question is,' said Alice, 'whether you **can** make words mean so many different things.'

'The question is,' said Humpty Dumpty, 'which is to be master – that's all.'

From *Through the Looking Glass*, Lewis Carroll

Taxonomy of Bacteria

The word 'species' has been used by scientists for many years; different people use it with different meanings, and in some cases individuals may use it with different meanings when they use it for different organisms. As in Humpty Dumpty, there have been many arguments over whether it is possible to be master of the word. The use of the word has been especially controversial in bacteria. In this review, we will see how the word species has been used in *Salmonella* taxonomy.

Humans have an inherent desire to classify objects in the world around them, in order to make sense of the apparently chaotic diversity that surrounds us. A small child, even at the age of a year or so, will obsessively sort objects such as marbles into piles according to size and colour. Biologists apply the same obsession to sorting the astonishing diversity of the living world into units called 'taxa'; the hope is that this will help us to understand that diversity. This classification of the living world, though begun by others such as Aristotle, was codified and extended by C. Linnaeus in the 1600s. According to Linnaeus, the living world can be classified into species that are monotypic, immutable and that breed true (Rosselló-Mora and Amann, 2001). The original system of Linnaeus had five ranks: species were divided into subspecies, and the species were grouped into higher ranks of organisms including genera, orders and classes.

Though Darwin used the term in the title *On the Origin of Species*, he recognized that it had a very different meaning when used by different people at different times, for he wrote 'I look at the term species as one arbitrarily given for the sake of convenience to a set of individuals closely resembling each other, and that it does not essentially differ from the term variety' (Darwin, 1859). Taxonomists may take up the view of monism or pluralism; species monists believe that one species concept is correct for all organisms, while pluralists believe

* Corresponding author, e-mail: kesander@ucalgary.ca

© CAB International 2013. *Salmonella in Domestic Animals, 2nd Edition* (eds P.A. Barrow and U. Methner)

that different concepts are correct for different organisms (Doolittle and Zhaxybayeva, 2009; Ereshefsky, 2010a). Clearly, the species in prokaryotes is not the same as that of eukaryotes, so some form of pluralism must be applied.

Yet there are good arguments for maintaining the use of the term 'species' in bacteria as well as in other organisms, as summarized by Doolittle and Zhaxybayeva (2009) and by Ereshefsky (2010a, b). The use of species names is important in bacteria in many fields, including agriculture, biotechnology, food safety, disease diagnosis, epidemiology and public health and bioterrorism. It is desirable to attempt to apply the species name in a consistent and defendable way. But even where there is general agreement about the taxa and their relationships, there may be disagreement on which strains should be given the rank of species and thus how many species should be named. Perhaps the most dramatic differences between taxonomists who are called 'splitters' (who separate taxa into many species) and those who are 'lumpers' (who designate a small number of separate species) are found in taxonomists for *Salmonella*, where the splitters consider each serotype to be a separate species, so there would now be over 2600 species in *Salmonella* (Kauffmann, 1961), while the lumpers, according to the scheme now widely used, designate only two species, *Salmonella enterica* and *S. bongori* (Le Minor and Popoff, 1987; Reeves *et al.*, 1989).

For those interested in understanding the diversity of *Salmonella*, determining and naming species is only part of the problem, because even within the serovar there is a startling variety of phage types, biotypes, electrophoretic types, sequence types, haplotypes etc., which represent real diversity in the population; this diversity must be understood in order to approach epidemiology in an informed way.

It is argued that successive speciation events created the tree of life; this is the notion that organismal diversity can be organized as 'groups within groups', which are formed as lineages successively separate, which yields a tree-like structure. However, this tree of life, first described by Darwin (1859), may not apply to bacteria where lateral gene transfer is an important mode of variation, so strains may have two quite distinct parents (Doolittle and Zhaxybayeva, 2009).

Introduction to *Salmonella*

Salmonella belongs to the family *Enterobacteriaceae*, and is a medically important pathogen for both humans and animals. Its main niche is the intestinal tract of humans and animals (Le Minor, 1991).

Salmonellosis in humans and animals can be broadly classified into two groups: enteric fever (typhoidal) and non-typhoidal salmonellosis (NTS) (Langridge *et al.*, 2008). The disease can manifest itself in five ways: enteric fever, gastroenteritis, bacteraemia, extra-intestinal focal infection and a carrier state (Langridge *et al.*, 2008) (Fig. 1.1).

The Kauffman–White scheme, first published in 1929, currently divides *Salmonella* into more than 2600 serotypes based on their serological reactions to somatic lipopolysaccharide (O), flagellar (H) and capsular (Vi) antigens (Grimont and Weill, 2007). However, these *Salmonella* serotypes can also be subdivided into the three following host range types that also influence clinical manifestations/presentations (Uzzau *et al.*, 2000; Stevens *et al.*, 2009): (i) host generalist (ubiquitous serovars) include *Salmonella enterica* serovar Typhimurium (*S.* Typhimurium) and *S.* Enteritidis that cause infections in diverse human and animal hosts; they produce a range of clinical symptoms but mainly acute and self-limiting gastroenteritis (Fig. 1.1) (Le Minor, 1991; Langridge *et al.*, 2008; Stevens *et al.*, 2009); (ii) host-adapted *Salmonella* (confined to a small number of hosts) such as *S.* Dublin in bovine animals and *S.* Choleraesuis in swine results in systemic infections, but these serovars can also infect humans and a limited number of other species (Le Minor, 1991; Langridge *et al.*, 2008; Stevens *et al.*, 2009); (iii) host-restricted *Salmonella* are associated with severe systemic infections in a single host: *S.* Typhi and *S.* Paratyphi cause enteric fever exclusively in man while *S.* Typhisuis causes paratyphoid in swine, *S.* Gallinarum causes typhoid in fowl and *S.* Abortusovis causes abortions in sheep (Le Minor, 1991; Stevens *et al.*, 2009) (Fig.1.1).

Like many other infectious diseases, the course and outcome of the infection depends on variable factors including the dose of inoculation, the immune status of the host (age, underlying disease) and the genetic

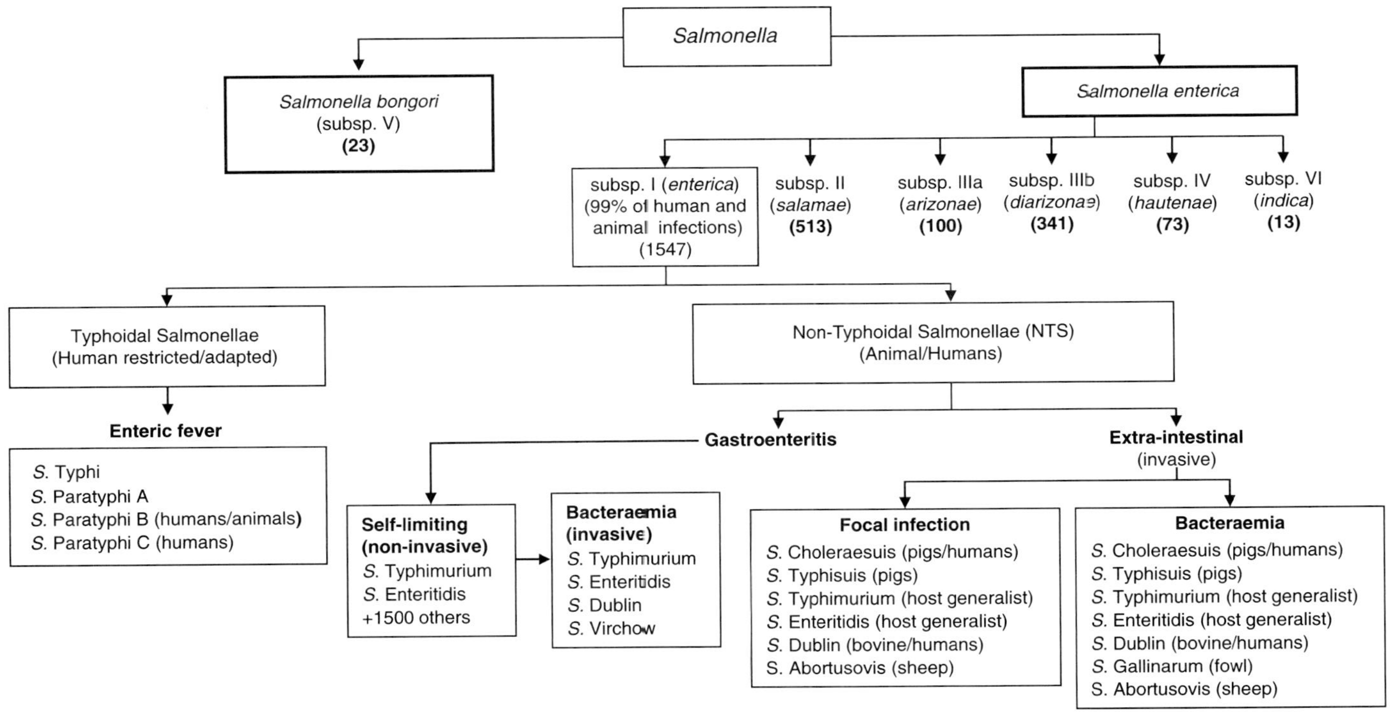

Fig. 1.1. Current scheme for classifying the genus *Salmonella*. Crosa *et al.* (1973) defined *Salmonella* to contain a single species, using DNA–DNA hybridization. A second species, designated *S. bongori*, was proposed by Reeves *et al.* (1989) using MLEE. *Salmonella* subspecies are defined by biotyping, DNA hybridization (Crosa *et al.*, 1973), 16sRNA analysis and MLEE (Reeves *et al.*, 1989). Serotyping is used to define serovars/serotypes within each subspecies. Numbers in brackets indicate the total number of serotypes included in each subspecies (Guibourdenche *et al.*, 2010). *Salmonella enterica* subsp. I is adapted to endotherms. Subspecies II is rarely found in humans but is commonly found in reptiles/ectotherms (Editorial team *et al.*, 2010). Subspecies IIIa and IIIb are naturally found in reptiles but human infections have increased in recent years due to reptiles being kept as pets (Schröter *et al.*, 2004; Editorial team *et al.*, 2010). Serotypes of subsp. IV and VI are rare and mainly found in reptiles; they seldom cause infections in humans (Editorial team *et al.*, 2010). *Salmonella bongori* is associated with ectotherms but has recently been isolated from endotherms (humans, birds) in Italy (Foti *et al.*, 2009). Common serotypes are listed, but other serotypes may cause bacteraemia or focal infections. Reproduced from Langridge, G.C., *et al.*, 2008. Invasive Salmonellosis in humans. Chapter 8.6.2.2 (revised version). In *EcoSal – Escherichia Coli and Salmonella: Cellular and Molecular Biology*. Böck, A., *et al.*, (eds). ASM Press, Washington, D.C., Figure 1.1. with permission from the American Society for Microbiology.

background of both the host and the infecting pathogen (e.g. virulence factors in the pathogen).

Species Concepts

We will consider, in our discussion of bacteria in general and of *Salmonella* in particular, three of the (several) species concepts that have been discussed in eukaryotes and also in bacteria (Doolittle and Zhaxybayeva, 2009; Ereshefsky, 2010a).

The ecotype species concept (ESC) (which yields the eco-species) was described by Cohan (2001); each cluster of strains corresponds to an ecotype, defined as a population of cells in the same ecological niche. The concept has roots in the history of microbiology, since bacteria were initially considered to be asexual clones; something resembling this concept was used to determine species in *Salmonella* starting in the 1880s, when species were named according to the disease they caused and the host they infected. The ecotype theory invokes periodic selection within the variants that arise by mutation in an asexual clone; the mutant that is selected will out-compete others in the population, and the genomes carrying the mutant will sweep to fixation along with the selected mutant (Cohan, 2001). Thus other diversity, that was neutral in the clone's members, will be purged. In this way, periodic selection limits variation in the genome and results in a population of cells that share a set of genes but are distinct from the population from which they were derived. Thus mutation (to produce variability) and selection both operate, but recombination has no role. In Cohan's view, the bacterial species as presently recognized are analogous to eukaryotic genera, rather than to eukaryotic species.

The second is the biological species concept (BSC) (which yields the bio-species), a concept developed by Ernst Mayr (1996) based on observations in higher animals. Since members of the bio-species reproduce by sexual mating and mate only (or preferentially) with members of the same species, they share a gene pool and the species maintains genetic cohesion. Bacteria were initially thought to be asexual; however, genetic recombination has been recognized in bacteria since the 1940s and 1950s (Lederberg and Tatum, 1946), but there are three differences between recombination in bacteria compared with those eukaryotes that reproduce sexually: reproduction in bacteria is due to binary fission, while sexual exchange if it occurs is (usually) rare and not linked to reproduction; there is only partial transfer of the genome of one parent, rather than fusion of gametes from both parents as in eukaryotes; genetic transfer in bacteria is unidirectional, with transfer from the donor to the recipient.

The total process of recombination in bacteria takes place in two steps; the first step is genetic transfer from donor to recipient to form a partial diploid zygote. The donor contribution may be a few kilobases in DNA-mediated transformation, or a few tens of kilobases in phage-mediated transduction, or up to hundreds of kilobases in plasmid-mediated conjugation (Snyder and Champness, 1997). The second step in the process is integration of the donor DNA into the recipient chromosome to restore the haploid state. (In some cases an intact replicon such as a plasmid is transferred, which does not have to integrate, but these cases are not further considered here.) Integration may occur by two different methods.

The first method is homologous recombination, which requires the RecA protein and occurs between regions of DNA in the donor and recipient that have a high degree of sequence identity: the allele from the donor replaces the allele of the recipient in a process called allelic replacement (Snyder and Champness, 1997). Thus, allelic replacement can insert genes from closely related bacteria but not from unrelated bacteria. Allelic replacement has the theoretical potential to form a gene pool with resulting genetic cohesion; members of this gene pool might form bio-species. We will see below that allelic replacement does occur in *S. enterica*.

The second method is site-specific recombination, which can insert fragments of DNA from the donor into the recipient chromosome by mechanisms that are not dependent on RecA protein and do not require DNA with high sequence identity (Nash, 1997). These site-specific mechanisms include insertion of prophages, transposons, or other DNA units. This results in lateral gene transfer (LGT) (also called horizontal gene transfer); it adds non-homologous blocks of DNA to the genome of a bacterium, in sizes ranging from a few kilobases to hundreds of kilobases. This process, like mutation, contributes to variation in the population, not to genetic cohesion as in allelic replacement, and therefore it would not contribute to forming bio-species. The consequence of LGT is that the genome of bacteria is composed of two types of genes: the core genome, which includes genes that are common to all the members of the group being studied, and the accessory genome, which includes genes that are missing from one or more of the members of the group being studied and which have resulted from LGT (Lan and Reeves, 2001). Thus, 89% of the genes of two serovars of *Salmonella*, Typhimurium strain LT2 (McClelland *et al.*, 2001) and Typhi strain CT18 (Parkhill *et al.*, 2001), are orthologues with nucleotide sequence identity usually higher than 99% (the core genome), while 11% of the genes do not have orthologues in the other member of the pair of serovars (the accessory genome). The core genome is not a fixed entity, but is determined by the strains being compared; as the number of strains in the comparison increases, the size of the core genome reduces and the size of the accessory genome increases. If all sequenced bacteria are included, the size of the core reduces to only about 20 genes, including only those involved in central processes such as replication and protein translation (Bapteste *et al.*, 2009). Taxonomic analysis usually studies the core genome, using sequence-based methods (such as multi-locus sequence typing, described below), though it can also study the accessory genome, using methods such as microarrays (Porwollik *et al.*, 2002).

The third concept is the phylogenetic species concept (PSC) that yields the phylo-species, in which the lineage of the cells is inferred from the degree of identity of nucleotide sequences. Strains that show >70% relatedness according to DNA–DNA hybridization (DDH) carried out under rigorously controlled conditions are placed in the same species according to many authorities including Staley (2006), though Crosa *et al.* (1973) consider >70% relatedness to indicate belonging to the genus *Salmonella*, and >80% belonging to the same species. Strains that have >97% identity in sequence of 16S rRNA are placed in the same species (Staley, 2006). Strains in which the average nucleotide identity (ANI) of all orthologues is >95% are considered members of the same species (Konstantinidis and Tiedje, 2005). Not surprisingly, use of different criteria such as 16S rRNA or ANI often yield a different answer as to where the species boundary should be placed. Whereas the eco-species is formed by the force of selection, and the bio-species is formed by the force of recombination (thus, each has a theoretical basis), the phylo-species is simply the result of a measurement of sequence divergence and does not, like the other two, have a theoretical basis. As we will see below, the genus *Salmonella* can be efficiently divided into a series of taxa with greater or lesser degrees of nucleotide sequence variation, but it is not clear how to separate these taxa into species. In practical terms, the system for designation of species that is actually used is a polyphasic system, in which more than one type of data is used, and sometimes more than one species concept is applied, especially with different strains of bacteria (Stackebrandt *et al.*, 2002).

It is not clear whether the concept of a tree of life, which is widely applied across the biological realm, can be applied to bacteria (Doolittle and Zhaxybayeva, 2009). If bacteria divided by binary fission, and no mutation, selection, or recombination occurred, the tree of life would look like a long narrow stick, with the very top of the stick being a homogeneous clone. If mutation by base pair change also occurred, but no selection or recombination, the tree would be flat-topped and featureless, because variation would be continuous and all the leaves on the flat top would be tiny clones. If mutation and selection occurred but no recombination, the flat top of the tree would be subdivided, as some variants are selected against while others survive; this is a simplified version of the ecotype theory, and the leaves of the tree would be eco-species. Finally, if genetic transfer also occurs, followed by homologous recombination and allelic exchange, it is possible that a bio-species of the type described in the BSC of higher animals might also be recognizable. A further complication is that genetic transfer may be followed by site-specific recombination and insertion of non-orthologous genes (i.e. by LGT) and not by homologous recombination and allelic exchange; in this case progeny have two quite unrelated parents, and the smoothly branching tree of life becomes a bush with many reticulations (Doolittle and Zhaxybayeva, 2009). The main objective of this review is to evaluate the application of these three species concepts to *Salmonella*.

Nomenclature in the Genus *Salmonella*

However, before going on to consider these three species concepts it is necessary to summarize the present situation of nomenclature in *Salmonella*. Le Minor and Popoff (1987) pointed out that the development of the taxonomy and nomenclature of the genus *Salmonella* may be considered to have evolved in four overlapping phases. The first taxonomy was based on the clinical role of *Salmonella* strains. The bacillus that causes typhoid was cultivated by Gaffky in 1884, after Eberth had observed the bacillus in spleen sections from a patient who died from typhoid (Grimont *et al.*, 2000). The strain we now recognize as the serotype Choleraesuis was isolated by Salmon and Smith from pigs, where it was thought to be the cause of hog cholera. Widal discovered that the serum of a typhoid patient agglutinated the typhoid bacillus; this led to development of the serodiagnostic 'Widal test' (Grimont *et al.*, 2000). In following years, *Salmonella* strains were isolated from many different clinical conditions and from many hosts; initially, these different isolates were often considered to be different species and given a range of names. But gradually it was realized that the same bacterium could cause similar, or sometimes different, clinical symptoms in different host species, and thereafter naming by host or clinical symptoms was largely abandoned.

In the second phase, taxonomy was based on antigenic specificities. Serological analysis emerged from the pioneering studies of White, amplified by Kauffmann to develop the Kauffmann–White scheme (Kauffmann, 1960). Each antigenically distinguishable *Salmonella* possesses a specific O (cell wall) and H (flagellar) antigen; many express alternate phase flagella of two antigenic types (H1 and H2) and a few produce Vi (capsular) antigen. Thus each *Salmonella* serotype is recognized by its unique combination of antigens (its antigenic formula) and each serotype was accorded species status (Kauffmann, 1961). For example, the antigenic formula for the serotype Typhimurium is 1,4,5,12:i:1,2. The four numbers before the colon indicate that the O-antigen has four antigenic factors; i indicates the antigenic factor of the phase 1 flagellar antigen and 1,2 the antigenic factors of the phase 2 flagellar antigen; the species name was *S. typhimurium*. Currently there are 67 O-antigens and 117 H-antigens that have been identified (Popoff, 2001; Grimont and Weill, 2007). Over 2600 serovars have been identified; the concept of 'one serovar-one species' became untenable because sometimes different serovars shared many traits and sometimes the serovar was found to be heterogeneous, thus the general opinion grew that serotypes do not merit species rank.

In the third phase, many taxonomists used a taxonomy based on biochemical tests. These tests include the ability to ferment sugars, or the presence of organic acids such as D-tartrate, or many other components. Typical biochemical reactions that are used for distinguishing species and subspecies are shown in Table 1.1 (Bale *et al.*, 2007). Using biochemical tests, three species were recognized by Borman *et al.* (1944), *S. choleraesuis*, *S. typhosa* and *S. kauffmannii* (with the last species including all serovars other than the first two). Kauffmann and Edwards (1952) made a similar proposal for three species, but replaced *S. kauffmannii* with *S. enterica*, and later Ewing replaced this over-arching species with the name *S. enteritidis* (Ewing, 1972). Kauffmann then divided the genus *Salmonella* on the basis of biochemical tests into four subgenera (I to IV), but continued to treat each serovar as a

Table 1.1. Typical biochemical reactions for species and subspecies differentiation (Bale *et al.*, 2007).

	S. enterica						
	Subspecies						*S. bongori*
Test or substrate	I	II	IIIa	IIIb	IV	VI	V
Dulcitol	+	+	–	–	–	d	+
Lactose	–	–	– (75%)	+ (75%)	–	d	–
ONPG	–	–	+	+	–	d	+
Salicin	–	–	–	–	+	–	–
Sorbitol	+	+	+	+	+	–	+
Malonate	–	+	+	+	–	–	–
Mucate	+	+	+	d	–	+	+
Gelatine	–	+	+	+	+	+	–
Growth in KCN	–	–	–	–	+	–	+

+: 90% or more positive reactions
–: 90% or more negative reactions
d: different reactions given by different serotypes

separate species. Le Minor *et al.* (1970) treated Kauffmann's subgenera as species *S. kauffmannii* (subgenus I), *S. salamae* (subgenus II), *S. arizonae* (subgenus III) and *S. houtenae* (subgenus IV). In 1980 the issue was further complicated, for the approved list of bacterial names included only *S. choleraesuis*, *S. enteritidis*, *S. typhi*, *S. typhimurium* (all members of subgenus I) and *S. arizonae* (Skerman *et al.*, 1980).

In the fourth phase, in recent years, taxonomy has been increasingly based on DNA relatedness. DDH studies showed that all *Salmonella* serovars that were tested formed a single DNA hybridization group, with all strains 70% to 100% related to each other, and much more closely related than to other genera; within this group seven subgroups were separated by studies of thermal stability of hybrids (Crosa *et al.*, 1973). There was good agreement between the DNA subgroups identified by DNA hybridization and the subgenera identified by Kauffmann based on biochemical tests, but subgenus III was separated into two groups. Assuming a strict interpretation of the Bacteriological Code, Le Minor *et al.* (1982) proposed the type species *S. choleraesuis* for the single *Salmonella* species and proposed six subspecies to which a seventh was shortly added.

It soon became obvious that this naming system suggested by Le Minor *et al.* (1982) based on knowledge current at the time, but also using a strict application of the Bacteriological Code, would lead to confusion when the species name (*choleraesuis*) was also used as a serovar name. For example, according to this system the name *S. choleraesuis* subsp. *choleraesuis* serovar Typhi refers to the serotype Typhi in subspecies I, which is limited to growth in humans where it causes a serious enteric infection, but the serovar Choleraesuis is quite different for it is adapted to growth in pigs where it causes acute infections but it also infects a range of animals including humans.

A proposal to emend the Code had been published and accepted, which defined a perilous name as 'a name, the application of which is likely to lead to accidents endangering health or life or both' (Rules Revision Committee, 1975). Le Minor and Popoff (1987) recognized that the name *S. choleraesuis*, which was being used as the name of the species to which most serovars belonged, would cause confusion not only for researchers but also for medical microbiologists and clinicians and could result in a health hazard. They therefore proposed that the species epithet should be changed to *Salmonella enterica;* this was not being used as a serovar name. This name had been suggested by Kauffmann and Edwards (1952) and was used by some but not all authorities in the years up to 1987.

Le Minor and Popoff (1987) also proposed that the type strain of *S. enterica* be represented by the well-known strain of serovar Typhimurium, LT2 (Lilleengen, 1948; Sanderson and Demerec, 1965), and they described the new species and the new type strain. Reeves *et al.* (1989), based primarily on data from multi-locus enzyme electrophoresis (MLEE), proposed that subspecies V be given the rank of species and be named *Salmonella bongori*.

Thus Le Minor and Popoff (1987) were proposing changes in the nomenclature of *Salmonella* and they were also asking that taxonomic interpretations be considered. Their request to recognize a single species, *S. enterica*, was not dealt with by the Judicial Commission because the Commission was empowered to act only on nomenclature, not on taxonomic questions. The Judicial Commission requested a reformulation of the Request for an Opinion, but such a modified request was not presented. There has been formal support for the proposal of *S. enterica* as the sole species (Euzeby, 1999), and there has been dissent from this proposal (Yabuuchi and Ezaki, 2000). However, during the period from the 1980s to the 2000s, the nomenclature and the taxonomic systems of Le Minor and Popoff (1987) was widely accepted in certain countries, despite the fact that these names had not been validly published and had no standing in nomenclature. Therefore in 2005 the Judicial Commission of the International Committee for Systematics of Prokaryotes ruled that the type species of the genus *Salmonella* is *S. enterica* and the type strain is strain LT2 (Judicial Commission of the International Committee on Systematics of Prokaryotes, 2005). The Commission made its decision based on the request from Euzeby (1999), using the description of *S. enterica* given by Le Minor and Popoff (1987). The Commission stated that though they can rule on nomenclature, and they did so, they do not have the authority to rule on taxonomy; however, they cited an accompanying article by Tindall *et al.* (2005) that supported the proposal that *Salmonella* be divided into two species, and that *S. enterica* be divided into six subspecies; they further pointed out that this would result in the taxonomy and nomenclature that was used at that time by the World Health Organization (WHO) and other organizations.

The Commission ruling created the subspecies *S. enterica* subsp. *enterica* Le Minor and Popoff 1987 (equivalent to subspecies I) (Fig. 1.1). Most published papers deal with members of this subspecies; if serovar Typhimurium is being discussed, most journals prefer that the name *S. enterica* serovar Typhimurium be presented on first use, and subsequent use can be the name *S.* Typhimurium. (Many journals do not require that the full name *Salmonella enterica* subsp. *enterica* serovar Typhimurium be presented; the assumption is that subsp. *enterica* is being considered.) The following subspecies names were also created: *S. enterica* subspecies *salamae* (=subspecies II); *S. enterica* subspecies *arizonae* (=subspecies IIIa); *S. enterica* subspecies *diarizonae* (=subspecies IIIb); *S. enterica* subspecies *houtenae* (=subspecies IV); and *S. enterica* subspecies *indica* (=subspecies VI).

Methods for Studying Local Epidemiology, or for Studying Global Epidemiology

There are, in general, two different types of problems in epidemiology. One type of problem is solved by outbreak analysis, which involves short-term or local epidemiology. Outbreak analysis can be studied efficiently by many methods, such as pulsed-field gel electrophoresis, ribotyping, phage typing and others. The second type of problem is long-term or global epidemiology; for this, methods that reveal microbial population structure and evolutionary patterns of strains isolated over a range of time and space are necessary. Methods that work well for outbreak analysis, which is often done on a local basis, may be unsuitable for studies of global epidemiology: the reagents and methods used may be hard to standardize between labs; it may be necessary to exchange living cells rather than DNA between labs to obtain data, which may be difficult or impossible. For global epidemiology it is important to have methods in which the data can be collected in digital form and can be readily shared between laboratories, usually using the Internet. DNA sequence data in which alleles of genes or total DNA sequences can be directly compared is an approach that can yield information on population structure and evolution. In this review, we will emphasize methods that are important for global epidemiology, though we recognize that methods for local epidemiology will often be practical and relevant.

Defining Taxonomy of *Salmonella* by the Phylogenetic Species Concept

In the sections above we described three concepts of the species in bacteria, the eco-species, the bio-species and the phylo-species. Data from a variety of methods are used to establish taxonomic groups, but the approach that seems to us to be the most useful at present for the population structure of taxa in *Salmonella* involves DNA sequence; this yields information on lineages and reveals the phylo-species. Therefore, this approach will be reviewed first; this will show how the strains have been grouped into taxa using the concept of the phylo-species. However, we recognize that though sequences allow subdivision of the genus into taxa, it is not clear when to apply the term 'species' to the different subdivisions. In later sections we will consider what has been the relevance of recombination (which yields the bio-species) and of selection (which yields the eco-species).

Defining the genus *Salmonella* using DDH, and using16S rRNA

In early studies it was not clear if the enteric bacteria form a spectrum of overlapping species, or if instead there are clear boundaries between groups. For example, the Tribe *Salmonelleae* within the family *Enterobacteriaceae* was at one time thought to be composed of the genera *Salmonella, Arizona* and *Citrobacter*; the species within these genera had been grouped on the basis of biochemical and serological tests (Edwards and Ewing, 1972). However, DDH at 60°C to DNA of Typhimurium LT2 showed that all *Salmonella* serovars that were tested formed a single DNA hybridization group, with DNA from *Salmonella* strains showing from 85% to 100% re-association with Typhimurium LT2 DNA (this was defined as DNA relatedness) (Crosa *et al.*, 1973). The strains previously placed in the genus *Arizona* were shown to be part of the genus *Salmonella* and composed of two groups, a monophasic, non-lactose fermenting group (now known as *S. enterica* subsp. *arizonae*, also called IIIa) and a diphasic, lactose fermenting group (now known as *S. enterica* subsp. *diarizonae*, also called IIIb); both groups gave from 70 to 80% DNA relatedness to Typhimurium LT2. Strains of *Citrobacter* and of *Escherichia coli* were 50% or less related to *Salmonella*, and members of other genera such as *Erwinia* and *Edwardsiella* were usually 40% or less related. The conclusions from DNA relatedness were confirmed by studies on the melting temperature of DNA hybrids (Crosa *et al.*, 1973). The average melting temperature of hybrids formed at 60°C between DNA from identical strains (e.g. Typhimurium LT2) were determined; these are about 85°C. Then the melting temperature of DNA from different hybrid combinations was tested; it was shown that DNA from other serovars in subspecies *enterica* with Typhimurium LT2 gave similar melting temperatures, no more than 2 to 3°C lower (this was called the ΔT_m). However, DNA from different genera such as *E. coli* gave a ΔT_m of 10–15°C. This indicated that the hybrid DNA that was formed from unrelated strains had many mismatches, and was readily melted.

Thus, the boundaries of the genus *Salmonella* have been defined through the use of DDH. However, the method is difficult to standardize and it is hard to share data electronically, so other DNA-based methods are more widely used. Small subunit rRNA sequences (16S rRNA in bacteria) have been used to determine the tree of life (Woese *et al.*, 1990) and are used to identify strains. However, the sequence conservation that has made 16S rRNA so suitable for determining relationships of very different genera makes it unsuitable for studies within a genus such as *Salmonella*; rRNA sequences within the genus do not have sufficient variation.

Microbes with 16S rRNA that are <98.7% identical are considered to be different species; these differences correlate with <70% DNA–DNA relatedness by DDH (Stackebrandt and Ebers, 2006). *Salmonella enterica* and *S. bongori* were clearly separated based on 16S sequence analysis (Christensen *et al.*, 1998; Grimont *et al.*, 2000). Within *S. enterica* the diphasic subspp. *enterica* and *indica* were separated from the monophasic *arizonae* and *houtenae* by 23S rRNA comparison (Christensen *et al.*, 1998). Based on 16S and 23S rRNA sequence comparison, the genus *Salmonella* is closely related to *E. coli*, *Shigella* and *Citrobacter* (Christensen *et al.*, 1998).

Defining taxa in *Salmonella* using nucleotide sequences yields information on population structure

Multi-locus enzyme electrophoresis (MLEE) was first used for population genetics studies in eukaryotes (Sage and Selander, 1975) and later applied to bacteria. In this method up to 24 enzymes for which activity can be detected in starch gel electrophoresis were assayed in cell extracts from many bacterial strains, and electromorphs with different electrophoretic mobility were equated with alleles for the structural gene locus corresponding to the enzyme (Beltran *et al.*, 1988). Thus, although the analysis is done on proteins, it yields data on nucleotide sequence. Those alleles with base pair changes that alter an amino acid in the protein to an amino acid with a different charge will produce a change in the electrophoretic mobility of the protein. Distinctive combinations of alleles were designated as electrophoretic types (ETs). Beltran *et al.* (1988, 1991) and Boyd *et al.* (1996) showed that in many serovars of *Salmonella*, separate isolates belonged to a single worldwide clone (i.e. the serovar was monophyletic), but they also showed that some serovars were polyphyletic, with isolates that were distantly related. Thus MLEE confirmed the value of serological data, but shows that serotyping does not reveal evolutionary relationships.

More detailed conclusions are available from nucleotide sequences, rather than from MLEE, although the data are of similar structure. Multi-locus sequence typing (MLST) was first described in detail by Maiden *et al.* (1998) for analysis of the sequence of ca. 500 bp fragments of 11 housekeeping genes of *Neisseria meningitidis*. MLST has advantages over other methods: the digital sequence data are (usually) unambiguous; the data are easily sharable between labs; and data can be collected from isolated DNA. These advantages have continued to expand in recent years as nucleotide sequencing becomes faster and cheaper and as exchange of data on the Internet becomes more efficient. Different housekeeping genes have been studied by investigators in *Salmonella*: Octavia and Lan (2006) used a set of four genes; McQuiston *et al.* (2008) used a different set of four genes; Sangal *et al.* (2010) and many other investigators used a different set of seven genes. Data on the latter set are maintained at University College, Cork, Ireland, and can be accessed at http://mlst.ucc.ie/mlst/dbs/Senterica. For each locus, alleles with different sequence were assigned arbitrary allele numbers; strains that differ in one or more alleles were assigned different sequence types (STs), and minimal-spanning trees were constructed based on the pairwise differences. Hu *et al.* (2006) sequenced intergenic regions in strains of *S.* Typhimurium.

To illustrate the type of information that can be derived from MLST in *Salmonella*, the report by Sangal *et al.* (2010) on *S.* Newport and related strains is represented in Plate 1. Over 330 Newport isolates, and representatives of other serovars from different geographic areas, were tested by MLST to determine evolution and population genetics; 49 STs were identified. The eBurst population genetics algorithm has been used in studying data from many species of bacteria; it calculates the distances based on the number of shared alleles. The minimal-spanning tree (MS_{Tree}) was calculated using principles similar to eBurst (Plate 1). Groups were defined as clusters of at least three STs with shared (identical) alleles in at least five out of seven alleles (i.e. double locus variants, DLVs); most strains shared six of the seven alleles (single locus variants, SLVs). The serovar Newport was revealed to be polyphyletic, with the isolates falling into three different groups, designated Newport I, II and III. However, the group Newport II seemed to consist of two subgroups, connected via an intermediate ST that shares only 5/7 alleles with STs in both of the subgroups. Some of the other serovars such as Paratyphi B are also polyphyletic, with 18 different STs in four distinct groups. But some serovars are apparently monophyletic; e.g. Typhimurium has over 350 isolates including 22 different STs, all but one clustered into a single group, and most strains of Enteritidis are also monophyletic in a single group (Plate 1). These data show that the serotype can sometimes reveal relationships, as in Typhimurium and Enteritidis, but in other cases such as Newport very unrelated bacteria are grouped together. Fricke *et al.* (2011) reported complete nucleotide sequences of 17 previously non-sequenced strains from subspecies *enterica*; this permitted sequence alignments of the 2.088-Mbp core chromosome shared by all 28 *Salmonella* strains for which sequence is now available. The serotype-based classification is supported for many pairs of isolates, but the Saintpaul and Newport serovars are two cases in which serotyping is not a good indication of evolutionary relationships based on whole-chromosome alignments.

The groups defined as described above are named Newport I, Newport II, Typhimurium etc., but it is not clear if groups such as Newport I and II are actually more related to each other than they are to members of other serovars. Therefore Sangal *et al.* (2010) have tentatively suggested that these different groups (which they call eBurst groups) should be given new numbers that do not link with the serovar name (Supplementary Table 9 in Sangal *et al.*, 2010). As more data accumulate, there may ultimately be agreement on a new naming/numbering system that would replace serovar names.

Defining taxa in *Salmonella* for groups with monomorphic structure

In most situations, analysis by MLST is successful in distinguishing many different STs within a serotype; these groups may be monophyletic, but still rather complex with many STs, as in Typhimurium (Kingsley *et al.*, 2009) and Enteritidis, or they may be polyphyletic, as in Newport (Sangal *et al.*, 2010). But in some situations, MLST with seven genes does not reveal enough variability to make meaningful distinctions within a serovar; these have been called monomorphic groups, and have been recognized in recently evolved pathogens such as *S.* Typhi and also in *Yersinia pestis* and *Mycobacterium tuberculosum* (Achtman, 2008; Achtman and Wagner, 2008). *Salmonella* Typhi had previously been shown to be homogeneous using MLEE methods (Selander *et al.*, 1990). For example, MLST for 26 *S.* Typhi strains showed limited variability, with only three polymorphic sites and a total of four STs; thus, adequate distinctions between strains could not be made (Kidgell *et al.*, 2002). Therefore, Roumagnac *et al.* (2006), using a method of mutation discovery, analysed Typhi strains from a range of geographic sources and identified 97 single nucleotide polymorphisms (SNPs). These SNPs were analysed within 483 different strains, and a total of 85 different haplotypes was identified (Plate 2). The distribution pattern of the SNPs in Typhi is unusual among MLST trees in that it is fully parsimonious, i.e. the tree suggests that each SNP is caused by a unique genetic event. The ancestral node was identified as haplotype 45 (H45), for this haplotype has the identical nucleotides as the eight sequenced genomes of *S. enterica* of other serovars; all other haplotypes result from mutations compared with that ancestral node. Many bridges between haplotypes are represented by extant haplotypes with a single SNP, indicating persistence of individual haplotypes in the population, even in this limited sample. Haplotypes and clusters of haplotypes were found in multiple continents (Africa, Asia and South America); it is not clear where H45, the ancestral node, evolved, since it is found in three continents indicating waves of global transmission. One of the haplotypes, H58, was widespread in South-east Asia (Roumagnac *et al.*, 2006) and has also been found in Kenya (Kariuki *et al.*, 2010).

The haplotypes defined in Roumagnac *et al.* (2006) can be further subdivided by detection of more SNPs. For example, Holt *et al.* (2010) used new sequencing methods to identify nearly 2000 SNPs, and then used the Illumina platform to type 1500 of these SNPs in 62 isolates of Typhi that were causing typhoid in Nepalese children. The H58 haplotype that was dominant in South-east Asia, and that made up a high proportion of the nalidixic acid-resistant isolates reported by Roumagnac *et al.* (2006), was the major haplotype in Nepal. The newly discovered SNPs permitted further subdivision of the H58 haplotype, thus giving greater sensitivity and resolution. The H58 haplotype was divided into lineages I and II, which were further subdivided to strain-specific sub-lineages H58-A, -B and -G. This type of subdivision allows identification of clonal origin and allows tracing of geographic movements of strains. Thus, using nucleotide sequencing the genus *Salmonella* can be subdivided into clades of diminishing differences, down to clones that differ in only a few SNPs.

Defining Taxonomy of *Salmonella* by the Biological Species Concept (Bio-species)

In the 1940s recombination was shown to occur in bacteria, but studies using MLEE in the 1980s indicated that the rate of recombination in bacterial strains is very low (Beltran *et al.*, 1988, 1991), i.e. that bacterial populations were primarily clonal, suggesting that recombination is rare in nature. However, through comparing DNA sequences, Smith *et al.* (1993) showed that recombination is sometimes common. They concluded that there were different types of bacterial populations, some of which (e.g. *Neisseria gonorrhoeae*) were fully sexual with much allelic exchange, other species were intermediate, but that *Salmonella* was entirely clonal, i.e. though recombination was detected in the laboratory, its rate in nature is low. However, it is now clear that recombination and allelic exchange occurs at a significant rate in wild-type strains of *Salmonella*.

There are three different approaches to determining whether homologous recombination and allelic exchange have been important in evolution of *Salmonella*. The first approach was developed by Dykhuisen and Green (1991) in *E. coli*. They showed that the pattern of evolution of alleles of different genes in *E. coli* was incongruent, i.e. comparisons of sequences showed that different genes have evolved at different rates and produced different gene trees. This was consistent with the notion that allelic exchange was involved; the allelic exchange occurred more frequently in some genes than others, thus explaining different results in different genes. Comparisons of genes in *E. coli* with those in *S.* Typhimurium showed that different gene trees have similar divergences, indicating that genetic exchange is not taking place between these two genera and the variation is due to mutation. Brown *et al.* (2002) also observed incongruence in different genes when they tested strains of *S. enterica*; this suggested that genetic exchange was also occurring in *Salmonella* strains.

A second approach analyses concatenated nucleotide sequences using the program Neighbor-net; an example of this is shown for *S.* Newport and related strains in Plate 3. The same sequence data, analysed for allelic differences rather than by using concatenated sequences, was shown earlier in Plate 1. The conclusions about the relationships of the strains, drawn from concatenated sequences (Plate 3), are similar to the conclusions drawn previously; Newport and Paratyphi B are polyphyletic, Typhimurium and Enteritidis are monophyletic. However, the Neighbor-net program marks conflicting signals in nucleotide sequences that arise by recombination or by recurrent mutations (homoplasies) as parallel paths in a phylogenetic network. Plate 3 shows that most STs from *S.* Enteritidis and *S.* Typhimurium radiated from a single point, indicating that diversity was mostly the result of mutations. But parallelograms were common in other groups, indicating a large amount of recombination; such parallelograms are seen within Newport II, and in the regions between the major groups. This suggests that allelic exchange has been common in the evolution of these groups.

A third approach was to examine the relative roles of recombination (R) and of mutation (M). The most complete data on genetic exchange and on the postulated formation of bio-species are found in *N. meningitidis*, where many strains have been analysed by MLST (Spratt *et al.*, 2001; Fraser *et al.*, 2007). Strains in which the ST varies at a single locus out of seven loci tested (a single locus variant, or SLV) are said to be part of a clonal complex. The frequency of homologous recombination within the clonal complexes in this species was estimated as follows. The alleles of different strains within this clonal complex were compared; alleles that differ by two or more adjacent base pairs are postulated to originate from recombination (R) (since two independent adjacent mutations are unlikely), whereas alleles that differ by a single base pair change are postulated to originate from mutation (M). In *N. meningitidis* the ratio of R/M=5 to 10, which indicates that more bases change by homologous recombination than change due to mutation (Spratt *et al.*, 2001), which indicates a major role for recombination. Bell *et al.* (2011) determined that R/M for strains in the *S. enterica* subsp. *enterica* was 1.4 if they measured per allele and 5.0 if they measured per site (several sites change in each allele due to recombination, only one due to mutation), which indicates a major role for recombination.

Thus, the three approaches above all indicate a significant role for allelic exchange in *Salmonella*. Falush *et al.* (2006) carried out MLST analysis of 207 strains of subspecies *enterica* of diverse serotypes along with 20 other strains of other subspecies and of *S. bongori*; these represented 108 different STs, mostly from subspecies *enterica*. Neighbour-joining trees of concatenated sequences showed each of the seven groups (six subspecies of *S. enterica*, and *S. bongori*) was monophyletic. Further analysis using the program STRUCTURE showed that substantial recombination has occurred within strains of *enterica*, revealed by a very highly mosaic pattern of ancestry of segments of genes, with alleles being shared between different strains within *enterica*. However, recombination between *enterica* and the other subspecies was rare, suggesting that there are barriers to allelic exchange between the different subspecies. Thus, the data follow the pattern that would be expected if there was extensive allelic exchange within the subspecies *enterica* (which might then be called a bio-species) and limited allelic exchange with strains from the other subspecies (which may represent other bio-species). Similarly, Brown *et al.* (2003) reported that strains in the SARB set (Salmonella Reference B), all of which are from the subspecies *enterica*, showed widespread allelic exchange, while strains from other subspecies that are represented in the SARC set (Salmonella Reference C) gave very little allelic exchange. Lan *et al.* (2009) also showed that recombination between strains of subspecies *enterica* is common.

In the BSC, different species are separated by a species barrier; in bacteria the barrier may be due to a lack of genetic transfer between the species, or by lack of allelic exchange between the DNA of the donor and the recipient. Sequence divergence results in a species barrier (Vulic *et al.*, 1997; Fraser *et al.*, 2007). Thus, two genera such as *Salmonella* and *Escherichia*, in which the sequences of orthologous genes have diverged by about 15% on average, have the recombination reduced by 1000-fold.

Thus, in summary, there is gathering evidence that allelic exchange between strains of *Salmonella* may be an important cohesive force. The data of Falush *et al.* (2006), Brown *et al.* (2003) and Lan *et al.* (2009) suggest that the subspecies of *Salmonella* may be the equivalent of bio-species.

Defining Taxonomy of *Salmonella* by the Ecotype Species Concept (Eco-species)

The ESC (which yields the eco-species) was described by Cohan (2001); each cluster of strains corresponds to an ecotype, defined as a population of cells in the same ecological niche. There is some evidence that serovars such as *S.* Typhi may be viewed as eco-species. Strains of this serovar are very distinct from other serovars when tested by MLEE (Selander *et al.*, 1990) and at the sequence level (Roumagnac *et al.*, 2006), and they constitute a relatively homogeneous group that was referred to above as monomorphic (Achtman, 2008). They are limited to growth in humans where they cause enteric fever (typhoid fever). There is little evidence for allelic exchange with other serovars of *Salmonella* in the seven genes of the MLST set (Falush *et al.*, 2006). However, an extensive set of genetic exchanges took place between *S.* Typhi and *S.* Paratyphi A at an earlier time, such that part of the genomes of the two serovars have diverged by 0.18% while part diverged by 1.2% (about the same amount of divergence as between other serovars), but again there was very little evidence of exchanges with other serovars of *Salmonella* (Didelot *et al.*, 2007). Clearly, according to the phylo-species concept, strains of *S.* Typhi are members of the species *S. enterica* subsp. *enterica* (Roumagnac *et al.*, 2006), but according to the eco-species concept they could be considered a different species. Sometimes issues of safety in clinical work are used, as in the continued use of the genus name *Shigella* to describe strains which cause diarrhoea in humans, though according to the criteria applied to other strains of *E. coli*, *Shigella* would clearly be part of the species *E. coli*.

Summary

At present, strains of *Salmonella* are normally classified first by serology, which allows separation into ca. 2600 serotypes. In the most widely used scheme, these strains are designated into two species, *S. enterica* and *S. bongori*, and *S. enterica* is further subdivided into six subspecies. Strains of *Salmonella* can be considered under three concepts, which have been called 'species concepts', though it is not always clear where the species boundaries should be placed when using these concepts. A very valuable concept is the PSC, in which the lineage of the cells is inferred from comparisons of the nucleotide sequences. The use of DDH, which yields an indirect measure of the nucleotide sequence similarity of two strains, revealed that all strains belonging to the genus *Salmonella* have >70% DNA relatedness, and thus helped to define the genus (Crosa *et al.*, 1973). The most widely used approach to classify strains within the genus, using this concept, is MLST. Analysis of sequence from seven genes allows strains to be separated into STs in which all seven genes have the same alleles, and into groups in which one or two of these alleles are different. The MLST data show that some serotypes are monophyletic (e.g. Typhimurium and Enteritidis) but other serotypes are polyphyletic (e.g. Newport and Paratyphi B) (Sangal *et al.*, 2010). This type of analysis can proceed to greater depth; analysis of strains of Typhi by MLST showed limited variability, but when large numbers of SNPs were detected and tested, strains could be subdivided into many different haplotypes (Roumagnac *et al.*, 2006; Holt *et al.*, 2010). In principle, one can identify a phylo-species in this way, but there is at present no theoretical basis for setting the boundaries of the species; strains with ANI >95% are said to be the same species, but the basis for the number is somewhat arbitrary.

The BSC usually applies to sexually reproducing higher animals. Thus, species of birds are recognizable as sharing a gene pool through mating, and through reproductive barriers against members of other species; these can be called bio-species. Bacteria can share genes through recombination, but the existence of bio-species that share a gene pool is not as clear as in higher animals. There is evidence for frequent allelic exchange between strains belonging to *S. enterica* subsp. *enterica* and for infrequent exchange with other subspecies of *S. enterica*; this suggests that members of the subspecies *enterica* constitute a bio-species. There are not yet enough data to conclude whether the other subspecies of *enterica* resemble separate bio-species. Unlike the phylo-species, the bio-species does have a theoretical basis, i.e. it is determined by the strains that can and do exchange genes through allelic exchange. The bio-species is based on study of orthologues in the core genome, which can undergo allelic exchange. Genes in the accessory genome, which enter by LGT and insert into the genome by site-specific recombination, are very important in determining the specific properties of different strains, but these cannot be used like the core genome to determine the bio-species.

In the ESC, each cluster of strains corresponds to an ecotype, defined as a population of cells in the same ecological niche. For example, *S.* Typhi occupies a specific ecological niche (tissues of humans) and causes a specific syndrome (enteric fever). It also is defined as a specific group by nucleotide sequencing. Thus it would seem definable as an eco-species, but many other serovars are not equally definable on an ecological basis. Some of the other host-restricted serovars (such as Typhisuis, Gallinarum and Abortusovis) might be considered in the same way.

The taxonomic system that is actually used must be stable, operational and predictive (Rosselló-Mora and Amann, 2001). The use of species names is important in bacteria in a number of fields: agriculture, biotechnology, food safety, disease diagnosis, epidemiology and public health and bioterrorism (Doolittle and Zhaxybayeva, 2009). Thus, since changes in the naming system cause considerable confusion, they must be very carefully considered before being made. Researchers in many fields, and the general public, have interests in the species names and the other designations that are used. It is likely that as it is recognized that the serovar is often polyphyletic, some renaming will ultimately be needed, but it is not clear what changes should be made and when. Thus, it is interesting to consider the theoretical basis for separating and naming species, but it is important that further changes not be made until clear advantages to science and to society can be demonstrated.

Abbreviations

ANI, average sequence identity; BSC, Biological Species Concept; DDH, DNA–DNA hybridization; ESC, Ecotype Species Concept; ET, electrophoretic type; LGT, lateral gene transfer; MLEE, multi-locus enzyme electrophoresis; MLST, multi-locus sequence typing; NTS, non-typhoidal salmonelloisis; PSC, Phylogenetic Species Concept; SLV, single locus variant; SNPs, single nucleotide polymorphisms; ST, sequence type.

Acknowledgements

The work was supported by a Discovery Grant from the Natural Sciences and Engineering Research Council of Canada.

References

Achtman, M. (2008) Evolution, population structure, and phylogeography of genetically monomorphic bacterial pathogens. *Annual Review of Microbiology* 62, 53–70.

Achtman, M. and Wagner, M. (2008) Microbial diversity and the genetic nature of microbial species. *Nature Reviews Microbiology* 6, 431–440.

Bale, J.A., de Pinna, E.M., Threlfall, E.J. and Ward, L.R. (2007) Kauffmann-White scheme-2007: *Salmonella* identification-serotypes and antigenic formulae. London, Health Protection Agency.

Bapteste, E., O'Malley, M.A., Beiko, R.G., Ereshefsky, M., Gogarten, J.P., Frankin-Hall, L., Lapointe, F.-J., Dupre, J., Dagan, T., Boucher, Y. and Martin, W. (2009) Prokaryotic evolution and the tree of life are two different things. *Biology Direct* 4, 34.

Bell, R.L., Gonzalez-Escalona, N., Stones, R. and Brown, E.W. (2011) Phylogenetic evaluation of the 'Typhimurium' complex of *Salmonella* strains using a seven-gene multi-locus sequence analysis. *Infection, Genetics and Evolution* 11, 83–91.

Beltran, P., Musser, J.M., Helmuth, R., Farmer, J.J. III, Frerichs, W.M., Wachsmuth, I.K., Ferris, K., McWhorter, A.C., Wells, J.G., Cravioto, A. and Selander, R.K. (1988) Towards a population genetic analysis of *Salmonella*: genetic diversity and relationships among strains of serovars *S. choleraesuis, S. derby, S. dublin, S. enteritidis, S. heidelberg, S. infantis, S. newport,* and *S. typhimurium*. *Proceedings of the National Academy of Sciences of the United States of America* 85, 7753–7757.

Beltran, P., Plock, S.A., Smith, N.H., Whittam, T.S., Old, D.C. and Selander, R.K. (1991) Reference collection of strains of the *Salmonella typhimurium* complex from natural populations. *Journal of General Microbiology* 137, 601–606.

Borman, E.K., Stuart, C.A. and Wheeler, K.M. (1944) Taxonomy of the Family *Enterobacteriaceae*. *Journal of Bacteriology* 48, 351–367.

Boyd, E.F., Wang, F.S., Whittam, T.S. and Selander, R.K. (1996) Molecular genetic relationships of the salmonellae. *Applied and Environmental Microbiology* 62, 804–808.

Brown, E.W., Kotewicz, M.L. and Cebula, T.A. (2002) Detection of recombination among *Salmonella enterica* strains using the incongruence length difference test. *Molecular Phylogenetics and Evolution* 24, 102–120.

Brown, E.W., Mammel, M.K., LeClerc, J.E. and Cebula, T.A. (2003) Limited boundaries for extensive horizontal gene transfer among *Salmonella* pathogens. *Proceedings of the National Academy of Sciences of the United States of America* 100, 15676–15681.

Christensen, H., Nordentoft, S. and Olsen, J.E. (1998) Phylogenetic relationships of *Salmonella* based on rRNA sequences. *International Journal of Systematic Bacteriology* 48, 605–610.

Cohan, F.M. (2001) Bacterial species and speciation. *Systematic Biology* 50, 513–524.

Crosa, J.F., Brenner, D.J., Ewing, W.H. and Falkow, S. (1973) Molecular relationships among Salmonellae. *Journal of Bacteriology* 115, 307–315.

Darwin, C. (1859) (1964) *On the Origin of Species: a Facsimile of the First Edition*. Harvard University Press, Cambridge, Massachusetts.

Didelot, X., Achtman, M., Parkhill, J., Thomson, N.R. and Falush, D. (2007) A bimodal pattern of relatedness between the *Salmonella* Paratyphi A and Typhi genomes: convergence or divergence by homologous recombination? *Genome Research* 17, 61–68.

Doolittle, W.F. and Zhaxybayeva, O. (2009) On the origin of prokaryotic species. *Genome Research* 19, 744–756.

Dykhuisen, D.E. and Green, L. (1991) Recombination in *Escherichia coli* and the definition of bacterial species. *Journal of Bacteriology* 173, 7257–7268.

Editorial Team (eurosurveillance@ecdc.europa.eu), Bertrand, S., Remhanen-Finne, R., Weill, F.-X., Rasch, W., Thornton, L., Perevoscikovs, J., vanPelt, W. and Heck, M. (2010) *Salmonella* infections associated with reptiles: the current situation in Europe. *Eurosurveillance* 13, 1–6.

Edwards, P.R. and Ewing, W.H. (1972) *Identification of Enterobacteriaceae*, 3rd edn. Burgess Publishing Company, Minneapolis, Minnesota.

Ereshefsky, M. (2010a) Microbiology and the species problem. *Biology and Philosophy* 25, 553–568.

Ereshefsky, M. (2010b) Mystery of mysteries: Darwin and the species problem. *Cladistics* 26, 1–13.

Euzeby, J.P. (1999) Revised *Salmonella* nomenclature: designation of *Salmonella enterica* (ex Kauffmann and Edwards 1952) LeMinor and Popoff 1987 sp. nov., nom. rev as the neotype species of the genus *Salmonella* Lignieres 1900 (Approved Lists 1980), rejection of the name *Salmonella choleraesuis* (Smith 1894) Weldin 1927 (Approved Lists 1980) and conservation of the name *Salmonella typhi* (Schroeter 1886) Warren and Scott 1930 (Approved Lists 1980). Request for an opinion. *Journal of Systematic Bacteriology* 49, 927–930.

Ewing, W.H. (1972) The nomenclature of *Salmonella*, its usage, and definitions for the three species. *Canadian Journal of Microbiology* 18, 1629–1637.

Falush, D., Torpdahl, M., Didelot, X., Conrad, D.F., Wilson, D.J. and Achtman, M. (2006) Mismatch induced speciation in *Salmonella*: model and data. *Philosophical Transactions of the Royal Society of London. Series B, Biological Sciences* 361, 2045–2063.

Foti, M., Daidone, A., Aleo, A., Pizzimenti, A., Giacopello, C. and Mammina, C. (2009) *Salmonella bongori* 48:z35:- in migratory birds in Italy. *Emerging Infectious Diseases* 15, 502–503.

Fraser, C., Hanage, W.P. and Spratt, B.G. (2007) Recombination and the nature of bacterial speciation. *Science* 315, 476–480.

Fricke, W.F., Mammel, M.K., McDermott, P.F., Tartera, C., White, D.G., LeClerc, J.E., Ravel, J. and Cebula, T.A. (2011) Comparative genomics of 28 *Salmonella enterica* isolates: evidence for CRISR-mediated adaptive sublineage evolution. *Journal of Bacteriology* 193, 3556–3568.

Grimont, P.A.D. and Weill, F.-X. (2007) Antigenic formulae of the *Salmonella* serovars. Paris, France: WHO Collaborating Centre for Reference and Research on *Salmonella*, Institut Pasteur. Available at: http://www.pasteur.fr/ip/portal/action/WebdriveActionEvent/oid/01s-000036-089 (accessed 5 March 2013).

Grimont, P.A.D., Grimont, F. and Bouvet, P. (2000) Taxonomy of the genus *Salmonella*. In: Wray, C. and Wray, A. (eds) Salmonella *in Domestic Animals*. CAB International, Wallingford, UK.

Guibourdenche, M., Roggentin, P., Mikoleit, M., Fields, P.I., Bockemühl, J., Grimont, P.A. and Weill, F.X. (2010) Supplement 2003-2007 (No.47) to the White-Kauffmann-Le Minor scheme. *Research in Microbiology* 161, 26–29.

Holt, K.E., Baker, S., Dongol, S., Basnyat, B., Adhirari, N., Thorson, S., Pulickal, A.S., Song, Y., Parkhill, J., Farrar, J.J., Murdoch, D.R., Kelly, D.F., Pollard, A.J. and Dougan, G. (2010) High-throughput bacterial SNP typing identifies distinct clusters of *Salmonella* Typhi causing typhoid in Nepalese children. *BMC Infectious Diseases* 10, 144.

Hu, H., Lan, R. and Reeves, P.R. (2006) Adaptation of multilocus sequencing for studying variation within a major clone: evolutionary relationships of *Salmonella enterica* Serovar Typhimurium. *Genetics* 172, 743–750.

Judicial Commission of the International Committee on Systematics of Prokaryotes (2005) The type species of the genus *Salmonella* Lignieres 1900 is *Salmonella enterica* (ex Kauffmann and Edwards 1952) Le Minor and Popoff 1987, with the type strain LT2^T, and conservation of the epithet *enterica* in *Salmonella enterica* over all earlier epithets that may be applied to this species. Opinion 80. *International Journal of Systematic and Evolutionary Microbiology* 55, 519–520.

Kariuki, S., Revathi, G., Kiiru, J., Mengo, D.M., Mwituria, J., Muyodi, J., Munyalo, A., Teo, Y.Y., Holt, K.E., Kingsley, R.A. and Dougan, G. (2010) Typhoid in Kenya is associated with a dominant multidrug-resistant *Salmonella enterica* serovar Typhi haplotype that is also widespread in Southeast Asia. *Journal of Clinical Microbiology* 48, 2171–2176.

Kauffmann, F. (1960) *The Bacteriology of Enterobacteriaceae*. Munksgaard, Copenhagen.

Kauffmann, F. (1961) The species definition in the *Enterobacteriaceae*. *International Bulletin of Bacteriological Nomenclature and Taxonomy* 11, 5–6.

Kauffmann, F. and Edwards, P.R. (1952) Classification and nomenclature of *Enterobacteriaceae*. *International Bulletin of Bacteriological Nomenclature and Taxonomy* 2, 2–8.

Kidgell, C., Reichard, U., Wain, J., Linz, B., Torpdahl, M., Dougan, G. and Achtman, M. (2002) *Salmonella typhi*, the causative agent of typhoid fever, is approximately 50,000 years old. *Infection Genetics and Evolution* 2, 39–45.

Kingsley, R.A., Msefula, C.L., Thomson, N.R., Kariuki, S., Holt, K.E., Gordon, M.A., Harris, D., Clarke, L., Whitehead, S., Sangal, V., Marsh, K., Achtman, M., Molyneux, M.E., Cormican, M., Parkhill, J., MacLennan, C.A., Heyderman, R.S. and Dougan, G. (2009) Epidemic multiple drug resistant *Salmonella typhimurium* causing invasive disease in sub-Saharan Africa have a distinct genotype. *Genome Research* 12, 2279–2287.

Konstantinidis, K.T. and Tiedje, J.M. (2005) Genomic insights that advance the species definition for prokaryotes. *Proceedings of the National Academy of Sciences of the United States of America* 102, 2567–2572.

Lan, R. and Reeves, P.R. (2001) When does a clone deserve a name? A perspective on bacterial species based on population genetics. *Trends in Microbiology* 9, 419–424.

Lan, R., Reeves, P.R. and Octavia, S. (2009) Population structure, origins and evolution of major *Salmonella enterica* clones. *Infection Genetics and Evolution* 9, 996–1005.

Langridge, G.C., Wain, J. and Nair, S. (2008) Invasive Salmonellosis in humans. Chapter 8.6.2.2 (revised version). In: Böck, A., Curtiss, R. III, Kaper, J.B., Neidhardt, F.C., Nyström, T., Rudd, K.E. and Squires, C.L. (eds) *EcoSal* – Escherichia coli *and* Salmonella*: Cellular and Molecular Biology.* ASM Press, Washington, DC.

Lederberg, J. and Tatum, E.L. (1946) Gene recombination in *Escherichia coli*. *Nature* 158, 558.

Le Minor, L. (1991) The genus *Salmonella*. In: Balow, H., Truper, H.G., Dworkin, M., Harder, W. and Schleifer, K.-H. (eds) *The Prokaryotes*, 2nd edn, vol. 3. Springer-Verlag, New York, pp. 2760–2774.

Le Minor, L. and Popoff, M.Y. (1987) Request for an opinion: designation of *Salmonella enterica* sp. nov., as the type and only species of the genus *Salmonella*. *International Journal of Systematic Bacteriology* 37, 465–468.

Le Minor, L., Rohde, R. and Taylor, J. (1970) Nomenclature des *Salmonella*. *Annales de l'Institut Pasteur (Paris)* 119, 206–210.

Le Minor, L., Veron, M. and Popoff, M. (1982) Proposition pour une nomenclature des *Salmonella*. *Annales de Microbiologie (Paris)* 133, 245–254.

Lilleengen, K. (1948) Typing of *Salmonella typhimurium* by means of bacteriophage. *Acta Pathologica et Microbiologica Scandinavica* Suppl. 77, 11–125.

Maiden, M.C.J., Bygraves, J.A., Feil, E., Morelli, G., Russell, J.E., Urwin, R., Zhang, Q., Zhou, J., Zurth, K., Caugant, D.A., Feavers, I.M., Achtman, M. and Spratt, B.G. (1998) Multilocus sequence typing: a portable approach to the identification of clones within populations of pathogenic microorganisms. *Proceedings of the National Academy of Sciences of the United States of America* 95, 3140–3145.

Mayr, E. (1996) What is a species, and what is it not? *Philosophy of Science* 63, 262–277.

McClelland, M., Sanderson, K.E., Spieth, J., Clifton, S.W., Latreille, P., Cortney, L., Porwollik, S., Ali, J., Dante, M., Du, F., Hou, S., Layman, D., Leonard, S., Nguyen, C., Scott, K., Holmes, A., Grewal, N., Mulvaney, E., Ryan, E., Sun, H., Florea, L., Miller, W., Stoneking, T., Nhan, M., Waterston, W. and Wilson, R.K. (2001) Complete genome sequence of *Salmonella enterica* serovar Typhimurium. *Nature* 413, 852–856.

McQuiston, J.R., Herrera-Leon, S., Wertheim, B.C., Doyle, J., Fields, P.I., Tauxe, R.V. and Logsdon, J.M. Jr (2008) Molecular phylogeny of the Salmonellae: relationship among *Salmonella* species and subspecies determined from four housekeeping genes and evidence of lateral gene transfer events. *Journal of Bacteriology* 190, 7060–7067.

Nash, H.A. (1997) Site-specific recombination: integration, excision, resolution, and inversion of defined DNA segments. In: Neidhardt, F.C. (ed.) Escherichia coli *and* Salmonella*: Cellular and Molecular Biology*, 2nd edn. ASM Press, Washington, DC, pp. 2363–2376.

Octavia, S. and Lan, R. (2006) Frequent recombination and low level of clonality within *Salmonella enterica* subspecies I. *Microbiology* 152, 1099–1108.

Parkhill, J., Dougan, G., James, K.D., Thomson, N.R., Pickard, D., Wain, J., Churcher, C., Mungall, K.L., Bentley, S.D., Holden, M.T., Sebaihia, M., Baker, S., Basham, D., Brooks, K., Chillingworth, T., Connerton, P., Cronin, A., Davis, P., Davies, R.M., Dowd, L., White, N., Farrar, J., Feltwell, T., Hamlin, N., Haque, A., Hien, T.T., Holroyd, S., Jagels, K., Krogh, A., Larsen, T.S., Leather, S., Moule, S., O'Gaora, P., Parry, C., Quail, M., Rutherford, K., Simmonds, M., Skelton, J., Stevens, K., Whitehead, S. and Barrell, B.G. (2001) Complete genome sequence of a multiple drug resistant *Salmonella enterica* serovar Typhi CT18. *Nature* 413, 848–852.

Popoff, M.Y. (2001) Antigenic formulas of the *Salmonella* serovars. 8 ed. Paris: WHO Collaborating Centre for Reference on *Salmonella*. Institute Pasteur, Paris, France.

Porwollik, S., Wong, R.M. and McClelland, M. (2002) Evolutionary genomics of *Salmonella*: gene acquisitions revealed by microarray analysis. *Proceedings of the National Academy of Sciences of the United States of America* 99, 8956–8961.

Reeves, M.W., Evins, G.M., Heiba, A.A., Plikaytis, B.D. and Farmer, J.J. III (1989) Clonal nature of *Salmonella typhi* and its genetic relatedness to other Salmonellae as shown by multilocus enzyme electrophoresis, and proposal of *Salmonella bongori* comb.nov. *Journal of Clinical Microbiology* 27, 313–320.

Rosselló-Mora, R. and Amann, R. (2001) The species concept for prokaryotes. *FEMS Microbiology Reviews* 25, 39–67.

Roumagnac, P., Weill, F.-X., Dolecek, C., Baker, S., Brisse, S., Nguyen, T.C., Thi, A.H.L., Acosta, C.J., Farrar, J., Dougan, G. and Achtman, M. (2006) Evolutionary history of Salmonella typhi. *Science* 314, 1301–1304.

Rules Revision Committee, Judicial Commission (1975) Proposal to emend the International Code of Nomenclature of Bacteria. *International Journal of Systematic Bacteriology* 35, 123.

Sage, R.D. and Selander, R.K. (1975) Trophic radiation through polymorphism in cichlid fishes. *Proceedings of the National Academy of Sciences of the United States of America* 72, 4669–4673.

Sanderson, K.E. and Demerec, M. (1965) The linkage map of *Salmonella typhimurium*. *Genetics* 51, 897–913.

Sangal, V., Harbottle, H., Mazzoni, C.J., Helmuth, R., Guerra, B., Didelot, X., Paglietti, B., Rabsch, W., Brisse, S., Weill, F-X., Roumagnac, P. and Achtman, M. (2010) Evolution and population structure of *Salmonella enterica* Serovar Newport. *Journal of Bacteriology* 192, 6465–6476.

Schröter, M., Roggentin, P., Hofmann, J., Hofmann, J., Speicher, A., Laufs, R. and Mack, D. (2004) Pet snakes as a reservoir for *Salmonella enterica* subsp. diarizonae (serogroup IIIa): a prospective study. *Applied and Environmental Microbiology* 70, 613–615.

Selander, R.K., Beltran, P., Smith, N.H., Helmuth, R., Rubin, F.A., Kopecko, D.J., Ferris, K., Tall, B.D., Cravioto, A. and Musser, J.M. (1990) Evolutionary genetic relationships of clones of Salmonella serovars that cause human typhoid and other enteric fevers. *Infection and Immunity* 58, 2262–2275.

Skerman, V.B.D., McGowan, V. and Sneath, P.H.A. (1980) Approved lists of bacterial names. *International Journal of Systematic Bacteriology* 30, 225–420.

Smith, J.M., Smith, N.H., O'Rourke, M. and Spratt. B.G. (1993) How clonal are bacteria? *Proceedings of the National Academy of Sciences of the United States of America* 90, 4384–4388.

Snyder, L. and Champness, W. (1997) *Molecular Genetics of Bacteria*. ASM Press, Washington.

Spratt, B.G., Hanage, W.P. and Feil, E.J. (2001) The relative contributions of recombination and point mutation to the diversification of bacterial clones. *Current Opinion in Microbiology* 4, 602–606.

Stackebrandt, E. and Ebers, E. (2006) Taxonomic parameters revisited: tarnished gold standards. *Microbiology Today* 33, 152–155.

Stackebrandt, E., Frederiksen, W., Garrity, G.M., Grimont, P.A.D., Kampfer, P., Maiden, M.C.J., Nesme, X., Rossello-Mora, R., Swings, J., Truper, H.G., Vauterin, L., Ward, A.C. and Whitman, W.B. (2002) Report of the ad hoc committee for the re-evaluation of the species definition in bacteriology. *International Journal of Systematic and Evolutionary Microbiology* 52, 1043–1047.

Staley, J.T. (2006) The bacterial species dilemma and the genomic-phylogenetic species concept. *Philosophical Transactions of the Royal Society B* 361, 1899–1909.

Stevens, M.P., Humphrey, T.J. and Maskell, D.J. (2009) Molecular insights into farm animal and zoonotic Salmonella infections. *Philosophical Transactions of the Royal Society B* 364, 2709–2723.

Tindall, B.J., Grimont, P.A.D., Garrity, G.M. and Euzeby, J.P. (2005) Nomenclature and taxonomy of the genus Salmonella. *International Journal of Systematic and Evolutionary Microbiology* 55, 521–524.

Uzzau, S., Brown, D.J., Wallis, T., Rubino, S., Leori, G., Casadusus, J., Platt, D.J. and Olsen, J.E. (2000) Host adapted serotypes of *Salmonella enterica*. *Epidemiology and Infection* 125, 229–255.

Vulic, M., Dionisio, F., Taddei, F. and Radman, M. (1997) Molecular keys to speciation: DNA polymorphism and the control of genetic exchange in enterobacteria. *Proceedings of the National Academy of Sciences of the United States of America* 94, 9763–9767.

Woese, C.R., Kandler, O. and Wheelis, M.L. (1990) Towards a natural system of organisms: proposal for the domains Archaea, Bacteria, and Eucarya. *Proceedings of the National Academy of Sciences of the United States of America* 87, 4576–4579.

Yabuuchi, E. and Ezaki, T. (2000) Arguments against the replacement of type species of the genus *Salmonella* from *Salmonella choleraesuis* to *Salmonella enterica* and the creation of the term neotype species, and for the conservation of *Salmonella choleraesuis*. *International Journal of Systematic and Evolutionary Microbiology* 50, 1693–1694.

After the chapter was written, the following paper was published:

Achtman, M., Wain, J., Weill, F.-X., Nair, S., Zhou, Z., Sangal, V., Kravland, M.G., Hale, J.L., Harbottle, H., Vesbeck, A., Dougan, G., Harrison, L.H., Brisse, S. and The *S. enterica* MLST Study Group (2012) Multilocus sequence typing as a replacement for serotyping in *Salmonella enterica*. PLoS Pathogens 8(6):e1002776, doi: 10.1371/journal.ppat.1002776.

2 Structure, Function and Synthesis of Surface Polysaccharides in *Salmonella*

Andrew N. Rycroft*
Royal Veterinary College, Hertfordshire, UK

Introduction

The surface polysaccharides of *Salmonella* spp. form the outermost components of the bacterial cell. They are in direct contact with the immediate environment of the organism and are therefore of great significance in the interaction of the organism with its habitat. For a bacterial pathogen such as *Salmonella*, which is able to exist in different habitats as it passes from the dry, external environment, through the acidity of the stomach, the lumen of the gut, the extracellular space of host tissues and the inside of the macrophage, the surface components provide a protective yet porous shield against the outside world. This chapter aims to review the chemical structure, biological function, biosynthesis and genetics of the surface polysaccharides found on the surface of *Salmonella*.

The Architecture of the Surface Structures of *Salmonella*

Much of what we understand about the nature of the outer envelope of Gram-negative bacteria has been derived from studies with *Escherichia coli* K-12 and *Salmonella enterica* serovar Typhimurium LT2. Essentially, there are three layers: the cytoplasmic membrane (CM; inner membrane), the peptidoglycan (P; murein) and the outer membrane (OM) (Fig. 2.1). The compartment between the two membranes, containing the peptidoglycan, is referred to as the periplasmic space.

The cytoplasmic membrane in *Salmonella* is composed of phospholipids and proteins. As in other Gram-negative bacteria, it transports nutrients, is the site of oxidative phosphorylation and the synthesis of phospholipid, peptidoglycan units and lipopolysaccharide (LPS). The cytoplasmic membrane is also the site of anchorage of the DNA during replication and has a role in the partitioning of daughter cells at cell division.

The peptidoglycan is a relatively thin layer in Gram-negative bacteria. It is composed of alternating residues of *N*-acetyl muramic acid and *N*-acetyl glucosamine forming long glycan chains, which are covalently cross-linked by peptide bridges. This forms a single bag-like molecule surrounding the cell protoplast, which serves to stabilize it against osmotic lysis. Approximately 3.5 atm pressure is thought to be exerted by the cytoplasm (Stock *et al.*, 1977).

The peptidoglycan confers rigidity and shape to the bacterial cell. Degrading the

* Author, e-mail: arycroft@rvc.ac.uk

© CAB International 2013. *Salmonella in Domestic Animals, 2nd Edition* (eds P.A. Barrow and U. Methner)

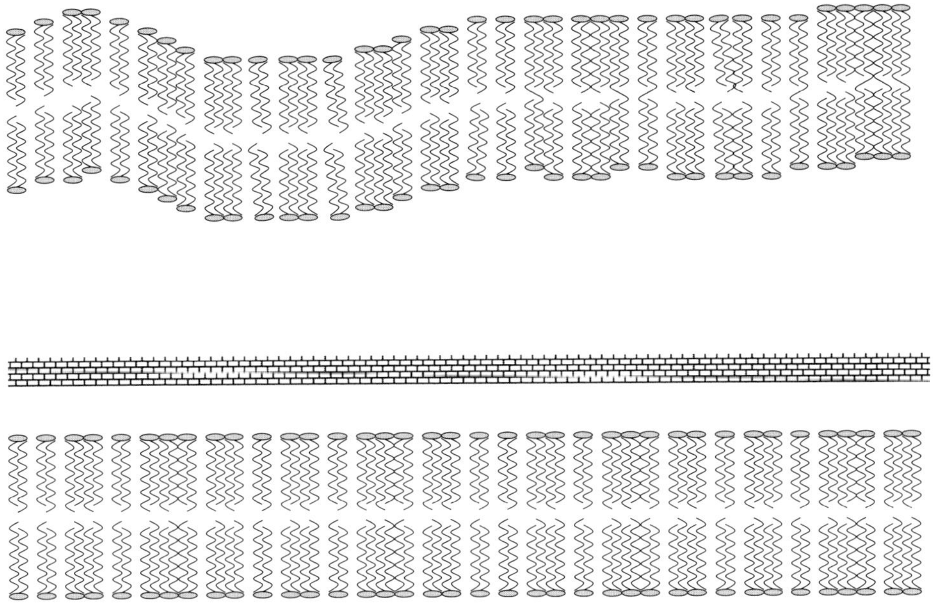

Fig. 2.1. Simplified representation of the envelope of *Salmonella*. Two lipid bilayers, the cytoplasmic membrane (CM) and the outer membrane (OM), are separated by the periplasmic space (P), in which the peptidoglycan provides tensile strength to support the cell against osmotic pressure.

peptidoglycan by first disrupting the outer membrane and then allowing lysozyme to penetrate and hydrolyse it, causes the cell to swell and lyse by the uptake of water through the cytoplasmic membrane into the cytosol. If this is prevented by immersion of the bacteria in a hypertonic medium such as 8% sucrose, the rod-shaped cells will round up to form osmotically fragile spheroplasts.

The periplasm contains the peptidoglycan and also numerous soluble proteins, which usually have one of three functions. These are: (i) catabolic functions, such as alkaline phosphatase, in which solutes for which no transport system exists are converted to a form that can be transported though the cytoplasmic membrane; (ii) binding proteins, which fasten on to nutrients such as amino acids, ions and sugars and assist their transport; and (iii) proteins, which degrade or modify harmful substances such as antibiotics, e.g. β-lactamase.

The two membranes are connected at various points known as zones of adhesion or Bayer bridges, first described by Bayer (1968). These sites of contact become visible by electron microscopy only when the inner membrane is plasmolysed or 'shrunk' away from the outer membrane by holding the organisms in hypertonic medium. These quasi-stable zones of adhesion are thought to facilitate the transport of hydrophobic materials such as LPS from the inner surface of the cytoplasmic membrane to the outer membrane and may be the site of synthesis of some outer membrane proteins.

The outer membrane is a highly complex lipid bilayer membrane structure, which surrounds the peptidoglycan layer and shields the periplasm from the external environment. It also prevents leakage of the periplasmic proteins away from the immediate environment of the cytoplasmic membrane. Electron microscopy has determined the thickness of the outer membrane to be like that of the cytoplasmic membrane, 7.5 nm. However, in composition and function it is quite different from the cytoplasmic membrane. It is composed primarily of phospholipid and protein but also LPS and lipoprotein. LPS is found exclusively in the outer leaflet of the outer membrane and the lipoprotein is present in the inner leaflet where it functions to anchor the outer membrane to the cell peptidoglycan. Enterobacterial common antigen is a minor component contributing only 0.2% of the cell's dry weight.

Since the natural habitat of *Salmonella* is the lower intestinal tract of animals of all kinds, it is logical to assume that the outer membrane functions to protect or assist the cell in this environment. In order to compete effectively with other microorganisms in the anaerobic, nutritionally sparse conditions of the gut, *Salmonella* need to be able to take up limiting nutrients effectively and to adapt to rapidly changing conditions. The outer membrane serves to allow the passive transport of selected molecules into the periplasm where they can be held and transported across the cytoplasmic membrane. At the same time, the outer membrane must serve to protect the delicate components of the cytoplasmic membrane from the detergent-like action of bile salts, fatty acids and glycerides. The intestinal lumen is replete with proteases and lipases, and these must be prevented from gaining access to the vicinity of the cytoplasmic membrane where they will cause damage to the membrane structures. Therefore, the outer membrane of *Salmonella* may be considered as a molecular sieve whose purpose is to allow required nutrients to access the periplasm while resisting the penetration of dangerous substances from the external environment.

Many Gram-negative bacteria such as *Escherichia coli*, *Klebsiella* or *Pasteurella* spp. possess a polysaccharide layer external to the outer membrane. *Salmonella enterica* is unusual among the enteric Gram-negative bacteria of mammals in that it usually possesses no capsular polysaccharide. The polysaccharide exposed at the surface is primarily the O side-chain of the LPS. The one exception to this is the Vi polysaccharide carried on the external surface of a very few strains of *Salmonella* such as some strains of *S.* Typhi and *S.* Dublin and which is present in addition to LPS.

Lipopolysaccharide

LPS is the molecule most closely associated with the surface of Gram-negative bacteria. It is also the immune-dominant antigen of the majority of Gram-negative bacteria. During the 1950s and 1960s a considerable research effort, due to the interest in LPS as a mediator of biological activity known as endotoxin activity, led to a wealth of information on their structure and biosynthesis. LPS is now recognized as a pathogen-associated molecular pattern (PAMP). Recognition of LPS by the Toll-like receptor 4 (TLR4) causes pro-inflammatory changes in host cell gene expression.

The structure of LPS has been elucidated over a number of years, investigations largely being conducted with *S.* Typhimurium LT2 and *E. coli* K-12 using a variety of techniques including biochemical analysis and examination of mutants deficient in LPS production. *Salmonella* has therefore come to be perceived as 'the norm' among Gram-negative bacteria although there is considerable variety of structure even within the genus.

LPS is amphipathic having both hydrophilic and hydrophobic components on the same molecule. Three regions of the molecule are recognized: the lipid A, the core oligosaccharide and the O side-chain repeating oligosaccharide. The core oligosaccharide is further subdivided into the inner and outer core regions (Fig. 2.2). The hydrophobic lipid A portion of the molecule resides within the outer leaflet of the outer membrane. The polysaccharide portion, which is hydrophilic, projects into the external environment.

Colonies of wild strains of *Salmonella* bacteria usually have a smooth appearance. This is associated with the presence of a full O side-chain, which is therefore termed the S form. Mutants of these that have lost their O side-chain, through natural occurrence or deliberate mutagenesis in the laboratory, often produce irregular-edged colonies with a dull surface. These are referred to as rough mutants and the LPS present in these bacteria as R form.

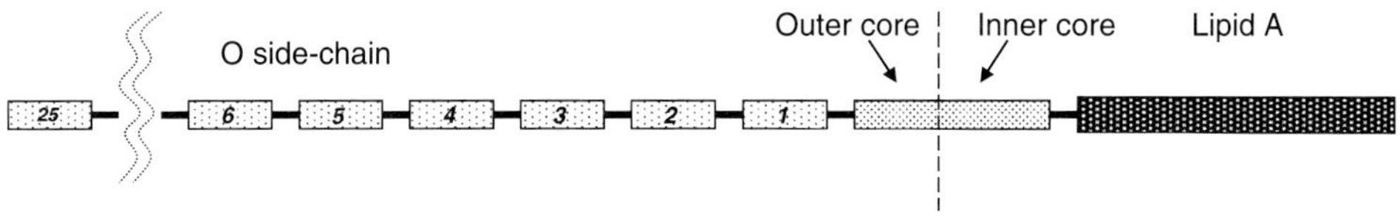

Fig. 2.2. Schematic representation of the structure of S-form lipopolysaccharide. Lipid A is joined, via the inner- and outer-core oligosaccharide, to the repeating oligosaccharide that forms the O side-chain. The length of the O side-chain is variable, but between 25 and 40 units is common in *Salmonella*.

Preparation and Purification of *Salmonella* Lipopolysaccharide

There are approximately 10^6 molecules of lipid A and 10^7 molecules of glycerophospholipid per bacterial cell (Goldman *et al.*, 1988). LPSs from *Salmonella* are often purified from the bacterial cells by one of two methods. S-form LPS is prepared by the phenol-water extraction method originally described by Westphal and Jann (1965). In this procedure, the bacteria are held at 65°C in 45% aqueous phenol. The S-form LPS, together with a proportion of the R-form LPS with a complete or nearly complete core oligosaccharide, is partitioned into the aqueous phase. For R-form LPS, the PCP method devised by Galanos *et al.* (1969) is preferable. This uses a mixture of 90% phenol, chloroform and petroleum ether to extract the bacteria at room temperature. LPS from deep rough mutants is only extracted using this method since it largely partitions into the hydrophobic phase. Other methods, which are intended to prepare purified LPS in both forms, have also been devised (Darveau and Hancock, 1983). Early studies with purified *Salmonella* LPS showed it to be highly variable in the O side-chain but conserved in structure in the core oligosaccharide and the lipid A.

Lipid A

Chemistry of lipid A

The structure of lipid A from *S. enterica* serovars is thought to be conserved. The lipid A component is embedded in the outer leaflet of the outer membrane of the organism, forming part of the lipid bilayer. It is responsible for the endotoxic properties of the LPS molecule (Raetz, 1993). While the general or approximate structure of lipid A was known for many years, the exact structure of lipid A was not finally established until 1983 in the laboratory of Ernst Rietschel, Otto Lüderitz and co-workers (Rietschel *et al.*, 1983). The delay in defining the structure was due to the complex structure of the molecule. This discovery opened the way to a fuller appreciation of the biosynthesis and pharmacology of lipid A endotoxin.

Enterobacteria such as *Salmonella* which are unable to synthesize lipid A are non-viable (Rick and Osborn, 1977; Rick and Young, 1982). The minimum requirement of the LPS molecule appears to be that found in Re mutants, in which the LPS comprises lipid A and two 3-deoxy-D-manno-octulosonic acid (KDO) residues (Fig. 2.3). The reasons why these components are essential for the bacteria to be viable are not fully understood, but deep rough mutants, lacking the heptose, are said to have a 'very deleterious' phenotype (Schnaitman and Klena, 1993).

Lipid A can be prepared from LPS by mild acid hydrolysis. Diphosphoryl lipid A (DPL) is obtained by treatment with 0.02 M sodium acetate, pH 4.5 at 100°C for 30 min. If harsher conditions are used (0.1 M HCl at 100°C for 30 min), monophosphoryl lipid A (MPL), lacking the phosphate group at the 1 position, is released.

Lipid A from *S.* Typhimurium, other *Salmonella* serovars and *E. coli* consists of two

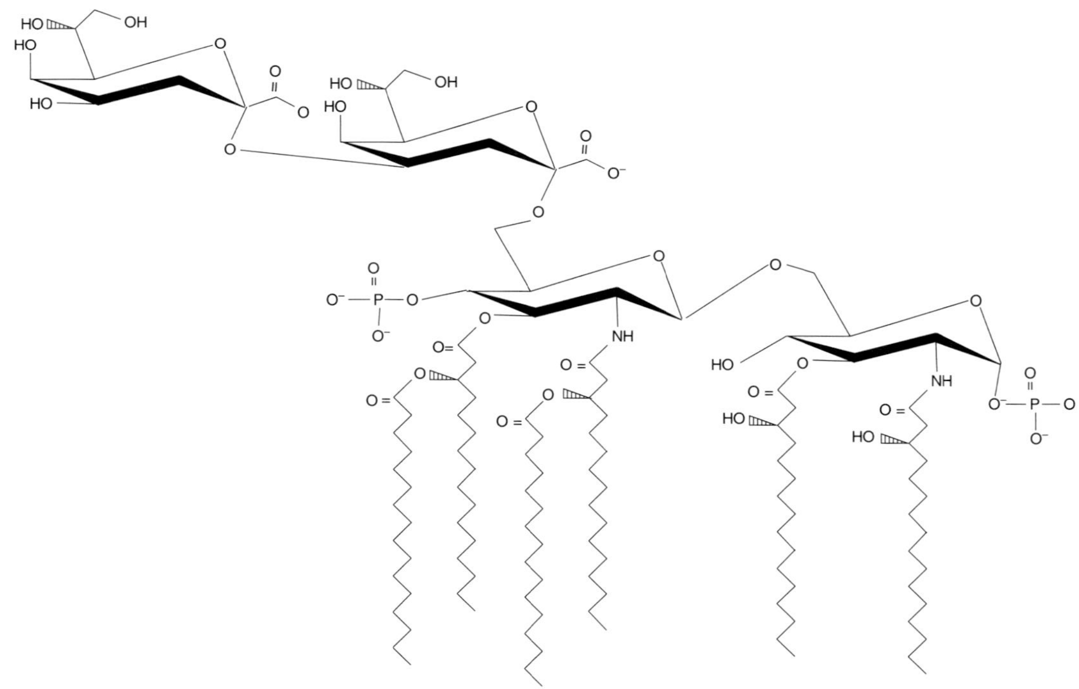

Fig. 2.3. The minimal Re chemotype lipopolysaccharide of *Salmonella*, sometimes known as KDO_2-lipid A. Two KDO residues are linked to the acetylated glucosamine disaccharide (lipid A). Linkage of the KDO to the glucosamine disaccharide involves the product of the *kdtA* gene.

glucosamine residues joined by a β(1-6) linkage, to which are substituted four fatty acid residues at positions 2 and 3 and 2′ and 3′. Those attached to positions 2 and 2′ are joined via amide links. The acyl moieties of lipid A are unusual because they are hydroxylated at carbon 3. They are also 2–6 carbons shorter than glycerophospholipids. Those hydroxylated fatty acids attached to positions 2′ and 3′ are further esterified, through the hydroxyls at C3, to additional fatty acyl residues giving six fatty acid chains in all.

Biological activities of lipid A

Lipid A has potent biological activity. Since lipid A has been a component of the Gram-negative cell envelope probably throughout the evolution of eukaryotes, the immune system of animals is exceedingly sensitive to it as a marker of infection. Lipid A has been known to induce pathophysiological effects such as endotoxic shock, pyrogenicity, activation of complement, coagulation and haemodynamic changes for many years. The dose of Re LPS from *Salmonella* Typhimurium producing a febrile response in 50% of rabbits is between 0.1 and 0.3 μg kg^{-1} body weight. Long recognized immunological effects include mitogenicity for B-lymphocytes and activation of macrophages, but it is only since the late 1990s that it has been known that these effects are mediated through the induction and release of numerous cytokines of monocyte and macrophage origin (interferon, tumour necrosis factor, colony stimulating factor and interleukin-1) through stimulation of the TLR4-MD2-CD14 pathway to activate the host defences during bacterial infection (Qureshi and Takayama, 1990; Poltorak *et al.*, 1998). It is through these activities that lipid A (endotoxin) contributes to the pathogenic or endotoxic shock activity of Gram-negative bacteria, including *Salmonella*. As an example of a substance that can modify or modulate an immune response, LPS is now considered to be a potent modulin (Henderson *et al.*, 1996).

Genetics of lipid A synthesis

The biosynthetic pathway of lipid A has been elucidated primarily in *E. coli* K-12. However, the genes and gene products required for this process seem to be identical for lipid A in *Salmonella*. Uridine diphosphate-*N*-acetyl glucosamine (UDP-GlcNAc) is a central precursor for the synthesis of both peptidoglycan and LPS. This leads to a group of phospholipids based not on glycerol, but on glucosamine. The only known function of these is as precursors of lipid A. Only four genes are known to be involved in lipid A synthesis and all of these are derived from studies with *E. coli*. These are *lpxA*, *lpxB*, *lpxC* and *lpxD*. These genes encode the enzymes that: (i) transfer β-hydroxymyristic acid from acyl carrier protein (ACP) to the 3-hydroxy group of UDP-GlcNAc (*lpxA*); (ii) remove the *N*-acetyl group from UDP-3-hydroxy myristoyl-GlcNAc (*lpxC*); (iii) transfer the β-hydroxymyristic acid from ACP to 2-amino group of deacylated GlcNAc to form UDP-2,3-dihydroxy myristoyl-glucosamine (*lpxD*); and (iv) form the β(1-6) bond between the glucosamines of one molecule of UDP-2,3-dihydroxy myristoyl-glucosamine and one of 2,3-dihydroxy myristoyl-glucosamine (lipid X) to form the lipid A disaccharide with four fatty acid residues and one phosphate group (*lpxB*) (Crowell *et al.*, 1987).

Core Oligosaccharide

The lipid A is linked through carbon 6′ of the glucosamine disaccharide to the core oligosaccharide. This link (α2-6) is made through a unique 8-carbon sugar called 3-deoxy-D-*manno*-octulosonic acid (KDO). A second, branch KDO (known as KDO II), is also added through an α(2-4) linkage. This structure is known as KDO_2-lipid A or Re endotoxin because it is the form of LPS seen in mutants with the Re chemotype – the minimal substructure for growth of the bacteria (Rick and Young, 1982). It is generally believed that a third KDO residue is added to KDO II at a late stage of core completion through a further α(2-4) linkage although this is not essential for viability in *Salmonella* (Lehmann *et al.*, 1971).

The core oligosaccharide consists of a conserved, non-repeating group of from six to eight sugars. In *Salmonella*, a single core oligosaccharide type (termed the Ra-core) is conserved throughout the genus (Holst and Brade, 1992). It consists of eight sugar residues in addition to the KDO residues which link it to the lipid A (Fig. 2.4). Two L-glycero-D-*manno*-heptose residues are attached to the KDO forming the so-called inner core. A third L-glycero-D-*manno*-heptose branches from the outermost heptose. This in turn is linked to 2 D-glucose, 2 D-galactose residues and *N*-acetyl glucosamine forming the outer core. In addition, *O*-pyrophosphorylethanolamine and *O*-phosphorylethanolamine are frequently substituted on to the L-glycero-D-*manno*-heptose and KDO residues, respectively.

Genetics of the Lipopolysaccharide Core Biosynthesis

The genetics of core biosynthesis have been extensively reviewed by Schnaitman and Klena (1993). The genes required for the production of core lipopolysaccharide belong primarily to the *rfa* gene cluster (Fig. 2.5). This was revised and a new system for the nomenclature of genes for polysaccharide biosynthesis was proposed by Reeves *et al.* (1996). The *rfa* gene cluster has largely been renamed the *waa* cluster (Table 2.1). While many of the genes are known from work with *S.* Typhimurium, others have only been identified in *E. coli* and their equivalent function in *Salmonella* is not known for certain. While the newer nomenclature is widely adopted, the original gene designations are still used in some cases, such as the genome annotation of *S.* Typhimurium, and so both systems remain in use to some extent.

Two *kds* genes (*kdsA* and *kdsB*) are required for synthesis of KDO. The KDO is then added to the glucosamine of lipid A disaccharide by the product of the *waaA* gene (previously *kdtA*), KDO transferase. KDO II is also added by this enzyme, and indirect evidence suggests that KDO III is further added by this enzyme at a late stage in synthesis of the core. The final steps in the acylation of lipid A are thought to be coupled to the attachment of KDO (Brozek and Raetz, 1990); however, the genes required for terminal acylation of lipid A are not yet known.

The synthesis of heptose and its conversion to L-glycero-D-manno-heptose involves *waaD* and *waaE* genes (previously *rfaD* and *rfaE*). Addition of the first heptose to KDO I requires a heptosyltransferase encoded by the *waaC* gene (previously *rfaC*), and completion of the inner core by addition of the second heptose requires *waaF* (*rfaF*). Mutants lacking these genes are said to exhibit a deep rough phenotype.

The first D-glucose of the outer core is attached by a glucosyl transferase, which is the product of the *waaG* gene (*rfaG*). The substrate, UDP-glucose, is cleaved to add the glucose residue to the second heptose

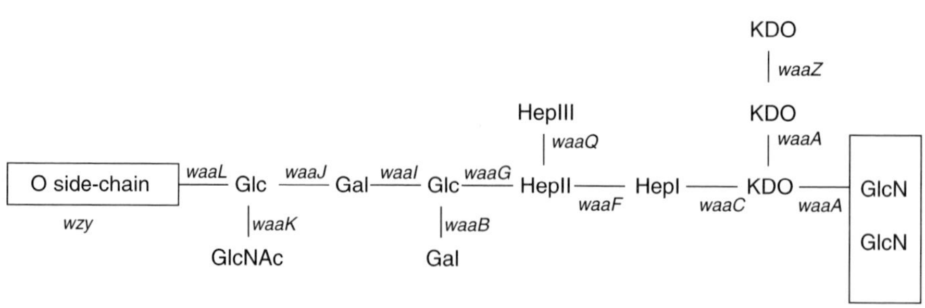

Fig. 2.4. The structure of the lipopolysaccharide core oligosaccharide of *Salmonella*. The genes known to be required for the synthesis of the core at various points are shown.

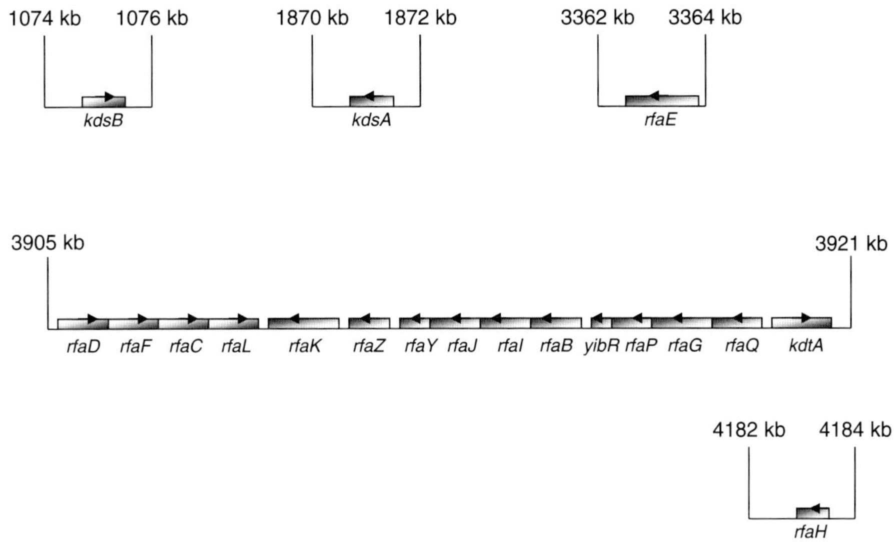

Fig. 2.5. Genomic arrangement of the *waa* (*rfa*) gene cluster and associated loci involved in the synthesis and attachment of the core O side-chain in *Salmonella* Typhimurium LT2 (Adapted from McClelland *et al.*, 2001).

Table 2.1. Genes involved in the synthesis of the lipopolysaccharide core in *Salmonella* Typhimurium.

Gene	Original designation	Function
kdsA		2-dehydro-3-deoxyphosphooctonate aldolase (KDO-8-phosphate synthesis).
kdsB		3-deoxy-manno-octulosonate cytidylyltransferase (CMP-KDO synthesis
waaA	*kdtA*	3-deoxy-D-manno-octulosonic-acid transferase (transfer of KDO to glucosamine)
yibR		Hypothetical inner membrane protein
waaE	*rfaE*	ADP heptose synthesis
gmhD	*rfaD*	Epimerization of ADP heptose to L-glycero-D-manno-heptose
waaC	*rfaC*	Heptosyltransferase: addition of heptose
waaF	*rfaF*	Addition of heptose II to complete the inner core
waaG	*rfaG*	Glucosyltransferase: addition of glucose to HepII
waaB	*rfaB*	Addition of branch D-galactose to glucose
waaI	*rfaI*	Galactosyltransferase: addition of D-galactose by (*waaJ*)
waaY	*rfaY*	Modification of heptose region of the core
waaJ	*rfaJ*	Addition of second D-glucose
waaK	*rfaK*	Transfer of branch *N*-acetyl glucosamine to some terminal glucose
rfaH	*rfaH*	Positive regulation of *waa*
waaQ	*rfaQ*	Addition of Hep III to core?
waaL	*rfaL*	'Ligase' addition of O-antigen to core
waaP	*rfaP*	Phosphorylation of HepI
waaZ	*rfaZ*	Addition of KdoIII to KdoII

Gene designations in the NCBI database remain in the original form. Many publications use the new nomenclature but both are still in use. For clarity therefore, both gene designations are given here.

(Hep II). Interestingly, mutants with a defective *waaG* gene produce neither flagella nor type 1 fimbriae. This suggests either a regulatory role for the WaaG protein or the synthesis of these surface appendages is dependent upon a certain degree of completion of the LPS core.

A D-galactose residue is then attached by an α(1-3) link to the D-glucose by a galactosyl transferase. This is the product of the *waaI* gene (*rfaI*). A branch D-galactose residue is also attached to the glucose in an α(1-6) link by the product of the *waaB* gene. The second, terminal α(1-2) linked D-glucose is then attached by the *waaJ* product and finally, completing the *Salmonella* core oligosaccharide, the *waaK* gene product transfers a branch *N*-acetyl glucosamine in α(1-2) linkage to a proportion of the terminal glucose residues.

The O-antigen

The serologically dominant and highly variable region of the LPS is the O side-chain. This is hydrophilic in nature and reaches out to the microenvironment of the bacterial cell (Fig. 2.2). It is a repeated tetra- or pentasaccharide, characterized by the inclusion of deoxy- and dideoxyhexoses. The number of repeats in the O side-chain varies from strain to strain and is dependent upon the prevailing growth conditions. The repeating nature and quantum variation of the O side-chain can be visualized by separation of S-form LPS on an SDS polyacrylamide gel and silver staining (Hitchcock and Brown, 1983). Each band in the 'ladder' represents a LPS molecule with one single oligosaccharide unit more or less than the one next to it. Between 25 and 40 units of the oligosaccharide is a common finding (Fig. 2.6).

The O side-chain in serological classification

The system that is used to differentiate the serovars of *Salmonella* (previously referred to as species) is based on the grouping of strains according to the structure of the O-antigenic side-chain polysaccharide coupled with determination of the serological specificity of the H (flagellar) antigen, which may be expressed in one of two phases. This is the White–Kauffmann–Le Minor scheme. Serological distinction of the O-antigens of *Salmonella* is made on the detection of particular antigens, which are designated by a number.

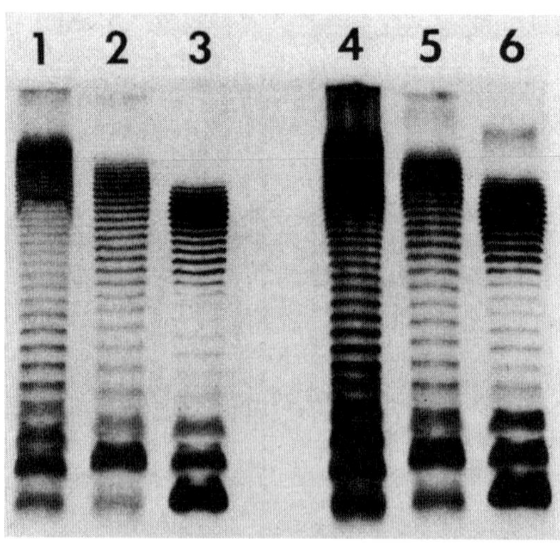

Fig. 2.6. Silver-stained polyacrylamide gel separation of *Salmonella* lipopolysaccharide showing ladder banding pattern derived from the stepwise change in length of O side-chain (from Peterson and McGroarty, 1985, with permission from the *Journal of Bacteriology*).

These factors are determined by the component sugars of the O side-chain. Thus, *S.* Typhimurium has the antigenic formula 1,4,5,12. Antigens 4 and 12 are found in all group B serovars although factor 12 is also found elsewhere. Factors 1 and 5 are additional factors, which assist in the definition of serological specificity of *S.* Typhimurium.

Synthesis and genetics of the O side-chain

The genes required for the biosynthesis of the O side-chain obviously vary from serotype to serotype since these contain different sugars and linkages in the repeating oligosaccharide. Nevertheless, there are basic similarities in these genes from those serotypes that have been examined. The group of genes involved in O side-chain synthesis is the 20 or so genes of the *wba* locus (previously *rfb*) (Fig. 2.7; Table 2.2), much of which maps near *his* at approximately 45 min on the *Salmonella* chromosome (Jiang *et al.*, 1991; McClelland *et al.*, 2001).

Among the enterobacteria, there are two systems of O-antigen synthesis based on the gene involved in attachment of the first sugar of the O side-chain to the undecaprenol phosphate antigen carrier lipid (ACL). Most *Salmonella* serotypes use the product of the *wbaP* (*rfbP*) gene rather than that of the alternative *wecA* (*rfe*) gene. These include O groups A, B, C2, D and E1. However, some serogroups (C1 and L) are *wecA*-dependent.

The O side-chain repeat unit of group B strains such as *Salmonella* Typhimurium has four or five sugars. The backbone sugars are the same in serogroups A, D and E1, comprising mannose, rhamnose and galactose whereas in group C2 this is Rha-Man-Man-Gal. In group B the mannose is substituted with abequose, a 3,6-dideoxy-galactose (which confers the O4 antigen factor) and the galactose is partially substituted with glucose. The abequose is further O-acetylated, which confers the O5 antigen. In other groups, the dideoxyhexose component is different: paratose in group A, abequose in B and C2, tyvelose in group D and none in E1.

Synthesis of group B O-antigen begins with the transfer of galactose phosphate to ACL by the product of the *wbaP* (*rfbP*) gene. The gene *wbaN* (*rfbN*) encodes the sugar transferase for addition of the rhamnose, while *wbaU* (*rfbU*) and *wbaV* (*rfbV*) encode the enzymes that attach rhamnose and abequose, respectively, using the sugar nucleotides as substrates. The glycosylation of galactose requires the *oafA* gene, which lies just outside the *rfb* cluster.

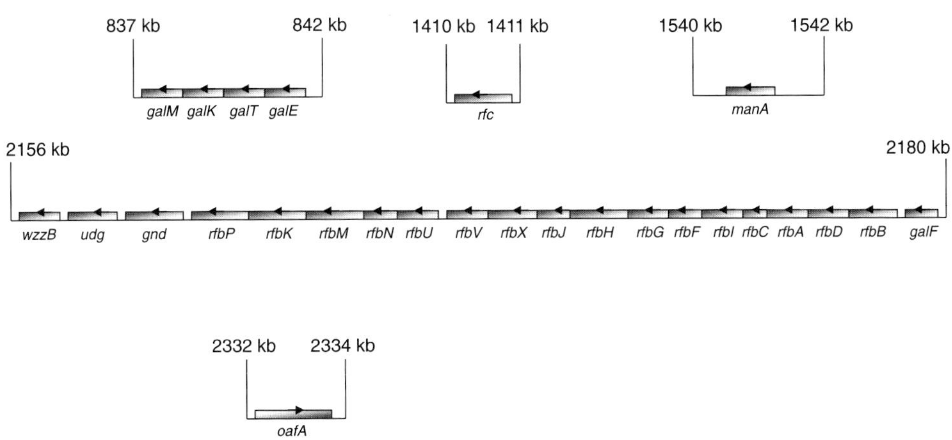

Fig. 2.7. Genomic arrangement of the *wba* (*rfb*) gene cluster and associated loci involved in the synthesis, attachment and regulation of the O side-chain in *Salmonella* Typhimurium LT2 (adapted from McClelland *et al.*, 2001).

Table 2.2. Genes involved in the synthesis of the lipopolysaccharide O antigen in *Salmonella* Typhimurium.

Gene	Original designation	Function
wbaBDAC	*rfbBDAC*	Synthesis of TDP-rhamnose
manB	*rfbKM*	Synthesis of GDP-mannose
ddhAB	*rfbFG*	Synthesis of CDP-4-keto-3,6-dideoxyglucose precursor
abe	*rfbJ*	Synthesis of CDP-abequose (group B)
prt	*rfbS*	Synthesis of CDP-paratose (group A)
tyv	*rfbE*	Synthesis of CDP-tyvelose (group D)
wbaP	*rfbP*	Initial step of attachment of Gal-P to ACL
wecA	*rfe*	Initial step of attachment of GlcNAc-P to ACL
wbaN	*rfbN*	Rhamnose transfer to galactose (groups A, B, D and E1)
wbaU	*rfbU*	Mannose transfer to rhamnose (groups A, B and D)
wbaV	*rfbV*	Abequose transfer to mannose (groups B and D)
wbaX	*rfbX*	O-antigen transferase
wbaH	*rfbH*	Lipopolysaccharide biosynthesis protein
wbaI	*rfbI*	CDP-6-deoxy-delta-3,4-glucose reductase
galF	*galF*	UTP-glucose-1-phosphate uridylyltransferase
galE	*galE*	UDP-galactose-4-epimerase
galT	*galT*	Galactose-1-phosphate uridylyltransferase
galK	*galK*	Galactokinase
galM	*galM*	Aldose 1-epimerase
wzzB	*wzzB*	Regulator of chain length of O-antigen component of LPS
udg	*udg*	UDP-glucose/GDP-mannose dehydrogenase
gnd	*gnd*	Formation of D-ribulose-5-phosphate
oafA	*oafA*	O-antigen acetylase
wzy	*rfc*	Polymerization of O side-chain units
waaL	*rfaL*	Attaches O side-chain to core oligosaccharide
wzz	*rol*	Regulates length of O side-chain

Mutants are known that produce the so-called semi-rough (SR) phenotype comprising a complete core and a single O-antigen subunit. The gene required for polymerization of multi-unit O-antigen molecules is *wzy* (*rfc*) encoding the O-antigen ligase. The LPS produced by this class of mutant has a high proportion of LPS chains substituted with a single O side-chain unit while the remainder have complete cores that carry no O-antigen. The proportion of LPS molecules with core only is approximately the same as that seen in strains with S-form LPS. Therefore it was recognized that these mutants can attach the first O-antigen unit but are defective in the polymerization step required to generate the repeating O side-chain. They are nevertheless able to ligate the first O unit to the core and efficiently transfer the resulting LPS to the surface of the outer membrane. The gene encoding this function is termed *wzy* (*rfc*) and it is located in the *wba* cluster in *Salmonella* strains of serogroups C1, C2 and E1. However, it is at a separate site in other serogroups such as B (Fig. 2.7). The Wzy protein is very hydrophobic, suggesting that it is a membrane protein. Attachment of the O-antigen to the core is carried out by the product of the *waaL* (*rfaL*) gene – also referred to as ligase (Kaniuk *et al.*, 2004). This gene is distantly located in the *rfa* locus (Fig. 2.5).

The mechanism by which O-antigen units are added to the growing O side-chain is still not entirely clear. The sugars of the oligosaccharide are transferred from sugar nucleotide phosphates to the carrier lipid molecule, the undecaprenol phosphate ACL, as illustrated in Fig. 2.8. Galactose, rhamnose and mannose are sequentially transferred to the ACL while it is in the inner face of the cytoplasmic membrane. Branch sugars, such as abequose of *S.* Typhimurium, are transferred to the mannose and galactose. This must then be transferred to the site of the lipid A core. As the ACL-trisaccharide reaches the outer leaflet of the cytoplasmic membrane, the galactosyl-phosphate bond of the ACL-trisaccharide is broken and the galactosyl bond is transferred to the terminal mannosyl residue of a second or acceptor lipid, forming an oligosaccharide lipid carrier. This is repeated several times, chain growth taking place by addition of oligosaccharide units to the reducing end of the polysaccharide chain. Therefore, the developing polysaccharide is always transferred to an ACL carrying an O-antigen unit. To recycle the ACL, a specific phosphorylase dephosphorylates the free ACL to the monophosphate derivative, which then returns to the inner cytoplasmic face to begin the addition of sugars to form an oligosaccharide unit (Fig. 2.8). In a few cases, e.g. *S.* Minneapolis and *S.* Typhimurium, certain branch sugars (glucose) are added not in the cytoplasm but after polymerization. Frequently when this is the case, substitution is incomplete. Similarly, O-acetylation is carried out once polymerization has taken place.

The completed polysaccharide O side-chain-ACL then interacts with the lipid A core. The transfer of the O side-chain polysaccharide from the ACL to the glucose of the *Salmonella* core is carried out by O-antigen LPS ligase. Once transferred, the LPS molecule must be relocated to the outer membrane. The flip-flop transfer of the LPS to the outer membrane is still not fully understood, but seems to involve outer-membrane proteins for which LPS has a strong affinity, as well as the Bayer-bridge adhesion points linking the inner and outer membranes.

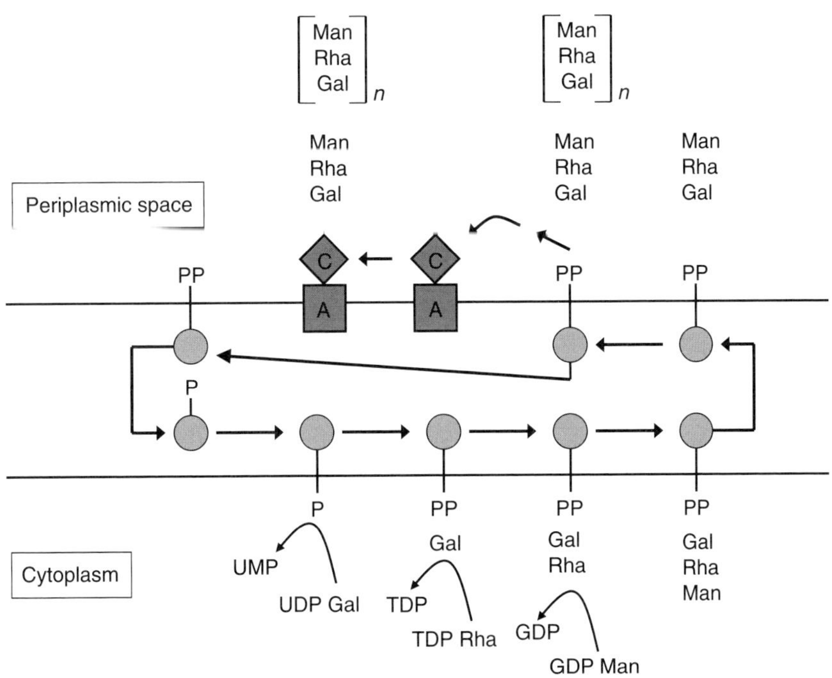

Fig. 2.8. Biosynthesis of O side-chain in *Salmonella*. At the inner face of the cytoplasmic membrane, the nucleotide sugars are transferred in sequence to the C55 polyisoprenoid phosphate carrier lipid. Following the transfer of the mannosylrhamnosylgalactose trisaccharide-carrier lipid to the outer face of the membrane, the trisaccharides polymerize, forming the lipid-linked O-antigen polymer, the polysaccharide portion of which is then passed to the lipid A core (AC). The liberated carrier lipid is then dephosphorylated and returned to the cytoplasmic face of the membrane.

The distribution of size of molecules of LPS can be seen on the characteristic laddering pattern in silver-stained polyacrylamide gels (Fig. 2.6). It is clear that, while there are a large number of molecules substituted with one, two or three O repeat units, this quickly decreases until there seem to be very few of intermediate size. As the size increases, the abundance once again increases to a maximum that is dependent upon the strain and its environmental conditions. Goldman and Hunt (1990) suggested that this distribution indicates a mechanism by which larger molecules are preferentially selected for ligation onto the LPS core. The O-antigen chain length regulator is *wzzB*, the final gene of the *rfb* cluster. This encodes an inner membrane protein belonging to the polysaccharide co-polymerase (PCP) family. Mutation of this gene caused an even distribution of chain lengths characteristic of random ligation and polymerization (Batchelor *et al.*, 1992).

The O side-chain in pathogenicity

The O-antigen component is also of importance in the interaction with the host in disease, particularly in evading the innate host defences. The structure and immunogenicity of the O side-chain may have profound effects on the ability of the humoral immune system to mount a response to infection and on the initial interaction with professional phagocytic cells.

Influence of Chemical Structure of Lipopolysaccharide on the Pathogenicity of *Salmonella*

LPS has long been recognized as contributing to virulence of *Salmonella* and survival of the organism in its natural habitat. Loss of the O-antigen in rough strains is associated with reduced virulence. The LPS is known to be required for colonization of the intestine (Nevola *et al.*, 1987), resistance to serum complement (Shaio and Rowland, 1985) and for contributing to invasion of, and survival in, macrophages (Murray *et al.*, 2006; Nagy *et al.*, 2006). Ilg *et al.* (2009) showed the presence of complete LPS is not essential for *in vitro* invasion or for inducing acute colitis, at least in streptomycin-pretreated mice. A Δ*wbaP* mutant (having no O-antigen) was attenuated in a competitive infection assay but still able to cause intestinal inflammation. The effect of stepwise loss of the O-antigen and core oligosaccharide was investigated by Kong *et al.* (2011). By introducing non-polar, defined deletion mutations into a strain of *S.* Typhimurium, the effects of deeper LPS mutants could be investigated. In general, mutants with truncated outer core and O-antigen were more sensitive to detergent (bile salts), polymyxin B and serum complement than wild-type. Less expected was the finding that the *waaG* mutant, with only the inner core, was as resistant to serum as the *waaL* mutant that produces a complete core and more resistant to serum than the *waaJ*, *rfaH* and *waaI* mutants.

The chemical nature of the O-antigen may also have direct influence on the pathogenicity of a strain or serotype. Differences in the virulence of serotypes and strains of *Salmonella* for animals are well known but this can result from differences other than those responsible for the serotype. In order to examine the importance and function of the O side-chain composition in an isogenic background, Valtonen and co-workers carried out genetic exchange experiments, using transduction, to alter a strain of *Salmonella* Typhimurium (serotype O-4,12) to carry the O-antigen of *S.* Enteritidis (O-9,12) or *S.* Montevideo (O-6,7) (Fig. 2.9). They clearly showed that the strain possessing the O-6,7 antigen was least virulent while the parent (O-4,12) showed the greatest virulence. The strain carrying the O-9,12 antigen was of intermediate virulence (Valtonen, 1970). These differences were shown to be manifest in immunosuppressed mice also, suggesting that the innate immunity of the animal was responsible for the differential response (Valtonen *et al.*, 1971). Subsequent experiments showed that when the O-9,12 serotype of a natural *S.* Enteritidis strain was replaced by transduction with the O-4,12 serotype of *S.* Typhimurium a statistically significant increase in virulence was observed (Valtonen

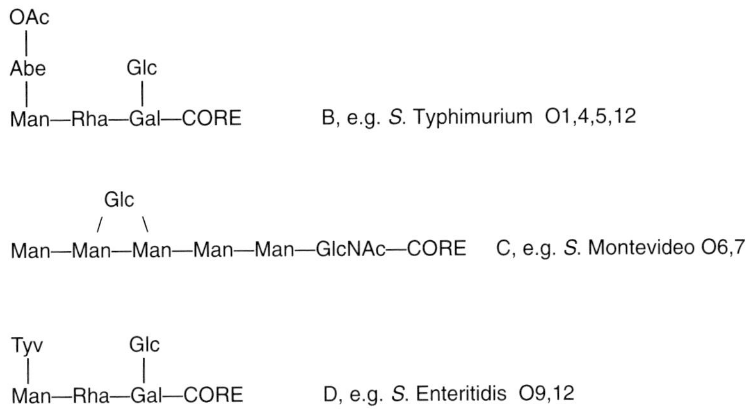

Fig. 2.9. Representative O side-chain repeat units from Salmonella Typhimurium (group B), S. Montevideo (group C1) and S. Enteritidis (group D).

et al., 1975). Since these strains were shown to differ little in their uptake by phagocytes both *in vitro* and *in vivo*, an O-6,7 strain was constructed to be isogenic with the O-4,12 strain and this correlated well with the clearance rates *in vivo*. However, neither strain was killed in an *in vitro* phagocytosis assay (Valtonen, 1977).

This work was continued by Liang-Takasaki *et al.* (1982). They found the rate of uptake of the isogenic strains by a macrophage-like cell line was inversely proportional to their mouse virulence. The differences in uptake were attributed to the differential affinity of the bacteria for the macrophages rather than the rate of uptake following the interaction. This was proposed as evidence for a receptor-mediated process. In addition, the uptake was shown to be complement-dependent and direct activation of complement by LPS was postulated as one important factor determining virulence. It was concluded that virulent bacteria may evade both complement killing and opsonophagocytosis by evolving LPS modified so as to reduce activation of complement. Later studies confirmed the differential activation of C3 by these strains and showed it to proceed primarily via the alternative pathway (Liang-Takasaki *et al.*, 1983a). Finally, these studies reverted to examining the strains in the whole animal and concluded that the difference in complement-dependent phagocytosis noted *in vitro* was the primary factor responsible for the observed virulence differences *in vivo* (Liang-Takasaki *et al.*, 1983b).

Enterobacterial Common Antigen

The enterobacterial common antigen (ECA) is an acidic cell surface glycolipid shared by essentially all members of the *Enterobacteriaceae* including *Salmonella* (Rick and Silver, 1996). It was considered to be of minor importance in the life of *Salmonella*. More recently, ECA has been shown to be required for resistance to bile salts. Mutations in the *wec* gene cluster, required for ECA synthesis, caused sensitivity to desoxocholate and significant reduction in virulence in a mouse oral infection model via the oral route but not the intraperitoneal route (Ramos-Morales *et al.*, 2003). They suggest that by protecting *Salmonella* from bile salts, ECA may enable colonization via the intestinal tract and virulence of the pathogen by the natural route of transmission.

ECA is found in two forms: the haptenic form and the immunogenic form (Mayer and Schmidt, 1979). The immunogenic form is covalently linked to the LPS core region of rough mutants. The haptenic form is not covalently linked to the LPS and it is found in both smooth and rough strains including those that produce the immunogenic form.

The serological specificity of ECA is governed by an amino sugar-containing heteropolysaccharide. This is primarily a trisaccharide repeating unit linear chain of 1-4 linked *N*-acetyl-D-glucosamine, *N*-acetyl-D-mannosaminuronic acid and *N*-acetylfucosamine residues.

The *wecA-E* (*rfe* and *rff*) gene cluster is required for biosynthesis of ECA. Products from the *rml* gene are known to be required for production of ECA as well as O side-chains. The products of the *mnaAB* and *fcnAB* genes are also required for ECA synthesis (such as synthesis of UDP-*N*-acetyl-D-mannosaminuronic acid). Strains of some *Salmonella* harbouring *wecA* mutations (e.g. *S.* Montevideo and *S.* Minnesota) cannot synthesize the O side-chain serogroup antigen or ECA while others (e.g. *S.* Typhimurium) with similar mutations fail to produce ECA. Biosynthesis involves transfer of the amino sugars to the carrier undecaprenyl phosphate in a manner similar to that for O-antigen side-chain and peptidoglycan components (Rick *et al.*, 1985). Polymerization of the trimers is followed by transfer of these to a phospholipid and incorporation into the outer membrane.

The Vi Antigen

The Vi antigen is the only true capsular polysaccharide produced by *Salmonella* spp. It was discovered in 1934 and was termed the Vi antigen because of its association with virulence. It is only produced by strains of *S.* Typhi and *S.* Paratyphi C together with a few strains of *S.* Dublin and *Citrobacter freundii*. As recognized with other enterobacteria bearing capsular polysaccharide, *Salmonella* carrying the Vi antigen are not agglutinable with anti-O antiserum. They therefore appear inagglutinable in slide agglutination tests until the bacteria have been heated (100°C, 60 min) to remove the masking effect of the capsule, revealing the O-specific antigen beneath. *In vivo*, the Vi polysaccharide prevents recognition of the *Salmonella* surface LPS by TLR4 (Wilson *et al.*, 2008). It inhibits C3b deposition at the bacterial surface to reduce opsonization and it reduces TLR-dependent interleukin-8 (IL-8) expression in the intestinal mucosa (Rafatellu *et al.*, 2005). Since few strains nfecting animals actually carry the Vi antigen, inagglutinability due to Vi is encountered very infrequently in clinical veterinary microbiology.

The Vi antigen is an unbranched homopolymer of α-1,4-(2-deoxy)-2-*N*-acetylgalactosaminuronic acid. It is O-acetylated in approximately 60% of the residues at the C3 position (Heynes and Kiessling, 1967). The Vi antigen is recognized as a group I polysaccharide in the scheme of Jann and Jann (1990). This scheme is based on chemical, physical and genetic criteria in which group I polysaccharides have high molecular mass and are thicker than type II polysaccharides, include hexuronic acid as the acidic component and are expressed along with LPS O-antigens.

Genes required for production of Vi are located on *viaB* on the 134 kb *Salmonella* pathogenicity island (SPI) 7, which is absent from most *Salmonella* serovars. The *tviBCDE* genes are involved in biosynthesis; export of the polysaccharide requires the genes *vexA-BCDE* (Virlogeux *et al.*, 1995; Pickard *et al.*, 2003). The *viaA* region is also present in certain Vi-negative bacteria such as *E. coli*. In this organism, a locus that is allelic to *viaA* is known by the designation *rcsB*. This is known to be a positive regulator of capsule biosynthesis, which is functional in *E. coli*. Therefore, transfer of the *viaB* locus to *E. coli* was shown to cause expression of Vi in *E. coli* (Johnson and Baron, 1969).

References

Batchelor, R.A., Alifano, P., Biffali, E., Hull, S.I. and Hull, R.A. (1992) Nucleotide sequence of the genes regulating O polysaccharide antigen chain length (*rol*) from *Escherichia coli* and *Salmonella typhimurium*: protein homology and functional complementation. *Journal of Bacteriology* 174, 5228–5236.

Bayer, M.E. (1968) Areas of adhesion between wall and membrane of *Escherichia coli*. *Journal of General Microbiology* 53, 395–404.

Brozek, K.A. and Raetz, C.R.H. (1990) Biosynthesis of lipid A in *Escherichia coli*. Acyl carrier protein-dependent incorporation of laurate and myristate. *Journal of Biological Chemistry* 265, 15410–15417.

Crowell, D.N., Reznikoff, W.S. and Raetz, C.R.H. (1987) Nucleotide sequence of the *Escherichia coli* gene for lipid A disaccharide synthetase. *Journal of Bacteriology* 169, 5727–5734.

Darveau, R.P. and Hancock, R.E.W. (1983) Procedure for isolation of bacterial lipopolysaccharides from both smooth and rough *Pseudomonas aeruginosa* and *Salmonella typhimurium* strains. *Journal of Bacteriology* 155, 831–838.

Galanos, C., Lüderitz, O. and Westphal, O. (1969) A new method for the extraction of R lipopolysaccharides. *European Journal of Biochemistry* 9, 245–249.

Goldman, R.C. and Hunt, F. (1990) Mechanism of O antigen distribution in lipopolysaccharide. *Journal of Bacteriology* 172, 5352–5359.

Goldman, R.C., Doran, C.C. and Capobianco, J.O. (1988) Analysis of lipopolysaccharide biosynthesis in *Salmonella typhimurium* and *Escherichia coli* by using agents which specifically block incorporation of 3-deoxy-D-manno-octulosonate. *Journal of Bacteriology* 170, 2185–2192.

Henderson, B., Poole, S. and Wilson, M. (1996) Bacterial modulins: a novel class of virulence factors which cause host tissue pathology by inducing cytokine synthesis. *Microbiological Reviews* 60, 316–341.

Heynes, K. and Kiessling, G. (1967) Strukturaufklarung des Vi-antigens aus *Citrobacter freundii* (*E. coli*) 5396/38. *Carbohydrate Research* 3, 340–352.

Hitchcock, P.J. and Brown, T.M. (1983) Morphological heterogeneity among Salmonella lipopolysaccharide chemotypes in silver-stained polyacrylamide gels. *Journal of Bacteriology* 154, 269–277.

Holst, O. and Brade, H. (1992) Chemical structure of the core region of lipopolysaccharides. In: Morrison, D.C. and Ryan, J.L. (eds) *Bacterial Endotoxic Lipopolysaccharides*, vol. 1. *Molecular Biochemistry and Cellular Biology of Lipopolysaccharides*. CRC Press, Boca Raton, Florida, pp. 135–169.

Ilg, K., Endt, K., Misselwitz, B., Stecher, B., Aebi, M. and Hardt, W.D. (2009) O-antigen-negative *Salmonella enterica* serovar Typhimurium is attenuated in intestinal colonization but elicits colitis in streptomycin-treated mice. *Infection and Immunity* 77, 2568–2575.

Jann, B. and Jann, K. (1990) Structure and biosynthesis of the capsular antigens of *Escherichia coli*. *Current Topics in Microbiology and Immunology* 150, 19–42.

Jiang, X.-M., Neal, B., Santiago, F., Lee, S.J., Romana, L.K. and Reeves, P.R. (1991) Structure and sequence of the *rfb* (O antigen) gene cluster of *Salmonella* serovar typhimurium (strain LT2). *Molecular Microbiology* 5, 695–713.

Johnson, E.M. and Baron, L.S. (1969) Genetic transfer of the Vi antigen from *Salmonella typhosa* to *Escherichia coli*. *Journal of Bacteriology* 99, 355–359.

Kaniuk, N.A., Vinogradov, E. and Whitfield, C. (2004) Investigation of the structural requirements in the lipopolysaccharide core acceptor for ligation of O antigens in the genus *Salmonella* - WaaL 'ligase' is not the sole determinant of acceptor specificity. *Journal of Biological Chemistry* 279, 36470–36480.

Kong, Q., Yang, J., Liu, Q., Alamuri, P., Roland, K.L. and Curtiss, R., 3rd (2011) Effect of deletion of genes involved in lipopolysaccharide core and O-antigen synthesis on virulence and immunogenicity of *Salmonella enterica* serovar Typhimurium. *Infection and Immunity* 79, 4227–4239.

Lehmann, V., Lüderitz, O. and Westphal, O. (1971) The linkage of pyrophosphorylethanolamine to heptose in the core of *Salmonella minnesota* lipopolysaccharides. *European Journal of Biochemistry* 21, 339–347.

Liang-Takasaki, C.-J., Makela, P.H. and Leive, L. (1982) Phagocytosis of bacteria by macrophages: changing the carbohydrate of lipopolysaccharide alters interaction with complement and macrophages. *Journal of Immunology* 128, 1229–1235.

Liang-Takasaki, C.-J., Grossman, N. and Leive, L. (1983a) Salmonellae activate complement differentially via the alternative pathway depending on the structure of their lipopolysaccharide O-antigen. *Journal of Immunology* 130, 1867–1870.

Liang-Takasaki, C.-J., Saxen, H., Makela, P.H. and Leive, L. (1983b) Complement activation by polysaccharide of lipopolysaccharide: an important virulence determinant of salmonellae. *Infection and Immunity* 41, 563–569.

Mayer, H. and Schmidt, G. (1979) Chemistry and biology of the enterobacterial common antigen (ECA). *Current Topics in Microbiology and Immunology* 85, 99–153.

McClelland, M., Sanderson, K.E., Spieth, J., Clifton, S.W., Latreille, P., Courtney, L., Porwollik, S., Ali, J., Dante, M., Du, F., Hou, S., Layman, D., Leonard, S., Nguyen, C., Scott, K., Holmes, A., Grewal, N., Mulvaney, E., Ryan, E., Sun, H., Florea, L., Miller, W., Stoneking, T., Nhan, M., Waterston, R. and Wilson,

R.K. (2001) Complete genome sequence of *Salmonella enterica* serovar Typhimurium LT2. *Nature* 413, 852–856.

Murray, G.L., Attridge, S.R. and Morona, R. (2006) Altering the length of the lipopolysaccharide O-antigen has an impact on the interaction of *Salmonella enterica* serovar Typhimurium with macrophages and complement. *Journal of Bacteriology* 188, 2735–2739.

Nagy, G., Danino, V., Dobrindt, U., Pallen, M., Chaudhuri, R., Emödy, L., Hinton, J.C. and Hacker, J. (2006) Down-regulation of key virulence factors makes the *Salmonella enterica* serovar Typhimurium *rfaH* mutant a promising live attenuated vaccine candidate. *Infection and Immunity* 74, 5914–5925.

Nevola, J.J., Laux, D.C. and Cohen, P.S. (1987) In vivo colonization of the mouse large intestine and in vitro penetration of intestinal mucus by an avirulent smooth strain of *Salmonella typhimurium* and its lipopolysaccharide-deficient mutant. *Infection and Immunity* 55, 2884–2890.

Peterson, A.A. and McGroarty, E.J. (1985) High-molecular-weight components in lipopolysaccharides of *Salmonella typhimurium, Salmonella minnesota,* and *Escherichia coli. Journal of Bacteriology* 162, 738–745.

Pickard, D., Wain, J., Baker, S., Line, A., Chohan, S., Fookes, M., Barron, A., Gaora, P.O., Chabalgoity, J.A., Thanky, N., Scholes, C., Thomson, N., Quail, M., Parkhill, J. and Dougan, G. (2003) Composition, acquisition, and distribution of the Vi exopolysaccharide-encoding *Salmonella enterica* pathogenicity island SPI-7. *Journal of Bacteriology* 185, 5055–5065.

Poltorak, A., He, X., Smirnova, I., Liu, M.Y., Van Huffel, C., Du, X., Birdwell, D., Alejos, E., Silva, M., Galanos, C., Freudenberg, M., Ricciardi-Castagnoli, P., Layton, B. and Beutler, B. (1998) Defective LPS signaling in C3H/HeJ and C57BL/10ScCr mice: mutations in Tlr4 gene. *Science* 282, 2085–2088.

Qureshi, N. and Takayama, K. (1990) Structure and function of lipid A. In: Inglewski B.H. and Clark, V.L. (eds) *The Bacteria*, vol. *XI. Molecular Basis of Bacterial Pathogenesis*. Academic Press, London, pp. 19–338.

Raetz, C.R.H. (1993) Bacterial endotoxins: extraordinary lipids that activate eukaryotic signal transduction. *Journal of Bacteriology* 175, 5745–5753.

Rafatellu, M., Chessa, D., Wilson, R.P., Dusold, R., Rubino, S. and Bäumler, A.J. (2005) The Vi capsule antigen of *Salmonella enterica* serotype Typhi reduces Toll-like receptor-dependent interleukin-8 expression in the intestinal mucosa. *Infection and Immunity* 73, 3367–3374.

Ramos-Morales, F., Prieto, A.I., Beuzón, C.R., Holden, D.W. and Casadesús, J. (2003) Role for *Salmonella enterica* enterobacterial common antigen in bile resistance and virulence. *Journal of Bacteriology* 185, 5328–5332.

Reeves, P.R., Hobbs, M., Valvano, M.A., Skurnik, M., Whitfield, C., Coplin, D., Kido, N., Klena, J., Maskell, D., Raetz, C.R. and Rick, P.D. (1996) Bacterial polysaccharide synthesis and gene nomenclature. *Trends in Microbiology* 4, 495–503.

Rick, P.D. and Osborn, M.J. (1977) Lipid A mutants of *Salmonella typhimurium*. Characterization of conditional lethal mutants in 3-deoxy-D-mannooctulosonate-8-phosphate synthetase. *Journal of Biological Chemistry* 252, 4895–4903.

Rick, P.D. and Silver, R.P. (1996) Enterobacterial common antigen and capsular polysaccharides. In: Neidhardt, F.C., Curtiss, R., III, Ingraham, J.L., Lin, E.C.C., Low, K.B., Magasanik, B., Reznikoff, W.S., Riley, M., Schaechter, M. and Umbarger, H.E. (eds) Escherichia coli *and* Salmonella*: Cellular and Molecular Biology*, 2nd edn. ASM Press, Washington, DC, pp. 104–122.

Rick, P.D. and Young, D.A. (1982) Isolation and characterization of a temperature-sensitive lethal mutant of *Salmonella typhimurium* that is conditionally defective in 3-deoxy-D-mannooctulosonate-8-synthetase. *Journal of Bacteriology* 150, 447–455.

Rick, P.D., Mayer, H., Neumeyer, B.A., Wolski, S. and Bitter-Suermann, D. (1985) Biosynthesis of enterobacterial common antigen. *Journal of Bacteriology* 162, 494–503.

Rietschel, E.T., Sidorczyk, Z., Zahringer, U., Wollenweber, H.-W. and Lüderitz, O. (1983) Analysis of the primary structure of lipid A. *ACS Symposium on Serology* 231, 214.

Schnaitman, C.A. and Klena, J.D. (1993) Genetics of lipopolysaccharide biosynthesis in enteric bacteria. *Microbiological Reviews* 57, 655–682.

Shaio, M.F. and Rowland, H. (1985) Bactericidal and opsonizing effects of normal serum on mutant strains of *Salmonella typhimurium*. *Infection and Immunity* 49, 647–653.

Stock, J.B., Rauch, B. and Roseman, S. (1977) Periplasmic space in *Salmonella typhimurium* and *Escherichia coli*. *Journal of Biological Chemistry* 252, 7850–7861.

Valtonen, M.V. (1977) Role of phagocytosis in mouse virulence of *Salmonella typhimurium* recombinants with O antigen 6,7 or 4,12. *Infection and Immunity* 18, 574–582.

Valtonen, M.V., Plosila, M., Valtonen, V.V. and Makela, P.H. (1975) Effect of the quality of the lipopolysaccharide on mouse virulence of *Salmonella enteritidis*. *Infection and Immunity* 12, 828–832.

Valtonen, V.V. (1970) Mouse virulence of *Salmonella* strains: the effect of different smooth-type O-side chains. *Journal of General Microbiology* 64, 255–268.

Valtonen, V.V., Aird, J., Valtonen, M.V., Makela, O. and Makela, P.H. (1971) Mouse virulence of *Salmonella*: antigen-dependent differences are demonstrable also after immunosuppression. *Acta Pathologica et Microbiologica Immunologica Scandinavica, Section B* 79, 715–718.

Virlogeux, I., Waxin, H., Ecobishon, C. and Popoff, M.Y. (1995) Role of the *viaB* locus in synthesis, transport and expression of *Salmonella typhi* Vi antigen. *Microbiology* 141, 3039–3047.

Westphal, O. and Jann, K. (1965) Bacterial lipopolysaccharide extraction with phenol water and further application of the procedure. *Methods in Carbohydrate Chemistry* 5, 83–91.

Wilson, R.P., Raffatellu, M., Chessa, D., Winter, S.E., Tükel, C. and Bäumler, A.J. (2008) The Vi-capsule prevents Toll-like receptor 4 recognition of *Salmonella*. *Cellular Microbiology* 10, 876–890.

3 Fimbriae and Flagella of *Salmonella enterica*

Dr Michael A. Jones*
School of Veterinary Medicine and Science, University of Nottingham, UK

Introduction

Fimbriae and flagella are proteinaceous surface components expressed by many bacteria. The terms fimbriae and pili were first used in 1955 and 1959, respectively, to describe non-flagella appendages of bacteria (Duguid *et al.*, 1955; Brinton, 1959). For consistency this group of proteins will be referred to as fimbriae, based on the argument set out by Ottow (1975). The bacterial flagellum is a multi-protein system composed of three main structures: the basal body, hook and filament. This chapter will discuss the role of fimbriae and flagella in the wider context of Salmonella biology but will refer to papers describing other genera where clear parallels can be drawn. Many studies have been carried out on *Escherichia coli* and the similarity between both the fimbrial operons and flagella apparatus between these and other members of the Enterobacteriaceae means that sensible conclusions can be drawn although some significant differences exist particularly in regulation of fimbriae.

Fimbriae

Fimbriae (Latin for 'thread'), also referred to as pili (Latin for 'hair'), are composed of a heterogeneous mix of proteins. They were identified on the surface of *E. coli* cells by electron microscopy (Houwink and van Iterson, 1950) and expression of fimbriae by *Salmonella* was first described over 50 years ago (Duguid and Gillies, 1958). Since this work a range of studies has been carried out on the structure, function and genetics of these surface components.

It is thought that fimbriae are important in overcoming repulsive electrostatic forces between the predominantly negatively charged bacteria and other negatively charged surfaces including other bacteria and tissues. The main structure is a 'fimbrial rod' composed of subunit proteins ranging between 15 and 25 kDa in size. The first functional role ascribed to fimbriae (pili) was as receptors for bacteriophage in 1949 (Anderson, 1949) and fimbriae were first recognized in electron micrographs of Gram-negative bacteria (Yanagawa *et al.*, 1968). Gillies and Duguid

* Author, e-mail: michael.a.jones@nottingham.ac.uk

© CAB International 2013. *Salmonella in Domestic Animals, 2nd Edition* (eds P.A. Barrow and U. Methner)

(1958) had previously observed that certain bacteria could agglutinate specific erythrocytes. Further studies showed that a differentiator of this agglutination was lectin–mannose interactions (Collier *et al.*, 1955; Duguid *et al.*, 1966). Since then, numerous fimbriae have been described in both Gram-negative and Gram-positive bacteria. The classification of fimbriae has become more complex as it has developed. Initial identification and separation was based on physical properties such as binding and antigenicity. The subsequent elucidation of the mechanism of formation of fimbriae has allowed for their classification based on their assembly pathways. This has been further enhanced by molecular analysis based on comparative sequence analysis. As sequencing became more widespread individual operons were sequenced and their presence across serovars determined using hybridization-based methods. More detailed separation of the fimbrial groups has now been proposed based on detailed comparative analysis of their component sequences. The following sections detail these classifications to aid the comparison of the literature from different historical periods in fimbrial research.

Structural classification of fimbriae in *Salmonella*

The fimbriae of the *Enterobacteriaceae* can be divided into two major classes based on whether they are mannose sensitive (MS) or mannose resistant (Salit and Gotschlich, 1977; Paranchych and Frost, 1988). Mannose sensitivity is based on the ability of the monosaccharide mannose to inhibit the adhesion of the fimbriae to erythrocytes (haemagglutination) (Salit and Gotschlich, 1977; Paranchych and Frost, 1988). Numerous other schemes have been used to classify the fimbriae since they were first identified, evolving into four major types.

Type 1 fimbriae

These were first defined as rigid filaments mediating mannose sensitive agglutination of bacteria (Duguid, 1959). The type 1 fimbriae mediate adhesion to a range of eukaryotic cells through their interactions with the mannosylated glycoprotein laminin on the host cells (Duguid *et al.*, 1966; Kukkonen *et al.*, 1993). The type 1 fimbriae are members of the chaperone usher group of fimbriae. They are found throughout the *Enterobacteriaceae* and present as peritrichous extensions of the bacterial surface. They have a diameter of ca. 6 nm and can extend up to 100 nm long (Korhonen *et al.*, 1980). During assembly the fimbrial subunits are secreted into the periplasmic space where they bind a chaperone to stop premature assembly. This subunit/chaperone complex then interacts with the usher protein in the outer membrane, which acts as a pore that allows transfers of the pilin to the growing filament (reviewed in detail by Kline *et al.*, 2010). Both F1 and SEF21 are type 1 fimbriae. SEF21 was first described on strains of *S.* Enteritis (Müller *et al.*, 1991).

Type II fimbriae

This group of fimbriae were first described as non-haemagglutinating variants of type 1 fimbriae in strains of *S.* Gallinarum and *S.* Pullorum, *S.* Paratyphi B and *S.* Dublin (Duguid and Gillies, 1958; Duguid *et al.*, 1966). Swenson *et al.* (1991) showed there was a close molecular similarity between type 1 and type II fimbriae and there is an antigenic similarity between and within the groups and between the type 1 and type II groups (Purcell *et al.*, 1987; Sojka *et al.*, 1996, 1998).

Type III fimbriae

Type III fimbriae are peritrichous and 3–5 nm in diameter. They mediate agglutination of tannic acid-treated erythrocytes in the presence of α-D-mannose (Duguid, 1959; Duguid *et al.*, 1966). These fimbrial filaments differ from type 1 as they are thinner, more numerous, with a strong mannose resistance. They include *mrkABCDF* in uropathogenic *E. coli* but these are not found in *Salmonella* (Duguid, 1959, 1968; Shedden, 1962). This group includes SEF18 and SEF14 and shares identity with the P and Cs31 fimbriae of *E. coli* and the Mrk fimbriae of *Klebsiella*. SEF14 are unique to certain group D serovars including all strains of *S.* Enteritidis and *S.* Dublin and were first described on strains of *S.* Enteritidis (Thorns *et al.*, 1990; Müller *et al.*, 1991). SEF14 fimbriae were originally described as displaying mannose-sensitive agglutination but apart from limited *N*-terminal homology they are significantly different from other type 1 fimbriae (Feutrier *et al.*, 1986).

Type IV fimbriae

These are extremely thin peritrichous mannose-resistant filaments. They have also been described as the GVVPQ fimbriae after the conserved *N*-terminal sequence of their main fimbrial subunit protein (Collinson *et al.*, 1992). First identified in *E. coli* as fimbriae that were serologically cross-reactive with SEF17 (17 kDa fimbriae of *S.* Enteritidis), these fimbriae are peritrichous with a tightly coiled appearance (Collinson *et al.*, 1992). SEF17 subunits are encoded for by *agfA* (aggregative fimbriae) and can be detected by serological methods and are in a number of the *Enterobacteriaceae* including some but not all *Salmonella* serovars (Doran *et al.*, 1993). The occurrence of *agf* appears to be variable within serovars; for example, only 50% of *S.* Typhimurium assessed being positive for the AgfA antigen (Doran *et al.*, 1993). Some bacteria that were negative by assessment for antigen were positive by DNA hybridization suggesting there is some epitope variation between strains (Doran *et al.*, 1993).

Classification by assembly pathway

Although morphological classification has been described as recently as 1988 (Paranchych and Frost, 1988), the understanding of the mechanisms of assembly and the introduction of rapid sequence analysis has led to the adoption of a classification system based on assembly and molecular phylogeny. However, the literature on the grouping of fimbriae is far from coordinated. The classification of the fimbriae of Gram-negative bacteria was rationalized by their splitting into four groups based on their mechanism of assembly. These groups are: (i) represented by the F fimbriae associated with conjunctive fertility (Tomoeda *et al.*, 1975; Eisenbrandt *et al.*, 1999; Lawley *et al.*, 2003); (ii) type IV fimbriae described above (Hobbs and Mattick, 1993; Strom and Lory, 1993; Nudleman and Kaiser, 2004); (iii) curli fimbriae, which are assembled by the extracellular nucleation/precipitation pathway (Hammar *et al.*, 1996); and (iv) the chaperone/usher dependent pathway (Jones *et al.*, 1992; Thanassi *et al.*, 1998; Sauer *et al.*, 2004; Vetsch *et al.*, 2006; Henderson *et al.*, 2011). Of these, three have been described in enteric pathogens, namely the chaperone usher pathway, the nucleator-dependent pathway and the type IV pathway.

The chaperone usher pathway functions by the secretion of fimbrial subunits through the inner membrane via the secretion apparatus (Yeg). Members of the chaperone-dependent pathway include *fim* (type-1 fimbriae), *lpf* (long polar fimbriae), *stf* (*S.* Typhimurium fimbriae), *bcf* (bovine colonization factor), *saf* (*Salmonella* fimbriae) and *pef* (plasmid-encoded fimbriae). Long polar fimbriae were identified when a *Salmonella* fimbrial operon was expressed in *E. coli* leading to the formation of fimbriae at the polar end of the expressing bacterium (Baümler and Heffron, 1995). The plasmid-encoded fimbriae (Pef) of *Salmonella* are so called because of their genomic localization when expressed in *E. coli* lead to profuse peritrichous fimbriae (Friedrich *et al.*, 1993; Woodward *et al.*, 1996).

Conservation between *Enterobacteriaceae*

Antigenic conservation can be observed with type 1 (Purcell *et al.*, 1987; Sojka *et al.*, 1996, 1998) and type 3 fimbriae between *Salmonella*, and other *Enterobacteriaceae Klebsiella* and *Yersinia* (Adegbola *et al.*, 1983; Old and Adegbola, 1985). However, conservation is not maintained across the different species and serovars and sequences do diverge so some sero-diagnosis can be used. Genomic hybridization studies have identified differences between strains and it was proposed this could account for some species-specific differences in behaviour *in vivo* (Clayton *et al.*, 2008). This hypothesis has been shown to be true in some cases (Morgan *et al.*, 2004) but due to the potential for redundancy in function the specific role of different fimbrial groups has been difficult to discern, as discussed below. The development of the diverse patterns of fimbrial operons within the genera of *Salmonella* has been attributed to both horizontal gene transfer and host-dependent selective deletion events (Baümler *et al.*, 1997a). The most complex to understand is the *lpf* operon, which appears to have undergone both positive and negative selection in different hosts (Baümler *et al.*, 1997a). Sef14 has been located on a pathogenicity islet in group D *Salmonella* (Thorns *et al.*, 1992; Turcotte and Woodward, 1993; Collinghan and Woodward, 2001).

Classification based on primary sequence

The sequencing of the *Salmonella* serovars has allowed the repertoires of the fimbrial operons in a range of serovars to be clearly defined (McClelland *et al.*, 2001), *S.* Enteritidis, *S.* Gallinarum (Thomson *et al.*, 2008), *S.* Typhi (Parkhill *et al.*, 2001) and *S.* Choleraesuis (Chiu *et al.*, 2005). Prior to the sequencing studies much of the data on distribution relied on hybridization and serological techniques, which indicated a wide distribution of fimbriae across the different enteric serotypes. These studies can now be reviewed alongside more detailed analysis using whole genome sequence information (Townsend *et al.*, 2001; Edwards *et al.*, 2002; Garaizar *et al.*, 2002; van Asten and van Dijk, 2005; Clayton *et al.*, 2008). This has the added information on the identity of operons that possess pseudogenes (Clayton *et al.*, 2008). Whilst the genome sequence has not been fully described for *S.* Pullorum, a similar genotype has been described for the different fimbrial operons (Clayton *et al.*, 2008). The loss of gene function in *S. enterica* genomes has been correlated with increased host specificity (Thomson *et al.*, 2008). In summary, *S.* Enteritidis PT4 has 13 chromosomal fimbrial operons, Typhimurium LT12 has 12 chromosomal operons and one plasmid-borne operon (*pef*), Choleraesuis SC-B67 has 11 operons and Typhi CT18 and Gallinarum 287/91 have 12 (McClelland *et al.*, 2001; Edwards *et al.*, 2002; Clayton *et al.*, 2008; Thomson *et al.*, 2008). There is disparity between descriptions of the fimbrial operon repertoire described by different authors, which has arisen due to the different methods of characterization. Hybridization studies lacked fidelity due to the nature of the comparative methods and have the potential to misrepresent operons based on physical or hybridization patterns. However, whole genome sequence analysis may miss variation between strains, a problem that might be circumvented by multiplex high throughput sequencing of further strains.

The subsequent sequencing of a number of *Salmonella* genomes combined with our molecular understanding of these operons has allowed further subclassification of these systems based on sequence homology and operon structure of the genes. This has the benefit that it allows direct classification of fimbrial genes from genome sequence data (Nuccio and Bäumler, 2007). This has led to the proposal of six groups (alpha, beta, gamma, kappa, pi and sigma) for the fimbrial usher family (FUP) (Nuccio and Bäumler, 2007). The gamma group is further subdivided into four γ_1, γ_2, γ_3 and γ_4. *Salmonella* has fimbrial operons in all the groups except sigma, alpha (*tcf*); beta (*stj*); gamma one, three and four (*bcf, sti, sth, saf, sef, stc, stb*); kappa (*pef, fae*) and pi (*stf, ste* and *std*) (Nuccio and Baümler, 2007).

Plasmid-encoded fimbriae

In addition to the chromosomal operons fimbrial operons vital to virulence are located on the *Salmonella* virulence plasmids (Rychlik *et al.*, 2006). These plasmid-encoded fimbriae (Pef) are in the chaperone usher group. The virulence plasmids encode a number of virulence-associated genes. Dissection of the specific function of *pef* requires care as the non-fimbrial *spv* genes on the plasmid are essential for virulence (Guiney and Fierer, 2011). Part of the virulence-associated phenotype of the plasmid is coded for by the plasmid-encoded fimbriae (*pef*) in serovars Enteritidis, Typhimurium and Choleraesuis (Friedrich *et al.*, 1993). The *pef* operon is absent in serovars Gallinarum and Dublin but replaced by the *fae* operon, which encodes for fimbriae closely related to those of the *E. coli* K88 fimbriae (Rychlik *et al.*, 2006). The evolution of these plasmids suggests that *pefA* has been essential during the development of the virulence plasmids. The virulence plasmids evolved from IncFIIA plasmid with the *spv* gene operon and is thought to have gained *pef* by fusion with another plasmid to introduce these genes into the lineages that later became Typhimurium, Enteritidis and Choleraesuis. It is hypothesized that these plasmids then underwent genomic reduction in *Salmonella* Enteritidis and Choleraesuis (Rychlik *et al.*, 2006).

The evolution of fimbrial operons in the genome is more complex. Comparative studies by DNA hybridization methods with members of *S.* Enteritidis have clear conservation and loss patterns between the serogroups (Table 3.1). This type of analysis has been refined by comparative studies between the genome sequences of different *Salmonella* serotypes leading to the identification of pseudogenes further defining the repertoire of fimbriae operons between strains (Clayton *et al.*, 2008). It is interesting to note that specific operons are conserved in the more host-adapted and typhoid-like strains, suggesting differing roles of fimbriae between serovars. Some variation is apparent in the data with specific serotype subtle variation between different types, for example Paratyphi appears to have the *tcf* operon while Paratyphi B and C do not (Table 3.1). This variation indicates that a more detailed study of some groups may be required to understand fully the role of fimbrial variation within serotypes.

Diagnostic tests

The variation in expression and presence of fimbriae in different *S. enterica* serovars has allowed for their use in the development of diagnostic tests. Simple latex agglutination tests have been developed that allow the identification of *S.* Enteritidis based on the presence of SEF14 (McLaren *et al.*, 1992; Thorns *et al.*, 1992, 1996). It has been proposed that this could be used for diagnoses of infected poultry as sero-conversion occurs within 10 days of infection and the IgG response persists for up to 4 weeks (Thorns *et al.*, 1996). While the advance of molecular typing appears to have bypassed the need for further development of antigen-based typing methods there may be value in serological testing of infected animals for rapid on-site diagnosis and typing.

In vitro studies

The first studies on the role of fimbriae were phenotypic in nature, looking at difference in fimbriation of isolates and their interaction with cells. Studies using cell culture and tissues have been used to model adherence but have not led to conclusive results regarding *in vivo* requirements (Mintz *et al.*, 1983; Old *et al.*, 1986). One of the problems in studying the *in vivo* process is the role that culture conditions may play in altering expression of the fimbriae and the potential differences in receptors on cells and tissues from different origins. However, *in vitro* studies have shown that disruption of fimbriae can impact on host cell interactions. Disruption of *lpf*, *fim* and *agf* (*csg*) reduce attachment of *S.* Typhimurium to epithelial cell lines *in vitro* (Tavendale *et al.*, 1983; Ernst *et al.*, 1990; Baümler *et al.*, 1996c; Sukupolvi *et al.*, 1997; Wilson *et al.*, 2000). Studies have also identified laminin and plasminogen receptors and an undefined 60 KDa glycoprotein receptor as targets for type 1 fimbriae (Kukkonen *et al.*, 1993, 1998; Ghosh *et al.*, 1996). The role of type 1 fimbriae and serotype-associated plasmid (SAP) mediated fimbriae in adhesion has also been described (Jones *et al.*, 1981, 1982).

The focus on fimbriae in attachment has often been investigated in isolation from other factors and it has become apparent in recent years that a more global approach is required to study the function of these genes. Infection by *Salmonella* is a multi-stage and multi-component process and the role of fimbriae has to be placed in this context. Fimbriae appear to play a role in establishing an initial adhesion, prior to a more permanent attachment by the

Table 3.1. Presence and absence of different fimbrial operons in selected *Salmonella enterica* serotypes.

	Identified by genome sequence and hybridization[1,2,3]					Identified by hybridization analysis[2,3]					
S. enterica serotype	Enteritidis	Typhimurium	Choleraesuis	Typhi	Gallinarum	Pullorum	Dublin	Derby	Paratyphi A	Paratyphi B	Paratyphi C
bcf	+	+	$+^{P}$	+	+	+	+	+	+	+	–
sti	$+^{s}$	+	$+^{*}$	–	$+^{v}$	+	–	–	–	–	–
or											
sta[†]	$+^{h}$	–	–	+	–	$+^{h}$	+	+	$+^{v}$	$+^{v}$	+
stf	+	+	$+^{s}$	–	$+^{P}$	...	...	...	...	...	...
saf	+	+	+	$+^{P}$	$+^{P}$	+	+	+	+	+	+
stb	+	+	+	+	$+^{P}$	+	+	+	+	+	–
tcf	–	–	+	+	–	–	–	–	+	–	–
fim	+	+	+	$+^{P}$	+	+	+	+	+	+	+
csg (agf)	+	+	+	$+^{P}$	+	+	+	+	+	+	+
peg	+	–	–	–	$+^{P}$	...	...	...	...	...	...
or											
stc	$-^{h}$	+	$+^{v}$	+	$-^{h}$	–	$+^{v}$	–	+	+	–
ste	$-^{s}+^{h}$	–	$-^{s}+^{h}$	$+^{P}$	+	+	+	+	+	+	+
std	+	+	+	+	$+^{v}$	+	+	–	+	+	–
lpf	+	+	$+^{PV}$	–	$+^{P}$	+	+	+	–	+	+
stg	$-^{s}+^{h}$	–	–	$+^{P}$	$-^{s}+^{h}$	+	$+^{v}$	–	–	–	–
sef	+	–	–	$+^{P}$	$+^{P}$	$+^{P}$	+	–	+	–	–
stj	–	+	–	–	–	...	–	...	–	–	–
sth	+	+	+	$+^{P}$	$+^{P}$	+	+	+	+	–	+
	Identified by hybridization[2,3]										
pef	+	+	$+^{v}$	–	–	–	–	–	–	+	+
bfp	+	+	+	–	+	+	+	...	...	...	...

[P] Pseudogenes as described by sequence; positive by both hybridization and sequence,[s] based on sequence data,[h] based on hybridization data; – not present; ... no data presented in cross serotype hybridizations; [v] variable data indicates that some mixed response for a specific serotype indication variation within serotypes; [*]data variable between some references. [†]*sti* is replaced in some serotypes as shown by sequence and hybridization[1,2] or hybridization.[2]
[1]Clayton *et al.*, 2008; [2]Townsend *et al.*, 2001; [3]van Asten and van Dijk, 2005.

type three section system 1 (TTSS-1) such that fimbrial adhesion could be considered reversible but that the TTSS-1 bind in an irreversible manner (Misselwitz *et al.*, 2011). However, *fim* mutants are defective in both attachment and invasion of a number of mammalian and avian cells (Bäumler *et al.*, 1996a; Guo *et al.*, 2009) and this study indicated that multiple factors were involved in the initial adhesion processes. Independent *lpfC* mutants were also shown to be defective in adhesion and invasion of Hep2 cells (Baümler *et al.*, 1996c), which seems to contradict other data that suggest that Pef, Lpf, Agf and Shd do not play a significant role in attachment of Hela cells (Misselwitz *et al.*, 2011). Shd is an outer membrane fibronectin-binding protein involved in faecal shedding in the mouse (Kingsley *et al.*, 2002). No clear data currently exist to identify if this discrepancy is due to host cell receptor differences. Data has been presented that indicate that preferential binding can occur and this can be dependent on specific fimbrial alleles (Guo *et al.*, 2009). The study compared binding of *Salmonella* to mammalian and avian cells and suggests that *fimH* alleles could enable preferential binding to different host cell types and may play a role in host specificity (Guo *et al.*, 2009). Thus it appears that fimbriae play specific roles and represent a group of adhesins with distinctive roles in the pathogen biology and therefore one may expect that expression is linked to specific niches or phases during infection.

Expression of fimbriae

The expression of fimbriae has been studied both *in vivo* and *in vitro* and for a number of fimbriae the conditions for expression have not been fully elucidated. Early studies on fimbriae were based on physical properties and antigenicity. Subsequent studies have tended to focus on the genes and regulation of expression for the type 1 fimbriae. These have three transcriptional regulators FimZ, FimY and FimW in its operon and a post-transcriptional tRNA regulator FimU. The gene *fimU* encodes a rare anticodon UCU for arginine and disruption of this gene abolishes SEF14 and disrupts SEF21 expression (Clouthier *et al.*, 1998). The regulation of type 1 fimbriae involves a number of interactions between these proteins and is also linked to other virulence properties of the bacteria through a positive interaction between FimZ and HilE, a repressor of SPI1 type three secretion (Saini *et al.*, 2009). FimW is a negative regulator acting on FimY (Tinker *et al.*, 2001). FimY acts a co-activator (Tinker and Clegg, 2000) along with FimZ, which is a positive regulator of the *fimAICDHF* operon (Yeh *et al.*, 2002). FimZ also has a self-regulatory role. However, this is not the only level of regulation and the leucine-responsive regulator Lrp has also been shown to have an indirect role as an activator of FimZ (McFarland *et al.*, 2008; Baek *et al.*, 2011). A further mechanism is involved in the phase variation, which can be observed for type 1 fimbriae of *E. coli* and *Salmonella* (Abraham *et al.*, 1985; Smith *et al.*, 1990). It has been well characterized in *E. coli* and involves the recombinases FimB and FimE, which mediate the recombination of the FimA promoter region and the orientation of transcription (Klemm, 1984; Abraham *et al.*, 1985). However, *S.* Typhimurium lacks homologues for FimB and FimE and there are not homologues for the *Salmonella* genes *FimZ*, *FimY* and *FimW* in the *E. coli* Fim operon.

The exact triggers for regulation are less well defined than the genetic components. It has been proposed that Lrp is involved in regulation in response to the nutritional state of the bacteria (Baek *et al.*, 2011) thus coordinating it with other virulence genes (Baek *et al.*, 2009). Nicholson and Low (2000) showed that transcription of *pef* could be modulated by DNA methylation in a Lrp-dependent manner. Similarly *std* fimbrial genes are regulated in part by DNA methylation (Jakomin *et al.*, 2008) suggesting that this plays a more widespread role in other fimbrial gene regulation. It has been proposed that there is a specific hierarchy and cross talk of regulation between flagella, type three secretion and fimbrial operons, such that the bacteria coordinate between the actions of moving, invading or persisting at specific points in their growth (Saini *et al.*, 2010). The data from this study were based on *in vitro* growth and only involved a single fimbrial system. Fimbriae of both *Salmonella* and *E. coli* are known to be poorly expressed during culture in laboratory media (Humphries *et al.*, 2003; Weening *et al.*, 2005; Low *et al.*, 2006), but the same fimbriae are induced in both the bovine and murine intestine and generate an antibody response in mice (Humphries *et al.*, 2003, 2005). These results highlight the limitations of *in vitro* experiments in understanding the regulation of these proteins in infection. The expression of fimbrial operons has been assessed in bacteria grown in calf ligated loops, indicating that expression of nine of the 12 operons could be detected: BcfA, FimA, LpfA, PefA, StbA, StcA, StdA, StfA and StiA (Humphries *et al.*, 2003). There also appears to be modulation of fimbrial expression during infection and up-regulation of the Stb operon has been observed for *Salmonella* Typhimurium in the intestine of the chicken gut compared to *in vitro* grown bacteria; again these studies are limited by the complex nature of stimuli that are likely to be involved (Harvey *et al.*, 2011).

Infection studies

The complexity of regulation is also reflected in the role of fimbriae during infection. The multiplicity of fimbrial operons has made them difficult to study. The defining of the specific role of fimbriae in infections has come through the study of individual and combination mutants of fimbrial genes. The role of type 1 fimbriae in adhesion to cells and agglutination has been used to support the argument that they play a role in intestinal colonization (Duguid *et al.*, 1966, 1976; Darekar and Eyer, 1973). This hypothesis was supported by a number of directed studies looking at binding of purified pili to cells (Korhonen *et al.*, 1980, 1981) and the effect of mutations on infections of mice (Tanaka and Katsube, 1978; Tanaka *et al.*, 1981).

Research has focused on the early interactions of *Salmonella* with the mucosal surface of the gut. The role of fimbriae in this interaction has been of interest to researchers since Takeuchi (1967) first observed fimbrial-like structures in the *in vivo* interactions of *Salmonella* with murine gut epithelium. However, the disruption of genes encoding individual fimbriae does not strongly reduce infection in murine infections with *S.* Typhimurium (Hohmann *et al.*, 1978; Lockman and Curtiss, 1992a, b). Infection studies with fimbrial mutants of *S.* Typhimurium, which did not express type 1 fimbriae, showed no effect on colonization. However, when combined with flagella mutations a ten-fold reduction in LD_{50} resulted compared to individual mutants alone, suggesting a combined role for flagella and fimbriae in infection (Lockman and Curtiss, 1992a, b). This highlights the problems of potential redundancy in these surface components during infection. However, it must be pointed out that subtle effects can be observed for individual fimbrial mutants. This redundancy of function has also been observed in studies that showed that disruption of the adhesins *fim*, *lpf*, *pef* and *agf* have synergistic effects in attenuating *S.* Typhimurium in mice (van der Velden *et al.*, 1998). Conversely, FimH has been associated with increased systemic infection of poultry with *S.* Gallinarum (Kuźmiźska-Bajor *et al.*, 2012).

Of the 13 fimbrial operons identified in *S.* Typhimurium, nine of these, *lpf*, *fim bcf*, *stb*, *stc*, *stc*, *std*, *sth*, *csg* and *pef*, have been associated with virulence in mice (van der Velden *et al.*, 1998; Tsolis *et al.*, 1999; Edwards *et al.*, 2000; Weening *et al.*, 2005; Lawley *et al.*, 2006; Clayton *et al.*, 2008). The *lpf*, *pef* and *agf* operons were shown to have a role in infections of susceptible BALB/c mice (Baümler *et al.*, 1996b, c, 1997b; van der Velden *et al.*, 1998). The fact that individual mutations have an attenuating effect suggests that they may have independent roles at specific points in the infection process.

The discussion of the role of fimbriae in infection is complicated by the differential results that can be achieved depending on the individual bacterial-host combination. The differences in fimbrial repertoire have been thought to be associated with host or niche specificity. The host-adapted typhoidal strains of *Salmonella* have reduced repertoires of genes (Clayton *et al.*, 2008), suggestive of the reduced requirement in systemic (typhoidal) disease compared to enteric colonization by less host-specific *Salmonella*.

In vivo data indicating a role in host specificity have come from the work of Morgan *et al.* (2004). This group infected both calves and chickens with matched random pools of *S.* Typhimurium signature-tagged mutants. Their data indicated that the mutations in *stb*, *fim*, *csg*, *sth*, *srg* and *orf7* did not affect colonization of calves, while colonization was reduced or eliminated in poultry. Conversely, mutations in the *pil* and flagellin operon did not attenuate colonization in the chicken but did so in calves (Morgan *et al.*, 2004). A separate study indicated that *saf* and *std* encoded fimbriae were required for infection of pigs (Carnell *et al.*, 2007).

A number of fimbriae, *lpfA-E*, *pefC*, *csgA* and *fimH*, but not *sthD* or *bcfF*, have been linked to the ability to form a biofilm on chicken intestinal mucosa *ex vivo* (Ledeboer *et al.*, 2006). However, *S.* Enteritidis mutants lacking *fimD*, *csgA*, *pefC*, *lpfC* and *sefA* invaded cell models (Thorns *et al.*, 1996; Allen-Vercoe *et al.*, 1999; Rajashekara *et al.*, 2000) and colonized the caeca at comparable levels to the parent strain in 1- to 5-day-old chickens (Allen-Vercoe and Woodward, 1999), suggesting they are unimportant or that other factors can compensate for their loss of function. In contrast, studies with *S.* Enteritidis looking at *stb*, *sti*, *stf*, *sth*, *bcf*, *csg* and *peg* found only the plasmid-encoded fimbriae (Pef) to have any significant effect on colonization delaying the caecal growth (Clayton *et al.*, 2008). Interestingly, parallel studies looking at adherence to cultured avian chicken kidney and Hep-2 cells did not show reduced adherence (Clayton *et al.*, 2008). This may reflect the source of the cells, which are not gut epithelial cells. In addition to cell adhesion and intestinal colonization two fimbriae, type I and curli, in *S.* Enteritidis have both been implicated in egg contamination although this may still be linked to processes of attachment and invasion (Cogan *et al.*, 2004; De Buck *et al.*, 2004).

Fimbrial vaccines

The role of fimbriae in colonization and infection has led to an interest in their use as vaccine targets. Fimbrial-based vaccines have provided protection for pigs against subsequent challenge with ETEC (Rutter and Jones, 1973). Similar approaches have not been attempted with *Salmonella*. Antibody is generated by attenuated *Salmonella* vaccine strains to fimbrial antigen (Cooper and Thorns, 1996) and Pef antigen in naturally infected birds (Woodward *et al.*, 1996). Given that natural infection leads to antibody generation it may be considered that this response is not protective, but studies delivering passive immunization with egg yolk antibody to SEF14 antigen have shown protection in murine challenge studies (Peralta *et al.*, 1994). Therefore, there may considerable scope to develop fimbrial-based vaccines.

Flagella

Bacterial flagella are filamentous multi-protein organelles that are responsible for bacterial motility. Flagella organelles were first studied by electron microscopy (Abram *et al.*, 1965, 1970; Cohen-Bazire and London, 1967). They are related through sequence and structural homology to the Type III secretion super-family. Flagella have three morphologically distinct substructures: the filament, hook and basal structure. The membrane-bound components of the flagella apparatus have much in common with the TTSS. The filament is assembled from single protein flagellin subunits and is used in the Kauffmann–White serotyping scheme for *Salmonella*. The flagella antigens were identified as heat-labile antigens and are used in conjunction with the thermostable 'O' antigens (Kauffmann, 1951). The simplicity of the flagella filament is not mirrored by the complexity of the other structures and genes required for flagella formation. There are upwards of 50 genes associated with their assembly and function. A number of these are involved in modification and correct formation of the structures and if mutated lead to changes in antigenic specificity and flagella shape (Iino and Mitani, 1966; Yamaguchi and Iino, 1969). The filament assembly is polar and processed by the sequential addition of subunits to the growing end (Asakura *et al.*, 1968; Emerson *et al.*, 1970). The flagella filament is sensitive to low pH, urea and other denaturing agents, which will lead to rapid disassociation (Abram and Koffler, 1964; Iino, 1969). It has been proposed that the flagellin subunits are transported through the growing filament through the central pore of the main multi-component export apparatus (Minamino and Macnab, 1999). Recent evidence indicates that the proton motive force is the main driver for export (Minamino *et al.*, 2011). The filaments extend to 16–22 μm in length. The hook structure is located at the base of the flagellum and is composed of a single polypeptide subunit with a molecular mass of 42,000 in *Salmonella* (Kagawa *et al.*, 1976). The physiochemical properties of the hook polymer and subunit protein are different from those of the flagellin subunit and the structure is much more resistant to low pH, urea and other denaturing agents than the flagella filament (Abram and Koffler, 1964). The basal structure of flagella is the most complex part of the structure, with multiple subunits (Ibuki *et al.*, 2011). The first structural images were of the *E. coli* basal body. The structural relatedness of this to the TTSS is readily apparent when comparing electron micrograph images of the two membrane-inserted structures. The outermost ring is referred to as the L-ring, the second ring as the P-ring as it is assumed to be associated with the peptidoglycan wall and the two inner rings are referred to as the S- and M-ring, which are directly in close contact with the plasma membrane and above the membrane, respectively (DePamphilis and Adler, 1971a, b, c). As with the hook the relative resistance of the basal body to disassociation means that it can be separated from the filament relatively easily (Hilmen *et al.*, 1974). The functional relationship between flagella and the TTSS has been further highlighted by work showing the potential for excretion of FliC through type three mechanisms (Lyons *et al.*, 2004; Sun *et al.*, 2007). A summary of the main proteins and their relatedness to Type-III apparatus is provided in Table 3.2.

Genetics of flagella

Genetic analysis of *S.* Typhimurium has shown that at least 50 genes are involved in flagellar apparatus formation and the majority of these are located in three regions of the chromosome, I, II and III (Kutsukake *et al.*,

Table 3.2. Homologues between type three export and flagellar proteins (based on Mcnab, 2004).

Flagellar protein	TSS protein homologue	Function in flagellum function
FliH	n.h. (YscL[a])	Regulator of FLiL activity
FliL	InvC	Export ATPase
FliJ	n.h.	General chaperon
FliK	InvJ	Hook length control
FlhA	InvA	Membrane component; interacts with soluble components
FlhB	SpaS	Membrane component; interacts with soluble components; specificity switching
FliO	n.h.	Membrane component; function unknown
FliP	YscR[a]	Membrane component; cleaved signal sequence
FliQ	SpaQ	Membrane component; function unknown
FliR	SpaR	Membrane component; function unknown
FliN	SpaO	C ring component, involved in motor function as well as export
FliF	HrpC[b]	MS ring protein; necessary for export; interacts with FlhA
FlgE	PrgI	Hook protein
FlgJ	n.h.	Muramidase and putative rod capping protein

n.h. No *Salmonella* Type III homologue
[a] *Yersinia enterocolitica*, gene homologue
[b] *Pseudomonas syringae*, presumed lipoprotein

1988, 1990). The phase-variable genes are in a separate H2 region (Kutsukake *et al.*, 1990).

The regulation of flagella expression is an ordered process requiring the coordination of a number of regulatory systems. The expression of genes can be divided based on their order of expression, the class I genes are the main regulatory genes (*flhDC*), which activate the structural genes of the basal body and hook (class II genes) (Kutsukake *et al.*, 1990; Liu and Matsumura, 1994; Prüss *et al.*, 2001), which are in turn controlled by cAMP-CAP complex and this operon is required for the control of all the other flagellar operons (Kutsukake *et al.*, 1990). The class II genes also encode for an alternative sigma factor, FliA (σ^{28}) and anti-sigma factor, FlgM (anti-σ^{28}). FliA is required to initiate subsequent transcription of the class III structural genes but is inhibited by the presence of FlgM. However, when the hook-basal body is complete it facilitates the release of FlgM from the cell so FliA becomes active (Ohnishi *et al.*, 1992). Thus flagella production is self-regulating and dependent on expression of the basal body prior to synthesis and assembly of the filament.

Alongside the auto-regulation of synthesis, a number of factors have been associated with the regulation of flagella. ClpX protease has been shown to regulate flagella function through both post-translational and transcriptional control involving FlhD/FlhC and flhDC (Kitagawa *et al.*, 2011). Bile salts and phospholipids have been shown to induce a range of genes in *Salmonella* including the TTSS on SPI-1 and class-III genes of flagella (Prouty *et al.*, 2004; Subramanian and Qadri, 2006).

The expression of flagella is not uniform across the different *Salmonella* serotypes and amongst those that express flagellin there are at least two distinct flagella antigens, H1 and H2, which relate to the phases of the flagella 1 and 2 respectively (Andrewes, 1922; Lederberg and Iino, 1956). Expression of flagellin is reduced in host-adapted serovars and the relevance of this is discussed below. This reduction of flagellum apparatus in avian-adapted 'typhoidal' serovars is due to deletion and rearrangement with pseudogenes in key genetic components (Thomson *et al.*, 2008). The rationale for infection for the loss of the flagellum is not clear but may relate to immune avoidance (Iqbal *et al.*, 2005; Chappell *et al.*, 2009). Data from the work of Morgan *et al.* (2004) would indicate that there are host-specific requirements for flagella function and chemotaxis in colonization of the intestinal tract.

The host immune response and flagella

Two major immunological considerations need to be discussed in relation to *Salmonella* flagella, its antigenicity and its role as an agonist for Toll-like receptor (TLR) 5.

Flagella are a major antigen of bacteria and are readily recognized by host adaptive immune systems. It is a major antigen for activated $CD4^+$ T cells in mice and poultry (Sbrogio-Almeida *et al.*, 2004). Challenge of mice with purified flagellin previously challenged with attenuated *S.* Typhimurium *aroA* strains stimulates the production of γ-IFN in a $CD4^+$ dependent manner leading to protective immunity against subsequent challenge with virulent *Salmonella* strains (Cookson and Bevan, 1997; McSorley *et al.*, 2000). The flagella antigens of *S. enterica* are phase variable and this phenomenon was first reported by Andrewes (1922) with the description of two distinct antigen populations in the serology of the bacteria, which were identified as flagella antigens (Lederberg and Iino, 1956). The frequency of transition between the phases is ca. 10^{-3}–10^{-5} per bacterium per generation (Lederberg and Iino, 1956). This phase variation is not observed in *Escherichia* and monophasic *Salmonella* species because *Salmonella* diverged from *E. coli* with the acquisition of the first pathogenicity island to form *S. bongori*. The subsequent addition of the second pathogenicity island formed *S. enterica* and its subspecies. At some point *S. enterica* acquired a second flagellin and the ability to phase vary led to the potential to separate *S. enterica* into monophasic and biphasic subspecies groups. The biphasic subspecies can alternate their gene expression between the flagellin subunit *fliC* (phase 1) and *fljB* (phase 2), which is mediated by the genes *fljA* and *hin* that flank *fljB* providing a 'flip-flop' regulatory mechanism to alternate expression of the phase 1 or phase 2 antigens (Szekely and Simon, 1983). This antigenic variation is achieved by varying the amino acids in the externalized hairpin structure of the flagellin subunit whilst the distal ends of the peptide are maintained since they are required to maintain flagella shape (Kanto *et al.*, 1991).

Flagella as an immune mediator

Salmonella flagellin is a potent immune stimulator and potent inducer of proinflammatory mediators both *in vivo* and *in vitro* in mammals and poultry (Hayashi *et al.*, 2001; Zeng *et al.*, 2003; Sbrogio-Almeida *et al.*, 2004). Flagellin is a pathogen-associated molecular pattern (PAMP), which can bind the TLR-5 and initiate an immune response (Hayashi *et al.*, 2001). This response triggers a signalling cascade, which leads to degradation of the regulatory protein IκB and the release of the transcription factor NFκB and its subsequent transfer to the nucleus (Tallant *et al.*, 2004). This NfκB signalling resulting from stimulation by a number of *Salmonella* PAMPs and type-III effector specific signalling is central to triggering enterocolitis (Elewaut *et al.*, 1999; Gewirtz *et al.*, 2000; Zeng *et al.*, 2003). Filaments of flagella will not stimulate TLR-5 and it is only the monomers that are immune-stimulatory (Hayashi *et al.*, 2001; Smith *et al.*, 2003). The binding to the toll receptor is independent of the variable domain of the flagellin and is linked to a conserved region (D1), which, when mutated, reduces the immune-stimulatory properties of the subunits drastically (Smith *et al.*, 2003). This hydrophobic motif is conserved in flagellin sequences of 377 various bacterial species (Jacchieri *et al.*, 2003). The role of flagella in initiating an immune response has been a topic of debate in the *Salmonella* field and also includes the debate on the role of different individual Toll receptors in initiating the immune response. In poultry TLR-5 and initiation of the inflammatory response is prominent (Iqbal *et al.*, 2005) and it has been argued that similar signalling is important in the stimulation of epithelial responses in other species (Zeng *et al.*, 2003). It has been argued that the lack of flagellin expression in the *Salmonella* serovars Gallinarum and Pullorum, which cause typhoidal infections in birds, is important in reducing the initiation of the immune response during early invasion and systemic spread (Kaiser *et al.*, 2000; Chappell *et al.*, 2009). However, other TLR receptors and their agonists will still be interacting during the infection, suggesting a degree of subtlety to the process of immune stimulation that has not yet been elucidated. Both host and bacterial factors affect the induction of immune responses by flagellin (Sbrogio-Almeida *et al.*, 2004). Flagella function and motility have been shown along with SPI-1 to impact on invasion in cell models (Shah *et al.*, 2011) and it has been suggested that regulation of these operons is linked (Jones *et al.*, 1981; Wang *et al.*, 2005).

During infections flagella have been shown to be important in the induction of colitis in mice (Stecher *et al.*, 2004). However, the role of flagella may be species-specific and mutation of *fljB* has been shown to have differential effects in calf and chick infection models along with a gene (*STM1557*) involved in chemotaxis and motility (Morgan *et al.*, 2004). Yet even within species there are differences between different flagella mutants, *fljA* (FliC repressor) is adherent for colonization of the pig while individual *fljB* mutant challenge was not affected in the same study (Carnell *et al.*, 2007). Flagella function is also not essential to all serovars as the non-flagellate *S.* Gallinarum and *S.* Pullorum are proficient in causing typhoid-like disease. It appears that this loss of flagella function is associated with typhoidal forms of disease and it has been suggested that the lack of flagella allows for a more stealthy approach to infection (Chappell *et al.*, 2009). The TLR stimulatory activity of *fliC* has led to the study of flagellin as a potential adjuvant and also as a carrier protein in the development of vaccines (Zhang *et al.*, 2011).

Other roles

Beyond their role in motility and the stimulation of immune responses through TLR-5 flagella have also been implicated in sensing the environment. It has been proposed that flagella can act as a wetness sensor with moisture affecting motility under different environmental conditions (Wang *et al.*, 2005). This function is mediated by moisture effects on secretion of FlgM, which leads to gene repression within the bacteria. Mechanical restrictions on flagella rotation in the *Enterobacteriaceae* may occur and studies with *Proteus* have shown that this could be mediated through the master regulator FldH (Furness *et al.*, 1997). Some subtle functions may exist that are less obvious than simple motility and attachment functions and the exact role of these in the infection process is unclear and will be difficult to determine as a result of this subtlety.

Concluding Remarks

The surface proteins of fimbriae and flagella both play a role in virulence of *Salmonella*. The fimbriae represent a diverse group of operons that are regulated at different stages of infection by a range of different environmental stimuli. Fimbriae appear to initiate interactions with cell surfaces and much of the data are in relation to epithelial cells. Flagella also have a multiplicity of roles in addition to motility. What is obvious is that both external components act in concert with other bacterial factors providing an overlapping range of functions to promote movement to, attachment to and eventual invasion of the cells. During this process these factors also interact with the host immune system with flagella stimulating inflammatory responses along other bacterial components. These proteins also represent an important group of surface antigens. The role of fimbriae in specific niches will require further analysis to provide an extension of our understanding of their multiple roles *in vivo*.

References

Abraham, J.M., Freitag, C.S., Clements, J.R. and Eisenstein, B.I. (1985) An invertible element of DNA controls phase variation of type 1 fimbriae of *Escherichia coli*. *Proceedings of the National Academy of Sciences of the United States of America* 82, 5724–5727.

Abram, D. and Koffler, H. (1964) *In vitro* formation of flagella like filaments and other structures from flagellin. *Journal of Molecular Biology* 9, 168–185.

Abram, D., Koffler, H. and Vatter, A.E. (1965) Basal structure and attachment of flagella in cells of *Proteus vulgaris*. *Journal of Bacteriology* 90, 1337–1354.

Abram, D., Mitchen, J.R., Koffler, H. and Vatter, A.E. (1970) Differentiation within the bacterial flagellum and isolation of the proximal hook. *Journal of Bacteriology* 101, 250–261.

Adegbola, R.A., Old, D.C. and Aleksić, S. (1983) Rare MR/K-like haemagglutinins (and type 3-like fimbriae) of *Salmonella* strains. *FEMS Microbiology Letters* 19, 233–238.

Allen-Vercoe, E. and Woodward, M.J. (1999) The role of flagella, but not fimbriae, in the adherence of *Salmonella enterica* serotype Enteritidis to chick gut explant. *Journal of Medical Microbiology* 48, 771–780.

Allen-Vercoe, E., Sayers, A.R. and Woodward, M.J. (1999) Virulence of *Salmonella enterica* serotype Enteritidis a-flagellate and a-fimbriate mutants in a day-old chick model. *Epidemiology and Infection* 122, 395–402.

Anderson, T.F. (1949) *Nature of the Bacterial Surface*. Oxford University Press, Oxford, UK.

Andrewes, F.W. (1922) Studies in group-agglutination I. The salmonella group and its antigenic structure. *Journal of Pathology and Bacteriology* 23, 505–521.

Asakura, S., Eguchi, G. and Iino, T. (1968) Unidirectional growth of *Salmonella* flagella *in vitro*. *Journal of Molecular Biology* 35, 227–236.

Baek, C.H., Wang, S., Roland, K.L. and Curtiss, R. III (2009) Leucine-responsive regulatory protein (Lrp) acts as a virulence repressor in *Salmonella enterica* serovar Typhimurium. *Journal of Bacteriology* 191, 1278–1292.

Baek, C.H., Kang, H.Y., Roland, K.L. and Curtiss, R. III (2011) Lrp acts as both a positive and negative regulator for type 1 fimbriae production in *Salmonella enterica* serovar Typhimurium. *PLoS One* 6, e26896.

Bäumler, A.J. and Heffron, F. (1995) Identification and sequence analysis of *lpfABCDE*, a putative fimbrial operon of *Salmonella typhimurium*. *Journal of Bacteriology* 177, 2087–2097.

Bäumler, A.J., Tsolis, R.M. and Heffron, F. (1996a) Contribution of fimbrial operons to attachment to and invasion of epithelial cell lines by *Salmonella typhimurium*. *Infection and Immunity* 64, 1862–1865.
Bäumler, A.J., Tsolis, R.M., Bowe, F., Kusters, J.G., Hoffmann, S. and Heffron, F. (1996b) The *pef* fimbrial operon of *Salmonella typhimurium* mediates adhesion to murine small intestine and is necessary for fluid accumulation in the infant mouse. *Infection and Immunity* 64, 61–68.
Bäumler, A.J., Tsolis, R.M. and Heffron, F. (1996c) The *lpf* fimbrial operon mediates adhesion of *Salmonella typhimurium* to murine Peyer's patches. *Proceedings of the National Academy of Sciences of the United States of America* 93, 279–283.
Bäumler, A.J., Gilde, A.J., Tsolis, R.M., van der Velden, A.W., Ahmer, B.M. and Heffron, F. (1997a) Contribution of horizontal gene transfer and deletion events to development of distinctive patterns of fimbrial operons during evolution of *Salmonella* serotypes. *Journal of Bacteriology* 179, 317–322.
Bäumler, A.J., Tsolis, R.M., Valentine, P.J., Ficht, T.A. and Heffron, F. (1997b) Synergistic effect of mutations in *invA* and *lpfC* on the ability of *Salmonella typhimurium* to cause murine typhoid. *Infection and Immunity* 65, 2254–2259.
Brinton, C.C. Jr (1959) Non-flagellar appendages of bacteria. *Nature* 183, 782–786.
Carnell, S.C., Bowen, A., Morgan, E., Maskell, D.J., Wallis, T.S. and Stevens, M.P. (2007) Role in virulence and protective efficacy in pigs of *Salmonella enterica* serovar Typhimurium secreted components identified by signature-tagged mutagenesis. *Microbiology* 153, 1940–1952.
Chappell, L., Kaiser, P., Barrow, P., Jones, M.A., Johnston, C. and Wigley, P. (2009) The immunobiology of avian systemic salmonellosis. *Veterinary Immunology and Immunopathology* 128, 53–59.
Chiu, C.H., Tang, P., Chu, C., Hu, S., Bao, Q., Yu, J., Chou, Y.Y., Wang, H.S. and Lee, Y.S. (2005) The genome sequence of *Salmonella enterica* serovar Choleraesuis, a highly invasive and resistant zoonotic pathogen. *Nucleic Acids Research* 33, 1690–1698.
Clayton, D.J., Bowen, A.J., Hulme, S.D., Buckley, A.M., Deacon, V.L., Thomson, N.R., Barrow, P.A., Morgan, E., Jones, M.A., Watson, M. and Stevens, M.P. (2008) Analysis of the role of 13 major fimbrial subunits in colonisation of the chicken intestines by *Salmonella enterica* serovar Enteritidis reveals a role for a novel locus. *BMC Microbiology* 8, 228.
Clouthier, S.C., Collinson, S.K., White, A.P., Banser, P.A. and Kay, W.W. (1998) tRNA(Arg) (*fimU*) and expression of SEF14 and SEF21 in *Salmonella enteritidis*. *Journal of Bacteriology* 180, 840–845.
Cogan, T.A., Jørgensen, F., Lappin-Scott, H.M., Benson, C.E., Woodward, M.J. and Humphrey, T.J. (2004) Flagella and curli fimbriae are important for the growth of *Salmonella enterica* serovars in hen eggs. *Microbiology* 150, 1063–1071.
Cohen-Bazire, G. and London, J. (1967) Basal organelles of bacterial flagella. *Journal of Bacteriology* 94, 458–465.
Collier, W.A., Wong, S.T. and De Miranda, J.C. (1955) Bacterien-Haemaglutination. II. Unspecifische hemming der Coli-Haemaglutination. *Antonie van Leeuwenhoek Journal of Microbiology and Serology* 21, 124–132.
Collighan, R.J. and Woodward, M.J. (2001) The SEF14 fimbrial antigen of *Salmonella enterica* serovar Enteritidis is encoded within a pathogenicity islet. *Vet Microbiology* 80, 235–245.
Collinson, S.K., Emödy, L., Trust, T.J. and Kay, W.W. (1992) Thin aggregative fimbriae from diarrheagenic *Escherichia coli*. *Journal of Bacteriology* 174, 4490–4495.
Cookson, B.T. and Bevan, M. (1997) Identification of a natural T cell epitope presented by *Salmonella*-infected macrophages and recognized by T cells from orally immunized mice. *Journal of Immunology* 158, 4310–4319.
Cooper, G.L. and Thorns, C.J. (1996) Evaluation of SEF14 fimbrial dot blot and flagellar western blot tests as indicators of *Salmonella enteritidis* infection in chickens. *Veterinary Record* 138, 149–153.
Darekar, M.R. and Eyer, H. (1973) The role of fimbriae in the processes of infection. Preliminary report. *Zentralbl Bakteriol Orig A* 225, 130–134.
De Buck, J., Van Immerseel, F., Haesebrouck, F. and Ducatelle, R. (2004) Effect of type 1 fimbriae of *Salmonella enterica* serotype Enteritidis on bacteraemia and reproductive tract infection in laying hens. *Avian Pathology* 33, 314–320.
DePamphilis, M.L. and Adler, J. (1971a) Purification of intact flagella from *Escherichia coli* and *Bacillus subtilis*. *Journal of Bacteriology* 105, 376–383.
DePamphilis, M.L. and Adler, J. (1971b) Attachment of flagellar basal bodies to the cell envelope: specific attachment to the outer, lipopolysaccharide membrane and the cytoplasmic membrane. *Journal of Bacteriology* 105, 396–407.
DePamphilis, M.L. and Adler, J. (1971c) Fine structure and isolation of the hook-basal body complex of flagella from *Escherichia coli* and *Bacillus subtilis*. *Journal of Bacteriology* 105, 384–395.

Doran, J.L., Collinson, S.K., Burian, J., Sarlós, G., Todd, E.C., Munro, C.K., Kay, C.M., Banser, P.A., Peterkin, P.I. and Kay, W.W. (1993) DNA-based diagnostic tests for *Salmonella* species targeting *agfA*, the structural gene for thin, aggregative fimbriae. *Journal of Clinical Microbiology* 31, 2263–2273.

Duguid, J.P. (1959) Fimbriae and adhesive properties in *Klebsiella* strains. *Journal of General Microbiology* 21, 271–286.

Duguid, J.P. (1968) The function of bacterial fimbriae. *Archivum Immunologiae et Therapia Experimentalis* 16, 173–188.

Duguid, J.P. and Gillies, R.R. (1958) Fimbriae and haemagglutinating activity in *Salmonella, Klebsiella, Proteus* and *Chormobacterium*. *Journal of Pathology and Bacteriology* 75, 519–520.

Duguid, J.P., Smith, I.W., Dempster, G. and Edmunds, P.N. (1955) Non-flagellar filamentous appendages (fimbriae) and haemagglutinating activity in Bacterium coli. *Journal of Pathology and Bacteriology* 70, 335–348.

Duguid, J.P., Anderson, E.S. and Campbell, I. (1966) Fimbriae and adhesive properties in *Salmonellae*. *Journal of Pathology and Bacteriology* 92, 107–138.

Duguid, J.P., Darekar, M.R. and Wheater, D.W. (1976) Fimbriae and infectivity in *Salmonella typhimurium*. *Journal of Medical Microbiology* 9, 459–473.

Edwards, R.A., Schifferli, D.M. and Maloy, S.R. (2000) A role for *Salmonella* fimbriae in intraperitoneal infections. *Proceedings of the National Academy of Sciences of the United States of America* 97, 1258–1262.

Edwards, R.A., Olsen, G.J. and Maloy, S.R. (2002) Comparative genomics of closely related *Salmonellae*. *Trends in Microbiology* 10, 94–99.

Eisenbrandt, R., Kalkum, M., Lai, E.M., Lurz, R., Kado, C.I. and Lanka, E. (1999) Conjugative pili of IncP plasmids, and the Ti plasmid T pilus are composed of cyclic subunits. *Journal of Biological Chemistry* 274, 22548–22555.

Elewaut, D., DiDonato, J.A., Kim, J.M., Truong, F., Eckmann, L. and Kagnoff, M.F. (1999) NF-κB is a central regulator of the intestinal epithelial cell innate immune response induced by infection with enteroinvasive bacteria. *Journal of Immunology* 163, 1457–1466.

Emerson, S.U., Tokuyasu, K. and Simon, M.I. (1970) Bacterial flagella: polarity of elongation. *Science* 169, 190–192.

Ernst, R.K., Dombroski, D.M. and Merrick, J.M. (1990) Anaerobiosis, type 1 fimbriae, and growth phase are factors that affect invasion of HEp-2 cells by *Salmonella typhimurium*. *Infection and Immunity* 58, 2014–2016.

Feutrier, J., Kay, W.W. and Trust, T.J. (1986) Purification and characterization of fimbriae from *Salmonella enteritidis*. *Journal of Bacteriology* 168, 221–227.

Friedrich, M.J., Kinsey, N.E., Vila, J. and Kadner, R.J. (1993) Nucleotide sequence of a 13.9 kb segment of the 90 kb virulence plasmid of *Salmonella typhimurium*: the presence of fimbrial biosynthetic genes. *Molecular Microbiology* 8, 543–558.

Furness, R.B., Fraser, G.M., Hay, N.A. and Hughes, C. (1997) Negative feedback from a *Proteus* class II flagellum export defect to the flhDC master operon controlling cell division and flagellum assembly. *Journal of Bacteriology* 179, 5585–5588.

Garaizar, J., Porwollik, S., Echeita, A., Rementeria, A., Herrera, S., Wong, R.M., Frye, J., Usera, M.A. and McClelland, M. (2002) DNA microarray-based typing of an atypical monophasic *Salmonella enterica* serovar. *Journal of Clinical Microbiology* 40, 2074–2078.

Gewirtz, A.T., Rao, A.S., Simon, P.O., Merlin, D., Carnes, D., Madara, J.L. and Neish, A.S. (2000) *Salmonella typhimurium* induces epithelial IL-8 expression via Ca2+-mediated activation of the NF-κB pathway. *Journal of Clinical Investigation* 105, 79–92.

Ghosh, S., Mittal, A., Vohra, H. and Ganguly, N.K. (1996) Interaction of a rat intestinal brush border membrane glycoprotein with type-1 fimbriae of *Salmonella typhimurium*. *Molecular and Cellular Biochemistry* 158, 125–131.

Gillies, R.R. and Duguid, J.P. (1958) The fimbrial antigens of *Shigella flexneri*. *Journal of Hygiene* 56, 303–318.

Guiney, D.G. and Fierer, J. (2011) The role of the *spv* genes in *Salmonella* pathogenesis. *Frontiers in Microbiology* 2, 129.

Guo, A., Cao, S., Tu, L., Chen, P., Zhang, C., Jia, A., Yang, W., Liu, Z., Chen, H. and Schifferli, D.M. (2009) FimH alleles direct preferential binding of *Salmonella* to distinct mammalian cells or to avian cells. *Microbiology* 155, 1623–1633.

Hammar, M., Bian, Z. and Normark, S. (1996) Nucleator-dependent intercellular assembly of adhesive curli organelles in *Escherichia coli*. *Proceedings of the National Academy of Sciences of the United States of America* 93, 6562–6566.

Harvey, P.C., Watson, M., Hulme, S., Jones, M.A., Lovell, M., Berchieri, A. Jr, Young, J., Bumstead, N. and Barrow, P. (2011) *Salmonella enterica* serovar *typhimurium* colonizing the lumen of the chicken intestine grows slowly and upregulates a unique set of virulence and metabolism genes. *Infection and Immunity* 79, 4105–4121.

Hayashi, F., Smith, K.D., Ozinsky, A., Hawn, T.R., Yi, E.C., Goodlett, D.R., Eng, J.K., Akira, S., Underhill, D.M. and Aderem, A. (2001) The innate immune response to bacterial flagellin is mediated by Toll-like receptor 5. *Nature* 410, 1099–1103.

Henderson, N.S., Ng, T.W., Talukder, I. and Thanassi, D.G. (2011) Function of the usher *N*-terminus in catalyzing pilus assembly. *Molecular Microbiology* 79, 954–967.

Hilmen, M., Silverman, M. and Simon, M. (1974) The regulation of flagellar formation and function. *Journal of Supramolecular Structure and Cellular Biochemistry* 2, 360–371.

Hobbs, M. and Mattick, J.S. (1993) Common components in the assembly of type 4 fimbriae, DNA transfer systems, filamentous phage and protein-secretion apparatus: a general system for the formation of surface-associated protein complexes. *Molecular Microbiology* 10, 233–243.

Hohmann, A.W., Schmidt, G. and Rowley, D. (1978) Intestinal colonization and virulence of *Salmonella* in mice. *Infection and Immunity* 22, 763–770.

Houwink, A.L. and van Iterson, W. (1950) Electron microscopical observations on bacterial cytology; a study on flagellation. *Biochimica et Biophysica Acta* 5, 10–44.

Humphries, A.D., Raffatellu, M., Winterk, S., Weening, E.H., Kingsley, R.A., Droleskey, R., Zhang, S., Figueiredo, J., Khare, S., Nunes, J., Adams, L.G., Tsolis, R.M. and Baümler, A.J. (2003) The use of flow cytometry to detect expression of subunits encoded by 11 *Salmonella enterica* serotype Typhimurium fimbrial operons. *Molecular Microbiology* 48, 1357–1376.

Humphries, A., Deridder, S. and Bäumler, A.J. (2005) *Salmonella enterica* serotype Typhimurium fimbrial proteins serve as antigens during infection of mice. *Infection and Immunity* 73, 5329–5338.

Ibuki, T., Imada, K., Minamino, T., Kato, T., Miyata, T. and Namba, K. (2011) Common architecture of the flagellar type III protein export apparatus and F- and V-type ATPases. *Nature Structural and Molecular Biology* 18, 277–282.

Iino, T. (1969) Genetics and chemistry of bacterial flagella. *Bacteriological Reviews* 33, 454–475.

Iino, T. and Mitani, M. (1966) Flagella-shape mutants in *Salmonella*. *Journal of General Microbiology* 44, 27–40.

Iqbal, M., Philbin, V.J., Withanage, G.S., Wigley, P., Beal, R.K., Goodchild, M.J., Barrow, P., McConnell, I., Maskell, D.J., Young, J., Bumstead, N., Boyd, Y. and Smith, A.L. (2005) Identification and functional characterization of chicken toll-like receptor 5 reveals a fundamental role in the biology of infection with *Salmonella enterica* serovar *typhimurium*. *Infection and Immunity* 73, 2344–2350.

Jacchieri, S.G., Torquato, R. and Brentani, R.R. (2003) Structural study of binding of flagellin by Toll-like receptor 5. *Journal of Bacteriology* 185, 4243–4247.

Jakomin, M., Chessa, D., Bäumler, A.J. and Casadesús, J. (2008) Regulation of the *Salmonella enterica std* fimbrial operon by DNA adenine methylation, SeqA, and HdfR. *Journal of Bacteriology* 190, 7406–7413.

Jones, C.H., Jacob-Dubuisson, F., Dodson, K., Kuehn, M., Slonim, L., Striker, R. and Hultgren, S.J. (1992) Adhesin presentation in bacteria requires molecular chaperones and ushers. *Infection and Immunity* 60, 4445–4451.

Jones, G.W., Richardson, L.A. and Uhlman, D. (1981) The invasion of HeLa cells by *Salmonella* typhimurium: reversible and irreversible bacterial attachment and the role of bacterial motility. *Journal of General Microbiology* 127, 351–360.

Jones, G.W., Rabert, D.K., Svinarich, D.M. and Whitfield, H.J. (1982) Association of adhesive, invasive, and virulent phenotypes of *Salmonella typhimurium* with autonomous 60-megadalton plasmids. *Infection and Immunity* 38, 476–486.

Kagawa, H., Owaribe, K., Asakura, S. and Takahashi, N. (1976) Flagellar hook protein from *Salmonella* SJ25. *Journal of Bacteriology* 125, 68–73.

Kaiser, P., Rothwell, L., Galyov, E.E., Barrow, P.A., Burnside, J. and Wigley, P. (2000) Differential cytokine expression in avian cells in response to invasion by *Salmonella typhimurium*, *Salmonella enteritidis* and *Salmonella gallinarum*. *Microbiology* 146, 3217–3226.

Kanto, S., Okino, H., Aizawa, S. and Yamaguchi, S. (1991) Amino acids responsible for flagellar shape are distributed in terminal regions of flagellin. *Journal of Molecular Biology* 219, 471–480.

Kauffmann, F. (1951) *Enterobacteriaceae*, 1st edn. Munksgaard, Copenhagen.

Kingsley, R.A., Santos, R.L., Keestra, A.M., Adams, L.G. and Baümler, A.J. (2002) *Salmonella enterica* serotype Typhimurium ShdA is an outer membrane fibronectin-binding protein that is expressed in the intestine. *Molecular Microbiology* 43, 895–905.

Kitagawa, R., Takaya, A. and Yamamoto, T. (2011) Dual regulatory pathways of flagellar gene expression by ClpXP protease in enterohaemorrhagic *Escherichia coli*. *Microbiology* 157, 3094–3103.

Klemm, P. (1984) The *fimA* gene encoding the type-1 fimbrial subunit of *Escherichia coli*. Nucleotide sequence and primary structure of the protein. *European Journal of Biochemistry* 143, 395–399.

Kline, K.A., Dodson, K.W., Caparon, M.G. and Hultgren, S.J. (2010) A tale of two pili: assembly and function of pili in bacteria. *Trends in Microbiology* 18, 224–232.

Korhonen, T.K., Lounatmaa, K., Ranta, H. and Kuusi, N. (1980) Characterization of type 1 pili of *Salmonella typhimurium* LT2. *Journal of Bacteriology* 144, 800–805.

Korhonen, T.K., Leffler, H. and Svanborg Edén, C. (1981) Binding specificity of piliated strains of *Escherichia coli* and *Salmonella typhimurium* to epithelial cells, *Saccharomyces cerevisiae* cells, and erythrocytes. *Infection and Immunity* 32, 796–804.

Kukkonen, M., Raunio, T., Virkola, R., Lähteenmäki, K., Mäkelä, P.H., Klemm, P., Clegg, S. and Korhonen, T.K. (1993) Basement membrane carbohydrate as a target for bacterial adhesion: binding of type I fimbriae of *Salmonella enterica* and *Escherichia coli* to laminin. *Molecular Microbiology* 7, 229–237.

Kukkonen, M., Saarela, S., Lähteenmäki, K., Hynönen, U., Westerlund-Wikström, B., Rhen, M. and Korhonen, T.K. (1998) Identification of two laminin-binding fimbriae, the type 1 fimbria of *Salmonella enterica* serovar *typhimurium* and the G fimbria of *Escherichia coli*, as plasminogen receptors. *Infection and Immunity* 66, 4965–4970.

Kutsukake, K., Ohya, Y., Yamaguchi, S. and Iino, T. (1988) Operon structure of flagellar genes in *Salmonella typhimurium*. *Molecular and General Genetics* 214, 11–15.

Kutsukake, K., Ohya, Y. and Iino, T. (1990) Transcriptional analysis of the flagellar regulon of *Salmonella typhimurium*. *Journal of Bacteriology* 172, 741–747.

Kuźmińska-Bajor, M., Kuczkowski, M., Grzymajło, K., Wojciech, L., Sabat, M., Kisiela, D., Wieliczko, A. and Ugorski, M. (2012) Decreased colonization of chicks by *Salmonella enterica* serovar Gallinarum expressing mannose-sensitive FimH adhesin from *Salmonella enterica* serovar Enteritidis. *Veterinary Microbiology* Feb 3, 158, 205–210.

Lawley, T.D., Klimke, W.A., Gubbins, M.J. and Frost, L.S. (2003) F factor conjugation is a true type IV secretion system. *FEMS Microbiology Letters* 224, 1–15.

Lawley, T.D., Chan, K., Thompson, L.J., Kim, C.C., Govoni, G.R. and Monack, D.M. (2006) Genome-wide screen for *Salmonella* genes required for long-term systemic infection of the mouse. *PLoS Pathogens* 2, e11.

Ledeboer, N.A., Frye, J.G., McClelland, M. and Jones, B.D. (2006) *Salmonella enterica* serovar Typhimurium requires the Lpf, Pef, and Tafi fimbriae for biofilm formation on HEp-2 tissue culture cells and chicken intestinal epithelium. *Infection and Immunity* 74, 3156–3169.

Lederberg, J. and Iino, T. (1956) Phase variation in *Salmonella*. *Genetics* 41, 743–757.

Liu, X. and Matsumura, P. (1994) The FlhD/FlhC complex, a transcriptional activator of the *Escherichia coli* flagellar class II operons. *Journal of Bacteriology* 176, 7345–7351.

Lockman, H.A. and Curtiss, R. III (1992a) Virulence of non-type 1-fimbriated and nonfimbriated nonflagellated *Salmonella typhimurium* mutants in murine typhoid fever. *Infection and Immunity* 60, 491–496.

Lockman, H.A. and Curtiss, R. III (1992b) Isolation and characterization of conditional adherent and non-type 1 fimbriated *Salmonella typhimurium* mutants. *Molecular Microbiology* 6, 933–945.

Low, A.S., Holden, N., Rosser, T., Roe, A.J., Constantinidou, C., Hobman, J.L., Smith, D.G., Low, J.C. and Gally, D.L. (2006) Analysis of fimbrial gene clusters and their expression in enterohaemorrhagic *Escherichia coli* O157:H7. *Environmental Microbiology* 8, 1033–1047.

Lyons, S., Wang, L., Casanova, J.E., Sitaraman, S.V., Merlin, D. and Gewirtz, A.T. (2004) *Salmonella typhimurium* transcytoses flagellin via an SPI2-mediated vesicular transport pathway. *Journal of Cell Science* 117, 5771–5780.

McClelland, M., Sanderson, K.E., Spieth, J., Clifton, S.W., Latreille, P., Courtney, L., Porwollik, S., Ali, J., Dante, M., Du, F., Hou, S., Layman, D., Leonard, S., Nguyen, C., Scott, K., Holmes, A., Grewal, N., Mulvaney, E., Ryan, E., Sun, H., Florea, L., Miller, W., Stoneking, T., Nhan, M., Waterston, R. and Wilson R.K. (2001) Complete genome sequence of *Salmonella enterica* serovar Typhimurium LT2. *Nature* 413, 852–856.

McFarland, K.A., Lucchini, S., Hinton, J.C. and Dorman, C.J. (2008) The leucine-responsive regulatory protein, Lrp, activates transcription of the *fim* operon in *Salmonella enterica* serovar Typhimurium via the *fimZ* regulatory gene. *Journal of Bacteriology* 190, 602–612.

McLaren, I.M., Sojka, M.G., Thorns, C.J. and Wray, C. (1992) An interlaboratory trial of a latex agglutination kit for rapid identification of *Salmonella enteritidis*. *Veterinary Record* 131, 235–236.

Macnab, R.M. (2004) Type III flagellar protein export and flagellar assembly. *Biochimica et Biophysica Acta* 1694, 207–217.

McSorley, S.J., Cookson, B.T. and Jenkins, M.K. (2000) Characterization of CD4+ T cell responses during natural infection with *Salmonella typhimurium*. *Journal of Immunology* 164, 986–993.

Minamino, T. and Macnab, R.M. (1999) Components of the *Salmonella* flagellar export apparatus and classification of export substrates. *Journal of Bacteriology* 181, 1388–1394.

Minamino, T., Morimoto, Y.V., Hara, N. and Namba, K. (2011) An energy transduction mechanism used in bacterial flagellar type III protein export. *Nature Communications* 2, 475.

Mintz, C.S., Cliver, D.O. and Deibel, R.H. (1983) Attachment of *Salmonella* to mammalian cells *in vitro*. *Canadian Journal of Microbiology* 29, 1731–1735.

Misselwitz, B., Kreibich, S.K., Rout, S., Stecher, B., Periaswamy, B. and Hardt, W.D. (2011) *Salmonella enterica* serovar Typhimurium binds to HeLa cells via Fim-mediated reversible adhesion and irreversible type three secretion system 1-mediated docking. *Infection and Immunity* 79, 330–341.

Morgan, E., Campbell, J.D., Rowe, S.C., Bispham, J., Stevens, M.P., Bowen, A.J., Barrow, P.A., Maskell, D.J. and Wallis, T.S. (2004) Identification of host-specific colonization factors of *Salmonella enterica* serovar Typhimurium. *Molecular Microbiology* 54, 994–1010.

Müller, K.H., Collinson, S.K., Trust, T.J. and Kay, W.W. (1991) Type 1 fimbriae of *Salmonella enteritidis*. *Journal of Bacteriology* 173, 4765–4772.

Nicholson, B. and Low, D. (2000) DNA methylation-dependent regulation of pef expression in *Salmonella typhimurium*. *Molecular Microbiology* 35, 728–742.

Nuccio, S.P. and Bäumler, A.J. (2007) Evolution of the chaperone/usher assembly pathway: fimbrial classification goes Greek. *Microbiology and Molecular Biology Reviews* 71, 551–575.

Nudleman, E. and Kaiser, D. (2004) Pulling together with type IV pili. *Journal of Molecular Microbiology and Biotechnology* 7, 52–62.

Ohnishi, K., Kutsukake, K., Suzuki, H. and Lino, T. (1992) A novel transcriptional regulation mechanism in the flagellar regulon of *Salmonella typhimurium*: an anti-sigma factor inhibits the activity of the flagellum-specific sigma factor, σF. *Molecular Microbiology* 6, 3149–3157.

Old, D.C. and Adegbola, R.A. (1985) Antigenic relationships among type-1 fimbriae of *Enterobacteriaceae* revealed by immuno-electronmicroscopy. *Journal of Medical Microbiology* 24, 21–28.

Old, D.C., Roy, A.I. and Tavendale, A. (1986) Differences in adhesiveness among type 1 fimbriate strains of *Enterobacteriaceae* revealed by an in vitro HEp2 cell adhesion model. *Journal of Applied Bacteriology* 61, 563–568.

Ottow, J.C. (1975) Ecology, physiology, and genetics of fimbriae and pili. *Annual Review of Microbiology* 29, 79–108.

Paranchych, W. and Frost, L.S. (1988) The physiology and biochemistry of pili. *Advances in Microbial Physiology* 29, 53–114.

Parkhill, J., Dougan, G., James, K.D., Thomson, N.R., Pickard, D., Wain, J., Churcher, C., Mungall, K.L., Bentley, S.D., Holden, M.T., Sebaihia, M., Baker, S., Basham, D., Brooks, K., Chillingworth, T., Connerton, P., Cronin, A., Davis, P., Davies, R.M., Dowd, L., White, N., Farrar, J., Feltwell, T., Hamlin, N., Haque, A., Hien, T.T., Holroyd, S., Jagels, K., Krogh, A., Larsen, T.S., Leather, S., Moule, S., O'Gaora, P., Parry, C., Quail, M., Rutherford, K., Simmonds, M., Skelton, J., Stevens, K., Whitehead, S. and Barrell, B.G. (2001) Complete genome sequence of a multiple drug resistant *Salmonella enterica* serovar Typhi CT18. *Nature* 413, 848–852.

Peralta, R.C., Yokoyama, H., Ikemori, Y., Kuroki, M. and Kodama, Y. (1994) Passive immunisation against experimental salmonellosis in mice by orally administered hen egg-yolk antibodies specific for 14-kDa fimbriae of *Salmonella enteritidis*. *Journal of Medical Microbiology* 41, 29–35.

Prouty, A.M., Brodsky, I.E., Manos, J., Belas, R., Falkow, S. and Gunn, J.S. (2004) Transcriptional regulation of *Salmonella enterica* serovar Typhimurium genes by bile. *FEMS Immunology and Microbiology* 41, 177–185.

Prüss, B.M., Liu, X., Hendrickson, W. and Matsumura, P. (2001) FlhD/FlhC-regulated promoters analyzed by gene array and *lacZ* gene fusions. *FEMS Microbiology Letters* 197, 91–97.

Purcell, B.K., Pruckler, J. and Clegg, S. (1987) Nucleotide sequences of the genes encoding type 1 fimbrial subunits of *Klebsiella pneumoniae* and *Salmonella typhimurium*. *Journal of Bacteriology* 169, 5831–5834.

Rajashekara, G., Munir, S., Alexeyev, M.F., Halvorson, D.A., Wells, C.L. and Nagaraja, K.V. (2000) Pathogenic role of SEF14, SEF17, and SEF21 fimbriae in *Salmonella enterica* serovar Enteritidis infection of chickens. *Applied Environmental Microbiology* 66, 1759–1763.

Rutter, J.M. and Jones, G.W. (1973) Protection against enteric disease caused by Escherichia coli – a model for vaccination with a virulence determinant? *Nature* 242, 531–532.

Rychlik, I., Gregorova, D. and Hradecka, H. (2006) Distribution and function of plasmids in *Salmonella enterica*. *Veterinary Microbiology* 12, 1–10.

Saini, S., Pearl, J.A. and Rao, C.V. (2009) Role of FimW, FimY, and FimZ in regulating the expression of type i fimbriae in *Salmonella enterica* serovar Typhimurium. *Journal of Bacteriology* 191, 3003–3010.
Saini, S., Slauch, J.M., Aldridge, P.D. and Rao, C.V. (2010) Role of cross talk in regulating the dynamic expression of the flagellar *Salmonella* pathogenicity island 1 and type 1 fimbrial genes. *Journal of Bacteriology* 192, 5767–5777.
Salit, I.E. and Gotschlich, E.C. (1977) Hemagglutination by purified type 1 *Escherichia coli* pili. *Journal of Experimental Medicine* 146, 1169–1181.
Sauer, F.G., Remaut, H., Hultgren, S.J. and Waksman, G. (2004) Fiber assembly by the chaperone-usher pathway. *Biochimica et Biophysica Acta* 1694, 259–267.
Sbrogio-Almeida, M.E., Mosca, T., Massis, L.M., Abrahamsohn, I.A. and Ferreira, L.C. (2004) Host and bacterial factors affecting induction of immune responses to flagellin expressed by attenuated *Salmonella* vaccine strains. *Infection and Immunity* 72, 2546–2555.
Shah, D.H., Zhou, X., Addwebi, T., Davis, M.A., Orfe, L., Call, D.R., Guard, J. and Besser, T.E. (2011) Cell invasion of poultry-associated *Salmonella enterica* serovar Enteritidis isolates is associated with pathogenicity, motility and proteins secreted by the type III secretion system. *Microbiology* 157, 1428–1445.
Shedden, W.I. (1962) Fimbriae and haemagglutinating activity in strains of *Proteus hauseri*. *Journal of General Microbiology* 28, 1–7.
Smith, K.D., Andersen-Nissen, E., Hayashi, F., Strobe, K., Bergman, M.A., Barrett, S.L., Cookson, B.T. and Aderem, A. (2003) Toll-like receptor 5 recognizes a conserved site on flagellin required for protofilament formation and bacterial motility. *Nature Immunology* 4, 1247–1253.
Smith, N.H., Beltran, P. and Selander, R.K. (1990) Recombination of *Salmonella* phase 1 flagellin genes generates new serovars. *Journal of Bacteriology* 172, 2209–2216.
Sojka, M.G., Dibb-Fuller, M. and Thorns, C.J. (1996) Characterisation of monoclonal antibodies specific to SEF 21 fimbriae of *Salmonella enteritidis* and their reactivity with other Salmonellae and Enterobacteria. *Veterinary Microbiology* 48, 207–221.
Sojka, M.G., Carter, M.A. and Thorns, C.J. (1998) Characterisation of epitopes of type 1 fimbriae of *Salmonella* using monoclonal antibodies specific for SEF21 fimbriae of *Salmonella enteritidis*. *Veterinary Microbiology* 59, 157–174.
Stecher, B., Hapfelmeier, S., Müller, C., Kremer, M., Stallmach, T. and Hardt, W.D. (2004) Flagella and chemotaxis are required for efficient induction of *Salmonella enterica* serovar Typhimurium colitis in streptomycin-pretreated mice. *Infection and Immunity* 72, 4138–4150.
Strom, M.S. and Lory, S. (1993) Structure-function and biogenesis of type IV pili. *Annual Review of Microbiology* 47, 565–596.
Subramanian, N. and Qadri, A. (2006) Lysophospholipid sensing triggers secretion of flagellin from pathogenic salmonella. *Nature Immunology* 7, 583–589.
Sukupolvi, S., Lorenz, R.G., Gordon, J.I., Bian, Z., Pfeifer, J.D., Normark, S.J. and Rhen, M. (1997) Expression of thin aggregative fimbriae promotes interaction of *Salmonella typhimurium* SR-11 with mouse small intestinal epithelial cells. *Infection and Immunity* 65, 5320–5325.
Sun, Y.H., Rolán, H.G. and Tsolis, R.M. (2007) Injection of flagellin into the host cell cytosol by *Salmonella enterica* serotype Typhimurium. *Journal of Biological Chemistry* 282, 33897–33901.
Swenson, D.L., Clegg, S. and Old, D.C. (1991) The frequency of *fim* genes among *Salmonella* serovars. *Microbial Pathogenesis* 10, 487–492.
Szekely, E. and Simon, M. (1983) DNA sequence adjacent to flagellar genes and evolution of flagellar-phase variation. *Journal of Bacteriology* 155, 74–81.
Takeuchi, A. (1967) Electron microscope studies of experimental *Salmonella* infection. I. Penetration into the intestinal epithelium by *Salmonella typhimurium*. *American Journal of Pathology* 50, 109–136.
Tallant, T., Deb, A., Kar, N., Lupica, J., de Veer, M.J. and DiDonato, J.A. (2004) Flagellin acting via TLR5 is the major activator of key signalling pathways leading to NF-kappa B and proinflammatory gene program activation in intestinal epithelial cells. *BMC Microbiology* 4, 33.
Tanaka, Y. and Katsube, Y. (1978) Infectivity of *Salmonella typhimurium* for mice in relation to fimbriae. *Nihon Juigaku Zasshi* 40, 671–681.
Tanaka, Y., Katsube, Y., Mutoh, T. and Imaizumi, K. (1981) Fimbriae of *Salmonella typhimurium* and their role in mouse intestinal colonization of the organism. *Nihon Juigaku Zasshi* 43, 51–62.
Tavendale, A., Jardine, C.K.H., Old, D.C. and Duguid, J.P. (1983) Haemagglutinins and adhesion of *Salmonella typhimurium* to HEp2 and HeLa cells. *Journal of Medical Microbiology* 16, 371–380.
Thanassi, D.G., Saulino, E.T. and Hultgren, S.J. (1998) The chaperone/usher pathway: a major terminal branch of the general secretory pathway. *Current Opinion in Microbiology* 1, 223–231.

Thomson, N.R., Clayton, D.J., Windhorst, D., Vernikos, G., Davidson, S., Churcher, C., Quail, M.A., Stevens, M., Jones, M.A., Watson, M., Barron, A., Layton, A., Pickard, D., Kingsley, R.A., Bignell, A., Clark, L., Harris, B., Ormond, D., Abdellah, Z., Brooks, K., Cherevach, I., Chillingworth, T., Woodward, J., Norberczak, H., Lord, A., Arrowsmith, C., Jagels, K., Moule, S., Mungall, K., Sanders, M., Whitehead, S., Chabalgoity, J.A., Maskell, D., Humphrey, T., Roberts, M., Barrow, P.A., Dougan, G. and Parkhill, J. (2008) Comparative genome analysis of *Salmonella* Enteritidis PT4 and *Salmonella* Gallinarum 287/91 provides insights into evolutionary and host adaptation pathways. *Genome Research* 18, 1624–1637.

Thorns, C.J., Sojka, M.G. and Chasey, D. (1990) Detection of a novel fimbrial structure on the surface of *Salmonella enteritidis* by using a monoclonal antibody. *Journal of Clinical Microbiology* 28, 2409–2414.

Thorns, C.J., Sojka, M.G., McLaren, I.M. and Dibb-Fuller, M. (1992) Characterisation of monoclonal antibodies against a fimbrial structure of *Salmonella enteritidis* and certain other serogroup D salmonellae and their application as serotyping reagents. *Research in Veterinary Science* 53, 300–308.

Thorns, C.J., Turcotte, C., Gemmell, C.G. and Woodward, M.J. (1996) Studies into the role of the SEF14 fimbrial antigen in the pathogenesis of *Salmonella enteritidis*. *Microbial Pathogenesis* 20, 235–246.

Tinker, J.K. and Clegg, S. (2000) Characterization of FimY as a coactivator of type 1 fimbrial expression in *Salmonella enterica* serovar Typhimurium. *Infection and Immunity* 68, 3305–3313.

Tinker, J.K., Hancox, L.S. and Clegg, S. (2001) FimW is a negative regulator affecting type 1 fimbrial expression in *Salmonella enterica* serovar *typhimurium*. *Journal of Bacteriology* 183, 435–442.

Tomoeda, M., Inuzuka, M. and Date, T. (1975) Bacterial sex pili. *Progress in Biophysics and Molecular Biology* 30, 23–56.

Townsend, S.M., Kramer, N.E., Edwards, R., Baker, S., Hamlin, N., Simmonds, M., Stevens, K., Maloy, S., Parkhill, J., Dougan, G. and Bäumler, A.J. (2001) *Salmonella enterica* serovar Typhi possesses a unique repertoire of fimbrial gene sequences. *Infection and Immunity* 69, 2894–2901.

Tsolis, R.M., Townsend, S.M., Miao, E.A., Miller, S.I., Ficht, T.A., Adams, L.G. and Baümler, A.J. (1999) Identification of a putative *Salmonella enterica* serotype Typhimurium host range factor with homology to IpaH and YopM by signature-tagged mutagenesis. *Infection and Immunity* 67, 6385–6393.

Turcotte, C. and Woodward, M.J. (1993) Cloning, DNA nucleotide sequence and distribution of the gene encoding the SEF14 fimbrial antigen of *Salmonella enteritidis*. *Journal of General Microbiology* 139, 1477–1485.

van Asten, A.J.A.M. and van Dijk, J.E. (2005) Distribution of 'classic' virulence factors among *Salmonella* spp. *FEMS Immunology and Medical Microbiology* 44, 251–259.

van der Velden, A.W.M., Baümler, A.J., Tsolis, R.M. and Heffron, F. (1998) Multiple fimbrial adhesins are required for full virulence of *Salmonella typhimurium* in mice. *Infection and Immunity* 66, 2803–2808.

Vetsch, M., Erilov, D., Moliere, N., Nishiyama, M., Ignatov, O. and Glockshuber, R. (2006) Mechanism of fibre assembly through the chaperone usher pathway. *EMBO Reports* 7, 734–738.

Wang, Q., Suzuki, A., Mariconda, S., Porwollik, S. and Harshey, R.M. (2005) Sensing wetness: a new role for the bacterial flagellum. *EMBO Journal* 24, 2034–2042.

Weening, E.H., Barker, J.D., Laarakker, M.C., Humphries, A.D., Tsolis, R.M. and Bäumler, A.J. (2005) The *Salmonella enterica* serotype Typhimurium *lpf*, *bcf*, *stb*, *stc*, *std*, and *sth* fimbrial operons are required for intestinal persistence in mice. *Infection and Immunity* 73, 3358–3366.

Wilson, R.L., Elthon, J., Clegg, S. and Jones, B.D. (2000) *Salmonella enterica* serovars gallinarum and pullorum expressing *Salmonella enterica* serovar Typhimurium type 1 fimbriae exhibit increased invasiveness for mammalian cells. *Infection and Immunity* 68, 4782–4785.

Woodward, M.J., Allen-Vercoe, E. and Redstone, J.S. (1996) Distribution, gene sequence and expression *in vivo* of the plasmid encoded fimbrial antigen of *Salmonella* serotype Enteritidis. *Epidemiology and Infection* 117, 17–28.

Yamaguchi, S. and Iino, T. (1969) Genetic determination of the antigenic specificity of flagellar protein in *salmonella*. *Journal of General Microbiology* 55, 59–74.

Yanagawa, R., Otsuki, K. and Tokui, T. (1968) Electron microscopy of fine structure of *Corynebacterium renale* with special reference to pili. *The Japanese Journal of Veterinary Research* 16, 31–37.

Yeh, K.S., Tinker, J.K. and Clegg, S. (2002) FimZ binds the *Salmonella* typhimurium *fimA* promoter region and may regulate its own expression with FimY. *Microbiology and Immunology* 46, 1–10.

Zeng, H., Carlson, A.Q., Guo, Y., Yu, Y., Collier-Hyams, L.S., Madara, J.L., Gewirtz, A.T. and Neish, A.S. (2003) Flagellin is the major proinflammatory determinant of enteropathogenic *Salmonella*. *Journal of Immunology* 171, 3668–3674.

Zhang, H., Liu, L., Wen, K., Huang, J., Geng, S., Shen, J., Pan, Z. and Jiao, X. (2011) Chimeric flagellin expressed by *Salmonella typhimurium* induces an ESAT-6-specific Th1-type immune response and CTL effects following intranasal immunization. *Cellular and Molecular Immunology* 8, 496–501.

4 Characterizing *Salmonella* Genomes

Muna F. Anjum[1]* and Nicholas R. Thomson[2]

[1]*Animal Health Veterinary Laboratories Agency, Addlestone, UK;* [2]*Wellcome Trust Sanger Laboratory, Hinxton, UK*

Introduction

The genus *Salmonella* is a diverse group of enteric pathogens, which infect humans and animals. It is a member of the family *Enterobacteriaceae* (enterics), which form a group of bacteria that take their name from the fact that they generally, but not exclusively, inhabit the gastrointestinal tract of animals. They were first observed in 1880 by Eberth in spleen sections and mesenteric lymph nodes from a patient who died from typhoid; subsequently the typhoid bacillus was cultivated in 1884 by Gaffky (Grimont *et al.*, 2000). The group includes many of the most important pathogens of humans and an array of different animals where they cause a spectrum of diseases leading to significant morbidity and mortality.

Salmonella are predominately pathogenic *Enterobacteriaceae* that are thought to have diverged from a common ancestor with *Escherichia coli* approximately 100 million years ago (Grimont *et al.*, 2000). Based on biochemical studies the genus *Salmonella* was divided into seven distinctive subspecies (Doolittle *et al.*, 1996; Brenner *et al.*, 2000). DNA hybridization and more recently multi-locus enzyme electrophoresis (MLEE), amplified fragment length polymorphism (AFLP) and multi-locus sequence typing (MLST) (Crosa *et al.*, 1973; Selander *et al.*, 1986; Torpdahl and Ahrens, 2004) and whole genome sequencing, has clarified these relationships showing that unlike *S. enterica*, *S. bongori* forms a tight cluster of highly related serotypes that are clearly separated from the majority of the salmonellae (Torpdahl and Ahrens, 2004; Falush *et al.*, 2006) (Plate 4). As a consequence *Salmonella* is currently divided into the two species *S. bongori* and *S. enterica*, with *S. enterica* being further subdivided into subspecies I, II, IIIa, IIIb, IV and VI, also known as *enterica*, *salamae*, *arizonae*, *diarizonae*, *indica* and *houtenae*, respectively (Crosa *et al.*, 1973; Le Minor *et al.*, 1982; Reeves *et al.*, 1989). In 1998 the White–Kauffmann–Le Minor scheme divided *Salmonella* according to antigenic structure or serovars. This classification scheme defines the serogroup according to expression of somatic lipopolysaccharide O antigens, and the serovar by expression of flagellar H antigens. It divided *Salmonella* into 2449 serovars, of which only 20 were in *S. bongori*. Of the remaining serovars 1443 were in *S. enterica* subsp. *enterica*, 488 in subsp. *salamae*, 94 in subsp. *arizonae*, 70 in subsp. *houtenae* and 11 in subsp. *indica*

* Corresponding author, e-mail: muna.anjum@ahvla.gsi.gov.uk

© CAB International 2013. *Salmonella in Domestic Animals, 2nd Edition* (eds P.A. Barrow and U. Methner)

(Le Minor *et al.*, 1986). However, these numbers are subject to regular review as more serovars are isolated and defined (Popoff *et al.*, 1998).

Only a small fraction of the thousands of *Salmonella* serovars regularly cause disease within humans and animals. Moreover, of those that do cause disease in warm-blooded animals 12 of the most prevalent serovars, all belonging to *S. enterica* subsp. *enterica*, have been shown to be responsible for more than 70% of all human infections (Centers for Disease Control and Prevention). The other subspecies, and serovars of *S. enterica* and *S. bongori*, are more closely associated with cold-blooded animals but do sporadically appear as human clinical infections largely from close contact with companion animals (pets), such as snakes, lizards and terrapins (Warwick *et al.*, 2001).

Within the serovars of *S. enterica* subsp. *enterica* that cause disease in warm-blooded animals there are examples of both promiscuous and host-adapted pathotypes. Those able to infect a broad range of hosts include *Salmonella enterica* subsp. *enterica* serovar Typhimurium, *Salmonella enterica* subsp. *enterica* serovar Enteritidis, and those that are host-restricted include *Salmonella enterica* subsp. *enterica* serovar Typhi and *Salmonella enterica* subsp. *enterica* serovar Gallinarum. From here on the nomenclature used for all serovars within *Salmonella enterica* subsp. *enterica* will be represented by *S.* Serovar, e.g. *S.* Typhimurium, *S.* Enteritidis, *S.* Typhi and *S.* Gallinarum, as defined by the National *Salmonella* Reference Laboratory at the Centers for Disease Control and Prevention (CDC) in the USA (Brenner *et al.*, 2000). Promiscuous serovars such as *S.* Enteritidis or *S.* Typhimurium, which are the most common causes of salmonellae-induced human food poisoning (Rodrigue *et al.*, 1990), are able to colonize the alimentary tract of a variety of animals, including humans, and cause gastroenteritis. Host-specific serovars such as *S.* Typhi and *S.* Gallinarum display a more invasive pathology causing systemic typhoid and typhoid-like disease in humans and poultry, respectively, and rarely cause enteritis in humans (Rodrigue *et al.*, 1990; Barrow *et al.*, 1994).

The *Salmonella* Genome

Plate 4 depicts the phylogenetic structure of the salmonellae showing a now characteristic star phylogeny for *S. enterica* subsp. *enterica*, the intermediate but distinct branching positions of the other *S. enterica* subspecies and clear separation from the only other true *Salmonella* species, *S. bongori*. It is clear from this figure that, despite there being significant substructure in the *S. bongori* tree (Plate 4 inset), how relatively conserved members of this species are compared to those falling within *S. enterica*.

Despite *Escherichia coli* and *Salmonella* having diverged millions of years ago, comparison of the genomes of *E. coli* K12 with *Salmonella* strains that phylogenetically span the genus shows a remarkable level of similarity including extensive regions of synteny (Plate 5). It is evident from Plate 5 that the conserved genomic regions or core regions are interspersed with sequences that are unique to one or other of the genomes. This is common in the *Enterobacteriaceae* where significant diversity has been driven by horizontal gene transfer set against a background of gradual genome sequence drift (Mandal, 1979). These observations have led to genes within bacterial genomes being classed as core, core variable or accessory functions. Core functions are present in the species and all close relatives (in this example between two genera within the same bacterial family). They are usually considered to be essential for growth and replication. Core variable functions are important for that species/lineage in that particular niche but are not necessarily universally present across all taxa. So-called accessory genes are functions that may confer an advantage to that particular isolate in that specific niche. Many of these accessory functions are shuttled into bacterial genomes by lysogenic phage or on transmissible plasmids and can be gained and lost rapidly.

In *Salmonella* many of its unique genes, compared to *E. coli*, are found on large discrete genomic islands that include prophage elements and specialized loci termed *Salmonella* pathogenicity islands (SPIs) (Plate 5) (McClelland *et al.*, 2000, 2001; Parkhill *et al.*, 2001). These *Salmonella*-specific functions include many genes required for the full expression of virulence. This chapter will aim to highlight the fluidity of the *Salmonella* genome (plasmids will not be considered here).

Tools for Defining the *Salmonella* Genome

Over the past few decades, major advances in the field of molecular biology, coupled with advances in genomic technologies, have led to an explosive growth in the biological information generated by the scientific community. The ultimate goal of the field is to gain new insight into the molecular basis of disease/pathogenesis, which can come from studying serovars associated with different disease outcomes or infecting different hosts, and the structural and functional gene homologues that they harbour. Differences between pathogens and commensals point to possible virulence determinants and disclose evolutionary histories that can be used to understand the extent of genetic variability within a natural population.

It has only been possible to fully assess and appreciate such diversity using genomic tools such as DNA microarray technology and whole genome sequencing. DNA microarrays, based on the genome sequence of a small number of representative members of this genus, allow the genome content of a relatively large number of bacterial isolates to be rapidly screened to assess the extent of genetic variability within a bacterial population to single gene resolution. Comparative genomic hybridization (CGH) DNA-based microarray studies involve genomic DNA from one or more reference strains and a test strain that are labelled with fluorescent dyes and hybridized to a microarray slide, containing probes representing all genes present in the reference strain spotted on the slide. These arrays are often supplemented with additional non-reference genes in an attempt to capture the 'pan-genome' of a particular species or genus and therefore expand their utility. In contrast, whole genome sequencing evaluates genomic differences in bacterial strains using indices of genome organization that vary both between species and within isolates of a species, e.g. the gene content (Anjum *et al.*, 2003; Schmidt and Hensel, 2004), G+C content (Thomson *et al.*, 2004), the occurrence and location of gene duplications, rearrangements, insertions (Sueoka, 1999) and horizontal gene transfer (Szpirer *et al.*, 1999; Brown *et al.*, 2003; Bischoff *et al.*, 2004). The following review discusses how whole genome sequencing and microarrays have been used to understand the relatedness of *Salmonella* strains and species, and provide information on genomic diversity.

Conservation in Architecture and Size of *Salmonella* Genomes

The rapid developments in output (measured in base pairs per run) from next-generation sequencing platforms such as ABI SOLiD or Illumina GAII, HiSeq and MiSeq and the gradual reduction in the costs of sequencing has meant that single genome sequencing projects have now given way to multi-genome projects. At the time of writing there were >30 complete or published genomes and over 300 ongoing (http://www.genomesonline.org). But even this is likely to be a dramatic underestimate of the amount of sequencing data that will be available for *Salmonella* over the coming months. These sequence data build upon a huge base of comparative array data from which several themes are developing in our understanding of the evolution and diversity of this bacterium. We will use a small number of *Salmonella* genomes or microarray studies to illustrate these themes.

Table 4.1 shows that despite differences in host range and disease severity of different *Salmonella enterica* subsp. *enterica* serovars there is a high degree of similarity between them. The examples shown include promiscuous serovars such as *S.* Typhimurium in addition to *S.* Choleraesuis, which has a broader host range (infecting pigs and occasionally humans) than the human-adapted *S.* Typhi

Table 4.1. Comparison of general genome features of selected sequenced *S. enterica* subsp. *enterica* I and *S. bongori.*

Common name	*S. bongori*	*S.* Typhi	*S.* Typhimurium	*S.* Enteritidis	*S.* Gallinarum	*S.* Choleraesuis	*S.* Paratyphi A
Subspecies	V	I	I	I	I	I	I
Strain	12419	CT18	LT2	P125109 (PT4)	287/91	SC-B67	SARB42
Size (kb)	4460	4809	4857	4685	4658	4755	4585
G + C content (%)	51.33	52.09	52.22	52.17	52.20	52.11	53.00
CDSs	3945	4599	4451	4320	4274	4445	4263
Pseudogenes	78	204	25	112	309	151	173
CDS density (%)	86.0	87.6	86.8	85.5	79.9	83.9	82.5
tRNAs	84	78	85	84	75	85	82
Prophage	5	7	6	1(5)	0(2)	5	3

and *S.* Paratyphi A, but a narrow host range compared to *S.* Typhimurium. This similarity in the general features of the genomes even extends to *S. bongori.*

An alignment of the genomes of *E. coli* and isolates representing both *Salmonella* species show they share a high degree of overall synteny, even these most distantly related *Salmonella* species being essentially co-linear. The exception is the large-scale rearrangement shown around the terminus of replication (shown in blue; Plate 5). This type of reciprocal inversion event around the terminus, or origin, of replication is a very common event that distinguishes closely related bacterial genomes and is evident in many published pairwise comparisons of other *Salmonella* serovar genomes (Boyd and Hartl, 1997; Liu and Sanderson, 1998; Eisen *et al.*, 2000; Tillier and Collins, 2000). It has been suggested that because chromosomal replication in many bacteria proceeds via bidirectional replication forks, starting at the origin and finishing at the terminus, that unpackaged DNA close to these symmetrical replication forks offers an ideal substrate for recombination to occur (Alokam *et al.*, 2002). Moreover, this type of recombination is thought to be more likely to be tolerated because reciprocal recombination maintains the gene order, orientation and distance with respect to the origin, as well as preserving the size of the replichores and the G/C bias of the leading strand (Tillier and Collins, 2000; Mackiewicz *et al.*, 2001; Rocha, 2004).

Other than reciprocal recombination events around the origin or terminus of replication, studies looking at multiple isolates of the same serovar have shown that the genome is relatively stably maintained with no or few further rearrangements (Bigot *et al.*, 2005). As might be expected there are exceptions and specific mutator strains of Typhimurium have been shown to undergo genomic rearrangements at *rrn* operons (Liu and Sanderson, 1995) and by microarray *S.* Typhimurium strains have been seen to stably amplify parts of their genome in non-mutator strains of *S.* Typhimurium (Liu *et al.*, 2003).

Defining the *Salmonella* Core and Accessory Genome

Clearly as the level of resolution increases with every new genome our understanding of the make-up of *Salmonella* genomes is redefined and refined. Comparisons of *S.* Typhimurium LT2, *S.* Enteritidis and *S.* Gallinarum showed that genes conserved between serovars show approximately 99% identity at the nucleotide level, whereas if this is broadened to comparisons of *S.* Typhimurium with either *S. bongori* or *E. coli* those figures fall to 91% and 80%, respectively (Porwollik *et al.*, 2004; Fookes *et al.*, 2011). With this high sequence identity it has been relatively straightforward, using reciprocal best top hit or clustering based approaches, to define the shared, or core gene set, and determine the number of unique genes present in each isolate, often referred to as the accessory genes (Plate 5). The core gene set shared by 35 genomes from across *Salmonella* is currently estimated to be 2811 gene families and the pan-genome to be greater than 10,000 genes (Plate 6) (Daubin and Ochman, 2004). Even between members of the same or closely related serovars we find between 1 and 5% of the genes to be strain-specific; these are largely prophage elements and to a lesser extent other mobile genetic elements and plasmids (Porwollik *et al.*, 2002; Thomson *et al.*, 2004; Kingsley *et al.*, 2009; Jacobsen *et al.*, 2011). However, in comparison to *E. coli*, which has a similar sized genome to *Salmonella* (~4.5–5.7 Mb), these figures are relatively conservative. Comparisons of two different *E. coli* pathovars with *E. coli* K12 showed they can carry an additional ~1.3–1.4 Mb of unique sequence (~1300 genes) (Porwollik *et al.*, 2002). Moreover, comparing between 17 and 57 *E. coli* genomes, representing multiple pathovars, has shown that the core genome could be as little as 1472 to 2200 genes and the pan-genome is open, composed of >13,000 genes as indicated by the discovery rate for novel genes of ~300 for every new genome added to the analysis (Fig. 4.1) (Perna *et al.*, 2001; Rasko *et al.*, 2008; Lukjancenko *et al.*, 2010).

So it is clear that the *Salmonella* genome, although conservative relative to *E. coli*, is still highly plastic. However, to begin to make sense of these gene acquisitions we must first determine when and at what point in the phylogenetic history of *Salmonella* these genes were gained. This will help differentiate those functions that are *Salmonella* genus-specific and likely to encode functions for a generic '*Salmonella*-type' enteric lifestyle from those that differentiate *Salmonella* lineages.

Vernikos *et al.* (2007) analysed the divergence of 11 *Salmonella* genomes from *E. coli* and *Shigella* and attempted to reconstruct the horizontal gene transfer (HGT) events on to a phylogenetic tree constructed using the sequence of the core conserved genes. Parsimony was used to infer the sequence of events that led to the currently observed genome structure of the *Salmonella*. What was most striking is that functional breakdown of the putative horizontally acquired (PHA) DNA shows that recent evolutionary time has been dominated by the integration of bacteriophage but earlier evolutionary events occurring in the salmonellae were dominated by the acquisition of metabolic and virulence functions. This is a slight distortion because the assumption is made that only genes that confer an advantage would be fixed in the genome over the longer term. This predicts that functions such as prophage structural genes would likely be rapidly gained and then lost and so are less likely to appear higher in the tree.

Looking at the PHA gene distribution across the *Salmonella* tree Vernikos *et al.* (2007) showed that approximately 35–40% of the PHA DNA, including many of the important SPIs (including SPI-1, SPI-5, SPI-4, *ttr* genes, 5′ region only of SPI-3), were ancient acquisition events, appearing at the base of the *Salmonella* lineage following the divergence from *E. coli* but before speciation into *S. bongori* and *S. enterica*. It was suggested that these genes were likely key early events that facilitated adaptation to a new niche(s).

Vernikos *et al.* also showed that cumulatively 60–70% of all the PHA DNA was acquired prior to the divergence of the *S. enterica* subspecies and so was shared by most members of the *S. enterica* lineage including SPI-1, SPI-2, SPI-3, SPI-4, SPI-5, SPI-6, SPI-10 (5′ region), SPI-16 and SPI-17. This suggests that, depending on whether *Salmonella* as a whole is referred to or *S. enterica* subspecies, with the exclusion of *S. bongori*, most of the genomic islands and SPIs that are commonly considered to be part of the accessory genome have been fixed within the genus for a considerable period of time,

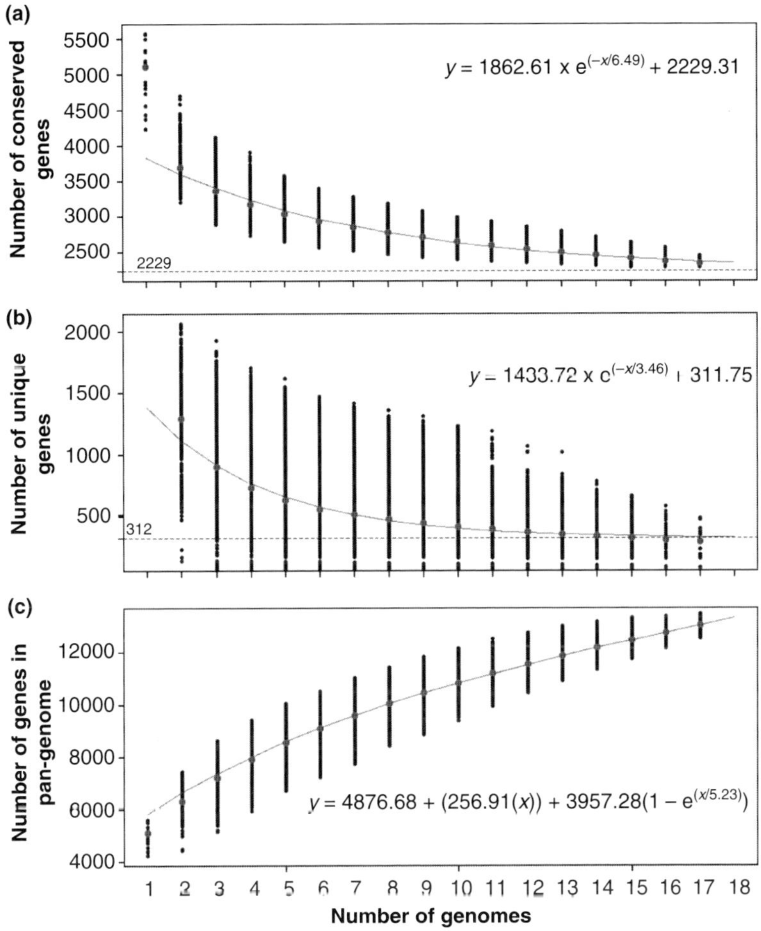

Fig. 4.1. Conserved core, unique and pan-genome calculations for *E. coli*. (a) Each point indicates the number of genes that are conserved in genomes. The curved line shows the exponential decay model based on the median value for conserved genes when increasing numbers of genomes were compared. (b) Decreasing number of unique genes in a genome with increasing number of genomes compared. The curved line shows the exponential decay model based on the median value for unique genes when increasing numbers of genomes were compared. (c) Pan-genome of the species *E. coli*. The extrapolated curve continues to increase, and thus *E. coli* has an open pan-genome. (Rasko *et al.*, Copyright © American Society for Microbiology, *Journal of Bacteriology*, Vol. 190 (No. 20) 2008, pp. 6881–6893.)

measured in tens of millions of years, and so should now be considered as part of the *Salmonella*, or alternatively *S. enterica*, core genome, and not accessory. This also explains why studies looking for differences in the SPI content of contemporary outbreak strains find little or no differences in the makeup of the classical *Salmonella* virulence genes they encode (Litrup *et al.*, 2010; Petersen *et al.*, 2011).

What is in the Core Genome of *Salmonella* and Why is this Useful to Know?

Many studies have looked at the core genome content because of the recognition that functions, including metabolic pathways that facilitate colonization and allow the exploitation of nutrients specific to a particular niche, are as important to pathogenicity as the more dedicated virulence functions. These core genes include most of the central and intermediary metabolism genes/pathways, e.g. citric acid cycle, fatty acid biosynthesis, pentose phosphate pathway and pyruvate metabolism (Anjum *et al.*, 2003; Chan *et al.*, 2003; Vernikos *et al.*, 2007). The conservation of these essential genes for metabolic function and virulence are discussed in the following section.

After this point, with so many studies defining core genomes and core functions it is worth keeping in mind what is meant by 'core' in each study and whether it refers to the enterobacterial core or that of *Salmonella* as a whole, *S. enterica* or the core shared between two closely related serotypes of *S. enterica* subsp. *enterica*. Each of these definitions has its own set of core functions, the significance of which requires careful interpretation. Clearly the extent of the cores can overlap but it is the differences between these broad and close comparisons that will highlight the alternative evolutionary paths taken by different lineages.

A recent study comparing the core genome metabolic maps of possibly the most distantly related members of the salmonellae, *S. bongori* and *S.* Typhi, showed them to be generally similar with a few interesting differences. Fookes *et al.* (2011) showed that all pathways known to be involved in the generation of precursor metabolites and energy for *S.* Typhi (30 pathways) are present in *S. bongori*. Only 8 of the 146 *S.* Typhi predicted biosynthetic pathways (including the biosynthesis of amino acids, carbohydrates, fatty acids and lipids) were missing from *S. bongori*. Of the 78 degradative pathways carried by *S.* Typhi, *S. bongori* shares 72 and possesses three unique pathways (with respect to *S.* Typhi). The metabolic differences of interest include vitamin B_{12} biosynthesis, which is thought to have been lost by *Salmonella* and then acquired by *S. enterica* following *Salmonella* speciation (Laurence and Roth, 1996). The ability to make endogenous vitamin B_{12} has recently been shown to be important for survival in macrophages (Lawrence and Roth, 1996), a niche in which *S. bongori* is not adapted to survive (Klumpp and Fuchs, 2007).

Conversely, *S. bongori* possesses the capacity to degrade lactose, which has been proposed to enable *E. coli* to colonize the gut of young mammals by the metabolism of milk sugar. The only other salmonellae that appear to contain the complete *lac* operon are *S. enterica* subspp. *arizonae* and *diarizonae*, but there is no strong conservation in genes or the site of insertion, suggesting independent acquisition events (Hansen-Wester *et al.*, 2004). In addition to presence and absence of pathways this analysis highlighted examples where a pathway present in *S. bongori* thought to represent the ancestral state had been replaced with another energetically more efficient but functionally analogous pathway in *S. enterica* lineages, thus providing evidence of metabolic streamlining.

Salmonella Metabolic Model; Mapping the Core

Various studies have used the core genome information to construct models of metabolic pathways to understand evolutionary differences in metabolic potential. Using the core genome identified from microarray studies the *Salmonella* metabolic model *i*MA945 was constructed (AbuOun *et al.*, 2009) and compared to the genes present in *E. coli* K12 (Feist *et al.*, 2007) and *S.* Typhimurium strains (Raghunathan *et al.*, 2009). The *i*MA945 model comprises 945 genes, 1964 reactions and 1036 metabolites, showing significant overlap with homologous genes present in *E. coli* MG1655 model *i*AF1260 (Fig. 4.2) (Feist *et al.*, 2007) and compares well with another *S.* Typhimurium strain LT2 *i*RR1083 metabolic model, which is also based on a wide range of *in vitro* conditions, but additionally includes host cell environmental conditions present during infection (Raghunathan *et al.*, 2009). To construct the *i*MA945 model, *in silico* growth simulations were compared to phenotypic data obtained from respiration/growth in different substrates using the OmniLog PhenotypeMicroarray technology system (Biolog); the *in silico* and *in vitro* results were generally in good agreement. In only 19 conditions of the 379 tested was *E. coli* K12

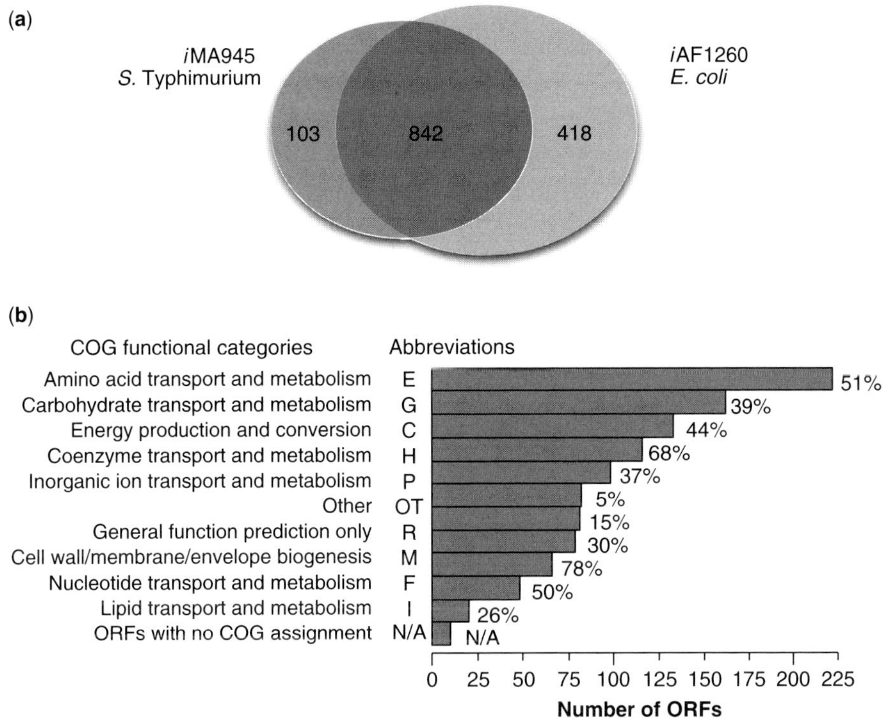

Fig. 4.2. A *Salmonella* genome scale model. (a) Venn diagram showing the homology overlap between the *S.* Typhimurium model *i*MA945 and the *E. coli* model *i*AF1260. (b) Classification of the ORFs included in *i*MA945 grouped into COG functional categories. The length of each bar represents the number of genes in each COG that is included in the model. The percentage assigned to each class refers to the coverage of the total number in the genome accounted for in the model. Some of the ORFs do not currently have a COG functional category assignment (here represented as N/A). Note that although each ORF is only counted once within each COG functional category, some ORFs have multiple COG category assignments (reproduced from AbuOun *et al.*, 2009).

unable to utilize substrates that *Salmonella* could utilize, including Tween 40 or 80, 1,2-propanediol, adonitol/ribitol and *p*-hydroxyphenylacetic acid. In 17 conditions, *E. coli* K12 was able to utilize substrates that the majority of *Salmonella* strains included in this study were unable to utilize, including lactulose, D-allose and L-tryptophan, consistent with the phylogenetically close relationship between these organisms. However, not all core genes are essential for virulence *in vivo*. The genome-scale metabolic network of *Salmonella* Typhimurium LT2 (iRR1083) developed by Raghunathan *et al.* (2009) was used to identify genes essential for conditions that mimic host cell environments, i.e. virulence *in vivo*. They compared these genes to those shown experimentally to be essential or non-essential for replication within the host cell showing that the *in silico* virulence predictions by iRR1083 overlapped with the *in vivo* virulence characterization by 92%. Examples of genes within this category include the aromatic amino acid biosynthesis genes *aroABCD*, which are well known to attenuate *Salmonella* serovars (Raghunathan *et al.*, 2009).

These metabolic models build on a wealth of experimental data that show how genes within the *Salmonella* core gene set that perform central metabolic functions are essential for virulence and colonization of its host. On reflection this makes perfect sense, but these functions are often ignored in favour of the 'smoking guns': Type III secretion systems etc. There are many studies reinforcing the role of various metabolic pathways in virulence including those using transcriptomic data. Antunes *et al.* (2012) noted from studies of *S.* Typhimurium that in the presence of murine bile many genes involved in central metabolism are affected, with the citric acid cycle being repressed and alternative respiratory systems being activated, and *phoP*, which is involved in *Salmonella* virulence, being repressed. Other transcriptome profiling studies of RNA extracted from *S.* Typhimurium present in the luminal contents of ceca of 1-day-old chicks have shown significant upregulation of a number of amino acid and carbohydrate utilization genes in comparison to *in vitro* cultures (Medalla *et al.*, 2011). Upregulated genes include, amongst others, genes from the *pdu* and *ttr* operon involved in anaerobic catabolism of 1,2-propanediol and ethanolamine in *Salmonella*; mutation in the *ttr* gene was found to significantly reduce colonization in chickens.

Understanding the pathways that *Salmonella* employs to survive and adapt within the host environment, and identifying genes that are essential components of these pathways, will ultimately be essential for the task of constructing avirulent mutants for vaccine development or identifying candidate pathways or reactions to block for therapeutic purposes.

Functional Gene Loss: Pseudogenes

Along with the wholesale acquisition of genes it is clear that gene loss plays an important role in the fluidity of the *Salmonella* genome (McClelland *et al.*, 2000; Parkhill *et al.*, 2001; Thomson *et al.*, 2006). The clearest picture for the role of functional gene loss in bacterial evolution comes from studying the presence and nature of pseudogenes. The working definition of a pseudogene in genome annotation is that the protein coding portion of the gene contains a premature stop codon(s), frameshift mutation(s) or internal deletion(s) or is disrupted by, for example, the insertion of an IS element, and so is not predicted to be transcribed or translated. Clearly there are always dangers associated with *in silico* prediction of pseudogenes: it is very difficult to predict the impact of changes in, for example, the promoter regions of genes, where the promoter has not been experimentally defined, and because there are known mechanisms that allow read-through of stop codons or the correction of reading frame by programmed ribosomal frame-shifting. Indeed, there are even dangers from assuming that a gene function has been lost when a significant part of the coding sequence has been deleted. However, increasingly through experimental studies that allow us to associate phenotype to genotype and by comparative genomics and/or transcriptomics, more confidence is being placed on predictions of non-functionality and the interpretations that have been made around their significance. With the above caveats, what is the extent and significance to our understanding of the biology, and evolution, of the strains that contain them?

Analysis of the genome of *S.* Typhi, which is restricted to human hosts and causes an acute febrile illness, revealed the presence of over 200 pseudogenes, compared to *S.* Typhimurium, which carries between 25 and 77 (Table 4.1; Parkhill *et al.*, 2001; Chiu *et al.*, 2005; Kingsley *et al.*, 2009). Looking at the distribution of the pseudogenes in *S.* Typhi it is apparent that the patterns of gene loss are non-random; pseudogenes are over-represented in genes that are specific to *S.* Typhi, or *Salmonella* in general, when for example compared to *E. coli*. What is more, many of the *S.* Typhi pseudogenes have intact counterparts involved in aspects of virulence or host interaction in broad host-range *Salmonellae* such as *S.* Typhimurium (McClelland *et al.*, 2001).

As more *Salmonella* are sequenced, similarities in the patterns of pseudogene formation can be observed with the same traits being lost independently in different *Salmonella* lineages (usually associated with limited host ranges and more acute invasive disease). *Salmonella* Paratyphi A causes a typhoid-like illness and possesses a significant number of mutations in genes also defunct in *S.* Typhi including those encoding the Type Three Secretion System (TTSS) effector proteins associated with diarrhoea or systemic disease: SopA, SlrP, SopD2 and SseJ (Parkhill *et al.*, 2001). Additionally, *S.* Paratyphi A carries mutations in *sifB* and *sspH2*, whilst *S.* Typhi has lost a functional copy of *sopE2*. Other important functions lost by *S.* Typhi and *S.* Paratyphi A include components of multiple chaperone-usher fimbrial systems and *tar* encoding a chemotaxis receptor protein, which, if deleted in *S.* Typhimurium, leads to a hyper-invasive phenotype (Jones *et al.*, 1992). Consequently, their loss may actually prolong and moderate the infection, thereby increasing transmission, and is consistent with *S.* Typhi and *S.* Paratyphi A rarely causing diarrhoea.

Similar patterns of gene loss are seen in *S.* Choleraesuis, which also rarely causes diarrhoea, and *S.* Gallinarum, which causes a typhoid-like disease in chickens, including pseudogenes involved in shedding and colonization of the gut (see below) as well as potential patho-adaptive mutations in chemotaxis signal transduction pathways that increase invasiveness of the bacterium (Jones *et al.*, 1992; Chiu *et al.*, 2005; Thomson *et al.*, 2008).

It is not just virulence genes that are found as pseudogenes in these salmonellae; *S.* Typhi, *S.* Paratyphi A and *S.* Gallinarum possess independent mutations in genes involved in common core metabolic pathways: cobalamin (vitamin B_{12}) biosynthesis, propanediol utilization pathway and tetrathionate respiration (Parkhill *et al.*, 2001; McClelland *et al.*, 2004; Thomson *et al.*, 2008; Holt *et al.*, 2009). Under anaerobic conditions *Salmonella* can produce endogenous B_{12}, which acts as a cofactor for the energetically efficient degradation of 1,2-propanediol, which proceeds with tetrathionate acting as a terminal electron acceptor (Roth *et al.*, 1996). In *S.* Typhimurium 1,2-propanediol is an important source of energy. *Salmonella* Typhimurium mutants unable to use 1,2- propanediol are significantly attenuated in their ability to grow in macrophages (Klumpp and Fuchs, 2007).

Moreover, the ability to use tetrathionate produced naturally in the lumen of the inflamed gut as an electron acceptor has been shown to confer a competitive advantage for *S.* Typhimurium by allowing it to outcompete normal microbiota (Winter *et al.*, 2010). In this situation tetrathionate respiration also enables *S.* Typhimurium to utilize ethanolamine as a nutrient. Ethanolamine supports little fermentative growth but is readily found in the intestine of healthy calves. It is the possession of these metabolic functions that is thought to allow *S.* Typhimurium to be competitive and successfully colonize the intestinal lumen (Thiennimitr *et al.*, 2011).

Interestingly, of the *S.* Paratyphi A (173) and *S.* Choleraesuis (151) pseudogenes only 28 and 17 are also disrupted in *S.* Typhi, respectively, indicating that they have arisen independently. Furthermore, most of the pseudogenes found in salmonellae are caused by single point mutations or deletions/insertions, suggesting that they have been inactivated relatively recently. Together, this suggests that the patterns of functional gene loss represent markers of convergent evolution, which are believed to be associated with host restriction and moving away from adaptation from a gut to a more systemic lifestyle.

Patterns of Recombination Provide Insights into the Order of Pseudogene Accumulation

More light was shed on the significance of pseudogene accumulation in salmonellae by looking for evidence of recombination in the genomes of *S.* Typhi and *S.* Paratyphi A. Didelot *et al.* (2007) looked at the levels of nucleotide variation in regions shared between *S.* Typhi and *S.* Paratyphi A and between *S.* Typhi and a range of other *S. enterica* serovars. They showed that when comparing *S.* Typhi and *S.* Paratyphi A regions of the genome essentially fell into two classes differentiated by differences in the level of sequence similarity: (i) around 77% of the genome showed a level of nucleotide diversity of 1.2%, roughly that seen between *S.* Typhi or *S.* Paratyphi A and any other serovar; and (ii) the other 23% of the *S.* Typhi genome showed a much lower diversity, around 0.18%, indicative of much more recent common ancestry. These low diversity regions were scattered around the genome in 124 blocks with average size of 6.4 kb. One interpretation of this data, put forward by the authors, was that *S.* Paratyphi A and *S.* Typhi diverged at the same time as the rest of the *S. enterica* group, but then subsequently exchanged around a quarter of their genomes, possibly by phage-mediated DNA transfer. This observation was taken further by Holt *et al.* (2009), who linked the recombination between these two serovars to the presence of pseudogenes with shared and independent mutations. By comparing multiple *S.* Paratyphi A and *S.* Typhi genomes, these authors differentiated pseudogenes into four groups: (i) those that were located in high divergence regions with shared mutations and considered to have been present in, and inherited from, a common ancestor; (ii) pseudogenes lying within low diversity regions with identical mutations, which were assumed to have been recently exchanged; (iii) pseudogenes with independent inactivating mutations, the majority of which were expected to have become pseudogenes after recombination; and (iv) pseudogenes that were strain-specific and so likely to be formed recently (evidence of ongoing functional gene loss).

Group 1 pseudogenes were described as being 'well tolerated' and showed a higher proportion of multiple mutations than other groups. Of the genes within this group 28 (out of 38) were putative phage or transposase genes or gene remnants and so it was suggested that their presence was unlikely to have an impact on the 'fitness' of these serovars. But within this group there were also pseudogenes, for example *sopD2*, which is known to play a role in virulence and remain intact in less invasive *S. enterica* serovars such as *S.* Typhimurium (Holt *et al.*, 2009). It was suggested that the loss of these genes may have been a prerequisite for subsequent adaptation to the systemic niche. The group 2 recombined genes also included type III secretion system effectors such as *sopA*, necessary for virulence in both murine systemic infections and bovine gastrointestinal infections by Typhimurium, the loss of which, the authors suggest, could have been significant factors in either restricting these two serovars or in their adaptation to a new systemic lifestyle. Of the group 3 pseudogenes, >100 were found to be specific to each serovar, 22 of which were present in both serovars with different inactivating mutations. These were considered to represent convergent gene loss and therefore likely to be good examples of patho-adaptive mutations associated with adaptation to the human host. These pseudogenes included *fhuA*, *fhuE*, *shdA*, *ratB* and *sivH*, all known to be involved or implicated in host interactions. Although the group 4 genes largely represent strain differences, Holt *et al.* (2009) showed that several of the pseudogenes in this group were found to have appeared sporadically in isolates from each of the two serovars and so were suggested to be glimpses of ongoing convergence.

As the authors also point out, although Paratyphi A and Typhi share 27 pseudogenes that were not present in their common ancestor, only five fall within recombination regions, suggesting that although recombination and pseudogene formation are linked they are largely independent processes in terms of their role in genetic convergence of these two serovars. But this phenomenon did allow the identification of the different groups of pseudogenes and for them to be placed at different time points in their evolution, perhaps giving us the first glimpse of a pathway to host adaptation.

The Variable Genome and its Source in *Salmonella*

Salmonella pathogenicity islands

The acquisition and loss of mobile elements through horizontal gene transfer results in the elasticity of bacterial genomes, which is a major driving force for their evolution, pathogenicity and adaptation to different environments (Kudva *et al.*, 2002; Jiang *et al.*, 2004). In *Salmonella*, horizontally acquired DNA sequences with functionally related genes, often referred to as pathogenicity islands or genomic islands (GIs), have been found with

1

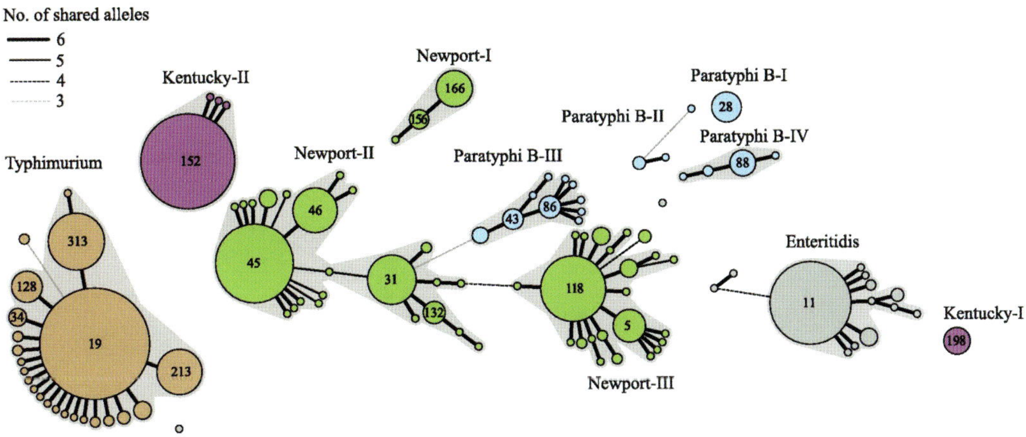

2

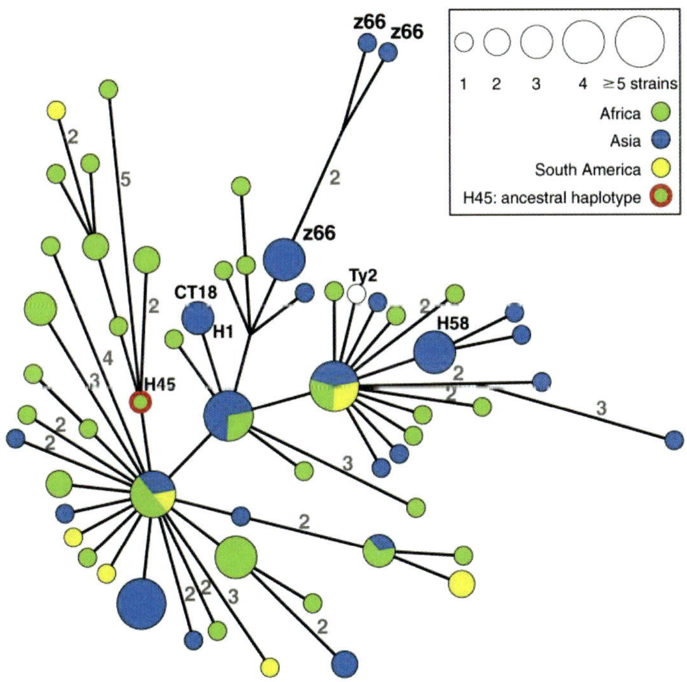

Plate 1. The minimal-spanning (MS) tree of the allelic profiles from seven house-keeping genes from strains representing serotypes of *Salmonella enterica*. The numbers in the circles are sequence type (ST) designations. The numbers of shared alleles of the different STs are shown in the top left corner. (From Sangal, V., *et al.* (2010) *Journal of Bacteriology* 192, 6465–6476, Fig. 3, with permission from the American Society for Microbiology).

Plate 2. Minimal-spanning (MS) tree of 105 isolates of *S.* Typhi based on sequence polymorphisms. The tree shows 59 haplotypes (nodes) based on 88 single nucleotide polymorphisms (SNPs). The continental origin of each haplotype is indicated by colours. The numbers on the edges indicate the number of SNPs that separate the nodes; unlabelled edges are single SNPs. z66 refers to a flagellar variant common in Indonesia. The numbers of a few of the haplotypes are shown (H45 and H58). (From Roumagnac, P., *et al.* (2006) *Science* 314, 1301–1304, Fig. 1, with permission from The American Association for the Advancement of Science).

3

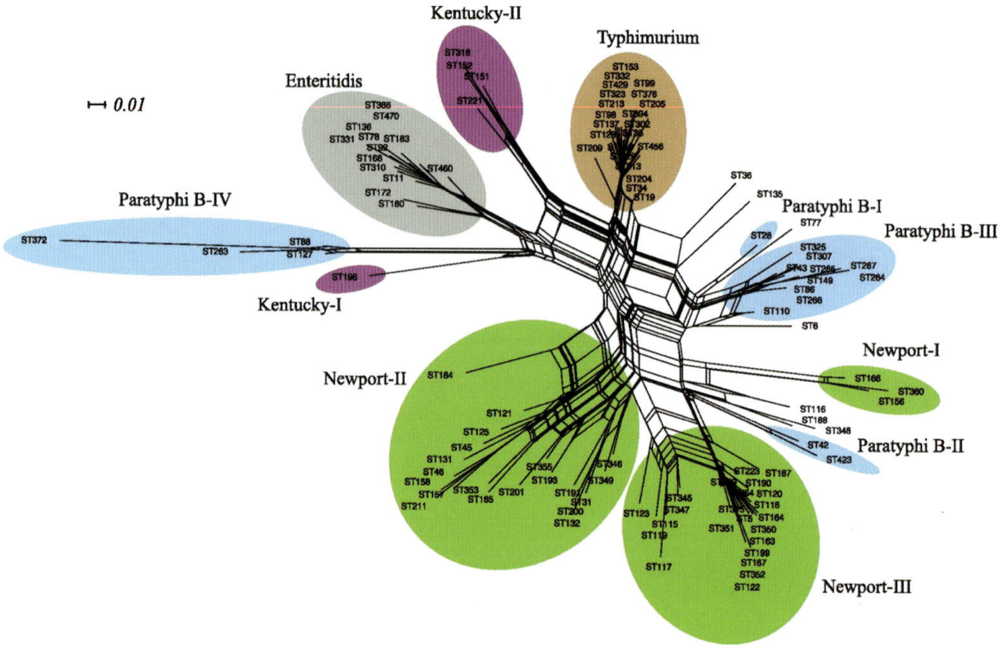

4

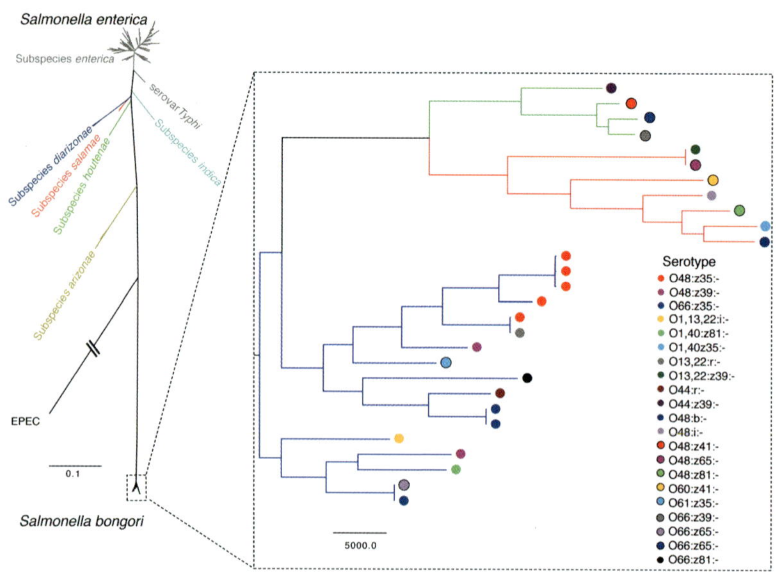

Plate 3. Neighbour-net analysis of concatenated sequence from seven house-keeping genes from strains representing serotypes of *Salmonella enterica.* The scale represents phylogenetic distances between sequence type (ST) designations. (From Sangal, V., *et al.* (2010) *Journal of Bacteriology* 192, 6465–6476, Fig. 2, with permission from the American Society for Microbiology).

Plate 4. Maximum likelihood phylogenetic tree of *Salmonella* based on concatenated MLST loci. The relationships of the isolates shown in the enlarged region were produced using a maximum likelihood phylogenetic tree of *S. bongori* based on the whole genome alignments produced by mapping sequence reads to the reference genome *S. bongori* 12419. The location of the root for the tree for the enlarged region was determined by using *S. arizonae* as an outgroup. The *S. bongori* isolates shown represent 21 different serotypes (SV), inferred by the coloured circles, the tree branches are coloured by BAPS cluster (taken from Fookes, M., *et al.* (2011), *PLoS Pathogens*, 7(8), e1002191. doi:10.1371/journal.ppat.1002191).

5

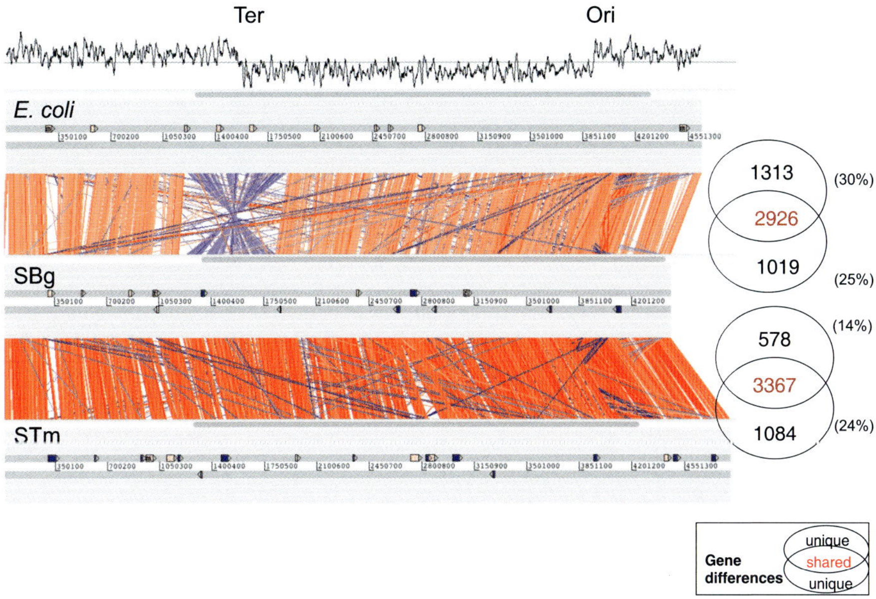

6

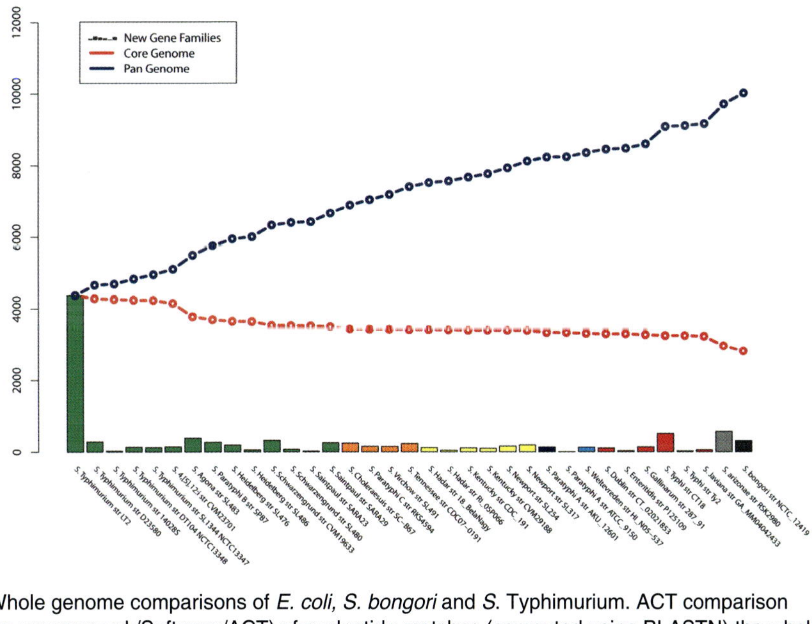

Plate 5. Whole genome comparisons of *E. coli, S. bongori* and *S.* Typhimurium. ACT comparison (http://www.sanger.ac.uk/Software/ACT) of nucleotide matches (computed using BLASTN) the whole genome sequences of *E. coli* K12 strain MG1655 (*E. coli*), *S. bongori* strain 12419 (SBg) and *S.* Typhimurium LT2 (STm). Forward and reverse strands of DNA are shown for each genome (dark grey lines). The red bars between the DNA lines represent individual TBLASTX matches, with inverted matches coloured blue. The position of all the *Salmonella* pathogenicity islands (SPIs) 1 to SPI-17 are marked on the DNA lines, where present, as coloured boxes (dark and light blue) as are the positions of prophage regions marked as coloured boxes (pink). The G-C skew (G+C/G-C) for the genome of *E. coli* K12 is shown with the positions of the origin (Ori) and terminus (Ter) of replication marked.

Plate 6. Pan- and core genome plots of 35 *Salmonella* strains. The red and blue lines show the progression in the core and pan-genomes as more and more genomes are considered, while the columns indicate the amount of novel gene families encountered. The colour of the columns represents the serogroup O:9 (red), O:8 (yellow), O:7 (orange), O:4 (green) and O:2 (blue) (Adapted with permission from Jacobsen, A., *et al.* (2011), *Microbial Ecology* 62,487 504).

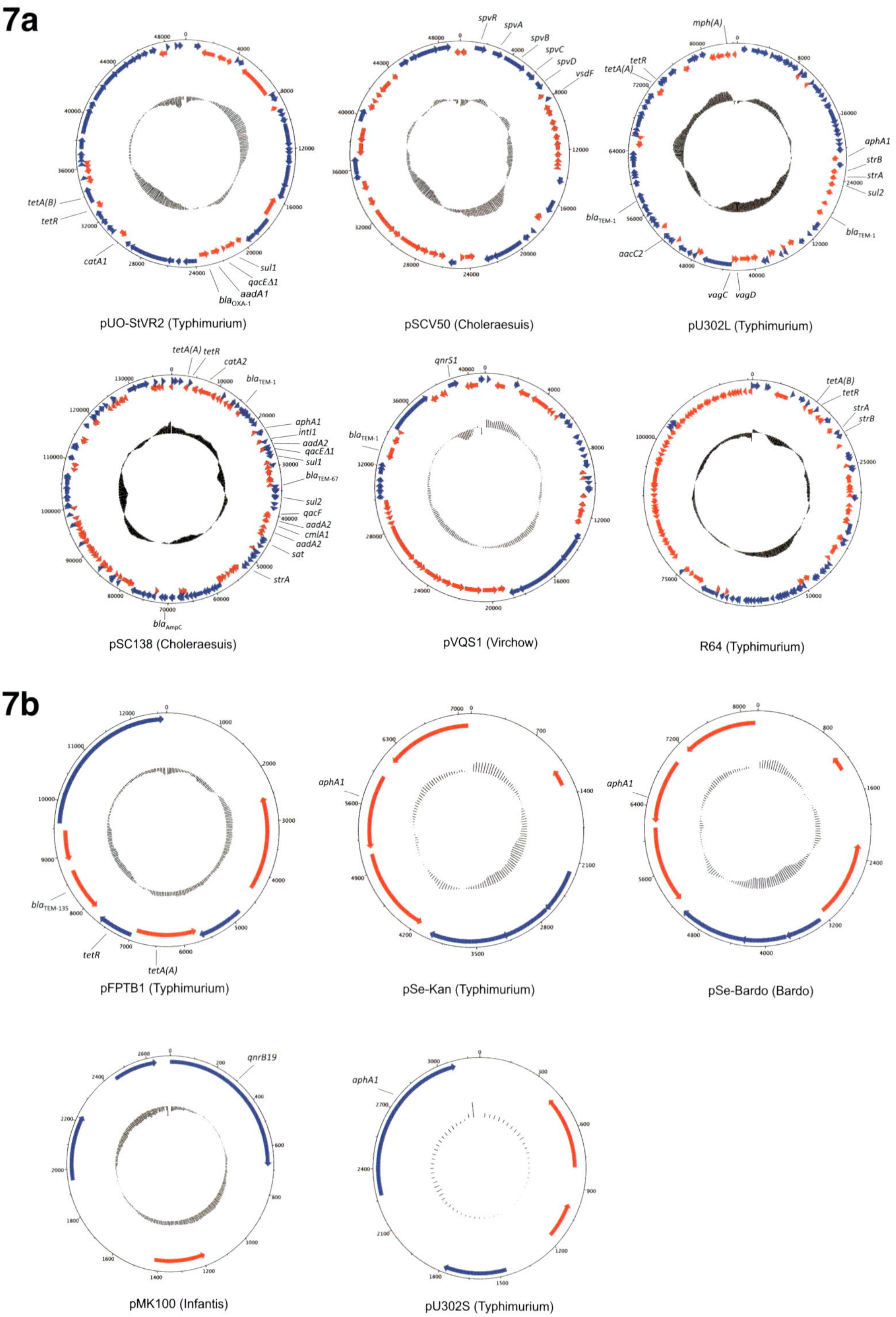

Plate 7. Genetic maps of a selection of (a) high- and (b) low-molecular weight plasmids, identified in serovars of *Salmonella* and whose sequences have been completely determined. Circular maps are shown (not drawn to scale) with antimicrobial resistance-encoding genes and other interesting determinants marked. The nucleotide sizes are marked at intervals around each map. Arrowheads represent the direction of transcription (blue, in the clockwise direction and red, in the counter-clockwise direction). The percentage GC content is shown as the inner core of each plasmid map.

limited phylogenetic distributions. This class of mobile elements shows common features such as being inserted alongside tRNA genes, have direct repeats (DRs) and mobility genes, e.g. integrase and transposase (Hacker *et al.*, 1997; Hacker and Kaper, 2000; Welch *et al.*, 2002). Traditionally, GIs in *Salmonella* that carry genes associated with virulence have been termed *Salmonella* pathogenicity islands (SPIs). It is apparent that most SPIs were acquired early on in the evolution of *S. enterica*, being present in all of the sequenced isolates and microarray analysis (Schmidt and Hensel, 2004). However, there are exceptions to this; SPI-7, SPI-8 and SPI-15 appear to be more recent acquisitions with, for example, SPI-7 being restricted to *S.* Typhi isolates, although it has also been found in some isolates of *S.* Paratyphi C and *S.* Dublin (Anjum *et al.*, 2005). SPI-7 comprises a 134 kb pathogenicity island, which is located between partially duplicated copies of the *pheU* tRNA genes and encodes the Vi-capsule, which is used as an antigenic component of human typhoid vaccines. However, this region is unstable and can be lost on storage of strains. Indeed, pulse-field gel electrophoresis (PFGE) of 120 wild-type strains of serovar Typhi showed a large deletion in the fragment that contains SPI-7, in eight strains. Further analysis by multiplex PCR and microarray showed seven of the eight strains had precise deletions of SPI-7, whilst part of SPI-7 had been retained in the eighth strain (Pickard *et al.*, 2003).

Other SPIs that show a punctuated distribution across the *Salmonella* phylogenetic tree include SPI-10 encoding a P4-like phage (ST46), the *sef/pef* fimbrial islet (Nair *et al.*, 2004; Bishop *et al.*, 2005), as well as a family of SPIs that encode four phylogenetically distinct type VI secretion systems (T6SS) encoded on SPI-6, SPI-19, SPI-20, SPI-21 and SPI-22 (Folkesson *et al.*, 2002; Thomson *et al.*, 2004; Blondel *et al.*, 2009). It is noteworthy that looking across the *Salmonella* genus as a whole there are representatives of each of the major T6SS phylogenetic groups, which may underline their long term and continued importance for *Salmonella*. T6SSs have been linked to a wide range of functions including adherence, cytotoxicity, host-cell invasion and biofilm formation to survival in phagocytic cells such as macrophages and amoeba (Fookes *et al.*, 2011).

The majority of the other SPIs are exceptional PIs, because many, such as SPI-13 and SPI-14, have few features associated with the classic GI definition (Hacker *et al.*, 1997; Hacker and Kaper, 2000; Schmidt and Hensel, 2004; Cascales, 2008). The fact that many SPIs lack identifiable repeat elements flanking their boundaries and mobility genes, e.g. integrases, suggests that either they have been mislabelled as GIs or in fact simply represent genomic material deleted in other lineages rather than acquired in the strain in which they have been identified. Conversely, these SPIs could represent mobile elements that have stably integrated in the *Salmonella* chromosome, but have over time lost their ability to mobilize and the features associated with mobilization (Hacker *et al.*, 1997).

Prophages and other variable elements

Bacterial viruses (bacteriophages) are one of the most important driving forces in pathogen evolution. After infecting the bacterial host some bacteriophages enter the lysogenic state by integrating into the host genome where they may remain stably maintained for many bacterial generations. All of the published *Salmonella* genomes are polylysogenic, carrying between 3 and 5 integrated bacteriophages (referred to as prophages) as well as several prophage remnants. As well as contributing to the overall DNA diversity, differentiating both *Salmonella* lineages and isolates, bacteriophages can also act as vectors carrying 'cargo genes', which can impinge directly on the pathogenic potential of their host, converting a non-pathogen into a pathogen, a process called lysogenic conversion (Wong *et al.*, 1998). *Salmonella* Typhimurium harbours several lysogenic bacteriophages: Gifsy-1, Gifsy-2, Fels-2 and SopE (Plate 5) (Frobisher and Brown, 1927; Figueroa-Bossi *et al.*, 2001). The genetic cargo of these prophages includes the *sopE* gene, encoding a TTSS effector protein shown to stimulate GDP/GTP nucleotide exchange in several Rho GTPases *in vitro* (Stanley *et al.*, 2000) and *sodCI*, a CuZn periplasmic superoxide dismutase that protects the host against oxidative stress (Hardt *et al.*, 1998). Many of the *S.* Typhimurium prophage cargo genes have been shown to increase the pathogenicity of *S.* Typhimurium in various models including mice, cattle and macrophages *in vitro* (Farrant *et al.*, 1997; Figueroa-Bossi and Bossi, 1999). Genome analysis has also shown evidence that prophages have also had a long term role in *Salmonella* evolution. Several *Salmonella* virulence determinants such as the T3SS effector protein SspH2 and the PhoPQ-activated genes *pagKMO* (Gunn *et al.*, 1998; Figueroa-Bossi *et al.*, 2001) and various LPS modification genes are surrounded by prophage gene remnants. SPI-16 is a typical example of this in that it is inserted alongside tRNA-*arg*, encodes three genes that are similar to LPS modification genes and carries a partial integrase. The whole element is delimited by direct repeats. Both the LPS modification CDSs and the direct repeat display a high sequence identity to bacteriophage P22 (Miao *et al.*, 1999; Pedulla *et al.*, 2003). It is thought that such sites mark ancient bacteriophage integration events where *sspH2* and *pagKMO* represent the genetic cargo carried by the phage. It is thought that the selective advantage conferred on the host by these cargo genes was sufficient for them to be selectively maintained while the phage vector was subsequently and sequentially deleted from the genome (Vernikos and Parkhill, 2006).

The observations made by whole genome comparisons have been augmented by comparative genome hybridization (CGH) using pan-*Salmonella* microarrays where the variable component of the *S. enterica* genome has been analysed in some detail. This includes the study by Porwollik *et al.* (Gunn *et al.*, 1998), where the gene content of 79 strains from 22 different serovars was studied. Overall, 867 *S.* Typhimurium LT2 chromosomal genes were found to be absent (or to have no close homologue) from at least one isolate of the representative set of strains from subspecies I included in this study. The majority of the polymorphic genes occurred in clusters, with a total of 85 polymorphic regions or clusters on the LT2 chromosomal backbone. Genetic elements that were frequently missing or divergent included the entire *rfb* locus, responsible for the lipopolysaccharide side chain structure, *rfc* (the O antigen polymerase), and the fimbrial operons *saf, stc, sti, stj* and *lpf*. In many cases isolates from the same serovar show a conserved genomic signature, such as *S.* Typhimurium, *S.* Typhi and *S.* Enteritidis and so are considered monophyletic. However, other *Salmonella* serovars show significant genome variation between isolates of the same serovar and, despite being co-classified by serology, the lineage is considered to be polyphyletic in nature (i.e. not all of the isolates of the same serovar show the same genomic signature). Serovars that appeared to be polyphyletic include Dublin, Saint Paul, Infantis, Muenster, Paratyphi B (Porwollik *et al.*, 2004) and Newport (McClelland *et al.*, 2004). Furthermore, CGH microarray studies comparing the genome of multidrug resistant *S.* Newport from cattle in the USA show that they are genetically closely related to the pan-susceptible strains from cattle in the UK, but contain three extra phage regions and a MDR plasmid. These strains were very different genomically to *S.* Newport poultry strains from the UK when compared by CGH microarray, PFGE and multi-locus sequencing studies (Wu *et al.*, 2010).

The real-time impact of phage on host diversity has been underlined in several recent studies using field strains. Epidemic serovar strains of *Salmonella* have emerged in different host species, regions and at different times. During the 1980s and 1990s *S.* Typhimurium definitive phage type 104 (DT104), associated with a multidrug resistance (MDR), emerged in cattle. Since 2000, cephalosporin-resistant MDR *S.* Newport has accounted for more than 90% of bovine *S.* Newport isolates. CGH microarray studies and suppression subtractive hybridization analyses, comparing the genome content of these MDR *Salmonella* with susceptible strains, revealed specific genes and gene loci that were conserved in recent and contemporary epidemic strains of *Salmonella* that were mainly related to mobile genetic elements (Saunders *et al.*, 2010). Pulse field gel electrophoresis patterns indicated that epidemic strains have been disseminated as a single clone or a small family of genetically related strains (Wu *et al.*, 2010). Work by Cooke *et al.* (2007), looking at the variation in the genomes of 61 *S.* Typhimurium isolates collected from a range of hosts (including cattle, crows, pigs and humans) from the same geographical region between 1996 and 2002, complements the previous findings. Their CHG microarray studies found six genomic regions differentiating the DT104 isolates; five were prophage and the sixth was *Salmonella* genomic island I (SGI-1), known to be largely restricted to *S.* Typhimurium DT104 isolates (Boyd *et al.*, 2002; Cooke *et al.*, 2007). Optical genetic mapping, which generates a physical map of the bacterial chromosome, has been used to differentiate between *S.* Typhimurium DT104 isolates collected pre- and during the epidemic period. The data corroborate with the findings of the studies mentioned above and show that strains of this phage type are largely clonal, with minor changes in SGI-1 and prophage content (Cooke *et al.*, 2007).

Work has also been performed using microarrays to interrogate *Salmonella* serovars such as *S.* Enteritidis, which is currently the most frequent cause of human salmonellosis and is transmitted to humans via poultry meat and eggs. In 1987, a phage typing scheme for *S.* Enteritidis was described to help trace the source of infection following outbreaks (Ward *et al.*, 1987). This scheme is based on differences in susceptibility to a panel of reference bacteriophages that separates most *S.* Enteritidis phage types (PTs) into two distinct lineages: PT4-like strains (including PT1, PT4, PT4b, PT6, PT6a, PT7 and PT24) and PT8-like strains (including PT2, PT8, PT13, PT13a and PT23). Microarray studies have also revealed genomic differences between these two groups. Several prophage regions are mainly responsible for the difference, and include a 38 kb ST64B region, an 18 kb Fels-2 region and a few genes belonging to prophages ST27 and ST35 (Porwollik *et al.*, 2005).

CGH microarray and partial genome sequencing studies by Morales (Morales *et al.*, 2005) and Olson (Olson *et al.*, 2007) to differentiate between strains from the highly prevalent subgroup PT13a for epidemiological trace-back studies following outbreaks, have shown that they are remarkably similar, although some differences could be characterized phenotypically such as formation of biofilms, and 20% difference in the ability to utilize compounds, as characterized by Omnilog Phenotype Microarray studies. A national 2-year survey was performed to determine the extent of *Salmonella* infection in poultry, following an epidemic outbreak of *S.* Enteritidis human infection in Uruguay, on sera from poultry and eggs. *Salmonella* Derby was found to be the most prevalent *Salmonella* isolated, followed by *S.* Gallinarum and *S.* Enteritidis. CGH microarray studies performed on *S.* Derby and *S.* Enteritidis revealed more than 350 genetic differences. *Salmonella* Derby lacked *Salmonella* pathogenicity islands 13 and 14 present in *S.* Enteritidis, the fimbrial *lpf* operon, and other regions encoding metabolic functions. Several of these regions are present not only in *S.* Enteritidis but also in all sequenced strains of *S.* Typhimurium, suggesting that these regions might be related to the capacity of *Salmonella* to cause foodborne disease (Betancor *et al.*, 2010).

In a study by Pan *et al.* (2009), *S.* Enteritidis phage types that are prevalent and commonly associated with human infections in Europe (PT4, PT6 and PT8) and the USA and Canada (PT8 and PT13a) were compared to a phage type (PT11) rarely associated with human infection, to assess genomic differences that may be attributed to human infection. The study showed that ~95% of the genome of the sequenced PT4 strain represented on the microarray was conserved within all *S.* Enteritidis strains tested. However, approximately 400 genes differentiated prevalent (PT4, 6, 8 and 13a) and sporadic (PT11) phage types. More than 75% of the genes that were unique to prevalent PTs were mobile genes, including plasmid genes such as *pefBCD* (plasmid-encoded fimbriae) genes, *srgC* (*SdiA* regulated gene), pSLT023–026 and conjugative transfer genes pSLT075–076. Prophage genes included a degenerate Gifsy-2 prophage region, a 12 kb prophage SE14 region and three genes identified within an unknown degenerate lysogenic bacteriophage region. Non-mobile element-associated genes included a group of putative amino acid ABC transporter genes. Omnilog Phenotype Microarray studies demonstrated that strains from prevalent PTs were less susceptible to urea stress and utilized a variety of amino acids more efficiently than PT11 strains. They were also better biofilm formers at the human body temperature of 37°C than at 28°C, whilst the converse was true for PT11 strains.

Salmonella Genomics: Epidemiological and Clinical Application

In the preceding sections the use of microarrays in comparative genomics to understand commonality and differences in the genome of *Salmonella* pathogens and their evolution were discussed. The knowledge gathered from characterization of their genomes can be applied to identification of *Salmonella* serovars in clinical diagnostic laboratories following outbreaks. There are numerous examples of the application of microarrays for epidemiological studies but two are highlighted here. The first includes an investigation of *S.* Enteritidis strains (PT 30 and 9c) that were isolated during three separate outbreaks associated with raw almonds, in the USA, Canada and in Sweden (Parker *et al.*, 2010). Molecular characterization, including microarrays, performed on *S.* Enteritidis PT30 and 9c strains recovered from different clinical, almond and orchard sites showed some differences in the almond-related PTs (30 and 9c) in comparison to other PTs but not within strains from the same PTs. Although all PT30 strains were genotypically identical, metabolic analysis using Biolog assays indicated that the clinical strains utilized certain amino acids more efficiently than the *S.* Enteritidis PT30 orchard strains, identifying possible important biochemical differences in the orchard strains, and allowing the use of biochemical characteristics to differentiate between strains from these different origins. The second was a study by Huehn *et al.* (2010), which compared the genotype of 148 strains from the emerging *S. enterica* serovar 4,[5],12:i:- from pig, pork and humans. Identical molecular traits such as PFGE profile and minor variations in microarray results indicated these strains from different origins to be highly related, showing their transmission along the food chain.

In fact non-typhoidal *S. enterica* serovars are easily passed from animals to humans, being classified as zoonotic pathogens. In addition to the risk presented by *Salmonella* serovars as potential farm and food-borne hazards, there has been a rapid emergence in recent years of multidrug-resistant *Salmonella*. This is due to the widespread use of many antimicrobials in human and veterinary medicine, which has led to extensive resistance to them. Resistances present within different isolates are usually characterized in diagnostic laboratories using phenotypic methods. Microarrays have been used to characterize resistant determinants in *Salmonella* isolated from farm animals and humans (Hopkins *et al.*, 2007; Batchelor *et al.*, 2008) to gain insight into the mechanisms of resistance and their spread through the food chain. The miniaturized microarrays, which are based on a linear multiplex amplification reaction using primers and incorporation of biotin-labelled dUTP, have also been applied for such epidemiological studies looking at antimicrobial resistance profiles within *Salmonella* isolated from livestock and humans, and the risk they pose to human health (Hopkins *et al.*, 2007; Batchelor *et al.*, 2008; Huehn *et al.*, 2010). These studies have shown that *Salmonella* isolates, especially those from *S.* Typhimurium, are highly likely to harbour multiple antimicrobial resistances that are present on mobile genetic elements such as plasmids and genomic islands, which are easily transferable by conjugation. Furthermore, isolates often carried more than one gene encoding resistance to the same class of antimicrobials.

The relative simplicity of the miniaturized oligonucleotide microarrays also make them suited for high-throughput use such as *Salmonella* serotyping. Currently most *Salmonella* reference laboratories use the antigenic formulae of the White–Kauffmann–Le Minor scheme to divide *Salmonella* isolates gathered from clinical and epidemiological submissions into serovars based on serological variation of the surface O-antigen of the lipopolysaccharide component and expression of the phase 1 and 2 flagellin antigens (Popoff *et al.*, 1998). Recently an array with molecular representation of the

White–Kauffmann–Le Minor *Salmonella* serotyping scheme using variability within the *rfb* gene cluster, the *fljB* and *fliC* flagellin genes and the capsular polysaccharide antigen (Vi) has been constructed for molecular serotyping of *Salmonella* strains (Franklin *et al.*, 2011). The aim of this array is to ultimately replace serological typing with molecular serogenotyping of the top 100 most prevalent *Salmonella* in North America and Europe (Franklin *et al.*, 2011).

However, epidemiological sequence-based typing, involving the direct interrogation of DNA sequences, is becoming more commonplace as the cost continues to fall. Performing whole genome sequencing using high-throughput next generation technologies such as 454 Sequencing™ on the Genome Sequencer FLX ™ System (Roche), Illumina (Solexa) Sequencer, Illumina HiSeq & MiSeq sequencers or the Ion Torrent (Life Technologies), are currently all over the literature. Several recent publications have shown how powerful these technologies are in interrogating the origin and evolution of bacterial pathogens following an outbreak. It includes the widely reported *E. coli* O104:H4 outbreak in Germany, which was one of the largest outbreaks of its kind (Mellmann *et al.*, 2011); a tuberculosis outbreak that occurred over 3 years in Canada and involved a medium-sized community (Gardy *et al.*, 2011); and the Amerithrax investigation, following the anthrax letter outbreak in 2001 (Rasko *et al.*, 2011). High-throughput genotyping has also been applied to tracing the evolution of *S.* Typhi in Jakarta, Indonesia. However, in this instance known nucleotide polymorphisms that are dispersed around the genome of this essentially clonal pathogen were used to determine the haplotype of 140 isolates associated with Indonesia (Baker *et al.*, 2008). In a recent publication, Leekitcharoenphon *et al.* (2012) analysed the whole genome sequence of 73 *S. enterica* isolates that were publicly available through NCBI and the Wellcome Trust Sanger Institute bacterial genome database. They identified a core of 2882 genes that were the core conserved genome and also the pan-genome representing the total genes present within *S. enterica*. A phylogenetic tree drawn using either the core or the pan-genome, which was not a sequence-based alignment tree but represents the presence or absence of gene clusters across *Salmonella* genomes, was similar and provided much better resolution than that from multilocus sequence typing (MLST) or using 16s rRNA, both of which are commonly used for epidemiological tracing. In future it seems likely that core or pan-genome based trees will be used rather than MLST to establish population structure and evolution of bacterial genomes within and between outbreak strains.

Concluding Remark

The availability of new, highly parallel sequencing technologies able to sequence whole genomes from a far greater number of isolates more rapidly and more cheaply than has ever been possible before has resulted in generating a burgeoning amount of data. The current challenge for scientists is to analyse these data using state-of-the-art computational approaches and marry that with classical microbiological and molecular knowledge of the salmonellae to provide important new information about the evolution of this genus and possibly identify new targets for pharmaceutical research with which to approach emerging problems of bacterial pan-antibiotic resistance.

References

AbuOun, M., Suthers, P.F., Jones, G.I., Carter, B.R., Saunders, M.P., Maranas, C.D., Woodward, M.J. and Anjum, M.F. (2009) Genome scale reconstruction of a *Salmonella* metabolic model: comparison of similarity and differences with a commensal *Escherichia coli* strain. *Journal of Biological Chemistry* 284, 29480–29488.

Alokam, S., Liu, S.L., Said, K. and Sanderson, K.E. (2002) Inversions over the terminus region in *Salmonella* and *Escherichia coli*: IS200s as the sites of homologous recombination inverting the chromosome of *Salmonella enterica* serovar typhi. *Journal of Bacteriology* 184, 6190–6197.

Anjum, M.F., Lucchini, S., Thompson, A., Hinton, J.C. and Woodward, M.J. (2003) Comparative genomic indexing reveals the phylogenomics of *Escherichia coli* pathogens. *Infection and Immunity* 71, 4674–4683.

Anjum, M.F., Marooney, C., Fookes, M., Baker, S., Dougan, G., Ivens, A. and Woodward, M.J. (2005) Identification of core and variable components of the *Salmonella enterica* subspecies I genome by microarray. *Infection and Immunity* 73, 7894–7905.

Antunes, L.C., Wang, M., Andersen, S.K., Ferreira, R.B., Kappelhoff, R., Han, J., Borchers, C.H. and Finlay, B.B. (2012) Repression of *Salmonella* phoP expression by small molecules from physiological bile. *Journal of Bacteriology* 194, 2286–2296.

Baker, S., Holt, K., van de Vosse, E., Roumagnac, P., Whitehead, S., King, E., Ewels, P., Keniry, A., Weill, F.X., Lightfoot, D., van Dissel, J.T., Sanderson, K.E., Farrar, J., Achtman, M., Deloukas, P. and Dougan, G. (2008) High-throughput genotyping of *Salmonella enterica* serovar Typhi allowing geographical assignment of haplotypes and pathotypes within an urban District of Jakarta, Indonesia. *Journal of Clinical Microbiology* 46, 1741–1746.

Barrow, P.A., Huggins, M.B. and Lovell, M.A. (1994) Host specificity of *Salmonella* infection in chickens and mice is expressed in vivo primarily at the level of the reticuloendothelial system. *Infection and Immunity* 62, 4602–4610.

Batchelor, M., Hopkins, K.L., Liebana, E., Slickers, P., Ehricht, R., Mafura, M., Aarestrup, F., Mevius, D., Clifton-Hadley, F.A., Woodward, M.J., Davies, R.H., Threlfall, E.J. and Anjum, M.F. (2008) Development of a miniaturised microarray-based assay for the rapid identification of antimicrobial resistance genes in Gram-negative bacteria. *International Journal of Antimicrobial Agents* 31, 440–451.

Betancor, L., Pereira, M., Martinez, A., Giossa, G., Fookes, M., Flores, K., Barrios, P., Repiso, V., Vignoli, R., Cordeiro, N., Algorta, G., Thomson, N., Maskell, D., Schelotto, F. and Chabalgoity, J.A. (2010) Prevalence of *Salmonella enterica* in poultry and eggs in Uruguay during an epidemic due to *Salmonella enterica* serovar Enteritidis. *Journal of Clinical Microbiology* 48, 2413–2423.

Bigot, S., Saleh, O.A., Lesterlin, C., Pages, C., El Karoui, M., Dennis, C., Grigoriev, M., Allemand, J.F., Barre, F.X. and Cornet, F. (2005) KOPS: DNA motifs that control *E. coli* chromosome segregation by orienting the FtsK translocase. *The EMBO Journal* 24, 3770–3780.

Bischoff, K.M., Edrington, T.S., Callaway, T.R., Genovese, K.J. and Nisbet, D.J. (2004) Characterization of antimicrobial resistant *Salmonella* Kinshasa from dairy calves in Texas. *Letters in Applied Microbiology* 38, 140–145.

Bishop, A.L., Baker, S., Jenks, S., Fookes, M., Gaora, P.O., Pickard, D., Anjum, M., Farrar, J., Hien, T.T., Ivens, A. and Dougan, G. (2005) Analysis of the hypervariable region of the *Salmonella enterica* genome associated with tRNA(leuX). *Journal of Bacteriology* 187, 2469–2482.

Blondel, C.J., Jimenez, J.C., Contreras, I. and Santiviago, C.A. (2009) Comparative genomic analysis uncovers 3 novel loci encoding type six secretion systems differentially distributed in *Salmonella* serotypes. *BMC Genomics* 10, 354.

Boyd, D., Cloeckaert, A., Chaslus-Dancla, E. and Mulvey, M.R. (2002) Characterization of variant *Salmonella* genomic island 1 multidrug resistance regions from serovars Typhimurium DT104 and Agona. *Antimicrobial Agents and Chemotherapy* 46, 1714–1722.

Boyd, E.F. and Hartl, D.L. (1997) Recent horizontal transmission of plasmids between natural populations of *Escherichia coli* and *Salmonella enterica*. *Journal of Bacteriology* 179, 1622–1627.

Brenner, F.W., Villar, R.G., Angulo, F.J., Tauxe, R. and Swaminathan, B. (2000) *Salmonella* nomenclature. *Journal of Clinical Microbiology* 38, 2465–2467.

Brown, E.W., Mammel, M.K., LeClerc, J.E. and Cebula, T.A. (2003) Limited boundaries for extensive horizontal gene transfer among *Salmonella* pathogens. *Proceedings of the National Academy of Sciences of the United States of America* 100, 15676–15681.

Cascales, E. (2008) The type VI secretion toolkit. *EMBO Reports* 9, 735–741.

Chan, K., Baker, S., Kim, C.C., Detweiler, C.S., Dougan, G. and Falkow, S. (2003) Genomic comparison of *Salmonella enterica* serovars and *Salmonella* bongori by use of an *S. enterica* serovar typhimurium DNA microarray. *Journal of Bacteriology* 185, 553–563.

Chiu, C.H., Tang, P., Chu, C., Hu, S., Bao, Q., Yu, J., Chou, Y.Y., Wang, H.S. and Lee, Y.S. (2005) The genome sequence of *Salmonella enterica* serovar Choleraesuis, a highly invasive and resistant zoonotic pathogen. *Nucleic Acids Research* 33, 1690–1698.

Cooke, F.J., Wain, J., Fookes, M., Ivens, A., Thomson, N., Brown, D.J., Threlfall, E.J., Gunn, G., Foster, G. and Dougan, G. (2007) Prophage sequences defining hot spots of genome variation in *Salmonella enterica* serovar Typhimurium can be used to discriminate between field isolates. *Journal of Clinical Microbiology* 45, 2590–2598.

Crosa, J.H., Brenner, D.J., Ewing, W.H. and Falkow, S. (1973) Molecular relationships among the salmonellae. *Journal of Bacteriology* 115, 307–315.

Daubin, V. and Ochman, H. (2004) Bacterial genomes as new gene homes: the genealogy of ORFans in *E. coli*. *Genome Research* 14, 1036–1042.

Didelot, X., Achtman, M., Parkhill, J., Thomson, N.R. and Falush, D. (2007) A bimodal pattern of relatedness between the *Salmonella* Paratyphi A and Typhi genomes: convergence or divergence by homologous recombination? *Genome Research* 17, 61–68.

Doolittle, R.F., Feng, D.F., Tsang, S., Cho, G. and Little, E. (1996) Determining divergence times of the major kingdoms of living organisms with a protein clock. *Science* 271, 470–477.

Eisen, J.A., Heidelberg, J.F., White, O. and Salzberg, S.L. (2000) Evidence for symmetric chromosomal inversions around the replication origin in bacteria. *Genome Biology* 1:research0011.0011 - 0011.0019.

Falush, D., Torpdahl, M., Didelot, X., Conrad, D.F., Wilson, D.J. and Achtman, M. (2006) Mismatch induced speciation in *Salmonella*: model and data. *Transactions of the Royal Society of London. Series B, Biological Sciences* 361, 2045–2053.

Farrant, J.L., Sansone, A., Canvin, J.R., Pallen, M.J., Langford, P.R., Wallis, T.S., Dougan, G. and Kroll, J.S. (1997) Bacterial copper- and zinc-cofactored superoxide dismutase contributes to the pathogenesis of systemic salmonellosis. *Molecular Microbiology* 25, 785–796.

Feist, A.M., Henry, C.S., Reed, J.L., Krummenacker, M., Joyce, A.R., Karp, P.D., Broadbelt, L.J., Hatzimanikatis, V. and Palsson, B.O. (2007) A genome-scale metabolic reconstruction for *Escherichia coli* K-12 MG1655 that accounts for 1260 ORFs and thermodynamic information. *Molecular Systems Biology* 3, 121.

Figueroa-Bossi, N. and Bossi, L. (1999) Inducible prophages contribute to *Salmonella* virulence in mice. *Molecular Microbiology* 33, 167–176.

Figueroa-Bossi, N., Uzzau, S., Maloriol, D. and Bossi, L. (2001) Variable assortment of prophages provides a transferable repertoire of pathogenic determinants in *Salmonella*. *Molecular Microbiology* 39, 260–271.

Folkesson, A., Lofdahl, S. and Normark, S. (2002) The *Salmonella enterica* subspecies I specific centisome 7 genomic island encodes novel protein families present in bacteria living in close contact with eukaryotic cells. *Research in Microbiology* 153, 537–545.

Fookes, M., Schroeder, G.N., Langridge, G.C., Blondel, C.J., Mammina, C., Connor, T.R., Seth-Smith, H., Vernikos, G.S., Robinson, K.S., Sanders, M., Petty, N.K., Kingsley, R.A., Baumler, A.J., Nuccio, S.P., Contreras, I., Santiviago, C.A., Maskell, D., Barrow, P., Humphrey, T., Nastasi, A., Roberts, M., Frankel, G., Parkhill, J., Dougan, G. and Thomson, N.R. (2011) *Salmonella bongori* provides insights into the evolution of the salmonellae. *PLoS Pathogens* 7:e1002191.

Franklin, K., Lingohr, E.J., Yoshida, C., Anjum, M., Bodrossy, L., Clark, C.G., Kropinski, A.M. and Karmali, M.A. (2011) Rapid genoserotyping tool for classification of *Salmonella* serovars. *Journal of Clinical Microbiology* 49, 2954–2965.

Frobisher, M. and Brown, J.H. (1927) Transmissable toxicogenicity of streptococci. *Bulletin of the Johns Hopkins Hospital* 41, 167.

Gardy, J.L., Johnston, J.C., Ho Sui, S.J., Cook, V.J., Shah, L., Brodkin, E., Rempel, S., Moore, R., Zhao, Y., Holt, R., Varhol, R., Birol, I., Lem, M., Sharma, M.K., Elwood, K., Jones, S.J., Brinkman, F.S., Brunham, R.C. and Tang, P. (2011) Whole-genome sequencing and social-network analysis of a tuberculosis outbreak. *The New England Journal of Medicine* 364, 730–739.

Grimont, P.A.D., Grimont, F. and Bouvet, P. (2000) Taxonomy of the Genus *Salmonella*. In: Wray, C. and Wray, A. (eds) Salmonella *in Domestic Animals*. CAB International, Wallingford, UK, pp. 1–18.

Gunn, J.S., Belden, W.J. and Miller, S.I. (1998) Identification of PhoP-PhoQ activated genes within a duplicated region of the *Salmonella typhimurium* chromosome. *Microbial Pathogenesis* 25, 77–90.

Hacker, J. and Kaper, J.B. (2000) Pathogenicity islands and the evolution of microbes. *Annual Review of Microbiology* 54, 641–679.

Hacker, J., Blum-Oehler, G., Muhldorfer, I. and Tschäpe, H. (1997) Pathogenicity islands of virulent bacteria: structure, function and impact on microbial evolution. *Molecular Microbiology* 23, 1089–1097.

Hansen-Wester, I., Chakravortty, D. and Hensel, M. (2004) Functional transfer of *Salmonella* pathogenicity island 2 to *Salmonella bongori* and *Escherichia coli*. *Infection and Immunity* 72, 2879–2888.

Hardt, W.D., Urlaub, H. and Galan, J.E. (1998) A substrate of the centisome 63 type III protein secretion system of *Salmonella typhimurium* is encoded by a cryptic bacteriophage. *Proceedings of the National Academy of Sciences of the United States of America* 95, 2574–2579.

Holt, K.E., Thomson, N.R., Wain, J., Langridge, G.C., Hasan, R., Bhutta, Z.A., Quail, M.A., Norbertczak, H., Walker, D., Simmonds, M., White, B., Bason, M., Mungall, M., Dougan, G. and Parkhill, J. (2009) Pseudogene accumulation in the evolutionary histories of *Salmonella enterica* serovars Paratyphi A and Typhi. *BMC Genomics* 10:36 doi:10.1186/1471-2164-10-36.

Hopkins, K.L., Batchelor, M.J., Anjum, M., Davies, R.H. and Threlfall, E.J. (2007) Comparison of antimicrobial resistance genes in nontyphoidal salmonellae of serotypes enteritidis, hadar, and virchow from humans and food-producing animals in England and Wales. *Microbial Drug Resistance* 13, 281–288.

Huehn, S., La Ragione, R.M., Anjum, M., Saunders, M., Woodward, M.J., Bunge, C., Helmuth, R., Hauser, E., Guerra, B., Beutlich, J., Brisabois, A., Peters, T., Svensson, L., Madajczak, G., Litrup, E., Imre, A., Herrera-Leon, S., Mevius, D., Newell, D.G. and Malorny, B. (2010) Virulotyping and antimicrobial resistance typing of *Salmonella enterica* serovars relevant to human health in Europe. *Foodborne Pathogens and Disease* 7, 523–535.

Jacobsen, A., Hendriksen, R.S., Aaresturp, F.M., Ussery, D.W. and Friis, C. (2011) The *Salmonella enterica* pan-genome. *Microbial Ecology* 62, 487–504.

Jiang, X., Rossanese, O.W., Brown, N.F., Kujat-Choy, S., Galan, J.E., Finlay, B.B. and Brumell, J.H. (2004) The related effector proteins SopD and SopD2 from *Salmonella enterica* serovar Typhimurium contribute to virulence during systemic infection of mice. *Molecular Microbiology* 54, 1186–1198.

Jones, B.D., Lee, C.A. and Falkow, S. (1992) Invasion by *Salmonella typhimurium* is affected by the direction of flagellar rotation. *Infection and Immunity* 60, 2475–2480.

Kingsley, R.A., Msefula, C.L., Thomson, N.R., Kariuki, S., Holt, K.E., Gordon, M.A., Harris, D., Clarke, L., Whitehead, S., Sangal, V., Marsh, K., Achtman, M., Molyneux, M.E., Cormican, M., Parkhill, J., MacLennan, C.A., Heyderman, R.S. and Dougan, G. (2009) Epidemic multiple drug resistant *Salmonella* Typhimurium causing invasive disease in sub-Saharan Africa have a distinct genotype. *Genome Research* 19, 2279–2287.

Klumpp, J. and Fuchs, T.M. (2007) Identification of novel genes in genomic islands that contribute to *Salmonella* typhimurium replication in macrophages. *Microbiology* 153, 1207–1220.

Kudva, I.T., Evans, P.S., Perna, N.T., Barrett, T.J., Ausubel, F.M., Blattner, F.R. and Calderwood, S.B. (2002) Strains of *Escherichia coli* O157:H7 differ primarily by insertions or deletions, not single-nucleotide polymorphisms. *Journal of Bacteriology* 184, 1873–1879.

Lawrence, J.G. and Roth, J.R. (1996) Evolution of coenzyme B12 synthesis among enteric bacteria: evidence for loss and reacquisition of a multigene complex. *Genetics* 142, 11–24.

Le Minor, L., Veron, M. and Popoff, M. (1982) [A proposal for *Salmonella* nomenclature]. *Annales de Microbiologie* 133, 245–254.

Le Minor, L., Popoff, M.Y., Laurent, B. and Hermant, D. (1986) [Characterization of a 7th subspecies of *Salmonella*: *S. choleraesuis* subsp. *indica* subsp. *nov.*]. *Annales de Microbiologie* 137B, 211–217.

Leekitcharoenphon, P., Lukjancenko, O., Friis, C., Aarestrup, F.M. and Ussery, D.W. (2012) Genomic variation in *Salmonella enterica* core genes for epidemiological typing. *BMC Genomics* 13, 88.

Litrup, E., Torpdahl, M., Malorny, B., Huehn, S., Helms, M., Christensen, H. and Nielsen, E.M. (2010) DNA microarray analysis of *Salmonella* serotype Typhimurium strains causing different symptoms of disease. *BMC Microbiology* 10, 96.

Liu, G.R., Edwards, K., Eisenstark, A., Fu, Y.M., Liu, W.Q., Sanderson, K.E., Johnston, R.N. and Liu, S.L. (2003) Genomic diversification among archival strains of *Salmonella enterica* serovar typhimurium LT7. *Journal of Bacteriology* 185, 2131–2142.

Liu, S.L. and Sanderson, K.E. (1995) I-CeuI reveals conservation of the genome of independent strains of *Salmonella typhimurium*. *Journal of Bacteriology* 177, 3355–3357.

Liu, S.L. and Sanderson, K.E. (1998) Homologous recombination between rrn operons rearranges the chromosome in host-specialized species of *Salmonella*. *FEMS Microbiology Letters* 164, 275–281.

Lukjancenko, O., Wassenaar, T.M. and Ussery, D.W. (2010) Comparison of 61 sequenced *Escherichia coli* genomes. *Microbial Ecology* 60, 708–720.

Mackiewicz, P., Mackiewicz, D., Gierlik, A., Kowalczuk, M., Nowicka, A., Dudkiewicz, M., Dudek, M.R. and Cebrat, S. (2001) The differential killing of genes by inversions in prokaryotic genomes. *Journal of Molecular Evolution* 53, 615–621.

Mandal, B.K. (1979) Typhoid and paratyphoid fever. *Clinical Gastroenterology* 8, 715–735.

McClelland, M., Florea, L., Sanderson, K., Clifton, S.W., Parkhill, J., Churcher, C., Dougan, G., Wilson, R.K. and Miller, W. (2000) Comparison of the *Escherichia coli* K-12 genome with sampled genomes of a *Klebsiella pneumoniae* and three *Salmonella enterica* serovars, Typhimurium, Typhi and Paratyphi. *Nucleic Acids Research* 28, 4974–4986.

McClelland, M., Sanderson, K.E., Spieth, J., Clifton, S.W., Latreille, P., Courtney, L., Porwollik, S., Ali, J., Dante, M., Du, F., Hou, S., Layman, D., Leonard, S., Nguyen, C., Scott, K., Holmes, A., Grewal, N., Mulvaney, E., Ryan, E., Sun, H., Florea, L., Miller, W., Stoneking, T., Nhan, M., Waterston, R. and Wilson, R.K. (2001) Complete genome sequence of *Salmonella enterica* serovar Typhimurium LT2. *Nature* 413, 852–856.

McClelland, M., Sanderson, K.E., Clifton, S.W., Latreille, P., Porwollik, S., Sabo, A., Meyer, R., Bieri, T., Ozersky, P., McLellan, M., Harkins, C.R., Wang, C., Nguyen, C., Berghoff, A., Elliott, G., Kohlberg, S., Strong, C., Du, F., Carter, J., Kremizki, C., Layman, D., Leonard, S., Sun, H., Fulton, L., Nash, W., Miner, T., Minx, P., Delehaunty, K., Fronick, C., Magrini, V., Nhan, M., Warren, W., Florea, L., Spieth, J. and Wilson, R.K. (2004) Comparison of genome degradation in Paratyphi A and Typhi, human-restricted serovars of *Salmonella enterica* that cause typhoid. *Nature Genetics* 36, 1268–1274.

Medalla, F., Sjolund-Karlsson, M., Shin, S., Harvey, E., Joyce, K., Theobald, L., Nygren, B.N., Pecic, G., Gay, K., Austin, J., Stuart, A., Blanton, E., Mintz, E.D., Whichard, J.M. and Barzilay, E.J. (2011) Ciprofloxacin-resistant *Salmonella enterica* Serotype Typhi, United States, 1999-2008. *Emerging Infectious Diseases* 17, 1095–1098.

Mellmann, A., Harmsen, D., Cummings, C.A., Zentz, E.B., Leopold, S.R., Rico, A., Prior, K., Szczepanowski, R., Ji, Y., Zhang, W., McLaughlin, S.F., Henkhaus, J.K., Leopold, B., Bielaszewska, M., Prager, R., Brzoska, P.M., Moore, R.L., Guenther, S., Rothberg, J.M. and Karch, H. (2011) Prospective genomic characterization of the German enterohemorrhagic *Escherichia coli* O104:H4 outbreak by rapid next generation sequencing technology. *PLoS One* 6:e22751.

Miao, E.A., Scherer, C.A., Tsolis, R.M., Kingsley, R.A., Adams, L.G., Baumler, A.J. and Miller, S.I. (1999) *Salmonella* typhimurium leucine-rich repeat proteins are targeted to the SPI1 and SPI2 type III secretion systems. *Molecular Microbiology* 34, 850–864.

Morales, C.A., Porwollik, S., Frye, J.G., Kinde, H., McClelland, M. and Guard-Bouldin, J. (2005) Correlation of phenotype with the genotype of egg-contaminating *Salmonella enterica* serovar Enteritidis. *Applied and Environmental Microbiology* 71, 4388–4399.

Nair, S., Alokam, S., Kothapalli, S., Porwollik, S., Proctor, E., Choy, C., McClelland, M., Liu, S.L. and Sanderson, K.E. (2004) *Salmonella enterica* serovar Typhi strains from which SPI7, a 134-kilobase island with genes for Vi exopolysaccharide and other functions, has been deleted. *Journal of Bacteriology* 186, 3214–3223.

Olson, A.B., Andrysiak, A.K., Tracz, D.M., Guard-Bouldin, J., Demczuk, W., Ng, L.K., Maki, A., Jamieson, F. and Gilmour, M.W. (2007) Limited genetic diversity in *Salmonella enterica* serovar Enteritidis PT13. *BMC Microbiology* 7, 87.

Pan, Z., Carter, B., Nunez-Garcia, J., Abuoun, M., Fookes, M., Ivens, A., Woodward, M.J. and Anjum, M.F. (2009) Identification of genetic and phenotypic differences associated with prevalent and non-prevalent *Salmonella* Enteritidis phage types: analysis of variation in amino acid transport. *Microbiology* 155, 3200–3213.

Parker, C.T., Huynh, S., Quinones, B., Harris, L.J. and Mandrell, R.E. (2010) Comparison of genotypes of *Salmonella enterica* serovar Enteritidis phage type 30 and 9c strains isolated during three outbreaks associated with raw almonds. *Applied and Environmental Microbiology* 76, 3723–3731.

Parkhill, J., Dougan, G., James, K.D., Thomson, N.R., Pickard, D., Wain, J., Churcher, C., Mungall, K.L., Bentley, S.D., Holden, M.T., Sebaihia, M., Baker, S., Basham, D., Brooks, K., Chillingworth, T., Connerton, P., Cronin, A., Davis, P., Davies, R.M., Dowd, L., White, N., Farrar, J., Feltwell, T., Hamlin, N., Haque, A., Hien, T.T., Holroyd, S., Jagels, K., Krogh, A., Larsen, T.S., Leather, S., Moule, S., O'Gaora, P., Parry, C., Quail, M., Rutherford, K., Simmonds, M., Skelton, J., Stevens, K., Whitehead, S. and Barrell, B.G. (2001) Complete genome sequence of a multiple drug resistant *Salmonella enterica* serovar Typhi CT18. *Nature* 413, 848–852.

Pedulla, M.L., Ford, M.E., Karthikeyan, T., Houtz, J.M., Hendrix, R.W., Hatfull, G.F., Poteete, A.R., Gilcrease, E.B., Winn-Stapley, D.A. and Casjens, S.R. (2003) Corrected sequence of the bacteriophage p22 genome. *Journal of Bacteriology* 185, 1475–1477.

Perna, N.T., Plunkett, G. 3rd, Burland, V., Mau, B., Glasner, J.D., Rose, D.J., Mayhew, G.F., Evans, P.S., Gregor, J., Kirkpatrick, H.A., Posfai, G., Hackett, J., Klink, S., Boutin, A., Shao, Y., Miller, L., Grotbeck, E.J., Davis,

N.W., Lim, A., Dimalanta, E.T., Potamousis, K.D., Apodaca, J., Anantharaman, T.S., Lin, J., Yen, G., Schwartz, D.C., Welch, R.A. and Blattner, F.R. (2001) Genome sequence of enterohaemorrhagic *Escherichia coli* O157:H7. *Nature* 409, 529–533.

Petersen, R.F., Litrup, E., Larsson, J.T., Torpdahl, M., Sorensen, G., Muller, L. and Nielsen, E.M. (2011) Molecular characterization of *Salmonella* Typhimurium highly successful outbreak strains. *Foodborne Pathogens and Disease* 8, 655–661.

Pickard, D., Wain, J., Baker, S., Line, A., Chohan, S., Fookes, M., Barron, A., Gaora, P.O., Chabalgoity, J.A., Thanky, N., Scholes, C., Thomson, N., Quail, M., Parkhill, J. and Dougan, G. (2003) Composition, acquisition, and distribution of the Vi exopolysaccharide-encoding *Salmonella enterica* pathogenicity island SPI-7. *Journal of Bacteriology* 185, 5055–5065.

Popoff, M.Y., Bockemuhl, J. and Brenner, F.W. (1998) Supplement 1997 (no. 41) to the Kauffmann-White scheme. *Research in Microbiology* 149, 601–604.

Porwollik, S., Wong, R.M. and McClelland, M. (2002) Evolutionary genomics of *Salmonella*: gene acquisitions revealed by microarray analysis. *Proceedings of the National Academy of Sciences of the United States of America* 99, 8956–8961.

Porwollik, S., Boyd, E.F., Choy, C., Cheng, P., Florea, L., Proctor, E. and McClelland, M. (2004) Characterization of *Salmonella enterica* subspecies I genovars by use of microarrays. *Journal of Bacteriology* 186, 5883–5898.

Porwollik, S., Santiviago, C.A., Cheng, P., Florea, L., Jackson, S. and McClelland, M. (2005) Differences in gene content between *Salmonella enterica* serovar Enteritidis isolates and comparison to closely related serovars Gallinarum and Dublin. *Journal of Bacteriology* 187, 6545–6555.

Raghunathan, A., Reed, J., Shin, S., Palsson, B. and Daefler, S. (2009) Constraint-based analysis of metabolic capacity of *Salmonella* typhimurium during host-pathogen interaction. *BMC Systems Biology* 3, 38.

Rasko, D.A., Rosovitz, M.J., Myers, G.S., Mongodin, E.F., Fricke, W.F., Gajer, P., Crabtree, J., Sebaihia, M., Thomson, N.R., Chaudhuri, R., Henderson, I.R., Sperandio, V. and Ravel, J. (2008) The pangenome structure of *Escherichia coli*: comparative genomic analysis of *E. coli* commensal and pathogenic isolates. *Journal of Bacteriology* 190, 6881–6893.

Rasko, D.A., Worsham, P.L., Abshire, T.G., Stanley, S.T., Bannan, J.D., Wilson, M.R., Langham, R.J., Decker, R.S., Jiang, L., Read, T.D., Phillippy, A.M., Salzberg, S.L., Pop, M., Van Ert, M.N., Kenefic, L.J., Keim, P.S., Fraser-Liggett, C.M. and Ravel, J. (2011) Bacillus anthracis comparative genome analysis in support of the Amerithrax investigation. *Proceedings of the National Academy of Sciences of the United States of America* 108, 5027–5032.

Reeves, M.W., Evins, G.M., Heiba, A.A., Plikaytis, B.D. and Farmer, J.J. 3rd (1989) Clonal nature of *Salmonella* typhi and its genetic relatedness to other salmonellae as shown by multilocus enzyme electrophoresis, and proposal of *Salmonella bongori* comb. *nov*. *Journal of Clinical Microbiology* 27, 313–320.

Rocha, E.P. (2004) The replication-related organization of bacterial genomes. *Microbiology* 150, 1609–1627.

Rodrigue, D.C., Tauxe, R.V. and Rowe, B. (1990) International increase in *Salmonella enteritidis*: a new pandemic? *Epidemiology and Infection* 105, 21–27.

Roth, J.R., Lawrence, J.G. and Bobik, T.A. (1996) Cobalamin (coenzyme B12): synthesis and biological significance. *Annual Review of Microbiology* 50, 137–181.

Saunders, M.P., Wu, G., Abuoun, M., Pan, Z., Anjum, M. and Woodward, M.J. (2010) Optical genetic mapping defines regions of chromosomal variation in serovars of *S. enterica* subsp. *enterica* of concern for human and animal health. *Epidemiology and Infection* 139, 1065–1074.

Schmidt, H. and Hensel, M. (2004) Pathogenicity islands in bacterial pathogenesis. *Clinical Microbiology Reviews* 17, 14–56.

Selander, R.K., Caugant, D.A., Ochman, H., Musser, J.M., Gilmour, M.N. and Whittam, T.S. (1986) Methods of multilocus enzyme electrophoresis for bacterial population genetics and systematics. *Applied and Environmental Microbiology* 51, 873–884.

Stanley, T.L., Ellermeier, C.D. and Slauch, J.M. (2000) Tissue-specific gene expression identifies a gene in the lysogenic phage Gifsy-1 that affects *Salmonella enterica* serovar typhimurium survival in Peyer's patches. *Journal of Bacteriology* 182, 4406–4413.

Sueoka, N. (1999) Two aspects of DNA base composition: G+C content and translation-coupled deviation from intra-strand rule of A=T and G=C. *Journal of Molecular Evolution* 49, 49–62.

Szpirer, C., Top, E., Couturier, M. and Mergeay, M. (1999) Retrotransfer or gene capture: a feature of conjugative plasmids, with ecological and evolutionary significance. *Microbiology* 145, 3321–3329.

Thiennimitr, P., Winter, S.E., Winter, M.G., Xavier, M.N., Tolstikov, V., Huseby, D.L., Sterzenbach, T., Tsolis, R.M., Roth, J.R. and Baumler, A.J. (2011) Intestinal inflammation allows *Salmonella* to use ethanolamine to compete with the microbiota. *Proceedings of the National Academy of Sciences of the United States of America* 108, 17480–17485.

Thomson, N., Baker, S., Pickard, D., Fookes, M., Anjum, M., Hamlin, N., Wain, J., House, D., Bhutta, Z., Chan, K., Falkow, S., Parkhill, J., Woodward, M., Ivens, A. and Dougan, G. (2004) The role of prophage-like elements in the diversity of *Salmonella enterica* serovars. *Journal of Molecular Biology* 339, 279–300.

Thomson, N.R., Howard, S., Wren, B.W., Holden, M.T., Crossman, L., Challis, G.L., Churcher, C., Mungall, K., Brooks, K., Chillingworth, T., Feltwell, T., Abdellah, Z., Hauser, H., Jagels, K., Maddison, M., Moule, S., Sanders, M., Whitehead, S., Quail, M.A., Dougan, G., Parkhill, J. and Prentice, M.B. (2006) The complete genome sequence and comparative genome analysis of the high pathogenicity *Yersinia enterocolitica* strain 8081. *PLoS Genetics* 2, e206.

Thomson, N.R., Clayton, D.J., Windhorst, D., Vernikos, G., Davidson, S., Churcher, C., Quail, M.A., Stevens, M., Jones, M.A., Watson, M., Barron, A., Layton, A., Pickard, D., Kingsley, R.A., Bignell, A., Clark, L., Harris, B., Ormond, D., Abdellah, Z., Brooks, K., Cherevach, I., Chillingworth, T., Woodward, J., Norberczak, H., Lord, A., Arrowsmith, C., Jagels, K., Moule, S., Mungall, K., Sanders, M., Whitehead, S., Chabalgoity, J.A., Maskell, D., Humphrey, T., Roberts, M., Barrow, P.A., Dougan, G. and Parkhill, J. (2008) Comparative genome analysis of *Salmonella* Enteritidis PT4 and *Salmonella* Gallinarum 287/91 provides insights into evolutionary and host adaptation pathways. *Genome Research* 18, 1624–1637.

Tillier, E.R.M. and Collins, R.A. (2000) Genome rearrangement by replication-directed translocation. *Nature Genetics* 26, 195–197.

Torpdahl, M. and Ahrens, P. (2004) Population structure of *Salmonella* investigated by amplified fragment length polymorphism. *Journal of Applied Microbiology* 97, 566–573.

Vernikos, G.S. and Parkhill, V. (2006) Interpolated variable order motifs for identification of horizontally acquired DNA: revisiting the *Salmonella* pathogenicity islands. *Bioinformatics* 22, 2196–2203.

Vernikos, G.S., Thomson, N.R. and Parkhill, J. (2007) Genetic flux over time in the *Salmonella* lineage. *Genome Biology* 8, R100.

Ward, L.R., de Sa, J.D. and Rowe, B. (1987) A phage-typing scheme for *Salmonella enteritidis*. *Epidemiology and Infection* 99, 291–294.

Warwick, C., Lambiris, A.J., Westwood, D. and Steedman, C. (2001) Reptile-related salmonellosis. *Journal of the Royal Society of Medicine* 94, 124–126.

Welch, R.A., Burland, V., Plunkett, G. 3rd, Redford, P., Roesch, P., Rasko, D., Buckles, E.L., Liou, S.R., Boutin, A., Hackett, J., Stroud, D., Mayhew, G.F., Rose, D.J., Zhou, S., Schwartz, D.C., Perna, N.T., Mobley, H.L., Donnenberg, M.S. and Blattner, F.R. (2002) Extensive mosaic structure revealed by the complete genome sequence of uropathogenic *Escherichia coli*. *Proceedings of the National Academy of Sciences of the United States of America* 99: 17020–17024.

Wong, K.K., McClelland, M., Stillwell, L.C., Sisk, E.C., Thurston, S.J. and Saffer, J.D. (1998) Identification and sequence analysis of a 27-kilobase chromosomal fragment containing a *Salmonella* pathogenicity island located at 92 minutes on the chromosome map of *Salmonella enterica* serovar *typhimurium* LT2. *Infection and Immunity* 66, 3365–3371.

Wu, G., AbuOun, M., Hackl, E., La Ragione, R.M., Fookes, M., Fenner, J., Pan, Z., Wenzl, P., Anjum, M.F. and Woodward, M.J. (2010) Epidemic multidrug-resistant (MDR-AmpC) *Salmonella enterica* serovar Newport strains contain three phage regions and a MDR resistance plasmid. *Environmental Microbiology Reports* 2, 228–235.

5 *Salmonella* Virulence Mechanisms and their Genetic Basis

Torsten Sterzenbach, Robert W. Crawford, Sebastian E. Winter and Andreas J. Bäumler*
Department of Medical Microbiology and Immunology, University of California at Davis, USA

Introduction

The genus *Salmonella* is named after the American veterinarian Daniel E. Salmon, who first isolated *Bacterium cholerae-suis* (*Salmonella enterica* serotype Choleraesuis abbreviated to *S. enterica* serotype Choleraesuis or *S.* Choleraesuis) from a pig (Salmon and Smith, 1885). The members of this genus are gram-negative facultative-anaerobic and peritrichously flagellated rods. *Salmonella* serotypes are distinguished from members of other genera of the *Enterobacteriaceae* by a combination of biochemical reactions, including the production of hydrogen sulfide, the use of tetrathionate as a terminal electron acceptor and others.

The genus *Salmonella* contains 2579 serotypes, which can be distinguished serologically based on antigenic properties of their lipopolysaccharide (LPS) sugar repeat units (O-antigens) and their structural protein subunits of flagella (H-antigens) (Grimont and Weill, 2007). Members of the genus *Salmonella* can be divided into two species, termed *Salmonella enterica* (Le Minor and Popoff, 1987), which contains 2557 serotypes, and *Salmonella bongori* (Reeves *et al.*, 1989), which comprises the remaining 22 serotypes. All *Salmonella* serotypes are considered potential pathogens of humans and/or animals (Kelterborn, 1967).

In a first approximation, diseases caused by *Salmonella* serotypes can be divided into two broad categories, those that remain localized to the intestinal tract (self-limiting gastroenteritis) and those that are associated with systemic dissemination of the bacteria. Localized and systemic infections are associated with different *Salmonella* serotypes. One goal of this overview is to illustrate that in immunocompetent hosts, these two different syndromes are a result of distinct virulence strategies being employed by the respective pathogens. Research on *Salmonella* pathogenesis suggests that these two distinct virulence strategies reflect differences in how the respective pathogens ensure their transmission to a new susceptible host. After a brief overview of the two major disease manifestations associated with *Salmonella* serotypes, this chapter will discuss the virulence factors responsible for host–pathogen interactions observed in both settings.

Clinical Manifestations

Gastroenteritis

The vast majority of *Salmonella* serotypes are capable of causing gastroenteritis in humans,

* Corresponding author, e-mail: ajbaumler@ucdavis.edu

© CAB International 2013. *Salmonella in Domestic Animals, 2nd Edition* (eds P.A. Barrow and U. Methner)

an infection that remains localized to the terminal ileum, colon and mesenteric lymph nodes (Zhang *et al.*, 2003). Bacterial invasion of these tissues leads to the development of inflammatory infiltrates that are dominated by neutrophils (McGovern and Slavutin, 1979; Murphy and Gorbach, 1982). Neutrophil influx in the terminal ileum and colon is accompanied by necrosis of the upper mucosa and the presence of neutrophils in the faeces (Harris *et al.*, 1972). The host inflammatory response is largely responsible for the characteristic symptoms produced during infection, which include diarrhoea, nausea, vomiting, intestinal cramping and fever. Importantly, host responses are elicited rapidly after ingestion of the organism, as indicated by an average incubation period of less than 1 day (Glynn and Palmer, 1992).

Localized infections that are similar to human gastroenteritis are caused by *Salmonella* serotypes in other large animal species, e.g. cattle and horses (Baker, 1970; Reynolds *et al.*, 1986). *Salmonella* serotypes associated with gastroenteritis transmit through the faecal–oral route, either directly or via contaminated food or water. This mode of transmission ensures circulation of these pathogens within their respective animal reservoirs, from where they can become introduced into the human food supply. While a large number of *Salmonella* serotypes can cause gastroenteritis, a select few serotypes account for the majority of cases in any given animal reservoir. In the case of humans, *S. enterica* serotypes Typhimurium and Enteritidis (*S.* Typhimurium and *S.* Enteritidis) are associated most frequently with this diarrheal disease (Rabsch *et al.*, 2001).

Systemic disease

Typhoid fever

A small number of *Salmonella* serotypes represent specialists that are associated with systemic infections in immunocompetent hosts. Perhaps the most infamous of these diseases is typhoid fever, which, in the absence of treatment, leads to a fatality rate of approximately 10%. Typhoid fever is caused by the strictly human-adapted *S. enterica* serotype Typhi (Raffatellu *et al.*, 2008b). After ingestion, the organism invades the mucosa of the small intestine, followed by its dissemination throughout the body. However, the initial spread of the pathogen does not evoke overt host responses, as indicated by the fact that typhoid fever has an average incubation period of 2 weeks (Olsen *et al.*, 2003).

Pathological changes in the intestine are characterized by a slow development of inflammatory infiltrates that are dominated by mononuclear cells (macrophages and dendritic cells) while neutrophils are scarce (Sprinz *et al.*, 1966; Mukawi, 1978; Kraus *et al.*, 1999; Nguyen *et al.*, 2004). The organism spreads to internal organs, most frequently the bone marrow, the liver and the spleen where it is found in histiocytic granulomas, known as typhoid nodules (Nasrallah and Nassar, 1978). Spread to the gall bladder or urinary bladder can lead to chronic carriage, which is important for human-to-human spread of the disease. Symptoms of typhoid fever are non-specific, commonly including fever and a slowed heart rate (bradycardia). Splenomegaly, hepatomegaly, or rose spots are encountered less frequently (Nasrallah and Nassar, 1978). Unlike gastroenteritis, typhoid fever is not considered a diarrhoeal disease, because this symptom develops late, after the onset of fever, in only a fraction (approximately one-third) of typhoid fever patients, while the remaining individuals remain either diarrhoea free or become constipated.

Salmonella Paratyphi A, and less frequently *S.* Paratyphi B and Paratyphi C, are associated with paratyphoid fever, a disease that is milder in its course but otherwise indistinguishable from typhoid fever. Together with *S.* Typhi, these pathogens are commonly referred to as typhoidal *Salmonella* serotypes.

Bacteraemia in humans

IMMUNOCOMPETENT INDIVIDUALS. Two non-typhoidal *Salmonella* serotypes can cause a systemic infection in immunocompetent humans that can be distinguished clinically from typhoid fever and has been termed bacteraemia (Saphra and Wassermann, 1954). These pathogens are *S.* Choleraesuis and *S.* Dublin (Saphra and Wassermann, 1954; Fang and Fierer, 1991). Bacteraemia in immunocompetent individuals is not a diarrhoeal disease and may manifest in the absence of enteric pathology. Similar to typhoid fever, only about one-third of bacteraemia patients develop diarrhoea (Saphra and Wassermann, 1954; Cherubin *et al.*, 1969; Fang and Fierer, 1991).

IMMUNOCOMPROMISED INDIVIDUALS. In immunocompromised humans, bacteraemia is a common complication of infections with non-typhoidal *Salmonella* serotypes that are normally associated with gastroenteritis in immunocompetent individuals (Gordon, 2008). The organisms most frequently associated with bacteraemia in immunocompromised individuals are *S.* Typhimurium and Enteritidis. Bacteraemia in immunocompromised individuals commonly develops in the absence of symptoms of gastroenteritis (Green and Cheesbrough, 1993; Brown and Eykyn, 2000). Knowledge about the specific immune defects that render individuals susceptible to bacteraemia with non-typhoidal *Salmonella* serotypes is instructive, as this information points to mucosal barrier functions that successfully prevent bacterial dissemination during gastroenteritis. Furthermore, *Salmonella* serotypes, such as *S.* Typhi, which are associated with systemic disease in immunocompetent hosts, are expected to possess specific virulence factors that enable them to overcome the mucosal barrier functions, which prevent bacterial dissemination during gastroenteritis.

Immune defects that increase the risk of developing bacteraemia include an advanced infection with human immunodeficiency virus (HIV) (Gordon *et al.*, 2001, 2002), severe paediatric malaria (Graham *et al.*, 2000; Walsh *et al.*, 2000), anaemia (Okuonghae *et al.*, 1993), neutropenia (Noriega *et al.*, 1994; Tumbarello *et al.*, 1995), interleukin (IL-)12/IL-23 deficiency (MacLennan *et al.*, 2004) and chronic granulomatous disease (Winkelstein *et al.*, 2000). Severe anaemia and advanced HIV infections are associated with a reduced microbiocidal activity of neutrophils (Humbert *et al.*, 1990; Coffey *et al.*, 1998; George *et al.*, 1998), while chronic granulomatous disease decreases the microbiocidal activity of phagocytes in general (Tauber *et al.*, 1983). Mutations in the shared p40 subunit of IL-12 and IL-23 increase the susceptibility to bacteraemia by an interferon (IFN)-γ-independent mechanism (MacLennan *et al.*, 2004), which could be related to the role of IL-23 in recruiting neutrophils to the intestinal mucosa during *S.* Typhimurium infection (Godinez *et al.*, 2009). Reduced neutrophil recruitment due to depletion in the intestinal mucosa of $CD4^+$ cells, specifically Th17 cells, has also been postulated to increase the risk of bacteraemia during advanced HIV disease (Raffatellu *et al.*, 2008a). Collectively, these clinical data point to an important role of neutrophils in preventing bacterial dissemination beyond the mesenteric lymph node during gastroenteritis.

Systemic infections in other host species

A small number of *Salmonella* serotypes are associated with systemic infections in immunocompetent animals. As is the case for the human-restricted serotype Typhi, these pathogens are considered host adapted and generally have a host range that is narrow compared to that of serotypes associated with gastroenteritis. For example, isolates of *S.* Gallinarum can be further subdivided into the biotypes Gallinarum and Pullorum, which cause systemic infections in poultry known as fowl typhoid and pullorum disease, respectively (Shivaprasad, 2000). *Salmonella* Choleraesuis and *S.* Dublin cause systemic disease in pigs and cattle, respectively (Turk *et al.*, 1992; Visser *et al.*, 1992). Systemic dissemination of *S.* Abortusequi and *S.* Abortusovi in horses and sheep, respectively, is not associated with overt signs of disease but manifests as abortion (Perrin *et al.*, 1950; Jack, 1968). Finally, a subset of *S.* Typhimurium strains can be distinguished by phage typing from strains associated with gastroenteritis in humans and are associated with systemic disease in pigeons (Rabsch *et al.*, 2002).

While the genetic basis for adaptation to different host species is poorly understood, the virulence strategies used by host-adapted *Salmonella* serotypes to spread systemically are likely to be variations of a common theme that involves an ability to overcome mucosal barrier functions and disseminate throughout the body. These virulence attributes are absent from *Salmonella* serotypes associated with gastroenteritis.

Virulence Factors Associated with Gastroenteritis

Invasion

The invasion-associated type III secretion system (T3SS-1)

Although gastroenteritis differs in important aspects from the systemic infections discussed above, *Salmonella* serotypes associated with either of these two different disease manifestations share a number of virulence strategies. Most importantly, all *Salmonella* serotypes enter the intestinal mucosa by actively invading the epithelial lining. This event occurs very early during host–pathogen interaction and is observed within 10 to 15 min after infection of ligated ileal loops (Frost *et al.*, 1997; Santos *et al.*, 2002). The use of tissue culture models to study invasion of epithelial cells led to the identified two virulence factors critical for this process, flagella-mediated motility (Liu *et al.*, 1988) and the type III secretion system (T3SS-1) (Galán and Curtiss III, 1989) encoded by genes located on *Salmonella* pathogenicity island 1 (SPI1) (Mills *et al.*, 1995) (Fig. 5.1).

T3SS-1-mediated invasion of polarized epithelial cells requires the function of the non-fimbrial adhesin SiiE, which is encoded by SPI4 (Gerlach *et al.*, 2008). Expression of the T3SS-1 apparatus and the SiiE adhesin is coordinately regulated through HilA, the master regulator of invasion genes encoded on SPI1 (Lee *et al.*, 1992; Ahmer *et al.*, 1999; De Keersmaecker *et al.*, 2005; Gerlach *et al.*, 2007; Thijs *et al.*, 2007; Main-Hester *et al.*, 2008). The main function of the SPI1-encoded T3SS-1 apparatus is to translocate proteins, termed effectors, into the host cell cytosol. Up to 15 effector proteins are known to be translocated by the T3SS-1 into host cells (Ibarra and Steele-Mortimer, 2009). These effector proteins are encoded by genes located either within SPI1 (e.g. *sipA*, *sipB*, *sipC*, *sipD* and *sptP*), on SPI5 (e.g. *sopB* (*sigD*)), on pathogenicity islets (e.g. *slrP*) or on bacteriophages (e.g. *sopE*).

A subset of these effector proteins, including SipA, SipC (SspC), SopA, SopB (SigD), SopD, SopE and SopE2 cooperate to induce actin rearrangements that promote bacterial entry into epithelial cells (Hardt *et al.*, 1998a; Hong and Miller, 1998; Hayward and Koronakis, 1999; Zhou *et al.*, 1999; Friebel *et al.*, 2001; Jepson *et al.*, 2001; McGhie *et al.*, 2001; Raffatellu *et al.*, 2005b). *In vivo*, invasion of the intestinal epithelium is accompanied by a rapid induction of inflammatory responses (Santos *et al.*, 2009). Inactivation of the T3SS-1 ameliorates or abrogates pathological changes at early time points after *S.* Typhimurium infection of calves (Watson *et al.*, 1998; Tsolis *et al.*, 1999a; Zhang *et al.*, 2002a, b) or streptomycin pre-treated mice (Hapfelmeier *et al.*, 2004). Only effector proteins contributing to epithelial invasion *in vitro* have been shown to contribute to the elicitation of inflammatory responses *in vivo* (Zhang *et al.*, 2002a, b; Hapfelmeier *et al.*, 2004).

Many of the genes involved in T3SS-1-mediated invasion are highly conserved among the genus *Salmonella* but are absent from the genomes of close relatives, such as *Escherichia coli*. This phylogenetic distribution is observed for SPI1 (Li *et al.*, 1995), SPI4 (Vernikos *et al.*, 2007), SPI5 (Mirold *et al.*, 2001), *sopE2* and *sopD* (Mirold *et al.*, 2001). The phylogenetic distribution of these genes explains why the ability to invade epithelial cells is a shared virulence strategy among *Salmonella* serotypes that distinguishes these pathogens from the closely related *E. coli* (Bäumler, 1997). Some T3SS-1 effector proteins are not conserved among *Salmonella* serotypes and may have accessory functions. For example, the *sopE* gene is encoded by a lysogenic bacteriophage (Hardt *et al.*, 1998b) that is only present in a small group of *S.* Typhimurium strains (Mirold *et al.*, 1999). Phage-mediated horizontal transfer of the

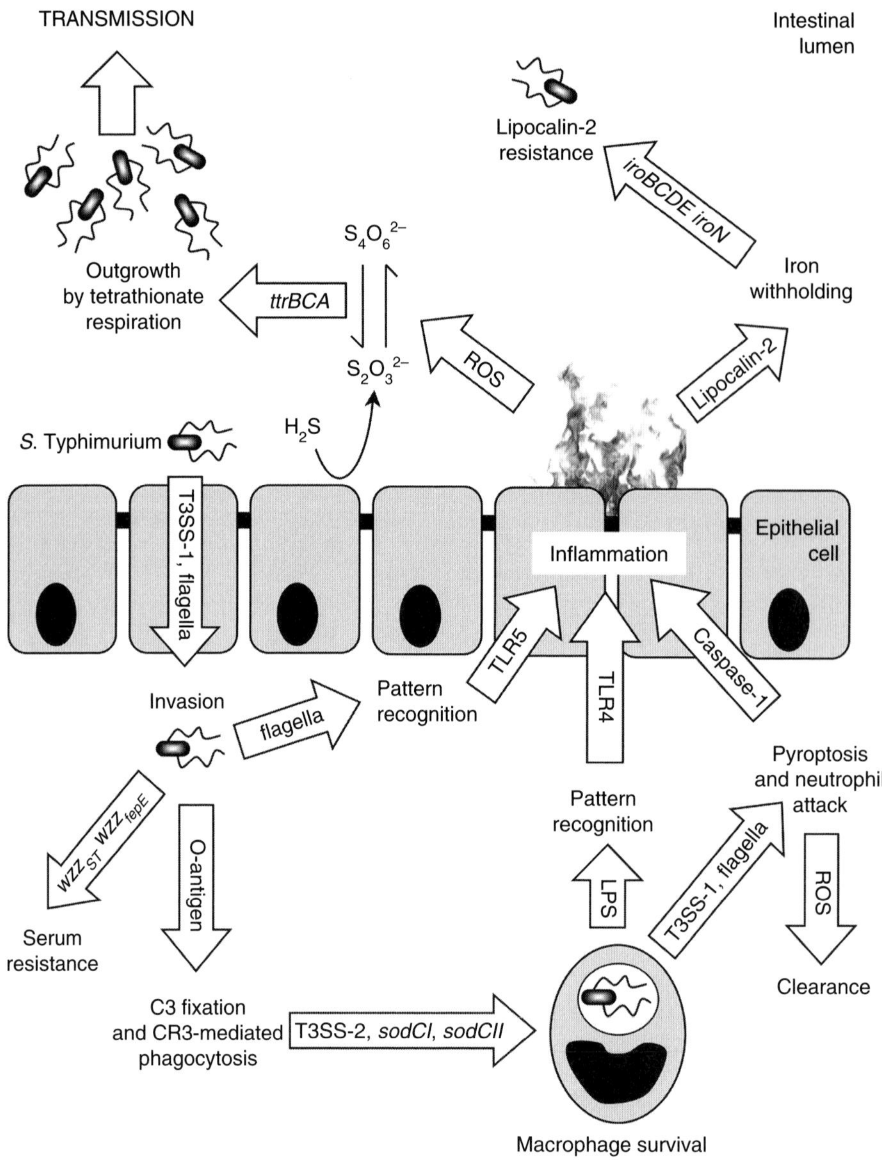

Fig. 5.1. Schematic representation of host–pathogen interactions that unfold during gastroenteritis. For explanation see text.

sopE gene may enable the pathogen to fine-tune the level of T3SS-1-dependent intestinal inflammation it elicits (Zhang *et al.*, 2002a). As discussed below, intestinal inflammation promotes transmission of *Salmonella* serotypes during gastroenteritis (Lawley *et al.*, 2008). By fine-tuning the level of intestinal inflammation, phage-mediated horizontal transfer of effector genes might optimize transmission, thereby giving rise to epidemic phage types. Consistent with this idea, phage-mediated horizontal transfer of the *sopE* gene gave rise to *S.* Typhimurium strains that were associated with epidemics in cattle (Mirold *et al.*, 1999).

Motility

A majority of studies has focused on eliciting the mechanisms by which the T3SS-1 contributes to bacterial invasion. However, a second factor, flagella, is of considerable importance during this process. The contribution of flagella to invasion might be largely indirect, by increasing bacterial contact with host cells. None the less, flagella-mediated motility contributes markedly to the efficiency of epithelial invasion by *Salmonella* serotypes *in vitro* (Khoramian-Falsafi *et al.*, 1990; Jones *et al.*, 1992; Van Asten *et al.*, 2000; Winter *et al.*, 2009a, b). Inactivation of flagella biosynthesis genes markedly reduces intestinal inflammation at early time points after *S.* Typhimurium infection of calves (Schmitt *et al.*, 2001; Winter *et al.*, 2009a) or in a murine colitis model (Stecher *et al.*, 2004). While the structural protein subunits of flagella (flagellin) can serve as a pathogen-associated molecular pattern (PAMP) that activates innate pathways of inflammation, motility *per se* contributes significantly to the ability of flagellated *S.* Typhimurium to trigger inflammation *in vivo* (Winter *et al.*, 2009a).

Expression of flagella is controlled in a hierarchical fashion by the master regulator FlhDC (Chiodini and Sundberg, 1981; Macnab, 2004). FlhDC activates transcription of genes encoding the alternative sigma factor FliA, the anti-sigma factor FlgM, the regulator FliZ, as well as genes required for hook-basal body formation. Secretion of FlgM through the completed hook-basal body frees FliA to induce expression of *fliC*, encoding phase 1 flagellin (H1-antigen) (Hughes *et al.*, 1993). FliZ controls expression of the T3SS-1 by activating *hilD*, a gene encoding a positive regulator of *hilA* expression in *S.* Typhimurium (Lucas *et al.*, 2000; Ellermeier *et al.*, 2005; Kage *et al.*, 2008). Thus FlhDC regulation ensures that two virulence factors critical for invasion of the epithelial lining, flagella and T3SS-1, are coordinately expressed during infection.

Survival in tissue

Serum resistance

After penetrating the epithelial lining, *Salmonella* serotypes become exposed to host defences encountered in the interstitial fluid, including complement. The complement system can be activated through various initiating events. However, all pathways rely on the fact that complement component 3 (C3) senses conserved microbial structures, such as the LPS of Gram-negative bacteria, and thus may serve as a pattern recognition event (Gasque, 2004; Winter *et al.*, 2010a). This results in the deposition of a C3 cleavage product (C3b) on the bacterial surface, a process known as C3 fixation. The mechanism of C3 fixation involves a reactive thioester group in C3b, which forms esters with free hydroxyl groups of LPS sugar moieties (Sahu *et al.*, 1994). C3 fixation has at least two consequences important for *Salmonella* infection.

One consequence of C3 fixation is the initiation of complement-mediated killing by triggering the formation of a membrane attack complex composed of the proteins C5b, C6, C7, C8 and C9 (Müller-Eberhard, 1986). *Salmonella* serotypes associated with gastroenteritis can withstand this killing mechanism, a property known as serum resistance. A key virulence factor in mediating serum resistance is the synthesis of long O-antigen chains in LPS, which is controlled by the wzz_{ST} and wzz_{fepE} genes (Bravo *et al.*, 2008; Holzer *et al.*, 2009) (Fig. 5.1). Long O-antigen chains reduce neither C3 fixation nor consumption of C5b, C6, C7, C8 and C9 (Joiner *et al.*, 1982a). Instead, long O-antigen chains confer serum resistance because the membrane attack complex forms at a great distance to the cell surface and fails to insert into the bacterial outer membrane (Joiner *et al.*, 1982b). In addition, *S.* Typhimurium possesses some accessory components that can further reduce the likelihood that the membrane attack complex reaches its target, the outer membrane. One of these accessory factors is Rck (Heffernan *et al.*, 1992a, b), an outer membrane protein encoded on the virulence plasmid, which binds complement regulatory protein factor H (fH), a protein preventing complement deposition on host cells (Ho *et al.*, 2010). However, in smooth strains with long O-antigen chains, Rck does not appear necessary. Another accessory factor is the outer membrane protease PgtE, which can cleave C3b, C4b and C5 when deposited close to the outer membrane, but a contribution of PgtE to serum resistance is only observed in strains lacking long O-antigen chains (Ramu *et al.*, 2007).

A second consequence of C3 fixation is the opsonization of bacteria, which promotes phagocytosis through complement receptor (CR) 3 (Fig. 5.1). *Salmonella* serotypes associated with gastroenteritis are serum resistant, but this virulence trait does not reduce C3 fixation (Joiner *et al.*, 1982a), presumably because deposition of C3b in the outer regions of the O-antigen remains unaffected by serum resistance mechanisms. An efficient C3 fixation may be one of the reasons why *Salmonella* serotypes associated with gastroenteritis remain susceptible to neutrophils, which can readily phagocytose these pathogens through CR3 (Joiner *et al.*, 1989; Troelstra *et al.*, 1999). While phagocytosis by neutrophils results in killing, *Salmonella* serotypes can survive when they become internalized by macrophages through CR3-dependent phagocytosis (Santos and Bäumler, 2004).

Macrophage survival

Salmonella Typhimurium is efficiently taken up by phagocytes in the intestinal mucosa and is observed microscopically in mononuclear cells (dendritic cells or macrophages) and neutrophils (Frost *et al.*, 1997; Santos *et al.*, 2002). A major bactericidal mechanism of phagocytes is the release of reactive oxygen intermediates (ROI) through the respiratory burst, followed later during infection by production of reactive nitrogen intermediates (RNI), a consequence of host cells producing high levels of inducible nitric oxide synthase (iNOS) (Vazquez-Torres and Fang, 2001). A certain level of intrinsic resistance to these killing mechanisms is required for survival in tissue. For example, the *sodCI* and *sodCII* genes of *S.* Typhimurium encode periplasmic superoxide dismutases, which scavenge superoxide radicals (O_2^-) and peroxynitrite ($OONO^-$). Both genes are required for full mouse virulence (De Groote *et al.*, 1997; Fang *et al.*, 1999). A mutation in *metL*, an enzyme involved in homocysteine biosynthesis, results in hypersusceptibility to nitric oxide (NO) and is required for mouse virulence (De Groote *et al.*, 1996).

Macrophages are the preferred intracellular niche for persistence of *Salmonella* serotypes in tissue (Santos and Bäumler, 2004). A key virulence factor required for survival in macrophages is the type III secretion system encoded by SPI2 (T3SS-2) (Ochman *et al.*, 1996). Genes on SPI2 that encode the T3SS-2 apparatus are present in all members of the species *S. enterica*, but are absent from *S. bongori* or *E. coli* (Ochman and Groisman, 1996; Hensel *et al.*, 1997). T3SS-2-mediated survival in macrophages is thus a shared virulence strategy among *S. enterica* serotypes and is found in pathogens associated with gastroenteritis as well as in serotypes associated with invasive disease (Bäumler, 1997) (Fig. 5.1). T3SS-2-mediated macrophage survival enhances the severity of intestinal inflammation and pathology in bovine and murine models of gastroenteritis (Tsolis *et al.*, 1999a; Coburn *et al.*, 2005).

The T3SS-2 translocates at least 16 effector proteins into the host cell cytosol, including SpiC, SseF, SseG, SlrP, SspH1, SspH2, SifA, SifB, SseI, SseJ, PipB, PipB2, SseK1, SseK2, GogB and SopD2 (Abrahams and Hensel, 2006). Although the molecular functions are known for some of these effector proteins, it remains unclear in most cases how they contribute to T3SS-2-mediated macrophage survival. One purpose of the T3SS-2 seems to be altering the properties of the *Salmonella* containing vacuole (SCV) by manipulating vesicular trafficking events (Uchiya *et al.*, 1999; Beuzon *et al.*, 2000; Vazquez-Torres *et al.*, 2000). For example, the T3SS-2 has been implicated in inhibiting phagolysosomal fusion of the SCV (Uchiya *et al.*, 1999), although this finding was later called into question (Drecktrah *et al.*, 2007). The T3SS-2 enables *S.* Typhimurium to evade the respiratory burst in macrophages (Vazquez-Torres *et al.*, 2000) by interfering with the assembly of the NADPH oxidase complex in the phagosomal membrane (Gallois *et al.*, 2001). As a result, *S.* Typhimurium prevents the production of superoxide radicals (O_2^-) in the SCV. While this process protects the pathogen in the SCV from oxidative damage, it does not reduce the overall superoxide production by macrophages (Vazquez-Torres *et al.*, 2000).

Some evidence suggests that the *spvRABCD* operon is also involved in the interaction of *Salmonella* serotypes with macrophages (Libby *et al.*, 2000). The *spvB* gene encodes an ADP-ribosyl transferase (Otto *et al.*, 2000), which is translocated into the host cell cytosol (Gotoh *et al.*, 2003) where it ADP-ribosylates actin (Tezcan-Merdol *et al.*, 2001), resulting in depolymerization of the actin cytoskeleton (Tezcan-Merdol *et al.*, 2005). The *spv* operon is required for full mouse virulence of *S.* Typhimurium (Gulig and Curtiss, 1987; Gulig *et al.*, 1992). Furthermore, inactivation of the *spv* operon reduces the number of bacteria recovered from the ileal mucosa of calves infected with *S.* Typhimurium (Tsolis *et al.*, 1999b).

The *spv* operon is located on virulence plasmids present in a small number of *S. enterica* subsp. *enterica* serotypes (Woodward *et al.*, 1989; Gulig, 1990; Rotger and Casadesus, 1999) or on the chromosome of *S. enterica* subsp. *arizonae* serotypes (Libby *et al.*, 2002). This limited phylogenetic distribution suggests that the *spv* operon is not part of a virulence strategy shared by all *Salmonella* serotypes associated with gastroenteritis.

Interaction with neutrophils

As discussed above, the actions of SopCI, SodCII and T3SS-2 confer some level of resistance to killing by ROI and contribute to macrophage survival of *S.* Typhimurium (De Groote *et al.*, 1997; Fang *et al.*, 1999; Vazquez-Torres *et al.*, 2000). However, patients with phagocyte oxidase deficiencies such as chronic granulomatous disease are defective in limiting systemic bacterial dissemination (Winkelstein *et al.*, 2000), which suggests that ROI-dependent killing mechanisms still constitute an effective barrier against the spread of *S.* Typhimurium. This ROI-dependent barrier function is likely mediated by neutrophils. Neutrophil depletion markedly increases the susceptibility to systemic dissemination of *S.* Typhimurium in humans (Noriega *et al.*, 1994; Tumbarello *et al.*, 1995; Fierer, 2001) and leads to the appearance of extracellular bacteria in tissue of mice (Conlan, 1996; Vassiloyanakopoulos *et al.*, 1998; Cheminay *et al.*, 2004). The extracellular stage observed in neutropenic mice might represent bacteria transiting from a deceased host cell to a new macrophage. Consistent with this idea, macrophage cell death, termed pyroptosis, is a known consequence of *S.* Typhimurium interaction with macrophages (Cookson and Brennan, 2001; Bergsbaken *et al.*, 2009) and the resulting release of bacteria leads to efficient clearance by ROI-dependent killing mechanisms of neutrophils (Miao *et al.*, 2010). These data suggest that the need to transit between host cells renders *S.* Typhimurium susceptible to neutrophil attack (Fig. 5.1).

C3 fixation results in efficient uptake of *S.* Typhimurium by neutrophils through CR3 (Joiner *et al.*, 1989), a process that is associated with the generation of a respiratory burst (Ross, 1986). A greater magnitude of the respiratory burst in neutrophils compared to resting macrophages may help explain why neutrophils have the capacity to prevent bacterial dissemination to internal organs. Macrophage survival is likely an important strategy to, at least temporarily, shelter *S.* Typhimurium from neutrophil killing mechanisms (Vassiloyanakopoulos *et al.*, 1998).

Intestinal colonization

Transmission

Gastroenteritis is a self-limiting infection with symptoms subsiding within less than 10 days. Invasion and colonization of intestinal tissue appears to be a dead end for *Salmonella* serotypes associated with gastroenteritis, because the pathogen is eventually cleared from intestinal tissues when adaptive immune responses develop (Mastroeni, 2002). However, the acute inflammatory response triggered by T3SS-1-mediated invasion and T3SS-2-mediated macrophage survival promotes the ability of *Salmonella* serotypes to colonize the lumen and increases their relative abundance in intestinal contents (Stecher *et al.*, 2007; Barman *et al.*, 2008). This luminal outgrowth of *Salmonella* serotypes during gastroenteritis is important for their transmission by the faecal–oral route (Lawley *et al.*, 2008).

Inactivation of T3SS-1 and T3SS-2 renders *S.* Typhimurium unable to trigger acute intestinal inflammation, prevents its outgrowth of the microbiota (Stecher *et al.*, 2007; Barman *et al.*, 2008) and blocks transmission in a mouse model (Lawley *et al.*, 2008). IL-10-deficient mice develop severe intestinal inflammation and support outgrowth of a T3SS-1/T3SS-2-deficient *S.* Typhimurium mutant (Stecher *et al.*, 2007). Thus, outgrowth of *Salmonella* serotypes in the lumen is driven by intestinal inflammation and the actions of T3SS-1 and T3SS-2 are required for inducing inflammation, but not subsequently for enhancing growth of the pathogen in the inflamed gut.

The picture emerging from these studies is that T3SS-1 and T3SS-2, the main virulence factors important for gastroenteritis, generate a luminal environment that tips the balance in the competition between *Salmonella* serotypes and the microbiota in favour of the pathogen. Furthermore, the overall pathogenic strategy of *Salmonella* serotypes associated with gastroenteritis appears to be an induction and subsequent exploitation of the host inflammatory response to enhance their transmission to a new host (Stecher and Hardt, 2008; Santos *et al.*, 2009; Winter *et al.*, 2010a).

Resistance to antimicrobials

One of the changes in the luminal environment during inflammation is the epithelial release of antimicrobials, including defensins and lipocalin-2 (Raffatellu *et al.*, 2007, 2009) (Fig. 5.1). Defensins are peptides exhibiting a membrane-targeted antimicrobial activity against a wide range of bacteria (Ouellette, 2006). PmrAB, a two-component regulatory system, controls expression of defensin resistance genes, which are involved in modifying LPS to reduce its negative charge by adding phosphoethanolamine or 4-amino-4-deoxy-*L*-arabinose moieties to phosphate groups in lipid A or the LPS core region (Gunn, 2008). Inactivation of *pmrAB* attenuates *S.* Typhimurium by the oral route of inoculation, but not when mice are infected by the peritoneal route (Gunn *et al.*, 2000). These data suggest that defensin resistance is primarily a requirement for survival in the intestine.

Lipocalin-2 is an antimicrobial protein whose secretion into the intestinal lumen is induced during inflammation (Raffatellu *et al.*, 2009). Lipocalin-2 prevents bacterial iron acquisition by binding enterobactin (Goetz *et al.*, 2002; Flo *et al.*, 2004; Berger *et al.*, 2006), a siderophore produced by *Salmonella* serotypes and many other *Enterobacteriaceae* (Pollack and Neilands, 1970; Pollack *et al.*, 1970). *Salmonella enterica* serotypes can synthesize a glycosylated derivative of enterobactin, termed salmochelin (Hantke *et al.*, 2003). Salmochelin is not bound by lipocalin-2 and its production therefore confers lipocalin-2 resistance (Fischbach *et al.*, 2006). The biosynthesis and uptake of salmochelin are encoded by the *iroBCDEN* gene cluster, which is present in all members of the species *S. enterica*, but absent from *S. bongori* and commensal *E. coli* isolates (Bäumler *et al.*, 1996, 1997, 1998). The presence of the *iroBCDEN* genes in *S.* Typhimurium confers a growth advantage in the intestinal lumen during inflammation, when large amounts of lipocalin-2 are released into the gut (Raffatellu *et al.*, 2009). However, the *iroBCDEN* genes confer no luminal growth advantage in the absence of intestinal inflammation or in lipocalin-2 deficient mice.

Outgrowth in the inflamed intestine

The above examples illustrate that *Salmonella* serotypes possess antimicrobial resistance mechanisms that contribute to intestinal colonization during gastroenteritis. A marked increase in the epithelial release of antimicrobials during inflammation might benefit *Salmonella* serotypes during their competition with commensal microbes that lack adequate resistance mechanisms. However, to a large part, the ability of *Salmonella* serotypes to outgrow the microbiota revolves around competition for nutrients.

Gastroenteritis is a diarrhoeal disease during which intestinal contents are removed from the intestinal lumen by flushing (Santos *et al.*, 2009). In this environment, microbes depend increasingly on nutrients present in the mucous layer for growth. Consistent with this idea, *S.* Typhimurium requires motility and chemotaxis towards mucous carbohydrates to increase its abundance in the intestinal lumen (Stecher *et al.*, 2008). The pathogen can colonize this niche using fimbrial adhesins that bind carbohydrate moieties present in the mucous layer (Chessa *et al.*, 2009). However, to outgrow the microbiota, the pathogen utilizes nutrients generated as a consequence of the host inflammatory response.

In the anaerobic environment of the gut, microbes rely on fermentation to produce energy for growth. Fermentation by the microbiota is accompanied by production of large quantities of hydrogen sulfide (H_2S), a highly cytotoxic compound. To protect itself from the toxic effects of hydrogen sulfide, host enterocytes produce enzymes that oxidize this compound to thiosulfate ($S_2O_3^{2-}$) (Levitt *et al.*, 1999; Furne *et al.*, 2001).

During gastroenteritis, neutrophils transmigrate into the intestinal lumen in large numbers, giving rise to an abundance of faecal leukocytes, which characterizes inflammatory diarrhoea (Harris *et al.*, 1972). The ROI produced during the respiratory burst of luminal neutrophils oxidize thiosulfate ($S_2O_3^{2-}$) into tetrathionate ($S_4O_6^{2-}$) (Winter *et al.*, 2010b) (Fig. 5.1). The *ttrBCA ttrRS* gene cluster enables *Salmonella* serotypes to use tetrathionate as a terminal electron acceptor (Hensel *et al.*, 1999). Through this mechanism, inflammation provides a respiratory electron acceptor for non-typhoidal *Salmonella* serotypes that enables these pathogens to use respiration instead of fermentation to produce energy for growth (Winter *et al.*, 2010b).

This strategy provides a considerable competitive growth advantage, since tetrathionate respiration enables *Salmonella* serotypes to utilize fermentation end products that cannot be consumed by the fermenting microbiota. Inactivation of genes required for tetrathionate respiration abrogates the ability of *S.* Typhimurium to outgrow the microbiota during intestinal inflammation (Winter *et al.*, 2010b). These data suggest that tetrathionate respiration is one of the main mechanisms enhancing outgrowth of *Salmonella* serotypes in the inflamed gut. The *ttrBCA ttrRS* genes are present in all *Salmonella* serotypes, but are absent from close relatives such as *E. coli* (Hensel *et al.*, 1997), illustrating that tetrathionate respiration is a virulence trait that is characteristic of the genus *Salmonella*. Interestingly, tetrathionate broth has been used since 1923 to enrich for *Salmonella* serotypes from biological samples containing competing microbes (Muller, 1923).

In summary, the principal pathogenic strategy of *Salmonella* serotypes associated with gastroenteritis is to use their virulence factors (T3SS-1, T3SS-2 and others) to elicit acute intestinal inflammation. This host response provides a new respiratory electron acceptor in the gut, enabling the pathogen to outgrow the microbiota in the lumen, thereby enhancing its transmission to the next host by faecal shedding of the organism (Fig. 5.1).

Virulence Factors Associated with Systemic Disease

Evasion of mucosal barrier functions and systemic dissemination

Invasion and entry into tissue

Although *Salmonella* serotypes are associated with systemic infections in a number of animal reservoirs, typhoid fever is the disease that has been studied most extensively and will be discussed in greater detail throughout this section.

T3SS-1 and T3SS-2, two major virulence factors important for gastroenteritis, are also key players during the pathogenesis of systemic infections in immunocompetent hosts (Fig. 5.2). However, while infection with *S.* Typhimurium causes symptoms of gastroenteritis within less than 1 day after infection (Glynn and Palmer, 1992), invasion by *S.* Typhi does not elicit overt intestinal host responses during the first 2 weeks after ingestion (Olsen *et al.*, 2003). Virulence factors that

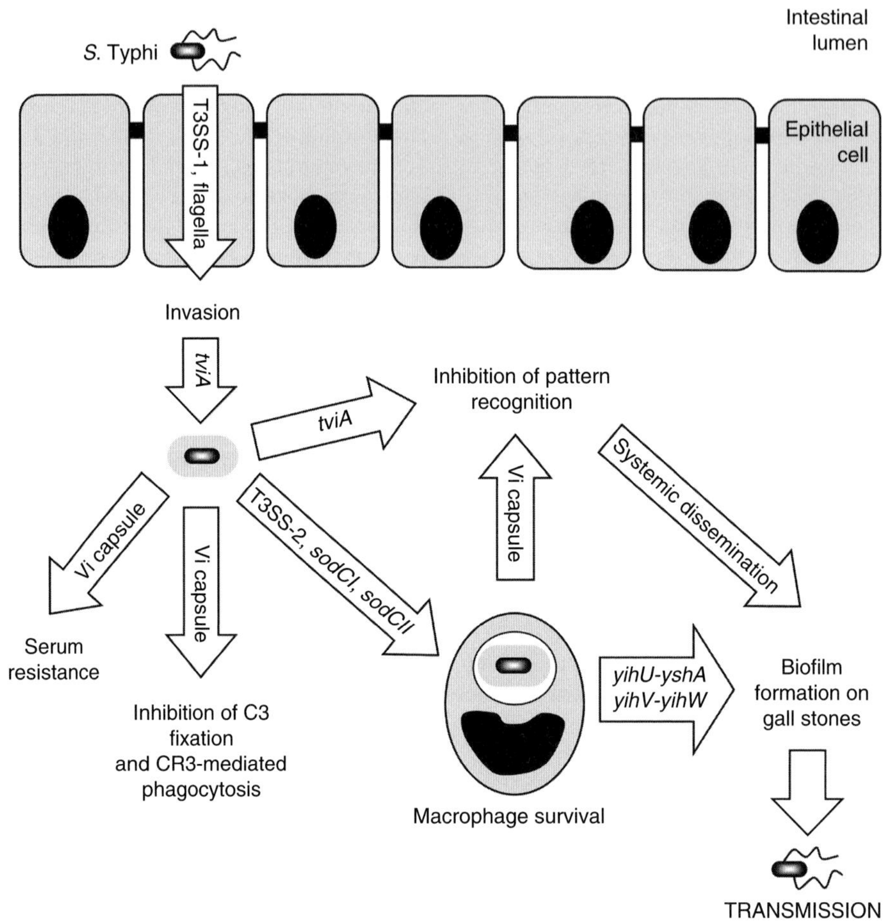

Fig. 5.2. Schematic representation of host–pathogen interactions that unfold during typhoid fever. For explanation see text.

enable *S.* Typhi to prevent the generation of host responses early after infection are encoded by the *viaB* locus, a DNA region located on SPI7 (Parkhill *et al.*, 2001). The *viaB* locus is absent from *Salmonella* serotypes associated with gastroenteritis and is only found in two other pathogens in the genus, *S.* Dublin and *S.* Paratyphi C, both of which are associated with systemic infections in immunocompetent hosts (Raffatellu *et al.*, 2006).

The *viaB* locus encodes genes for the positive regulation (*tviA*), the biosynthesis (*tviBCDE*) and the export (*vexABCDE*) of the virulence (Vi) capsular polysaccharide (Virlogeux *et al.*, 1995). TviA is thought to form hetero-dimers with the response regulator RcsB, thereby increasing its affinity for promoter regions (Virlogeux *et al.*, 1996). The RcsCDB phosphorelay system represses *flhDC* (Cano *et al.*, 2002), encoding a positive regulator of flagella and T3SS-1 in *Salmonella* serotypes (Frye *et al.*, 2006). Expression of *tviA* is controlled by the two-component system EnvZ/OmpR, which responds to changes in osmolarity. As a result, *tviA* is repressed at an osmolarity encountered in the intestinal lumen (approximately 300 mM) but expression is induced under osmotic conditions encountered in tissue (150 mM). In the absence of *tviA* (e.g. in *S.* Typhimurium), RcsB represses *flhDC* transcription in an osmolarity-independent fashion. By sensing the availability of TviA, RcsB incorporates a new regulatory signal, osmolarity, into the RcsCDB regulon of *S.* Typhi (Winter *et al.*, 2009b).

The presence of a new regulatory protein, TviA, in *S.* Typhi has important consequences for host–pathogen interaction. Since TviA is not expressed under high osmolarity, *S.* Typhi remains invasive, motile and non-capsulated while it resides in the intestinal lumen. However, TviA expression is induced at tissue osmolarity, resulting in production of the Vi capsule and a rapid repression of T3SS-1 and flagella gene expression when the pathogen transits through the intestinal epithelium (Tran *et al.*, 2010; Winter *et al.*, 2010c). One of the functions of the intestinal epithelium is to serve as a sentinel for microbial translocation from the gut lumen by expressing Toll-like receptor (TLR) 5 on its basolateral surface (Gewirtz *et al.*, 2001). TLR5 is a pattern recognition receptor of the innate immune system whose stimulation by its cognate PAMP, flagellin, initiates inflammatory responses leading to the recruitment of neutrophils. By repressing flagellin expression during the transition through the intestinal epithelium, TviA enables *S.* Typhi to evade this sentinel function and to increase its dissemination to internal organs (Winter *et al.*, 2010c) (Fig. 5.2).

Evasion of C3 fixation and opsonophagocytosis

A second consequence of TviA-mediated gene regulation is that the Vi capsule is expressed during the transition of *S.* Typhi through the intestinal epithelium (Tran *et al.*, 2010), which ensures that the pathogen is Vi-capsulated when it encounters complement. Vi-capsulated *S.* Typhi isolates deposit less C3b on their surface than non-capsulated isolates (Looney and Steigbigel, 1986), which can arise during laboratory passage by a spontaneous loss of SPI7 (Bueno *et al.*, 2004; Nair *et al.*, 2004). These data suggest that the Vi capsule is a virulence factor that prevents C3 fixation (Fig. 5.2). The Vi capsule is a homopolymer of (1→4)-2-acetamido-3-*O*-acetyl-2-deoxy-α-D-galacturonic acid (Heyns and Kiessling, 1967), a structure that does not contain free hydroxyl groups available for complement deposition. The lack in the Vi polysaccharide of free hydroxyl groups may explain why expression of this surface structure inhibits C3 fixation. An inhibition of C3 fixation is a property that distinguishes *S.* Typhi from *Salmonella* serotypes associated with gastroenteritis and helps explain differences in the disease manifestations between localized and systemic infections.

Vi-capsulated *S.* Typhi isolates are internalized more efficiently by phagocytes than non-capsulated isolates (Looney and Steigbigel, 1986), presumably because inhibition of C3 fixation prevents phagocytosis through CR3. Furthermore, inhibition of CR3-mediated phagocytosis by Vi-capsulated *S.* Typhi isolates prevents the generation of a respiratory burst in neutrophils (Miller *et al.*, 1972; Kossack *et al.*, 1981; Looney and Steigbigel, 1986). These properties likely contribute to the ability of *S.* Typhi to overcome a neutrophil barrier and spread beyond the mesenteric lymph node. *Salmonella* Dublin, which causes an invasive infection in cattle and can express the Vi capsular antigen (Hashimoto and Khan, 1997), exits from the mesenteric lymph node into the efferent lymphatics extracellularly (Pullinger *et al.*, 2007). This extracellular phase may render the pathogen susceptible to neutrophil attack and may therefore necessitate the use of antiphagocytic mechanisms, such as expression of the Vi capsular antigen, to ensure successful dissemination from the lymph node into the bloodstream. Such an extracellular phase during the initial dissemination of *S.* Typhi would explain why antibody responses elicited by vaccination with purified Vi capsular polysaccharide are protective in humans, because a defect in CR3-mediated clearance can now be compensated for by Fc receptor-mediated phagocytosis (Robbins and Robbins, 1984; Tacket *et al.*, 1986; Klugman *et al.*, 1987).

Anti-inflammatory properties of the Vi capsule

The Vi capsule attenuates inflammatory responses generated by TLR4, a pattern recognition receptor, which recognizes the lipid A moiety of LPS (Hirose *et al.*, 1997; Raffatellu *et al.*, 2005a; Wilson *et al.*, 2008) (Fig. 5.2). Furthermore, expression of the Vi capsule reduces intestinal inflammation and neutrophil recruitment in bovine and murine models of gastroenteritis (Raffatellu *et al.*, 2007; Haneda *et al.*, 2009). These anti-inflammatory properties of the Vi capsule might be a consequence of its ability to impair C3 fixation. An important role for complement in triggering LPS-induced inflammatory responses has surfaced in a number of previous studies. While TLR4 is necessary for triggering inflammatory responses to intraperitoneally administered LPS in mice, complement is crucial for fully inducing these responses *in vivo* (Li *et al.*, 2005; Perlik *et al.*, 2005; Zhang *et al.*, 2007). Similarly, while LPS-induced gene expression in macrophages is TLR4-dependent, TLR4 is not sufficient and requires CR3 to facilitate signalling *in vitro* (Perera *et al.*, 2001; Vogel *et al.*, 2001; Noubir *et al.*, 2004). During the interaction of *S.* Typhimurium with phagocytes, TLR4-dependent responses are attenuated when phagocytosis is blocked using anti-CR3 antibodies. In contrast, a TLR4-blocking peptide attenuates TLR4-dependent responses without reducing uptake of *S.* Typhimurium (van Bruggen *et al.*, 2007). These data point to a sequential interaction of bacteria with CR3 and TLR4, which might explain why opsonophagocytosis is necessary for triggering TLR4-dependent responses.

In summary, evasion of C3 fixation by the Vi capsule helps to explain a number of clinical differences between typhoid fever and gastroenteritis (Raffatellu *et al.*, 2006; Tsolis *et al.*, 2008). First, the Vi capsule attenuates intestinal inflammatory responses triggered by bacterial invasion, which likely contributes to the long incubation period of typhoid fever and the scarcity of neutrophils in intestinal infiltrates. Second, the Vi capsule prevents phagocytosis and ROI-mediated killing by neutrophils, which likely promotes systemic dissemination during typhoid fever. However, the *viaB* locus is absent from a number of *Salmonella* serotypes associated with systemic diseases and the mechanisms by which these pathogens overcome mucosal barrier functions remain to be discovered.

Chronic carriage

The ability to disseminate throughout the host and take residence in internal organs provides access to new potential routes of transmission. The utilization of such new routes of transmission is a common trait among *Salmonella* serotypes associated with systemic infections and this property distinguishes these pathogens from *Salmonella* serotypes associated with gastroenteritis. For example, the most important route of transmission in fowl typhoid and pullorum disease is transovarian infection resulting in vertical spread via the egg and to the chick or poult (Shivaprasad, 2000). In cattle, long-term *S.* Dublin carrier animals contribute to transmission of the pathogen within infected herds by periodically shedding bacteria through faeces or milk (Nielsen *et al.*, 2004).

The human-restricted serotype Typhi can establish chronic carriage in the gall bladder or urinary bladder of a fraction of patients and the respective individuals, termed 'typhoid Marys', are important reservoirs for transmission within the human population. The initial colonization of the urinary bladder during typhoid fever is associated with the passing of turbid urine, indicative of bacteria being present at concentrations above 10^8 bacteria ml^{-1} (Horton-Smith, 1900). This disease manifestation develops in the absence of symptoms of cystitis, which illustrates the stealthy design of *S.* Typhi. Colonization of the urinary bladder has become rare since the advent of antibiotic therapy. As a result, chronic gall bladder carriage is currently the main route of transmission through chronic carriers.

The estimated age of the *S.* Typhi lineage is approximately 50,000 years (Kidgell *et al.*, 2002), suggesting that the pathogen evolved when the human population existed in the form of small groups of hunters and gatherers. Transmission through 'typhoid Marys' was likely essential for maintaining the infection within groups of some 100 to 200 individuals that existed during this time and enabled the pathogen to become strictly human adapted (Kingsley and Bäumler, 2000).

The mechanisms important for establishing a chronic carrier status are largely unknown. The formation of gallstones increases the risk of developing chronic gall bladder carriage after recovering from typhoid fever. Colonization of gallstones involves biofilm formation of *S.* Typhi (Crawford *et al.*, 2010). An O-antigen capsule encoded by the *yihU-yshA* and *yihV-yihW* genes (Snyder *et al.*, 2006), which is distinct from the Vi capsular polysaccharide, is required for biofilm formation on gallstones (Crawford *et al.*, 2008), and thus may contribute to transmission success (Fig. 5.2).

Pseudogene formation during host adaptation

The genome of *S.* Typhi contains more than 200 pseudogenes, compared to only 39 present in *S.* Typhimurium (McClelland *et al.*, 2001; Parkhill *et al.*, 2001). Pseudogene formation in the *S.* Typhi lineage may reflect, at least in part, a loss of genes no longer required because of changes in the mode of transmission. For example, genes that promote intestinal colonization, which is important for transmission during gastroenteritis, include fimbrial operons, many of which contain pseudogenes in *S.* Typhi (Townsend *et al.*, 2001). Furthermore, one pseudogene found in *S.* Typhi strain CT18 is *ttrS*, encoding a regulator of tetrathionate respiration genes (Parkhill *et al.*, 2001). An elevated number of pseudogenes is also detected in the genomes of host-adapted *S.* Gallinarum and *S.* Choleraesuis and correlates with a host range that is more restricted than that of *Salmonella* serotypes associated with gastroenteritis (Chiu *et al.*, 2005; Thomson *et al.*, 2008).

In summary, the principal pathogenic strategy of *Salmonella* serotypes associated with systemic disease in immunocompetent hosts builds on an approach common to host–pathogen interactions of all *S. enterica* serotypes. This common approach includes a T3SS-1-mediated invasion of the intestinal epithelium followed by a T3SS-2-mediated macrophage survival. However, *Salmonella* serotypes associated with systemic disease have acquired additional virulence mechanisms that enable them to overcome mucosal barrier functions and spread systemically throughout the body. Systemic dissemination results in colonization of internal organs, which is essential for their transmission (Fig. 5.2).

While this overall virulence strategy is shared by all *Salmonella* serotypes associated with systemic disease in immunocompetent hosts, each pathogen has evolved different approaches to transmit from its respective reservoirs in internal organs to the next host. These include horizontal transmission from reservoirs in the gall bladder or urinary bladder, vertical transmission from reservoirs in the udder or the ovaries, or horizontal transmission from reservoirs in the placenta through abortion.

Acknowledgements

TS was supported by a postdoctoral fellowship from the Deutsche Forschungsgemeinschaft. Work in AJB's laboratory is supported by Public Health Service Grants AI040124, AI044170, AI073120, AI076246, AI079173 and AI088122.

References

Abrahams, G.L. and Hensel, M. (2006) Manipulating cellular transport and immune responses: dynamic interactions between intracellular *Salmonella enterica* and its host cells. *Cellular Microbiology* 8, 728–737.

Ahmer, B.M., van Reeuwijk, J., Watson, P.R., Wallis, T.S. and Heffron, F. (1999) *Salmonella* SirA is a global regulator of genes mediating enteropathogenesis. *Molecular Microbiology* 31, 971–982.

Baker, J.R. (1970) Salmonellosis in the horse. *British Veterinary Journal* 126, 100–105.

Barman, M., Unold, D., Shifley, K., Amir, E., Hung, K., Bos, N. and Salzman, N. (2008) Enteric salmonellosis disrupts the microbial ecology of the murine gastrointestinal tract. *Infection and Immunity* 76, 907–915.

Bäumler, A.J. (1997) The record of horizontal gene transfer in *Salmonella*. *Trends in Microbiology* 5, 318–322.

Bäumler, A.J., Tsolis, R.M., van der Velden, A.W.M., Stojiljkovic, I., Anic, S. and Heffron, F. (1996) Identification of a new iron regulated locus of *Salmonella typhi*. *Gene* 193, 207–213.

Bäumler, A.J., Heffron, F. and Reissbrodt, R. (1997) Rapid detection of *Salmonella enterica* with primers specific for *iroB*. *Journal of Clinical Microbiology* 35, 1224–1230.

Bäumler, A.J., Norris, T.L., Lasco, T., Voigt, W., Reissbrodt, R., Rabsch, W. and Heffron, F. (1998) IroN, a novel outer membrane siderophore receptor characteristic of *Salmonella enterica*. *Journal of Bacteriology* 180, 1446–1453.

Berger, T., Togawa, A., Duncan, G.S., Elia, A.J., You-Ten, A., Wakeham, A., Fong, H.E., Cheung, C.C. and Mak, T.W. (2006) Lipocalin 2-deficient mice exhibit increased sensitivity to *Escherichia coli* infection but not to ischemia-reperfusion injury. *Proceedings of the National Academy of Sciences of the United States of America* 103, 1834–1839.

Bergsbaken, T., Fink, S.L. and Cookson, B.T. (2009) Pyroptosis: host cell death and inflammation. *Nature Reviews Microbiology* 7, 99–109.

Beuzon, C.R., Meresse, S., Unsworth, K.E., Ruiz-Albert, J., Garvis, S., Waterman, S.R., Ryder, T.A., Boucrot, E. and Holden, D.W. (2000) *Salmonella* maintains the integrity of its intracellular vacuole through the action of SifA. *The EMBO Journal* 19, 3235–3249.

Bravo, D., Silva, C., Carter, J.A., Hoare, A., Alvarez, S.A., Blondel, C.J., Zaldivar, M., Valvano, M.A. and Contreras, I. (2008) Growth-phase regulation of lipopolysaccharide O-antigen chain length influences serum resistance in serovars of *Salmonella*. *Journal of Medical Microbiology* 57, 938–946.

Brown, M. and Eykyn, S.J. (2000) Non-typhoidal *Salmonella* bacteraemia without gastroenteritis: a marker of underlying immunosuppression. Review of cases at St. Thomas' Hospital 1970-1999. *Journal of Infection* 41, 256–259.

Bueno, S.M., Santiviago, C.A., Murillo, A.A., Fuentes, J.A., Trombert, A.N., Rodas, P.I., Youderian, P. and Mora, G.C. (2004) Precise excision of the large pathogenicity island, SPI7, in *Salmonella enterica* serovar Typhi. *Journal of Bacteriology* 186, 3202–3213.

Cano, D.A., Dominguez-Bernal, G., Tierrez, A., Garcia-del Portillo, F. and Casadesus, J. (2002) Regulation of capsule synthesis and cell motility in *Salmonella enterica* by the essential gene igaA. *Genetics* 162, 1513–1523.

Cheminay, C., Chakravortty, D. and Hensel, M. (2004) Role of neutrophils in murine salmonellosis. *Infection and Immunity* 72, 468–477.

Cherubin, C.E., Fodor, T., Denmark, L.I., Master, C.S., Fuerst, H.T. and Winter, J.W. (1969) Symptoms, septicemia and death in salmonellosis. *American Journal of Epidemiology* 90, 285–291.

Chessa, D., Winter, M.G., Jakomin, M. and Bäumler, A.J. (2009) *Salmonella enterica* serotype Typhimurium Std fimbriae bind terminal alpha(1,2)fucose residues in the cecal mucosa. *Molecular Microbiology,* 71, 864–875.

Chiodini, R.J. and Sundberg, J.P. (1981) Salmonellosis in reptiles: a review. *American Journal of Epidemiology* 113, 494–499.

Chiu, C.H., Tang, P., Chu, C., Hu, S., Bao, Q., Yu, J., Chou, Y.Y., Wang, H.S. and Lee, Y.S. (2005) The genome sequence of *Salmonella enterica* serovar Choleraesuis, a highly invasive and resistant zoonotic pathogen. *Nucleic Acids Research* 33, 1690–1698.

Coburn, B., Li, Y., Owen, D., Vallence, B.A. and Finlay, B.B. (2005) *Salmonella enterica* serovar Typhimurium pathogenicity island 2 is necessary for complete virulence in a mouse model of infectious enterocolitis. *Infection and Immunity* 73, 3219–3227.

Coffey, M.J., Phare, S.M., George, S., Peters-Golden, M. and Kazanjian, P.H. (1998) Granulocyte colony-stimulating factor administration to HIV-infected subjects augments reduced leukotriene synthesis and anticryptococcal activity in neutrophils. *Journal of Clinical Investigations* 102, 663–670.

Conlan, J.W. (1996) Neutrophils prevent extracellular colonization of the liver microvasculature by *Salmonella typhimurium*. *Infection and Immunity* 64, 1043–1047.

Cookson, B.T. and Brennan, M.A. (2001) Pro-inflammatory programmed cell death. *Trends in Microbiology* 9, 113–114.

Crawford, R.W., Gibson, D.L., Kay, W.W. and Gunn, J.S. (2008) Identification of a bile-induced exopolysaccharide required for *Salmonella* biofilm formation on gallstone surfaces. *Infection and Immunity* 76, 5341–5349.

Crawford, R.W., Rosales-Reyes, R., Ramirez-Aguilar Mde, L., Chapa-Azuela, O., Alpuche-Aranda, C. and Gunn, J.S. (2010) Gallstones play a significant role in *Salmonella* spp. gallbladder colonization and carriage. *Proceedings of the National Academy of Sciences of the United States of America* 107, 4353–4358.

De Groote, M.A., Testerman, T., Xu, Y., Stauffer, G. and Fang, F.C. (1996) Homocysteine antagonism of nitric oxide-related cytostasis in *Salmonella typhimurium*. *Science* 272, 414–417.

De Groote, M.A., Ochsner, U.A., Shiloh, M.U., Nathan, C., McCord, J.M., Dinauer, M.C., Libby, S.J., Vazquez, T.A., Xu, Y. and Fang, F.C. (1997) Periplasmic superoxide dismutase protects *Salmonella* from products of phagocyte NADPH-oxidase and nitric oxide synthase. *Proceedings of the National Academy of Sciences of the United States of America* 94, 13997–14001.

De Keersmaecker, S.C., Marchal, K., Verhoeven, T.L., Engelen, K., Vanderleyden, J. and Detweiler, C.S. (2005) Microarray analysis and motif detection reveal new targets of the *Salmonella enterica* serovar Typhimurium HilA regulatory protein, including hilA itself. *Journal of Bacteriology* 187, 4381–4391.

Drecktrah, D., Knodler, L.A., Howe, D. and Steele-Mortimer, O. (2007) *Salmonella* trafficking is defined by continuous dynamic interactions with the endolysosomal system. *Traffic* 8, 212–225.

Ellermeier, C.D., Ellermeier, J.R. and Slauch, J.M. (2005) HilD, HilC and RtsA constitute a feed forward loop that controls expression of the SPI1 type three secretion system regulator hilA in *Salmonella enterica* serovar Typhimurium. *Molecular Microbiology* 57, 691–705.

Fang, F.C. and Fierer, J. (1991) Human infection with *Salmonella dublin*. *Medicine (Baltimore)* 70, 198–207.

Fang, F.C., De Groote, M.A., Foster, J.W., Bäumler, A.J., Ochsner, U., Testerman, T., Bearson, S., Giard, J.C., Xu, Y., Campbell, G. and Laessig, T. (1999) Virulent *Salmonella typhimurium* has two periplasmic Cu, Zn-superoxide dismutases. *Proceedings of the National Academy of Sciences of the United States of America* 96, 7502–7507.

Fierer, J. (2001) Polymorphonuclear leukocytes and innate immunity to *Salmonella* infections in mice. *Microbes and Infection/Institut Pasteur* 3, 1233–1237.

Fischbach, M.A., Lin, H., Zhou, L., Yu, Y., Abergel, R.J., Liu, D.R., Raymond, K.N., Wanner, B.L., Strong, R.K., Walsh, C.T., Aderem, A. and Smith, K.D. (2006) The pathogen-associated iroA gene cluster mediates bacterial evasion of lipocalin 2. *Proceedings of the National Academy of Sciences of the United States of America* 103, 16502–16507.

Flo, T.H., Smith, K.D., Sato, S., Rodriguez, D.J., Holmes, M.A., Strong, R.K., Akira, S. and Aderem, A. (2004) Lipocalin 2 mediates an innate immune response to bacterial infection by sequestrating iron. *Nature* 432, 917–921.

Friebel, A., Ilchmann, H., Aepfelbacher, M., Ehrbar, K., Machleidt, W. and Hardt, W.D. (2001) SopE and SopE2 from *Salmonella typhimurium* activate different sets of RhoGTPases of the host cell. *Journal of Biological Chemistry* 276, 34035–34040.

Frost, A.J., Bland, A.P. and Wallis, T.S. (1997) The early dynamic response of the calf ileal epithelium to *Salmonella typhimurium*. *Veterinary Pathology* 34, 369–386.

Frye, J., Karlinsey, J.E., Felise, H.R., Marzolf, B., Dowidar, N., McClelland, M. and Hughes, K.T. (2006) Identification of new flagellar genes of *Salmonella enterica* serovar Typhimurium. *Journal of Bacteriology* 188, 2233–2243.

Furne, J., Springfield, J., Koenig, T., Demaster, E. and Levitt, M.D. (2001) Oxidation of hydrogen sulfide and methanethiol to thiosulfate by rat tissues: a specialized function of the colonic mucosa. *Biochemical Pharmacology* 62, 255–259.

Galán, J.E. and Curtiss III, R. (1989) Cloning and molecular characterization of genes whose products allow *Salmonella typhimurium* to penetrate tissue culture cells. *Proceedings of the National Academy of Sciences of the United States of America* 86, 6383–6387.

Gallois, A., Klein, J.R., Allen, L.A., Jones, B.D. and Nauseef, W.M. (2001) *Salmonella* pathogenicity island 2-encoded type III secretion system mediates exclusion of NADPH oxidase assembly from the phagosomal membrane. *Journal of Immunology* 166, 5741–5748.

Gasque, P. (2004) Complement: a unique innate immune sensor for danger signals. *Molecular Immunology* 41, 1089–1098.

George, S., Coffey, M., Cinti, S., Collins, J., Brown, M. and Kazanjian, P. (1998) Neutrophils from AIDS patients treated with granulocyte colony-stimulating factor demonstrate enhanced killing of *Mycobacterium avium*. *Journal of Infectious Diseases* 178, 1530–1533.

Gerlach, R.G., Jackel, D., Stecher, B., Wagner, C., Lupas, A., Hardt, W.D. and Hensel, M. (2007) *Salmonella* Pathogenicity Island 4 encodes a giant non-fimbrial adhesin and the cognate type 1 secretion system. *Cellular Microbiology* 9, 1834–1850.

Gerlach, R.G., Claudio, N., Rohde, M., Jackel, D., Wagner, C. and Hensel, M. (2008) Cooperation of *Salmonella* pathogenicity islands 1 and 4 is required to breach epithelial barriers. *Cellular Microbiology* 10, 2364–2376.

Gewirtz, A.T., Navas, T.A., Lyons, S., Godowski, P.J. and Madara, J.L. (2001) Cutting edge: bacterial flagellin activates basolaterally expressed TLR5 to induce epithelial proinflammatory gene expression. *Journal of Immunology* 167, 1882–1885.

Glynn, J.R. and Palmer, S.R. (1992) Incubation period, severity of disease, and infecting dose: evidence from a *Salmonella* outbreak. *American Journal of Epidemiology* 136, 1369–1377.

Godinez, I., Raffatellu, M., Chu, H., Paixao, T.A., Haneda, T., Santos, R.L., Bevins, C.L., Tsolis, R.M. and Bäumler, A.J. (2009) Interleukin-23 orchestrates mucosal responses to *Salmonella enterica* serotype Typhimurium in the intestine. *Infection and Immunity* 77, 387–398.

Goetz, D.H., Holmes, M.A., Borregaard, N., Bluhm, M.E., Raymond, K.N. and Strong, R.K. (2002) The neutrophil lipocalin NGAL is a bacteriostatic agent that interferes with siderophore-mediated iron acquisition. *Molecular Cell* 10, 1033–1043.

Gordon, M.A. (2008) *Salmonella* infections in immunocompromised adults. *Journal of Infection* 56, 413–422.

Gordon, M.A., Walsh, A.L., Chaponda, M., Soko, D., Mbvwinji, M., Molyneux, M.E. and Gordon, S.B. (2001) Bacteraemia and mortality among adult medical admissions in Malawi – predominance of non-typhi salmonellae and *Streptococcus pneumoniae*. *Journal of Infection* 42, 44–49.

Gordon, M.A., Banda, H.T., Gondwe, M., Gordon, S.B., Boeree, M.J., Walsh, A.L., Corkill, J.E., Hart, C.A., Gilks, C.F. and Molyneux, M.E. (2002) Non-typhoidal *Salmonella* bacteraemia among HIV-infected Malawian adults: high mortality and frequent recrudescence. *Aid* 16, 1633–1641.

Gotoh, H., Okada, N., Kim, Y.G., Shiraishi, K., Hirami, N., Haneda, T., Kurita, A., Kikuchi, Y. and Danbara, H. (2003) Extracellular secretion of the virulence plasmid-encoded ADP-ribosyltransferase SpvB in *Salmonella*. *Microbial Pathogenesis* 34, 227–238.

Graham, S.M., Walsh, A.L., Molyneux, E.M., Phiri, A.J. and Molyneux, M.E. (2000) Clinical presentation of non-typhoidal *Salmonella* bacteraemia in Malawian children. *Transactions of the Royal Society of Tropical Medicine and Hygiene* 94, 310–314.

Green, S.D. and Cheesbrough, J.S. (1993) *Salmonella* bacteraemia among young children at a rural hospital in western Zaire. *Annals of Tropical Paediatrics* 13, 45–53.

Grimont, P.A.D. and Weill, F.-X. (2007) *Antigenic formulae of the Salmonella serovars*. WHO Collaborating Centre for Reference and Research on *Salmonella*, Paris.

Gulig, P.A. (1990) Virulence plasmids of *Salmonella typhimurium* and other salmonellae. *Microbial Pathogenesis* 8, 3–11.

Gulig, P.A. and Curtiss, R. (1987) Plasmid-associated virulence of *Salmonella typhimurium*. *Infection and Immunity* 55, 2891–2901.

Gulig, P.A., Caldwell, A.L. and Chiodo, V.A. (1992) Identification, genetic analysis and DNA sequence of a 7.8-kb virulence region of the *Salmonella typhimurium* virulence plasmid. *Molecular Microbiology* 6, 1395–1411.

Gunn, J.S. (2008) The *Salmonella* PmrAB regulon: lipopolysaccharide modifications, antimicrobial peptide resistance and more. *Trends in Microbiology* 16, 284–290.

Gunn, J.S., Ryan, S.S., van Velkinburgh, J.C., Ernst, R.K. and Miller, S.I. (2000) Genetic and functional analysis of a PmrA-PmrB-regulated locus necessary for lipopolysaccharide modification, antimicrobial peptide resistance, and oral virulence of *Salmonella enterica* serovar Typhimurium. *Infection and Immunity* 68, 6139–6146.

Haneda, T., Winter, S.E., Butler, B.P., Wilson, R.P., Tukel, C., Winter, M.G., Godinez, I., Tsolis, R.M. and Bäumler, A.J. (2009) The capsule-encoding viaB locus reduces intestinal inflammation by a *Salmonella* pathogenicity island 1-independent mechanism. *Infection and Immunity* 77, 2932–2942.

Hantke, K., Nicholson, G., Rabsch, W. and Winkelmann, G. (2003) Salmochelins, siderophores of *Salmonella enterica* and uropathogenic *Escherichia coli* strains, are recognized by the outer membrane receptor IroN. *Proceedings of the National Academy of Sciences of the United States of America* 100, 3677–3682.

Hapfelmeier, S., Ehrbar, K., Stecher, B., Barthel, M., Kremer, M. and Hardt, W.D. (2004) Role of the *Salmonella* pathogenicity island 1 effector proteins SipA, SopB, SopE, and SopE2 in *Salmonella enterica* subspecies 1 serovar Typhimurium colitis in streptomycin-pretreated mice. *Infection and Immunity* 72, 795–809.

Hardt, W.D., Chen, L.M., Schuebel, K.E., Bustelo, X.R. and Galan, J.E. (1998a) *Salmonella typhimurium* encodes an activator of Rho GTPases that induces membrane ruffling and nuclear responses in host cells. *Cell* 93, 815–826.

Hardt, W.D., Urlaub, H. and Galan, J.E. (1998b) A substrate of the centisome 63 type III protein secretion system of *Salmonella typhimurium* is encoded by a cryptic bacteriophage. *Proceedings of the National Academy of Sciences of the United States of America* 95, 2574–2579.

Harris, J.C., Dupont, H.L. and Hornick, R.B. (1972) Fecal leukocytes in diarrheal illness. *Annals of Internal Medicine* 76, 697–703.

Hashimoto, Y. and Khan, A.Q. (1997) Comparison of ViaB regions of Vi-positive organisms. *FEMS Microbiology Letters* 157, 55–57.

Hayward, R.D. and Koronakis, V. (1999) Direct nucleation and bundling of actin by the SipC protein of invasive *Salmonella*. *The EMBO Journal* 18, 4926–4934.

Heffernan, E.J., Harwood, J., Fierer, J. and Guiney, D. (1992a) The *Salmonella typhimurium* virulence plasmid complement resistance gene *rck* is homologous to a family of virulence related outer membrane protein genes including pagC and ail. *Journal of Bacteriology* 174, 84–91.

Heffernan, E.J., Reed, S., Hackett, J., Fierer, J., Roudier, C. and Guiney, D. (1992b) Mechanism of resistance to complement-mediated killing of bacteria encoded by the *Salmonella typhimurium* virulence plasmid gene *rck*. *Journal of Clinical Investigation* 90, 953–964.

Hensel, M., Shea, J.E., Bäumler, A.J., Gleeson, C., Blattner, F. and Holden, D.W. (1997) Analysis of the boundaries of *Salmonella* pathogenicity island 2 and the corresponding chromosomal region of *Escherichia coli* K-12. *Journal of Bacteriology* 179, 1105–1111.

Hensel, M., Hinsley, A.P., Nikolaus, T., Sawers, G. and Berks, B.C. (1999) The genetic basis of tetrathionate respiration in *Salmonella typhimurium*. *Molecular Microbiology* 32, 275–287.

Heyns, K. and Kiessling, G. (1967) Strukturaufklarung des Vi-antigens aus Citrobacter freundii (*E. coli*) 5396/38. *Carbohydrate Research* 3, 340–353.

Hirose, K., Ezaki, T., Miyake, M., Li, T., Khan, A.Q., Kawamura, Y., Yokoyama, H. and Takami, T. (1997) Survival of Vi-capsulated and Vi-deleted *Salmonella typhi* strains in cultured macrophage expressing different levels of CD14 antigen. *FEMS Microbiology Letters* 147, 259–265.

Ho, D.K., Jarva, H. and Meri, S. (2010) Human complement factor H binds to outer membrane protein Rck of *Salmonella*. *Journal of Immunology* 185, 1763–1769.

Holzer, S.U., Schlumberger, M.C., Jackel, D. and Hensel, M. (2009) Effect of the O-antigen length of lipopolysaccharide on the functions of Type III secretion systems in *Salmonella enterica*. *Infection and Immunity* 77, 5458–5470.

Hong, K.H. and Miller, V.L. (1998) Identification of a novel *Salmonella* invasion locus homologous to *Shigella* ipgDE. *Journal of Bacteriology* 180, 1793–1802.

Horton-Smith, P. (1900) The Goulstonian Lectures on the typhoid bacillus and typhoid fever. Lecture II. *Lancet* 1, 910–920.

Hughes, K.T., Gillen, K.L., Semon, M.J. and Karlinsey, J.E. (1993) Sensing structural intermediates in bacterial flagellar assembly by export of a negative regulator. *Science* 262, 1277–1280.

Humbert, J.R., Winsor, E.L., Githens, J.M. and Schmitz, J.B. (1990) Neutrophil dysfunctions in sickle cell disease. *Biomedicine & Pharmacotherapy* 44, 153–158.

Ibarra, J.A. and Steele-Mortimer, O. (2009) *Salmonella* – the ultimate insider. *Salmonella* virulence factors that modulate intracellular survival. *Cellular Microbiology* 11, 1579–1586.

Jack, E.J. (1968) *Salmonella abortus ovis* – an atypical *Salmonella* serovar. *Veterinary Record* 82, 558.

Jepson, M.A., Kenny, B. and Leard, A.D. (2001) Role of sipA in the early stages of *Salmonella typhimurium* entry into epithelial cells. *Cellular Microbiology* 3, 417–426.

Joiner, K.A., Hammer, C.H., Brown, E.J., Cole, R.J. and Frank, M.M. (1982a) Studies on the mechanism of bacterial resistance to complement-mediated killing. I. Terminal complement components are deposited and released from *Salmonella minnesota* S218 without causing bacterial death. *Journal of Experimental Medicine* 155, 797–808.

Joiner, K.A., Hammer, C.H., Brown, E.J. and Frank, M.M. (1982b) Studies on the mechanism of bacterial resistance to complement-mediated killing. II. C8 and C9 release C5b67 from the surface of *Salmonella minnesota* S218 because the terminal complex does not insert into the bacterial outer membrane. *Journal of Experimental Medicine* 155, 809–819.

Joiner, K.A., Ganz, T., Albert, J. and Rotrosen, D. (1989) The opsonizing ligand on *Salmonella typhimurium* influences incorporation of specific, but not azurophil, granule constituents into neutrophil phagosomes. *Journal of Cell Biology* 109, 2771–2782.

Jones, B.D., Lee, C.A. and Falkow, S. (1992) Invasion of *Salmonella typhimurium* is affected by the direction of flagellar rotation. *Infection and Immunity* 60, 2475–2480.

Kage, H., Takaya, A., Ohya, M. and Yamamoto, T. (2008) Coordinated regulation of expression of *Salmonella* pathogenicity island 1 and flagellar type III secretion systems by ATP-dependent ClpXP protease. *Journal of Bacteriology* 190, 2470–2478.

Kelterborn, E. (1967) *Salmonella-Species. First isolations, names and occurrence.* S. Karl-Marx-Stadt, Hirzel Verlag, Leipzig.

Khoramian-Falsafi, T., Harayama, S., Kutsukake, K. and Pechere, J.C. (1990) Effect of motility and chemotaxis on the invasion of *Salmonella typhimurium* into HeLa cells. *Microbial Pathogenesis* 9, 47–53.

Kidgell, C., Reichard, U., Wain, J., Linz, B., Torpdahl, M., Dougan, G. and Achtman, M. (2002) *Salmonella typhi*, the causative agent of typhoid fever, is approximately 50,000 years old. *Infection, Genetics and Evolution* 2, 39–45.

Kingsley, R.A. and Bäumler, A.J. (2000) Host adaptation and the emergence of infectious disease: the *Salmonella* paradigm. *Molecular Microbiology* 36, 1006–1014.

Klugman, K.P., Gilbertson, I.T., Koornhof, H.J., Robbins, J.B., Schneerson, R., Schulz, D., Cadoz, M. and Armand, J. (1987) Protective activity of Vi capsular polysaccharide vaccine against typhoid fever. *Lancet* 2, 1165–1169.

Kossack, R.E., Guerrant, R.L., Densen, P., Schadelin, J. and Mandell, G.L. (1981) Diminished neutrophil oxidative metabolism after phagocytosis of virulent *Salmonella typhi. Infection and Immunity* 31, 674–678.

Kraus, M.D., Amatya, B. and Kimula, Y. (1999) Histopathology of typhoid enteritis: morphologic and immunophenotypic findings. *Modern Pathology* 12, 949–955.

Lawley, T.D., Bouley, D.M., Hoy, Y.E., Gerke, C., Relman, D.A. and Monack, D.M. (2008) Host transmission of *Salmonella enterica* serovar Typhimurium is controlled by virulence factors and indigenous intestinal microbiota. *Infection and Immunity* 76, 403–416.

Le Minor, L. and Popoff, M.Y. (1987) Designation of *Salmonella enterica* sp. nov., nom. rev., as the type and only species of the genus *Salmonella*. *International Journal of Systematic and Evolutionary Microbiology* 37, 465–468.

Lee, C.A., Jones, B.D. and Falkow, S. (1992) Identification of a *Salmonella typhimurium* invasion locus by selection for hyperinvasive mutants. *Proceedings of the National Academy of Sciences of the United States of America* 89, 1847–1851.

Levitt, M.D., Furne, J., Springfield, J., Suarez, F. and Demaster, E. (1999) Detoxification of hydrogen sulfide and methanethiol in the cecal mucosa. *Journal of Clinical Investigation* 104, 1107–1114.

Li, J., Ochman, H., Groisman, E.A., Boyd, E.F., Solomon, F., Nelson, K. and Selander, R.K. (1995) Relationship between evolutionary rate and cellular location among the Inv/Spa invasion proteins of *Salmonella enterica*. *Proceedings of the National Academy of Sciences of the United States of America* 92, 7252–7256.

Li, S., Boackle, S.A., Holers, V.M., Lambris, J.D. and Blatteis, C.M. (2005) Complement component c5a is integral to the febrile response of mice to lipopolysaccharide. *Neuroimmunomodulation* 12, 67–80.

Libby, S.J., Lesnick, M., Hasegawa, P., Weidenhammer, E. and Guiney, D.G. (2000) The *Salmonella* virulence plasmid *spv* genes are required for cytopathology in human monocyte-derived macrophages. *Cellular Microbiology* 2, 49–58.

Libby, S.J., Lesnick, M., Hasegawa, P., Kurth, M., Belcher, C., Fierer, J. and Guiney, D.G. (2002) Characterization of the spv locus in *Salmonella enterica* serovar Arizona. *Infection and Immunity* 70, 3290–3294.

Liu, S.L., Ezaki, T., Miura, H., Matsui, K. and Yabuuchi, E. (1988) Intact motility as a *Salmonella* typhi invasion-related factor. *Infection and Immunity* 56, 1967–1973.

Looney, R.J. and Steigbigel, R.T. (1986) Role of the Vi antigen of *Salmonella typhi* in resistance to host defense in vitro. *Journal of Laboratory and Clinical Medicine* 108, 506–516.

Lucas, R.L., Lostroh, C.P., Dirusso, C.C., Spector, M.P., Wanner, B.L. and Lee, C.A. (2000) Multiple factors independently regulate hilA and invasion gene expression in *Salmonella enterica* serovar *typhimurium*. *Journal of Bacteriology* 182, 1872–1882.

MacLennan, C., Fieschi, C., Lammas, D.A., Picard, C., Dorman, S.E., Sanal, O., MacLennan, J.M., Holland, S.M., Ottenhoff, T.H., Casanova, J.L. and Kumararatne, D.S. (2004) Interleukin (IL)-12 and IL-23 are key cytokines for immunity against *Salmonella* in humans. *Journal of Infectious Diseases* 190, 1755–1757.

Macnab, R.M. (2004) Type III flagellar protein export and flagellar assembly. *Biochimica et Biophysica Acta* 1694, 207–217.

Main-Hester, K.L., Colpitts, K.M., Thomas, G.A., Fang, F.C. and Libby, S.J. (2008) Coordinate regulation of *Salmonella* pathogenicity island 1 (SPI1) and SPI4 in *Salmonella enterica* serovar Typhimurium. *Infection and Immunity* 76, 1024–1035.

Mastroeni, P. (2002) Immunity to systemic *Salmonella* infections. *Current Molecular Medicine* 2, 393–406.

McClelland, M., Sanderson, K.E., Spieth, J., Clifton, S.W., Latreille, P., Courtney, L., Porwollik, S., Ali, J., Dante, M., Du, F., Hou, S., Layman, D., Leonard, S., Nguyen, C., Scott, K., Holmes, A., Grewal, N., Mulvaney, E., Ryan, E., Sun, H., Florea, L., Miller, W., Stoneking, T., Nhan, M., Waterston, R. and Wilson, R.K. (2001) Complete genome sequence of *Salmonella enterica* serovar Typhimurium LT2. *Nature* 413, 852–856.

McGhie, E.J., Hayward, R.D. and Koronakis, V. (2001) Cooperation between actin-binding proteins of invasive *Salmonella*: SipA potentiates SipC nucleation and bundling of actin. *The EMBO Journal* 20, 2131–2139.

McGovern, V.J. and Slavutin, L.J. (1979) Pathology of salmonella colitis. *American Journal of Surgical Pathology* 3, 483–490.

Miao, E.A., Leaf, I.A., Treuting, P.M., Mao, D.P., Dors, M., Sarkar, A., Warren, S.E., Wewers, M.D. and Aderem, A. (2010) Caspase-1-induced pyroptosis is an innate immune effector mechanism against intracellular bacteria. *Nature Immunology* 11, 1136–1142.

Miller, R.M., Garbus, J. and Hornick, R.B. (1972) Lack of enhanced oxygen consumption by polymorphonuclear leucocytes on phagocytosis of virulent *Salmonella typhi*. *Science* 175, 1010–1011.

Mills, D.M., Bajaj, V. and Lee, C.A. (1995) A 40kb chromosomal fragment encoding *Salmonella typhimurium* invasion genes is absent from the corresponding region of the *Escherichia coli* K-12 chromosome. *Molecular Microbiology* 15, 749–759.

Mirold, S., Rabsch, W., Rohde, M., Stender, S., Tschäpe, H., Russmann, H., Igwe, E. and Hardt, W.D. (1999) Isolation of a temperate bacteriophage encoding the type III effector protein SopE from an epidemic *Salmonella typhimurium* strain. *Proceedings of the National Academy of Sciences of the United States of America* 96, 9845–9850.

Mirold, S., Ehrbar, K., Weissmuller, A., Prager, R., Tschäpe, H., Russmann, H. and Hardt, W.D. (2001) *Salmonella* host cell invasion emerged by acquisition of a mosaic of separate genetic elements, including *Salmonella* pathogenicity island 1 (SPI1), SPI5, and sopE2. *Journal of Bacteriology* 183, 2348–2358.

Mukawi, T.J. (1978) Histopathological study of typhoid perforation of the small intestines. *Southeast Asian Journal of Tropical Medicine and Public Health* 9, 252–255.

Muller, L. (1923) Un nouveau milieu d'enrichissement pour la recherche du Bacille Typhique at Paratyphique. *Comptes Rendus des Seances de la Societe de Biologie et de ses Filiales* 89, 434–437.

Müller-Eberhard, H.J. (1986) The membrane attack complex of complement. *Annual Review of Immunology* 4, 503–528.

Murphy, T.F. and Gorbach, S.L. (1982) *Salmonella* colitis. *New York State Journal of Medicine* 82, 1236–1238.

Nair, S., Alokam, S., Kothapalli, S., Porwollik, S., Proctor, E., Choy, C., McClelland, M., Liu, S.L. and Sanderson, K.E. (2004) *Salmonella enterica* serovar Typhi strains from which SPI7, a 134-kilobase island with genes for Vi exopolysaccharide and other functions, has been deleted. *Journal of Bacteriology* 186, 3214–3223.

Nasrallah, S.M. and Nassar, V.H. (1978) Enteric fever: a clinicopathologic study of 104 cases. *American Journal of Gastroenterology* 69, 63–69.

Nguyen, Q.C., Everest, P., Tran, T.K., House, D., Murch, S., Parry, C., Connerton, P., Phan, V.B., To, S.D., Mastroeni, P., White, N.J., Tran, T.H., Vo, V.H., Dougan, G., Farrar, J.J. and Wain, J. (2004) A clinical, microbiological, and pathological study of intestinal perforation associated with typhoid fever. *Clinical Infectious Diseases* 39, 61–67.

Nielsen, L.R., Schukken, Y.H., Grohn, Y.T. and Ersboll, A.K. (2004) *Salmonella* Dublin infection in dairy cattle: risk factors for becoming a carrier. *Preventive Veterinary Medicine* 65, 47–62.

Noriega, L.M., van der Auwera, P., Daneau, D., Meunier, F. and Aoun, M. (1994) *Salmonella* infections in a cancer center. *Supportive Care in Cancer* 2, 116–122.

Noubir, S., Hmama, Z. and Reiner, N.E. (2004) Dual receptors and distinct pathways mediate interleukin-1 receptor-associated kinase degradation in response to lipopolysaccharide. Involvement of CD14/TLR4, CR3, and phosphatidylinositol 3-kinase. *Journal of Biological Chemistry* 279, 25189–25195.

Ochman, H. and Groisman, E.A. (1996) Distribution of pathogenicity islands in *Salmonella* spp. *Infection and Immunity* 64, 5410–5412.

Ochman, H., Soncini, F.C., Solomon, F. and Groisman, E.A. (1996) Identification of a pathogenicity island for *Salmonella* survival in host cells. *Proceedings of the National Academy of Sciences of the United States of America* 93, 7800–7804.

Okuonghae, H.O., Nwankwo, M.U. and Offor, E.C. (1993) Pattern of bacteraemia in febrile children with sickle cell anaemia. *Annals of Tropical Paediatrics* 13, 55–64.

Olsen, S.J., Bleasdale, S.C., Magnano, A.R., Landrigan, C., Holland, B.H., Tauxe, R.V., Mintz, E.D. and Luby, S. (2003) Outbreaks of typhoid fever in the United States, 1960-99. *Epidemiology and Infection* 130, 13–21.

Otto, H., Tezcan-Merdol, D., Girisch, R., Haag, F., Rhen, M. and Koch-Nolte, F. (2000) The spvB gene-product of the *Salmonella enterica* virulence plasmid is a mono(ADP-ribosyl)transferase. *Molecular Microbiology* 37, 1106–1115.

Ouellette, A.J. (2006) Paneth cell alpha-defensin synthesis and function. *Current Topics in Microbiology and Immunology* 306, 1–25.

Parkhill, J., Dougan, G., James, K.D., Thomson, N.R., Pickard, D., Wain, J., Churcher, C., Mungall, K.L., Bentley, S.D., Holden, M.T., Sebaihia, M., Baker, S., Basham, D., Brooks, K., Chillingworth, T., Connerton, P., Cronin, A., Davis, P., Davies, R.M., Dowd, L., White, N., Farrar, J., Feltwell, T., Hamlin, N., Haque, A., Hien, T.T., Holroyd, S., Jagels, K., Krogh, A., Larsen, T.S., Leather, S., Moule, S., O'Gaora, P., Parry, C., Quail, M., Rutherford, K., Simmonds, M., Skelton, J., Stevens, K., Whitehead, S. and Barrell, B.G. (2001) Complete genome sequence of a multiple drug resistant *Salmonella enterica* serovar Typhi CT18. *Nature* 413, 848–852.

Perera, P.Y., Mayadas, T.N., Takeuchi, O., Akira, S., Zaks-Zilberman, M., Goyert, S.M. and Vogel, S.N. (2001) CD11b/CD18 acts in concert with CD14 and Toll-like receptor (TLR) 4 to elicit full lipopolysaccharide and taxol-inducible gene expression. *Journal of Immunology* 166, 574–581.

Perlik, V., Li, Z., Goorha, S., Ballou, L.R. and Blatteis, C.M. (2005) LPS-activated complement, not LPS per se, triggers the early release of PGE2 by Kupffer cells. *American Journal of Physiology. Regulatory, Integrative and Comparative Physiology* 289, R332–R339.

Perrin, G., Saurat, P. and Verge, J. (1950) New aspects of infection of Equidae by *Salmonella* abortus equi. *Recueil de médecine vétérinaire* 126, 321–328.

Pollack, J.R. and Neilands, J.B. (1970) Enterobactin, an iron transport compound from *Salmonella typhimurium*. *Biochemical and Biophysical Research Communications* 38, 989–992.

Pollack, J.R., Ames, B.N. and Neilands, J.B. (1970) Iron transport in *Salmonella typhimurium:* Mutants blocked in the biosynthesis of enterobactin. *Journal of Bacteriology* 104, 635–639.

Pullinger, G.D., Paulin, S.M., Charleston, B., Watson, P.R., Bowen, A.J., Dziva, F., Morgan, E., Villarreal-Ramos, B., Wallis, T.S. and Stevens, M.P. (2007) Systemic translocation of *Salmonella enterica* serovar Dublin in cattle occurs predominantly via efferent lymphatics in a cell-free niche and requires type III secretion system 1 (T3SS-1) but not T3SS-2. *Infection and Immunity* 75, 5191–5199.

Rabsch, W., Tschäpe, H. and Bäumler, A.J. (2001) Non-typhoidal salmonellosis: emerging problems. *Microbes and Infection/Institut Pasteur* 3, 237–247.

Rabsch, W., Andrews, H.L., Kingsley, R.A., Prager, R., Tschäpe, H., Adams, L.G. and Bäumler, A.J. (2002) *Salmonella enterica* serotype Typhimurium and its host-adapted variants. *Infection and Immunity* 70, 2249–2255.

Raffatellu, M., Chessa, D., Wilson, R.P., Dusold, R., Rubino, S. and Bäumler, A.J. (2005a) The Vi capsular antigen of *Salmonella enterica* serotype Typhi reduces Toll-like receptor-dependent interleukin-8 expression in the intestinal mucosa. *Infection and Immunity* 73, 3367–3374.

Raffatellu, M., Wilson, R.P., Chessa, D., Andrews-Polymenis, H., Tran, Q.T., Lawhon, S., Khare, S., Adams, L.G. and Bäumler, A.J. (2005b) SipA, SopA, SopB, SopD and SopE2 contribute to *Salmonella enterica* serotype Typhimurium invasion of epithelial cells. *Infection and Immunity* 73, 146–154.

Raffatellu, M., Chessa, D., Wilson, R.P., Tukel, C., Akcelik, M. and Bäumler, A.J. (2006) Capsule-mediated immune evasion: a new hypothesis explaining aspects of typhoid fever pathogenesis. *Infection and Immunity* 74, 19–27.

Raffatellu, M., Santos, R.L., Chessa, D., Wilson, R.P., Winter, S.E., Rossetti, C.A., Lawhon, S.D., Chu, H., Lau, T., Bevins, C.L., Adams, L.G. and Bäumler, A.J. (2007) The capsule encoding viaB locus reduces IL-17 expression and mucosal innate responses in the bovine intestinal mucosa during infection with *Salmonella enterica* serotype Typhi. *Infection and Immunity* 75, 4342–4350.

Raffatellu, M., Santos, R.L., Verhoeven, D.E., George, M.D., Wilson, R.P., Winter, S.E., Godinez, I., Sankaran, S., Paixao, T.A., Gordon, M.A., Kolls, J.K., Dandekar, S. and Bäumler, A.J. (2008a) Simian immunodeficiency virus-induced mucosal interleukin-17 deficiency promotes *Salmonella* dissemination from the gut. *Nature Medicine* 14, 421–428.

Raffatellu, M., Wilson, R.P., Winter, S.E. and Bäumler, A.J. (2008b) Clinical pathogenesis of typhoid fever. *Journal of Infection in Developing Countries* 2, 260–266.

Raffatellu, M., George, M.D., Akiyama, Y., Hornsby, M.J., Nuccio, S.P., Paixao, T.A., Butler, B.P., Chu, H., Santos, R.L., Berger, T., Mak, T.W., Tsolis, R.M., Bevins, C.L., Solnick, J.V., Dandekar, S. and Bäumler, A.J. (2009) Lipocalin-2 resistance confers an advantage to *Salmonella enterica* serotype Typhimurium for growth and survival in the inflamed intestine. *Cell Host & Microbe* 5, 476–486.

Ramu, P., Tanskanen, R., Holmberg, M., Lahteenmaki, K., Korhonen, T.K. and Meri, S. (2007) The surface protease PgtE of *Salmonella enterica* affects complement activity by proteolytically cleaving C3b, C4b and C5. *FEBS Letters* 581, 1716–1720.

Reeves, M.W., Evins, G.M., Heiba, A.A., Plikaytis, B.D. and Farmer III, J.J. (1989) Clonal nature of *Salmonella typhi* and its genetic relatedness to other salmonellae as shown by multilocus enzyme electrophoresis, and proposal of *Salmonella bongori* comb. nov. *Journal of Clinical Microbiology* 27, 313–320.

Reynolds, D.J., Morgan, J.H., Chanter, N., Jones, P.W., Bridger, J.C., Debney, T.G. and Bunch, K.J. (1986) Microbiology of calf diarrhoea in southern Britain. *Veterinary Record* 119, 34–39.

Robbins, J.D. and Robbins, J.B. (1984) Reexamination of the protective role of the capsular polysaccharide (Vi antigen) of *Salmonella typhi*. *Journal of Infectious Diseases* 150, 436–449.

Ross, G.D. (1986) Clinical and laboratory features of patients with an inherited deficiency of neutrophil membrane complement receptor type 3 (CR3) and the related membrane antigens LFA-1 and p150, 95. *Journal of Clinical Immunology* 6, 107–113.

Rotger, R. and Casadesus, J. (1999) The virulence plasmids of *Salmonella*. *International Microbiology* 2, 177–184.

Sahu, A., Kozel, T.R. and Pangburn, M.K. (1994) Specificity of the thioester-containing reactive site of human C3 and its significance to complement activation. *Biochemical Journal* 302, 429–436.

Salmon, D.E. and Smith, T. (1885) Report on Swine Plague. United States Department of Agriculture, Washington, DC.

Santos, R.L. and Bäumler, A.J. (2004) Cell tropism of *Salmonella enterica*. *International Journal of Medical Microbiology* 294, 225–233.

Santos, R.L., Zhang, S., Tsolis, R.M., Bäumler, A.J. and Adams, L.G. (2002) Morphologic and molecular characterization of *Salmonella typhimurium* infection in neonatal calves. *Veterinary Pathology* 39, 200–215.

Santos, R.L., Raffatellu, M., Bevins, C.L., Adams, L.G., Tukel, C., Tsolis, R.M. and Bäumler, A.J. (2009) Life in the inflamed intestine, *Salmonella* style. *Trends in Microbiology* 17, 498–506.

Saphra, I. and Wassermann, M. (1954) *Salmonella cholerae suis:* a clinical and epidemiological evaluation of 329 infections identified between 1940 and 1954 in the New York *Salmonella* Center. *American Journal of the Medical Sciences* 228, 525–533.

Schmitt, C.K., Ikeda, J.S., Darnell, S.C., Watson, P.R., Bispham, J., Wallis, T.S., Weinstein, D.L., Metcalf, E.S. and O'Brien, A.D. (2001) Absence of all components of the flagellar export and synthesis machinery differentially alters virulence of *Salmonella enterica* serovar Typhimurium in models of typhoid fever, survival in macrophages, tissue culture invasiveness, and calf enterocolitis. *Infection and Immunity* 69, 5619–5625.

Shivaprasad, H.L. (2000) Fowl typhoid and pullorum disease. *Revue Scientifique et Technique (International Office of Epizootics)* 19, 405–424.

Snyder, D.S., Gibson, D., Heiss, C., Kay, W. and Azadi, P. (2006) Structure of a capsular polysaccharide isolated from *Salmonella enteritidis*. *Carbohydrate Research* 341, 2388–2397.

Sprinz, H., Gangarosa, E.J., Williams, M., Hornick, R.B. and Woodward, T.E. (1966) Histopathology of the upper small intestines in typhoid fever. Biopsy study of experimental disease in man. *American Journal of Digestive Diseases* 11, 615–624.

Stecher, B. and Hardt, W.D. (2008) The role of microbiota in infectious disease. *Trends in Microbiology* 16, 107–114.

Stecher, B., Hapfelmeier, S., Muller, C., Kremer, M., Stallmach, T. and Hardt, W.D. (2004) Flagella and chemotaxis are required for efficient induction of *Salmonella enterica* serovar Typhimurium colitis in streptomycin-pretreated mice. *Infection and Immunity* 72, 4138–4150.

Stecher, B., Robbiani, R., Walker, A.W., Westendorf, A.M., Barthel, M., Kremer, M., Chaffron, S., MacPherson, A.J., Buer, J., Parkhill, J., Dougan, G., von Mering, C. and Hardt, W.D. (2007) *Salmonella enterica* serovar *typhimurium* exploits inflammation to compete with the intestinal microbiota. *PLoS Biology* 5, 2177–2189.

Stecher, B., Barthel, M., Schlumberger, M.C., Haberli, L., Rabsch, W., Kremer, M. and Hardt, W.D. (2008) Motility allows *S.* Typhimurium to benefit from the mucosal defence. *Cellular Microbiology* 10, 1166–1180.

Tacket, C.O., Ferreccio, C., Robbins, J.B., Tsai, C.M., Schulz, D., Cadoz, M., Goudeau, A. and Levine, M.M. (1986) Safety and immunogenicity of two *Salmonella* typhi Vi capsular polysaccharide vaccines. *Journal of Infectious Diseases* 154, 342–345.

Tauber, A.I., Borregaard, N., Simons, E. and Wright, J. (1983) Chronic granulomatous disease: a syndrome of phagocyte oxidase deficiencies. *Medicine (Baltimore)* 62, 286–309.

Tezcan-Merdol, D., Nyman, T., Lindberg, U., Haag, F., Koch-Nolte, F. and Rhen, M. (2001) Actin is ADP-ribosylated by the *Salmonella enterica* virulence-associated protein SpvB. *Molecular Microbiology* 39, 606–619.

Tezcan-Merdol, D., Engstrand, L. and Rhen, M. (2005) *Salmonella enterica* SpvB-mediated ADP-ribosylation as an activator for host cell actin degradation. *International Journal of Medical Microbiology* 295, 201–212.

Thijs, I.M., de Keersmaecker, S.C., Fadda, A., Engelen, K., Zhao, H., McClelland, M., Marchal, K. and Vanderleyden, J. (2007) Delineation of the *Salmonella enterica* serovar Typhimurium HilA regulon through genome-wide location and transcript analysis. *Journal of Bacteriology* 189, 4587–4596.

Thomson, N.R., Clayton, D.J., Windhorst, D., Vernikos, G., Davidson, S., Churcher, C., Quail, M.A., Stevens, M., Jones, M.A., Watson, M., Barron, A., Layton, A., Pickard, D., Kingsley, R.A., Bignell, A., Clark, L., Harris, B., Ormond, D., Abdellah, Z., Brooks, K., Cherevach, I., Chillingworth, T., Woodward, J., Norberczak, H., Lord, A., Arrowsmith, C., Jagels, K., Moule, S., Mungall, K., Sanders, M., Whitehead, S., Chabalgoity, J.A., Maskell, D., Humphrey, T., Roberts, M., Barrow, P.A., Dougan, G. and Parkhill, J. (2008) Comparative genome analysis of *Salmonella* Enteritidis PT4 and *Salmonella* Gallinarum 287/91 provides insights into evolutionary and host adaptation pathways. *Genome Research* 18, 1624–1637.

Townsend, S.M., Kramer, N.E., Edwards, R., Baker, S., Hamlin, N., Simmonds, M., Stevens, K., Maloy, S., Parkhill, J., Dougan, G. and Bäumler, A.J. (2001) *Salmonella enterica* serotype Typhi possesses a unique repertoire of fimbrial gene sequences. *Infection and Immunity* 69, 2894–2901.

Tran, Q.T., Gomez, G., Khare, S., Lawhon, S.D., Raffatellu, M., Bäumler, A.J., Ajithdoss, D., Dhavala, S. and Adams, L.G. (2010) The *Salmonella enterica* serotype Typhi Vi capsular antigen is expressed after the bacterium enters the ileal mucosa. *Infection and Immunity* 78, 527–535.

Troelstra, A., de Graaf-Miltenburg, L.A., van Bommel, T., Verhoef, J., van Kessel, K.P. and van Strijp, J.A. (1999) Lipopolysaccharide-coated erythrocytes activate human neutrophils via CD14 while subsequent binding is through CD11b/CD18. *Journal of Immunology* 162, 4220–4225.

Tsolis, R.M., Adams, L.G., Ficht, T.A. and Bäumler, A.J. (1999a) Contribution of *Salmonella typhimurium* virulence factors to diarrheal disease in calves. *Infection and Immunity* 67, 4879–4885.

Tsolis, R.M., Townsend, S.M., Miao, E.A., Miller, S.I., Ficht, T.A., Adams, L.G. and Bäumler, A.J. (1999b) Identification of a putative *Salmonella enterica* serotype *typhimurium* host range factor with homology to IpaH and YopM by signature-tagged mutagenesis. *Infection and Immunity* 67, 6385–6393.

Tsolis, R.M., Young, G.M., Solnick, J.V. and Bäumler, A.J. (2008) From bench to bedside: stealth of enteroinvasive pathogens. *Nature Reviews Microbiology* 6, 883–892.

Tumbarello, M., Tacconelli, E., Caponera, S., Cauda, R. and Ortona, L. (1995) The impact of bacteraemia on HIV infection. Nine years experience in a large Italian university hospital. *Journal of Infection* 31, 123–131.

Turk, J.R., Fales, W.H., Maddox, C., Miller, M., Pace, L., Fischer, J., Kreeger, J., Johnson, G., Turnquist, S., Ramos, J.A. *et al.* (1992) Pneumonia associated with *Salmonella choleraesuis* infection in swine: 99 cases (1987-1990). *Journal of the American Veterinary Medical Association* 201, 1615–1616.

Uchiya, K., Barbieri, M.A., Funato, K., Shah, A.H., Stahl, P.D. and Groisman, E.A. (1999) A *Salmonella* virulence protein that inhibits cellular trafficking. *The EMBO Journal* 18, 3924–3933.

Van Asten, F.J., Hendriks, H.G., Koninkx, J.F., van der Zeijst, B.A. and Gaastra, W. (2000) Inactivation of the flagellin gene of *Salmonella enterica* serotype *enteritidis* strongly reduces invasion into differentiated Caco-2 cells. *FEMS Microbiology Letters* 185, 175–179.

Van Bruggen, R., Zweers, D., van Diepen, A., van Dissel, J.T., Roos, D., Verhoeven, A.J. and Kuijpers, T.W. (2007) Complement receptor 3 and Toll-like receptor 4 act sequentially in uptake and intracellular killing of unopsonized *Salmonella enterica* serovar Typhimurium by human neutrophils. *Infection and Immunity* 75, 2655–2660.

Vassiloyanakopoulos, A.P., Okamoto, S. and Fierer, J. (1998) The crucial role of polymorphonuclear leukocytes in resistance to *Salmonella dublin* infections in genetically susceptible and resistant mice. *Proceedings of the National Academy of Sciences of the United States of America* 95, 7676–7681.

Vazquez-Torres, A. and Fang, F.C. (2001) Oxygen-dependent anti-*Salmonella* activity of macrophages. *Trends in Microbiology* 9, 29–33.

Vazquez-Torres, A., Xu, Y., Jones-Carson, J., Holden, D.W., Lucia, S.M., Dinauer, M.C., Mastroeni, P. and Fang, F.C. (2000) *Salmonella* pathogenicity island 2-dependent evasion of the phagocyte NADPH oxidase. *Science* 287, 1655–1658.

Vernikos, G.S., Thomson, N.R. and Parkhill, J. (2007) Genetic flux over time in the *Salmonella* lineage. *Genome Biology* 8, R100.

Virlogeux, I., Waxin, H., Ecobichon, C. and Popoff, M.Y. (1995) Role of the viaB locus in synthesis, transport and expression of *Salmonella* typhi Vi antigen. *Microbiology* 141, 3039–3047.

Virlogeux, I., Waxin, H., Ecobichon, C., Lee, J.O. and Popoff, M.Y. (1996) Characterization of the *rcsA* and *rcsB* genes from *Salmonella* typhi: rcsB through tviA is involved in regulation of Vi antigen synthesis. *Journal of Bacteriology* 178, 1691–1698.

Visser, I.J., Veen, M. and van der Giessen, J.W. (1992) *Salmonella dublin* infections in cattle, a review. *Tijdschrift voor Diergeneeskunde* 117, 730–734.

Vogel, S., Hirschfeld, M.J. and Perera, P.Y. (2001) Signal integration in lipopolysaccharide (LPS)-stimulated murine macrophages. *Journal of Endotoxin Research* 7, 237–241.

Walsh, A.L., Phiri, A.J., Graham, S.M., Molyneux, E.M. and Molyneux, M.E. (2000) Bacteremia in febrile Malawian children: clinical and microbiologic features. *The Pediatric Infectious Disease Journal* 19, 312–318.

Watson, P.R., Galyov, E.E., Paulin, S.M., Jones, P.W. and Wallis, T.S. (1998) Mutation of invH, but not stn, reduces salmonella-induced enteritis in cattle. *Infection and Immunity* 66, 1432–1438.

Wilson, R.P., Raffatellu, M., Chessa, D., Winter, S.E., Tukel, C. and Bäumler, A.J. (2008) The Vi-capsule prevents Toll-like receptor 4 recognition of *Salmonella*. *Cellular Microbiology* 10, 876–890.

Winkelstein, J.A., Marino, M.C., Johnston, R.B., Jr, Boyle, J., Curnutte, J., Gallin, J.I., Malech, H.L., Holland, S.M., Ochs, H., Quie, P., Buckley, R.H., Foster, C.B., Chanock, S.J. and Dickler, H. (2000) Chronic granulomatous disease. Report on a national registry of 368 patients. *Medicine (Baltimore)* 79, 155–169.

Winter, S.E., Thiennimitr, P., Nuccio, S.P., Haneda, T., Winter, M.G., Wilson, R.P., Russell, J.M., Henry, T., Tran, Q.T., Lawhon, S.D., Gomez, G., Bevins, C.L., Russmann, H., Monack, D.M., Adams, L.G. and Bäumler, A.J. (2009a) Contribution of flagellin pattern recognition to intestinal inflammation during *Salmonella enterica* serotype *typhimurium* infection. *Infection and Immunity* 77, 1904–1916.

Winter, S.E., Winter, M.G., Thiennimitr, P., Gerriets, V.A., Nuccio, S.P., Russmann, H. and Bäumler, A.J. (2009b) The TviA auxiliary protein renders the *Salmonella enterica* serotype Typhi RcsB regulon responsive to changes in osmolarity. *Molecular Microbiology* 74, 175–193.

Winter, S.E., Keestra, A.M., Tsolis, R.M. and Bäumler, A.J. (2010a) The blessings and curses of intestinal inflammation. *Cell Host & Microbe* 8, 36–43.

Winter, S.E., Thiennimitr, P., Winter, M.G., Butler, B.P., Huseby, D.L., Crawford, R.W., Russell, J.M., Bevins, C.L., Adams, L.G., Tsolis, R.M., Roth, J.R. and Bäumler, A.J. (2010b) Gut inflammation provides a respiratory electron acceptor for *Salmonella*. *Nature* 467, 426–429.

Winter, S.E., Winter, M.G., Godinez, I., Yang, H.-J., Russmann, H., Andrews-Polymenis, H.L. and Bäumler, A.J. (2010c) A rapid change in virulence gene expression during the transition from the intestinal lumen into tissue promotes systemic dissemination of *Salmonella*. *PLoS Pathogens* 6, e10001060.

Woodward, M.J., McLaren, I. and Wray, C. (1989) Distribution of virulence plasmids within salmonellae. *Journal of General Microbiology* 135, 503–511.

Zhang, S., Santos, R.L., Tsolis, R.M., Mirold, S., Hardt, W.-D., Adams, L.G. and Bäumler, A.J. (2002a) Phage mediated horizontal transfer of the *sopE1* gene increases enteropathogenicity of *Salmonella enterica* serotype Typhimurium for calves. *FEMS Microbiology Letters* 217, 243–247.

Zhang, S., Santos, R.L., Tsolis, R.M., Stender, S., Hardt, W.-D., Bäumler, A.J. and Adams, L.G. (2002b) SipA, SopA, SopB, SopD and SopE2 act in concert to induce diarrhea in calves infected with *Salmonella enterica* serotype Typhimurium. *Infection and Immunity* 70, 3843–3855.

Zhang, S., Kingsley, R.A., Santos, R.L., Andrews-Polymenis, H., Raffatellu, M., Figueiredo, J., Nunes, J., Tsolis, R.M., Adams, L.G. and Bäumler, A.J. (2003) Molecular pathogenesis of *Salmonella enterica* serotype *typhimurium*-induced diarrhea. *Infection and Immunity* 71, 1–12.

Zhang, X., Kimura, Y., Fang, C., Zhou, L., Sfyroera, G., Lambris, J.D., Wetsel, R.A., Miwa, T. and Song, W.C. (2007) Regulation of Toll-like receptor-mediated inflammatory response by complement in vivo. *Blood* 110, 228–236.

Zhou, D., Mooseker, M.S. and Galan, J.E. (1999) Role of the S. *typhimurium* actin-binding protein SipA in bacterial internalization. *Science* 283, 2092–2095.

6 Host Genetic Susceptibility/Resistance

Pete Kaiser* and Mark Stevens
The Roslin Institute and Royal (Dick) School of Veterinary Studies, University of Edinburgh, UK

Introduction

Salmonella enterica is an animal and zoonotic pathogen of worldwide importance. Infections can result in acute enteritis to systemic typhoid fever, depending on pathogen- and host-specific factors (Stevens *et al.*, 2009). Human non-typhoidal salmonellosis is frequently acquired from food-producing animals, and an estimated 93.8 million cases and 155,000 deaths occur worldwide each year (Majowicz *et al.*, 2010). Infections tend to be self-limiting, confined to the intestines and associated with serovars with a broad host range. By contrast, host-restricted serovars typically elicit more severe systemic disease in specific hosts. For example, serovars Typhi and Paratyphi cause an estimated 21.6 million cases of human typhoid fever with a 1% fatality rate (Crump *et al.*, 2004), and other host-restricted serovars exert substantial welfare and economic costs on livestock and poultry farmers worldwide. To begin to control non-typhoidal salmonellosis in the human population, an obvious approach would be to reduce the levels of *Salmonella* colonization in animals used to produce food. The availability of complete or partial genome sequences for a range of *S. enterica* serovars and their hosts revolutionizes our ability to design more effective vaccines and to identify genes associated with host resistance. This article reviews our knowledge of the genetic basis of resistance to salmonellosis in food-producing animals toward control of zoonotic and systemic infections. We recognize that a plethora of other factors influence host susceptibility to infection, including immune status, diet, intestinal microbiota, stress and husbandry practices, but this chapter focuses on host genetics.

Resistance to *Salmonella* Infection in Chickens

Poultry meat and eggs are key sources of human non-typhoidal salmonellosis owing to the ability of selected *S. enterica* serovars to colonize the avian intestinal and reproductive tracts. Other serovars are restricted to poultry and elicit systemic disease. Indeed, devastating outbreaks of fowl typhoid and pullorum disease, caused by serovars Gallinarum and Pullorum, respectively, continue to afflict the poultry industry in many countries (reviewed in Barrow and Freitas Neto, 2011). In the European Community, regulations compel

* Corresponding author, e-mail: pete.kaiser@roslin.ed.ac.uk

© CAB International 2013. *Salmonella in Domestic Animals, 2nd Edition* (eds P.A. Barrow and U. Methner)

poultry producers to control *Salmonella* in breeders and layers (Zoonosis Directive EC/92/117). However antibiotic prophylaxis is prohibited in broilers and vaccines are not used. In this context, selection of birds with improved resistance to avian salmonellosis is desirable. Such an approach is particularly feasible with poultry, as the genetics of the vast majority of chickens reared worldwide each year are controlled by just four breeding companies. The Food and Agriculture Organization estimated that there were global stocks of 19 billion poultry in 2009; therefore enormous potential for the rational improvement of broilers and layers exists.

Studies on resistance to salmonellosis in the chicken have focused on three main models: resistance to systemic salmonellosis (whether reliant on use of host-restricted serovars or administration of ubiquitous serovars via parenteral routes or to neonatal chicks), resistance to initial intestinal colonization (typically the first few days after oral inoculation) and resistance to the long-term carrier state (often several weeks after infection; reviewed in Calenge *et al.*, 2010). As discussed below, distinct traits appear to influence resistance to avian systemic salmonellosis and intestinal colonization; however, it is unclear whether the phenotypes arising from the latter two models are separate or linked. The degree of initial colonization of a bird may affect the propensity for the carrier state, and thus it would not be surprising if, as research in this area increases, there were found to be resistance genes in common for both models.

Avian resistance to systemic salmonellosis

Differences in susceptibility to systemic avian salmonellosis have been known for many years, early work being restricted to outbred lines (Hutt and Scholes, 1941; Smith, 1956). Avian resistance to systemic salmonellosis has been studied using inbred lines of white leghorn chicken that exhibit heritable differences in resistance to oral and intravenous *S.* Typhimurium infection (Bumstead and Barrow, 1988) and oral and intramuscular inoculation with serovars Gallinarum, Pullorum or Enteritidis, implying that the resistance was expressed in the tissues post-invasion (Bumstead and Barrow, 1993). The level of resistance was in some cases profound: the intramuscular LD_{50} in a susceptible line was $\log_{10}$ <1.0 and in a resistant line was >8.0. In addition to different *Salmonella* serovars the same lines were resistant or susceptible to *Mycobacterium avium* (Barrow and Bumstead, unpublished results). As such lines differ in resistance to a range of serovars and infection routes, it could be inferred that a common resistance mechanism may exist. Resistance in such lines is autosomal, dominant, not linked to sex or major histocompatibility complex (MHC) haplotype, and is associated with control of *Salmonella* by macrophages (Wigley *et al.*, 2002) and heterophils (Swaggerty *et al.*, 2005; Redmond *et al.*, 2011). Moreover, the nature, magnitude and timing of cytokine responses of cells from such lines differ (Swaggerty *et al.*, 2004, 2006, 2008; Wigley *et al.*, 2006), and it is reasonable to assume that such responses are under genetic control. Using a first generation backcross of line 6_1 (resistant) and 15I (susceptible) birds, resistance of chicks to intravenous *S.* Typhimurium infection was linked to a ca. 2 cM locus (*SAL1*) on chromosome 5 by analysis of the segregation of 124 microsatellite markers (Mariani *et al.*, 2001). Independent studies also linked resistance to systemic salmonellosis to this region (Kaiser and Lamont, 2002; Tilquin *et al.*, 2005).

The advent of the chicken genome sequence (International Chicken Genome Sequencing Consortium, 2004), the ability to map single-nucleotide polymorphisms (SNPs) (Wong *et al.*, 2004) and ongoing genome annotation (http://www.ensembl.org/Gallus_gallus) has helped to fine map the *SAL1* locus. Analysis of SNPs spanning *SAL1* in a sixth generation congenic backcross population of line 6_1 and 15I birds has resolved the resistance-associated region to 54.0–54.8 Mb on the long arm of chromosome 5 ($F = 8.72$, $P = 0.00475$) (Fife *et al.*, 2009). This region encodes just 14 genes, including two striking candidates, *AKT1* and *SIVA1* (Fig. 6.1). Next-generation sequencing of the genomes of line 6_1 and 15I birds has revealed further variation within and proximal to these genes (Kaiser *et al.*, unpublished observations).

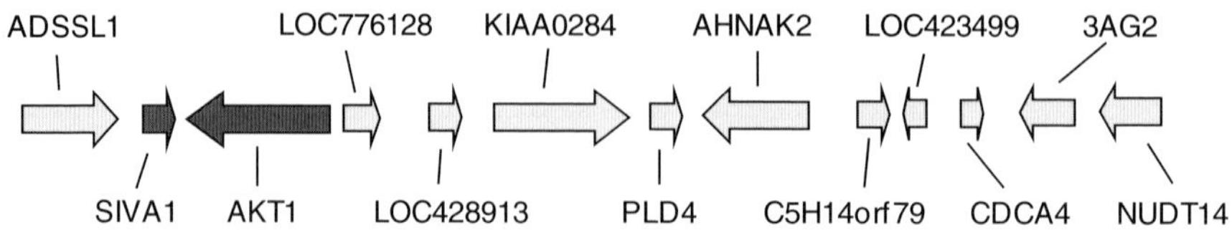

Fig. 6.1. Schematic diagram of the *SAL1* locus on chicken chromosome 5 (Fife *et al.*, 2009).

Recent analysis of SNPs associated with the ability of heterophils from advanced inter-cross chickens to control *S.* Enteritidis *ex vivo* independently associated both *AKT1* and *SIVA1* with differential resistance (Redmond *et al.*, 2011). Moreover, a case-control study of polymorphisms in a single population of outbred commercial layers exposed to a fowl typhoid outbreak in the field has independently confirmed the importance of *SAL1* polymorphisms in resistance to *S.* Gallinarum (Fife *et al.*, unpublished observations). This finding independently confirmed the importance of *SAL1* polymorphisms in resistance to *S.* Gallinarum, indicating that marker-assisted selection of protective quantitative trait loci (QTL) has the potential to protect birds against natural exposure to *Salmonella*. The mechanism by which *SAL1*-encoded alleles and particular SNPs exert their effect remains to be elucidated. *AKT1* and *SIVA1* are considered in more detail below, though it remains possible that other *SAL1*-encoded genes may contribute to the resistance observed in inbred lines and cells isolated from such lines.

AKT (also known as protein kinase B) is a serine/threonine kinase that modulates multiple processes, in particular apoptosis, cell proliferation and development (reviewed in Hers *et al.*, 2011). In humans, three isoforms exist that share similar structures but differ in tissue distribution and function. Aberrant loss or gain of AKT activation is associated with type-2 diabetes, cancer and other disorders. AKT is an excellent functional and positional candidate for resistance to systemic salmonellosis in chickens as *Salmonella*-induced activation of AKT1 protects mammalian epithelial cells from apoptosis (Knodler *et al.*, 2005). Moreover, inhibitors of AKT1 activation can eradicate intracellular *Salmonella* in a manner reversible by ectopic expression of AKT1 (Kuijl *et al.*, 2007; Chiu *et al.*, 2009). One such inhibitor (AR-12) prolonged life and reduced replication of *Salmonella* in the organs of mice (Chiu *et al.*, 2009). Another isoform in mammals, AKT2, protects mice against *Salmonella*-induced enteritis and colonization (Kum *et al.*, 2011). AKT2$^{-/-}$ mice exhibit elevated levels of *S.* Typhimurium, neutrophils and pro-inflammatory cytokines in their intestines relative to control mice (Kum *et al.*, 2011). Consistent with its role as a pro-survival kinase, *S.* Typhimurium-infected AKT2$^{-/-}$ mice had higher numbers of annexin V^{+} and terminal transferase dUTP nick-end labelling-positive (TUNEL^{+}) apoptotic cells in the intestinal mucosa (Kum *et al.*, 2011). It is noteworthy, however, that species-specific differences may exist, as no obvious homologue of AKT2 exists in the draft chicken genome sequence at the time of writing. Depending on the cell type and stage of infection, apoptosis may play both positive and negative roles in control of *Salmonella* infection (reviewed in Fink and Cookson, 2007). For example, *S.* Typhimurium requires caspase-1 to colonize the murine intestines and translocate to visceral organs (Monack *et al.*, 2000), yet caspase-1-dependent pro-inflammatory cell death (pyroptosis) is considered an effective means of control of intracellular bacterial pathogens by effector cells of the innate response (Miao *et al.*, 2010). Further studies are therefore needed to evaluate whether the nature and frequency of apoptosis differs in inbred lines that differ in resistance to systemic salmonellosis.

At a cellular level, AKT1 may facilitate intracellular net replication of *Salmonella* not only by promoting host cell survival, but by modulating bacterial entry and maturation of the *Salmonella*-containing vacuole (SCV).

AKT1 is activated at the plasma membrane by the *Salmonella* type III secreted effector SopB (also known as SigD), which exhibits phosphoinositide phosphatase activity (Steele-Mortimer *et al.*, 2000; Patel *et al.*, 2009). SopB promotes rearrangements of subcortical actin and membrane fission during bacterial entry (Terebiznik *et al.*, 2002) and inhibits SCV-lysosome fusion (Hernandez *et al.*, 2004). Analysis of the impact of AKT1 inhibitors on these processes indicated that activated AKT1 targets the kinase PAK4, which in turn modulates the activity of a guanine nucleotide exchange factor that controls RhoA and Rac1 GTPases involved in actin assembly (Kuijl *et al.*, 2007). Activated AKT1 also phosphorylates the GTPase-activating protein AS160, preventing its recruitment to phagosome membranes leading to activation of RAB14, which in turn inhibits SCV-lysosome fusion (Kuijl *et al.*, 2007). The importance of SopB-mediated activation of AKT during *Salmonella* infection is evidenced by the fact that $AKT2^{-/-}$ and control mice show comparable resistance to *Salmonella*-induced enteritis and colonization by a *sopB* null mutant (Kum *et al.*, 2011). One may predict that if AKT polymorphisms explain the differential resistance of inbred lines, a *sopB* mutant incapable of activating AKT would colonize the organs of such lines to a comparable extent. Given the potential for AKT to modulate the intracellular fate of *Salmonella*, research is needed to define whether bacterial trafficking and net intracellular replication differ between birds that vary in resistance. The advent of novel fluorescence-based methods to follow *Salmonella* net replication in individual cells and tissues holds promise in this regard (Helaine *et al.*, 2010).

SIVA1 is encoded adjacent to AKT1 and is a pro-apoptotic factor that binds the cytoplasmic tail of CD27 (a member of the tumour necrosis factor receptor superfamily) and induces cell death via a caspase-dependent pathway in human and murine cells (Py *et al.*, 2004; Prasad *et al.*, 1997). SIVA1 also binds to Bcl-x(L) and Bcl2 and inhibits their anti-apoptotic activity (Xue *et al.*, 2002; Chu *et al.*, 2004). SIVA1 also associates with (and may be phosphorylated by) non-receptor tyrosine kinases such as ABL1 in the apoptotic response to reactive oxygen species (Cao *et al.*, 2001). It has been proposed that differences in the expression or function of SIVA1 in the progeny of advanced inter-cross chicken lines may explain differences in the ability of heterophils from such birds to release heterophil extracellular traps (HETs) via an apoptosis-like pathway (Redmond *et al.*, 2011). No evidence yet exists that SIVA1 is expressed in heterophils (or the mammalian equivalent, the neutrophil), that it influences HET formation, or that HETs control *Salmonella* infection *in vivo*. SIVA1 can also inhibit activation of NF-κB (Gudi *et al.*, 2006) whereas AKT1 can activate NF-κB by regulation of I-κB kinase (Madrid *et al.*, 2000). Such regulation may be significant in *SAL1*-mediated resistance, as cells from inbred lines differ in the timing and magnitude of cytokine responses to *Salmonella* (Wigley *et al.*, 2006).

Several other intracellular bacterial pathogens are believed to activate AKT to delay apoptosis and support net replication, including *Mycobacterium tuberculosis* (Kuijl *et al.*, 2007), *Coxiella burnetii* (Voth and Heinzen, 2009) and *Chlamydia trachomatis* (Verbeke *et al.*, 2006). AKT1 also aids entry of avian leukosis viruses (Feng *et al.*, 2011), delays apoptosis and induces inflammation during avian reovirus infection (Lin *et al.*, 2010) and supports replication of infectious bursal disease virus (Wei *et al.*, 2011). Induction of a SIVA1-dependent apoptotic pathway has been reported to support influenza A virus infection (Shiozaki *et al.*, 2011). In selecting for resistance associated with *SAL1*, potential therefore exists to improve control of a range of poultry diseases; however, researchers must be alert to the potential for deleterious effects on resistance to other avian pathogens since there was no correlation between the resistance of different lines to *Salmonella* and to other pathogens including *Escherichia coli*, *Eimeria* spp. and viruses such as infectious bronchitis and infectious bursal disease (Bumstead *et al.*, 1991).

Early studies on resistance to systemic salmonellosis in inbred white leghorn chicken lines (Bumstead and Barrow, 1988, 1993) also identified linkage with chicken NRAMP1 (natural resistance-associated macrophage protein 1, also known as SLC11A1) and Toll-like receptor 4 (TLR4) (Hu *et al.*, 1997), both of which have been implicated in resistance in murine typhoid models (reviewed in Dougan *et al.*, 2011). These two loci accounted for 33% of the differences in early resistance to systemic *S.* Typhimurium infection observed between the inbred lines Wl and C. However, there were no polymorphisms in NRAMP1 between other inbred lines which differed greatly in resistance to systemic salmonellosis.

Avian resistance to early intestinal colonization

Oral infection of 6-week-old inbred lines, which had been inoculated with a standardized gut flora within 24 h of hatching, with *S.* Typhimurium indicated a heritable difference in extent of colonization within days of infection. The increased resistance was dominant and not sex-linked. It was not related to any inhibitory effect of the flora and there was no correlation with resistance to systemic infection mediated by the *SAL1* locus or to MHC or *NRAMP1*. Resistant lines had significantly higher numbers of circulating heterophils (Barrow *et al.*, 2003). The same lines also showed increased resistance to colonization by *Campylobacter jejuni* (Boyd *et al.*, 2005). Several studies have sought to associate resistance to early intestinal colonization with polymorphisms in candidate genes.

Among the candidate genes significantly associated with caecal load 7 days after oral inoculation of 3-week-old chickens with *S.* Enteritidis were those encoding SLC11A1, inhibitor of apoptosis protein 1 (IAP1), prosaposin (PSAP), caspase-1 (CASP1), inducible nitric oxide production (iNOS), interleukin-2 (IL-2), immunoglobulin light chain (IGL), and transforming growth factors-β2 and -β4 (TGF-β2 and -β4) (Kramer *et al.*, 2003). In the same study, SLC11A1, CASP1, IL-2, IGL and TGF-β4 were also associated with the bacterial load in the liver, whereas TGF-β3 was associated with the splenic load of *S.* Enteritidis (Kramer *et al.*, 2003). Polymorphisms affecting the genes encoding avian β-defensins clustered on chicken chromosome 3, including *AvBD3, AvBD11, AvBD12* and *AvBD13,* have also been associated with caecal bacterial load in chickens orally infected with *S.* Enteritidis, while *AvBD5* was associated with spleen bacterial load (Hasenstein and Lamont, 2007). Genetic variation in *TRAIL, TGFβ3, CD28, MD-2, IL-10* and *MAPKAPK2* has also been associated with caecal and/or splenic bacterial load (Malek and Lamont, 2003; Malek *et al.*, 2004; Ghebremicael *et al.*, 2008) and the *TLR4* gene has been linked to resistance to infection with *S.* Typhimurium in chickens (Leveque *et al.*, 2003). The MHC complex has been associated with the antibody response to *S.* Enteritidis vaccine (Zhou and Lamont, 2003).

As with studies on the genetic basis of avian resistance to systemic salmonellosis, inbred lines of chicken, and crosses between such, have proven useful in mapping QTL associated with intestinal colonization. Unlike previous studies that used a candidate gene approach or low density genome-wide screens, a recent study with a backcross experimental design on the inbred chicken lines 6_1 (resistant) and N (susceptible) exploited 1255 high-density genome-wide SNP markers to identify QTL associated with resistance to initial caecal colonization by *S.* Typhimurium (Fife *et al.*, 2011). Analysis of log transformed caecal bacterial levels between the parental lines revealed a significant difference on all 4 days post-infection ($P<0.05$). Analysis of the genotypes of the backcross (F1 × N) population ($n=288$) revealed four QTL on chromosomes 2, 3, 12 and 25 for the two traits examined in the study: log transformed bacterial counts in the caeca and presence of a hardened caseous caecal core. These two traits were selected as the highest numbers of bacteria in chickens orally infected with *S.* Typhimurium are typically found in the caeca (Barrow *et al.*, 1987) and the presence of caseous cores in the caeca is an indication of the severity of inflammation of the caeca, or typhlitis (Wray *et al.*, 1996). Among the four QTL identified in this study was one genome-wide significant QTL on chromosome 2 at 20 Mb and three additional QTL, on chromosomes 3, 12 and 25 at 96 Mb, 15 Mb and 1 Mb, respectively, which were significant at the chromosome wide level ($P<0.05$).

In a previous independent study on a line 6_1 and N backcross, a QTL associated with *S*. Enteritidis gut colonization was identified on chromosome 2 at 22.6 Mb (Tilquin *et al*., 2005; Calenge *et al*., 2009). Fife *et al*. (2011) identified a QTL associated with the presence of hardened caseous caecal cores on chromosome 2 at 20 Mb, thus confirming a locus with effects on *Salmonella* gut colonization levels and severity at this location. The innate immune genes for myeloid differentiation primary response 88 (MyD88) and interleukin-6 (IL-6) genes are located on chromosome 2 at 4.7 Mb and 30.9 Mb, respectively. However, since the QTL peak with a 1-LOD drop ranges from 12.8 to 22.3 Mb (Fife *et al*., 2011), these genes, located outside this range, are unlikely to contribute to the QTL. The gene for neuropilin-1 precursor (NRP1), which acts as a membrane-bound co-receptor to a tyrosine kinase receptor for both vascular endothelial growth factor (VEGF) and semaphorin, at 13.8 Mb lies within the 1-LOD drop peak (12.8–22.3 Mb). Whether this is the causative gene for this QTL merits further investigation. The lack of significance at this QTL for bacterial levels in the caeca may be indicative of a role for the QTL in disease severity as a trait, rather than the magnitude of bacterial colonization.

A QTL associated with caecal levels of *S*. Typhimurium was also identified on chromosome 3 with a peak centred at 96 Mb and ranging from 88.4 to 108.3 Mb (1-LOD drop). Several genes involved in innate immunity are located just outside the 1-LOD drop range: IL-17A and IL-17F are at 110.36 and 110.37 Mb respectively; and AvBD1–14 are located between 110.2 and 110.27 Mb. Analyses of polymorphism in AvBD3, 5, 11, 12 and 13 have previously shown associations with *Salmonella* load in poultry (Hasenstein *et al*., 2006; Hasenstein and Lamont, 2007). No previous QTL or candidate genes were identified under the peaks for the QTL on chromosomes 12 and 25.

Although these QTL show significance at either the genome-wide or chromosome-wide level, the resolution is insufficient to accurately identify the causative genes. The ranges of the QTL are 19.9 Mb on chromosome 3, 9.5 Mb on chromosome 2 and 5.7 Mb on chromosome 12. The true location of the gene(s) responsible for resistance to *Salmonella* colonization will only become apparent when additional recombination is introduced in order to break down the extensive linkage disequilibrium (LD) present in these layer lines (Aerts *et al*., 2007). This may be accomplished with additional backcrossing of the lines, or with the use of advanced inter-cross lines (AIL) or outbred populations to fine map the resistance QTL. It is noteworthy that a number of the QTL identified in populations derived from crosses between lines 6_1 and N have also been associated with resistance to intestinal colonization by *Salmonella* in commercial birds (Tilquin *et al*., 2005; Calenge *et al*., 2009).

Avian resistance to the carrier state

From a food safety viewpoint, resistance to the carrier state is a key trait for selective breeding. In chickens, apart from the first few days post-hatch, infection with broad-host-range serovars of *Salmonella*, for example Typhimurium or Enteritidis, does not elicit severe pathology. However, infected animals may progress to become asymptomatic carriers that cannot be easily identified and removed from the food chain, resulting in contamination of meat and eggs. Understanding resistance to the carrier state in chickens and selecting for increased resistance will therefore be an important tool towards the goal of reducing the number of cases of zoonotic infection caused by *Salmonella*. Intestinal colonization is a complex virulence feature involving both bacterial and host characteristics and long-term persistence inevitably involves the immune response to the intestinal infection. How variation between lines in the persistent carrier state relates to differences in short-term colonization remains unclear.

As with the other resistance models discussed above, two different approaches have been used to understand resistance to the carrier state: candidate gene approaches (Beaumont *et al*., 2003) and attempts to map QTLs by genome-wide analysis (Yunis *et al*., 2002;

Tilquin *et al.*, 2005; Kaiser *et al.*, 2008). The latter has moved from the use of microsatellites (Yunis *et al.*, 2002) to SNPs and whole genome microarrays as sophisticated post-genomic resources and the appropriate technologies have become available. It has also been shown in principle that it is feasible to select for increased resistance to *S.* Enteritidis carrier state (Beaumont *et al.*, 2009).

Assessment of the carrier state involves measurement of the persistence of *Salmonella* in infected chickens several weeks post-infection, as opposed to assessment of colonization that occurs in the first few days post-infection. Models to follow development of the *S.* Enteritidis carrier state in young birds used day-old chicks (Guillot *et al.*, 1995) or week-old chicks (Duchet-Suchaux *et al.*, 1995, 1997) and measured the persistence of bacteria in different organs for several weeks post-infection. The carrier state in adult chickens is less well characterized, although there are reports of the persistence of bacteria in different organs following infection of birds at the peak of lay (Lindell *et al.*, 1994; Protais *et al.*, 1996).

Many candidate genes have been suggested or tested for a role in resistance to the carrier state. *NRAMP1* had an effect on spleen contamination in lines inoculated orally at peak of lay and killed four weeks later (Beaumont *et al.*, 2003) but in this study a role for *TLR4* was not observed. Other candidate genes tested included *IAP1*, *PSAP*, *MHC Class I* and, again, *NRAMP1* (Lamont *et al.*, 2002; Liu *et al.*, 2003). Whole genome microarray studies have identified a plethora of genes that are either differentially expressed before and after *S.* Enteritidis infection (Cheeseman *et al.*, 2007; van Hemert *et al.*, 2007; Zhang *et al.*, 2008) or differentially expressed between different lines infected with *S.* Enteritidis (van Hemert *et al.*, 2006a, b; Zhou and Lamont, 2007; Chiang *et al.*, 2008). Post-genome, the simplified identification of specific immune response genes and our greater understanding of the role they play in avian immunity have helped researchers to focus on the role of specific gene families in resistance to the carrier state, such as Toll-like receptors (Abasht *et al.*, 2008, 2009; Mackinnon *et al.*, 2009), other innate immune response genes (Sadeyen *et al.*, 2006) and cytokines (Kaiser *et al.*, 2006; Redmond *et al.*, 2009).

Relatively few genome-wide QTL studies have been carried out to identify genes involved in the resistance to the carrier state in the chicken. Using backcross and F2 progeny from the same inbred lines of chickens (6_1 and N) used by Fife *et al.* (2011) to map QTL for resistance to colonization, Tilquin *et al.* (2005) identified QTL for resistance to the carrier state. The $(N \times 6(1)) \times N$ backcross progeny were inoculated at 6 weeks of age with *S.* Typhimurium and bacteria enumerated on cloacal swabs collected at weekly intervals from 1 to 4 weeks post-infection. Forty-six backcross progeny were selectively genotyped for 135 microsatellite markers respectively and non-parametric interval mapping using least-squares mapped a genome-wide significant QTL on chromosome 1 at 2 weeks post-infection and a QTL with chromosome-wide significance on chromosome 15 (Tilquin *et al.*, 2005). The progeny of the F2 cross were inoculated at 1 week of age with *S.* Enteritidis and cloacal swabs were sampled at 4 and 5 weeks post-inoculation and caecal loads were assessed 1 week later. A total of 33 F2 progeny were selectively genotyped for 103 microsatellite markers and a genome-wide significant QTL mapped on chromosome 2 and chromosome-wide significant QTL mapped on chromosomes 2, 5 and 16 (Tilquin *et al.*, 2005). Different QTLs were found for cloacal loads and bacterial numbers in the caecal contents. Some QTLs were specific for the different progenies, probably due to differences in experimental details (the progenies themselves, serotypes of bacteria used, time of infection and time of sampling). The two QTL on chromosomes 2 and 16 were confirmed in a subsequent analysis including all animals, while those on chromosomes 1 and 16 were replicated in an independent population of a commercial line of layers (Calenge *et al.*, 2009). QTL and candidate genes have also been confirmed in adult chickens and chicks from a commercial line (Beaumont *et al.*, 2009). Interestingly, these differed between the adult birds and the chicks, suggesting genetic control of resistance to the *Salmonella* carrier state differs according to the age of the bird.

A more powerful QTL analysis was carried out recently (Calenge *et al.*, 2011) using a higher number of animals (~400) genotyped with a higher number of markers (480 SNPs). Using this approach, a more extended genome scan was performed, which identified novel QTLs on several microchromosomes, not previously covered in other analyses. Among them, one QTL on microchromosome 14 was significant at the genome-wide level. However, although half of the phenotypic data used were the same as in previous analyses (Tilquin *et al.*, 2005; Calenge *et al.*, 2009), several of the QTLs previously observed were not detected in the new analysis, including the genome-wide significant QTL on chromosome 2 (Tilquin *et al.*, 2005).

Practical implementation of knowledge on resistance genes or QTLs requires their use in selection for increased resistance in commercial flocks of birds. Legarra *et al.* (2011) recently investigated the feasibility of a genomic selection approach to increase resistance to the carrier state in commercial layers. The study used lines divergently selected for resistance to the carrier state as young chicks and as adults at the peak of lay. A total of 831 informative SNPs were used to type 600 birds that were infected with *S.* Enteritidis, and then phenotyped 28 days (young animals) or 38 days (adults) post-infection. Variance component analysis of the SNP data showed that the set of SNPs used captured a large part of the genetic variation. This confirmed that genomic selection for resistance to the *Salmonella* carrier state in laying hens is promising, but that denser SNP coverage on more animals will be required to fully assess its potential.

Resistance to *Salmonella* Infection in Pigs

In comparison to poultry, resistance to *Salmonella* infection in pigs is more poorly characterized, despite the fact that *Salmonella* in pigs represents a major food safety problem. Indeed, it was recently estimated that more than 50% of pig herds in the USA are *Salmonella*-positive (APHIS, 2009), with 7% of pig carcasses sampled between 1998 and 2000 in the USA contaminated with the bacterium (Rigney *et al.*, 2004).

As in the chicken, early work on resistance to *Salmonella* infection in the pig focused on candidate genes identified in studies using murine models. Although pig NRAMP1 (Sun *et al.*, 1998; Zhang *et al.*, 2000) is strongly expressed in macrophages and neutrophils following LPS stimulation (Zhang *et al.*, 2000), it has yet to have a role ascribed to it in porcine *Salmonella* infection (Zhang *et al.*, 2000). Pig TLR5 and TLR9, both of which recognize pathogen-associated molecular patterns on bacteria, are both up-regulated after challenge of pigs with *S.* Typhimurium and *S.* Choleraesuis (Burkey *et al.*, 2007), but again they have not been associated with resistance.

Analysis of immune parameters associated with resistance to systemic *S.* Choleraesuis infection in a reference family of pigs indicated that resistance was associated with higher number of circulating neutrophils and enhanced neutrophil function, but a lower mitogenic response of lymphocytes both pre- and post-infection and a lower antibody response (van Diemen *et al.*, 2002). Recruitment of neutrophils to the intestines and stimulation of their oxidative responses is believed to play a protective role in the response to *S.* Typhimurium infection in gnotobiotic piglets induced by pre-oral inoculation with live vaccine strains 24 h earlier (Foster *et al.*, 2003, 2005). The impact of circulating immune cells is less clear, as a recent independent study has suggested that shedding of *S.* Typhimurium by intranasally-dosed pigs is positively correlated with serum IFN-γ levels at 2 days post-infection (dpi), and that IFN-γ levels are in turn positively associated with higher levels of banded neutrophils (at 2 dpi), circulating neutrophils (at 7 and 14 dpi), monocytes (at 7 dpi) and white blood cells (at 7, 14 and 20 dpi) (Uthe *et al.*, 2009). The authors of the same report also associated shedding levels with a polymorphism in *CCT7*, a gene of ill-defined function that is up-regulated in pigs infected with *S.* Typhimurium (Uthe *et al.*, 2009). Further analysis of the association of genetic variation in candidate genes with faecal excretion or tissue colonization by *Salmonella* in pigs, informed by porcine transcriptional responses to infection, has linked shedding levels to SNPs in thirteen genes, including *GNG3, NCF2, TAP1, VCL, AMT, CCR1, CD163, CCT7, EMP1* and *ACP2* (Uthe *et al.*, 2011a). The authors further validated the approach of focusing on genes that are differentially expressed during *Salmonella* infection, and subject to natural variation as determined by bioinformatic analysis, in further study of the association of SNPs associated with shedding (Uthe *et al.*, 2011b).

Few genome-wide searches for QTL associated with resistance to *Salmonella* in pigs exist at the time of writing. Using the same resource population of pigs challenged with *S.* Choleraesuis as described by van Diemen *et al.* (2002), 14 different chromosomal regions were significantly associated with susceptibility by mapping of amplified fragment length polymorphism (AFLP) markers (Galina-Pantoja *et al.*, 2009). More than one linked marker was found on chromosomes 1, 7, 13, 14 and 18. Regions on chromosomes 1, 7 and 14 were significantly associated with *Salmonella* counts in the liver and regions on chromosomes 11, 13 and 18 with counts in spleen (Galina-Pantoja *et al.*, 2009). Further research is now needed to confirm the relevance of the QTL, genes and SNPs in wider populations, and to understand how they exert their effect.

Other Mammalian Species

In comparison to poultry and pigs, little research has been done on resistance to *Salmonella* infection in the other main farm animal species, cattle and sheep.

Despite the availability of the cattle genome sequence and the associated post-genomics technologies and tools, and the fact that cattle are both a source of human salmonellosis and suffer economic loss through *S.* Dublin infection, remarkably little has been published on genetic resistance to *Salmonella* infection in cattle. There are very few reports of differential resistance to salmonellosis between different breeds of cattle, although Jersey calves are more susceptible to *S.* Typhimurium infection than Friesian calves (Wray and Sojka, 1978). Heritability estimates for susceptibility or resistance to salmonellosis in cattle have yet to be made (Berry *et al.*, 2011) and resistance QTL have yet to be identified. Bovine *NRAMP1* has been cloned (Feng *et al.*, 1996), identified as a candidate gene for resistance to bovine brucellosis (Harmon *et al.*, 1985, 1989; Qureshi *et al.*, 1996) and associated with resistance to *S.* Dublin and *S.* Typhimurium *in vitro* in macrophages from cattle genetically resistant to infection with *Brucella abortus* (Qureshi *et al.*, 1996).

In sheep, genetic resistance to *S.* Abortusovis was first demonstrated in 1995 (Lantier *et al.*, 1995). Sheep *NRAMP1* was cloned as a candidate gene for this resistance soon afterwards (Bussmann *et al.*, 1998). More detailed analysis of traits involved in resistance to *S.* Abortusovis vaccination (specifically humoral immune response, number of bacteria in the lymph nodes and spleen, weight of these organs, and body weight loss between vaccination and slaughter), using a large experimental population of more than 1200 lambs from 30 sires of the Inra401 sheep, showed statistically significant heritabilities of between 0.10 and 0.64 (Moreno *et al.*, 2003), leading the authors to conclude that resistance to *Salmonella* infection in the sheep, as in other species, is under genetic control. Correlations between the traits were in agreement with known immune mechanisms. No link was seen in the same population between *Salmonella* resistance and PrP genotype (Vitezica *et al.*, 2007). Although this population would be ideal to identify QTL associated with *Salmonella* resistance, no reports have yet been published.

Perspectives

Mapping resistance QTLs for *Salmonella* resistance is already realistic for all farm animal livestock species, even for the sheep where the genome sequence is still to be completed. The next step is to characterize the resistance genes themselves and eventually the causative nucleotide change, or quantitative trait nucleotide (QTN). Currently, this is a more realistic prospect for the chicken, due to the combined availability of a relatively complete, well-annotated genome sequence, more than 12 million SNPs identified through the comprehensive resequencing of over 30 lines of chickens (commercial, inbred and rare-breeds), whole genome microarrays, whole genome copy number variation arrays and a newly developed 650K whole genome SNP array. However, most of these resources will be available for the other farm animal species within the next 2 to 5 years. Perhaps the greater advantage for the chicken still lies in the fact that it is by far the most studied of the farm animal livestock species for resistance to *Salmonella*, although further progress will still rely on accurate and comprehensive phenotypic measurements, particularly in commercial lines of birds, and definition of the distribution of protective QTL/QTN in pedigree populations.

Ultimately, identification of resistance genes and the causative QTN will require definitive biological proof of phenotype, best generated by ablating function of the candidate gene. This can be achieved through the use of lentiviral vectors to knock-down gene expression in chickens and potentially in pigs. There is also the realistic prospect of creating defined gene knock-out mutants in poultry, since the development of primordial germ cell technology (van de Lavoir *et al.*, 2006). The ability to derive transgenic animals is already available for several farm animal species, and animals could be engineered to possess resistance alleles to chosen pathogens or to express short hair-pin RNAs, delivered by lentiviral vectors, such as recently used by Lyall *et al.* (2011) to suppress avian influenza expression in genetically modified chickens. There is always the option, of course, once resistance markers, genes or QTN are identified, to select for more resistant animals using conventional breeding techniques.

References

Abasht, B., Kaiser, M.G. and Lamont, S.J. (2008) Toll-like receptor gene expression in cecum and spleen of advanced intercross line chicks infected with *Salmonella enterica* serovar Enteritidis. *Veterinary Immunology and Immunopathology* 123, 314–323.

Abasht, B., Kaiser, M., van der Poel, J. and Lamont, S. (2009) Genetic lines differ in Toll-like receptor gene expression in spleens of chicks inoculated with *Salmonella enterica* serovar Enteritidis. *Poultry Science* 88, 744–749.

Aerts, J., Megens, H.J., Veenendaal, T., Ovcharenko, I., Crooijmans, R., Gordon, L., Stubbs, L. and Groenen, M. (2007) Extent of linkage disequilibrium in chicken. *Cytogenetics and Genome Research* 117, 338–345.

APHIS (2009) APHIS info sheet. *Salmonella* on US swine sites – prevalence and antimicrobial susceptibility. Available at: http://www.aphis.usda.gov/vs/ceah/ncahs/nahms/swine/swine2006/Swine2006_salmonella_infosheet.pdf (accessed on 1 December 2010).

Barrow, P.A. and Freitas Neto, O.C. (2011) Pullorum disease and fowl typhoid – new thoughts on old diseases: a review. *Avian Pathology* 40, 1–13.

Barrow, P.A., Huggins, M.B., Lovell, M.A. and Simpson, J.M. (1987) Observations on the pathogenesis of experimental *Salmonella typhimurium* infection in chickens. *Research in Veterinary Science* 42, 194–199.

Barrow, P.A., Bumstead, N., Marston, K., Lovell, M.A. and Wigley, P. (2003) Faecal shedding and intestinal colonization of *Salmonella enterica* in in-bred chickens: the effect of host-genetic background. *Epidemiology and Infection* 132, 117–126.

Beaumont, C., Protais, J., Pitel, F., Leveque, G., Malo, D., Lantier, F., Plisson-Petit, F., Colin, P., Protais, M., Le Roy, P., Elsen, J.M., Milan, D., Lantier, I., Neau, A., Salvat, G. and Vignal, A. (2003) Effect of two candidate genes on the *Salmonella* carrier state in fowl. *Poultry Science* 82, 721–726.

Beaumont, C., Chapuis, H., Protais, J., Sellier, N., Menanteau, P., Fravalo, P. and Velge, P. (2009) Resistance to *Salmonella* carrier state: selection may be efficient but response depends on animal's age. *Genetics Research* 91, 161–169.

Berry, D.P., Bermingham, M.L., Good, M. and More, S.J. (2011) Genetics of animal health and disease in cattle. *Irish Veterinary Journal* 64, 5.

Boyd, Y., Herbert, E.G., Marston, K.L., Jones, M.A. and Barrow, P.A. (2005) Host genes affect intestinal colonisation of newly-hatched chickens by *Campylobacter jejuni*. *Immunogenetics* 57, 248–253.

Bumstead, N. and Barrow, P.A. (1988) Genetics of resistance to *Salmonella typhimurium* in newly hatched chicks. *British Poultry Science* 29, 521–530.

Bumstead, N. and Barrow, P.A. (1993) Resistance to *S. gallinarum, S. pullorum* and *S. enteritidis* in inbred lines of chickens. *Avian Diseases* 37, 717–726.

Bumstead, N., Millard, B.M., Barrow, P.A. and Cook, J.K.A. (1991) The genetic basis of disease resistance in chickens. In: Owen, J.B. and Axford, R.F.E. (eds) *Breeding for Disease Resistance in Farm Animals*. CAB International, Wallingford, UK, pp. 10–23.

Burkey, T.E., Skjolaas, K.A., Dritz, S.S. and Minton, J.E. (2007) Expression of Toll-like receptors, interleukin 8, macrophage migration inhibitory factor, and osteopontin in tissues from pigs challenged with *Salmonella enterica* serovar Typhimurium or serovar Choleraesuis. *Veterinary Immunology and Immunopathology* 115, 309–319.

Bussmann, V., Lantier, I., Pitel, F., Patri, S., Nau, F., Gros, P., Elsen, J.M. and Lantier, F. (1998) cDNA cloning, structural organisation, and expression of the sheep *NRAMP1* gene. *Mammalian Genome* 9, 1027–1031.

Calenge, F., Lecerf, F., Demars, J., Feve, K., Vignoles, F., Pitel, F., Vignal, A., Velge, P., Sellier, N. and Beaumont, C. (2009) QTL for resistance to *Salmonella* carrier state confirmed in both experimental and commercial chicken lines. *Animal Genetics* 40(5), 590–597.

Calenge, F., Kaiser, P., Vignal, A. and Beaumont, C. (2010) Genetic control of resistance to salmonellosis and to *Salmonella* carrier-state in fowl: a review. *Genetics, Selection, Evolution* 42, 11.

Calenge, F., Vignal, A., Demars, J., Feve, K., Menanteau, P., Velge, P. and Beaumont, C. (2011) New QTL for resistance to *Salmonella* carrier-state identified on fowl microchromosomes. *Molecular Genetics and Genomics* 285, 237–243.

Cao, C., Ren, X., Kharbanda, S., Koleske, A., Prasad, K.V. and Kufe, D. (2001) The ARG tyrosine kinase interacts with Siva-1 in the apoptotic response to oxidative stress. *Journal of Biological Chemistry* 276, 11465–11468.

Cheeseman, J., Kaiser, M., Ciraci, C., Kaiser, P. and Lamont, S. (2007) Breed effect on early cytokine mRNA expression in spleen and cecum of chickens with and without *Salmonella enteritidis* infection. *Developmental and Comparative Immunology* 31, 52–60.

Chiang, H., Swaggerty, C., Kogut, M., Dowd, S., Li, X., Pevzner, I. and Zhou, H. (2008) Gene expression profiling in chicken heterophils with *Salmonella enteritidis* stimulation using a chicken 44K Agilent microarray *BMC Genomics* 9, 526.

Chiu, H.C., Kulp, S.K., Soni, S., Wang, D., Gunn, J.S., Schlesinger, L.S. and Chen, C.S. (2009) Eradication of intracellular *Salmonella enterica* serovar Typhimurium with a small-molecule, host cell-directed agent. *Antimicrobial Agents and Chemotherapy* 53, 5236–5244.

Chu, F., Borthakur, A., Sun, X., Barkinge, J., Gudi, R., Hawkins, S. and Prasad, K.V. (2004) The Siva-1 putative amphipathic helical region (SAH) is sufficient to bind to BCL-XL and sensitize cells to UV radiation induced apoptosis. *Apoptosis* 9, 83–95.

Crump, J.A., Luby, S.P. and Mintz, E.D. (2004) The global burden of typhoid fever. *Bulletin of the World Health Organisation* 82, 346–353.

Dougan, G., John, V., Palmer, S. and Mastroeni, P. (2011) Immunity to salmonellosis. *Immunological Reviews* 240, 196–210.

Duchet-Suchaux, M., Léchopier, P., Marly, J., Bernardet, P., Delaunay, R. and Pardon, P. (1995) Quantification of experimental *Salmonella enteritidis* carrier state in B13 leghorn chicks. *Avian Diseases* 39, 796–803.

Duchet-Suchaux, M., Mompart, F., Berthelot, F., Beaumont, C., Léchopier, P. and Pardon, P. (1997) Differences in frequency, level and duration of cecal carriage between four outbred chicken lines infected orally with *Salmonella enteritidis*. *Avian Diseases* 41, 559–567.

Feng, J., Li, Y., Hashad, M., Schurr, E., Gros, P., Adams, L.G. and Templeton, J.W. (1996) Bovine natural resistance associated macrophage protein 1 (*NRAMP1*) gene. *Genome Research* 6, 956–964.

Feng, S.Z., Cao, W.S. and Liao, M. (2011) The PI3K/Akt pathway is involved in early infection of some exogenous avian leukosis viruses. *Journal of General Virology* 92, 1688–1697.

Fife, M., Salmon, N., Hocking, P. and Kaiser, P. (2009) Fine mapping of the chicken salmonellosis resistance locus (SAL1). *Animal Genetics* 40, 871–877.

Fife, M.S., Howell, J., Salmon, N., van Diemen, P.M., Jones, M.A., Hocking, P.M., Stevens, M.P. and Kaiser, P. (2011) Genome-wide SNP analysis identifies major QTL for *Salmonella* colonisation in the chicken. *Animal Genetics* 42, 134–140.

Fink, S.L. and Cookson, B.T. (2007) Pyroptosis and host cell death responses during *Salmonella* infection. *Cellular Microbiology* 9, 2562–2570.

Foster, N., Lovell, M.A., Marston, K.L., Hulme, S.D., Frost, A.J., Bland, P. and Barrow, P.A. (2003) Rapid protection of gnotobiotic pigs against experimental salmonellosis following induction of polymorphonuclear leukocytes by avirulent *Salmonella enterica*. *Infection and Immunity* 71, 2182–2191.

Foster, N., Hulme, S., Lovell, M., Reed, K. and Barrow, P. (2005) Stimulation of gp91 phagocytic oxidase and reactive oxygen species in neutrophils by an avirulent *Salmonella enterica* serovar Infantis strain protects gnotobiotic piglets from lethal challenge with serovar Typhimurium strain F98 without inducing intestinal pathology. *Infection and Immunity* 73, 4539–4547.

Galina-Pantoja, L., Siggens, K., van Schriek, M.G. and Heuven, H.C. (2009) Mapping markers linked to porcine salmonellosis susceptibility. *Animal Genetics* 40, 795–803.

Ghebremicael, S.B., Hasenstein, J.R. and Lamont, S.J. (2008) Association of interleukin-10 cluster genes and *Salmonella* response in the chicken. *Poultry Science* 87, 22–26.

Gudi, R., Barkinge, J., Hawkins, S., Chu, F., Manicassamy, S., Sun, Z., Duke-Cohan, J.S. and Prasad, K.V. (2006) Siva-1 negatively regulates NF-kappaB activity: effect on T-cell receptor-mediated activation-induced cell death (AICD). *Oncogene* 25, 3458–3462.

Guillot, J., Beaumont, C., Bellatif, F., Mouline, C., Lantier, F., Colin, P. and Protais, J. (1995) Comparison of resistance of various poultry lines to infection by *Salmonella enteritidis*. *Veterinary Research* 26, 81–86.

Harmon, B.G., Templeton, J.W., Crawford, R.P., Heck, F.C., Williams, J.D. and Adams, L.G. (1985) Macrophage function and immune response of *Brucella abortus* naturally resistant and susceptible cattle. In: Skamene, E. (ed.) *Genetic Control of Host Resistance to Infection and Malignancy*. Alan R. Liss, New York, pp. 345–354.

Harmon, B.G., Adams, L.G., Templeton, J.W. and Smith, R. III (1989) Macrophage function in mammary glands of *Brucella abortus*-infected cows and cows that resisted infection after inoculation of *Brucella abortus*. *American Journal of Veterinary Research* 50, 459–465.

Hasenstein, J.R. and Lamont, S.J. (2007) Chicken gallinacin gene cluster associated with *Salmonella* response in advanced intercross line. *Avian Diseases* 51, 561–567.

Hasenstein, J.R., Zhang, G. and Lamont, S.J. (2006) Analyses of five gallinacin genes and the *Salmonella enterica* serovar Enteritidis response in poultry. *Infection and Immunity* 74, 3375–3380.

Helaine, S., Thompson, J.A., Watson, K.G., Liu, M., Boyle, C. and Holden, D.W. (2010) Dynamics of intracellular bacterial replication at the single cell level. *Proceedings of the National Academy of Sciences of the United States of America* 107, 3746–3751.

Hernandez, L.D., Hueffer, K., Wenk, M.R. and Galán, J.E. (2004) *Salmonella* modulates vesicular traffic by altering phosphoinositide metabolism. *Science* 304, 1805–1807.

Hers, I., Vincent, E.E. and Tavaré, J.M. (2011) mAkt signalling in health and disease. *Cellular Signalling* 23, 1515–1527.

Hu, J., Bumstead, N., Barrow, P., Sebastiani, G., Olien, L., Morgan, K. and Malo, D. (1997) Resistance to salmonellosis in the chicken is linked to *NRAMP1* and TNC. *Genome Research* 6, 693–704.

Hutt, F.B. and Scholes, J.C. (1941) Genetics of the fowl. XIII. Breed differences in susceptibility to *Salmonella pullorum*. *Poultry Science* 20, 342–352.

International Chicken Genome Sequencing Consortium (2004) Sequence and comparative analysis of the chicken genome provide unique perspectives on vertebrate evolution. *Nature* 432, 695–716.

Kaiser, M.G. and Lamont, S.J. (2002) Microsatellites linked to *Salmonella enterica* serovar Enteritidis burden in spleen and cecal content of young F1 broiler-cross chicks. *Poultry Science* 81, 657–663.

Kaiser, M., Cheeseman, J., Kaiser, P. and Lamont, S. (2006) Cytokine expression in chicken peripheral blood mononuclear cells after in vitro exposure to *Salmonella enterica* serovar Enteritidis. *Poultry Science* 85, 1907–1911.

Kaiser, P., Howell, J., Fife, M., Sadeyen, J.R., Salmon, N., Rothwell, L., Young, J., van Diemen, P., Stevens, M., Poh, T.Y., Jones, M., Barrow, P., Swaggerty, C., Kogut, M., Smith, J. and Burt, D. (2008) Integrated immunogenomics in the chicken: deciphering the immune response to identify disease resistance genes. *Developments in Biologicals (Basel)* 132, 57–66.

Knodler, L.A., Finlay, B.B. and Steele-Mortimer, O. (2005) The *Salmonella* effector protein SopB protects epithelial cells from apoptosis by sustained activation of Akt. *Journal of Biological Chemistry* 280, 9058–9064.

Kramer, J., Malek, M. and Lamont, S.J. (2003) Association of twelve candidate gene polymorphisms and response to challenge with *Salmonella enteritidis* in poultry. *Animal Genetics* 34, 339–348.

Kuijl, C., Savage, N.D., Marsman, M., Tuin, A.W., Janssen, L., Egan, D.A., Ketema, M., van den Nieuwendijk, R., van den Eeden, S.J., Geluk, A., Poot, A., van der Marel, G., Beijersbergen, R.L., Overkleeft, H., Ottenhoff, T.H. and Neefjes, J. (2007) Intracellular bacterial growth is controlled by a kinase network around PKB/AKT1. *Nature* 450, 725–730.

Kum, W.W., Lo, B.C., Yu, H.B. and Finlay, B.B. (2011) Protective role of Akt2 in *Salmonella enterica* serovar Typhimurium-induced gastroenterocolitis. *Infection and Immunity* 79, 2554–2566.
Lamont, S., Kaiser, M. and Liu, W. (2002) Candidate genes for resistance to *Salmonella enteritidis* colonization in chickens as detected in a novel genetic cross. *Veterinary Immunology and Immunopathology* 87, 423–428.
Lantier, F., Pitel, F., Berthon, P., Lantier, I., Gautier, A., Boivin, R., Weisbecker, J.L., Brunel, J.C., Francois, D., Gellin, J., Vu Tien, J. and Elsen, J.-M. (1995) Contrôle genetique de la resistance aux *Salmonellae* chez les ovins. *Rencontres Autour des Recherches sur les Ruminants* 2, 311–316.
Legarra, A., Calenge, F., Mariani, P., Velge, P. and Beaumont, C. (2011) Use of a reduced set of single nucleotide polymorphisms for genetic evaluation of resistance to *Salmonella* carrier state in laying hens. *Poultry Science* 90, 731–736.
Leveque, G., Forgetta, V., Morroll, S., Smith, A.L., Bumstead, N., Barrow, P., Loredo-Osti, J.C., Morgan, K. and Malo, D. (2003) Allelic variation in TLR4 is linked to susceptibility to *Salmonella enterica* serovar Typhimurium infection in chickens. *Infection and Immunity* 71, 1116–1124.
Lin, P.Y., Liu, H.J., Liao, M.H., Chang, C.D., Chang, C.I., Cheng, H.L., Lee, J.W. and Shih, W.L. (2010) Activation of PI 3-kinase/Akt/NF-κB and Stat3 signaling by avian reovirus S1133 in the early stages of infection results in an inflammatory response and delayed apoptosis. *Virology* 400, 104–114.
Lindell, K., Saeed, A. and McCabe, G. (1994) Evaluation of resistance of four strains of commercial laying hens to experimental infection with *Salmonella enteritidis* phage type eight. *Poultry Science* 73, 757–762.
Liu, W., Kaiser, M. and Lamont, S. (2003) Natural resistance-associated macrophage protein 1 gene polymorphisms and response to vaccine against or challenge with *Salmonella enteritidis* in young chicks. *Poultry Science* 82, 259–266.
Lyall, J., Irvine, R.M., Sherman, A., McKinley, T.J., Núñez, A., Purdie, A., Outtrim, L., Brown, I.H., Rolleston-Smith, G., Sang, H. and Tiley, L. (2011) Suppression of avian influenza transmission in genetically modified chickens. *Science* 331, 223–226.
MacKinnon, K.M., He, H., Nerren, J.R., Swaggerty, C.L., Genovese, K.J. and Kogut, M.H. (2009) Expression profile of toll-like receptors within the gastrointestinal tract of 2-day-old *Salmonella enteriditis*-infected broiler chickens. *Veterinary Microbiology* 137, 313–319.
Madrid, L.V., Wang, C.Y., Guttridge, D.C., Schottelius, A.J., Baldwin, A.S. Jr and Mayo, M.W. (2000) Akt suppresses apoptosis by stimulating the transactivation potential of the RelA/p65 subunit of NF-κB. *Molecular and Cellular Biology* 20, 1626–1638.
Majowicz, S.E., Musto, J., Scallan, E., Angulo, F.J., Kirk, M., O'Brien, S.J., Jones, T.F., Fazil, A. and Hoekstra, R.M.; International Collaboration on Enteric Disease 'Burden of Illness' Studies (2010) The global burden of nontyphoidal *Salmonella* gastroenteritis. *Clinical Infectious Diseases* 50, 882–889.
Malek, M. and Lamont, S.J. (2003) Association of INOS, TRAIL, TGF-beta2, TGF-beta3, and IgL genes with response to *Salmonella enteritidis* in poultry. *Genetics, Selection, Evolution* 35, S99–S111.
Malek, M., Hasenstein, J.R. and Lamont, S.J. (2004) Analysis of chicken TLR4, CD28, MIF, MD-2, and LITAF genes in a *Salmonella enteritidis* resource population. *Poultry Science* 83, 544–549.
Mariani, P., Barrow, P.A., Cheng, H.H., Groenen, M.M., Negrini, R. and Bumstead, N. (2001) Localization to chicken chromosome 5 of a novel locus determining salmonellosis resistance. *Immunogenetics* 53, 786–791.
Miao, E.A., Leaf, I.A., Treuting, P.M., Mao, D.P., Dors, M., Sarkar, A., Warren, S.E., Wewers, M.D. and Aderem, A. (2010) Caspase-1-induced pyroptosis is an innate immune effector mechanism against intracellular bacteria. *Nature Immunology* 11, 1135–1142.
Monack, D.M., Hersh, D., Ghori, N., Bouley, D., Zychlinsky, A. and Falkow, S. (2000) *Salmonella* exploits caspase-1 to colonize Peyer's patches in a murine typhoid model. *Journal of Experimental Medicine* 192, 249–258.
Moreno, C.R., Lantier, F., Bertho, P., Gautier-Bouchardon, A.V., Boivin, R., Lantier, I., Brunel, J.C., Weisbecker, J.L., Francois, D., Bouix, J. and Elsen, J.M. (2003) Genetic parameters for resistance to the *Salmonella abortusovis* vaccinal strain Rv6 in sheep. *Genetics, Selection and Evolution* 35, 199–217.
Patel, J.C., Hueffer, K., Lam, T.T. and Galán, J.E. (2009) Diversification of a *Salmonella* virulence protein function by ubiquitin-dependent differential localization. *Cell* 137, 283–294.
Prasad, K.V., Ao, Z., Yoon, Y., Wu, M.X., Rizk, M., Jacquot, S. and Schlossman, S.F. (1997) CD27, a member of the tumor necrosis factor receptor family, induces apoptosis and binds to Siva, a proapoptotic protein. *Proceedings of the National Academy of Sciences USA* 94, 6346–6351.

Protais, J., Colin, P., Beaumont, C., Guillot, J., Lantier, F., Pardon, P. and Bennejean, G. (1996) Line differences in resistance to *Salmonella enteritidis* PT4 infection. *British Poultry Science* 37, 329–339.

Py, B., Slomianny, C., Auberger, P., Petit, P.X. and Benichou, S. (2004) Siva-1 and an alternative splice form lacking the death domain, Siva-2, similarly induce apoptosis in T lymphocytes via a caspase-dependent mitochondrial pathway. *Journal of Immunology* 172, 4008–4017.

Qureshi, T., Templeton, J.W. and Adams, L.G. (1996) Intracellular survival of *Brucella abortus, Mycobacterium bovis* bcg, *Salmonella Dublin*, and *Salmonella typhimurium* in macrophages from cattle genetically resistant to *Brucella abortus*. *Veterinary Immunology and Immunopathology* 50, 55–65.

Redmond, S., Chuammitri, P., Andreasen, C., Palic, D. and Lamont, S. (2009) Chicken heterophils from commercially selected and non-selected genetic lines express cytokines differently after exposure to *Salmonella enteritidis*. *Veterinary Immunology and Immunopathology* 132, 129–134.

Redmond, S.B., Chuammitri, P., Andreasen, C.B., Palić, D. and Lamont, S.J. (2011) Genetic control of chicken heterophil function in advanced intercross lines: associations with novel and with known *Salmonella* resistance loci and a likely mechanism for cell death in extracellular trap production. *Immunogenetics* 63, 449–458.

Rigney, C.P., Salamone, B.P., Anandaraman, N., Rose, B.E., Umholtz, R.L., Ferris, K.E., Parham, D.R. and James, W. (2004) *Salmonella* serotypes in selected classes of food animal carcasses and raw ground products, January 1998 through December 2000. *Journal of the American Veterinary Medical Association* 224, 524–530.

Sadeyen, J.-R., Trotereau, J., Protais, J., Beaumont, C., Sellier, N., Salvat, G., Velge, P. and Lalmanach, A.-C. (2006) *Salmonella* carrier-state in hens: study of host resistance by a gene expression approach. *Microbes and Infection* 8, 1308–1314.

Shiozaki, T., Iwai, A., Kawaoka, Y., Takada, A., Kida, H. and Miyazaki, T. (2011) Requirement for Siva-1 for replication of influenza A virus through apoptosis induction. *Journal of General Virology* 92, 315–325.

Smith, H.W. (1956) The susceptibility of different breeds of chickens to experimental *Salmonella Gallinarum* infection. *British Poultry Science* 35, 701–705.

Steele-Mortimer, O., Knodler, L.A., Marcus, S.L., Scheid, M.P., Goh, B., Pfeifer, C.G., Duronio, V. and Finlay, B.B. (2000) Activation of Akt/protein kinase B in epithelial cells by the *Salmonella* Typhimurium effector SigD. *Journal of Biological Chemistry* 275, 37718–37724.

Stevens, M.P., Humphrey, T.J. and Maskell, D.J. (2009) Molecular insights into farm animal and zoonotic *Salmonella* infections. *Philosophical Transactions of the Royal Society of London B Biological Sciences* 364, 2709–2723.

Sun, H.S., Wang, L., Rothschild, M.F. and Tuggle, C.K. (1998) Mapping of the natural resistance-associated macrophage protein 1 (NRAMP1) gene to pig chromosome 15. *Animal Genetics* 29, 138–140.

Swaggerty, C.L., Kogut, M.H., Ferro, P.J., Rothwell, L., Pevzner, I.Y. and Kaiser, P. (2004) Differential cytokine mRNA expression in heterophils isolated from *Salmonella*-resistant and -susceptible chickens. *Immunology* 113, 139–148.

Swaggerty, C.L., Ferro, P.J., Pevzner, I.Y. and Kogut, M.H. (2005) Heterophils are associated with resistance to systemic *Salmonella enteritidis* infections in genetically distinct chicken lines. *FEMS Immunology and Medical Microbiology* 43, 149–154.

Swaggerty, C.L., Kaiser, P., Rothwell, L., Pevzner, I.Y. and Kogut, M.H. (2006) Heterophil cytokine mRNA profiles from genetically distinct lines of chickens with differential heterophil-mediated innate immune responses. *Avian Pathology* 35, 102–108.

Swaggerty, C., Pevzner, I., Kaiser, P. and Kogut, M. (2008) Profiling pro-inflammatory cytokine and chemokine mRNA expression levels as a novel method for selection of increased innate immune responsiveness. *Veterinary Immunology and Immunopathology* 126, 35–42.

Terebiznik, M.R., Vieira, O.V., Marcus, S.L., Slade, A., Yip, C.M., Trimble, W.S., Meyer, T., Finlay, B.B. and Grinstein, S. (2002) Elimination of host cell PtdIns(4,5)P(2) by bacterial SigD promotes membrane fission during invasion by *Salmonella*. *Nature Cell Biology* 4, 766–773.

Tilquin, P., Barrow, P.A., Marly, J., Pitel, F., Plisson-Petit, F., Velge, P., Vignal, A., Baret, P.V., Bumstead, N. and Beaumont, C. (2005) A genome scan for quantitative trait loci affecting the *Salmonella* carrier-state in the chicken. *Genetics Selection Evolution* 37, 539–561.

Uthe, J.J., Wang, Y., Qu, L., Nettleton, D., Tuggle, C.K. and Bearson, S.M. (2009) Correlating blood immune parameters and a CCT7 genetic variant with the shedding of *Salmonella enterica* serovar Typhimurium in swine. *Veterinary Microbiology* 135, 384–388.

Uthe, J.J., Bearson, S.M., Qu, L., Dekkers, J.C., Nettleton, D., Rodriguez Torres, Y., O'Connor, A.M., McKean, J.D. and Tuggle, C.K. (2011a) Integrating comparative expression profiling data and association of SNPs with *Salmonella* shedding for improved food safety and porcine disease resistance. *Animal Genetics* 42, 521–534.

Uthe, J.J., Qu, L., Couture, O., Bearson, S.M., O'Connor, A.M., McKean, J.D., Torres, Y.R., Dekkers, J.C., Nettleton, D. and Tuggle, C.K. (2011b) Use of bioinformatic SNP predictions in differentially expressed genes to find SNPs associated with *Salmonella* colonization in swine. *Journal of Animal Breeding and Genetics* 128, 354–365.

van de Lavoir, M.C., Diamond, J.H., Leighton, P.A., Mather-Love, C., Heyer, B.S., Bradshaw, R., Kerchner, A., Hooi, L.T., Gessaro, T.M., Swanberg, S.E., Delany, M.E. and Etches, R.J. (2006) Germline transmission of genetically modified primordial germ cells. *Nature* 441, 766–769.

van Diemen, P.M., Kreukniet, M.B., Galina, L., Bumstead, N. and Wallis, T.S. (2002) Characterisation of a resource population of pigs screened for resistance to salmonellosis. *Veterinary Immunology and Immunopathology* 88, 183–196.

van Hemert, S., Hoekman, A., Smits, M. and Rebel, J. (2006a) Early host gene expression responses to a *Salmonella* infection in the intestine of chickens with different genetic background examined with cDNA and oligonucleotide microarrays. *Comparative Biochemistry and Physiology Part D Genomics Proteomics* 1, 292–299.

van Hemert, S., Hoekman, A., Smits, M. and Rebel, J. (2006b) Gene expression responses to a *Salmonella* infection in the chicken intestine differ between lines. *Veterinary Immunology and Immunopathology* 114, 247–258.

van Hemert, S., Hoekman, A., Smits, M. and Rebel, J. (2007) Immunological and gene expression responses to a *Salmonella* infection in the chicken intestine. *Veterinary Research* 38, 51–63.

Verbeke, P., Welter-Stahl, L., Ying, S., Hansen, J., Häcker, G., Darville, T. and Ojcius, D.M. (2006) Recruitment of BAD by the *Chlamydia trachomatis* vacuole correlates with host-cell survival. *PLoS Pathogens* 2, e45.

Vitezica, Z.G., Moreno, C.R., Lantier, F., Lantier, I., Schibler, L., Roig, A., Francois, D., Bouix, J., Allain, D., Brunel, J.C., Barillet, F. and Elsen, J.M. (2007) Quantitative trait loci linked to *PRNP* gene controlling health and production traits in INRA 401 sheep. *Genetics, Selection and Evolution* 39, 421–430.

Voth, D.E. and Heinzen, R.A. (2009) Sustained activation of Akt and Erk1/2 is required for *Coxiella burnetii* antiapoptotic activity. *Infection and Immunity* 77, 205–213.

Wei, L., Zhu, S., Ruan, G., Hou, L., Wang, J., Wang, B. and Liu, J. (2011) Infectious bursal disease virus activates the phosphatidylinositol 3-kinase (PI3K)/Akt signaling pathway by interaction of VP5 protein with the p85α subunit of PI3K. *Virology* 417, 211–220.

Wigley, P., Hulme, S.D., Bumstead, N. and Barrow, P.A. (2002) *In vivo* and *in vitro* studies of genetic resistance to systemic salmonellosis in the chicken encoded by the SAL1 locus. *Microbes and Infection* 4, 1111–1120.

Wigley, P., Hulme, S., Rothwell, L., Bumstead, N., Kaiser, P. and Barrow, P. (2006) Macrophages isolated from chickens genetically resistant or susceptible to systemic salmonellosis show magnitudinal and temporal differential expression of cytokines and chemokines following *Salmonella enterica* challenge. *Infection and Immunity* 74, 1425–1430.

Wong, G.K., Liu, B., Wang, J., Zhang, Y., Yang, X., Zhang, Z., Meng, Q., Zhou, J., Li, D., Zhang, J., Ni, P., Li, S., Ran, L., Li, H., Zhang, J., Li, R., Li, S., Zheng, H., Lin, W., Li, G., Wang, X., Zhao, W., Li, J., Ye, C., Dai, M., Ruan, J., Zhou, Y., Li, Y., He, X., Zhang, Y., Wang, J., Huang, X., Tong, W., Chen, J., Ye, J., Chen, C., Wei, N., Li, G., Dong, L., Lan, F., Sun, Y., Zhang, Z., Yang, Z., Yu, Y., Huang, Y., He, D., Xi, Y., Wei, D., Qi, Q., Li, W., Shi, J., Wang, M., Xie, F., Wang, J., Zhang, X., Wang, P., Zhao, Y., Li, N., Yang, N., Dong, W., Hu, S., Zeng, C., Zheng, W., Hao, B., Hillier, L.W., Yang, S.P., Warren, W.C., Wilson, R.K., Brandström, M., Ellegren, H., Crooijmans, R.P., van der Poel, J.J., Bovenhuis, H., Groenen, M.A., Ovcharenko, I., Gordon, L., Stubbs, L., Lucas, S., Glavina, T., Aerts, A., Kaiser, P., Rothwell, L., Young, J.R., Rogers, S., Walker, B.A., van Hateren, A., Kaufman, J., Bumstead, N., Lamont, S.J., Zhou, H., Hocking, P.M., Morrice, D., de Koning, D.J., Law, A., Bartley, N., Burt, D.W., Hunt, H., Cheng, H.H., Gunnarsson, U., Wahlberg, P., Andersson, L., Kindlund, E., Tammi, M.T., Andersson, B., Webber, C., Ponting, C.P., Overton, I.M., Boardman, P.E., Tang, H., Hubbard, S.J., Wilson, S.A., Yu, J., Wang, J. and Yang, H.; International Chicken Polymorphism Map Consortium (2004) A genetic variation map for chicken with 2.8 million single-nucleotide polymorphisms. Nature 432, 717–722.

Wray, C. and Sojka, W.J. (1978) Experimental *Salmonella typhimurium* infection in calves. *Research in Veterinary Science* 25, 139–143.

Wray, C., Davies, R.H. and Corkish, J.D. (1996) Enterobacteriaceae. In: Jordan, F.T.W. and Pattison, M. (eds) *Poultry Diseases*. W.B. Saunders, Cambridge, UK, pp. 9–43.

Xue, L., Chu, F., Cheng, Y., Sun, X., Borthakur, A., Ramarao, M., Pandey, P., Wu, M., Schlossman, S.F. and Prasad, K.V. (2002) Siva-1 binds to and inhibits BCL-X(L)-mediated protection against UV radiation-induced apoptosis. *Proceedings of the National Academy of Sciences USA* 99, 6925–6930.

Yunis, R., Heller, E., Hillel, J. and Cahaner, A. (2002) Microsatellite markers associated with quantitative trait loci controlling antibody response to *Escherichia coli* and *Salmonella enteritidis* in young broilers. *Animal Genetics* 33, 407–414.

Zhang, G., Wu, H., Ross, C.R., Minton, J.E. and Blecha, F. (2000) Cloning of porcine *Nramp1* and its induction by lipopolysaccharide, tumor necrosis factor alpha, and interleukin-1β: role of CD14 and mitogen-activated protein kinases. *Infection and Immunity* 68, 1086–1093.

Zhang, S., Lillehoj, H., Kim, C., Keeler, C.J., Babu, U. and Zhang, M. (2008) Transcriptional response of chicken macrophages to *Salmonella enterica* serovar Enteritidis infection. *Developments in Biologicals (Basel)* 132, 141–151.

Zhou, H. and Lamont, S.J. (2003) Chicken MHC class I and II gene effects on antibody response kinetics in adult chickens. *Immunogenetics* 55, 133–140.

Zhou, H. and Lamont, S. (2007) Global gene expression profile after *Salmonella enterica* serovar *enteritidis* challenge in two F8 advanced intercross chicken lines. *Cytogenetics and Genome Research* 117, 131–138.

7 Antimicrobial Resistance in *Salmonella*

Geovana Brenner Michael,[1] Ruth Hall,[2] Séamus Fanning[3] and Stefan Schwarz[1]*

[1]*Institute of Farm Animal Genetics, Friedrich-Loeffler-Institut (FLI), Germany;* [2]*School of Molecular Bioscience, The University of Sydney, Australia;* [3]*UCD Centre for Food Safety, School of Public Health, Physiotherapy & Population Science, UCD Veterinary Sciences Centre, University College Dublin, Ireland*

Introduction

Under the selective pressure imposed by the use of antimicrobial agents, members of the genus *Salmonella* have acquired a wide variety of genes, gene complexes or have developed mutations that confer resistance to antimicrobial agents. Many of the currently known resistance genes are located on mobile genetic elements such as transposons, integrons and gene cassettes, plasmids and genomic islands. As a consequence such resistance genes are exchanged between bacteria living in the same habitat, e.g. the *Enterobacteriaceae* in the gastrointestinal tract of humans and animals (Schwarz and Chaslus-Dancla, 2001). In this regard, bacteria of the genus *Salmonella* may play an important role as either acceptors or donors of resistance genes and thus are of relevance for the dissemination of resistance genes.

Antimicrobial multi-resistance has been documented in various *Salmonella enterica* subsp. *enterica* serovars and numerous antimicrobial resistance genes have been identified by molecular approaches, including hybridization and PCR analysis (Aarts *et al*., 2001). However, the results obtained may be biased by the use of different gene probes and PCR primers for detection of the resistance genes. Thus, sequence data appear to be the most reliable approach to confirm the presence of a resistance gene. In this chapter, we summarize which genes and mutations associated with resistance to the different classes of antimicrobial agents are currently known to occur in *Salmonella* isolates, particularly the ones whose sequences have been deposited in the databases. Furthermore, the location of resistance genes on mobile elements and co-location with other resistance markers are discussed.

Resistance of *Salmonella* to Different Classes of Antimicrobial Agents

The following subsections are intended to provide an overview of the genes that confer resistance to antimicrobial agents in *S. enterica* subsp. *enterica*. Due to the wealth of data obtained from the analysis of the various serovars, it is impossible to list every serovar in which each resistance gene has been

* Corresponding author, e-mail: stefan.schwarz@fli.bund.de

© CAB International 2013. *Salmonella in Domestic Animals, 2nd Edition* (eds P.A. Barrow and U. Methner)

detected. Instead, examples of the presence of the resistance genes are given, and referencing relies on an earlier review (Michael *et al.*, 2006) supplemented with new information that has been published since then.

Resistance to tetracyclines

Although more than 40 different tetracycline resistance genes have been described, only five of them – *tetA*(A), *tetA*(B), *tetA*(C), *tetA*(D) and *tetA*(G) – have been reported in *Salmonella* isolates via sequences deposited in publicly available databases. All of these *tetA* genes encode an efflux protein consisting of 12 transmembrane segments that transports tetracycline, oxytetracycline, chlortetracycline and doxycycline. TetA(B) can also export minocycline. The five *tetA* genes are associated with different elements: *tetA*(G) has exclusively been detected as a component of the *Salmonella* Genomic Island 1 (SGI1)- or 2 (SGI2)-associated multi-resistance gene clusters (see Fig. 7.1 and section 3, below). The *tetA*(A) and *tetA*(B) genes are associated with transposons Tn*1721* and Tn*10*, respectively. Tn*10* is widespread among different *Salmonella* serovars, and truncated copies of both transposons have been identified on large multi-resistance plasmids, and on plasmids conferring resistance to tetracyclines alone; tetracyclines + penicillins; or tetracyclines + streptomycin. Plasmids carrying *tetA*(C) or *tetA*(D) genes have been identified only infrequently. In rare cases, more than one *tetA* gene has been seen in the same isolate (Michael *et al.*, 2006).

Resistance to phenicols

The molecular basis of bacterial resistance to chloramphenicol and its fluorinated derivative florfenicol has been reviewed (Schwarz

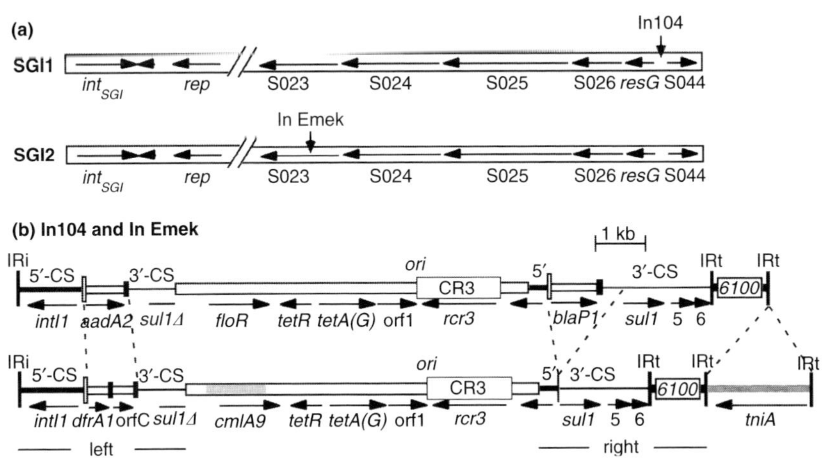

Fig. 7.1. (a) Schematic representation of the derivation of SGI1 and SGI2 from ancestral components. The SGI1 backbone is an open box with hatches surrounding the part that is not shown and arrows indicating orientation and length of genes and open reading frames. Vertical arrows indicate the position of the integrons. (b) The integrons In104 from SGI1 and In Emek from SGI2 are drawn from GenBank accession nos AF261825 and AY963803. Lines of different thickness represent regions with different origins, e.g. the 5′-CS, 3′-CS and *tni* regions of class 1 integrons. Tall open boxes represent the *attI1* sites and gene cassettes are open boxes with a black bar, indicating the *attC* site, at one end. CR3 and IS*6100* are represented by open boxes labelled with the element's designation. The central region that is not integron-derived is represented as a narrower open box. The position and orientation of genes and open reading frames, which are named or numbered, are indicated by arrows below. Dashed lines join regions that are replaced or only present in one integron.

et al., 2004). In *Salmonella*, enzymatic inactivation by type A or type B chloramphenicol acetyltransferases (Cat), as well as the export of chloramphenicol or chloramphenicol/florfenicol by specific efflux proteins, are the dominant resistance mechanisms. Two *catA* genes, *catA1* and *catA2*, have so far been detected in *Salmonella* isolates. The Tn*9*- or Tn*2670*-borne gene *catA1* has been detected in a wide variety of serovars whereas *catA2* is present only in a few serovars. Three *catB* genes, *catB2*, *catB3* and *catB8*, are known to occur in *Salmonella*. They are all located in gene cassettes mainly in class 1 multi-resistance integrons. The chloramphenicol exporter gene *cmlA1* and a close relative, *cmlA4*, are also cassette-borne genes found in plasmid-linked class 1 integrons (Michael *et al.*, 2005). Other relatives of the *cmlA*-encoded efflux proteins, encoded by the *floR* (also designated *flo*, flo_{St}, *pp-flo*, or *cmlA*-like) and *cmlA9* genes can also export florfenicol. These genes are also a part of the SGI1- and SGI2-associated multi-resistance gene clusters (see Fig. 7.1). In addition, *floR* has been identified on a conjugative R55-related plasmid from *S.* Newport and together with the β-lactamase gene bla_{CMY-2} on multi-resistance plasmids in *S.* Typhimurium and *S.* Newport (Doublet *et al.*, 2004b). The presence of more than one phenicol resistance gene in the same *Salmonella* isolate appears to be rare, and involves genes specifying different resistance mechanisms, such as *catA1* + *floR* in *S.* Typhimurium var. Copenhagen or *catA2* + *cmlA1* in *S.* Choleraesuis (Michael *et al.*, 2006).

Resistance to aminoglycosides and aminocyclitols

In *Salmonella*, as in most other bacteria, resistance to aminoglycosides is most frequently mediated by aminoglycoside-modifying enzymes, O-adenyltransferases, N-acetyltransferases and O-phosphotransferases. For each of these three classes, numerous members are known which differ in the position they modify and more or less extensively in their structure. A recent review provided a summary of the various aminoglycoside-modifying enzymes and their substrate profiles identified in bacteria (Ramirez and Tolmasky, 2010). The use of two different nomenclature systems for the genes coding for each aminoglycoside-modifying enzyme confuses this area. The original designations are *aadA*, *aadB*, *aacA*, *aacC* and *aphA*, *B*, *C* etc., where A, B, C etc. indicated the position modified and numbers indicated the specific gene. A more recent and now outmoded system uses designations such as *aph(3″)-Ib* indicating the type of modification (*aph* for aminoglycoside phosphotransferase), the position where the modification is introduced (3″) and I, II, II etc. indicating the substrate profile, and a letter (*b*) the specific gene.

Resistance to streptomycin and spectinomycin

Resistance to streptomycin and the aminocyclitol spectinomycin is conferred by *aadA* genes encoding aminoglycoside-O-adenyltransferases whose products act at the 3″ position (also called *ant(3″)* aminoglycoside-O-nucleotidyltransferase genes). At least ten defined *aadA* genes, *aadA1*, *aadA2*, *aadA5*, *aadA6*, *aadA7*, *aadA12*, *aadA21*, *aadA22*, *aadA23* and *aadA24*, have been sequenced from various *Salmonella* serovars (Michael *et al.*, 2006; Egorova *et al.*, 2007; Rodríguez *et al.*, 2008; Wiesner *et al.*, 2009). All of these *aadA* genes are in gene cassettes in class 1 or class 2 integrons, with some of the integrons located on plasmids whilst others are part of the SGI1-associated multi-resistance gene cluster (Fig. 7.1).

The genes *strA* (also known as *aph(3″)-Ib*) and *strB* (*aph(6)-Id*) both encode phosphotransferases and confer resistance to streptomycin only. These genes are part of Tn*5393* where they are linked (Cain and Hall, 2011). However, the *strA–strB* end of Tn*5393* is frequently associated with the sulfonamide resistance gene *sul2* and how this can occur has recently been described (Yau *et al.*, 2010). The *strA–strB* genes have been detected in the chromosomal DNA and on plasmids of many *Salmonella* serovars (Michael *et al.*, 2006).

Resistance to other aminoglycosides

The cassette-borne *aadB* gene (occasionally *ant(2″)-Ia*), which confers resistance to gentamicin, kanamycin and tobramycin via an aminoglycoside-2″-O-adenyltransferase, was found together with either *aadA1* or *aadA2* in the same integron in single isolates of serovars Heidelberg, Saintpaul, Senftenberg and Typhimurium (Michael *et al.*, 2006).

Genes encoding *N*-acetyltransferases that acetylate positions 3 (*aacC, aac(3)*), and 6′ (*aacA, aac(6′)*) have been detected in gentamicin-resistant *Salmonella* isolates. Several gene cassette-associated *aacC* genes, *aacC-A1* (*aac(3)-Ia*), *aacC-A2* (*aac(3)-Ib*), *aacC-A4* (*aac(3)-Id*) and *aacC-A5* (also called *aac(3)-Id*), have been identified as part of integrons in various *Salmonella* serovars (Levings *et al.*, 2005b). They are found in plasmids and in SGI1 variants. Various cassette-associated *aacA* (*aac(6′)*) genes, such as *aacA4* (*aac(6′)-Ib* and amino acid substitution variants *aac(6′)-IIc, aac(6′)-Ib-cr*), *aac(6′)-I30*, *aac(6′)-Iy*, and *aac(6′)-Iaa* have been listed to occur in *Salmonella* (Ramirez and Tolmasky, 2010). In addition, the *aacC2* gene conferring resistance to gentamicin and tobramycin has been found in an SGI1 relative from *S.* Virchow (Wilson and Hall, 2010), and the *aacC4* (*aac(3)-IV*) gene which confers resistance to apramycin as well as gentamicin, netilmicin, tobramycin was detected in *S.* Typhimurium isolates (Chaslus-Dancla *et al.*, 1991). The *aacC4* gene with an adjacent *hph* gene, conferring resistance to hygromycin, was also identified in an IncA/C plasmid from serovars Senftenberg and Ohio (Evershed *et al.*, 2009).

Five different classes of phosphotransferase genes (*aph*) have been described, but only those whose gene products phosphorylate the aminoglycoside at positions 3′ have so far been identified in *Salmonella* isolates. An *aph(3′)-Ia*, *aph(3′)-Ib* and *aph(3′)-Ic* gene responsible for resistance to kanamycin and neomycin has been found on large multiresistance plasmids from *S.* Choleraesuis (Chiu *et al.*, 2005) and *S.* Typhimurium (Chen *et al.*, 2007; Cain and Hall, 2011; Plate 7a). The Tn*5*-borne *aph(3′)-IIa* gene (also known as *kan*, *neo*, or *aphA2*) was detected by PCR in single isolates of serovars Derby, Enteritidis, Haardt and Typhimurium (Michael *et al.*, 2006).

Recently, the Tn*1548*-associated gene *armA* coding for a 16S rRNA methylase that confers high-level resistance to all clinically available aminoglycosides (except streptomycin) has been sequenced from *S.* Stanley and *S.* Paratyphi B (Folster *et al.*, 2009; Du *et al.*, 2012). In the latter case the *armA* gene was co-located on a ca. 71.8 kb plasmid that also harboured a number of other resistance genes: *dfrA1*, *aadA5*, *sul1*, *msr*(E) (referred to as *mel*), *mph*(E) (referred to as *mph2*), *qnrB2*, *aac(6′)-Ib-cr* and $bla_{CTX\text{-}M\text{-}3}$ (Du *et al.*, 2012). Of the five genes *rmtA–rmtE* that code for a 16S rRNA methylase with a similar substrate spectrum as ArmA, only the *rmtC* gene has been identified in *Salmonella* so far (Folster *et al.*, 2009).

Resistance to trimethoprim

High-level trimethoprim resistance in *Enterobacteriaceae* is mainly due to the replacement of a trimethoprim-sensitive dihydrofolate reductase by a plasmid-, transposon- or cassette-borne trimethoprim-resistant dihydrofolate reductase. So far, more than 30 different trimethoprim resistance-mediating dihydrofolate reductase (*dfr*) genes have been identified. These are subdivided on the basis of their structure into two major types, which are referred to as *dfrA* and *dfrB* (Recchia and Hall, 1995).

A total of 16 different *dfrA* genes, mostly cassette-borne and located in class 1 or class 2 integrons, have been sequenced from various *Salmonella* serovars. These include: *dfrA1, dfrA3, dfrA5, dfrA7, dfrA10, dfrA12, dfrA13, dfrA14, dfrA15b, dfrA16, dfrA17, dfrA19, dfrA21, dfrA23, dfrA25* and *dfrA32* (Agerso *et al.*, 2006; Michael *et al.*, 2006; Krauland *et al.*, 2010). The *dfrA1* gene was detected most frequently, and it is also a component of the SGI1-associated multiresistance gene clusters in serovars Albany and Emek (Hall, 2010). The *dfrA10* gene was detected in the SGI1 variant of *S.* Agona (Boyd *et al.*, 2002) and in serovar Kiambu (Levings *et al.*, 2005a). In a number of studies, integrons containing *dfrA* gene cassettes have been found on multi-resistance plasmids (see Cain *et al.*, 2010).

Only a single cassette-borne *dfrB* gene, *dfrB6*, was detected together with an *aadA1* cassette in a class 1 integron in clonally related *S.* Infantis isolates (Levings *et al.*, 2006b).

Resistance to sulfonamides

Three sulfonamide resistance genes, *sul1*, *sul2*, and *sul3*, all of which encode sulfonamide-resistant dihydropteroate synthases have been identified and all have been found in *Salmonella* (Michael *et al.*, 2006). The *sul1* gene is part of the 3′-conserved segment (3′-CS) of class 1 integrons. Although numerous reports identify the gene cassettes located in class 1 integrons, whether the *sul1* gene is also present has rarely been investigated (Cain *et al.*, 2010). The *sul2* gene is normally associated with the small mobile element CR2 (Partridge and Hall, 2003), but is also often physically linked with the streptomycin resistance genes *strA–strB* (Cain *et al.*, 2010; Yau *et al.*, 2010). The more recently described *sul3* gene is usually found in a region that replaces the 3′-CS of class 1 integrons, but it has been detected together with *sul1* on a large multi-resistance plasmid from *S.* Choleraesuis (Chiu *et al.*, 2005). This gene is widespread in various serovars (Guerra *et al.*, 2004).

Resistance to penicillins and cephalosporins

Bacterial resistance to β-lactam antibiotics (including penicillins and cephalosporins) in *Salmonella* is mainly mediated by β-lactamase enzymes, which inactivate the antibiotics. The β-lactamases identified in *Salmonella* constitute a diverse group of enzymes encoded by a large repertoire of genes. Database searches identified at least 11 different subgroups of β-lactamase genes (*bla*) coding for TEM, SHV, PSE, OXA, PER, CTX-M, CMY, ACC, DHA, KPC or SCO types. A few examples of different β-lactamases identified in *Salmonella* are given below (for further references see Michael *et al.*, 2006).

The TEM-type β-lactamases are all products of variants of a single gene, bla_{TEM}, that is part of Tn2. Those encoded by bla_{TEM-1} and $bla_{TEM-135}$ represent broad-spectrum penicillinases. Other bla_{TEM} variants, such as bla_{TEM-3}, bla_{TEM-4}, bla_{TEM-20}, bla_{TEM-27}, bla_{TEM-52}, bla_{TEM-63}, $bla_{TEM-131}$, $bla_{TEM-138}$ (Chouchani *et al.*, 2006) and $bla_{TEM-188}$, code for extended-spectrum β-lactamases (ESBLs), which can also inactivate oxyiminocephalosporins and monobactams. The SHV-type β-lactamases are also all products of variants of a single gene, and those found in *Salmonella*, bla_{SHV-2}, bla_{SHV-2a}, bla_{SHV-5}, bla_{SHV-9}, and bla_{SHV-12}, encode ESBLs. The PSE-1 or CARB-2 β-lactamase is a penicillinase that hydrolyses carbenicillin. The cassette-borne *blaP1* or bla_{PSE-1} gene is in the SGI1 multi-resistance gene cluster (*blaP1* in Fig. 7.1) and is most frequently found in *Salmonella* strains harbouring SGI1. A closely related gene bla_{CARB-8} was detected in a gene cassette in a multi-resistance integron. Several OXA-type β-lactamases, which exhibit enhanced activity against oxacillin and cloxacillin, have been identified in *Salmonella*. Examples include bla_{OXA-1}, bla_{OXA-2}, bla_{OXA-9}, bla_{OXA-10} (formerly known as bla_{PSE-2}), bla_{OXA-30} and bla_{OXA-53}. These bla_{OXA} genes are also commonly cassette-borne and widely distributed among Gram-negative bacteria. Two types of PER β-lactamases, PER-1 and PER-2, classified as ESBLs have been identified in *Salmonella*. The bla_{PER-1} and bla_{PER-2} genes are often located on multi-resistance plasmids. A wide range of CTX-M β-lactamases, all of which are ESBLs, are currently known. In *Salmonella*, the following genes coding for these enzymes have been detected: $bla_{CTX-M-2}$, $bla_{CTX-M-3}$, $bla_{CTX-M-4}$, $bla_{CTX-M-5}$, $bla_{CTX-M-6}$, $bla_{CTX-M-7}$, $bla_{CTX-M-9}$, $bla_{CTX-M-14}$, $bla_{CTX-M-15}$, $bla_{CTX-M-17}$ or $bla_{CTX-M-18}$, $bla_{CTX-M-27}$, $bla_{CTX-M-28}$, $bla_{CTX-M-32}$, $bla_{CTX-M-53}$ (Doublet *et al.*, 2009c), $bla_{CTX-M-61}$, $bla_{CTX-M-65}$ + $bla_{CTX-M-90}$, and $bla_{CTX-M-83}$ to $bla_{CTX-M-86}$ (Cui *et al.*, 2009).

AmpC β-lactamases, such as CMY-, AAC- and DHA-β-lactamases, have also been identified in *Salmonella*. These cephalosporinases can hydrolyse all β-lactams except carbapenems. Three different types of CMY β-lactamases determined by bla_{CMY-2}, bla_{CMY-4} and bla_{CMY-7} genes have been detected in various *S. enterica* serovars with bla_{CMY-2} being most common. Only one representative of the bla_{ACC-1}, bla_{SCO-1} and bla_{DHA-1} genes is known in *Salmonella* (Ktari *et al.*, 2009). Finally, the KPC-2 carbapenemase has recently been detected as the first representative of this class of β-lactamases in *Salmonella* isolates.

Resistance to quinolones and fluoroquinolones

In *Salmonella*, mutations that result in quinolone/fluoroquinolone resistance are located in the quinolone resistance-determining region (QRDR) of the genes *gyrA*, *gyrB*, *parC* and/or *parE*, which code for subunits of the DNA gyrase or the topoisomerase IV (reviewed by Cloeckaert and Chaslus-Dancla, 2001; Piddock, 2002; Hopkins *et al.*, 2005). Single or double mutations resulting in amino acid exchanges most frequently affect the positions Ser-83 or Asp-87 in GyrA, Ser80 in ParC, Ser-464 in GyrB, whereas alterations in ParE are rarely observed.

Currently, there are three types of transferable quinolone resistance genes associated with plasmids and integrons, including: (i) five different *qnr* gene families, *qnrA1-7*; *qnrB1-72*; *qnrC*; *qnrD* and *qnrS1-8*, whose products protect the DNA topoisomerases from the inhibitory effects of quinolones/fluoroquinolones (Jacoby *et al.*, 2008); (ii) a variant form of the cassette-associated *aacA4* aminoglycoside acetyltransferase gene, *aac(6')-Ib-cr*, that confers cross-resistance to ciprofloxacin (Robicsek *et al.*, 2006); and (iii) *qepA* encoding a substrate-specific efflux pump (Yamane *et al.*, 2007). Various *qnr* genes (*qnrA1, qnrB2, qnrB4, qnrB5, qnrB6, qnrB12, qnrB19, qnrS1, qnrS4, qnrD*) and the *aac(6')-Ib-cr* gene have been identified in *Salmonella* serovars (Torpdahl *et al.*, 2009; Sjölund-Karlsson *et al.*, 2010; Veldman *et al.*, 2011). In particular *qnrS1*, *qnrB2* and *qnrB19* are often located on plasmids, which can also harbour additional resistance genes (Hopkins *et al.*, 2007; Kehrenberg *et al.*, 2007; García-Fernández *et al.*, 2009).The *qepA* gene has not been detected yet in *Salmonella*.

Miscellaneous resistance properties

The sequences of large multi-resistance plasmids or multi-resistance integrons have revealed several unexpected resistance genes. Since *Salmonella* and other *Enterobacteriaceae* are commonly resistant to clinically achievable levels of macrolides, it was surprising to find genes such as *mph*(A) coding for a macrolide phosphotransferase on pU302L from *S.* Typhimurium (Chen *et al.*, 2007), *ere*(A) specifying a macrolide esterase in *S.* Wien (AY827837), *msr*(E) (also named *mel*) and *mph*(E) (also named *mph2*) coding for an ABC transporter involved in macrolide resistance and a macrolide phosphotransferase, respectively, on pXD1 from *S.* Paratyphi B (Du *et al.*, 2012), and the cassette-borne lincosamide nucleotidyltransferase gene *linG* in *S.* Stanley (Levings *et al.*, 2006a).

The *sat* or *sat2* genes, coding for streptothricin acetyltransferases, are also detected occasionally in *Salmonella* isolates (Ahmed *et al.*, 2005; Chiu *et al.*, 2005). The location of *ere*(A), *sat* and *sat2* in gene cassettes in class 1 or in class 2 integrons (usually as part of Tn7) might explain how they are acquired by *Salmonella* isolates.

Finally, it may be relevant in terms of co-selection of resistances to antimicrobials and heavy metals that multi-resistance plasmids such as pSC138 from *S.* Choleraesuis (Chiu *et al.*, 2005), pU302L (Chen *et al.*, 2007) and pSRC26 and pSRC125 from *S.* Typhimurium (Cain *et al.*, 2010) and also SGI1K from *S.* Kentucky (Levings *et al.*, 2007) and some of its variants, all carry *mer* operons conferring resistance to mercury compounds.

SGI-type genomic islands

In several *Salmonella* serovars multiple antibiotic resistance is due to the presence of a genomic island that harbours resistance genes. The best understood of these genomic resistance islands are those that are found in a specific location in the chromosome, at the end of the *thdF* gene. The first island of this type (Fig. 7.1) was found in *S.* Typhimurium DT104 isolates resistant to ampicillin, chloramphenicol, florfenicol, streptomycin, spectinomycin, sulfonamides and tetracycline and was named SGI1 for *Salmonella* genomic island 1 (Boyd *et al.*, 2001; Mulvey *et al.*, 2006). However, a related but independently derived island, SGI2, was subsequently found in *S.* Emek isolates that are resistant to chloramphenicol, florfenicol, sulfonamides, tetracycline and trimethoprim (Levings *et al.*, 2008; Wilson and Hall, 2010). SGI1 and relatives carrying different sets of genes that confer resistance to more, fewer or different antibiotics have since been found in other *Salmonella* serovars (including Agona, Albany, Cerro, Derby, Düsseldorf, Haifa, Infantis, Kedougou, Kentucky, Kiambu, Kingston, Meleagredis, Newport, Paratyphi B, Tallahassee) and also in *Proteus mirabilis* (for details see Hall, 2010). However, there is often a clear association between the variant type and serovar. For example, SGI1 is found in serovars Typhimurium, Meleagredis and Paratyphi B dT^{+} (Djordjevic *et al.*, 2009; Hall, 2010), whereas SGI1-A, is seen in serovars Agona (Boyd *et al.*, 2002; Doublet *et al.*, 2004a) and Kiambu (Levings *et al.*, 2005a) and SGI1-K is found in serovar Kentucky (Levings *et al.*, 2007; Le Hello *et al.*, 2011). SGI2 and relatives have so far only been found in serovars Emek (Levings *et al.*, 2008; Vo *et al.*, 2010) and Virchow (Doublet *et al.*, 2009a; Chu *et al.*, 2012). This is consistent with limited horizontal transfer events and extensive clonal expansion. However, SGI1 is mobilizable but cannot transfer itself into a new host unless an IncA/C plasmid is present to facilitate transfer (Doublet *et al.*, 2005; Douard *et al.*, 2010). Hence, these genomic islands are integrative mobilizable elements.

SGI1 (42.4 kb) and SGI2 (43.2 kb) both carry a complex class 1 integron, which contains the resistance genes. In104 in SGI1 is located between *resG* and S044 near one end of the island backbone and InEmek in SGI2 is located within S023 (Fig. 7.1a). A gene, int_{SGI} (on the left in Fig. 7.1a) in the backbone encodes a tyrosine recombinase family site-specific recombinase. $IntI_{SGI}$ can excise the SGI from the chromosome and re-insert it at preferred sites (Doublet *et al.*, 2005). The main chromosomal integration site is located close to the 3′-end of the *thdF* gene, but a preferred secondary integration site has also been found (Doublet *et al.*, 2008a). In all *Salmonella* serovars except Typhimurium, *thdF* is adjacent to *yidY*, and linkage of markers internal to the SGI to these genes is often used to identify isolates carrying an SGI (Boyd *et al.*, 2002; Levings *et al.*, 2005a; Djordjevic *et al.*, 2009; Wilson and Hall, 2010). Linkage of markers in the integron to ones in the island backbone distinguish SGI1 from SGI2 (Levings *et al.*, 2005a; Wilson and Hall, 2010).

The antibiotic resistance genes are all found in the class 1 integrons belonging to the In4 family. In104 includes five resistance genes (Fig. 7.1b). Two cassette-associated genes, *aadA2* (streptomycin and spectinomycin resistance) and *blaP1* (bla_{PSE-1}) (resistance to ampicillin) are found on the left and right, respectively (as in Fig. 7.1b), and a complete *sul1* sulfonamide resistance gene is located in the longer 3′-CS on the right. The *tetA*(G) tetracycline resistance gene and *floR* gene, a *cmlA1* homologue, both encode efflux proteins. They are located between the two class 1 integron-derived regions (labelled left and right in Fig. 7.1b) and next to the small mobile element CR3. In Emek has a similar structure (Fig. 7.1b), but contains the *dfrA1* (trimethoprim resistance) and orfC cassettes on the left and *sul1* but no cassette on the right due to a deletion that removed the cassette integration site (*attI*) (Levings *et al.*, 2005a). The configuration between the integron-derived segments is the same as in In104, except that part of the *floR* gene has been replaced by an allelic variant to create *cmlA9* (Levings *et al.*, 2008). The remaining difference is the presence of part of a *tni* module that is related but not identical to that of Tn*402* (Wilson and Hall, 2010).

Simple variant forms of SGI1 and SGI2

Homologous recombination can generate variants of SGI1 and SGI2 with different resistance genes. SGI1 variants, that harbour an integron between *resG* and S044 (as shown in Fig. 7.1a), in which one or both of the gene cassettes have been replaced by other cassettes conferring resistance to different antibiotics have been identified (see Tables 1 and 2 in Hall, 2010). These can arise via homologous recombination with another class 1 integron if recombination occurs in both the 5′-CS and 3′-CS on the same side of the complex integron. For example, SGI1-F and SGI1-I are the same as SGI1 except that the *dfrA1*-orfC cassette array has replaced the cassette on the left and right, respectively (Doublet *et al.*, 2003). The *dfrA10* trimethoprim resistance gene, in association with CR1 and part of the 3′-CS, is seen as an addition to SGI1 (SGI1-A) (Doublet *et al.*, 2004a; Levings *et al.*, 2005a). This configuration can also arise via homologous recombination between the resident and incoming copies of the *sul1* gene.

SGI1, the variants of SGI1 carrying different gene cassettes described above, or SGI2 can lose the region between the two copies of either the 5′-CS or the 3′-CS. The resulting variants have lost the *floR* or *cmlA9* and *tetA*(G) genes and one of the cassette-encoded resistance genes. The variants named SGI1-B and SGI1-C derived from SGI1 retain *blaP1* or *aadA2*, respectively. They arise spontaneously (Djordjevic *et al.*, 2009) and are found among SGI-containing isolates from humans and animals (for references see Djordjevic *et al.*, 2009 and Hall, 2010). Equivalent derivatives of SGI2 have also been detected (Levings *et al.*, 2008; Wilson and Hall, 2010; Chu *et al.*, 2012).

The SGI1-H/SGI1-K/SGI1-L group

Most studies have not determined whether the complete backbone of the island is present in the various SGI variants. However, a modified backbone is found in the SGI1-H/SGI1-L/SGI1-K group (Doublet *et al.*, 2009b; Wilson and Hall, 2010). These three variant types confer resistance to gentamicin and to streptomycin and spectinomycin due to a pair of gene cassettes, *aacCA5-aadA7* (Doublet *et al.*, 2004c; Levings *et al.*, 2005b). SGI1-H found in *S.* Newport has the simplest configuration with an integron identical to In104 except that the *aacCA5-aadA7* cassettes are found on the left (Doublet *et al.*, 2004c). SGI1-H is likely to be the ancestor of a set of the more complex SGI1 variants SGI1-K and SGI1-L.

SGI1-K (accession no.: AY463797) was found in a *S.* Kentucky isolate resistant to ampicillin, gentamicin, streptomycin, spectinomycin, sulfonamides and tetracycline (Levings *et al.*, 2007). The integron in SGI1-K includes only the *aacCA5-aadA7* cassette array and *sul1* (Levings *et al.*, 2007). It also includes a *mer* module conferring resistance to mercuric ions (Hg(II)) that is a hybrid of the ones found in Tn*501* and Tn*21* (Levings *et al.*, 2007). Tetracycline resistance was due to a *tetA*(A) determinant instead of *tetA*(G), ampicillin resistance was conferred by the bla_{TEM} gene and streptomycin resistance by the *strAB* genes (Levings *et al.*, 2005b). The *tetA*(A), *strAB* and bla_{TEM} genes are found in a 13.1 kb region located between the *mer* module and a remnant of S044 (Doublet *et al.*, 2008b). This region consists of fragments of transposons Tn*1721*, Tn*5393* and Tn*2* supplying the resistance genes and two copies of IS*26*. A number of variants, some of which have lost all of the antibiotic resistance genes, have arisen via deletions or rearrangements caused by IS*26* and have been seen in *S.* Kentucky isolates (Doublet *et al.*, 2008b; Le Hello *et al.*, 2011).

The SGI1-L variant SGI1-L1 (Doublet *et al.*, 2009b) contains an arrangement that is likely to be an intermediate between SGI1-H and SGI1-K. In SGI1-L1, the integron containing the *aacAC5-aadA7* and *blaP1* cassettes are in the same position as in SGI1-H, namely nearest to *resG* and S044, respectively. A third integron region containing the *dfrA15* trimethoprim resistance gene cassette is located between them together with the region containing the *mer*, *strA-strB*, *tetA*(A) and bla_{TEM} genes found in SGI1-K. SGI1-K can be generated from SGI1-L1 by the action of IS*26*. SGI1-H and SGI1-L1 and their variants are found in *S.* Newport (Doublet *et al.*, 2009b), suggesting that evolution occurred in this serovar.

Further SGI1 variants

The variant SGI1-S found in *S.* Virchow SL491 (accession no.: ABFH02000001; draft genome) contains an unusual arrangement with both an integron and the mercuric ion resistance transposon Tn*512* both inserted between *resG* and S044 (Wilson and Hall, 2010). Within the integron are the *dfrA1*-orfC cassette pair, the *sul1* gene and two aminoglycoside resistance genes *rmtC*, which confers resistance to gentamicin, kanamycin, tobramycin and amikacin, and *aacC2*, which confers resistance to gentamicin and tobramycin. A few cases where the IS*6100* has caused deletions in In104 or relatives have been documented.

Resistance Plasmids in *Salmonella*

Plasmids play an important role in the horizontal transfer of resistance genes between *Salmonella* and other bacteria. Moreover, they can undergo recombination, integration and co-integrate formation, processes giving rise to new plasmids that carry parts of each 'parental' plasmid. To better understand how multidrug resistance plasmids of *Salmonella* evolve and to improve our knowledge of the epidemiology of the associated resistance markers, complete sequence analysis of resistance plasmids is indispensable. Selected examples are provided below that highlight the importance of horizontal gene transfer as well as recombination, integration and co-integrate formation in the evolution of resistance plasmids in *Salmonella*.

High molecular weight plasmids in *Salmonella*

Some representative large plasmids of >40 kb from various serovars that have been completely sequenced are shown in Plate 7a. These broadly represent a backbone structure noted in large plasmids, consisting of those genes necessary to maintain and in some cases transfer the plasmid between bacteria. In addition, there are accessory regions, which are variable and may contain resistance and/or virulence-encoding genes.

Plasmid UO-StVR2 (49,507 bp, accession no.: AM991977) is an example of a hybrid virulence-resistance plasmid from *S.* Typhimurium (Herrero *et al.*, 2008). This plasmid was derived from the serovar-specific virulence plasmid pSLT, following the acquisition of a complex resistance island, flanked by regions containing toxin-antitoxin and iron-uptake systems. Plasmid UO-StVR2 (Plate 7a) confers resistance to ampicillin (encoded by the bla_{OXA-1}), chloramphenicol (*catA1*), streptomycin/spectinomycin (*aadA1*), sulfonamides (*sul1*) and tetracycline (*tetA*(B)). These genes are clustered on a resistance island of 28,756 bp. Both the bla_{OXA-1} and the *aadA1* genes are contained within the variable gene cassette region of an integron denoted as InH. Several pSLT-associated virulence genes, such as *spvC*, *rck* and *samA* among others, are also located on this plasmid. Further virulence/resistance hybrid plasmids, which – like pUO-StVR2 – allow for the co-selection of virulence and antimicrobial resistance genes have recently been described in *Salmonella* serovar 4,[5],12:i:- (García *et al.*, 2011) and *S.* Enteritidis (Rodríguez *et al.*, 2011).

From a *S.* Typhimurium PT U302 isolate, designated as G8430, two plasmids, one large denoted as pU302L (81,514 bp, accession no.: AY333434, Plate 7a) and a smaller 3208 bp plasmid, pU302S (accession no.: AY333433, Plate 7b) were identified (Chen *et al.*, 2007). The former is an F-like plasmid with two replication regions consisting of a functional *oriS* (from RepF1A) and an inactive *oriV* (of RepF1B). Several interesting plasmid-encoded genes were noted including a post-segregational killing system (encoded by *hok/sok*), along with four toxin-antitoxin systems (including *ccdA/B*; *pemI/K* and two *vagC/D* loci) and a plasmid partitioning system (*sopA/B/C*). Since pU302L lacked *oriT*, it is incapable of conjugal transfer. Furthermore it possesses 14 IS elements, along with several truncated transposons and other similar features. Interestingly the locus between 21,660 and 29,080 bp in pU302L contained a resistance-encoding gene cluster with the following composition: IS*26*-*strB*-*strA*-*sul2*-[---]-IS*26*-bla_{TEM-1}-IS*1294*. This arrangement (apart from the distally located IS*1294*, which is replaced by IS*26* in other plasmids) has been detected previously on a number of plasmids including pHCM1 from *S.* Typhi (Wain *et al.*, 2003) and an IncHI2 plasmid from *S.* Typhimurium (Cain *et al.*, 2010), and an IncI plasmid from *S.* Enteritidis and on the chromosome of *S.* Typhimurium DT193 (Daly *et al.*, 2005), suggesting that it may move *en bloc* among enteric bacteria. The smaller pU302S (Plate 7b) contained a ColE1-like origin, along with an *oriT*, *mobA* and *aphA1* genes. No virulence markers were associated with either pU302L or pU302S.

A plasmid, denoted as pSC138 (138,742 bp, accession no.: AY509004) and the serovar-specific virulence plasmid SCV50 (49,558 bp, accession no.: AY509003) were identified in the complete genome of *S.* Choleraesuis SC-B67 (Chiu *et al.*, 2005). Plasmid pSC138 was re-annotated recently and found to contain 177 ORFs, of which 60% have known functions. It contains several examples of mobile genetic elements, including two integrons, seven IS elements, eight transposons and a truncated prophage. The plasmid can be divided into three distinguishable regions of similar size (Ye *et al.*, 2011). The first of these is a 50 kb DNA sequence containing a Tn*21*-like transposon, denoted as Tn*6088*. A second region of approximately 30 kb contains the transfer/maintenance genes, in addition to a specific IS*Ecp1*-bla_{AmpC}-*blc*-*sugE*-structure inserted into a *finQ* gene. The latter gene array was also recognized in other *Salmonella* serovars including Choleraesuis and other *Enterobacteriaceae*. The bla_{AmpC} gene confers resistance to extended-spectrum β-lactams while the roles of both *blc* and *sugE* remain to be determined, though the former is thought to encode an outer membrane lipoprotein. A Rep_3 replication region is located in the third region that contained a truncated Qin prophage sequence along with a toxin-antitoxin gene combination *relE-relB* and an *int2* phage integrase gene. pSCV50 is the smallest known virulence plasmid in *Salmonella* and does not carry any antimicrobial resistance genes.

A streptomycin and tetracycline resistance plasmid of group IncI1, denoted as pR64 (120,826 bp, accession no.: AP005147, Plate 7a), was isolated from *S.* Typhimurium some time ago (Furuichi *et al.*, 1984). Although the sequence of the conjugation transfer region was determined earlier, the DNA sequence of the entire plasmid has been recently completed (Sampei *et al.*, 2010). Plasmid R64 contains 126 ORFs. Five major regions are recognized, one of which accounts for antimicrobial resistance. The antimicrobial resistance determinants are located in a region of 27.7 kb contained within two transposons. Tetracycline resistance is mediated by a Tn*10*-borne *tetA*(C) gene whilst streptomycin resistance is based on the genes *strA-strB* located within Tn*6082*. Both of these transposons are flanked by IS2 elements, with an additional IS*1133* located within this locus. Interestingly these transposons are found inserted into the *arsA1* gene part of an arsenic-resistance operon.

Recently a resistance plasmid was identified in a *S.* Virchow isolate (Karczmarczyk *et al.*, 2012). Plasmid pVQS1 (40,995 bp, Plate 7a) contained 49 ORFs, divided into regions associated with plasmid replication, maintenance, conjugation and antimicrobial resistance. Within the latter region, a complete Tn3 structure, including $bla_{\text{TEM-1}}$, was located distal to a *qnrS1* determinant; an arrangement that has been observed previously on plasmid pINF5 from avian *S.* Infantis (Kehrenberg *et al.*, 2006). With the exception of the resistance-encoding region, the remainder of pVQS1 was 98% similar at the nucleotide sequence level to the IncN group plasmids R46 (accession no.: AY046276) and MUR050 (accession no.: AY522431). Plasmid VQS1 could be transferred at high-frequency to *E. coli*, a feature that could account for the dissemination of its resistance determinants.

Low molecular weight plasmids in *Salmonella*

In contrast to the data available for large *Salmonella* plasmids, comparatively little information is available describing low molecular weight plasmids, despite the fact that an estimated 10% of *Salmonella* field isolates contain these genetic elements (Rychlik *et al.*, 2006).

The *strA-strB-sul2*-carrying plasmid RSF1010 is found in *Salmonella* (Yau *et al.*, 2010). Recently, small pU302S-related plasmids, which carried a unique *aph(3')-I* gene, were isolated from *S.* Typhimurium, *S.* Newport and *S.* Bardo (Chen *et al.*, 2011). Of these, pSe-Kan (7,132 bp, accession no.: HQ230976) and pSe-Bardo (8,198 bp, accession no.: HQ230977) were sequenced and annotated (Plate 7b). Both were almost identical, with pSe-Bardo possessing a few additional features, including an extra copy of IS*930*. No mobilization genes were identified on either plasmid. When pSe-Kan was compared to pU302S, similarities were mainly confined to the RNA I/II and *rom*-encoding regions

(Chen *et al.*, 2011). Interestingly, based on the sequence identities of the IS*930* elements compared with those contained in pKPN2 and pKPN3 from *Klebsiella pneumoniae*, *Salmonella* isolates may have acquired these genetic elements more recently from *K. pneumoniae* that shared the same ecological niche.

Genes encoding resistance to tetracycline and β-lactams in Gram-negative bacteria have been associated with transposons. The tetracycline resistance gene of hybridization class A (*tetA*(A)) is associated with the Tn*1721* transposon. Complete structures and derivatives thereof were noted in a wide range of conjugative and mobilizable plasmids in Gram-negative bacteria of human, animal, plant and environmental origin (for details see Pasquali *et al.*, 2005). Similarly, genes encoding TEM-type β-lactamases are prevalent also among these bacteria, being detected on conjugative and non-conjugative plasmids and on the chromosome. Plasmid pFPTB1 (12,656 bp, accession no.: AJ634602) was purified from a *S.* Typhimurium PT U302 isolate cultured from a rabbit. This plasmid contains a replication region that is very similar to pJHCMW1 of *K. pneumoniae*, suggesting that the replication of pFPTB1 is mediated by RNA molecules (Pasquali *et al.*, 2005). The plasmid also possessed two transposon-related parts elaborating resistance to ampicillin and tetracycline. A Tn3-like transposon of 4,950 bp encodes a novel β-lactamase gene, $bla_{\text{TEM-135}}$. The second transposon, a Tn*1721*-like structure, contains the *tetA*(A) and *tetR* genes coding for resistance to tetracycline. The evolution of this plasmid structure is of interest, as it represents an example of a co-integrate structure formed between resistance-mediating transposons. Should the Tn3-Tn*1721* structure be disseminated as a unit then this could contribute to the simultaneous spread of resistance to two important classes of antimicrobial compound used in veterinary medicine.

A *qnrS1* gene was reported in 2006 in a *S.* Infantis isolate of avian origin (Kehrenberg *et al.*, 2006), wherein, it was located close to a Tn3-like element carrying a $bla_{\text{TEM-1}}$ gene on a non-conjugative plasmid, denoted as pINF5. This Tn3-*qnrS1* arrangement was identified also on a plasmid, pAH0376 (accession no.: AB187515) from *Shigella flexneri* and more recently in *S.* Virchow cultured from an individual returning from a visit to a foreign country (Karczmarczyk *et al.*, 2012). The genetic organization of these loci is suggestive of the independent acquisition of each marker. The *qnrS1* determinant alone was also identified and characterized, on a 10,066 bp plasmid (pTPqnrS-1a, accession no.: AM746977) from a multi-resistant *S.* Typhimurium. Interestingly, *S.* Typhimurium cultured from a human, in Taiwan between 2003 and 2006, contained a plasmid of 10,107 bp denoted as pST728/06-2 (accession no.: EU715253), that shared 99% nucleic acid sequence identity with pTPqnrS-1a (Wu *et al.*, 2008).

The *qnrB19* allele was also prevalent, with this variant being most often associated with *Salmonella* of different serovars from several European countries. The latter marker was originally characterized on a small ColE-like plasmid (pSGI5, accession no.: FN428572) contained in a *S.* Typhimurium that exhibited the penta-resistance profile, typical of DT104 (Hammerl *et al.*, 2010). An identical plasmid, designated pMK100 (2,699 bp, accession no.: HM070379, Plate 7b), together with a small variant were identified in *Salmonella* serovars Infantis, Uganda and 6,7:d- from Colombia (Karczmarczyk *et al.*, 2010). These isolates were recovered from a chicken and three unrelated food samples. Moreover, similar plasmids were reported in commensal microbial communities cultured from healthy children in Peru and Bolivia (Pallecchi *et al.*, 2009), highlighting the successful dissemination of this genetic element among diverse bacterial populations.

Conclusions

Salmonella enterica continues to accumulate antimicrobial resistance genes contributing to bacterial resistance to all major classes of active compounds. Dynamic evolution of regions containing these genes has culminated in a remarkable genetic redundancy. The repertoire of resistance markers found in *Salmonella* has disseminated via a range of mobile genetic elements, and the extent of clustering of several resistance genes in resistance islands, such as SGI1 and -2 seen on the *Salmonella* chromosome, or on multi-resistance plasmids has been revealed as larger regions are sequenced. Further novel clusters are likely to emerge in the future.

Understanding the relationship between selection pressure imposed as antimicrobial compounds are used, and the emergence of resistance genes and the resistance gene clusters they reside in is essential. This knowledge will be critical to the development of strategies to limit the continued evolution of drug resistance and the preservation of the current arsenal of compounds.

References

Aarts, H.J., Boumedine, K.S., Nesme, X. and Cloeckaert, A. (2001) Molecular tools for the characterisation of antibiotic-resistant bacteria. *Veterinary research* 32, 363–380.

Ageros, Y., Peirano, G. and Aarestrup, F.M. (2006) *dfrA25*, a novel trimethoprim resistance gene from *Salmonella* Agona isolated from a human urine sample in Brazil. *Journal of Antimicrobial Chemotherapy* 58, 1044–1047.

Ahmed, A.M., Nakano, H. and Shimamoto, T. (2005) Molecular characterization of integron in non-typhoid *Salmonella* serovars in Japan: description of an unusual class 2 integron, *Journal of Antimicrobial Chemotherapy* 55, 371–374.

Boyd, D., Peters, G.A., Cloeckaert, A., Boumedine, K.S., Chaslus-Dancla, E., Imberechts, H. and Mulvey, M.R. (2001) Complete nucleotide sequence of a 43-kilobase genomic island associated with the multidrug resistance region of *Salmonella enterica* serovar Typhimurium DT104 and its identification in phage type DT120 and serovar Agona. *Journal of Bacteriology* 183, 5725–5732.

Boyd, D., Cloeckaert, A., Chaslus-Dancla, E. and Mulvey, M.R. (2002) Characterization of variant *Salmonella* genomic island 1 multidrug resistance regions from serovars Typhimurium DT104 and Agona. *Antimicrobial Agents and Chemotherapy* 46, 1714–1722.

Cain, A.K. and Hall, R.M. (2011) Transposon Tn*5393*e carrying an *aphA1*-containing transposon upstream of *strAB* does not confer resistance to streptomycin. *Microbial Drug Resistance* 17, 389–394.

Cain, A.K., Liu, X., Djordjevic, S.P. and Hall, R.M. (2010) Transposons related to Tn*1696* in IncHI2 plasmids in *Salmonella enterica* serovar Typhimurium from Australian animals. *Microbial Drug Resistance* 16, 197–202.

Chaslus-Dancla, E., Pohl, P., Meurisse, M., Marin, M. and Lafont, J.P. (1991) High genetic homology between plasmids of human and animal origins conferring resistance to the aminoglycosides gentamicin and apramycin. *Antimicrobial Agents and Chemotherapy* 35, 590–593.

Chen, C.Y., Nace, G.W., Solow, B. and Fratamico, P. (2007) Complete nucleotide sequences of 84.5- and 3.2-kb plasmids in the multi-antibiotic resistant *Salmonella enterica* serovar Typhimurium U302 strain G8430. *Plasmid* 57, 29–43.

Chen, C.Y., Strobaugh, T.P., Jr, Lindsey, R.L., Frye, J.G. and Uhlich, G. (2011) Sequence analysis of a group of low molecular-weight plasmids carrying multiple IS*903* elements flanking a kanamycin resistance *aph* gene in *Salmonella enterica* serovars. *Plasmid* 65, 246–252.

Chiu, C.H., Tang, P., Chu, C., Hu, S., Bao, Q., Yu, J., Chou, Y.Y., Wang, H.S. and Lee, Y.S. (2005) The genome sequence of *Salmonella enterica* serovar Choleraesuis, a highly invasive and resistant zoonotic pathogen. *Nucleic Acids Research* 33, 1690–1698.

Chouchani, C., Berlemont, R., Masmoudi, A., Galleni, M., Frere, J.M., Belhadj, O. and Ben-Mahrez, K. (2006) A novel extended-spectrum TEM-type beta-lactamase, TEM-138, from *Salmonella enterica* serovar Infantis. *Antimicrobial Agents and Chemotherapy* 50, 3183–3185.

Chu, C., Doublet, B., Lee, Y.L., Cloeckaert, A., Chiou, C.S., Chen, S.W., Lin, C.W. and Chiu, C.H. (2012) *Salmonella* genomic island 1-J variants associated with change in the antibiotic resistance gene cluster in multidrug-resistant *Salmonella enterica* serovar Virchow isolated from humans, Taiwan, 2004-2006. *Clinical Microbiology and Infection* 18, 47–53.

Cloeckaert, A. and Chaslus-Dancla, E. (2001) Mechanisms of quinolone resistance in *Salmonella*. *Veterinary Research* 32, 301–310.

Cui, S., Li, J., Sun, Z., Hu, C., Jin, S., Li, F., Guo, Y., Ran, L. and Ma, Y. (2009) Characterization of *Salmonella enterica* isolates from infants and toddlers in Wuhan, China. *Journal of Antimicrobial Chemotherapy* 63, 87–94.

Daly, M., Villa, L., Pezzella, C., Fanning, S. and Carattoli, A. (2005) Comparison of multidrug resistance gene regions between two geographically unrelated *Salmonella* serotypes. *Journal of Antimicrobial Chemotherapy* 55, 558–561.

Djordjevic, S.P., Cain, A.K., Evershed, N.J., Falconer, L., Levings, R.S., Lightfoot, D. and Hall, R.M. (2009) Emergence and evolution of multiply antibiotic-resistant *Salmonella enterica* serovar Paratyphi B D-tartrate-utilizing strains containing SGI1. *Antimicrobial Agents and Chemotherapy* 53, 2319–2326.

Douard, G., Praud, K., Cloeckaert, A. and Doublet, B. (2010) The *Salmonella* genomic island 1 is specifically mobilized in trans by the IncA/C multidrug resistance plasmid family. *PLoS ONE* 5, e15302.

Doublet, B., Lailler, R., Meunier, D., Brisabois, A., Boyd, D., Mulvey, M.R., Chaslus-Dancla, E. and Cloeckaert, A. (2003) Variant *Salmonella* genomic island 1 antibiotic resistance gene cluster in *Salmonella enterica* serovar Albany. *Emerging Infectious Diseases* 9, 585–591.

Doublet, B., Butaye, P., Imberechts, H., Collard, J.M., Chaslus-Dancla, E. and Cloeckaert, A. (2004a) *Salmonella* Agona harboring genomic island 1-A. *Emerging Infectious Diseases* 10, 756–758.

Doublet, B., Caratolli, A., Whichard, J.M., White, D.G., Baucheron, S., Chaslus-Dancla, E. and Cloeckaert, A. (2004b) Plasmid-mediated florfenicol and ceftriaxone resistance encoded by the *floR* and $bla_{CMY\text{-}2}$ genes in *Salmonella enterica* serovars Typhimurium and Newport isolated in the United States. *FEMS Microbiology Letters* 15, 301–305.

Doublet, B., Weill, F.-X., Fabre, L., Chaslus-Dancla, E. and Cloeckaert, A. (2004c) Variant *Salmonella* genomic island 1 antibiotic resistance gene cluster containing a novel 3′-*N*-aminoglycoside acetyltransferase gene cassette, *aac(3)-Id*, in *Salmonella enterica* serovar Newport. *Antimicrobial Agents and Chemotherapy* 48, 3806–3812.

Doublet, B., Boyd, D., Mulvey, M.R. and Cloeckaert, A. (2005) The *Salmonella* genomic island 1 is an integrative mobilizable element. *Molecular Microbiology* 55, 1911–1924.

Doublet, B., Golding, G.R., Mulvey, M.R. and Cloeckaert, A. (2008a) Secondary chromosomal attachment site and tandem integration of the mobilizable *Salmonella* genomic island 1. *PLoS ONE* 3, e2060.

Doublet, B., Praud, K., Bertrand, S., Collard, J.M., Weill, F.X. and Cloeckaert, A. (2008b) Novel insertion sequence- and transposon-mediated genetic rearrangements in genomic island SGI1 of *Salmonella enterica* serovar Kentucky. *Antimicrobial Agents and Chemotherapy* 52, 3745–3754.

Doublet, B., Chu, C., Chiu, C.H., Fan, Y.C. and Cloeckaert, A. (2009a) Truncated *tni* module adjacent to the complex integron of *Salmonella* genomic island 1 in *Salmonella enterica* serovar Virchow. *Antimicrobial Agents and Chemotherapy* 53, 824–827.

Doublet, B., Praud, K., Weill, F.X. and Cloeckaert, A. (2009b) Association of IS*26*-composite transposons and complex In4-type integrons generates novel multidrug resistance loci in *Salmonella* genomic island 1. *Journal of Antimicrobial Chemotherapy* 63, 282–289.

Doublet, B., Granier, S.A., Robin, F., Bonnet, R., Fabre, L., Brisabois, A., Cloeckaert, A. and Weill, F.X. (2009c) Novel plasmid-encoded ceftazidime-hydrolyzing CTX-M-53 extended-spectrum beta-lactamase from *Salmonella enterica* serotypes Westhampton and Senftenberg. *Antimicrobial Agents and Chemotherapy* 53, 1944–1951.

Du, X.D., Li, D.X., Hu, G.Z., Wang, Y., Shang, Y.H., Wu, C.M., Liu, H.B. and Li, X.S. (2012) Tn*1548*-associated *armA* is co-located with *qnrB2*, *aac(6′)-Ib*-cr and $bla_{CTX\text{-}M\text{-}3}$ on an IncFII plasmid in a *Salmonella enterica* subsp. *enterica* serovar Paratyphi B strain isolated from chickens in China. *Journal of Antimicrobial Chemotherapy* 67, 246–248.

Egorova, S., Kaftyreva, L., Grimont, P.A. and Weill, F.X. (2007) Prevalence and characterization of extended-spectrum cephalosporin-resistant nontyphoidal *Salmonella* isolates in adults in Saint Petersburg, Russia (2002-2005). *Microbial Drug Resistance* 13, 102–107.

Evershed, N.J., Levings, R.S., Wilson, N.L., Djordjevic, S.P. and Hall, R.M. (2009) Unusual class 1 integron-associated gene cassette configuration found in IncA/C plasmids from *Salmonella enterica*. *Antimicrobial Agents and Chemotherapy* 53, 2640–2642.

Folster, J.P., Rickert, R., Barzilay, E.J. and Whichard, J.M. (2009) Identification of the aminoglycoside resistance determinants *armA* and *rmtC* among non-Typhi *Salmonella* isolates from humans in the United States. *Antimicrobial Agents and Chemotherapy* 53, 4563–4564.

Furuichi, T., Komano, T. and Nisioka, T. (1984) Physical and genetic analyses of the Inc-I alpha plasmid R64. *Journal of Bacteriology* 158, 997–1004.

García, P., Guerra, B., Bances, M., Mendoza, M.C. and Rodicio, M.R. (2011) IncA/C plasmids mediate antimicrobial resistance linked to virulence genes in the Spanish clone of the emerging *Salmonella enterica* serotype 4,[5],12:i:-. *Journal of Antimicrobial Chemotherapy* 66, 543–549.

García-Fernández, A., Fortini, D., Veldman, K., Mevius, D. and Carattoli, A. (2009) Characterization of plasmids harbouring *qnrS1*, *qnrB2* and *qnrB19* genes in *Salmonella*. *Journal of Antimicrobial Chemotherapy* 63, 274–281.

Guerra, B., Junker, E. and Helmuth, R. (2004) Incidence of the recently described sulfonamide resistance gene *sul3* among German *Salmonella enterica* strains isolated from livestock and food. *Antimicrobial Agents and Chemotherapy* 48, 2712–2715.

Hammerl, J.A., Beutlich, J., Hertwig, S., Mevius, D., Threlfall, E.J., Helmuth, R. and Guerra, B. (2010) pSGI15, a small ColE-like *qnrB19* plasmid of a *Salmonella enterica* serovar Typhimurium strain carrying *Salmonella* genomic island 1 (SGI1). *Journal of Antimicrobial Chemotherapy* 65, 173–175.

Hall, R.M. (2010) *Salmonella* genomic islands and antibiotic resistance in *Salmonella enterica*. *Future Microbiology* 5, 125–138.

Herrero, A., Mendoza, M.C., Rodicio, R. and Rodicio, M.R. (2008) Characterization of pUO-StVR2, a virulence-resistance plasmid evolved from the pSLT virulence plasmid of *Salmonella enterica* serovar Typhimurium. *Antimicrobial Agents and Chemotherapy* 52, 4514–4517.

Hopkins, K.L., Davies, R.H. and Threlfall, E.J. (2005) Mechanisms of quinolone resistance in *Escherichia coli* and *Salmonella*: Recent developments. *International Journal of Antimicrobial Agents* 25, 358–373.

Hopkins, K.L., Wootton, L., Day, M.R. and Threlfall, E.J. (2007) Plasmid-mediated quinolone resistance determinant *qnrS1* found in *Salmonella enterica* strains isolated in the UK. *Journal of Antimicrobial Chemotherapy* 59, 1071–1075.

Jacoby, G., Cattoir, V., Hooper, D., Martinez-Martinez, L., Nordmann, P., Pascual, A., Poirel, L. and Wang, M. (2008) *qnr* gene nomenclature. *Antimicrobial Agents and Chemotherapy* 52, 2297–2299.

Karczmarczyk, M., Martins, M., McCusker, M., Mattar, S., Amaral, L., Leonard, N., Aarestrup, F.M. and Fanning, S. (2010) Characterization of antimicrobial resistance in *Salmonella enterica* food and animal isolates from Colombia: identification of a *qnrB19*-mediated quinolone resistance marker in two novel serovars. *FEMS Microbiology Letters* 313, 10–19.

Karczmarczyk, M., Stephan, R., Hächler, H. and Fanning, S. (2012) Complete nucleotide sequence of pVQS1 containing a quinolone resistance determinant from *Salmonella enterica* serotype Virchow associated with foreign travel. *Journal of Antimicrobial Chemotherapy* 67, 1861–1864.

Kehrenberg, C., Friederichs, S., de Jong, A., Michael, G.B. and Schwarz, S. (2006) Identification of the plasmid-borne quinolone resistance gene *qnrS* in *Salmonella enterica* serovar Infantis. *Journal of Antimicrobial Chemotherapy* 58, 18–22.

Kehrenberg, C., Hopkins, K.L., Threlfall, E.J. and Schwarz, S. (2007) Complete nucleotide sequence of a small *qnrS1*-carrying plasmid from *Salmonella enterica* subsp. *enterica* Typhimurium DT193. *Journal of Antimicrobial Chemotherapy* 60, 903–905.

Krauland, M., Harrison, L., Paterson, D. and Marsh, J. (2010) Novel integron gene cassette arrays identified in a global collection of multi-drug resistant non-typhoidal *Salmonella enterica*. *Current Microbiology* 60, 217–223.

Ktari, S., Arlet, G., Verdet, C., Jaoua, S., Kachrid, A., Ben Redjeb, S., Mahjoubi-Rhimi, F. and Hammami, A. (2009) Molecular epidemiology and genetic environment of acquired bla_{ACC-1} in *Salmonella enterica* serotype Livingstone causing a large nosocomial outbreak in Tunisia. *Microbial Drug Resistance* 15, 279–286.

Le Hello, S., Hendriksen, R.S., Doublet, B., Fisher, I., Nielsen, E.M., Whichard, J.M., Bouchrif, B., Fashae, K., Granier, S.A., Jourdan-Da Silva, N., Cloeckaert, A., Threlfall, E.J., Angulo, F.J., Aarestrup, F.M., Wain, J. and Weill, F.X. (2011) International spread of an epidemic population of *Salmonella enterica* serotype Kentucky ST198 resistant to ciprofloxacin. *The Journal of Infectious Diseases* 204, 675–684.

Levings, R.S., Lightfoot, D., Partridge, S.R., Hall, R.M. and Djordjevic, S.P. (2005a) The genomic island SGI1, containing the multiple antibiotic resistance region of *Salmonella enterica* serovar Typhimurium DT104 or variants of it, is widely distributed in other *S. enterica* serovars. *Journal of Bacteriology* 187, 4401–4409.

Levings, R.S., Partridge, S.R., Lightfoot, D., Hall, R.M. and Djordjevic, S.P. (2005b) A new integron-associated gene cassette encoding a 3-*N*-aminoglycoside acetyltransferase. *Antimicrobial Agents and Chemotherapy* 49, 1238–1241.

Levings, R.S., Hall, R.M., Lightfoot, D. and Djordjevic, S.P. (2006a) *linG*, a new integron-associated gene cassette encoding a lincosamide nucleotidyltransferase. *Antimicrobial Agents and Chemotherapy* 50, 3514–3515.

Levings, R.S., Lightfoot, D., Elbourne, L.D., Djordjevic, S.P. and Hall, R.M. (2006b) New integron-associated gene cassette encoding a trimethoprim-resistant DfrB-type dihydrofolate reductase. *Antimicrobial Agents and Chemotherapy* 50, 2863–2865.

Levings, R.S., Partridge, S.R., Djordjevic, S.P. and Hall, R.M. (2007) SGI1-K, a variant of the SGI1 genomic island carrying a mercury resistance region, in *Salmonella enterica* serovar Kentucky. *Antimicrobial Agents and Chemotherapy* 51, 317–323.

Levings, R.S., Djordjevic, S.P. and Hall, R.M. (2008) SGI2, a relative of *Salmonella* genomic island SGI1 with an independent origin. *Antimicrobial Agents and Chemotherapy* 52, 2529–2537.

Michael, G.B., Cardoso, M. and Schwarz, S. (2005) Class1 integron-associated gene cassettes in *Salmonella enterica* subsp. *enterica* serovar Agona isolated from pig carcasses in Brazil. *Journal of Antimicrobial Chemotherapy* 55, 776–779.

Michael, G.B., Butaye, P., Cloeckaert, A. and Schwarz S. (2006) Genes and mutations conferring antimicrobial resistance in *Salmonella*: an update. *Microbes and Infection* 8, 1898–1914.

Mulvey, M.R., Boyd, D.A., Olson, A.B., Doublet, B. and Cloeckaert, A. (2006) The genetics of *Salmonella* genomic island 1. *Microbes and Infection* 8, 1915–1922.

Pallecchi, L., Riccobono, E., Mantella, A., Bartalesi, F., Sennati, S., Gamboa, H., Gotuzzo, E., Bartoloni, A. and Rossolini, G.M. (2009) High prevalence of *qnr* genes in commensal enterobacteria from healthy children in Peru and Bolivia. *Antimicrobial Agents and Chemotherapy* 53, 2632–2635.

Partridge, S.R. and Hall, R.M. (2003) In34, a complex In5 family class 1 integron containing orf513 and *dfrA10*. *Antimicrobial Agents and Chemotherapy* 47, 342–349.

Pasquali, F., Kehrenberg, C., Manfreda, G. and Schwarz, S. (2005) Physical linkage of Tn*3* and part of Tn*1721* in a tetracycline and ampicillin resistance plasmid from *Salmonella* Typhimurium. *Journal of Antimicrobial Chemotherapy* 55, 562–565.

Piddock, L.J.V. (2002) Fluoroquinolone resistance in *Salmonella* serovars isolated from humans and food animals. *FEMS Microbiology Reviews* 26, 3–16.

Ramirez, M.S. and Tolmasky, M.E. (2010) Aminoglycoside modifying enzymes. *Drug Resistance Updates* 13, 151–171.

Recchia, G.D. and Hall, R.M. (1995) Gene cassettes: a new class of mobile element. *Microbiology* 141, 3015–3027.

Robicsek, A., Strahilevitz, J., Jacoby, G.A., Macielag, M., Abbanat, D., Park, C.H., Bush, K. and Hooper, D.C. (2006) Fluoroquinolone-modifying enzyme: a new adaptation of a common aminoglycoside acetyltransferase. *Nature Medicine* 12, 83–88.

Rodríguez, I., Rodicio, M.R., Herrera-Leon, S., Echeita, A. and Mendoza, M.C. (2008) Class 1 integrons in multidrug-resistant non-typhoidal *Salmonella enterica* isolated in Spain between 2002 and 2004. *International Journal of Antimicrobial Agents* 32, 158–164.

Rodríguez, I., Guerra, B., Mendoza, M.C. and Rodicio, M.R. (2011) pUO-SeVR1 is an emergent virulence-resistance complex plasmid of *Salmonella enterica* serovar Enteritidis. *Journal of Antimicrobial Chemotherapy* 66, 218–220.

Rychlik, I., Gregorova, D. and Hradecka, H. (2006) Distribution and function of plasmids in *Salmonella enterica*. *Veterinary Microbiology* 112, 1–10.

Sampei, G., Furuya, N., Tachibana, K., Saitou, Y., Suzuki, T., Mizobuchi, K. and Komano, T. (2010) Complete genome sequence of the incompatibility group I1 plasmid R64. *Plasmid* 64, 92–103.

Schwarz, S. and Chaslus-Dancla, E. (2001) Use of antimicrobials in veterinary medicine and mechanisms of resistance. *Veterinary Research* 32, 201–225.

Schwarz, S., Kehrenberg, C., Doublet, B. and Cloeckaert A. (2004) Molecular basis of bacterial resistance to chloramphenicol and florfenicol. *FEMS Microbiology Reviews* 28, 519–542.

Sjölund-Karlsson, M., Howie, R., Rickert, R., Krueger, A., Tran, T.T., Zhao, S., Ball, T., Haro, J., Pecic, G., Joyce, K., Fedorka-Cray, P.J., Whichard, J.M. and McDermott, P.F. (2010) Plasmid-mediated quinolone resistance among non-Typhi *Salmonella enterica* isolates, USA. *Emerging Infectious Diseases* 16, 1789–1791.

Torpdahl, M., Hammerum, A.M., Zachariasen, C. and Nielsen, E.M. (2009) Detection of *qnr* genes in *Salmonella* isolated from humans in Denmark. *Journal of Antimicrobial Chemotherapy* 63, 406–408.

Veldman, K., Cavaco, L.M., Mevius, D., Battisti, A., Franco, A., Botteldoorn, N., Bruneau, M., Perrin-Guyomard, A., Cerny, T., De Frutos Escobar, C., Guerra, B., Schroeter, A., Gutierrez, M., Hopkins, K., Myllyniemi, A.L., Sunde, M., Wasyl, D. and Aarestrup, F.M. (2011) International collaborative study on the occurrence of plasmid-mediated quinolone resistance in *Salmonella enterica* and *Escherichia coli* isolated from animals, humans, food and the environment in 13 European countries. *Journal of Antimicrobial Chemotherapy* 66, 1278–1286.

Vo, A.T.T., Van Duijkeren, E., Gaastra, W. and Fluit, A.C. (2010) Antimicrobial Resistance, class 1 integrons, and genomic island 1 in *Salmonella* isolates from Vietnam. *PLoS ONE* 5, e9440.

Wain, J., Diem Nga, L.T., Kidgell, C., James, K., Fortune, S., Song Diep, T., Ali, T., Ó Gaora, P., Parry, C., Parkhill, J., Farrar, J., White, N.J. and Dougan, G. (2003) Molecular analysis of incHI1 antimicrobial resistance plasmids from *Salmonella* serovar Typhi strains associated with typhoid fever. *Antimicrobial Agents and Chemotherapy* 47, 2732–2739.

Wiesner, M., Zaidi, M.B., Calva, E., Fernandez-Mora, M., Calva, J.J. and Silva, C. (2009) Association of virulence plasmid and antibiotic resistance determinants with chromosomal multilocus genotypes in Mexican *Salmonella enterica* serovar Typhimurium strains. *BMC Microbiology* 9, 131.

Wilson, N.L. and Hall, R.M. (2010) Unusual class 1 integron configuration found in *Salmonella* genomic island 2 from *Salmonella enterica* serovar Emek. *Antimicrobial Agents and Chemotherapy* 54, 513–516.

Wu, J.J., Ko, W.C., Chiou, C.S., Chen, H.M., Wang, L.R. and Yan, J.J. (2008) Emergence of Qnr determinants in human *Salmonella* isolates in Taiwan. *Journal of Antimicrobial Chemotherapy* 62, 1269–1272.

Yamane, K., Wachino, J., Suzuki, S., Kimura, K., Shibata, N., Kato, H., Shibayama, K., Konda, T. and Arakawa, Y. (2007) New plasmid-mediated fluoroquinolone efflux pump, QepA, found in an *Escherichia coli* clinical isolate. *Antimicrobial Agents and Chemotherapy* 51, 3354–3360.

Yau, S., Liu, X., Djordjevic, S.P. and Hall, R.M. (2010) Persistence of RSF1010-like plasmids and origin of their *sul2-strA-strB* antibiotic resistance gene cluster. *Microbial Drug Resistance* 16, 249–252.

Ye, J., Su, L.H., Chen, C.L., Hu, S., Wang, J., Yu, J. and Chiu, C.H. (2011) Analysis of pSC138, the multidrug resistance plasmid of *Salmonella enterica* serotype Choleraesuis SC-B67. *Plasmid* 65, 132–140.

8 Immunity to *Salmonella* in Farm Animals and Murine Models of Disease

Neil Foster[1]* and Angela Berndt[2]
[1]*School of Veterinary Medicine and Science, University of Nottingham, UK;*
[2]*Friedrich Loeffler Institute, Germany*

Introduction

In comparison with the increasingly detailed information becoming available on the cellular and humoral responses to *Salmonella* infection in mice, our knowledge of how the host responds to different types of infections seen in cattle, pigs and poultry is more limited. Recent reviews of avian immunology include those by Van Immerseel *et al.* (2005), Wigley *et al.* (2006a), Lillehoj *et al.* (2007), Smith and Beal (2008) and Chappell *et al.* (2009). Similar reviews on bovine (Zhang *et al.*, 2003a; Santos and Bäumler, 2004) immunology have also been compiled. Nevertheless, very important information has been obtained from murine models of infection and these have informed vaccine research and development. Pigs have also been used to model human infection and in this review it therefore seems appropriate initially to compare the immune response to *Salmonella* in mice and pigs prior to discussing salmonellosis of cattle and poultry.

Comparative Study of Salmonellosis in Pigs and Mice

Between 1996 and 2000 over 73,000 cases of salmonellosis were reported in the UK and *Salmonella* was attributed to most fatalities that resulted from food-borne infection (Adak *et al.*, 2005). In this latter survey pork and pig products (ham and bacon) were found to be important sources of human food-borne disease, whilst another survey has shown that *Salmonella* serovars (such as *S.* Typhimurium and *S.* Derby) were isolated from the caeca of 23% of all pigs slaughtered in UK abattoirs (Ivanek *et al.*, 2004) and entry of *Salmonella* into the human food chain results largely from carcass contamination. In pigs, clinical disease may occur in the post-weaning period or, less frequently, in the neonatal pig, manifesting in clinical signs of diarrhoea and vomiting, which are most often mild. However, *S.* Choleraesuis, which is much more host-adapted to pigs, can cause significant disease and subsequent economic loss. Intestinal colonization

* Corresponding author, e-mail: n.foster@nottingham.ac.uk

© CAB International 2013. *Salmonella in Domestic Animals, 2nd Edition* (eds P.A. Barrow and U. Methner)

versus systemic infection is also seen in experimental infection of pigs with *S.* Typhimurium whereas systemic infection with peripheral organ dissemination occurs in pigs infected with *S.* Choleraesuis (Reed *et al.*, 1986). Much of the knowledge accrued regarding *Salmonella*–host interaction has been born out of studies using mice as an infection model. These studies have yielded valuable information, although salmonellosis of mice manifests very differently to the disease in pigs. Therefore, studies of immunity to *Salmonella* in pigs have several benefits since it is the target host for the development of vaccines to reduce endemic *Salmonella* infection and therefore reduce the load in the human food chain, while control of *S.* Choleraesuis is important for the prevention of disease in pigs and subsequent economic loss to the pig industry. Furthermore, infection studies in pigs relate more closely to human disease in terms of anatomical size and haemodynamics.

Since *S.* Typhimurium and *S.* Choleraesuis have very different pathological effects in pigs, a comparative review of the immune response to these pathogens in pigs will be discussed below. These will also be compared to the immune response to *S.* Typhimurium in the murine infection model.

Production of inflammatory cytokines following *S.* Typhimurium and *S.* Choleraesuis infection

Initial recognition of *Salmonella* invasion occurs via pathogen recognition receptors that recognize pathogen-associated molecular patterns (PAMPs). The best studied of these PAMPs are the Toll-like receptors (TLRs). Ten TLRs are now known and of these TLR4 (which recognizes lipopolysaccharide) and TLR5 (which recognizes bacterial flagellin) are essential in the recognition and immune response to *Salmonella* (reviewed by Carpenter and O'Neill, 2007). This initial recognition results in the production of inflammatory mediators such as cytokines, which activate innate immune cells, and chemokines, which stimulate migration of more immune cells to the site of infection. Numerous studies, over many years, have discovered a large number of important genes required for *Salmonella* invasion and maintenance within this harsh host environment. In most cases these studies have been performed in mice. These have shown that genes within the cluster known as *Salmonella* pathogenicity island 1 (SPI-1) are required for invasion of epithelial cells *in vitro* (Galán and Curtiss, 1989) but complete invasion into deeper murine tissues is not prevented by SP-1 mutations *in vivo*. Similarly in pigs, mutation in SPI-1 genes inhibits intestinal colonization but does not prevent colonization of tonsillar tissue, which provides an infectious route (Boyen *et al.*, 2006a). However, murine salmonellosis has a completely different disease profile compared to that seen in pigs infected with either *S.* Typhimurium or *S.* Choleraesuis. In susceptible mice *S.* Typhimurium does not reside in the intestinal tissues in great numbers and induces little inflammation and no diarrhoea. Instead, *S.* Typhimurium quickly invades the mesenteric lymph nodes and disseminates to the liver and spleen inducing symptoms more akin to typhoid than gastroenteritis (reviewed by Tsolis *et al.*, 1999a). This is correlated with a significant increase in many inflammatory cytokines in serum, including TNF-α and IFN-γ, which are essential in activating antimicrobial killing pathways in innate immune cells but which, if not controlled, lead to an overwhelming systemic inflammatory response and sepsis (Jotwani *et al.*, 1995).

In pigs, *in vivo* studies have shown that *S.* Typhimurium DT104 also induces an inflammatory immune response. This also manifests in elevated levels of pro-inflammatory cytokines in serum, such as IL-8 and TNF-α (Collado-Romero *et al.*, 2010) and increased mRNA expression of TNF-α, IFN-γ and IL-8 in the serum/ileum (Trebichavsky *et al.*, 1997, 2003). A longitudinal study by Uthe *et al.* (2009) reported that inflammatory mediators, such as TNF-α, in the ileo-caecal and mesenteric lymph nodes and blood of post-weaned pigs infected with *S.* Typhimurium χ4232 initially increased within 48 h post-infection but then decreased to control levels shortly after this time. In comparison, *S.* Choleraesuis induced an extended up-regulation of mRNA over a 21 day experimental period (Uthe *et al.*, 2009). One study by Paulin *et al.* (2007) has shown that these differences observed in pigs infected with *S.* Typhimurium and *S.* Choleraesuis may have a bearing on the relative pathogenesis of these different serovars in the pig. This study reported that *S.* Typhimurium 4/74 (SL1344) replicates rapidly within the ileal wall of pigs and this stimulates a rapid inflammatory response with greater induction of TNF-α, IL-8 and IL-18 mRNA when compared to *S.* Choleraesuis, which has a slower replication rate. Therefore, although both *S.* Typhimurium and *S.* Choleraesuis induce the production of pro-inflammatory cytokines in pig tissues, this appears to be more prolonged for *S.* Choleraesuis, which replicates more slowly but disseminates to the blood and peripheral organs compared to a rapid and very robust cytokine response to *S.* Typhimurium, which may (directly or indirectly) have a protective effect by inhibiting dissemination of the bacteria to the blood and peripheral organs.

The innate immune response to *Salmonella* in pigs and mice

Neutrophils

Following the production of chemokines by *Salmonella*-infected porcine enterocytes, phagocytic cells infiltrate the intestine probably to suppress the *Salmonella* population early after infection before large numbers of bacteria become established. Neutrophils represent the first wave of innate immune cells to enter intestinal tissues of pigs infected with *Salmonella*. Our studies have shown that, in highly susceptible 5-day-old gnotobiotic (germ-free) piglets, neutrophils infiltrate the intestine within a few hours post-infection with *S.* Typhimurium F98 (data not shown) and inoculation and colonization of these piglets 24 h earlier with an avirulent rough mutant of *S.* Infantis 1326/28 can be used to protect pigs against subsequent challenge with virulent *S.* Typhimurium and which prevents enteritis and dissemination to peripheral organs (Foster *et al.*, 2003a). This protection appears mainly to be the result of the induction of neutrophilia by the avirulent strain prior to challenge, and the subsequent oxidative killing of bacteria via neutrophil NADPH phagocytic oxidase pathways (Foster *et al.*, 2003a, 2005). As stated earlier, *Salmonella* induce rapid production of high concentrations of IL-8 from intestinal enterocytes and since IL-8 is firmly established as an important neutrophil chemo-attractant (Ben-Baruch *et al.*, 1995; Cassatella, 1999) this is most likely the reason for the rapid neutrophilia observed in pigs. IL-8-induced neutrophil migration across human colonic carcinoma cell line (T84) monolayers is stimulated by the *S.* Typhimurium flagellin assembly protein FliE (Reed *et al.*, 2002) and this may also be a major stimulant in porcine intestine, although this has yet to be reported. Similarly, a correlation between IL-8 production and extensive intestinal neutrophilia has also been shown in pigs infected with *S.* Choleraesuis (Hyland *et al.*, 2006) and resistance to *S.* Choleraesuis is correlated with greater numbers of circulating neutrophils, which also have greater killing efficiency (van Diemen *et al.*, 2002).

In murine infection with *S.* Typhimurium, infiltration of the intestine by phagocytes occurs due to monocyte/macrophages rather than neutrophils (Shirai *et al.*, 1979) and probably reflects the difference in disease profile in these two hosts. However, if the antibiotic streptomycin is administered to mice prior to oral inoculation with *S.* Typhimurium, the *Salmonella* persist in the intestinal tissues and stimulate a very significant neutrophil migration into the intestine, resulting in colitis (Barthel *et al.*, 2003). This may suggest that in mice the presence of a gut flora inhibits invasion of intestinal enterocytes by *S.* Typhimurium and this probably results in invasion via other routes. Studies have shown that in mice these include: microfold (M) cells residing on follicle-associated epithelium (Jones *et al.*, 1994), CD18+ macrophages, which carry *Salmonella* into blood (Vasquez-Torres *et al.*, 1999) or dendritic cells (DCs), which may capture and carry *Salmonella* to draining lymph nodes (Rescigno *et al.*, 2001). It is possible that this utilization of the murine immune response by *S.* Typhimurium to infect deeper tissues may be the reason for the different disease profile observed in mice.

Macrophages

Macrophages from a number of different host species are known to express genes (natural resistance-associated macrophage proteins, NRAMPs) that confer innate host resistance to *Salmonella*, encoding proteins required for transporting metal ions across the phagosome (Vidal *et al.*, 1993). Other important early host responses include the production of IL-12 from infected macrophages, which stimulate development of IFN-γ-producing Type 1 CD4+ lymphocytes (Th1 cells) and production of TNF-α from these cells, both of which potentiate macrophage killing pathways (reviewed by Lalmanach and Lantier, 1999).

However, the ability of *S.* Typhimurium to survive, replicate and kill macrophages determines virulence in mice (Lindgren *et al.*, 1996) and once *Salmonella* enter the macrophage phagosome they alter various biochemical structures recognized by the host cell (Trent *et al.*, 2001; Prost and Miller, 2008). This is achieved by proteins produced by the two-component *phoP/Q* regulon (Miller, 1991) and the *Salmonella* pathogenicity island 2 (SPI-2) gene cluster (Cirillo *et al.*, 1998). Initially, *Salmonella* survive within the phagosome of murine macrophages (Alpuche-Aranda *et al.*, 1992) where they are resistant to, or inhibit, various cell-killing pathways such as oxidative burst (De Groote *et al.*, 1997; Foster *et al.*, 2003b) and resistant *S.* Typhimurium strains also inhibit production of both IFN-γ and TNF-α by these macrophages (Lalmanach and Lantier, 1999).

The importance of wild-type SPI-2 genes in *Salmonella* virulence has now been shown in many studies. For example, mutation of the SPI-2 gene *sseD*, needed for translocation of effector proteins in the acidic host phagosome (Nikolaus *et al.*, 2001), inhibits *S.* Typhimurium replication in murine macrophages (Hölzer and Hensel, 2010), and in pigs, *S.* Typhimurium DT104 virulence is also attenuated via *sseD* mutation (Brumme *et al.*, 2007). However, there are also differences between relevant SPI-2 virulence genes in mice and pigs, with the two-component SPI-2 genes *ssrA/ssrB* being required for macrophage survival and virulence in mice but not in pigs (Boyen *et al.*, 2008). However, SPI-1 genes have also been shown to be important for the killing of murine macrophages by *S.* Typhimurium (Lundberg *et al.*, 1999), including SipB-dependent caspase-induced apoptosis (Hersh *et al.*, 1999). Wild-type SipB (and the products of other SPI-1 genes such as *hilA* and *sipA*) increase *S.* Typhimurium invasion of porcine macrophages and are also involved in the early intra-cellular establishment of the bacteria in macrophages, being involved in both the formation of spacious phagosomes and early cytotoxicity (Boyen *et al.*, 2006b). This latter study, however, found no difference in IL-8 or reactive oxygen species due to SPI-1 mutation. Pavlova *et al.* (2011) have also shown that wild-type SPI-1 (*hilA*, *sipA* and *sipB*) genes increases invasion of porcine alveolar macrophages by *S.* Typhimurium but in addition they report that these genes down-regulate mRNA expression for many inflammatory cytokines such as TNF-α and IL-8. While considering possible differences in the role of SPI-1 and SPI-2 in host-adapted and non-adapted *Salmonella* it is pertinent to highlight a recent study by Forest *et al.* (2010) who have shown that complete deletion of the SPI-2 type three secretion system in *S.* Typhi (the cause of human typhoid) has no effect on survival of the *Salmonella* in human macrophages.

Macrophages, in addition to neutrophils, migrate into intestinal tissue of pigs infected with *Salmonella*, and in 5-day-old gnotobiotic piglets infected with *S.* Typhimurium F98, neutrophilia into the villi occurs within 24 h and at this time significant numbers of macrophages are observed in the sub-mucosa (Foster *et al.*, 2003a), suggesting that the initial neutrophil phase is possibly followed by macrophages. However, it is debatable whether the ability of *Salmonella* to survive inside macrophages determines virulence in pigs since non-host-adapted *S.* Typhimurium survives in much greater numbers in porcine alveolar macrophages when compared with host-adapted (and highly virulent) *S.* Choleraesuis and both serovars kill macrophages in which they survive (Watson *et al.*, 2000). However, in pigs *S.* Typhimurium does not normally react with pig alveolar macrophages (unless systemic infection occurs) and so this study may not truly reflect the survival dynamics occurring *in vivo*. Conversely, the study may suggest that the relationship between *Salmonella* in porcine macrophages differs from that observed in mice.

Defensins in pigs and their role in infection

Very little has been done on characterizing the defensins of species other than the mouse and nothing so far which might suggest in a concrete way that defensins contribute to resistance in the pig. β-defensin 1 and 2 expression has been studied in the pig in relation to *Salmonella* infection. Although there is differential expression of the two defensins in different regions of the gut, *S.* Typhimurium infection appeared to have little or no effect on expression (Veldhuizen *et al.*, 2007).

The adaptive immune response to *Salmonella* in pigs and mice

As previously discussed, the innate immune response to *Salmonella* is essential for early suppression of the *Salmonella* population but adaptive immunity is essential for resolution of *Salmonella* infection. Therefore, another important function of the innate immune system is its role in stimulating adaptive immunity via antigen presentation to lymphocytes. Amongst the antigen-presenting cells (APCs), dendritic cells (DCs) are able to present orders of magnitude more antigen than macrophages and are the only APCs capable of presentation to naive lymphocytes (reviewed by Mellman *et al.*, 1998). Murine DCs present *Salmonella* antigen in association with either major histocompatibility complex (MHC) class I (MHC I) or MHC II to CD4+ or CD8+ T lymphocytes, respectively (reviewed by Sundquist *et al.*, 2004). However, studies have also reported that *Salmonella* can inhibit antigen presentation by DCs to T lymphocytes via a SPI-2-dependent mechanism that prevents intra-cellular degradation required for subsequent antigen presentation (Tobar *et al.*, 2006). This may be a host-specific phenomenon since only *S.* Typhi can do this in human cells, whereas *S.* Typhimurium cannot (reviewed by Bueno *et al.*, 2007). Intra-cellular *S.* Typhimurium also down-regulates expression of FliC in mice, which inhibits presentation of flagellin to cognate T lymphocytes (Cummings *et al.*, 2005), which are significantly numerous (McSorley *et al.*, 2002). This would suggest that the effect of a very important T cell population is negated and may have an important effect on prolonged *Salmonella* maintenance.

However, the adaptive immune response does eventually resolve infection and Nauciel (1990) showed that this was due to CD4+ lymphocytes. The importance of lymphocytes in *Salmonella* clearance was also reported in a study by Sinha *et al.* (1997) in which high mortality was observed in athymic mice challenged with *aroA* and *htrA* mutants, while these proved avirulent in wild-type mice which quickly cleared them. Successful long-term vaccination against *Salmonella* in mice requires the induction of memory CD4+ Th1 lymphocytes, which produce pro-inflammatory cytokines, as well as antibody-producing B lymphocytes/plasma cells (Mastroeni and Ménager, 2003). *Salmonella* outer membrane protein A (OmpA) has been shown to activate murine DCs to produce IL-12 and increase expression of MHC I, MHC II and co-stimulatory molecules (Lee *et al.*, 2010). This latter study also showed that DCs pulsed with OmpA polarized mixed lymphocyte populations towards an IFN-γ-producing (Th1) phenotype due to OmpA-stimulated IL-12. Although DCs are certainly important in directing the T lymphocyte response during *Salmonella* infection, B lymphocytes are essential in the early polarization of Th1 phenotypes in mice (Ugrinovic *et al.*, 2003). This occurs via B cell myD88, whereas the development of Th1 memory cells occurs via B cell antigen presentation and MHC II (Barr *et al.*, 2010). B cells are also important in recall of antibody responses against *Salmonella*. For example, in mice serum IgG directed against O-specific polysaccharide (Robbins *et al.*, 1992) and *Salmonella* Omps (Singh *et al.*, 1996; Secundino *et al.*, 2006) protects against re-infection, possibly by *Salmonella* agglutination, thus preventing dissemination of the *Salmonella* to the peripheral tissues but also via opsonization and increased innate cell clearance. The importance of IgA has also been shown in a study by Michetti *et al.* (1992) in which mice were protected from infection by *Salmonella* by pre-administration of a *Salmonella*-specific monoclonal IgA.

Comparatively little is known about adaptive immunity during salmonellosis in pigs. However, Gray *et al.* (1995) showed that protective immunity in pigs infected with *S.* Choleraesuis was associated with increased serum T lymphocyte numbers and an increased concentration of systemic and intestinal antibodies (IgM, IgG and IgA). Chu *et al.* (2007) have reported the successful use of a live (virulence plasmid-cured) *S.* Choleraesuis vaccine. This study showed that vaccination of sows induced high maternal antibody titres, which were associated with protection in piglets, while vaccination of piglets induced *Salmonella*-specific T lymphocyte proliferation following challenge. A similar study also showed that sows vaccinated with a *S.* Typhimurium *cpxR* deletion mutant conferred protection to suckling piglets via passive transfer of IgG and IgA (Hur and Lee, 2010), while cross protection was also observed in pigs vaccinated with attenuated *S.* Choleraesuis SC54 prior to challenge with a virulent *S.* Typhimurium field strain, isolated from septic pigs (Letellier *et al.*, 2001). In this case a significant reduction in *Salmonella* numbers isolated from the mesenteric lymph nodes and ileum was correlated with high intestinal IgA titres. This latter study suggests that antibodies recognized shared epitopes (possibly epitopes such as found in Omps or other major surface antigens) between different serovars and may suggest that protection of piglets by passive immunity could be successful against various strains within the same serovar or between different serovars using the same antigens. In comparison, a study by Trebichavsky *et al.* (1997) also reported that cross protection in gnotobiotic piglets to *S.* Typhimurium LT2 (inoculated 1 week prior to challenge with a rough mutant *S.* Typhimurium SF1591 strain) was associated with intestinal infiltration by αβ T lymphocytes and an increased IgA response, once again suggesting the importance of both T and B lymphocytes in protection against *Salmonella*. However, this study also showed that pigs inoculated with *S.* Typhimurium SF1591 were not protected against challenge with *S.* Minnesota mR595 (Trebichavsky *et al.*, 1997), suggesting that O-antigens may continue to be important and that cross protection may be more difficult to achieve in conventional vaccines in weaned pigs.

Cattle

In cattle, *Salmonella* Dublin and *Salmonella* Typhimurium are the most important *Salmonella* serovars (Hirsh *et al.*, 2004). The course of the infection in cattle depends, as with other animals, on age, husbandry conditions, host immune status, *Salmonella* serovar, infection dose and the route of infection. Calves infected with *Salmonella* Dublin become weak and dehydrated and commonly develop diarrhoea. Pneumonia and septicaemia without diarrhoea may also occur (Rings, 1985). *Salmonella* Dublin is the more invasive serovar compared to *S.* Typhimurium and may also produce meningo-encephalitis, septic arthritis, and septic physitis with or without enteric disease (Mee, 1995; Mohler *et al.*, 2009) and, after recovering from infection, some cattle may develop into carriers (Wallis, 2006). In contrast, oral infection of calves with *S.* Typhimurium results in an enteric disease (Tsolis *et al.*, 1999b; Zhang *et al.*, 2003a) and closely approximates the *S.* Typhimurium-induced enterocolitis in humans (Zhang *et al.*, 2003a).

Most of our knowledge about the pathogenesis and immunology of bovine salmonellosis *in vivo* originates from studies using ligated ileal loop models in calves. A prerequisite for the development of illness is the capacity of *Salmonella* organisms to migrate into the intestinal tissue. *Salmonella* Typhimurium seems not to prefer any specific cell type to invade into the gut mucosa, but enters the epithelial cells at the tips of absorptive villi as well as the follicle-associated epithelial cells of the domed villi in Peyer's patches. Accordingly, *S.* Typhimurium has been observed in all epithelial cell types of the gastrointestinal tract of calves (Santos *et al.*, 2002a). Invasion has been shown to be more rapid via M cells covering the domed villi than via enterocytes of the regular epithelium (Frost *et al.*, 1997; Santos and Bäumler, 2004). However, M cells appear not to be the main cell type of *Salmonella* entry (Bolton *et al.*, 1999). After migration into the gut tissue, *Salmonella* organisms are located intra-cellularly in macrophages, dendritic cells or neutrophils but not in fibroblasts or other mesenchymal cells of the mucosal lamina propria (Santos *et al.*, 2002a; Santos and Bäumler, 2004). In the systemic *S.* Dublin infection, the bacteria emigrate from the ileum to the mesenteric lymph nodes and periphery by way of the draining lymphatics (Paulin *et al.*, 2002; Pullinger *et al.*, 2007).

Granulocytes

At 1 h after *S.* Typhimurium inoculation of bovine ligated ileal loops, neutrophils begin to penetrate into the intestinal mucosa. After 3 h, large numbers of granulocytes are observable in tissue together with necrosis and epithelial detachment at the tips of absorptive villi of gut (Santos *et al.*, 2001). A positive correlation between neutrophil tissue infiltration and fluid secretion into the intestinal lumen has been postulated (Santos *et al.*, 2001). The granulocytes induce a loss of epithelial integrity of the gut mucosa and, thus, contribute to an enhanced liquid flow into the gut lumen and diarrhoea (Zhang *et al.*, 2003a). Accordingly, a decrease of the serum protein concentration is detectable in blood samples of calves infected orally with *S.* Typhimurium (Santos *et al.*, 2002b). The neutrophil influx is typically triggered by distinct chemo-attractant cytokines of the CXC subfamily containing an *N*-terminal glutamate-leucine-arginine (ELR) sequence motif (Zhang *et al.*, 2003a). There are five CXC chemokines with an ELR motif in cattle. These include IL-8, granulocyte chemotactic protein 2 (GCP-2, or CXCL6/GCP-2), growth-related oncogene α (GRO-α, CXCL1/GRO-α, or melanoma growth stimulatory activity (MGSA)), GRO-β (or CXCL2/GRO-β) and GRO-γ (or CXCL3/GRO-γ) (Morsey *et al.*, 1996; Modi *et al.*, 1998; Zhang *et al.*, 2003a). The enormous infiltration of neutrophils into the affected intestine after *S.* Typhimurium infection of bovine ligated loops correlates with an increased expression of IL-8, GRO-α and -γ and GCP-2 in Peyer's patches (Santos *et al.*, 2002a; Zhang *et al.*, 2003a). GRO-γ expression appears after only 1 h while the other chemokines are expressed at around 3 h after *Salmonella* exposure (Santos *et al.*, 2002a). Additionally, enhanced transcription of the pro-inflammatory cytokines IL-1, IL-4 and the IL-1 receptor antagonist IL-1Rα has been demonstrated, but the expression of IL-18, IL-10 and TNF-α is unchanged in bovine gut after *S.* Typhimurium infection (Santos *et al.*, 2002a). In serum of *S.* Takoradi-infected lactating dairy cows, the bioactivity of IL-1β and IL-6 but not TNF-α is significantly increased (Konnai *et al.*, 2001). These results underline the inflammatory character of the enteric *Salmonella* infection in cattle. However, the pro-inflammatory cytokines IL-1β and TNF-α seem only to be poorly correlated with the presence or absence of neutrophils, as the representative cells of inflammation, in tissue (Nunes *et al.*, 2010). Instead, GRO-α is considered to be the most important stimulus for the tissue influx of neutrophils into the bovine intestinal mucosa after *Salmonella* exposure (Zhang *et al.*, 2003b). The role of neutrophils in the pathogenesis of bovine non-typhoidal salmonellosis has hardly been analysed *in vivo*. However, neutrophils seem to be effective killers of intra-cellular *S.* Typhimurium (Santos *et al.*, 2002a). In a recent study, calves with a naturally occurring bovine leukocyte adhesion deficiency (BLAD; $CD18^-$ calves) mutation, whose neutrophils are unable to extra-vasate and infiltrate the extra-vascular matrix, were used to address this question. The data from this study revealed that the infection of $CD18^-$ calves with *S.* Typhimurium results in no significant tissue infiltration by neutrophils, less tissue damage, reduced luminal fluid accumulation and increased bacterial invasion in comparison with the $CD18^+$ control calves (Nunes *et al.*, 2010).

Salmonella flagellin

The protein monomer of the flagellar filament, flagellin, is considered to be the main attribute of *Salmonella* strains to induce inflammation and innate immune mechanisms after infection. In *S.* Typhimurium-infected ligated loops of calves, flagellin recognition induces increased expression of macrophage inflammatory protein 3α (MIP-3α) mRNA as well as more fluid accumulation (Winter *et al.*, 2009). Winter *et al.* (2009) postulated in their studies that flagellin promotes intestinal inflammation in calf but not in mice due to differences in the expression of pattern recognition receptors (PRRs), as the TLR5, in intestinal tissue. Werling *et al.* (2006) have already shown that bovine macrophages express TLR5 (the receptor for flagellin) (Werling *et al.*, 2006) and bind flagellin and respond with potent CXCL8 expression (Metcalfe *et al.*, 2010).

Macrophages and dendritic cells

The interactions of macrophages or dendritic cells with *Salmonella* organisms and possible different functions of these cells are not well understood in bovine enteric salmonellosis. In peripheral blood of cattle infected with *S.* Takoradi, the number of MHC II-positive cells increases significantly (Konnai *et al.*, 2001). Normally, MCH II can be expressed by macrophages, DCs and monocytes but also by activated T cells and B lymphocytes. Bovine peripheral blood-derived DCs infected with *S.* Typhimurium up-regulate the expression of surface molecules such as MHC I and MHC II as well as CD40, CD80 and CD86 (Norimatsu *et al.*, 2003). In contrast, macrophages show only a marginal increase in CD40 expression. Following infection, both DCs and macrophages increase transcription of TNF-α, IL-1β, IL-6 and iNOS, while DCs amplify their mRNA expression of IL-10 and granulocyte-macrophage colony-stimulating factor (GM-CSF) and macrophages show elevated IL-12p40 transcription in consequence of *S.* Typhimurium exposure (Norimatsu *et al.*, 2003). However, live bacteria induce greater up-regulation of CD40 and CD86 expression and increased transcription of IL-6, IL-12 when compared with stimulation of DCs with killed bacteria (Norimatsu *et al.*, 2004).

T cells

Acute salmonellosis in calves is typically associated with lymphocyte depletion in Peyer's patch follicles (Santos *et al.*, 2002a). A significant decline in the areas of lymphoid follicles and domes has been found to be due to a depletion of B lymphocytes in jejunal and ileal Peyer's patches following *S.* Dublin inoculation. The occurrence of intraepithelial lymphocytes in follicle-associated epithelium changes from predominantly B cells in control calves to $CD8^+$ lymphocytes in infected animals (Liebler *et al.*, 1994). Similarly, the ratio of $CD4^+$ T cells to $CD8^+$ T cells decreases in favour of the $CD8^+$ lymphocytes in blood of *S.* Takoradi-infected lactating dairy cows (Konnai *et al.*, 2001). These facts suggest the development of a cell-mediated, rather than humoral, immune response in cattle with salmonellosis. Hedges *et al.* (2007) have also shown that the number of $CD8^+$ lymphocytes increases at inflammatory sites following infection and that gamma/delta T cells derived from lymphatic ducts draining the gut mucosa are activated as shown by an increased IL-2Rα expression on these cells in *S.* Typhimurium-inoculated calves.

Defensins

As with pigs there is an increasing amount of information on β-defensins in cattle (Selsted *et al.*, 1993; Gallagher *et al.*, 1995), but as yet very little work has been done on any association between differential expression and *Salmonella* infection.

Poultry

Salmonella organisms infect poultry, as with mammals, mainly via the faecal–oral route. To induce gastroenteritis, the pathogen must first reach the distal ileum and caecum where it must out-compete the resident microbial flora and penetrate the mucus and mucosal epithelium. In fact, the intestinal epithelium is not only the physical barrier but also the initiator of the innate immune response to

Salmonella. Specialized epithelial cells can produce bactericidal peptides, and the encounter between bacteria and epithelial cells rapidly stimulates the release of pro-inflammatory interleukins and chemokines that attract innate immune cells such as granulocytes, macrophages and immature dendritic cells. These cells constitute the first line of immune cell defence and are able to phagocytose and kill pathogens non-specifically prior to triggering a wide range of immune reactions. However, innate immune mechanisms alone are insufficient to eliminate *Salmonella* infection and an adaptive immune response, with highly specific T and B cells, is elicited to completely eradicate the pathogen.

For effective removal of harmful agents in the gastrointestinal tract, a highly specialized lymphoid tissue exists separately in gut (gut-associated lymphoid tissue, GALT). An attribute of GALT is the formation of a characteristic epithelium covering the lymphoid tissue and containing M cells perfectly equipped for the uptake of particular antigens from the intestinal lumen. In contrast to the well-organized GALT in mammals, the avian counterpart does not always develop such a specialized epithelium and most of the avian gut tissue is separated from the lumen by absorptive epithelium. Some distinctive tissues such as the two caecal tonsils (located at the ileo-caecal junctions), up to six Peyer's patches and Meckel's diverticulum (the remnant of the yolk sac) have some similarity with the corresponding epithelium found in mammals (Befus *et al.*, 1980; Burns and Maxwell, 1986). In chicken, the small intestine is the main site of *Salmonella* invasion, which does not possess separate lymph nodes but simply some diffuse lymphoid aggregates overlaid by M cells. The role of M cells in *Salmonella* invasion in chicken is not known (Smith and Beal, 2008).

A lot of work has been done to find genetic reasons for the different resistance/susceptibility of specific chicken lines against different *Salmonella* serovars (summarized by Wigley, 2004 and Calenge *et al.*, 2010). Genetic resistance of chickens to systemic salmonellosis seems to be associated with genomic regions carrying the candidate genes *NRAMP1* (natural resistance-associated macrophage protein, now *SLC11A1*), MHC, *TLR4* and the quantitative trait locus *SAL1* (Hu *et al.*, 1997; Mariani *et al.*, 2001; Wigley *et al.*, 2001, 2002a; Wigley, 2004; Calenge *et al.*, 2010). Different studies on the resistance of chickens to salmonellosis, and the *Salmonella* carrier state in fowl, demonstrate that the genetic control differs between different chicken lines, the trait assessed and the chicken's age (Calenge *et al.*, 2010).

Most of our knowledge on the immune response against non-host-specific *Salmonella* infections originates from investigations with *S.* Typhimurium-infected mice. Unfortunately, the mouse model is not very representative of infection in birds because a typhoid-like infection is produced in mice that differs from the gastrointestinal infection found in chickens following *S.* Typhimurium inoculation. Moreover, the immune system of avian species is different from that of the mammalians in several ways (Smith and Beal, 2008). The avian immune system shows properties indicating a phylogenetically intermediate position of the birds between reptiles and mammals. Thus, there is a considerable interest in the nature of avian immune defence mechanisms against *Salmonella* infection in poultry species. Accordingly, an increasing number of publications dealing with different aspects of the avian immune system have been generated during the last 10 years (summarized by Davison *et al.*, 2008).

Salmonellosis produced by *Salmonella* Gallinarum or Pullorum in poultry

At least two types of *Salmonella* infection in poultry need to be considered: (i) primarily an infection of the reticulo-endothelial system, with little or no initial intestinal involvement; and (ii) an extensive intestinal infection by an organism with varying degrees of systemic dissemination. In the first case, the infection is induced by the host-adapted *S.* Gallinarum and Pullorum in fowl. In the second case, the disease is caused by non-host-specific *Salmonella* strains, the most important serovars being *S.* Enteritidis and Typhimurium.

The immunobiology of the avian systemic salmonellosis produced by *S.* Gallinarum or Pullorum has been recently described by Chappell *et al.* (2009). The authors specify three distinct phases of avian systemic salmonellosis during each of which there is significant interaction with the immune system. The first phase represents the intestinal invasion but how exactly the *Salmonella* strains enter the gut mucosa is unclear since the absence of flagella in both of these serovars might hamper the penetration of the mucous layer normally covering the gut mucosa. There is some evidence that the bacteria enter the systemic body systems via enterocytes and lymphatic tissue structures in gut, such as Peyer's patches and caecal tonsils (Barrow and Duchet-Suchaux, 1997; Withanage *et al.*, 2005). The contribution of the *Salmonella* pathogenicity island (SPI)-1 type III secretion system (TTSS) of the *Salmonella* strains is unclear and under discussion, but does seem to be of some importance in *S.* Pullorum virulence (Wigley *et al.*, 2002b). An immunological hallmark of the *S.* Gallinarum and *S.* Pullorum infection is the absence of an inflammatory response within the intestinal mucosa, with no significant influx of heterophil granulocytes (Henderson *et al.*, 1999). In parallel with this phenomenon is the observation that the transcription of the main chemoattractants for granulocytes and monocytes, namely chCXCLi1 and chCXCLi2 (see below), are found to be down-regulated after infection (Hughes *et al.*, 2007; Chappell *et al.*, 2009).

The second phase of the *S.* Gallinarum and *S.* Pullorum infection is characterized by the initiation of a systemic infection. At first, the serovars are internalized by macrophages and dendritic cells underlying the mucosal epithelium and probably transported to spleen, liver, ovaries and bone marrow (Wigley *et al.*, 2001). A prerequisite for the development of a systemic infection is the ability of the *Salmonella* strains to survive in macrophages. Like other *Salmonella* strains, *S.* Gallinarum and *S.* Pullorum possess a SPI-2 TTSS that enables the pathogens to better survive within the cells by preventing the fusion of phagosome and lysosome or by detoxification of reactive oxygen or nitrogen intermediates (Cheminay *et al.*, 2005; Jones *et al.*, 2007). However, Chadfield *et al.* (2003) reported that host-specific *Salmonella* serovars Gallinarum or Pullorum did not survive better than non-host-specific *S.* Typhimurium in avian macrophages.

The elicited immune response during the third phase of infection determines the fate of the infected birds and is characterized by the production of high amounts of specific antibodies and T-cell proliferation (Wigley *et al.*, 2005). There are significantly reduced levels of production of the inflammatory cytokines IL-18 and IFN-γ in the spleens of birds infected with *S.* Pullorum when compared with *S.* Enteritidis-infected chickens and these authors proposed that unlike *S.* Enteritidis, which generated a Th1-type response, *S.* Pullorum induced a response that more closely resembled the Th2 response in mammals (Chappell *et al.*, 2009). Surviving chickens remain *Salmonella* carriers for the rest of their lives (Wigley *et al.*, 2001) and this is more often observed following infection with *S.* Pullorum than *S.* Gallinarum, which may therefore be explained by the immune-modulating properties of this serovar (Chappell *et al.*, 2009). In the case of chickens that are carriers of *S.* Pullorum, the bacteria persist within macrophages in the spleen and liver (Wigley *et al.*, 2001).

Infection with non-host-specific *Salmonella* serovars in poultry

The infection with non-host-specific *Salmonella* serovars (enteric *Salmonella* strains) leads to an enteric disease in chickens. *Salmonella* serovars Enteritidis and Typhimurium are the most frequently found serovars in fowl and are responsible for the majority of food-borne enteritis in humans, predominantly caused by poultry products as chicken meat, eggs and egg products. The immune response in *Salmonella*-positive chickens produces an intensive reaction in caecum, spleen, bursa of Fabricus and blood, characterized by a significant influx of immune cells such as granulocytes, macrophages, T and B cells (Berndt and Methner, 2001, 2004; Beal *et al.*, 2004a, 2005; Berndt *et al.*, 2006, 2007) as well as antigen-specific antibody production (IgG, IgA, IgM) (Zhang-Barber *et al.*, 1999; Beal *et al.*, 2006a) and transcriptional up-regulation of various pro-inflammatory cytokines, chemokines, and mediators of the innate or adaptive immune response (Beal *et al.*, 2004a, 2005; Withanage *et al.*, 2004, 2005; Berndt *et al.*, 2007; Cheeseman *et al.*, 2007; Fasina *et al.*, 2008; Pieper *et al.*, 2011). Furthermore, as a result of infection with *S.* Enteritidis, changes in immune cell composition have also been observed in the ovary and oviduct (Withanage *et al.*, 1998; Barua and Yoshimura, 2004).

Chicks younger than 3 days are very susceptible to infection with enteric *Salmonella* strains, and severe illnesses accompanied by systemic infection are possible. Older chickens and turkeys, ducks and geese are more resistant (Barrow *et al.*, 1987, 1999; Pomeroy *et al.*, 1989; Holt *et al.*, 1999; Beal *et al.*, 2004a; Yu *et al.*, 2008). There is experimental evidence that older chickens show a more competent T-cell immunity in gut and stronger T-cell responses after *S.* Typhimurium infection compared to very young birds (Beal *et al.*, 2004b, 2005). However, *Salmonella* can colonize and persist for many weeks in the ilea and caeca of older chickens without clinical symptoms (Barrow, 2000; Beal *et al.*, 2004b). Additionally, a small proportion of *Salmonella* organisms are able to penetrate the gut mucosa and invade deeper organs such as the liver and spleen (Barrow, 2000).

The role of avian intestinal epithelial cells as a barrier against invading salmonellae in poultry

Intestinal epithelial cells are not only a physical barrier for invading salmonellae but are also the first initiators of host innate immune defence against *Salmonella*. A very important pattern recognition receptor, the Toll-like receptor-5 (TLR5), is situated at the basolateral site of these cells (Gewirtz *et al.*, 2001). Generally, TLRs sense the presence of PAMPs commonly found on a wide range of microorganisms and trigger innate immune mechanisms (Akira and Takeda, 2004; Keestra *et al.*, 2008). The main ligand for TLR5 is flagellin, which in avian species has an orthologous gene structure to that found in mammals (Groenen *et al.*, 2000; Schmid *et al.*, 2000; Fukui *et al.*, 2001), and it has also been shown that avian TLR5 responds to flagellin (Kogut *et al.*, 2005; He *et al.*, 2006). A role for this receptor in restricting the entry of flagellated *Salmonella* into the systemic circulation of chickens has been postulated (Iqbal *et al.*, 2005). In consequence of the recognition of flagellated *Salmonella* strains by TLR5, the cells are stimulated to produce cytokines such as inflammatory IL-1β and the chemokine IL-8. Increased IL-1β transcription, which induces the expression of genes associated with inflammation, has been described following *Salmonella* infection of poultry (Withanage *et al.*, 2004; Fasina *et al.*, 2008).

The role of avian granulocytes in *Salmonella*-infected poultry

The regulatory properties of IL-1 promote the infiltration of inflammatory cells such as granulocytes and other immune competent cells into the extra-vascular space (Dinarello, 2003), whereas IL-8 is best known as a chemotactic protein (chemokine CXCL8) that attracts granulocytes. In chickens, two different CXCL8-like chemokines have been described: the chicken (ch) CXCLi1 (CAF/IL-8, previously described as 9E3/-CEF4) and CXCLi2 (K60). Both chemokines are similar to human IL-8 (Sick *et al.*, 2000). At low concentrations, chCAF is chemotactic for monocytes/macrophages and lymphocytes (Martins-Green and Feugate, 1998). K60 was identified later than CAF and is more efficient in attracting granulocytes (Kaiser and Stäheli, 2008). Up-regulation of CXCLi1 and CXCLi2 transcription accompanied by an elevated number of macrophages and granulocytes was shown in caecum of young chicks following infection with *S.* Enteritidis and *S.* Typhimurium (Kogut, 2002; Berndt *et al.*, 2007; Cheeseman *et al.*, 2008).

Heterophils, the avian counterparts of mammalian neutrophils, are considered crucial in the initial effector response against

Salmonella in young poultry and large numbers of heterophils are rapidly recruited into the caecal mucosa after oral infection of day-old chicks with *S.* Enteritidis or *S.* Typhimurium (Kogut *et al.*, 1994; Berndt *et al.*, 2007; Cheeseman *et al.*, 2008). At the site of infection, heterophils can influence the acute inflammatory response by unspecific uptake of mucosal or luminal pathogens and production of toxic reactive oxygen species, proteolytic enzymes and other peptides with antimicrobial activity (Kogut *et al.*, 2001; Swaggerty *et al.*, 2003; Hasenstein and Lamont, 2007; van Dijk *et al.*, 2009). Studies have also correlated increased heterophil influx into the site of infection with increased resistance against *S.* Enteritidis infection in neonatal chickens (Swaggerty *et al.*, 2005; He *et al.*, 2007). Furthermore, a relationship between heterophil function, increased pro-inflammatory cytokine mRNA expression and increased resistance to *S.* Enteritidis in day-old chicks has also been postulated (Ferro *et al.*, 2004; Swaggerty *et al.*, 2006). In day-old and 14-day-old commercial turkeys and layer chickens, heterophil function has been shown to be poor and to correlate with increased susceptibility to infection with *Salmonella* pathogens (Lowry *et al.*, 1997; Genovese *et al.*, 2000). Kogut *et al.* (2003) demonstrated that avian granulocytes are capable of transcriptional activity and protein synthesis. Evidence of transcription of cytokines/chemokines as IL-6, CXCLi2, TGF-β4 or the T-helper-1 (Th1)-associated cytokine IL-18 by heterophils (Swaggerty *et al.*, 2006) indicates the potential of these cells to influence the fate of the immune response after *Salmonella* infection of chicks. Chicken heterophils also constitutively express a range of different TLRs, for instance the TLR1/6/10, TLR2, 3, 4, 5 and 7 (Kogut *et al.*, 2005). Stimulation with *Salmonella*-derived flagellin directly induces oxidative burst and an up-regulation of the transcription of pro-inflammatory cytokines such as IL-1β, IL-6 and IL-8 in heterophils (Kogut *et al.*, 2005). Recent studies have also reported an avian-specific TLR (TLR15), which may have evolved to be expressed on heterophils as a broad-spectrum TLR involved in the immune response to bacteria that have the potential to cause diseases in chickens (Nerren *et al.*, 2010). In comparison between resistant and susceptible chickens, non-stimulated heterophils isolated from *Salmonella*-resistant chickens express greater TLR15 and stronger TLR15 up-regulation after *S.* Enteritidis stimulation (Nerren *et al.*, 2009).

The role of avian macrophages in *Salmonella*-infected poultry

Like granulocytes, macrophages are crucial cells of the innate immune response during *Salmonella* infection. Macrophages are regulatory cells that are important not only in innate immune surveillance but also in stimulating adaptive immune mechanisms. The functional features of these professional phagocytes to recognize, engulf and kill *Salmonella* organisms as well as the capability of *Salmonella* to survive within these cells determine the development of either a predominantly local or a more systemic infection. The peak of the number of macrophages is reached shortly after that of the granulocytes in the caecal mucosa of *S.* Enteritidis- or *S.* Typhimurium-infected day-old chicks (Berndt *et al.*, 2007). *In vitro* studies showed, on the one hand, that avian macrophages possess very efficient bactericidal functions against *Salmonella* (Dil and Qureshi, 2003). On the other hand, *Salmonella* is capable of survival within cultured chicken macrophages (Desmidt *et al.*, 1998; Garcia-del Portillo, 2001). *In vivo*, however, only a limited number of bacteria of the *Salmonella* serovars Enteritidis and Typhimurium were found to be co-localized with avian caecal macrophages (Berndt *et al.*, 2007). Thus, the possibility of an extracellular dissemination in the gut mucosa and of extracellular virulence mechanisms of *Salmonella* strains *in vivo* cannot be ruled out.

Avian macrophages have been shown to express TLR4 (Dil and Qureshi, 2002), which is activated via LPS-bound CD14 receptors, by help of the CD14 molecule. Following activation of intra-cellular pathways, and subsequent binding of transcription factors to DNA promoter sequences, a variety of pro-inflammatory cytokines (such as IL-6 and IL-1) and cytotoxic molecules including reactive oxygen and nitrogen intermediates such as ROS and NO are produced. *Salmonella* Typhimurium and *S.* Enteritidis infection of the avian macrophage line HD11 cells enhances NO production (Babu *et al.*, 2006). The addition of IFN-γ, as the most important macrophage-stimulating mediator, to cell-cultured peripheral blood mononuclear cell-derived macrophages results in significantly fewer surviving *S.* Enteritidis than *S.* Typhimurium. Moreover, *S.* Typhimurium shows higher potential to necrotize macrophages (Okamura *et al.*, 2005), demonstrating different host–pathogen interactions between distinct *Salmonella* serovars.

In avian enteric salmonellosis, macrophages make an essential contribution to the cocktail of cytokines and mediators, secreted as a consequence of infection in the intestine and, by doing so, are important in determining the progress of the innate- and the development of adaptive immune responses. Wigley *et al.* (2006b) reported that macrophages respond to *Salmonella* infection by producing significantly increased transcription of IL-6, IL-1β, CCLi2 and CXCLi1 mRNA but differences were reported between different chicken lines and *Salmonella* serovars. As stated by the authors, these cytokines lead to increased pro-inflammatory activity including an enhanced influx of polymorphonuclear cells, elevated macrophage activation and, in the case of IL-6, in an activation of lymphocytes.

A more recent study used gene expression profiling microarrays to explore the genome-wide transcriptome profiles of chicken macrophages stimulated with *Salmonella*-derived endotoxin. The work demonstrates that endotoxin exposure significantly affects mRNA expression of IL-1β, IL-6, IL-8 and TLR15 but not IL-10 or IFN-γ in HD11 macrophages (Ciraci *et al.*, 2010) and, thus, indicates the contribution of macrophages to promote an inflammatory response.

The role of avian defensins in *Salmonella*-infected poultry

The defensins are a class of three subtypes of small cationic antimicrobial peptides α-, β- and θ- of which only the β-defensins exist in birds. More than 30 different β-defensins have been identified in avian species, with only avian β-defensin (AvBD)1–14 in chickens: the AvBD1 to 14 (Evans *et al.*, 1994; Harwig *et al.*, 1994; Zhao *et al.*, 2001; Lynn *et al.*, 2004; Xiao *et al.*, 2004; Higgs *et al.*, 2005) plus others have been described in other birds. Our knowledge of their biological function is limited. They are synthesized largely by heterophils and epithelial cells and in a wide range of tissues including the gut. It is therefore expected that they will play a role in defence and resistance as they have increasingly been found to do in mammals.

Infection with *Salmonella* either systemically, including the reproductive tract, or in the gut has been shown to have an effect on β-defensin expression. Following systemic infection the effects have been found to be variable. At 3 and 5 days after oral *S.* Typhimurium infection of day-old female broiler chicks, the β-defensins AvBD1, 2, 4 and 6 are significantly increased in caecal tonsils (Akbari *et al.*, 2008). In contrast, male brown newly hatched chicks did not respond to *S.* Enteritidis by augmented gallinacin 1, 2, 4 and 6 (AvBD1, 2, 4, 6) expression in caecum at 4 and 10 days after infection (Crhanova *et al.*, 2011). Ramasamy *et al.* (2012) quantified the mRNA expression levels of AvBD1–14 in gastrointestinal tissues of 3-day-old broiler chicks after 24 h of oral infection with *S.* Pullorum and revealed significant up-regulation of AvBD3, 4, 5, 6 and 12 as well as significant down-regulation of the expression of AvBD10, 11, 13 and 14 in one or only few tissues examined. In the ovary of sexually mature 52-week-old *S.* Enteritidis-infected chickens, AvBD4, 5, 7, 11 and 12 transcription is up-regulated, while the infection shows no significant influence on the expression of these genes in aged 104-week-old birds (Michailidis *et al.*, 2012). Correlation between levels of defensin expression and resistance/susceptibility are difficult currently to unravel because of the interfering effect of different bacterial numbers in the gut.

The adaptive immune response in the *Salmonella* infection of poultry

The eradication of non-host-specific *Salmonella* infection is effected by the help of a strong adaptive immune reaction. While strong B-cell reaction, including IgA response in gut, is induced after primary and secondary infection, the antibody production does not always correlate with *Salmonella* resistance in chickens (reviewed by Beal and Smith, 2007). Surprisingly, B cells, as the indicators of humoral immune mechanisms, are not found to be the essential factors for clearance of enteric *S.* Typhimurium in chickens (Beal *et al.*, 2006b). Instead, *Salmonella* removal seems to require a cell-mediated Th1-immune response although *S.* Pullorum appears to modulate this towards a Th2-type response characterized by low IFN-γ and higher IL-4 levels (Chappell *et al.*, 2009), which appears to promote the carrier state as indicated above. Therefore, considerable effort has been undertaken to explore avian cellular immune defence in different organs, such as gut, spleen, liver and blood. Changes in number, distribution and antigen-specific proliferation of T cells (Sasai *et al.*, 2000; Berndt and Methner, 2001; Asheg *et al.*, 2002; Babu *et al.*, 2003; Beal *et al.*, 2004a, b, 2005; Okamura *et al.*, 2004; Berndt *et al.*, 2007; Van Hemert *et al.*, 2007; Holt *et al.*, 2010; Pieper *et al.*, 2011) as well as delayed-type hypersensitivity response have been observed (Hassan and Curtiss, 1994). A predominance of $CD8^+$ T cells, as the representative population of a cell-mediated immune response, was shown in blood, caecum, bursa of Fabricus and spleen after primary *Salmonella* infection of young chicks (Berndt and Methner, 2001; Beal *et al.*, 2005). Additionally, higher numbers of γδ T cells were shown to appear after *Salmonella* infection of young chicks (Berndt and Methner, 2001). The relevance of these unique T lymphocytes in immune defence against *Salmonella* organisms has not yet been fully understood. A role as a link between the innate and adaptive immune response has been proposed for human and mice γδ T lymphocytes (Scotet *et al.*, 2008; Bonneville *et al.*, 2010). Some efforts have been undertaken to characterize better these numerically small lymphocyte populations in *Salmonella*-treated and non-treated birds. Based on the CD8α antigen expression of γδ T cells, three main avian γδ T-cell subgroups were identified: CD8α-negative ($CD8\alpha^-$), CD8α-diminished ($CD8\alpha^{+dim}$) and CD8α-highly positive ($CD8\alpha^{+high}$) γδ T lymphocytes (Berndt *et al.*, 2006). The $CD8\alpha^{+high}$ population additionally consists of the CD8αα homodimer-bearing and the CD8αβ heterodimer-bearing γδ T-cell subtype (Tregaskes *et al.*, 1995; Berndt *et al.*, 2006). The subset composition of γδ T cells varies according to their localization in the avian body as well as the age of the chickens (Pieper *et al.*, 2008). *Salmonella* immunization and infection of very young chicks is accompanied by an increase of $CD8\alpha\alpha^+$ T cells in peripheral blood, caecum and spleen (Berndt *et al.*, 2006; Pieper *et al.*, 2011). In *S.* Typhimurium-exposed chickens, the $CD8\alpha\alpha^+$ and $CD8\alpha\beta^+$ γδ T cells, but not the $CD8\alpha^-$ γδ T cells of blood and spleen, induce activation of Th1-related proteins such as Fas, FasL, IL-2Rα and IFN-γ. The avian $CD8\alpha\alpha^+$ lymphocytes constitute the proportionally major subset within the $CD8\alpha^{+high}$ T-cell population of blood, caecum and spleen and produce significant IFN-γ mRNA expression following *S.* Typhimurium infection of day-old chicks (Pieper *et al.*, 2011).

In parallel to investigations of T-cell composition, the transcription rates of several immune-relevant cytokines, chemokines or proteins and receptors have been analysed in the gastrointestinal tract and spleens of chickens following *Salmonella* infection or vaccination. Generally, gene expression responses to *Salmonella* infection in the intestine differ between chicken lines (Van Hemert *et al.*, 2006). *Salmonella* exposure significantly increases intestinal and splenic IL-12, IL-18 and IFN-γ transcription (Berndt *et al.*, 2007; Cheeseman *et al.*, 2007, 2008; Abasht *et al.*, 2008; González-Carvajal *et al.*, 2008) and, thus, underlines the importance of cell-mediated immune mechanisms for the eradication of pathogenic *Salmonella* organisms. Additionally, transcriptional up-regulation of T-cell-attracting chemokines such as lymphotactin and MIB-1β was found in the caeca of *Salmonella*-infected young chicks (Berndt *et al.*, 2007).

T-cell responsiveness is suppressed at onset of lay in the female, presumably by the high concentrations of circulating sex hormones at this time. In *S.* Pullorum-infected chickens this results in a resurgent infection and spread of the small number of bacteria to the reproductive tract with vertical transmission (Wigley *et al.*, 2005).

Vaccination to control *Salmonella* infection in poultry

Vaccination is used to control *Salmonella* infection in poultry flocks. Various vaccines, including live and killed preparations of *S.* Enteritidis and *S.* Typhimurium, have been applied to better defend poultry flocks from a *Salmonella* infection. Compared to live-attenuated vaccines, killed vaccines are considered as poor inducers of cell-mediated immunity (Babu *et al.*, 2004; Van Immerseel *et al.*, 2005). Nevertheless, Okamura *et al.* (2004) demonstrated an increased production of IFN-γ and IL-2 by antigen-stimulated splenocytes following vaccination of chickens with a commercially available killed vaccine. After vaccination of day-old chicks with live-attenuated *Salmonella* vaccines, a clear immune response with increased influx of $CD3^+$ and $CD8^+$ was detected (Berndt and Methner, 2001; Babu *et al.*, 2003; González-Carvajal *et al.*, 2008). However, the levels of change were lower in vaccine-treated chickens than those found in *Salmonella* wild-type-infected birds (Berndt and Methner, 2001; Berndt *et al.*, 2006). Generally, the degree of protection obtained after priming with a virulent *Salmonella* strain was shown to be greater than the level of defence induced by the use of attenuated vaccine strains in chickens (Barrow *et al.*, 1987; Beal *et al.*, 2004b). Studies evaluating the impact of live and killed *Salmonella* vaccines on *S.* Enteritidis clearance suggest that live vaccines protect against *S.* Enteritidis probably by enhancing cell-mediated immunity (Babu *et al.*, 2004). Furthermore, immune lymphokines produced by *S.* Enteritidis-immunized chickens significantly reduces horizontal transmission of *Salmonella* in young turkey and broiler chicks, indicating a prospective novel prevention strategy against *Salmonella* that could be implemented in the poultry industry (Lowry *et al.*, 1999).

The essential immune reactions required for enhanced protection against *Salmonella* organisms after challenge of primarily infected or vaccinated chickens have not been fully elucidated as yet. Secondary infection of birds is restricted to the gastrointestinal tract and is of shorter duration than primary infection (Beal *et al.*, 2004a). After secondary *Salmonella* challenge, a rapid expression of a macrophage inflammatory protein (MIP) family chemokines (IL-6, IL-12 and IFN-γ) occurs in addition to a lymphocyte influx (Withanage *et al.*, 2004; González-Carvajal *et al.*, 2008) and strong protection against intestinal colonization have been described (Withanage *et al.*, 2004).

Conclusion

In conclusion, a wealth of data has now been published regarding immunity to salmonellosis in mice. In some cases these data can be applied to salmonellosis in pigs, cattle and chickens, in particular when livestock become infected with typhoidal *Salmonella* serovars, and this may inform new therapeutics and vaccines for use in livestock. However, much less has been published regarding actual salmonellosis in livestock and to a certain extent this has been hampered by a lack of essential (species-specific) reagents. As these reagents become more readily available, more immunological studies are being reported in veterinary species, which may lead to important future discoveries.

References

Abasht, B., Kaiser, M.G. and Lamont, S.J. (2008) Toll-like receptor gene expression in cecum and spleen of advanced intercross line chicks infected with *Salmonella enterica* serovar Enteritidis. *Veterinary Immunology and Immunopathology* 123, 314–323.

Adak, G.K., Meakins, S.M., Yip, H., Lopman, B.A. and O'Brien, S.J. (2005) *Centers for Disease Control and Prevention Publication* 11, 3–5.

Akbari, M.R., Haghighi, H.R., Chambers, J.R., Brisbin, J., Read, L.R. and Sharif, S. (2008) Expression of antimicrobial peptides in cecal tonsils of chickens treated with probiotics and infected with *Salmonella enterica* serovar Typhimurium. *Clinical and Vaccine Immunology* 15, 1689–1693.

Akira, S. and Takeda, K. (2004) Toll-like receptor signalling. *Nature Reviews Immunology* 4, 499–511.

Alpuche-Aranda, C.M., Swanson, J.A., Loomis, W.P. and Miller, S.I. (1992) *Salmonella typhimurium* activates virulence gene transcription within acidified macrophage phagosomes. *Proceedings of the National Academy of Sciences USA* 89, 10079–10083.

Asheg, A., Levkut, M., Revajova, V., Sevcikova, Z., Kolodzieyski, L. and Pistl, J. (2002) T lymphocyte subpopulations and B lymphocyte cells in caecum and spleen of chicks infected with *Salmonella enteritidis*. *Acta Histochemica* 104, 435–439.

Babu, U., Scott, M., Myers, M.J., Okamura, M., Gaines, D., Yancy, H.F., Lillehoj, H., Heckert, R.A. and Raybourne, R.B. (2003) Effects of live attenuated and killed *Salmonella* vaccine on T-lymphocyte mediated immunity in laying hens. *Veterinary Immunology and Immunopathology* 91, 39–44.

Babu, U., Dalloul, R.A., Okamura, M., Lillehoj, H.S., Xie, H., Raybourne, R.B., Gaines, D. and Heckert, R.A. (2004) *Salmonella enteritidis* clearance and immune response in chickens following *Salmonella* vaccination and challenge. *Veterinary Immunology and Immunopathology* 101, 251–257.

Babu, U.S., Gaines, D.W., Lillehoj, H. and Raybourne, R.B. (2006) Differential reactive oxygen and nitrogen production and clearance of *Salmonella* serovars by chicken and mouse macrophages. *Developmental & Comparative Immunology* 30, 942–953.

Barr, T.A., Brown, S., Mastroeni, P. and Gray, D. (2010) TLR and B cell receptor signals to B cells differentially program primary and memory Th1 responses to *Salmonella* enterica. *The Journal of Immunology* 185, 2783–2789.

Barrow, P.A. (2000) The paratyphoid *Salmonellae*. *Revue scientifique et technique de l'Office International des Epizooties* 19, 351–375.

Barrow, P.A. and Duchet-Suchaux, M. (1997) *Salmonella* carriage and the carrier state. *Proceedings of the 2nd International Symposium on* Salmonella *and Salmonellosis*, Ploufragan, France.

Barrow, P.A., Huggins, M.B., Lovell, M.A. and Simpson, J.M. (1987) Observations on the pathogenesis of experimental *Salmonella typhimurium* infection in chickens. *Research in Veterinary Science* 4, 194–199.

Barrow, P.A., Lovell, M.A., Murphy, C.K. and Page, K. (1999) *Salmonella* infection in a commercial line of ducks; experimental studies on virulence, intestinal colonisation and immune protection. *Epidemiology and Infection* 123, 121–132.

Barthel, M., Hapfelmeier, S., Quintanilla-Martinez, L., Kremer, M., Rohde, M., Hogardt, M., Pfeffer, K., Rüssmann, H. and Dietrich-Hardt, W. (2003) Pretreatment of mice with streptomycin provides a *Salmonella enterica* serovar Typhimurium colitis model that allows analysis of both pathogen and host. *Infection and Immunity* 71, 2839–2858.

Barua, A. and Yoshimura, Y. (2004) Ovarian cell-mediated immune response to *Salmonella* enteritidis infection in laying hens (*Gallus domesticus*). *Poultry Science* 83, 997–1002.

Beal, R.K. and Smith, A.L. (2007) Antibody response to *Salmonella*: its induction and role in protection against avian enteric salmonellosis. *Expert Review of Anti-infective Therapy* 5, 873–881.

Beal, R.K., Powers, C., Wigley, P., Barrow, P.A. and Smith, A.L. (2004a) Temporal dynamics of the cellular, humoral and cytokine responses in chickens during primary and secondary infection with *Salmonella enterica* serovar Typhimurium. *Avian Pathology* 33, 25–33.

Beal, R.K., Wigley, P., Powers, C., Hulme, S.D., Barrow, P.A. and Smith, A.L. (2004b) Age at primary infection with *Salmonella enterica* serovar Typhimurium in the chicken influences persistence of infection and subsequent immunity to re-challenge. *Veterinary Immunology and Immunopathology* 100, 151–164.

Beal, R.K., Powers, C., Wigley, P., Barrow, P.A., Kaiser, P. and Smith, A.L. (2005) A strong antigen-specific T-cell response is associated with age and genetically dependent resistance to avian enteric salmonellosis. *Infection and Immunity* 73, 7509–7516.

Beal, R.K., Wigley, P., Powers, C., Barrow, P.A. and Smith, A.L. (2006a) Cross-reactive cellular and humoral immune responses to *Salmonella enterica* serovars Typhimurium and Enteritidis are associated with protection to heterologous re-challenge. *Veterinary Immunology and Immunopathology* 114, 84–93.

Beal, R.K., Powers, C., Davison, T.F., Barrow, P.A. and Smith, A.L. (2006b) Clearance of enteric *Salmonella enterica* Serovar Typhimurium in chickens is independent of B-cell function. *Infection and Immunity* 74, 1442–1444.

Befus, D.A., Johnston, N., Leslie, G.A. and Bienenstock, J. (1980) Gut associated lymphoid tissue in the chicken. I. Morphology, ontogeny, and some functional characteristics of Peyer's patches. *The Journal of Immunology* 125, 2626–2632.

Ben-Baruch, A., Michiel, D.F. and Oppenheim, J.J. (1995) Signals and receptors involved in recruitment of inflammatory cells. *The Journal of Biological Chemistry* 270, 11703–11706.

Berndt, A. and Methner, U. (2001) Gamma/delta T cell response of chickens after oral administration of attenuated and non-attenuated *Salmonella typhimurium* strains. *Veterinary Immunology and Immunopathology* 78, 143–161.

Berndt, A. and Methner, U. (2004) B cell and macrophage response in chicks after oral administration of *Salmonella typhimurium* strains. *Comparative Immunology, Microbiology & Infectious Diseases* 27, 235–246.

Berndt, A., Pieper, J. and Methner, U. (2006) Circulating gamma delta T cells in response to *Salmonella enterica* serovar Enteritidis exposure in chickens. *Infection and Immunity* 74, 3967–3978.

Berndt, A., Wilhelm, A., Jugert, Ch., Pieper, J., Sachse, K. and Methner, U. (2007) Chicken cecum immune response to *Salmonella enterica* serovars of different levels of invasiveness. *Infection and Immunity* 75, 5993–6007.

Bolton, A., Osborne, M.P., Wallis, T.S. and Stephen, J. (1999) Interaction of *Salmonella cholerasuis*, *Salmonella dublin* and *Salmonella typhimurium* with porcine and bovine terminal ileum in vivo. *Microbiology* 145, 2431–2441.

Bonneville, M., O'Brien, R.L. and Born, W.K. (2010) T cell effector functions: a blend of innate programming and acquired plasticity. *Nature Reviews Immunology* 10, 467–489.

Boyen, F., Pasmans, F., Van Immerseel, F., Morgan, E., Adriaensen, C., Hernalsteens, J.P., Decostere, A., Ducatelle, R. and Haesebrouck, F. (2006a) *Salmonella* Typhimurium SPI-1 genes promote intestinal but not tonsillar colonization in pigs. *Microbes and Infection* 8, 2899–2907.

Boyen, F., Pasmans, F., Donné, E., Van Immerseel, F., Adriaensen, C., Hernalsteens, J.P., Ducatelle, R. and Haesebrouck, F. (2006b) Role of SPI-1 in the interactions of *Salmonella* Typhimurium with porcine macrophages. *Veterinary Microbiology* 113, 35–44.

Boyen, F., Pasmans, F., Van Immerseel, F., Morgan, E., Botteldoorn, N., Heyndrickx, M., Volf, J., Favoreel, H., Hernalsteens, J.P., Ducatelle, R. and Haesebrouck, F. (2008) A limited role for SsrA/B in persistent *Salmonella* Typhimurium infections in pigs. *Veterinary Microbiology* 128, 364–373.

Brumme, S., Arnold, T., Sigmarsson, H., Lehmann, J., Scholz, H.C., Hardt, W.D., Hensel, A., Truyen, U. and Roesler, U. (2007) Impact of *Salmonella* Typhimurium DT104 virulence factors invC and sseD on the onset, clinical course, colonization patterns and immune response of porcine salmonellosis. *Veterinary Microbiology* 124, 274–285.

Bueno, S.M., González, P.A., Schwebach, J.R. and Kalergis, A.M. (2007) T cell immunity evasion by virulent *Salmonella* enterica. *Immunology Letters* 111, 14–20.

Burns, R.B. and Maxwell, M.H. (1986) Ultrastructure of Peyer's patches in the domestic fowl and turkey. *Journal of Anatomy* 147, 235–243.

Calenge, F., Kaiser, P., Vignal, A. and Beauont, C. (2010) Genetic control of resistance to salmonellosis and to *Salmonella* carrier-state in fowl: a review. *Genetics Selection Evolution* 42, 11–22.

Carpenter, S. and O'Neill, L.A. (2007) How important are Toll-like receptors for antimicrobial responses? *Cellular Microbiology* 9, 1891–1901.

Cassatella, M.A. (1999) Neutrophil derived proteins: selling cytokines by the pound. *Advances in Immunology* 73, 369–509.

Chadfield, M.S., Brown, D.J., Aabo, S., Christensen, J.P. and Olsen, J.E. (2003) Comparison of intestinal invasion and macrophage response of *Salmonella* Gallinarum and other host-adapted *Salmonella* enterica serovars in the avian host. *Veterinary Microbiology* 92, 49–64.

Chappell, L., Kaiser, P., Barrow, P., Jones, M.A., Johnston, C. and Wigley, P. (2009) The immunobiology of avian systemic salmonellosis. *Veterinary Immunology and Immunopathology* 128, 53–59.

Cheeseman, J.H., Kaiser, M.G., Ciraci, C., Kaiser, P. and Lamont, S.J. (2007) Breed effect on early cytokine mRNA expression in spleen and cecum of chickens with and without *Salmonella* enteritidis infection. *Developmental & Comparative Immunology* 31, 52–60.

Cheeseman, J.H., Levy, N.A., Kaiser, P., Lillehoj, H.S. and Lamont, S.J. (2008) *Salmonella* Enteritidis-induced alteration of inflammatory CXCL chemokine messenger-RNA expression and histologic changes in the ceca of infected chicks. *Avian Diseases* 52, 229–234.

Cheminay, C., Mohlenbrink, A. and Hensel, M. (2005) Intracellular *Salmonella* inhibit antigen presentation by dendritic cells. *The Journal of Immunology* 174, 2892–2899.

Chu, C.Y., Wang, S.Y., Chen, Z.W., Chien, M.S., Huang, J.P., Chen, J.J., Hong, L.S., Shiau, A.L., Tsai, J.L. and Wu, C.L. (2007) Heterologous protection in pigs induced by a plasmid-cured and *crp* gene-deleted *Salmonella choleraesuis* live vaccine. *Vaccine* 25, 7031–7040.

Ciraci, C., Tuggle, C.K., Wannemuehler, M.J., Nettleton, D. and Lamont, S.J. (2010) Unique genome-wide transcriptome profiles of chicken macrophages exposed to *Salmonella*-derived endotoxin. *BMC Genomics* 11, 545–556.

Cirillo, D.M., Valdivia, R.H., Monack, D.M. and Falkow, S. (1998) Macrophage-dependent induction of the *Salmonella* pathogenicity island 2 type III secretion system and its role in intracellular survival. *Molecular Microbiology* 30, 175 188.

Collado-Romero, M., Arce, C., Ramírez-Boo, M., Carvajal, A. and Garrido, J.J. (2010) Quantitative analysis of the immune response upon *Salmonella typhimurium* infection along the porcine intestinal gut. *Veterinary Research* 41, 23–24.

Crhanova, M., Hradecka, H., Faldynova, M., Matulova, M., Havlickova, H., Sisak, F. and Rychlik, I. (2011) Immune response of chicken gut to natural colonization by gut microflora and to *Salmonella enterica* serovar Enteritidis infection. *Infection and Immunity* 79, 2755–2763.

Cummings, L.A., Barrett, S.L., Wilkerson, W.D., Fellnerova, I. and Cookson, B.T. (2005) FliC-specific CD4+ T cell responses are restricted by bacterial regulation of antigen expression. *The Journal of Immunology* 174, 7929–7938.

Davison, F., Kaspers, B. and Schat, K.A. (eds) (2008) *Avian Immunology*. Elsevier, Amsterdam.

De Groote, M.A., Ochsner, U.A., Shiloh, M.U., Nathan, C., McCord, J.M., Dinauer, M.C., Libby, S.J., Vazquez-Torres, A., Xu, Y. and Fang, F.C. (1997) Periplasmic superoxide dismutase protects *Salmonella* from products of phagocyte NADPH-oxidase and nitric oxide synthase. *Proceedings of the National Academy of Sciences of the United States of America* 94, 13997–14001.

Desmidt, M., Ducatelle, R., Mast, J., Goddeeries, B.M., Kaspers, B. and Haesebrouck, F. (1998) Role of the humoral immune system in *Salmonella enteritidis* phage type for infection in chickens. *Veterinary Immunology and Immunopathology* 63, 355–367.

Dil, N. and Qureshi, M.A. (2002) Differential expression of inducible nitric oxide synthase is associated with differential Toll-like receptor-4 expression in chicken macrophages from different genetic backgrounds. *Veterinary Immunology and Immunopathology* 84, 191–207.

Dil, N. and Qureshi, M.A. (2003) Interleukin-1beta does not contribute to genetic strain-based differences in iNOS expression and activity in chicken macrophages. *Developmental & Comparative Immunology* 27, 137–146.

Dinarello, Ch.A. (2003) Interleukine-1 Family (I-1F1, F2). In: Thomson, A.W. and Lotze, M.T. (eds) *The Cytokine Handbook*, 4th edn. Academic Press, Amsterdam.

Evans, E.W., Beach, G.G., Wunderlich, J. and Harmon, B.G. (1994) Isolation of antimicrobial peptides from avian heterophils. *Journal of Leukocyte Biology* 56, 661–665.

Fasina, Y.O., Holt, P.S., Moran, E.T., Moore, R.W., Conner, D.E. and McKee, S.R. (2008) Intestinal cytokine response of commercial source broiler chicks to *Salmonella* Typhimurium infection. *Poultry Science* 87, 1335–1346.

Ferro, P.J., Swaggerty, C.L., Kaiser, P., Pevzner, I.Y. and Kogut, M.H. (2004) Heterophils isolated from chickens resistant to extra-intestinal *Salmonella enteritidis* infection express higher levels of pro-inflammatory cytokine mRNA following infection than heterophils from susceptible chickens. *Epidemiology and Infection* 132, 1029–1037.

Forest, C.G., Ferraro, E., Sabbagh, S.C. and Daigle, F. (2010) Intracellular survival of *Salmonella* enterica serovar Typhi in human macrophages is independent of *Salmonella* pathogenicity island (SPI)-2. *Microbiology* 156, 3689–3698.

Foster, N., Lovell, M.A., Marston, K.L., Hulme, S.D., Frost, A.J., Bland, P. and Barrow, P.A. (2003a) Rapid protection of gnotobiotic pigs against experimental salmonellosis following induction of polymorphonuclear leukocytes by avirulent *Salmonella* enterica. *Infection and Immunity* 71, 2182–2191.

Foster, N., Hulme, S.D. and Barrow, P.A. (2003b) Induction of antimicrobial pathways during early-phase immune response to *Salmonella* spp. in murine macrophages: gamma interferon (IFN-gamma) and upregulation of IFN-gamma receptor alpha expression are required for NADPH phagocytic oxidase gp91-stimulated oxidative burst and control of virulent *Salmonella* spp. *Infection and Immunity* 71, 4733–4741.

Foster, N., Hulme, S., Lovell, M., Reed, K. and Barrow, P.A. (2005) Stimulation of gp91 phagocytic oxidase and reactive oxygen species in neutrophils by an avirulent *Salmonella* enterica serovar infantis strain protects gnotobiotic piglets from lethal challenge with serovar Typhimurium strain F98 without inducing intestinal pathology. *Infection and Immunity* 73, 4539–4547.

Frost, A.J., Bland, A.P. and Wallis, T.S. (1997) The early dynamic response of the calf ileal epithelium to *Salmonella typhimurium*. *Veterinary Pathology* 34, 369–386.

Fukui, A., Inoue, N., Matsumoto, M., Nomura, M., Yamada, K., Matsuda, Y., Toyoshima, K. and Seya, T. (2001) Molecular cloning and functional characterization of chicken toll-like receptors. A single chicken toll covers multiple molecular patterns. *The Journal of Biological Chemistry* 276, 47143–47149.

Galán, J.E. and Curtiss III, R. (1989) Cloning and molecular characterization of genes whose products allow *Salmonella typhimurium* to penetrate tissue culture cells. *Proceedings of the National Academy of Sciences USA* 86, 6383–6387.

Gallagher, D.S., Jr, Ryan, A.M., Diamond, G., Bevins, C.L. and Womack, J.E. (1995) Somatic cell mapping of beta-defensin genes to cattle syntenic group U25 and fluorescence in situ localization to chromosome 27. *Mammalian Genome* 6, 554–556.

Garcia-del Portillo, F. (2001) *Salmonella* intracellular proliferation: where, when and how? *Microbes and Infection* 3, 1305–1311.

Genovese, L.L., Lowry, V.K., Genovese, K.J. and Kogut, M.H. (2000) Longevity of augmented phagocytic activity of heterophils in neonatal chickens following administration of *Salmonella enteritidis*-immune lymphokines to chickens. *Avian Pathology* 29, 117–122.

Gewirtz, A.T., Navas, T.A., Lyons, S., Godowski, P.J. and Madara, J.L. (2001) Cutting edge: bacterial flagellin activates basolaterally expressed TLR5 to induce epithelial proinflammatory gene expression. *The Journal of Immunology* 167, 1882–1885.

González-Carvajal, B., Methner, U., Pieper, J. and Berndt, A. (2008) Effects of *Salmonella enterica* serovar Enteritidis on cellular recruitment and cytokine gene expression in caecum of vaccinated chickens. *Vaccine* 26, 5423–5433.

Gray, J.T., Fedorka-Cray, P.J., Stabel, T.J. and Ackermann, M.R. (1995) Influence of inoculation route on the carrier state of *Salmonella choleraesuis* in swine. *Veterinary Microbiology* 47, 43–59.

Groenen, M.A., Cheng, H.H., Bumstead, N., Benkel, B.F., Briels, W.E., Burke, T., Burt, D.W., Crittenden, L.B., Dodgson, J., Hillel, J., Lamont, S., de Leon, A.P., Soller, M., Takahaschi, H. and Vignal, A. (2000) A consensus linkage map of the chicken genome. *Genome Research* 10, 137–147.

Harwig, S.S.L., Swiderek, K.M., Kokryakov, V.N., Tan, L., Lee, T.D., Panyutich, E.A., Aleshina, G.M., Shamova, O.V. and Lehrer, R.I. (1994) Gallinacins: cysteine-rich antimicrobial peptides of chicken leukocytes. *FEBS Letters* 342, 281–325.

Hasenstein, J.R. and Lamont, S.J. (2007) Chicken gallinacin gene cluster associated with *Salmonella* response in advanced intercross line. *Avian Diseases* 51, 561–567.

Hassan, J.O. and Curtiss III, R. (1994) Virulent *Salmonella typhimurium*-induced lymphocyte depletion and immunosuppression in chickens. *Infection and Immunity* 62, 2027–2036.

He, H., Genovese, K.J., Nisbet, D.J. and Kogut, M.H. (2006) Profile of Toll-like receptor expressions and induction of nitric oxide synthesis by Toll-like receptor agonists in chicken monocytes. *Molecular Immunology* 43, 783–789.

He, H., Genovese, K.J., Swaggerty, C.L., Nisbet, D.J. and Kogut, M.H. (2007) In vivo priming heterophil innate immune functions and increasing resistance to *Salmonella* Enteritidis infection in neonatal chickens by immune stimulatory CpG oligodeoxynucleotides. *Veterinary Immunology and Immunopathology* 117, 275–283.

Hedges, J.F., Buckner, D.L., Rask, K.M., Kerns, H.M.M., Jackiw, L.O., Trunkle, T.C., Pascual, D.W. and Jutila, M.A. (2007) Mucosal lymphatic-derived T cells respond early to experimental *Salmonella* enterocolitis by increasing expression of IL-2R. *Cellular Immunology* 246, 8–16.

Henderson, S.C., Bounous, D.I. and Lee, M.D. (1999) Early events in the pathogenesis of avian salmonellosis. *Infection and Immunity* 67, 3580–3586.

Hersh, D., Monack, D.M., Smith, M.R., Ghori, N., Falkow, S. and Zychlinsky, A. (1999) The *Salmonella* invasin SipB induces macrophage apoptosis by binding to caspase-1. *Proceedings of the National Academy of Sciences USA* 96, 2396–2401.

Higgs, R., Lynn, D.J., Gaines, S., McMahon, J., Tierney, J., James, T., Lloyd, A.T., Mulcahy, G. and O'Farrelly, C. (2005) The synthetic form of a novel chicken β-defensin identified *in silico* is predominantly active against intestinal pathogens. *Immunogenetics* 57, 90–98.

Hirsh, D.C., MacLachlan, N.J. and Walker, R.L. (eds) (2004) *Veterinary Microbiology*, 2nd edn. Blackwell Publishing, Ames, Iowa.

Holt, P.S., Gast, R.K., Porter, R.E. and Stone, H.D. (1999) Hyporesponsiveness of the systemic and mucosal humoral immune systems in chickens infected with *Salmonella enterica* serovar *enteritidis* at one day of age. *Poultry Science* 78, 1510–1519.

Holt, P.S., Vaughn, L.E. and Gast, R.K. (2010) Flow cytometric characterization of Peyer's patch and cecal tonsil T lymphocytes in laying hens following challenge with *Salmonella enterica* serovar Enteritidis. *Veterinary Immunology and Immunopathology* 133, 276–281.

Hölzer, S.U. and Hensel, M. (2010) Functional dissection of translocon proteins of the *Salmonella* pathogenicity island 2-encoded type III secretion system. *BMC Microbiology* 10, 104.

Hu, J., Bumstead, N., Barrow, P., Sebastiani, G., Olien, L., Morgan, K. and Malo, D. (1997) Resistance of salmonellosis in the chicken is linked to NRAMP1 and TNC. *Genome Research* 7, 693–704.

Hughes, S., Poh, T.Y., Bumstead, N. and Kaiser, P. (2007) Re-evaluation of the chicken MIP family of chemokines and their receptors suggests that CCL5 is the prototypic MIP family chemokine, and that different species have developed different repertoires of both the CC chemokines and their receptors. *Developmental and Comparative Immunology* 3, 72–86.

Hur, J. and Lee, J.H. (2010) Immunization of pregnant sows with a novel virulence gene deleted live *Salmonella* vaccine and protection of their suckling piglets against salmonellosis. *Veterinary Microbiology* 143, 270–276.

Hyland, K.A., Kohrt, L., Vulchanova, L. and Murtaugh, M.P. (2006) Mucosal innate immune response to intragastric infection by *Salmonella* enterica serovar Choleraesuis. *Molecular Immunology* 43, 1890–1899.

Iqbal, M., Philbin, V.J., Withanage, G.S., Wigley, P., Beal, R.K., Goodchild, M.J., Barrow, P., McConnell, I., Maskell, D.J., Young, J., Bumstead, N., Boyd, Y. and Smith, A.L. (2005) Identification and functional characterization of chicken toll-like receptor 5 reveals a fundamental role in the biology of infection with *Salmonella enterica* serovar typhimurium. *Infection and Immunity* 73, 2344–2350.

Ivanek, R., Snary, E.L., Cook, A.J. and Grohn, Y.T. (2004) A mathematical model for the transmission of *Salmonella* Typhimurium within a grower-finisher pig herd in Great Britain. *Journal of Food Protection* 67, 2403–2409.

Jones, B.D., Ghori, N. and Falkow, S. (1994) *Salmonella typhimurium* initiates murine infection by penetrating and destroying the specialized epithelial M cells of the Peyer's patches. *The Journal of Experimental Medicine* 180, 15–23.

Jones, M.A., Hulme, S.D., Barrow, P.A. and Wigley, P. (2007) The *Salmonella* pathogenicity island 1 and *Salmonella* pathogenicity island 2 type III secretion systems play a major role in pathogenesis of systemic disease and gastrointestinal tract colonization of *Salmonella enterica* serovar Typhimurium in the chicken. *Avian Pathology* 36, 199–203.

Jotwani, R., Tanaka, Y., Watanabe, K., Tanaka, K., Kato, N. and Ueno, K. (1995) Cytokine stimulation during *Salmonella* typhimurium sepsis in Itys mice. *Journal of Medical Microbiology* 42, 348–352.

Kaiser, P. and Stäheli, P. (2008) Avian cytokines and chemokines. In: Davison, F., Kaspers, B. and Schat, K.A. (eds) *Avian Immunology*, 1st edn. Elsevier, Amsterdam.

Keestra, A.M., de Zoete, M.R., van Aubel, R.A.M.H. and van Putten, J.P.M. (2008) Functional characterization of chicken TLR5 reveals species-specific recognition of flagellin. *Molecular Immunology* 45, 1298–1307.

Kogut, M.H. (2002) Dynamics of a protective avian inflammatory response: the role of an IL-8-like cytokine in the recruitment of heterophils to the site of organ invasion by *Salmonella enteritidis*. *Comparative Immunology, Microbiology & Infectious Diseases* 25, 159–172.

Kogut, M.H., Tellez, G.I., McGruder, E.D., Hargis, B.M., Williams, J.D., Corrier, D.E. and DeLoach, J.R. (1994) Heterophils are decisive components in the early responses of chickens to *Salmonella enteritidis* infections. *Microbial Pathogenesis* 16, 141–151.

Kogut, M.H., Genovese, K.J. and Lowry, V.K. (2001) Differential activation of single transduction pathways mediating phagocytosis, oxidative burst, and degranulation by chicken heterophils in response to stimulation with opsonized *Salmonella enteritidis*. *Inflammation* 25, 7–15.

Kogut, M.H., Rothwell, L. and Kaiser, P. (2003) Differential regulation of cytokine gene expression by avian heterophils during receptor-mediated phagocytosis of opsonized *Salmonella enteritidis*. *Journal of Interferon and Cytokine Research* 23, 319–327.

Kogut, M.H., Iqbal, M., He, H., Philbin, V., Kaiser, P. and Smith, A. (2005) Expression and function of Toll-like receptors in chicken heterophils. *Developmental & Comparative Immunology* 29, 791–808.

Konnai, S., Ohtsuka, H., Sakamoto, T., Nakaoka, Y., Kiku, Y., Koiwa, M., Takahaschi, J., Yokomizo, Y. and Yoshino, T. (2001) Inflammatory cytokines and antigen-responsive mononuclear cells in peripheral blood of cattle infected with *Salmonella* Takoradi. *The Journal of Veterinary Medical Science* 63, 859–865.

Lalmanach, A.-C. and Lantier, F. (1999) Host cytokine response and resistance to *Salmonella* infection. *Microbes and Infection* 1, 719–726.

Lee, J.S., Jung, I.D., Lee, C.M., Park, J.W., Chun, S.H., Jeong, S.K., Ha, T.K., Shin, Y.K., Kim, D.J. and Park, Y.M. (2010) Outer membrane protein a of *Salmonella enterica* serovar Typhimurium activates dendritic cells and enhances Th1 polarization. *BMC Microbiology* 15, 263.

Letellier, A., Messier, S., Lessard, L., Chénier, S. and Quessy, S. (2001) Host response to various treatments to reduce *Salmonella* infections in swine. *Canadian Journal of Veterinary Research* 65, 168–172.

Liebler, E.M., Press, C.McL. and Landsverk, T. (1994) Lymphocyte subpopulations in jejunal and ileal Peyer's patches of calves with experimental *Salmonella dublin* infection. *Journal of Veterinary Medicine* 41, 1–10.

Lillehoj, H.S., Kim, C.H., Keeler, C.L. Jr and Zhang, S. (2007) Immunogenomic approaches to study host immunity to enteric pathogens. *Poultry Science* 86, 1491–1500.

Lindgren, S.W., Stojiljkovic, I. and Heffron, F. (1996) Macrophage killing is an essential virulence mechanism of *Salmonella* typhimurium. *Proceedings of the National Academy of Sciences USA* 93, 4197–4201.

Lowry, V.K., Genovese, K.J., Bowden, L.L. and Kogut, M.H. (1997) Ontogeny of the phagocytic and bactericidal activities of turkey heterophils and their potential by *Salmonella* enteritidis-immune lymphokines. *FEMS Immunology and Medical Microbiology* 19, 95–100.

Lowry, V.K., Tellez, G.I., Nisbet, D.J., Garcia, G., Urquiza, O., Stanker, L.H. and Kogut, M.H. (1999) Efficacy of *Salmonella* enteritidis-immune lymphokines on horizontal transmission of *S.* arizonae in turkeys and *S.* gallinarum in chickens. *International Journal of Food Microbiology* 48, 139–148.

Lundberg, U., Vinatzer, U., Berdnik, D., von Gabain, A. and Baccarini, M. (1999) Growth phase-regulated induction of *Salmonella*-induced macrophage apoptosis correlates with transient expression of SPI-1 genes. *Journal of Bacteriology* 181, 3433–3437.

Lynn, D.J., Higgs, R., Gaines, S., Tierney, J., James, T., Lloyd, A.T., Fares, M.A., Mulcahy, G. and O'Farrelly, C. (2004) Bioinformatic discovery and initial characterisation of nine novel antimicrobial peptide genes in the chicken. *Immunogenetics* 56, 170–177.

Mariani, P., Barrow, P.A., Cheng, H.H., Groenen, M.M., Negrini, R. and Bumstead, N. (2001) Localization of chicken chromosome 5 of a novel locus determining salmonellosis resistance. *Immunogenetics* 53, 786–791.

Martins-Green, M. and Feugate, J.E. (1998) The 9E3/CEF4 gene product is a chemotactic and angiogenic factor that can initiate the wound-healing cascade *in vivo*. *Cytokine* 10, 522–535.

Mastroeni, P. and Ménager, N. (2003) Development of acquired immunity to Salmonella. *Journal of Medical Microbiology* 52, 453–459.

McSorley, S.J., Asch, S., Costalonga, M., Reinhardt, R.L. and Jenkins, M.K. (2002) Tracking *Salmonella*-specific CD4 T cells *in vivo* reveals a local mucosal response to a disseminated infection. *Immunity* 16, 365–377.

Mee, J.F. (1995) Terminal gangrene and ositis in calves attributed to *Salmonella*-Dublin infection. *Irish Veterinary Journal* 48, 22–28.

Mellman, I., Turley, S.J. and Steinman, R.M. (1998) Antigen processing for amateurs and professionals. *Trends in Cell Biology* 8, 231–237.

Metcalfe, H.J., Best, A., Kanellos, T., La Ragione, R.M. and Werling, D. (2010) Flagellin expression enhances *Salmonella* accumulation in TLR5-positive macrophages. *Developmental & Comparative Immunology* 34, 997–804.

Michailidis, G., Avdi, M. and Argiriou, A. (2012) Transcriptional profiling of antimicrobial peptides avian β-defensins in the chicken ovary during sexual maturation and in response to *Salmonella* Enteritidis infection. *Research in Veterinary Science* 92, 60–65.

Michetti, P., Mahan, M.J., Slauch, J.M., Mekalanos, J.J. and Neutra, M.R. (1992) Monoclonal secretory immunoglobulin A protects mice against oral challenge with the invasive pathogen *Salmonella* Typhimurium. *Infection and Immunity* 60, 1786–1792.

Miller, S.I. (1991) PhoP/PhoQ: macrophage-specific modulators of *Salmonella* virulence? *Molecular Microbiology* 5, 2073–2078.

Modi, W.S., Amarante, M.R., Hanson, M., Womack, J.E. and Chidambaram, A. (1998) Assignment of the mouse and cow CXC chemokine genes. *Cytogenetics and Cell Genetics* 81, 213–216.

Mohler, V.L., Izzo, M.M. and House, J.K. (2009) *Salmonella* in calves. *Veterinary Clinics of North America – Food Animal Practice* 25, 37–54.

Morsey, M.A., Popowych, Y., Kowalski, J., Gerlach, G., Godson, D., Campos, M. and Babiuk, L.A. (1996) Molecular cloning and expression of bovine interleukin-8. *Microbial Pathogenesis* 20, 203–212.

Nauciel, C. (1990) Role of CD4+ T cells and T-independent mechanisms in acquired resistance to *Salmonella* typhimurium infection. *The Journal of Immunology* 145, 1265–1269.

Nerren, J.R., Swaggerty, C.L., MacKinnon, K.M., Genovese, K.J., He, H., Pevzner, I. and Kogut, M.H. (2009) Differential mRNA expression of the avian-specific toll-like receptor 15 between heterophils from *Salmonella*-susceptible and -resistant chickens. *Immunogenetics* 61, 71–77.

Nerren, J.R., Genovese, H.H.K. and Kogut, M.H. (2010) Expression of the avian-specific toll-like receptor 15 in chicken heterophils is mediated by Gram-negative and Gram-positive bacteria, but not TLR agonists. *Veterinary Immunology and Immunopathology* 136, 151–156.

Nikolaus, T., Deiwick, J., Rappl, C., Freeman, J.A., Schröder, W., Miller, S.I. and Hensel, M. (2001) SseBCD proteins are secreted by the type III secretion system of *Salmonella* pathogenicity island 2 and function as a translocon. *Journal of Bacteriology* 183, 6036–6045.

Norimatsu, M., Harris, J., Chance, V., Dougan, G., Howard, C.J. and Villarreal-Ramos, B. (2003) Differential response of bovine monocyte-derived macrophages and dendritic cells to infection with *Salmonella typhimurium* in a low-dose model *in vitro*. *The Journal of Immunology* 108, 55–61.

Norimatsu, M., Chance, V., Dougan, G., Howard, C.J. and Villarreal-Ramos, B. (2004) Live *Salmonella enterica* serovar Typhimurium (*S.* Typhimurium) elicit dendritic cell responses that differ from those induced by killed *S.* Typhimurium. *Veterinary Immunology and Immunopathology* 98, 193–201.

Nunes, J.S., Lawhon, S.D., Rossetti, C.A., Khare, S., Figueiredo, J.F., Gull, T., Burghardt, R.C., Bäumler, A.J., Tsolis, R.M., Andrews-Polymenis, H.L. and Adams, L.G. (2010) Morphologic and cytokine profile characterization of *Salmonella enterica* serovar Typhimurium infection in calves with bovine leukocyte adhesion deficiency. *Veterinary Pathology* 47, 322–333.

Okamura, M., Lillehoj, H.S., Raybourne, R.B., Babu, U.S. and Heckert, R.A. (2004) Cell-mediated immune responses to a killed *Salmonella* enteritidis vaccine: lymphocyte proliferation, T-cell changes and interleukin-6 (IL-6), IL-1, IL-2, and IFN-gamma production. *Comparative Immunology, Microbiology & Infectious Diseases* 27, 255–272.

Okamura, M., Lillehoj, H.S., Raybourne, R.B., Babu, U.S., Heckert, R.A., Tani, H., Sasai, K., Baba, E. and Lillehoj, E.P. (2005) Differential responses of macrophages to *Salmonella enterica* serovars Enteritidis and Typhimurium. *Veterinary Immunology and Immunopathology* 107, 327–335.

Paulin, S.M., Watson, P.R., Benmore, A.R., Stevens, M.P., Jones, P.W., Villareal-Ramos, B. and Walis, T.S. (2002) Analysis of *Salmonella enteric* serotype-host specificity in calves: avirulence of *S. enterica* serotype Gallinarum correlates with bacterial dissemination from mesenteric lymph nodes and persistence *in vivo*. *Infection and Immunity* 70, 6788–6797.

Paulin, S.M., Jagannathan, A., Campbell, J., Wallis, T.S. and Stevens, M.P. (2007) Net replication of *Salmonella* enterica serovars Typhimurium and Choleraesuis in porcine intestinal mucosa and nodes is associated with their differential virulence. *Infection and Immunity* 75, 3950–3960.

Pavlova, B., Volf, J., Ondrackova, P., Matiasovic, J., Stepanova, H., Crhanova, M., Karasova, D., Faldyna, M. and Rychlik, I. (2011) SPI-1-encoded type III secretion system of *Salmonella* enterica is required for the suppression of porcine alveolar macrophage cytokine expression. *Veterinary Research* 42, 16–18.

Pieper, J., Methner, U. and Berndt, A. (2008) Heterogeneity of avian γδ T cells. *Veterinary Immunology and Immunopathology* 124, 241–252.

Pieper, J., Methner, U. and Berndt, A. (2011) Characterization of avian γδ T-cells subsets after *Salmonella* Typhimurium infection of chicks. *Infection and Immunity* 79, 822–829.

Pomeroy, B.S., Nagaraja, K.V., Ausherman, L.T., Peterson, I.L. and Friendshuh, K.A. (1989) Studies on feasibility of producing *Salmonella*-free turkeys. *Avian Diseases* 33, 1–7.

Prost, L.R. and Miller, S.I. (2008) The *Salmonella*e PhoQ sensor: mechanisms of detection of phagosome signals. *Cellular Microbiology* 10, 576–582.

Pullinger, G.D., Paulin, S.M., Charleston, B., Watson, P.R., Bowen, A.J., Dziva, F., Morgan, E., Villarreal-Ramos, B., Wallis, T.S. and Stevens, M.P. (2007) Systemic Translocation of *Salmonella enterica* serovar Dublin in cattle occurs predominantly via efferent lymphatics in a cell-free niche and requires type III secretion system 1 (T3SS-1) but not T3SS-2. *Infection and Immunity* 75, 5191–5199.

Ramasamy, K.T., Verma, P. and Reddy, M.R. (2012) Differential gene expression of antimicrobial peptides β defensins in the gastrointestinal tract of *Salmonella* serovar Pullorum infected broiler chickens. *Veterinary Research Communications* 36, 57–62.

Reed, K.A., Hobert, M.E., Kolenda, C.E., Sands, K.A., Rathman, M., O'Connor, M., Lyons, S., Gewirtz, A.T., Sansonetti, P.J. and Madara, J.L. (2002) The *Salmonella* typhimurium flagellar basal body protein FliE is required for flagellin production and to induce a proinflammatory response in epithelial cells. *The Journal of Biological Chemistry* 277, 13346–13353.

Reed, W.M., Olander, H.J. and Thacker, H.L. (1986) Studies on the pathogenesis of *Salmonella typhimurium* and *Salmonella choleraesuis* var *kunzendorf* infection in weanling pigs. *American Journal of Veterinary Research* 47, 75–83.

Rescigno, M., Urbano, M., Valzasina, B., Francolini, M., Rotta, G., Bonasio, R., Granucci, R., Kraehenbuhl, J.P. and Ricciardi-Castagnoli, P. (2001) Dendritic cells express tight junction proteins and penetrate gut epithelia monolayers to sample bacteria. *Nature Immunology* 2, 361–367.

Rings, D.M. (1985) Salmonellosis in calves. *Veterinary Clinics of North America - Food Animal Practice* 1, 529–539.

Robbins, J.B., Chu, C. and Schneerson, R. (1992) Hypothesis for vaccine development: protective immunity to enteric diseases caused by nontyphoidal *Salmonellae* and shigellae may be conferred by serum IgG antibodies to the O-specific polysaccharide of their lipopolysaccharides. *Clinical Infectious Diseases* 15, 346–361.

Santos, R.L. and Bäumler, A.J. (2004) Cell tropism of *Salmonella enterica*. *International Journal of Medical Microbiology* 294, 225–233.

Santos, R.L., Tsolis, R.M., Zhang, S., Ficht, T.A., Bäumler, J. and Adams, L.G. (2001) *Salmonella*-induced cell death is not required for enteritis in calves. *Infection and Immunity* 79, 4610–4617.

Santos, R.L., Zhang, S., Tsolis, R.M., Bäumler, A.J. and Adams, L.G. (2002a) Morphologic and molecular characterization of *Salmonella typhimurium* infection in neonatal calves. *Veterinary Pathology* 39, 200–215.

Santos, R.L., Tsolis, R.M., Bäumler, A.J. and Adams, L.G. (2002b) Dynamics of hematologic and blood chemical changes in *Salmonella typhimurium* infected calves. *American Journal of Veterinary Research* 63, 1145–1150.

Sasai, K., Aita, M., Lillehoj, H.S., Miyamoto, T., Fukata, T. and Baba, E. (2000) Dynamics of lymphocyte subpopulation changes in the cecal tonsils of chickens infected with *Salmonella enteriditis*. *Veterinary Microbiology* 74, 345–351.

Scotet, E., Nedellec, S., Devilder, M.-C., Allain, S. and Bonneville, M. (2008) Bridging innate and adaptive immunity through γδ T-dendritic cell crosstalk. *Frontiers in Bioscience* 13, 6872–6885.

Schmid, M., Nanda, I., Guttenbach, M., Steinlein, C., Hoehn, M., Schartl, M., Haaf, T., Weigend, S., Fries, R., Buerstedde, J.M., Wimmers, K., Burt, D.W., Smith, J., A'Hara, S., Law, A., Griffin, D.K., Bumstead, N., Kaufman, J., Thomson, P.A., Burke, T., Groenen, M.A., Crooijmans, R.P., Vignal, A., Fillon, V., Morisson, M., Pitel, F., Tixier-Boichard, M., Ladjali-Mohammedi, K., Hillel, J., Mäki-Tanila, A., Cheng, H.H., Delany, M.E., Burnside, J. and Mizuno, S. (2000) First report on chicken genes and chromosomes. *Cytogenetics and Cell Genetics* 90, 169–218.

Secundino, I., Lopez-Macias, C., Cervantes-Barragan, L., Gil-Cruz, C., Rios-Sarabia, N., Pastelin-Palacios, R., Villasis-Keever, M.A., Becker, I., Puente, J.L., Calva, E. and Isibasi, A. (2006) *Salmonella* porins induce a sustained, lifelong specific bactericidal antibody memory response. *Immunology* 117, 59–60.

Selsted, M.E., Tang, Y.-Q., Morris, W.L., McGuire, P.A., Novotny, M.J., Smith, W., Henschen, A.H. and Cullor, J.S. (1993) Purification, primary structures, and antibacterial activities of beta-defensins, a new family of antimicrobial peptides from bovine neutrophils. *The Journal of Biological Chemistry* 268, 6641–6648.

Shirai, Y., Sunakawa, K, Chihashi, Y. and Yamaguchi, H. (1979) A morphological study in germfree mice (*Salmonella* infection). *Experimental Pathology* 17, 158–166.

Sick, C., Schneider, K., Staeheli, P. and Weining, K.C. (2000) Novel chicken CXC and CC chemokines. *Cytokine* 12, 181–186.

Singh, S.P., Williams, Y.U., Benjamin, W.H., Klebba, P.E. and Boyd, D. (1996) Immunoprotection by monoclonal antibodies to the porins and lipopolysaccharide of *Salmonella* Typhimurium. *Microbial Pathogenesis* 21, 249–263.

Sinha, K., Mastroeni, P., Harrison, J., de Hormaeche, R.D. and Hormaeche, C.E. (1997) *Salmonella* typhimurium aroA, htrA, and aroD htrA mutants cause progressive infections in athymic (nu/nu) BALB/c mice. *Infection and Immunity* 65, 1566–1569.

Smith, A.L. and Beal, R. (2008) The avian enteric immune system in health and disease – Bacterial infections of the gut – *Salmonella*. In: Davison, F., Kaspers, B. and Schat, K.A. (eds) *Avian Immunology*. Academic Press, London, pp. 243–271.

Sundquist, M., Rydström, A. and Wick, M.J. (2004) Immunity to *Salmonella* from a dendritic point of view. *Cellular Microbiology* 6, 1–11.

Swaggerty, C.L., Pevzner, I.Y., Lowry, V.K., Farnell, M.B. and Kogut, M.H. (2003) Functional comparison of heterophils isolated from commercial broiler chickens. *Avian Pathology* 32, 95–102.

Swaggerty, C.L., Ferro, P.J., Pevzner, I.Y. and Kogut, M.H. (2005) Heterophils are associated with resistance to systemic *Salmonella* enteritidis infections in genetically distinct chicken lines. *FEMS Immunology & Medical Microbiology* 43, 149–154.

Swaggerty, C.L., Kaiser, P., Rothwell, L., Pevzner, I.Y. and Kogut, M.H. (2006) Heterophil cytokine mRNA profiles from genetically distinct lines of chickens with differential heterophil-mediated innate immune responses. *Avian Pathology* 35, 102–108.

Tobar, J.A., Carreño, L.J., Bueno, S.M., González, P.A., Mora, J.E., Quezada, S.A. and Kalergis, A.M. (2006) Virulent *Salmonella* enterica serovar typhimurium evades adaptive immunity by preventing dendritic cells from activating T cells. *Infection and Immunity* 74, 6438–6448.

Trebichavsky, I., Dlabac, V., Rehakova, Z., Zahradnickova, M. and Splichal, I. (1997) Cellular changes and cytokine expression in the ilea of gnotobiotic piglets resulting from peroral *Salmonella* typhimurium challenge. *Infection and Immunity* 65, 5244–5249.

Trebichavsky, I., Splichal, I., Splichalova, A., Muneta, Y. and Mori, Y. (2003) Systemic and local cytokine response of young piglets to oral infection with *Salmonella enterica* serotype Typhimurium. *Folia Microbiologica* 48, 403–407.

Tregaskes, C.A., Kong, F.-K., Paramithiotis, E., Chen, C.-L.H., Ratcliffe, M.J.H., Davison, F. and Young, J.R. (1995) Identification and analysis of the expression of CD8 alpha beta and CD8 alpha alpha isoforms in chickens reveals a major TCR-gamma delta CD8 alpha beta subset of intestinal intraepithelial lymphocytes. *The Journal of Immunology* 154, 4485–4494.

Trent, M.S., Pabich, W., Raetz, C.R. and Miller, S.I. (2001) A PhoP / PhoQ-induced Lipase (PagL) that catalyzes 3-O-deacylation of lipid A precursors in membranes of *Salmonella* typhimurium. *The Journal of Biological Chemistry* 276, 9083–9092.

Tsolis, R.M., Kingsley, R.A., Townsend, S.M., Ficht, T.A., Adams, L.G. and Baumler, A.J. (1999a) Of mice, calves, and men: comparison of the mouse typhoid model with other *Salmonella* infections. *Advances in Experimental Medicine and Biology* 473, 261–274.

Tsolis, R.M., Adams, L.G., Ficht, T.A. and Bäumler, A.J. (1999b) Contribution of *Salmonella enterica* serovar Typhimurium virulence factors to diarrheal disease in calves. *Infection and Immunity* 67, 4879–4885.

Ugrinovic, S., Ménager, N., Goh, N. and Mastroeni, P. (2003) Characterization and development of T-Cell immune responses in B-cell-deficient (Igh-6(-/-)) mice with *Salmonella* enterica serovar Typhimurium infection. *Infection and Immunity* 71, 6808–6819.

Uthe, J.J., Wang, Y., Qu, L., Nettleton, D., Tuggle, C.K. and Bearson, S.M. (2009) Correlating blood immune parameters and a CCT7 genetic variant with the shedding of *Salmonella enterica* serovar Typhimurium in swine. *Veterinary Microbiology* 135, 384–388.

Van Diemen, P.M., Kreukniet, M.B., Galina, L., Bumstead, N. and Wallis, T.S. (2002) Characterisation of a resource population of pigs screened for resistance to salmonellosis. *Veterinary Immunology and Immunopathology* 88, 183–196.

Van Dijk, A., Tersteeg-Zijderveld, M.H.G., Tjeerdesma-van Bikhoven, J.L.M., Jansman, A.J.M., Veldhuizen, E.J.A. and Haagsman, H.P. (2009) Chicken heterophils are recruited to the site of *Salmonella* infection and release antibacterial mature Cathelicidin-2 upon stimulation with LPS. *Molecular Immunology* 46, 1517–1526.

Van Hemert, S., Hoekman, J.W.A., Smits, M.A. and Rebel, J.M.J. (2006) Gene expression responses to a *Salmonella* infection in the chicken intestine differ between lines. *Veterinary Immunology and Immunopathology* 114, 247–258.

Van Hemert, S., Hoekman, J.W.A., Smits, M.A. and Rebel, J.M.J. (2007) Immunological and gene expression responses to a *Salmonella* infection in the chicken intestine. *Veterinary Research* 38, 51–63.

Van Immerseel, F., Methner, U., Rychlik, I., Nagy, B., Velge, P., Martin, G., Foster, N., Ducatelle, R. and Barrow, P.A. (2005) Vaccination and early protection against non-host-specific *Salmonella* serotypes in poultry: exploitation of innate immunity and microbial activity. *Epidemiology and Infection* 133, 959–978.

Vasquez-Torres, A., Jones-Carson, J., Bäumler, A.J., Falkow, S., Valdivia, R., Brown, W., Le, M., Berggren, R., Parks, W.T. and Fang, F.C. (1999) Extra intestinal dissemination of *Salmonella* by CD18-expressing phagocytes. *Nature* 401, 804–808.

Veldhuizen, E.J., van Dijk, A., Tersteeg, M.H., Kalkhove, S.I., van der Meulen, J., Niewold, T.A. and Haagsman, H.P. (2007) Expression of beta-defensins pBD-1 and pBD-2 along the small intestinal tract of the pig: lack of upregulation *in vivo* upon *Salmonella* typhimurium infection. *Molecular Immunology* 44, 276–283.

Vidal, S.M., Malo, D., Vogan, K., Skamene, E. and Gros, P. (1993) Natural resistance to infection with intracellular parasites: isolation of a candidate for *Bcg*. *Cell* 73, 469–485.

Wallis, T.S. (2006) Host-specificity of *Salmonella* infections in animal species. In: Mastroeni, P. and Maskell, D. (eds) Salmonella *Infections, Clinical, Immunological and Molecular Aspects*. Cambridge University Press, Cambridge, pp. 89–116.

Watson, P.R., Paulin, S.M., Jones, P.W. and Wallis, T.S. (2000) Interaction of *Salmonella* serotypes with porcine macrophages in vitro does not correlate with virulence. *Microbiology* 146, 1639–1649.

Werling, D., Piercy, J. and Coffey, T.J. (2006) Expression of TOLL-like receptors (TLR) by bovine antigen-presenting cells-potential role in pathogen discrimination? *Veterinary Immunology and Immunopathology* 112, 2–11.

Wigley, P. (2004) Genetic resistance to *Salmonella* infection in domestic animals. *Research in Veterinary Science* 76, 165–169.

Wigley, P., Berchieri Jr, A., Page, K.L., Smith, A.L. and Barrow, P.A. (2001) *Salmonella enterica* serovar Pullorum persist in splenic macrophages and in the reproductive tract during persistent, disease-free carriage in chickens. *Infection and Immunity* 69, 7873–7879.

Wigley, P., Hulme, S.D., Bumstead, N. and Barrow, P.A. (2002a) *In vivo* and *in vitro* studies of genetic resistance to systemic salmonellosis in the chicken encoded by the SAL1 locus. *Microbes and Infection* 4, 1111–1120.

Wigley, P., Jones, M.A. and Barrow, P.A. (2002b) *Salmonella enterica* serovar Pullorum requires the *Salmonella* pathogenicity island 2 type III secretion system for virulence and carriage in the chicken. *Avian Pathology* 31, 501–506.

Wigley, P., Hulme, S.D., Powers, C., Beal, R.K., Berchieri Jr, A., Smith, A. and Barrow, P. (2005) Infection of the reproductive tract and eggs with *Salmonella enterica* serovar pullorum in the chicken is associated with suppression of cellular immunity at sexual maturity. *Infection and Immunity* 73, 2986–2990.

Wigley, P., Barrow, P. and Villareal-Ramis, B. (2006a) Immunity to *Salmonella* in domestic (food animal) species. In: Mastroeni, P. and Maskell, D. (eds) Salmonella *Infections, Clinical, Immunological and Molecular Aspects*. Cambridge University Press, Cambridge, pp. 299–321.

Wigley, P., Hulme, S., Rothwell, L., Bumstead, N., Kaiser, P. and Barrow, P. (2006b) Macrophages isolated from chickens genetically resistant or susceptible to systemic salmonellosis show magnitudinal and temporal differential expression of cytokines and chemokines following *Salmonella enterica* challenge. *Infection and Immunity* 74, 1425–1430.

Winter, S.E., Thiennimitr, P., Nuccio, S.-P., Haneda, T., Winter, M.G., Wilson, R.P., Russell, J.M., Henry, T., Henry, T., Tran, Q.T., Lawhon, S.D., Gomez, G., Bevins, C.L., Rüssmann, H., Monack, D.M., Adams, L.G. and Bäumler, A.J. (2009) Contribution of flagellin pattern recognition to intestinal inflammation during *Salmonella enterica* serotype Typhimurium infection. *Infection and Immunity* 77, 1904–1910.

Withanage, G.S., Sasai, K., Fukata, T., Miyamoto, T., Baba, E. and Lillehoj, H.S. (1998) T lymphocytes, B lymphocytes and macrophages in the ovaries and oviducts of laying hens experimentally infected with *Salmonella enteritidis*. *Veterinary Immunology and Immunopathology* 66, 173–184.

Withanage, G.S., Kaiser, P., Wigley, P., Wigley, P., Powers, C., Mastroeni, P., Brooks, Barrow, P., Smith, A., Maskell, D. and McConnell, I. (2004) Rapid expression of chemokines and proinflammatory cytokines in newly hatched chickens infected with *Salmonella enterica* serovar Typhimurium. *Infection and Immunity* 72, 2152–2159.

Withanage, G.S., Wigley, P., Kaiser, P., Mastroeni, P., Brooks, H., Powers, C., Beal, R., Barrow, P., Maskell, D. and McConnell, I. (2005) Cytokine and chemokine responses associated with clearance of a primary *Salmonella enterica* serovar Typhimurium infection in the chicken and in protective immunity to rechallenge. *Infection and Immunity* 73, 5173–5182.

Xiao, Y., Hughes, A.L., Ando, J., Matsuda, Y., Cheng, J.F., Skinner-Noble, D. and Zhang, G. (2004) A genome-wide screen identifies a single beta-defensin gene cluster in the chicken: implications for the origin and evolution of mammalian defensins. *BMC Genomics* 5, 56.

Yu, C.-Y., Chu, C., Chou, S.-J., Chao, M.-R., Yeh, C.-M., Lo, D.-Y., Su, Y.-C., Horng, Y.-M., Weng, B.-C., Tsay, J.-G. and Huang, K.-C. (2008) Comparison of the association of age with the infection of *Salmonella* and *Salmonella* enterica serovar Typhimurium in Peking ducks and Roman geese. *Poultry Science* 87, 1544–1549.

Zhang, S., Kingsley, R.A., Santos, R.L., Andrews-Polymenis, H., Raffatellu, M., Figueiredo, J., Nunes, J., Tsolis, R.M., Adams, L.G. and Bäumler, A.J. (2003a) Molecular pathogenesis of *Salmonella enterica* serotype Typhimurium-induced diarrhea. *Infection and Immunity* 71, 1–12.

Zhang, S., Adams, L.G., Nunes, J., Khare, S., Tsolis, R.M. and Bäumler, A.J. (2003b) Secreted effector proteins of *Salmonella enterica* serotype typhimurium elicit host-specific chemokine profiles in animal models of typhoid fever and enterocolitis. *Infection and Immunity* 71, 4795–4803.

Zhao, C., Nguyen, T., Liu, L., Sacco, R.E., Brogden, K.A. and Lehrer, R.I. (2001) Gallinacin-3, an inducible epithelial beta-defensin in the chicken. *Infection and Immunity* 69, 2684–2691.

Zhang-Barber, L., Turner, A.K. and Barrow, P.A. (1999) Vaccination for control of *Salmonella* in poultry. *Vaccine* 17, 2538–2545.

9 *Salmonella* Infections in the Domestic Fowl

H.L. Shivaprasad,[1]* Ulrich Methner[2] and Paul A. Barrow[3]

[1]*California Animal Health and Food Safety Laboratory System, University of California, USA;* [2]*Institute of Bacterial Infections and Zoonoses at the Friedrich-Loeffler-Institute, Federal Research Institute for Animal Health, Germany;* [3]*School of Veterinary Medicine and Science, University of Nottingham, UK*

Introduction

Salmonellosis is a group of acute or chronic diseases of fowl caused by one or more members of the genus *Salmonella*. It is of great economic significance to all phases of the poultry industry throughout the world. Domestic fowl constitute one of the largest reservoirs of *Salmonella* and is important as a risk to public health through consumption of contaminated eggs and meat.

Four diseases caused by *Salmonella* are important in poultry; pullorum disease caused by *Salmonella enterica* serovar Pullorum, fowl typhoid caused by *S.* Gallinarum, paratyphoid caused by several serovars and subspecies of *Salmonella* most notably *S.* Enteritidis, *S.* Typhimurium, *S.* Heidelberg to name a few and arizonosis caused by *S. enterica* subsp. *arizonae*.

Historical Perspective

Pullorum disease (PD), caused by *S.* Pullorum, was first described by Rettger (1900), who named the pathogen *Bacterium pullorum* (Rettger, 1909). Fowl typhoid in poultry (FT), caused by *S.* Gallinarum, was first described in England in 1888 (Klein, 1889). Both diseases have a worldwide distribution (Pomeroy, 1984). During the first five to six decades of the 20th century, the main issues with respect to salmonellosis in fowl was worldwide prevalence of PD and FT in chickens and turkeys, associated with high mortality and which hindered the expansion of the poultry industry until the development and widespread application of testing and control measures (Rettger, 1909; Hewitt, 1928; Schaffer *et al.*, 1931; Hinshaw and McNeil, 1940; Moore, 1946; Chase, 1947; McDermott, 1947; Bullis, 1977; Pomeroy, 1984; Snoeyenbos, 1984). A voluntary National Poultry Improvement Program (NPIP), aimed at preventing disease transmission to progeny by testing of breeder flocks, became operative in the USA in 1935 (Shivaprasad and Barrow, 2008). These measures finally resulted in a much reduced prevalence of these diseases in most of the developed countries in the 1950s and 1960s (Shivaprasad, 2000; Shivaprasad and Barrow, 2008). Canada, the USA and several European

* Corresponding author, e-mail: hlshivaprasad@ucdavid.edu

© CAB International 2013. *Salmonella in Domestic Animals, 2nd Edition* (eds P.A. Barrow and U. Methner)

countries have recently reported absence or a low prevalence of PD and FT (Thain and Blandford, 1981; Johnson *et al.*, 1992; Salem *et al.*, 1992; Erbeck *et al.*, 1993). However, both diseases still occur as major economic problems in countries in Eastern Europe, Central and South America (Silva *et al.*, 1981), Africa (Bouzoubaa and Nagaraja, 1984) and Asia (Chishti *et al.*, 1985; Kaushik *et al.*, 1986). Pullorum disease is diagnosed occasionally in backyard chicken flocks in the USA, posing a potential risk to the commercial poultry industry (Shivaprasad and Barrow, 2008). Fowl typhoid was diagnosed both in commercial as well as in backyard layer chickens in 2005 and 2006 in the UK (Barrow and Freitas Neto, 2011). Both PD and FT have been reported in chickens in various countries in Europe during the 2000s (Barrow and Freitas Neto, 2011).

In the last six to seven decades, there has been a rapid increase in the isolation of the non-host specific *Salmonella* serovars from humans and fowl as the industry has expanded (Galton *et al.*, 1964; Guthrie, 1992). This was particularly the case with *S.* Typhimurium, which until more recently has been the most prevalent serovar isolated from humans and animals including fowl in many countries (Kelterborn, 1967; McCoy, 1975; Bullis, 1977; Wray, 1985; Lior, 1989; Ferris and Miller, 1990; Rodrigue *et al.*, 1990; Kühn *et al.*, 1993; Hargrett-Bean and Potter, 1995). Poultry and poultry products have been the main sources of non-host-specific *Salmonella* infecting humans (Schaaf, 1936; Edwards, 1958; Galton *et al.*, 1964; Seeliger and Maya, 1964; McCoy, 1975; Laszlo *et al.*, 1985; Humphrey *et al.*, 1988; St Louis *et al.*, 1988); other food sources have also been associated with zoonotic infection.

According to the Centers for Disease Control and Prevention (CDC) the incidence of human *Salmonella* infections in the USA in 2010 was higher than any other food-borne pathogen (CDC, 2011). It has been found that more than 70% of human salmonellosis in the USA has been attributed to the consumption of contaminated chicken, turkey or eggs (CDC, 2011). The most widespread human salmonellosis is due to *S.* Enteritidis. Outbreaks occur in many countries including a large occurrence in the USA in 2010 resulting in recall of more than half a billion eggs (Kuehn, 2010). *Salmonella* Enteritidis accounted for 32% of all human salmonellosis between 1996 and 1998 and 19.2% for the year 2009 even though their rates declined from 1999 to 2003 in USA (Foley *et al.*, 2011).

An increase in human infections due to *S.* Enteritidis was also observed with a concomitant increase in the isolations from poultry-related sources occurred between 2007 and 2010 in British Colombia, Canada (Taylor *et al.*, 2012). *Salmonella* Enteritidis constituted 72.8% among the *Salmonella* isolated from cloacal swabs from chickens in Zimbabwe (Makaya *et al.*, 2012). *Salmonella* Infantis has been observed to be common in both layers and broiler chickens in Japan (Iwabuchi *et al.*, 2011). In Australia some serotypes have become endemic or have increased in incidence such as *S.* Sofia and *S.* Typhimurium (Mellor *et al.*, 2010; Wales and Davies, 2011). Other *Salmonella* serotypes implicated in international spread including the USA include *S.* Kentucky and *S.* Schwarzengrund and, specifically in USA, *S.* Heidelberg and *S.* Typhimurium (Aarestrup *et al.*, 2007; Foley *et al.*, 2011; Le Hello *et al.*, 2011).

Infections of Domestic Fowl

Infections caused by *Salmonella* Gallinarum and *Salmonella* Pullorum

Salmonella Pullorum and *S.* Gallinarum are non-motile, host-specific salmonellae, which cause PD and FT, respectively, diseases specific to chickens, turkeys and other avian species (Klein, 1889; Rettger, 1900).

Fowl typhoid

The first described outbreak of FT was characterized by high mortality, especially during the first 2 months of the outbreak. The descriptions of the disease at that time summarize well the signs and pathology of the disease. The chickens appeared normal until about 24–36 h before death. The signs of disease began with yellow-to-green diarrhoea with the birds dying a day or so later (Klein, 1889). Other signs included huddling, laboured breathing and gasping, seen in newly-hatched to 5-day-old chicks and seen also in 21- and 28-day-old chickens (Kaushik *et al.*, 1986).

Post-mortem signs include enlargement of the spleen and liver, which may have a greenish bronze colour and whitish necrotic foci distributed uniformly on its surface, a much enlarged spleen with embedded whitish necrotic foci, catarrhal enteritis, an enlarged heart with small pinhead-sized white foci on the myocardium, haemorrhages in the pericardial fat, the endocardium and the proventriculus, severely congested lungs and enlarged and congested kidneys (Klein, 1889; Chishti *et al.*, 1985; Kaushik *et al.*, 1986; Shivaprasad and Barrow, 2008). Histological examination reveals fatty degeneration of the liver and diffuse parenchymatous hepatitis with focal areas of necrosis and mononuclear infiltration in the periportal areas, severe hyperplasia of the reticulo-endothelial cells in the spleen, occasionally accompanied by areas of necrosis disintegration of muscle fibres and infiltration of mononuclear cells in the myocardium, congestion and infiltration by mononuclear cells sub-epithelially in the mesobronchus of the lungs and congestion and perivascular infiltration of mononuclear cells in the kidneys (Kaushik *et al.*, 1986; Shivaprasad and Barrow, 2008).

The disease affects chickens, turkeys and guinea-fowl and birds of all ages and breeds. Historically, FT and PD often tended not to occur simultaneously on the same farm and appeared to persist on farms from year to year (Moore, 1946).

Pullorum disease

Pullorum disease was first described as 'fatal septicaemia' or 'white diarrhoea' by Rettger (1900, 1909), who reported on a disease of young chickens involving high mortality with loss of appetite and diarrhoea and sometimes with chickens being found dead a few days after hatching. Convalescent animals sometimes remain stunted for weeks afterwards. Similar findings, also with runting, swollen joints and lameness, have been reported by others (Salem *et al.*, 1992; Erbeck *et al.*, 1993).

Pullorum disease tends to occur in younger chickens than FT. In a study of 200 chickens with grossly enlarged livers and spleens, in chickens below 4 weeks of age, of 4–8 weeks of age, of 9–24 weeks of age and above 24 weeks of age, the isolation rates of *S.* Pullorum were 38.9%, 2.3%, 7.9% and 13.0%, respectively, whereas *S.* Gallinarum isolations were made from 1.1%, 31.8%, 10.5% and 4.3% of chickens of these age-groups, respectively (Chishti *et al.*, 1985).

Pullorum disease in laying hens causes reduced egg production, fertility and hatchability (Bullis, 1977) with the organism frequently isolated from the ovaries and a large percentage of the ova from infected ovaries never maturing. Such birds lay some fully developed eggs capable of hatching, containing the organism, from which infected chicks develop (Berchieri *et al.*, 2001). These infected hatchlings transmit the infection readily by the horizontal route. In general, *S.* Pullorum in adult hens produces no noticeable symptoms although occasionally a fatal septicaemia may occur in a few birds. The disease was historically most prevalent during the 4 months from March to June (Hewitt, 1928). Chilling of chicks during transport or crowding, overheating or chilling during the critical first week of brooding aggravates PD in young chicks and was frequently associated in the past with transport of hatchlings by train.

Some breeds of chickens, especially the white leghorn, are more resistant to PD and simultaneously to FT than are others (Hutt and Scholes, 1941; Bumstead and Barrow, 1993), which is related to the recently identified *SAL1* locus on chromosome 5 (Mariani *et al.*, 2001).

The whole-blood test, employing killed *S.* Pullorum bacteria stained with crystal violet as the antigen (Schaffer *et al.*, 1931), has been used widely and successfully in chickens to identify birds that are carrying the organism. Birds identified in this way may be removed from the flock. This is possible since carrier birds do not excrete the organism in the faeces (Gast, 1997). Newer approaches with pen-side ELISAs may also be used for this purpose (Barrow *et al.*, 1992; Berchieri *et al.*, 1995).

In recent years, most of the PD outbreaks in the USA have been reported in small or backyard poultry flocks, which may serve as potential reservoirs for disease transmission to commercial flocks (Erbeck *et al.*, 1993) and this is likely to be the situation in much of the rest of the world where countries have experienced gradual intensification of their industry.

Typical epidemiology is demonstrated by relatively recent experience in the USA. A large outbreak of PD occurred among Delaware roasters. The outbreak involved 19 breeder flocks and more than 261 grown-out premises in five states in the USA (Johnson *et al.*, 1992; Salem *et al.*, 1992). Twenty-two parents (multiplier) breeder flocks became infected. The transmission occurred vertically through the egg and horizontally by contact in the hatcheries and by placement of chicks on contaminated litter (Johnson *et al.*, 1992).

The clinical pathology of the disease has been described in detail recently (Lister and Barrow, 2008; Shivaprasad and Barrow, 2008). Chickens affected by PD are emaciated and anaemic, with pale livers and intestines, and with the alimentary tract almost empty or with the caeca nearly filled with a caseous material and the yolk sacs unabsorbed (Rettger, 1900, 1909). Severe articular and periarticular swelling, especially of the hock joints and also the wing joints, may be observed (Salem *et al.*, 1992; Shivaprasad, 2000). The livers are enlarged and show multiple small white foci and petechial haemorrhages. Hydropericardium and turbid pericardial fluid, and white nodular lesions that look like tumours may be found in the heart and gizzard. The spleens are mottled or pale with brown nodules in the lungs of some of the birds.

Histologically, separation of muscle fibres and infiltrations of macrophages, lymphocytes, plasma cells and heterophils are seen in the heart and gizzard muscles. Lesions in the liver consist of hepatocellular coagulative necrosis, small foci of mixed heterophil-mononuclear cells, enlarged portal lymphoid nodules and foci of extramedullary granulocytopoiesis. An acute, severe lymphocytic depletion is seen in the spleen, and acute cortical lymphocyte loss and medullary expansion may be observed in multiple thymic lobes. The joint lesions consist of acute synovitis and extensive infiltration of the synovial membrane by plasma cells. A bronchopneumonia, with consolidation and filling of tertiary bronchi with mononuclear cells and heterophils, may be observed in some birds (Salem *et al.*, 1992; Shivaprasad, 2000).

After isolation of the organism from hepatic blood it was described by Rettger (1900) as an 'active motile, aerobic and facultative anaerobic bacillus'. *Salmonella* Pullorum has long been considered to lack flagella and found to be non-motile. However, recently it has been shown that *S.* Pullorum reacted with *Salmonella* anti-flagellar antisera (Ibrahim *et al.*, 1986), genes encoding flagella in *S.* Pullorum have been identified (Kilger and Grimont, 1993) and motility has been reported to be induced and observed in 39 of 44 *S.* Pullorum strains examined (Holt and Chaubal, 1997).

Arizonosis

Arizonosis caused by *S. enterica* subsp. *arizonae* is an egg-transmitted disease primarily of young turkey poults that still occurs sporadically in commercial flocks and which may also infect and unusually cause disease in chickens or other species of birds (Crespo *et al.*, 2004; Shivaprasad *et al.*, 2006; Shivaprasad and Barrow, 2008). Reptiles can be a source of *S. arizonae* for birds and for man. The bacteria tend to localize in the ovary and oviduct of breeder turkeys and the poults hatched from infected breeders develop disease. The disease is characterized by diarrhoea with pasting of faeces in the vent, anorexia, huddling near the heat source and increased mortality sometimes approaching 50%. In poults from 1 to 3 weeks of age some birds develop ataxia, opisthotonus, torticollis and blindness with corneal opacity. Pathology includes omphalitis, typhlitis, hepatitis, meningitis, ophthalmitis and otitis interna (Shivaprasad *et al.*, 2006; Shivaprasad and Barrow, 2008). The bacteria can be readily isolated from the yolk sac, caeca, liver, brain and eyes. For further details on the disease, diagnosis, treatment, prevention and eradication refer to Shivaprasad (2008).

Infections caused by other *Salmonella* serovars

Poultry may be infected with a wide variety of *Salmonella* serovars with the infection largely confined to the gastrointestinal tract with faecal excretion.

Pathogenesis

Infection of chickens more than 3–4 days old results in no clinical disease although the faecal excretion is of public health concern (see below). The increase in resistance seen at this age is attributed to increasing maturity in cells of the macrophage-monocyte series although heterophil activity is also likely to be involved.

Experimental *S.* Typhimurium infection in newly hatched chickens showed that, after invasion from the gut, the bacteria are transported to and multiply in liver and spleen followed by spread to other organs as the animals become ill. The cause of death is probably a combination of anorexia and dehydration resulting from general malaise and diarrhoea. Invasiveness is thought to be the virulence determinant of overriding importance in chicks of this age (Barrow *et al.*, 1987). Following oral inoculation of *S.* Enteritidis in 1-day-old chicks, the organisms spread rapidly from the caeca and crop to internal tissues. The incidence of invasion decreases rapidly with age. Intraluminal phagocytosis of *Salmonella* bacteria may be observed occasionally. A few organisms may be seen in close association with the epithelial brush border in the lower ileal lumina. In 1-day-old birds, the mode of entry appears to be translocation and an early mucosal heterophil response was noted in the intestines but not in the crop. Phagocytosis was not observed in the epithelium but was seen occasionally in the lamina propria of the ileocaecal junction and of the caeca. Intra-tissue *Salmonella* were seen occasionally in the caeca of 2-week-old birds but were not detected in adult birds (Turnbull and Snoeyenbos, 1973).

Many factors influence the occurrence of salmonellosis in the domestic fowl. These include the following.

Age and dose

A correlation exists between the age of the chicken and the extent of faecal shedding. Experimental oral infection of chickens aged 2 days and 1, 2, 4 and 8 weeks with 10^2, 10^4, 10^6, 10^8 or 10^{10} *S.* Typhimurium bacteria showed that 10^2 *S.* Typhimurium bacteria induced infection in all the 2-day-old chicks and two-thirds of the 1- and 2-week-old birds. Similarly, 10^4 bacteria induced infection in all 2-day-old and 1-week-old chicks but in only about 25% of chicks 2, 4 and 8 weeks old. Even 10^6 bacteria were insufficient to induce infection in half of the 8-week-old chickens and a quarter of the 4-week-olds. Mortality occurred only between 2 and 12 days post-infection (p.i.) in chicks infected when 2 days old (Sadler *et al.*, 1969). These results were similar to the correlation between recovery from the tissues and the level of circulating antibody detected by ELISA (Barrow, 1992).

Others found similar results with *S.* Enteritidis (Gast and Beard, 1990; Barrow and Lovell, 1991; Humphrey *et al.*, 1991a, b; Cooper *et al.*, 1994a). After oral inoculation of various food-poisoning *Salmonella* serovars, the number of chickens excreting *Salmonella* bacteria in their faeces gradually declined over a period of at least 4 weeks. In contrast, serovars adapted to other animal hosts, such as *S.* Choleraesuis and *S.* Abortusovis, were excreted for no longer than a few days (Barrow *et al.*, 1988).

Route of infection

Chicks are more susceptible to *Salmonella* infection by inhalation and parenteral routes than via the oral route (Barrow *et al.*, 1987; Poppe and Gyles, 1987; Baskerville *et al.*, 1992; Poppe *et al.*, 1993b; Cooper *et al.*, 1994b).

Serovar and strain

The extent of colonization of the alimentary tract of chickens depends on the *Salmonella* serovar. Early work by Smith and Tucker (1980) showed that chickens experimentally challenged with *S.* Typhimurium or *S.* Menston excreted both strains in the faeces for weeks, whereas *S.* Choleraesuis, a serovar host-specific for pigs, was eliminated within a short time. Later work analysing the distribution of these serovars in the alimentary tract of newly-hatched or 3-week-old chickens confirmed these findings (Barrow *et al.*, 1988). When chicks 1 and 7 days old were given feed contaminated artificially with 30–200 organisms g^{-1} of either *S.* Typhimurium or *S.* Kedougou, *S.* Typhimurium was recovered from caeca, lungs, liver, spleen and kidneys but *S.* Kedougou only from the caeca. *Salmonella* Kedougou was a more efficient intestinal colonizer than *S.* Typhimurium in the young chicks, while the reverse was true in the older birds (Xu *et al.*, 1988). In general, the less invasive the serovar the more extensive is the colonization, involving shedding or larger numbers of bacteria over longer periods (Barrow *et al.*, 1988).

Invasiveness of Salmonella *strains*

Strain differences in the *in vivo* invasiveness of *S.* Typhimurium (Barrow *et al.*, 1987) or *S.* Enteritidis appeared to be not PT- but strain-related (Timoney *et al.*, 1989; Poppe *et al.*, 1993b; Gast and Benson, 1996). Less invasive serovars such as *S.* Infantis and *S.* Montevideo colonize the gut better and are excreted in the faeces for longer than highly invasive serovars such as *S.* Typhimurium and *S.* Enteritidis. Whether this is the result of the stronger immune response induced by the more invasive strains, as seems likely, is unknown.

Other studies have shown that strains with a wrinkled colony and which have greater amounts of high molecular weight LPS are more virulent for chickens, when inoculated parenterally, in terms of bacterial counts in the spleen, localization in the reproductive tract and percentage of contaminated eggs (Petter, 1993; Guard-Petter *et al.*, 1995; Cox, 1996) but also more tolerant to heat, acid and hydrogen peroxide than non-wrinkled colonies (Humphrey *et al.*, 1996). There does also appear to be a degree of organ specificity so that otherwise identical PT13 strains originally isolated from the ovary or blood showed differences in their isolation from liver, spleen and caeca after experimental oral inoculation; the ovarian isolate was not re-isolated (Poppe *et al.*, 1993a). However, the ovarian isolate formed an entire and smooth colony, whereas the blood isolate developed a corrugated colony appearance after 2 days of growth at room temperature on Luria Bertani broth (LB) agar (C. Poppe, unpublished data).

Some authors have reported that strains of *S.* Enteritidis PT4 were more invasive for young chicks than strains of PT7, 8 and 13a, and they suggested that the increased invasiveness of PT4 may be one of the factors that contributed to the establishment of *S.* Enteritidis PT4 in the UK (Hinton *et al.*, 1990a). The same authors also found that more recent isolates of *S.* Enteritidis PT4 were more invasive than strains isolated in previous years and suggested that recent isolates of PT4 may have an enhanced virulence for chickens (Hinton *et al.*, 1990b). Other authors have found no difference in invasiveness or colonization ability between different phage types (Barrow, 1991).

Breed of chicken

Partially inbred and outbred lines of chickens can show pronounced differences in mortality following challenge of newly hatched chicks with *S.* Typhimurium (Barrow *et al.*, 1987; Bumstead and Barrow, 1988). These differences were observed with a range of five strains of *S.* Typhimurium of differing degrees of virulence and following both oral and intramuscular challenge. Mendelian genetics indicated that it was consistent with the inheritance of a dominant autosomal resistance gene. There was no evidence of association with the major histocompatibility complex. The same lines were resistant to *S.* Gallinarum, *S.* Pullorum and *S.* Enteritidis, indicating a common mechanism (Bumstead and Barrow, 1993). The resistance is related to the recently identified *SAL1* locus on chromosome 5 (Mariani *et al.*, 2001).

Additional studies also showed consistent differences between inbred lines in the extent to which *S.* Typhimurium and *S.* Enteritidis colonized the gut of chickens (Duchet-Suchaux *et al.*, 1997; Barrow *et al.*, 2003). This was not related to differences in gut flora between batches of birds or individual birds. Standard Mendelian genetics also showed this to be a dominant autosomal trait (Barrow *et al.*, 2003). Again, interestingly, the same lines were also more resistant to colonization by *Campylobacter jejuni* (Boyd *et al.*, 2005).

Virulence factors and immune dynamics

Evidence is accumulating on the various microbial factors associated with colonization, invasion and dissemination of *Salmonella* in poultry and the effect on the host response (Berndt *et al.*, 2007; Jones *et al.*, 2007; Fasina *et al.*, 2008; Chappell *et al.*, 2009; Dunkley *et al.*, 2009; Setta *et al.*, 2012a, b).

In vitro incubation of *Salmonella* with mammalian tissue cells has shown that invasion of epithelial cells is complex and involves several genetic loci and host factors as stated above (Wallis and Galyov, 2000). Large genetic elements, termed *Salmonella* pathogenicity islands (SPI), contribute to virulence in a variety of ways including invasion (SPI-1) and enteritis (SPI-5), intra-cellular survival (SPI-2) and colonization (SPI-3) (see Chapter 5). SPI-2 is required for both systemic and gastrointestinal colonization of *S.* Typhimurium infection of 1-day-old and 1-week-old chicks (Jones *et al.*, 2007). Random mutagenesis studies to identify colonization genes have indicated the involvement of genes associated with host-interaction, metabolism and stress responses resulting from survival in an environment to which *Salmonella* are not, in all probability, ideally adapted (Turner *et al.*, 1998; Morgan *et al.*, 2004). Similar studies using *S.* Gallinarum also identified well known virulence genes (Shah *et al.*, 2005). Gene expression studies using microarrays also indicated that unique metabolic pathways required for catabolism of degeneration products of host gut membranes (1,2-propanediol, propionate and ethanolamine) and host-attachment via fimbrial genes were important *in vivo* (Harvey *et al.*, 2011).

Infection of very young chickens with *S.* Typhimurium or *S.* Enteritidis where most pathological changes occur is characterized by massive inflammatory responses in the intestine associated with infiltration of heterophil granulocytes, macrophages, B cells and CD4+ and CD8+ lymphocytes into the lamina propria (Withanage *et al.*, 2003; Berndt *et al.*, 2007). Up-regulation of RNA expression for a number of chemokines including IL-1β, IL-8, K60 (a CXC chemokine) and MIP 1β was observed (Withanage *et al.*, 2004). Up-regulation of IL-6 and INFγ mRNA was also observed whereas IL-10 mRNA expression decreased (Fasina *et al.*, 2008). The findings are indicative of a strong Th1-type response against these highly virulent serovars. Other serovars, including *S.* Pullorum, *S.* Infantis and *S.* Hadar, have also been studied albeit in less detail to determine whether different responses are associated with different aspects of their infection biology. *Salmonella* Enteritidis infection in newly hatched birds stimulated the expression of CXCLi1 and CXCLi2 chemokines in the caecal tonsils, while *S.* Gallinarum up-regulated the expression of LITAF. In older chickens, *S.* Enteritidis infection resulted in a significantly higher expression of CXCLi2, iNOS, LITAF and IL-10 while *S.* Pullorum appeared to down-regulate CXCLi1 expression in the caecal tonsils (Berndt *et al.*, 2007; Setta *et al.*, 2012a).

In vitro Salmonella serovars Typhimurium, Enteritidis, Hadar and Infantis showed a greater level of invasion and/or uptake characters when compared with *S.* Pullorum or *S.* Gallinarum. Nitrate and reactive oxygen species were greater in *Salmonella*-infected macrophages with the expression of iNOS and NF-κB by chicken macrophages infected with both systemic and broad host-range serovars. There was higher mRNA gene expression for CXCLi2, IL-6 and iNOS genes in response to *S.* Enteritidis infection when compared to *S.* Pullorum-infected cells. *Salmonella* Typhimurium- and *S.* Hadar-infected HD11 showed higher gene expression for CXCLi2 versus *S.* Pullorum-infected cells. Higher mRNA gene expression levels of pro-inflammatory cytokine IL-6, chemokines CXCLi1 and CXCLi2 and iNOS genes were detected in *S.* Typhimurium- and *S.* Enteritidis-infected chicken epithelial cells followed by *S.* Hadar and *S.* Infantis while no significant changes were observed in *S.* Pullorum or *S.* Gallinarum-infected cells (Setta *et al.*, 2012b). There is some evidence from *in vivo* studies that *S.* Pullorum produces a response that closely resembles a Th2-type response with lower IFNγ and IL-12 and higher IL-4 levels on the spleen (Chappell *et al.*, 2009).

Diagnosis

Signs and pathology

These are rarely pathognomic. Lesions associated with FT (above) are highly indicative, but without isolation of the organism they can be misleading. Salmonellosis in broilers due to *S.* Typhimurium infection has been characterized by growth retardation, blindness, twisted necks, lameness and mortality and cull rates that varied between 1.7% and 10.6% in flocks during the first 2 weeks of age (Padron, 1990). Affected young chicks may exhibit symptoms including anorexia, adipsia, depression, ruffled feathers, huddling together in groups, reluctance to move, drowsiness, somnolence, dehydration, white diarrhoea and stained or pasted vents (Schaaf, 1936; McIlroy *et al.*, 1989; Baskerville *et al.*, 1992). During the second week of life, chicks infected with *S.* Enteritidis PT4 failed to grow and had a stunted appearance (O'Brien, 1988). Clinical signs are sometimes found in laying hens infected with *S.* Enteritidis. Increased mortality (1.6% per month) and decreased egg production (8% over a period of 6 weeks) have been found in a large commercial laying flock infected with *S.* Enteritidis PT4 (Kinde *et al.*, 1996).

Serology

Serological tests do not reliably detect birds with intestinal infection with *Salmonella*. Agglutination tests with *S.* Typhimurium and *S.* Pullorum antigens did not dependably detect infection in 4-week-old white leghorn chickens infected orally with 10^6 *S.* Typhimurium (Olesiuk *et al.*, 1969). Similarly, 6-month-old SPF brown leghorn cockerels inoculated orally with 10^{10} *S.* Typhimurium were colonized 1 day p.i., but a rising agglutinating titre against the H antigen or a monophasic *S.* Typhimurium strain was only noted during 3–6 days p.i. and reached a peak at 9 days p.i., after which it persisted at moderate level until the end of the experiment 45 days p.i. at which time none of the birds were still colonized with *Salmonella*. Development of a titre depends on the occurrence of a systemic infection (Brown *et al.*, 1975). A similar study of cockerels infected with *S.* Infantis showed that the serological response was lower, fell more quickly and frequently became negative 3–6 weeks p.i. (Brown *et al.*, 1976).

More recent use of the more sensitive ELISA to some extent confirms these findings. Using either LPS or a sonicated antigen high titres of circulating specific IgG can be detected for many months after infection (Hassan *et al.*, 1990). In some cases high titres can be observed in the absence of detectable faecal excretion indicating infection. Specific IgA and IgM can also be detected in the serum and, in the case of IgA, in the gut (Hassan *et al.*, 1991). Although there is some correlation between the titre observed and the infecting dose (Humphrey *et al.*, 1991b; Barrow, 1992) the presence of antibodies is not an absolute indicator of infection of any individual bird and all serological tests must be regarded as flock tests. In the cases of *S.* Enteritidis examination of a number of flocks always indicated the presence of a small number of birds with very high levels of antibody (McLeod and Barrow, 1992). The incorporation of flagella antigen in the tests allows for differentiation between flagellate group D serovars (*S.* Enteritidis) and the non-flagellated *S.* Pullorum and *S.* Gallinarum (Berchieri *et al.*, 1995).

The microantiglobulin test, employing stained *S.* Enteritidis PT4 antigen, and an ELISA, using LPS antigen from *S.* Enteritidis, were both more sensitive than the slide and tube agglutination tests, detected more infected birds that were negative by the rapid slide and tube agglutination tests and showed high titres in some birds from which *Salmonella* could not be isolated post-mortem. Sera from two flocks that had a history of natural *S.* Enteritidis infection were evaluated by all the tests; evidence of infection was found with the microantiglobulin and ELISA tests but not with the other tests (Cooper *et al.*, 1989). The pullorum test, which uses a common O antigen with *S.* Enteritidis, appears to detect only a low proportion of infected birds (Hopper and Mawer, 1988). The ability to raise an immune response is influenced by the age of the hens. Hens of 20 weeks infected orally with *S.* Enteritidis developed high titres of antibodies of the immunoglobulin

M (IgM) class, while those that were 1 year old at infection developed relatively little antibody (Humphrey *et al.*, 1991a).

Culture

Numerous methods for the isolation of *Salmonella* have been described. Cultural methods have been reviewed regularly (Barrow, 1995; Tietjen and Fung, 1995).

Molecular techniques

For rapid, accurate, economical diagnosis of multiple serotypes of *Salmonellae* molecular techniques have become available and are beginning to revolutionize the diagnosis of salmonellosis in poultry. For techniques such as ribotyping, differentiation by genes, PCR, multiplex PCR see Shivaprasad and Barrow (2008), Barrow and Freitas Neto (2011), Kang *et al.* (2011), Akiba *et al.* (2011) and Singh *et al.* (2012). In one study by the use of multiplex PCR, seven serovars, Enteritidis, Typhimurium, Hadar, Choleraesuis, Dublin, Infantis and Gallinarum, were rapidly identified with sufficient specificity (Akiba *et al.*, 2011) although a few false-positive results for closely related serovars occurred. Another technique that has become available for identification of *Salmonella* serovars is multilocus sequence typing (Singh *et al.*, 2012). The availability of the whole genome sequences for a number of serovars may begin to facilitate serovar and strain differentiation (Barrow and Freitas Neto, 2011; Feng *et al.*, 2012).

Epidemiology

Prevalent serovars

Most of the information regarding the prevalence of *Salmonella* has been based on passive laboratory-based *Salmonella* surveillance (Faddoul and Fellows, 1966; Sojka *et al.*, 1975). Often no distinction has been made between symptomatic and asymptomatic infection. Such surveillance systems have inherent biases (Galton *et al.*, 1964; Bynoe and Yurack, 1964). A number of factors, including intensity of surveillance (Galton *et al.*, 1964), submission for serotyping (Sojka *et al.*, 1975), severity of illness and association with a recognized outbreak in the human population (Philbrook *et al.*, 1960; Telzak *et al.*, 1990; van de Giessen *et al.*, 1992; Altekruse *et al.*, 1993) and lack of a systematic method of reporting (Edwards, 1958), affect whether an infection will be reported. This results in the number of cases of both animal and human salmonellosis being substantially underestimated. However, the surveillance data allow broad comparisons and identification of trends, reservoirs and routes of transmission of *Salmonella* serovars to be made.

There is considerable variation in the occurrence of serovars in domestic fowl in different countries and at different times. Serovars become widespread in a country or geographical area for a given period and may then decrease in incidence (Faddoul and Fellows, 1966; Borland, 1975). *Salmonella* Typhimurium was generally the most common serovar isolated from poultry in many countries, between the 1950s until the late 1970s (Faddoul and Fellows, 1966). In 1948, a list of the commonest serovars in chickens and turkeys in the USA ranked in declining order included *S.* Typhimurium, *S.* Anatum, *S.* Derby, *S.* Bareilly, *S.* Meleagridis, *S.* Oranienburg, *S.* Give, *S.* Bredeney, *S.* Newport and *S.* Montevideo (Bullis, 1977). In 1976, the commonest serovars isolated from chickens and turkeys in the USA ranked in declining order were *S.* Typhimurium, *S.* Heidelberg, *S.* Saintpaul, *S.* Infantis, *S.* Thompson, *S.* Montevideo, *S.* Worthington, *S.* Johannesburg, *S.* Enteritidis and *S.* Anatum (Bullis, 1977). *Salmonella* Typhimurium was the commonest *Salmonella* serovar isolated from poultry and other birds in the UK during the period 1968–1973; it accounted for 41.1% of all isolates and was followed, in decreasing frequency of isolation, by *S.* Enteritidis (6.2%), *S.* Pullorum (3.9%) and *S.* Gallinarum (2.8%) (Sojka *et al.*, 1975).

Similar changes have taken place in other countries. In the UK in addition to the dominance of *S.* Typhimurium, *S.* Agona was isolated from UK broilers in the 1950s and replaced by *S.* Hadar in turkeys with spread into broilers in the 1970s, when all three serovars were eclipsed by the *S.* Enteritidis epidemic in the 1980s.

A study in the Netherlands in 1989 to determine the presence of *Salmonella* in 49 and 52 randomly selected layer and broiler flocks showed that *S.* Infantis and *S.* Virchow were each isolated from 30.9% of the flocks, while *S.* Typhimurium, *S.* Enteritidis and *S.* Hadar were isolated from 25%, 20.6%, and 17.6% of the flocks, respectively. *Salmonella* were isolated from the faecal samples of 47% of the layer and 94% of the broiler flocks. *Salmonella* Enteritidis was isolated from nine of the 49 (18.4%) layer flocks and from six of the 52 (11.5%) broiler flocks (van de Giessen *et al.*, 1991).

Nationwide studies were carried out in Canada in 1989–1990 to determine the prevalence of *Salmonella* in randomly selected layer, broiler and turkey flocks. Faecal samples and/or scrapings from egg belts from 52.9% of 295 layer flocks were contaminated with *Salmonella*. Thirty-five different *Salmonella* serovars were isolated. The most prevalent serovars were *S.* Heidelberg, *S.* Infantis, *S.* Hadar and *S.* Schwarzengrund; they were isolated from samples of 20%, 6.1%, 5.8% and 5.1% of the flocks, respectively. *Salmonella* Enteritidis was isolated from 2.7% of the layer flocks; *S.* Enteritidis PT8 was isolated from five flocks, PT13a from two flocks and PT13 from one flock (Poppe *et al.*, 1991a). A similar study of 294 broiler flocks showed that environmental samples (litter and/or water) from 76.9% of the flocks were contaminated by *Salmonella*. Fifty different serovars were isolated. The most prevalent serovars were *S.* Hadar, *S.* Infantis and *S.* Schwarzengrund; they were isolated from samples of 33.3%, 8.8% and 7.1% of the flocks, respectively. *Salmonella* Enteritidis was isolated from 3.1% of the flocks; *S.* Enteritidis PT8 was isolated from seven flocks and PT13a from two flocks (Poppe *et al.*, 1991b).

In the USA, in 1990 a survey of spent laying hens was conducted over a period of 3 months to estimate the prevalence and distribution of *S.* Enteritidis in commercial egg-production flocks. It showed that any *Salmonella* serovar and *S.* Enteritidis were isolated from 24% and 3%, respectively, of 23,431 pooled caecal samples collected from 406 layer houses. Regionally, the estimated prevalence of *S.* Enteritidis-positive houses (i.e. at least one positive sample found in a house) for the northern, south-eastern and central/western regions was 45%, 3% and 17%, respectively. Overall, the prevalence of *Salmonella*-positive houses was 86% (Ebel *et al.*, 1992).

During the last 20–25 years, *S.* Enteritidis has replaced *S.* Typhimurium as the commonest serovar in poultry in many countries worldwide. This has been associated with a pandemic in human enteritis (Rodrigue *et al.*, 1990). A comprehensive monograph on all aspects of *S.* Enteritidis has been published (Saeed, 1999). In England and Wales, the percentage of *S.* Enteritidis isolates from poultry rose from 3.3% of all *Salmonella* serovars in 1985, to 6.9% in 1986, to 22.3% in 1987, to 47.8% in 1988 and to 48.3% in 1989. The most frequently reported *S.* Enteritidis phage type (PT) was PT4, which accounted for 71% of the isolates from poultry in 1988 (McIlroy and McCracken, 1990). However, more recently, there has been a reduction in the isolation rates of *S.* Enteritidis in the UK: the number of isolations from chickens declined from 823 in 1993 to 17 in 2010.

Currently the most commonly identified serotypes among clinical and environmental samples submitted for identification in 2010 in the USA were *S.* Enteritidis, *S.* Kentucky, *S.* Heidelberg, *S.* Senftenberg, *S.* Typhimurium and *S.* Mbandaka in chickens (Morningstar-Shaw *et al.*, 2012).

More recent surveys have been conducted in many countries around the world with interesting results. In China Liu *et al.* (2011) found serovars such as *S.* Babelsberg and *S.* Fresno in live chickens and feed, Lu *et al.* (2011) found *S.* Indiana with high frequency whereas Yang *et al.* (2010) in northern China identified 24 serovars including Enteritidis (31.5% of isolates), which was the most common, followed by Typhimurium (13.4%), Shubra (10.0%), Indiana (9.7%), Derby (9.5%) and Djugu (7.0%). In Nigeria *S.* Virchow was a dominant serovar with rare serovars such as *S.* Apapa, *S.* Mouschaui, *S.* Jukestown, *S.* Oritamerin and *S.* Onireke also isolated from both humans and chickens (Fashae *et al.*, 2010).

To gain information on the prevalence of *Salmonella* to support the EU comprehensive *Salmonella* control strategy in poultry and pigs (EU, 2003a, b), baseline studies were carried out starting in 2004 for laying hens, in 2005 for broilers and 2006 for turkeys. In laying hens, despite the very high variation in the prevalence between the member states ranging from 0% to 62.2%, the most frequently isolated serovar was by far *S.* Enteritidis, which was isolated in 18 countries and accounted for 50.8% of the reported isolates during the baseline study (EFSA, 2006). *Salmonella* Infantis was the second most encountered serovar (8.3%) followed by *S.* Typhimurium (5.2%); both were detected in 14 member states. In broilers, the baseline study revealed a *Salmonella* spp. EU weighted flock prevalence of 23.7% (EFSA, 2007). The prevalence of broiler flocks positive to *S.* Enteritidis and/or *S.* Typhimurium was 11.0%, however, differences between member states were considerable. These changes have been accompanied by a relative rise in the incidence of *S.* Infantis and *S.* Mbandaka in some countries.

Sources of Infection and Routes of Transmission

The sources of *Salmonella* infection for domestic fowl are numerous. Poultry and many other animals are often carriers, latently infected or, less frequently, clinically ill, and they may excrete *Salmonella* in their faeces and form a large reservoir and source of contamination for other animals, humans and the environment. Poultry often become infected via horizontal transmission by litter, faeces, feed, water, fluff, dust, shavings, straw, insects, equipment and other fomites contaminated with *Salmonella* and by contact with other chicks or poults, rodents, pets, wild birds, other domestic and wild animals and personnel contaminated with *Salmonella*. Vertical transmission to progeny occurs when the ovary is infected or the developing eggs become infected in the oviduct.

Management practices can have a significant influence on the extent of transmission of *Salmonella*. Many of the factors that influence horizontal and vertical transmission are interrelated.

Horizontal transmission

In the hatchery

Horizontal spread of *Salmonella* occurs during hatching. This was shown when experimentally contaminated and *Salmonella*-free eggs were incubated together resulting in an infection rate of 44% of digestive tracts of hatched control chicks that had not been artificially contaminated (Cason *et al.*, 1994).

Air

Poultry may become infected by aerosols containing *Salmonella*. Laying hens exposed to aerosols containing 10^3 or 10^5 but not those given 10^2 *S.* Enteritidis PT4 bacteria were shown to develop diarrhoea and lose weight with some deaths (Baskerville *et al.*, 1992).

Litter

Chicks or poults in barns often contaminate the litter with faeces containing *Salmonella*, and contaminated litter is an important source and means of transmission of *Salmonella*. Poultry often ingest *Salmonella* by picking at faecal and caecal droppings of littermates. *Salmonella* have been found to spread rapidly from infected day-old chicks to pen-mates reared on litter (Snoeyenbos *et al.*, 1969; Rigby and Pettit, 1979). Infection of contact chicks reached about 100% within 7 days of contact (Snoeyenbos *et al.*, 1969). *Salmonella* have been isolated from 30% of litter samples in 55% of broiler chicken houses (Long *et al.*, 1980). Another study of contamination of the environment of broilers showed that *Salmonella* were commonly isolated from litter: 47.4% of 3534 litter samples contained *Salmonella* and one or more litter samples of 223 of 294 (75.9%) broiler flocks were positive for *Salmonella* (Poppe *et al.*, 1991b). Chickens on litter transmit *Salmonella* more readily than when in wire cages (Brownell *et al.*, 1969; Rigby and Pettit, 1979). Placing chicks infected orally with *S.* Typhimurium in wire cages accelerated the age-related decline in faecal excretion of *S.* Typhimurium (Rigby and Pettit, 1979), presumably by reducing reinfection.

However, litter can also have a negative effect on infection spread. The infectivity and mortality rate among chicks were higher on fresh litter than on built-up litter (Botts *et al.*, 1952). Several studies have shown that *S.* Pullorum, *S.* Gallinarum, *S.* Infantis and *S.* Typhimurium persist longer in fresh litter than in built-up litter (Botts *et al.*, 1952; Tucker, 1967; Fanelli *et al.*, 1970). *Salmonella* Pullorum and *S.* Gallinarum persisted for 11 weeks in new litter but for only 3 weeks in built-up litter. Similarly, *S.* Thompson survived for 8–20 weeks in new litter, but for only 4–5 weeks in old litter. When the infected pens were left unoccupied, the survival time of *Salmonella* bacteria in both types of litter increased to more than 30 weeks (Tucker, 1967). Cycling of *Salmonella* bacteria between litter and the intestinal tract appeared to be more evident in unchanged new litter than in built-up litter or in fresh litter changed periodically (Fanelli *et al.*, 1970).

The water content of litter is important (Tucker, 1967). Water activity was positively correlated with *Salmonella*-positive drag swabs of litter in broiler chicken houses (Opara *et al.*, 1992). Increased moisture and a high pH as a result of dissolved ammonia were shown to be the cause of the higher bactericidal activity of old or built-up litter compared with new litter (Turnbull and Snoeyenbos, 1973).

Water

Contaminated drinking-water has long been known to facilitate the spread of *Salmonella* (Gauger and Greaves, 1946). In a study of contamination in broiler flocks, *Salmonella* were isolated from 108 of 875 (12.3%) water samples and one or more water samples from 63 of 292 (21.6%) flocks were positive for *Salmonella* (Poppe *et al.*, 1991b). Chicks and poults often defecate in the drinkers and contaminate the drinking-water with their beaks and by stepping or walking in the drinkers. This happens particularly with young chicks or poults before the drinkers are raised from the floor of the barn. There is a significantly greater risk of contamination of drinking-water with *Salmonella* from trough drinkers and plastic bell drinkers than from nipple drinkers (Renwick *et al.*, 1992). Laying hens inoculated with 10^5 *S.* Enteritidis PT4 spread the infection via drinking-water to other uninoculated hens in 1–5 days (Nakamura *et al.*, 1994).

Feed

The role of feed in *Salmonella* infection together with approaches for its control has been reviewed (Williams, 1981) and is discussed in depth in Chapter 19. The feed may contain *Salmonella* and form a source of infection for poultry. Serovars of *Salmonella* found in broilers have been traced to feeds, water and the breeder flocks from which the broilers originated (Morris *et al.*, 1969). In the study of nine broiler flocks, the frequency of contamination of feed was lower than that of litter, water and dust (Higgins *et al.*, 1982). Likewise, *Salmonella* contamination of the environment of layer flocks' feed samples were less often contaminated with *Salmonella* than were egg-belt scrapings: *Salmonella* were isolated from 7.2% of feed samples and 25.7% of egg belt-samples (Poppe *et al.*, 1991a). Examination of environmental samples from broiler flocks showed that 13.4% of feed samples, 12.3% of water samples and 47.7% of litter samples were contaminated with *Salmonella* (Poppe *et al.*, 1991b).

Rodents

Rodents play an important role in the epidemiology of *Salmonella* infection in poultry (Henzler and Opitz, 1992; Anon., 1995). A microbiological survey of ten mice-infested poultry farms showed than, on five farms where no *S.* Enteritidis was isolated, 29.5% of 696 environmental samples and 6% of 232 mice were culture-positive for other *Salmonella* serovars. On another five farms on which *S.* Enteritidis was isolated, *Salmonella* of any serovar were isolated from 41.4% of 1407 environmental samples and from 31.8% of 483 mice, and *S.* Enteritidis from 7.5% of

1407 environmental samples and from 24% of the 483 mice. A bacterial count from the faeces of a mouse yielded more than 10^5 *S.* Enteritidis bacteria per faecal pellet (Henzler and Opitz, 1992). There is a correlation between the level of infestation and transmission to layers (Carrique-Mas *et al.*, 2009; Lapuz *et al.*, 2012). Clearance from flocks is also sometimes associated with elimination of rodents (Carrique-Mas *et al.*, 2009).

Stress

The stress of induced moulting in ageing hens is well known to increase the shedding of *Salmonella*. Intestinal levels of *S.* Enteritidis increased 100–1000-fold in moulted compared with unmoulted hens on day 7 and day 14 post experimental infection (Holt and Porter, 1992). *Salmonella* Enteritidis was transmitted more rapidly to unchallenged hens in cages adjacent to moulted infected hens than to those in cages adjacent to unmoulted infected hens (Holt, 1995). Short-term exposure to environmental stress, such as the introduction of young chickens in the same rearing room and the removal of feed and water for 2 days, may also result in an increase in the shedding rate of *S.* Enteritidis by laying hens (Nakamura *et al.*, 1994). It is now known that stress leads to increase levels of neuroendocrine stress hormones such as noradrenaline and norepinephrine in the gut, which can stimulate increased expression of a number of bacterial virulence determinants (Methner *et al.*, 2008).

Housing

The manner in which chickens are kept may influence the percentage of infected hens within a flock. Thus open-sided housing is likely to lead to increase environmental contamination. Similarly, the provision of new housing with improved environmental control will lead to reduced levels of environmental infection providing management is at a high level. Investigation of an outbreak of *S.* Enteritidis PT4 among 176,000 laying hens showed a lower prevalence among caged than among free-range hens (1.6 versus 50%) (Kinde *et al.*, 1996). In an experiment where laying hens housed in four different housing systems were infected with *S.* Enteritidis, bird to bird transmission and contaminated eggs were higher in birds housed in the aviary and floor systems compared to those housed in conventional and furnished cage systems (De Vylder *et al.*, 2011). Windowless houses, moulting and in-line egg processing were also risk factors for *Salmonella* infection in laying-hen farms in a study conducted in Japan (Sasaki *et al.*, 2012).

Penetration of the eggshell

The mechanism of egg infection has been reviewed recently by Gantois *et al.* (2009). Contamination of the egg contents may occur by contamination of the eggshell with faeces from hens excreting *Salmonella* (Schaaf, 1936; Williams *et al.*, 1968; Borland, 1975; Timoney *et al.*, 1989). Hens may have only an enteric infection and the *Salmonella* in the faeces may penetrate the eggshell pores as the egg cools and before the establishment on its surface of the proteinaceous cuticular barrier, which prevents bacterial invasion of the egg (Board, 1966; Forsythe *et al.*, 1967; Williams *et al.*, 1968). Alternatively, faecal matter adherent to the shell may contaminate the egg contents when the eggs have cracks or when the eggs are broken open for the preparation of food products (Borland, 1975). There appears to be a link between the shedding of high numbers of *S.* Enteritidis bacteria and contamination of eggs. When cloacal tissues were heavily contaminated with *S.* Enteritidis, the eggs were culture-positive, whereas, if these tissues had a low rate of infection, the eggs were culture-negative (Keller *et al.*, 1995).

Vertical transmission of *Salmonella* through eggs

Transmission of *Salmonella* via hatching eggs may occur as a result of infection of the ovary and oviduct. For an oophoritis to occur, the bird must have experienced a systemic infection. The poultry-specific serovars, *S.* Pullorum and *S.* Gallinarum, are the main serovars transmitted vertically. Other serovars that may cause a transovarian infection include

S. Typhimurium, *S.* Enteritidis, *S.* Heidelberg and *S.* Menston (Schaaf, 1936; Gordon and Tucker, 1965; Snoeyenbos *et al.*, 1969; Hopper and Mawer, 1988; Cooper *et al.*, 1989; Humphrey *et al.*, 1989b; McIlroy *et al.*, 1989; Timoney *et al.*, 1989; Gast and Beard, 1990; Barnhart *et al.*, 1991; Hoop and Pospischil, 1993; Corkish *et al.*, 1994; Keller *et al.*, 1995).

Salmonella Enteritidis strains not uncommonly colonize the reproductive tract, which results in eggs containing *Salmonella*. Examination of 1119 eggs from two small flocks of 35 hens contained *Salmonella* bacteria. The production of infected eggs was clustered, though intermittent. The positive eggs were produced by ten of the 35 hens (Humphrey *et al.*, 1989b). Inoculation of approximately 10^6 *S.* Enteritidis into the crop of adult hens was followed by a bacteraemia with infection of many body sites, including peritoneum, ovules and oviduct, in the majority of the hens (Timoney *et al.*, 1989). The organisms were present in the yolk and albumen of eggs of about 10% of the hens shortly after infection and again 10 days later, which is evidence for egg or transovarian transmission of the infection. The finding that the albumen, but not yolk samples, of some of the eggs were positive suggests that some eggs became infected in the oviduct (Timoney *et al.*, 1989).

Examination of 37 laying hens from three small flocks with a naturally acquired infection showed that in six hens the ovaries and in ten hens the oviduct were colonized by *S.* Enteritidis PT4. By immune-histochemical labelling, *S.* Enteritidis was demonstrated in seven of eight culture-positive hens on the surface of and within the epithelial cells in the lumen and in the tuberine glands of the oviduct and intracellularly in the follicular epithelium of the ovary (Hoop and Pospischil, 1993). When adult laying hens were inoculated orally with 10^8 *S.* Enteritidis, the microorganisms were isolated 2 days p.i. from the spleen, liver, heart, gall bladder and intestinal tissues and from various sections of the ovary and oviduct (Keller *et al.*, 1995). Detection of microorganisms by immuno-histochemical staining was rare for most tissues, despite their culture-positive status, but they could be detected in oviduct tissues associated with forming eggs, indicating a heavier colonization in the egg during its development. Forming eggs taken from the oviduct were culture-positive at a rate of c. 30%, while freshly laid eggs in the same experiment were positive at a rate of less than 0.6%, suggesting that forming eggs are colonized in the reproductive tract but that factors within the eggs significantly control the pathogen before the eggs are laid. When the cloacal tissues were heavily contaminated with *S.* Enteritidis the eggs were culture-positive, whereas if these tissues had a low rate of infection, the eggs were culture-negative. It was concluded that, prior to eggshell deposition, forming eggs are subject to descending infections from colonized ovarian tissue, lateral infection from colonized upper oviduct tissues and ascending infections from colonized vaginal and cloacal tissues (Keller *et al.*, 1995).

Examination of the attachment and invasion of chicken ovarian granulosa cells by *S.* Enteritidis PT8 showed that the organism can invade and multiply in these cells. The bacteria were found, with or without a surrounding membrane, in the cytoplasm of granulosa cells. It was suggested that the granulosa cell layer of the pre-ovulatory follicles may be a preferred site for the colonization of the chicken ovaries by invasive strains of *S.* Enteritidis (Thiagarajan *et al.*, 1994, 1996). More recent work has suggested that *S.* Enteritidis strains are also able to adhere to isthmus via secretions which may be significant in this being its predominant site of colonization of the oviduct (De Buck *et al.*, 2003).

A study was conducted in which ten hens were taken from each of three flocks naturally infected with *S.* Enteritidis and from one flock naturally infected with *S.* Typhimurium (Cooper *et al.*, 1989). In the first flock, *Salmonella* could not be isolated by cloacal swab or by the culture of 78 eggs, whilst *S.* Enteritidis PT4 was isolated on post-mortem examination from three birds, from the caeca, the oviduct and/or the ovary. In the second flock, *S.* Enteritidis was isolated by cloacal swab on one occasion and from a pooled sample of two eggs on one occasion from a total of 39 eggs, but it was not isolated post-mortem from any organ. In the third flock, *Salmonella* spp. could not be isolated by cloacal swab or by the culture of 47 eggs; however, three unshelled yolks taken from one bird yielded *S.* Enteritidis PT1, four hens had congested ovaries, shrunken follicles and evidence of inspissation and six birds yielded *S.* Enteritidis PT1 from the reproductive organs. In the fourth block, infected with *S.* Typhimurium, the organism could not be isolated from 32 eggs and no gross pathological changes were observed on post-mortem in any of the hens (Cooper *et al.*, 1989). Likewise, others observed ovarian infection, congestion of ovules, misshapen ovules and egg peritonitis in hens from a laying flock infected with *S.* Enteritidis PT4 (Hopper and Mawer, 1988), and a diffuse yellow fibrinous peritonitis, internal laying of soft-shelled eggs, clots of inspissated yolk in the peritoneal cavity and/or the oviduct and shrunken thick-walled congested follicles containing coagulated yolk in hens of another layer flock infected with *S.* Enteritidis PT4 (Read *et al.*, 1994).

In one comparative study it was found that *S.* Enteritidis had increased ability to colonize the vaginal epithelium of laying hens than other serovars: *S.* Agona, *S.* Infantis, *S.* Hadar, *S.* Heidelberg, *S.* Montevideo and *S.* Typhimurium (Mizumoto *et al.*, 2005). The authors suggested that the lipopolysaccharide (LPS) type 09 of *S.* Enteritidis may play an important and essential role in tropism of the reproductive tract. It has been suggested that immune responses to *Salmonella* play an important and significant role in the infection of reproductive tract and eggs.

One study on immunological responses during the carrier state and through the onset of laying in hens infected with *S.* Pullorum showed that both the T-cell response to the bacteria and nonspecific responses to mitogenic stimulation fell sharply in both infected and non-infected birds at point of lay (Wigley *et al.*, 2005). This coincided with the increase in numbers of *S.* Pullorum in the spleen and reproductive tract, but the bacterial numbers declined and T-cell response began to increase 3 weeks after the onset of laying in infected birds. These findings suggest that suppression of immune responses at the onset of lay plays a major role in the ability of *S.* Pullorum to infect the reproductive tract, leading to transmission of the bacteria to eggs (Wigley *et al.*, 2005).

Environmental Considerations

The faecal excretion of *Salmonella* by poultry, the transportation and disposal of slurry and manure from poultry houses and barns, the transportation of slaughter offal to rendering plants, the cross-contamination of rendered meat meal and other poultry and animal by-products by dust and contaminated conveyor belts in the rendering department of slaughtering plants and in feed mills, hoppers, bins, and trucks transporting feed to poultry barns all contribute to spreading *Salmonella* in the environment (further details will be found in Chapters 19 and 20). Pigeons, sparrows, other birds, rodents, cats, dogs and insects may be contaminated by contact with or the ingestion of spilled meat meal, feather meal and other animal by-products outside rendering department at slaughtering plants and at poultry houses from conveyor belts, hoppers and open trucks. This may lead to contamination of effluents, surface waters, creeks, rivers, lakes, pastures and soil, to the colonization of birds, cattle, pigs, sheep, horses, rodents and other animals or to contamination of animal feeds or many contribute directly to the recolonization of farm animals (Tannock and Smith, 1971; Borland, 1975; Diesch, 1978; Morse, 1978; Oosterom, 1991; Kirkwood *et al.*, 1994).

Treatment

Many antibiotics have been used either singly, in combination with other antimicrobial agents or in conjunction with the administration of caecal competitive exclusion (CE) flora from adult birds to prevent *Salmonella* infection or to treat chickens with clinical salmonellosis (Seuna *et al.*, 1985). However, administration of antimicrobials to chickens is often followed by the development of resistance and prolonged excretion of *Salmonella* (Smith and Tucker, 1975; Barrow, 1989; Manning *et al.*, 1994). Gentamicin and enrofloxacin have been used to eliminate *Salmonella* from layer-type hatching eggs artificially infected with *S.* Enteritidis (Hafez *et al.*, 1992). However, this practice is discouraged and not generally used as result of concerns over increased pressure for selection of resistance in the *Salmonella* and other enteric bacteria likely to be present. When groups of chicks and turkey poults experimentally infected orally with various doses of *S.* Typhimurium var. Copenhagen and treated for 6–10 days per os with water containing enrofloxacin (dosage 50 ppm of the aqueous solution), the *Salmonella* were eliminated from the faeces for a short period of time, after which they were again excreted, albeit at lower numbers (Guillot and Millemann, 1992). These results are reminiscent of similar studies by Smith and Tucker (1975) and work in humans (Neill *et al.*, 1991), where treatment with tetracycline or streptomycin in chickens and ciprofloxacin in humans failed to completely curtail excretion of *Salmonella*.

In the Netherlands, part of the *S.* Enteritidis eradication programme in poultry breeder flocks during the period 1989–1992 involved elimination by slaughter of elite, grandparent and other breeder flocks that were positive for *S.* Enteritidis followed by treatment with enrofloxacin, followed by two treatments with CE flora (Nurmi and Rantala, 1973). Four *S.* Enteritidis PT4-positive flocks (in total approximately 100,000 birds) became serologically negative after treatment (Edel, 1994). The use of CE treatment following antibiotic use is designed to replace the flora eliminated by the antimicrobials, which itself is the cause of the resurgence in excretion following cessation of treatment indicated above.

Levels of resistance to antibiotics vary hugely around the world. Relatively low levels of resistance are observed in EU countries albeit with relatively higher levels against sulfonamides in Germany and the Baltic States and to quinolones in a number of countries including the UK, Ireland and Spain (EFSA, 2007).

The picture in much of the world reflects extensive use of antimicrobials in poultry rearing although whether this is for therapy, control of colonization or blanket prophylaxis against a variety of pathogens is unclear. The latter is most likely.

Thus in a recent study in the USA 31% of *Salmonella* isolated were resistant to three antibiotics and 21% resistant to ceftiofur (M'ikanatha *et al.*, 2010). In contrast, levels can be very high with *S.* Paratyphi B variant Java and *S.* Heidelberg from chickens in Colombia being resistant to between 2 and 15 antimicrobials with 15% of isolates resistant to nine drugs and 40% resistant to tetracycline, cephalosporins and quinolones (Donado-Godoy *et al.*, 2012). In Brazil 250 *Salmonella* strains tested were resistant to one or more antibiotics, 53.2% of which were multidrug resistant. Strains of *S.* Heidelberg were resistant to ceftriaxone (75.0%) and to ceftiofur (43.8%) (Medeiros *et al.*, 2011). In some countries levels of resistance can be very high. In Nigeria a high frequency of resistance to tetracycline (93% of isolates), nalidixic acid (81%) and sulfamethoxazole (87%) was observed amongst isolates from chickens (Fashae *et al.*, 2010). In one study in China more than 80% of the *S.* Indiana isolates were highly resistant to ampicillin (97.7% of isolates), amoxicillin/clavulanic acid (87.9%), cephalothin (87.9%), ceftiofur (85.7%), chloramphenicol (84.9%), florfenicol (90.9%), tetracycline (97.7%), doxycycline (98.5%), kanamycin (90.2%), and gentamicin (92.5%) with approximately 60% resistant to enrofloxacin (65.4%), norfloxacin (78.9%), and ciprofloxacin (59.4%). Of the *S.* Enteritidis isolates, 73% were resistant to ampicillin, 33.1% to amoxicillin/clavulanic acid, 66.3% to tetracycline and 65.3% to doxycycline (Lu *et al.*, 2011).

Isolates of *S.* Gallinarum are also not infrequently resistant where antibiotics are freely available and used indiscriminately. In South Korea 94.3% of isolates were resistant to nalidixic acid and resistant/intermediately resistant to fluoroquinolones, and 63.8% were resistant to three or more antimicrobials (Kang *et al.*, 2010). High levels have also been found in Algeria (Bounar-Kechih *et al.*, 2012).

Prevention

Competitive exclusion

Nurmi and Rantala (1973) demonstrated that oral administration of caecal bacterial flora from adult birds to newly hatched chickens increased the chick's resistance to *Salmonella* infection. Evaluations under field conditions were carried out in several countries; CE treatment of 88 broiler units in Germany showed that 42% of the 38 treated flocks were colonized with *Salmonella* bacteria, whereas 48% of the 50 untreated flocks were colonized (Huttner *et al.*, 1981). Trials in Sweden, involving 2.86 million broilers, were colonized versus 1.5% of the untreated broilers (Wierup *et al.*, 1987), whereas trials in the Netherlands with 284 flocks consisting of 8 million broilers showed that 14.7% of the treated flocks and 0.9% of the treated broilers were colonized with *Salmonella* bacteria versus 24.1% of untreated flocks and 3.5% of untreated broilers (Goren *et al.*, 1988). However, examination of faeces collected from the broiler transport crates and skin samples from the broilers after slaughter showed that the differences between treated and untreated flocks and broilers were minimal (Goren *et al.*, 1988). Studies on the control of *S.* Enteritidis colonization in broiler and leghorn chicks with dietary lactose and a defined caecal flora maintained as a continuous-flow (CF) culture showed that treatment with a defined cultures of caecal and dietary lactose had an increased protective effect when compared with treatment with either caecal culture or dietary lactose alone (Corrier *et al.*, 1992). Competitive exclusion products have been used in combination with other products although gut flora preparations have been found to have the greatest effect (Revolledo *et al.*, 2009). Further information can be found in Chapter 21.

Vaccines

Live, attenuated *S.* Enteritidis, *S.* Gallinarum and *S.* Typhimurium strains and bacterins have been used with the aim of reducing the colonization of liver, spleen, ovaries and caeca in chickens and lowering the shedding of *S.* Enteritidis and other serovars in faeces and eggs. Barrow *et al.* (1990a) found that oral infection with *S.* Typhimurium induced a strong immune protection against the same serovar, which might act as a gold standard in terms of expected levels of protection. An *aroA* or undefined rough mutant also induced protection although the level of protection was not as high as that produced by the parent strain. An *aroA* mutant of *S.* Enteritidis was also found to generate immunity against localization in the ovary, liver and spleen. The *S.* Gallinarum 9R vaccine was even more protective (Barrow *et al.*, 1990b, 1991) and has been used extensively in layers for this purpose although there are claims of reversion to virulence in the vaccine. The 9R strain was, however, isolated from the ovaries through the period of examination, whereas the *aroA* strain was not. One advantage of the 9R vaccine is that it will not induce the production of specific antibodies against LPS and so ELISA and other assays may continue to be used in vaccinated birds. Oral vaccination of newly hatched chickens with another *aroA* *S.* Enteritidis strain also generated a reduction of colonization of spleens, livers and caeca of vaccinated chickens compared with unvaccinated controls. Inclusion of an intramuscular (i.m.) booster to the first intravenous (i.v.) vaccination gave increased protection to the ovary, although the vaccine strain was isolated on one occasion from a batch of eggs laid at 20 weeks old (Cooper *et al.*, 1994b).

Another approach was the use of a stable, live, avirulent, genetically modified Δ*cya* Δ*crp* *S.* Typhimurium vaccine strain, X3985. Oral vaccination of chickens at 1 and 14 days of age with 10^8 cfu of X3985 protected against invasion of spleen, ovary and bursa of Fabricius and colonization of the ileum and caeca in chickens challenged with 10^6 cfu of virulent homologous *Salmonella* strains from the serogroup B. Chickens challenged with heterologous *Salmonella* strains from the serogroups C, D and E were also reportedly protected, however this work has since been discredited. Chickens from vaccinated hens had significantly higher antibody responses than did the progeny of non-vaccinated hens after oral infection with *Salmonella* strains (Hassan and Curtiss, 1994, 1996).

In contrast to live, attenuated vaccines, killed *Salmonella* vaccines have not produced convincing levels of protection against wild-type *Salmonella* challenge (Truscott, 1981; Barrow *et al.*, 1990a, b; Gast *et al.*, 1992, 1993), although others have seen protection when chickens were challenged via the i.v. or i.m. route (Timms *et al.*, 1990), which would tend to produce a bias in favour of the vaccine. There is also evidence from the field that killed vaccines have some effect against faecal excretion. Given that under these circumstances some birds will be infected with small doses it may be these birds where some protection occurs.

Claims for cross protection against different serogroups have been made on several occasions (Dueger *et al.*, 2003) with protection in some cases as a result of the relatively short period between vaccination and challenge such that innate immunity or competitive exclusion by the vaccine strain may have been responsible. The generation of protection between serogroups remains a subject of study and speculation. Further detailed information on vaccines will be found in Chapter 22.

Public Health Aspects

Sources of infection

In the early years of the *S*. Enteritidis pandemic many human infections were traced to contaminated eggs and to the laying hens at the farm that supplied the eggs (Telzak *et al.*, 1990; CDC, 1992; van de Giessen *et al.*, 1992; Altekruse *et al.*, 1993; Henzler *et al.*, 1994). Shell eggs, cooked eggs or egg products have all been implicated in outbreaks of *S*. Enteritidis infection (Anon., 1988; Coyle *et al.*, 1988; Humphrey *et al.*, 1988; Paul and Batchelor, 1988; Perales and Audicana, 1988; Cowden *et al.*, 1989; Mawer *et al.*, 1989; Stevens *et al.*, 1989; Hennessy *et al.*, 1996).

These large outbreaks were associated with egg or egg product consumption. It seemed likely at the time that the broiler industry was similarly infected as was found to be the case. Thus *S*. Enteritidis infections in humans have also been associated with the consumption of meat (Humphrey *et al.*, 1988; Reilly *et al.*, 1988). People may become infected with *S*. Enteritidis as a result of infected broiler breeder flocks producing infected broiler rearing flocks and contamination of broilers at slaughter (McIlroy *et al.*, 1989; Corkish *et al.*, 1994). Broilers may exhibit a pericarditis due to *S*. Enteriditis infection, and pure cultures of *S*. Enteritidis have been obtained from such infections (O'Brien, 1988; Rampling *et al.*, 1989). In the UK, *S*. Enteritidis PT4 has been isolated from 16–21% of chilled and frozen chicken (Roberts, 1991). In another study in the UK, *S*. Enteritidis was isolated from 51% of raw chicken and from 23% of giblet samples (Plummer *et al.*, 1995).

Other serovars have also been identified as a cause of food-borne infections associated with the consumption of insufficiently cooked or raw eggs, egg white or yolk or food products containing such ingredients, including *S*. Typhimurium infection which has been found to be implicated and was recovered from some of the eggs (Philbrook *et al.*, 1960). Raw eggs used to make the icing of a birthday cake, vanilla slices made by mixing ingredients in a mixing bowl also used for mixing the contents of raw shelled eggs, and raw eggs used to make savoury quiche, banana pie, fruit pie, fruit flan and meringues were all associated with outbreaks of *S*. Typhimurium PT141 in the 1980s (Chapman *et al.*, 1988). More recently other serovars have become relatively more prevalent in poultry flocks as a result of the introduction of measures to control *S*. Enteritidis and *S*. Typhimurium. Serovars, such as *S*. Infantis, have also been found to be associated with egg contamination (Rivoal *et al.*, 2009), both in Europe and Japan (Noda *et al.*, 2010). Given the low invasiveness of *S*. Infantis, this would seem to be largely the result of faecal contamination.

Prevention

The global significance of the *S*. Enteritidis problem in poultry for human health (Rodrigue *et al.*, 1990) led to several early recommendations to eliminate or curtail salmonellosis in humans and thereby poultry. The tracing of outbreak-associated eggs to farms where laying hens were infected with *S*. Enteritidis led the US Department of Agriculture to implement a national programme to control the spread of *S*. Enteritidis in commercial layer flocks (Hedberg *et al.*, 1993).

After a large nosocomial infection in New York City (Telzac *et al.*, 1990), all health care facilities in New York State were directed to eliminate raw or undercooked eggs from the diets of persons who are institutionalized, elderly and/or immunocompromised. People immunocompromised by the human immunodeficiency virus were shown to be particularly vulnerable to recurrent septicaemia caused by *S.* Enteritidis, *S.* Typhimurium and *S.* Dublin, but not by *S.* Heidelberg (Levine *et al.*, 1991). It has been recommended to pasteurize eggs for use in nursing homes, in other institutional settings and in commercial foods that may not be adequately cooked before eating (Telzak *et al.*, 1990; Hedberg *et al.*, 1993).

Consumers were advised to avoid eating raw or undercooked eggs and to avoid eating foods that contain raw eggs, e.g. home-made products, such as Caesar salad, egg-nog, mayonnaise and ice-cream (Steinert *et al.*, 1990; Buckner *et al.*, 1994). Strains of *S.* Enteritidis, *S.* Typhimurium and *S.* Senftenberg inoculated into the yolk of shell eggs were found to survive forms of cooking where some of the yolk remained liquid (Humphrey *et al.*, 1989a). Consumers were also advised to refrigerate eggs (Humphrey, 1990). It was found that several *S.* Enteritidis phage types, *S.* Typhimurium and other *Salmonella* serovars did not grow in the egg or egg yolk when stored below 10°C (Humphrey, 1990; Saeed and Koons, 1993). *Salmonella* remained viable but did not multiply in the egg white at 20°C or 30°C and many died out 4°C (Bradshaw *et al.*, 1990; Lock and Board, 1992). Other recommendations were not to microwave dishes containing raw eggs but to cook them (Evans *et al.*, 1995), in order to prevent cross-contamination from raw eggs to other foods, to wash hands, cooking utensils and food-preparation surfaces with soap and water after contact with raw eggs, not to sample food products containing raw egg, such as biscuit batter, and to promptly refrigerate foods containing eggs (Humphrey *et al.*, 1994; CDC, 1996).

Many European countries individually introduced measures to increase surveillance and introduce interventions, which became incorporated into EU legislation (EU, 1992).

In the EU, in 2003 a modified and comprehensive *Salmonella* control strategy in poultry and pig populations was introduced (EU, 2003a, b). To gain comparable information on the prevalence of *Salmonella*, baseline studies were carried out starting in 2004 for laying hens, in 2005 for broilers and 2006 for turkeys. Data on the prevalence of *Salmonella* in breeding birds of *Gallus gallus* were available according to the previous Zoonoses Directive (EU, 1992). On the basis of these prevalence data, targets for the reduction of *Salmonella* for each animal population were set and the member states had to implement national control programmes to achieve the targets (see also Chapter 23). The targets established for breeding flocks of *G. gallus* cover the five most frequent *Salmonella* serovars in human salmonellosis, *S.* Enteritidis, *S.* Typhimurium, *S.* Infantis, *S.* Virchow and *S.* Hadar. The Community targets established for laying hens, broilers and turkeys cover *S.* Enteritidis and *S.* Typhimurium (EU, 2003a).

After establishing control programmes in the member states the prevalences of *Salmonella* in different poultry populations decreased (EFSA, 2012). In *G. gallus* breeding flocks the prevalence of the five targeted serovars (*S.* Enteritidis, *S.* Typhimurium, *S.* Infantis, *S.* Virchow and *S.* Hadar) was 0.7% in 2010 and decreased compared with 2009 (1.2%) and 2008 (1.3%) (EFSA, 2010, 2011, 2012). The most common of the targeted serovars in breeding flocks was *S.* Enteritidis. In laying hens the member states reported between 0% and 13.2% samples as positive with the targeted serovars *S.* Enteritidis and *S.* Typhimurium in 2010. The reported *S.* Enteritidis and *S.* Typhimurium prevalence in the EU has continued to decline from 3.5% in 2008 and 3.2% in 2009 to 1.9% in 2010 (EFSA, 2012). In broilers, the member states reported 4.1% of the tested flocks as *Salmonella*-positive and 0.4% positive for the two target serovars (*S.* Enteritidis, *S.* Typhimurium) compared with 5.0% and 0.7%, respectively, in 2009.

The NPIP contains a US *S.* Enteritidis monitored programme intended to reduce the incidence of *Salmonella* organisms in hatching eggs and chicks through a sanitation programme at the breeder farm and the hatchery. It lists requirements to sample meconium from chick boxes and chicks that died within 7 days hatching and for the samples to be sent to an authorized laboratory. It also states requirements regarding the pelletizing and heating of feed and its components and the environmental samples to be taken to verify if they contain group D *Salmonella*, regulates the use of a federally licenced vaccination in multiplier breeding flocks provided that they were examined serologically and bacteriologically after having reached the age of 4 months, states that hatching eggs may be incubated only at hatcheries meeting the NPIP provisions, stipulates sampling plans for flocks from which *S.* Enteritidis have been isolated to determine if they are eligible under the programme, and stipulates the conditions for hatcheries to meet the requirements of the programme.

Practices to control *Salmonella* have been instituted and promoted by the poultry industry in several other countries. A 'Canadian Egg Industry Code of Practice' and 'Best Management Practices for Turkey Production' to prevent and control *Salmonella* have been produced by the Canadian Egg Marketing Agency and the Canadian Turkey Marketing Agency, respectively. Management practices to reduce the risk of *Salmonella* infection in broilers and turkeys in the USA were described by Holder (1993) and Nagaraja and Halvorson (1993). After depopulation of the flock infected with *Salmonella*, a cleansing and disinfection procedure must be carried out before the premises may be repopulated. Procedures to disinfect and to sample poultry houses after cleansing and disinfection and before placing chicks or hens have been described (Davies and Wray, 1996a; Davison *et al.*, 1996), but complete elimination of *Salmonella* and rodents carrying the pathogen will always be difficult to achieve (Davies and Wray, 1996b).

In the USA, the Food and Drug Administration (FDA) issued a final rule that required shell egg producers to implement measures to prevent *S.* Enteritidis from contaminating eggs on the farm and from further growth during storage and transportation, and requires the producers to maintain records concerning their compliance with the rule and to register with FDA. The FDA took this action because *S.* Enteritidis is among the leading bacterial causes of food-borne illness in the USA, and shell eggs are a primary source of human infections. The final rule will reduce *S.* Enteritidis-associated illnesses and deaths by reducing the risk that shell eggs are contaminated. The final rule was effective 8 September 2009 (CFR, 2009). The rule requires that measures designed to prevent *S.* Enteritidis be adopted by virtually all egg producers with 3000 or more laying hens whose shell eggs are not processed with a treatment, such as pasteurization, to ensure their safety.

References

Aarestrup, F.M., Hendriksen, R.S., Lockett, J., Gay, K., Teates, K., McDermott, P.F., White, D.G., Hasman, H., Sørensen, G., Bangtrakulnonth, A., Pornreongwong, S., Pulsrikarn, C., Angulo, F.J. and Gerner-Smidt, P. (2007) International spread of multidrug-resistant *Salmonella* Schwarzengrund in food products. *Emerging Infectious Diseases* 13, 726–731.

Akiba, M., Kusumoto, M. and Iwata, T. (2011) Rapid identification of *Salmonella enterica* serovars, Typhimurium, Choleraesuis, Infantis, Hadar, Enteritidis, Dublin and Gallinarum, by multiplex PCR. *Journal of Microbiological Methods* 85, 9–15.

Altekruse, S., Koehler, J., Hickman-Brenner, R., Tauxe, R.V. and Ferris, K. (1993) A comparison of *Salmonella enteritidis* phage types from egg-associated outbreaks and implicated laying flocks. *Epidemiology and Infection* 110, 17–22.

Anonymous (1988) *Salmonella enteritidis* phage type 4: chicken and egg. *Lancet* ii, 720–722.

Anonymous (1995) Salmonella *Enteritidis Pilot Project Progress Report.* A cooperative effort of the Pennsylvania Poultry Producers, Pennsylvania Poultry Federation, Egg Association of America, Pennsylvania

Department of Agriculture, Pennsylvania State University, and the United States Department of Agriculture, Washington, DC, pp. 48–49.

Barnhart, H.M., Dreesen, D.W., Bastien, R. and Pancorbo, O.C. (1991) Prevalence of *Salmonella enteritidis* and other serovars in ovaries of layer hens at time of slaughter. *Journal of Food Protection* 54, 488–491.

Barrow, P.A. (1989) Further observations on the effect of feeding diets containing avoparcin on the excretion of salmonellas by experimentally infected chickens. *Epidemiology and Infection* 102, 239–252.

Barrow, P.A. (1991) Experimental infection of chickens with *Salmonella enteritidis*. *Avian Pathology* 20, 145–153.

Barrow, P.A. (1992) Further observations on the serological response to experimental *Salmonella typhimurium* in chickens measured by ELISA. *Epidemiology and Infection* 108, 231–241.

Barrow, P.A. (1995) Recent Progress *in the Diagnosis and Control of* Salmonella *Infections in Poultry*. Document 63 SG/10A, Office International des Epizooties, Paris, 12

Barrow, P.A. and Freitas Neto, O.C. (2011) Pullorum disease and fowl typhoid – new thoughts on old diseases: a review. *Avian Pathology* 40, 1–13.

Barrow, P.A. and Lovell, M.A. (1991) Experimental infection of egg-laying hens with *Salmonella enteritidis*. *Avian Pathology* 20, 339–352.

Barrow, P.A., Huggins, M.B., Lovell, M.A. and Simpson, J.M. (1987) Observations on the pathogenesis of experimental *Salmonella typhimurium* infection in chickens *Research in Veterinary Science* 42, 194–199.

Barrow, P.A., Simpson, J.M. and Lovell, M.A. (1988) Intestinal colonisation in the chicken by food-poisoning *Salmonella* serovars, microbial characteristics associated with faecal excretion. *Avian Pathology* 17, 571–588.

Barrow, P.A., Hassan, J.O. and Berchieri, A. Jr (1990a) Reduction in faecal excretion by chickens of *Salmonella typhimurium* by immunization with avirulent mutants of *S. typhimurium*. *Epidemiology and Infection* 104, 413–426.

Barrow, P.A., Lovell, M.A. and Berchieri, A. (1990b) Immunisation of laying hens against *Salmonella enteritidis* with live attenuated vaccines. *Veterinary Record* 126, 241–242.

Barrow, P.A., Berchieri, A. Jr and Al-Haddad, O. (1992) The serological response of chickens to infection with *Salmonella gallinarum-pullorum* detected by ELISA. *Avian Diseases* 36, 227–236.

Barrow, P.A., Bumstead, N., Marston, K., Lovell, M.A. and Wigley, P. (2003) Faecal shedding and intestinal colonisation of *Salmonella enterica* in in-bred chickens; the effect of host-genetic background. *Epidemiology and Infection* 132, 117–126.

Baskerville, A., Humphrey, T.J., Fitzgeorge, R.B., Cook, R.W., Chart, H., Rowe, B. and Whitehead, A. (1992) Airborne infection of laying hens with *Salmonella enteritidis* phage type 4. *Veterinary Record* 130, 395–398.

Berchieri, A. Jr, Iba, A.M. and Barrow, P.A. (1995) Examination by ELISA of sera obtained from chicken breeder and layer flocks showing evidence of fowl typhoid or pullorum disease. *Avian Pathology* 24, 411–420.

Berchieri, A. Jr, Murphy, C.K., Marston, K. and Barrow, P.A. (2001) Observations on the persistence and vertical transmission of *Salmonella enterica* serovars Pullorum and Gallinarum in chickens; effect of bacterial and host genetic background. *Avian Pathology* 30, 229–239.

Berndt, A., Wilhelm, A., Jugert, C., Pieper, J., Sachse, K. and Methner, U. (2007) Chicken cecum immune response to *Salmonella enterica* serovars of different levels of invasiveness. *Infection and Immunity* 75, 5993–6007.

Board, R.G. (1966) The course of microbial infection of the hen's eggs. *Journal of Applied Bacteriology* 29, 319–341.

Borland, E.D. (1975) *Salmonella* infection in poultry. *Veterinary Record* 97, 406–408.

Botts, C.W., Ferguson, L.C., Birkeland, J.M. and Winter, A.R. (1952) The influence of litter on the control of *Salmonella* infections in chicks. *American Journal of Veterinary Research* 13, 562–565.

Bounar-Kechih, S., Hamdi, T.M., Mezali, L., Assaous, F. and Rahal, K. (2012) Antimicrobial resistance of 100 *Salmonella* strains isolated from *Gallus gallus* in 4 wilayas of Algeria. *Poultry Science* 91, 1179–1185.

Bouzoubaa, K. and Nagaraja, K.V. (1984) Epidemiological studies on the incidence of salmonellosis in chicken breeder/hatchery operations in Morocco. In: Snoeyenbos, G.H. (ed.) *Proceedings of the International Symposium on Salmonella*. American Association of Avian Pathologists, Kennett Square, Pennsylvania, p. 337.

Boyd, Y., Herbert, E.G., Marston, K.L., Jones, M.A. and Barrow, P.A. (2005) Host genes affect intestinal colonisation of newly-hatched chickens by *Campylobacter jejuni*. *Immunogenetics* 57, 248–253.

Bradshaw, J.G., Shah, D.B., Forney, E. and Madden, J.M. (1990) Growth of *Salmonella enteritidis* in yolk of shell eggs from normal and seropositive hens. *Journal of Food Protection* 53, 1033–1036.

Brown, D.D., Ross, J.G. and Smith, A.F. (1975) Experimental infection of cockerels with *Salmonella typhimurium. Research in Veterinary Science* 18, 165–170.

Brown, D.D., Ross, J.G. and Smith, A.F. (1976) Experimental infection of poultry with *Salmonella infantis. Research in Veterinary Science* 20, 237–243.

Brownell, J.R., Sadler, W.W. and Fanelli, M.J. (1969) Factors influencing the intestinal infection of chickens with *Salmonella typhimurium. Avian Diseases* 13, 804–816.

Buckner, P., Ferguson, D., Anzalone, F., Anzalone, D., Taylor, J., Hlady, W.G. and Hopkins, R.S. (1994) Outbreak of *Salmonella enteritidis* associated with homemade ice-cream - Florida, 1993. *Morbidity and Mortality Weekly Report* 43, 669–671.

Bullis, K.L. (1977) The history of avian medicine in the US II. Pullorum disease and fowl typhoid. *Avian Diseases* 21, 422–429.

Bumstead, N. and Barrow, P.A. (1988) Genetics of resistance to *Salmonella typhimurium* in newly hatched chicks. *British Poultry Science* 29, 521–529.

Bumstead, N. and Barrow, P.A. (1993) Resistance to *Salmonella gallinarum, S. pullorum* and *S. enteritidis* in inbred lines of chickens. *Avian Diseases* 37, 189–193.

Bynoe, E.T. and Yurack, J.A. (1964) Salmonellosis in Canada. In: van Oye, E. (ed.) *The World Problem of Salmonellosis*. W Junk Publishers, The Hague, pp. 397–420.

Carrique-Mas, J.J., Breslin, M., Snow, L., McLaren, I., Sayers, A.R. and Davies, R.H. (2009) Persistence and clearance of different *Salmonella* serovars in buildings housing laying hens. *Epidemiology and Infection* 137, 837–846.

Cason, J.A., Cox, N.A. and Bailey, J.S. (1994) Transmission of *Salmonella typhimurium* during hatching of broiler chicks. *Avian Diseases* 38, 583–588.

CDC (1992) Outbreak of *Salmonella enteritidis* infection associated with consumption of raw shell eggs, 1991. *Morbidity and Mortality Weekly Report* 41, 369–372.

CDC (1996) Outbreaks of *Salmonella* serovar *Enteritidis* infection associated with consumption of raw shell egg - United States, 1994-1995. *Morbidity and Mortality Weekly Report* 45, 737–742.

CDC (2011) Centers for Disease Control and Prevention. Vital signs: incidence and tends of infection with pathogens transmitted commonly through food-borne diseases active surveillance network, 10 US sites, 1996-2010. *Morbidity and Mortality Weekly Report* 60, 749–755.

CFR (2009) Code of Federal Regulations of United States of America; 21 CFR 118.8 as of 8 September 2009.

Chapman, P.A., Rhodes, P. and Rylands, W. (1988) *Salmonella typhimurium* phage type 141 infections in Sheffield during 1984 and 1985: association with hens' eggs. *Epidemiology and Infection* 101, 75–82.

Chappell, L., Kaiser, P., Barrow, P., Jones, M.A., Johnston, C. and Wigley, P. (2009) The immunobiology of avian systemic salmonellosis. *Veterinary Immunology and Immunopathology* 128, 53–59.

Chase, F.E. (1947) *Salmonella* studies in fowl. *Canadian Journal of Public Health* 38, 82–83.

Chishti, M.A., Khan, M.Z. and Siddique, M (1985) Incidence of salmonellosis in chicken in and around Faisalabad. *Pakistan Veterinary Journal* 5, 79–82.

Cooper, G.L., Nicholas, R.A. and Bracewell, C.D. (1989) Serological and bacteriological investigations of chickens from flocks naturally infected with *Salmonella enteritidis. Veterinary Record* 125, 567–572.

Cooper, G.L., Venables, L.M., Woodward, M.J. and Hormaeche, C.E. (1994a) Invasiveness and persistence of *Salmonella enteritidis, Salmonella typhimurium*, and a genetically defined S. *enteritidis aroA* strain in young chicks. *Infection and* Immunity 62, 4739–4746.

Cooper, G.L., Venables, L.M., Woodward, M.J. and Hormaeche, C.E. (1994b) Vaccination of chickens with strain CVL30, a genetically defined *Salmonella enteritidis aroA* live oral vaccine candidate. *Infection and Immunity* 62, 4747–4754.

Corkish, J.D., Davies, R.H., Wray, C. and Nicholas, R.A.J. (1994) Observations on a broiler breeder flock naturally infected with *Salmonella enteritidis* phage type 4. *Veterinary Record* 134, 591–594.

Corrier, D.E., Snodgrass, J.D., Hinton, A. Jr and Deloach, J.R. (1992) Effect of anaerobic cecal microflora and dietary lactose on *Salmonella* colonization in bobwhite quail (*Colinus virginianus*). *Poultry Science* 71, 2022–2026.

Cowden, J.D., Chisholm, D., O'Mahony, M., Lynch, D., Mawer, S.L., Spain, G.E., Ward, L. and Rowe, B. (1989) Two outbreaks of *Salmonella enteritidis* phage type 4 infection associated with the consumption of fresh shell-egg products. *Epidemiology and Infection* 103, 47–52.

Cox, J.M. (1996) What makes *Salmonella enteritidis* stick in chickens? *World Poultry-Misset* May, 22–23.

Coyle, E.F., Palmer, S.R., Ribeiro, C.D., Jones, H.I., Howard, A.J., Ward, L. and Rowe, B. (1988) *Salmonella enteritidis* phage type 4 infection- association with hens' eggs. *Lancet* ii, 1295–1297.

Crespo, R., Jeffrey, J., Chin, R.P., Senties-Cue, G. and Shivaprasad, H.L. (2004) Genotypic and phenotypic characterization of *Salmonella arizonae* from an integrated turkey operation. *Avian Diseases* 48, 344–350.

Davies, R.H. and Wray, C. (1996a) Determination of an effective sampling regime to detect *Salmonella enteritidis* in the environment of poultry units. *Veterinary Microbiology* 50, 117–127.

Davies, R.H. and Wray, C. (1996b) Studies of contamination of three broiler breeder houses with *Salmonella enteritidis* before and after cleansing and disinfection. *Avian Diseases* 40, 626–633.

Davison, S., Benson, C.E. and Eckroade, R.J. (1996) Evaluation of disinfectants against *Salmonella enteritidis. Avian Diseases* 40, 272–277.

De Buck, J., Van Immerseel, F., Meulemans, G., Haesebrouck, F. and Ducatelle, R. (2003) Adhesion of *Salmonella enterica* serotype Enteritidis isolates to chicken isthmal glandular secretions. *Veterinary Microbiology* 93, 223–233.

De Vylder, J., Dewulf, J., Van Hoorebeke, S., Pasmans, F., Haesrbrouck, F., Ducatella, R. and Van Immerseel, F. (2011) Horizontal transmission of *Salmonella enteritidis* in groups of experimentally infected laying hens housed in different housing systems. *Poultry Science* 90, 1391–1396.

Diesch, S.L. (1978) Environmental aspects of salmonellosis. In: *Proceedings National Salmonellosis Seminar.* United States Animal Health Association and co-sponsors, Washington, DC, 11 pp.

Donado-Godoy, P., Gardner, I., Byrne, B.A., Leon, M., Perez-Gutierrez, E., Ovalle, M.V., Tafur, M.A. and Miller, W. (2012) Prevalence, risk factors, and antimicrobial resistance profiles of *Salmonella* from commercial broiler farms in two important poultry-producing regions of Colombia. *Journal of Food Protection* 75, 874–883.

Duchet-Suchaux, M., Mompart, F., Berthelot, F., Beaumont, C., Léchopier, P. and Pardon, P. (1997) Differences in frequency, level, and duration of cecal carriage between four outbred chicken lines infected orally with *Salmonella enteritidis*. *Avian Diseases* 41, 559–567.

Dueger, E.L., House, J.K., Heithoff, D.M. and Mahan, M.J. (2003) *Salmonella* DNA adenine methylase mutants prevent colonization of newly hatched chickens by homologous and heterologous serovars. *International Journal of Food Microbiology* 80, 153–159.

Dunkley, K.D., Callaway, T.R., Chalova, V.I., McReynolds, J.L., Hume, M.E., Dunkley, C.S., Kubena, L.F., Nisbet, D.J. and Ricke, S.C. (2009) Foodborne *Salmonella* ecology in the avian gastrointestinal tract. *Anaerobe* 15, 26–35.

Ebel, E.D., David, M.J. and Mason, J. (1992) Occurrence of *Salmonella enteritidis* in the US commercial egg industry report on a national spent hen survey. *Avian Diseases* 36, 646–654.

Edel, W. (1994) *Salmonella enteritidis* eradication programme in poultry breeder flocks in The Netherlands. *International Journal of Food Microbiology* 21, 171–178.

Edwards, P.R. (1958) Salmonellosis observations on incidence and control. *Annals of the New York Academy of Sciences* 70, 598–613.

EFSA (2006) Analysis of the baseline study on the prevalence of *Salmonella* in laying hen flocks of *Gallus gallus*. *The EFSA Journal* 81, 1–71.

EFSA (2007) Report of the task force on zoonoses data collection on the analysis of the baseline survey on the prevalence of *Salmonella* in broiler flocks of *Gallus gallus* in the EU 2005-2006. *The EFSA Journal* 98, 1–85.

EFSA (2010) The Community Summary Report on Trends and Sources of Zoonoses, Zoonotic agents and Foodborne Outbreaks in the European Union in 2008. *The EFSA Journal* 1496, 1–288.

EFSA (2011) The European Union Summary Report on Trends and Sources of Zoonoses, Zoonotic agents and Foodborne Outbreaks in 2009. *The EFSA Journal* 9, 2090, 1–378.

EFSA (2012) The European Union Summary Report on Trends and Sources of Zoonoses, Zoonotic agents and Foodborne outbreaks in 2008. *The EFSA Journal* 10, 2579, 1–442.

Erbeck, D.H., McLaughlin, B.G. and Singh, S.N. (1993) Pullorum disease with unusual signs in two backyard chicken flocks. *Avian Diseases* 31, 895–897.

EU (1992) Council Directive 92/117/EEC of 17 December 1992 concerning measures for protection against specified zoonoses and specified zoonotic agents in animals and products of animal origin in order to prevent outbreaks of food-borne infections and intoxications. *Official Journal of the European Union* L 62, 15.3.1993, 38–48.

EU (2003a) Regulation (EC) No 2160/2003 of the European Parliament and of the Council of 17 November 2003 on the control of *Salmonella* and other specified food-borne zoonotic agents. *Official Journal of the European Union* L 325, 12.12.2003, 1–15.

EU (2003b) Directive 2003/99/EC of the European Parliament and of the Council of 17 November 2003 on the monitoring of zoonoses and zoonotic agents. *Official Journal of the European Union* L 325, 12.12.2003, 31–40.

Evans, M.R., Parry, S.M. and Ribeiro, C.D. (1995) *Salmonella* outbreak from microwave cooked food. *Epidemiology and Infection* 115, 227–230.

Faddoul, G.P. and Fellows, G.W. (1966) A five-year survey of the incidence of salmonellae in avian species. *Avian Diseases* 10, 296–304.

Fanelli, M.J., Sadler, W.W. and Brownell, J.R. (1970) Preliminary studies on persistence of salmonellae in poultry litter. *Avian Diseases* 14, 131–141.

Fashae, K., Ogunsola, F., Aarestrup, F.M. and Hendriksen, R.S. (2010) Antimicrobial susceptibility and serovars of *Salmonella* from chickens and humans in Ibadan, Nigeria. *Journal of Infection in Developing Countries* 4, 484–494.

Fasina, Y.O., Holt, P.S., Moran, E.T., Moore, R.W., Conner, D.E. and McKee, S.R. (2008) Intestinal cytokine response of commercial source broiler chicks to *Salmonella typhimurium* infection. *Poultry Science* 87, 1335–1346.

Feng, Y., Xu, H.F., Li, Q.H., Zhang, S.Y., Wang, C.X., Zhu, D.L., Cao, F.L., Li, Y.G., Johnston, R.N., Zhou, J., Liu, G.R. and Liu, S.L. (2012) Complete genome sequence of *Salmonella enterica* serovar pullorum RKS5078. *Journal of Bacteriology* 194, 744.

Ferris, K.E. and Miller, D.A. (1990) *Salmonella* serovars from animals and related sources reported during July 1988-June 1989. In: *Proceedings of the 93rd Annual Meeting of the United States Animal Health Association*. Carter Printing, Richmond, Virginia, pp. 521–538.

Foley, S.L., Nayak, R., Hanning, I.B., Johnson, T.J., Han, J. and Ricke, S.C. (2011) Population dynamics of *Salmonella enterica* serotypes in commercial egg and poultry production. *Applied and Environmental Microbiology* 77, 4273–4279.

Forsythe, R.H., Ross, W.J. and Ayres, J.C. (1967) Salmonellae recovery following gastro-intestinal and ovarian inoculation in the domestic fowl. *Poultry Science* 46, 849–855.

Galton, M.M., Steele, J.H. and Newell, K.W. (1964) Epidemiology of salmonellosis in the United States. In: van Oye, E. (ed.) *The World Problem of Salmonellosis*. W Junk Publishers, The Hague, pp. 421–444.

Gantois, I., Ducatelle, R., Pasmans, F., Haesebrouck, F., Gast, R., Humphrey, T.J. and Van Immerseel, F. (2009) Mechanisms of egg contamination by *Salmonella* Enteritidis. *FEMS Microbiology Reviews* 33, 718–738.

Gast, R.K. (1997) Detecting infections of chickens with recent *Salmonella pullorum* isolates using standard serological methods. *Poultry Science* 76, 17–23.

Gast, R.K. and Beard, C.W. (1990) Production of *Salmonella enteritidis*-contaminated eggs by experimentally infected hens. *Avian Diseases* 34, 438–446.

Gast, R.K. and Benson, S.T. (1996) Intestinal colonization and organ invasion in chicks experimentally infected with *Salmonella enteritidis* phage type 4 and other phage types isolated from poultry in the United States. *Avian Diseases* 40, 853–857.

Gast, R.K., Stone, H.D., Holt, P.S. and Beard, C.W. (1992) Evaluation of the efficacy of oil-emulsion bacterins for protecting chickens against *Salmonella enteritidis*. *Avian Diseases* 37, 1085–1091.

Gast, R.K., Stone, H.D. and Holt, P.S. (1993) Evaluation of the efficacy of oil-emulsion bacterins for reducing faecal shedding of *Salmonella enteritidis* by laying hens. *Avian Diseases* 36, 992–999.

Gauger, H.C. and Greaves, R.E. (1946) Isolations of *Salmonella typhimurium* from drinking water in an infected environment. *Poultry Science* 25, 476–478.

Gordon, R.F. and Tucker, J.F. (1965) The epizootiology of *Salmonella menston* infection of fowls and the effect of feeding poultry food artificially infected with *Salmonella*. *British Poultry Science* 6, 251–264.

Goren, E., de Jong, W.A., Doornenbal, P., Bolder, N.M., Mulder, R.W.A.W. and Jansen, A. (1988) Reduction of *Salmonella* infection of broilers by spray application of intestinal microflora – a longitudinal study. *Veterinary Quarterly* 10, 249–255.

Guard-Petter, J., Lakshmi, B., Carlson, R. and Ingram, K. (1995) Characterization of lipopolysaccharide heterogeneity in *Salmonella enteritidis* by an improved gel electrophoresis method. *Applied and Environmental Microbiology* 61, 2845–2851.

Guillot, J.F. and Millemann, Y. (1992) Intestinal colonization of chickens and turkeys by *Salmonella* and antibiotic decontamination. In: *Reports and Communications, International Symposium on* Salmonella *and Salmonellosis*. Ploufragan/Saint-Brieuc, France, pp. 413–420.

Guthrie, R.K. (1992) Salmonella. CRC Press, Boca Raton, Florida, pp. 1–20.

Hafez, H.M., Jodas, S., Kosters, J. and Schmidt, H. (1992) Treatment of *Salmonella ententidis* artificially contaminated eggs with pressure-differential-dipping (PDD) using antibiotics. In: *Reports and Communications, International Symposium on* Salmonella *and Salmonellosis*. Ploufragan/Saint-Brieuc, France, pp. 421–427

Hargrett-Bean, N.A. and Potter, M.E. (1995) *Salmonella* serovars from human sources, January 1992 through December 1992. In: *Proceedings of the 98th Annual* Meeting *of the United States Animal Health Association*. Promiter Communications and Spectrum Press, Richmond, Virginia, pp. 439–442.

Harvey, P.C., Watson, M., Hulme, S., Jones, M.A., Lovell, M., Berchieri, A. Jr, Young, J., Bumstead, N. and Barrow, P. (2011) *Salmonella enterica* Serovar Typhimurium Colonizing the Lumen of the Chicken Intestine Grows Slowly and Upregulates a Unique Set of Virulence and Metabolism Genes. *Infection and Immunity* 79, 4105–4121.

Hassan, J.O. and Curtiss III, R. (1994) Development and evaluation of an experimental vaccination program using a live avirulent *Salmonella typhimurium* strain to protect immunized chickens against challenge with homologous and heterologous *Salmonella* serovars. *Infection and* Immunity 62, 5519–5527.

Hassan, J.O. and Curtiss III, R. (1996) Effect of vaccination of hens with an avirulent strain of *Salmonella typhimurium* on immunity of progeny challenged with wild-type *Salmonella* strains. *Infection and Immunity* 64, 938–944.

Hassan, J.O., Barrow, P.A., Mockett, A.P.A. and McLeod, S. (1990) Antibody response to experimental *Salmonella typhimurium* infection in chickens measured by ELISA. *Veterinary Record* 126, 519–522.

Hassan, J.O., Mockett, A.P.A., Catty, D. and Barrow, P.A. (1991) Infection and reinfection of chickens with *Salmonella typhimurium*; bacteriology and immune responses. *Avian Diseases* 35, 809–819.

Hedberg, C.W., David, M.J., White, K.E., MacDonald, K.L. and Osterholm, M.T. (1993) Role of egg consumption in sporadic *Salmonella enteritidis* and *Salmonella typhimurium* infections in Minnesota. *Journal of Infectious Diseases* 167, 107–111.

Hennessy, T.W., Hedberg, C.W., Slutsker, L., White, K.E., Besser-Wiek, J.M., Moen, M.E., Feldman, J., Coleman, W.W., Edmonson, L.M., MacDonald, K.L., Osterholm, M.T. and the investigation team (1996) A national outbreak of *Salmonella enteritidis* infections from ice-cream. *New England Journal of Medicine* 334, 1281–1286.

Henzler, D.J. and Opitz, H.M. (1992) The role of mice in the epizootiology of *Salmonella enteritidis* infection on chicken layer farms. *Avian Diseases* 36, 625–631.

Henzler, D.J., Ebel, E., Sanders, J., Kradel, D. and Mason, J. (1994) *Salmonella enteritidis* in eggs from commercial chicken layer flocks implicated in human outbreaks. *Avian Diseases* 38, 37–43.

Hewitt, E.A. (1928) Bacillary white diarrhoea in baby turkeys Cornell. *Veterinarian* 18, 272–276.

Higgins, R., Malo, R., Rene-Roberge, E. and Gauthier, R. (1982) Studies on the dissemination of *Salmonella* in nine broiler-chicken flocks. *Avian Diseases* 26, 26–33.

Hinshaw, W.R. and McNeil, E. (1940) Eradication of pullorum disease from turkey poults. In: *Proceedings of the 44th Annual Meeting of the United States Livestock Sanitary Association*, Chicago, Illinois, pp. 178–194.

Hinton, M., Threlfall, E.J. and Rowe, B. (1990a) The invasive potential of *Salmonella enteritidis* phage types for young chickens. *Letters of Applied Microbiology* 10, 237–239.

Hinton, M., Threlfall, E.J. and Rowe, B. (1990b) The invasiveness of different strains of *Salmonella enteritidis* phage type 4 for young chickens. *FEMS Microbiology Letters* 70, 193–196.

Holder, T. (1993) Best management practices for *Salmonella* risk reduction in broilers. In: *Proceedings of the 97th Annual Meeting of the United States Animal Health Association*. Carter Printing, Richmond, Virginia, pp. 486–504.

Holt, P.S. (1995) Horizontal transmission of *Salmonella enteritidis* in molted and unmolted laying chickens. *Avian Diseases* 39, 239–249.

Holt, P.S. and Chaubal, L.H. (1997) Detection of motility and putative synthesis of flagellar proteins in *Salmonella pullorum* cultures. *Journal of Clinical Microbiology* 35, 1016–1020.

Holt, P.S. and Porter, R.E. (1992) Microbiological and histopathological effects of an induced-molt fasting procedure on a *Salmonella enteritidis* infection in chickens. *Avian Diseases* 36, 610–618.

Hoop, R.K. and Pospischil, A. (1993) Bacteriological, serological, histological and immunohistochemical findings in laying hens with naturally acquired *Salmonella enteritidis* phage type 4 infection. *Veterinary Record* 133, 391–393.

Hopper, S.A. and Mawer, S. (1988) *Salmonella enteritidis* in a commercial layer flock. *Veterinary Record* 123, 351.

Humphrey, T.J. (1990) Growth of salmonellas in intact shell eggs, influence of storage temperature. *Veterinary Record* 126, 292.

Humphrey, T.J., Mead, G.C. and Rowe, B. (1988) Poultry meat as a source of human salmonellosis in England and Wales. *Epidemiology and Infection* 100, 175–184.

Humphrey, T.J., Greenwood, M., Gilbert, R.J., Rowe, B. and Chapman, P.A. (1989a) The survival of salmonellas in shell eggs cooked under simulated domestic conditions. *Epidemiology and Infection* 103, 35–45.

Humphrey, T.J., Baskerville, A., Mawer, S., Rowe, B. and Hopper, S. (1989b) *Salmonella enteritidis* phage type 4 from the contents of intact eggs, a study involving naturally infected hens. *Epidemiology and Infection* 103, 415–523.

Humphrey, T.J., Chart, H., Baskerville, A. and Rowe, B. (1991a) The influence of age on the response of SPF hens to infection with *Salmonella enteritidis* PT4. *Epidemiology and Infection* 106, 33–43.

Humphrey, T.J., Baskerville, A., Chart, H., Rowe, B. and Whitehead, A. (1991b) *Salmonella enteritidis* PT4 infection m specific pathogen free hens: influence of infecting dose. *Veterinary Record* 129, 482–485.

Humphrey, T.J., Martin, K.W. and Whitehead, A. (1994) Contamination of hands and work surfaces with *Salmonella enteritidis* PT4 during the preparation of egg dishes. *Epidemiology and Infection* 113, 403–409.

Humphrey, T.J., Williams, A., McAlpine, K., Lever, M.S., Guard-Petter, J. and Cox, J.M. (1996) Isolates of *Salmonella enterica* Enteritidis PT4 with enhanced heat and acid tolerance are more virulent in mice and more invasive in chickens. *Epidemiology and Infection* 117, 79–88.

Hutt, F.B. and Scholes, R.D. (1941) Genetics of the fowl. XIII. Breed differences in susceptibility to *Salmonella pullorum*. *Poultry Science* 20, 324–352.

Huttner, B., Landgraf, H. and Vielitz, E. (1981) Kontrolle der Salmonelleninfectionen in Mastelterntier-Bestanden durch Verabreichung von SPR-Darmflora on Eintagsküken. *Deutsche Tierärtzliche Wochenschrift* 88, 527–532.

Ibrahim, G.F., Lyons, M.J., Walker, R.A. and Fleet, G.H. (1986) Rapid detection of salmonellae in foods using immunoassay systems. *Journal of Food Protection* 49, 92–98.

Iwabuchi, E., Maruyama, N., Hara, A., Nishimura, M., Muramatsu, M., Ochiai, T. and Hirai, K. (2011) Nationwide survey of salmonella prevalence in environmental dust from layer farms in Japan. *Journal of Food Protection* 73, 1993–2000.

Johnson, D.C., David, M. and Goldsmith, S. (1992) Epizootiological investigation of an outbreak of pullorum disease in an integrated broiler operation. *Avian Diseases* 36, 770–775.

Jones, M.A., Hulme, S.D., Barrow, P.A. and Wigley, P. (2007) The *Salmonella* pathogenicity island 1 and *Salmonella* pathogenicity island 2 type III secretion systems play a major role in pathogenesis of systemic disease and gastrointestinal tract colonization of *Salmonella enterica* serovar Typhimurium in the chicken. *Avian Pathology* 36, 199–203.

Kang, M.S., Kim, A., Jung, B.Y., Her, M., Jeong, W., Cho, Y.M., Oh, J.Y., Lee, Y.J., Kwon, J.H. and Kwon, Y.K. (2010) Characterization of antimicrobial resistance of recent *Salmonella enterica* serovar Gallinarum isolates from chickens in South Korea. *Avian Pathology* 39, 201–205.

Kang, M.S., Kwon, Y.K., Jung, B.Y., Kim, A., Lee, K.M., An, B.K., Song, E.A., Kwon, J.H. and Chung, G.S. (2011) Differential identification of *Salmonella enterica* subsp. enterica serovar Gallinarum biovars Gallinarum and Pullorum based on polymorphic regions of glgC and speC genes. *Veterinary Microbiology* 147, 181–185.

Kaushik, R.K., Singh, J., Kumar, S. and Kulshreshtha, R.C. (1986) Fowl typhoid in a few poultry farms of Haryana state. *Indian Journal of Animal Sciences* 56, 511–514.

Keller, L.H., Benson, C.E., Krotec, K. and Eckroade, R.J. (1995) *Salmonella enteritidis* colonization of the reproductive tract and forming and freshly laid eggs of chickens. *Infection and Immunity* 63, 2443–2449.

Kelterborn, E. (1967) Salmonella *Species. First Isolations, Names, and Occurrence*. W Junk, The Hague, the Netherlands, pp. 20, 140–141, 377–379.

Kilger, G. and Grimont, P.A.D. (1993) Differentiation of *Salmonella* phase flagellar antigen types by restriction of the amplified *fhC* gene. *Journal of Clinical Microbiology* 31, 1108–1110.

Kinde, H., Read, D.H., Chin, R.P., Bickford, A.A., Walker, R.L., Ardans, A., Breitmeyer, R.E., Willoughby, D., Little, H.E., Kerr, D. and Gardner, I.A. (1996) *Salmonella enteritidis*, phage type 4 infection in a commercial layer flock in Southern California – bacteriologic and epidemiological findings. *Avian Diseases* 40, 665–671.

Kirkwood, J.K., Cunningham, A.A., Macgregor, S.K., Thornton, S.M. and Duff, J.P. (1994) *Salmonella enteritidis* excretion by carnivorous animals fed on day-old chicks. *Veterinary Record* 134, 683.

Klein, E. (1889) Ueber eine epidemische Krankheit der Hühner, verursacht durch einen Bacillus – *Bacillus gallinarum*. *Zentralblatt für Bakteriologie und Parasitenkunde* 5, 689–693.

Kuehn, B.M. (2010) Salmonella cases traced to egg producers: findings recall of more than 500 million eggs. *The Journal of the American Medical Association* 304, 1316.

Kühn, H., Rabsch, W., Gericke, B. and Reissbrodt, R. (1993) Infektionsepidemiologische Analysen von Salmonellosen, Shigellosen und anderen Enterobacteriaceae-Infektionen. *Bundesgesundheitsblatt* 36, 324–333.

Lapuz, R.R., Umali, D.V., Suzuki, T., Shirota, K. and Katoh, H. (2012) Comparison of the prevalence of *Salmonella* infection in layer hens from commercial layer farms with high and low rodent densities. *Avian Diseases* 56, 29–34.

Laszlo, V.G., Csorian, E.S. and Paszti, J. (1985) Phage types and epidemiological significance of *Salmonella enteritidis* strains in Hungary between 1976 and 1983. *Acta Microbiologica Hungarica* 32, 321–340.

Le Hello, S., Hendriksen, R.S., Doublet, B., Fisher, I., Nielsen, E.M., Whichard, J.M., Bouchrif, B., Fashae, K., Granier, S.A., Jourdan-Da Silva, N., Cloeckaert, A., Threlfall, E.J., Angulo, F.J., Aarestrup, F.M., Wain, J. and Weill, F.X. (2011) International spread of an endemic population of *Salmonella enterica* serotype Kentucky ST198 resistant to ciprofloxacin. *Journal of Infectious Diseases* 204, 675–684.

Levine, W.C., Buehler, J.W., Bean, N.H. and Tauxe, R.V. (1991) Epidemiology of nontyphoidal *Salmonella* bacteraemia during the human immunodeficiency virus epidemic. *Journal of Infectious Diseases* 164, 81–87.

Lior, H. (1989) Isolations of enteric pathogens from people in Canada. *Safety Watch* 14, 3.

Lister, S.A. and Barrow, P.A. (2008) Enterobacteriaceae. In: Pattison, M., McMullin, P.F., Bradbury, J.M. and Alexander, D.J. (eds) *Poultry Diseases*, 6th edn. Butterworth Heinemann, Oxford, UK, pp. 110–145.

Liu, W.B., Liu, B., Zhu, X.N., Yu, S.J. and Shi, X.M. (2011) Diversity of Salmonella isolates using serotyping and multilocus sequence typing. *Microbiology* 28, 1182–1189.

Lock, J.L. and Board, R.G. (1992) Persistence of contamination of hens' egg albumen in vitro with *Salmonella* serovars. *Epidemiology and Infection* 108, 389–396.

Long, J.R., DeWitt, W.E. and Ruet, J.L. (1980) Studies on *Salmonella* from floor litter of 60 broiler chicken houses in Nova Scotia Canadian. *Veterinary Journal* 21, 91–94.

Lu, Y., Wu, C.M., Wu, G.J., Zhao, H.Y., He, T., Cao, X.Y., Dai, L., Xia, L.N., Qin, S.S. and Shen, J.Z. (2011) Prevalence of antimicrobial resistance among *Salmonella* isolates from chicken in China. *Foodborne Pathogens and Disease* 8, 45–53.

Makaya, P.V., Matope, G. and Pfukenyl, D.M. (2012) Distribution of *Salmonella* serovars and antimicrobial susceptibility of *Salmonella* Enteritidis from poultry in Zimbabwe. *Avian Pathology* 41, 221–226.

Manning, J.G., Hargis, B.M., Hinton, A., Corner, D.E., DeLoach, J.R. and Creger, C.R. (1994) Effect of selected antibiotics and anticoccidials on *Salmonella enteritidis* caecal colonization and organ invasion in Leghorn chicks. *Avian Diseases* 38, 256–261.

Mariani, P., Barrow, P.A., Cheng, H.H., Groenen, M.M., Negrini, R. and Bumstead, N. (2001) Localization to chicken Chromosome 5 of a novel locus determining salmonellosis resistance. *Immunogenetics* 53, 786–791.

Mawer, S.L., Spain, G.E. and Rowe, B. (1989) *Salmonella enteritidis* phage type 4 and hens' eggs. *Lancet* i, 280–281.

McCoy, J.H. (1975) Trends in salmonella food poisoning in England and Wales 1941-72. *Journal of Hygiene (Cambridge)* 74, 271–282.

McDermott, L.A. (1947) The K formula stained antigen in the detection of standard and Younie types of *Salmonella pullorum* infection. *Canadian Journal of Public Health* 38, 83–84.

McIlroy, S.G. and McCracken, R.M. (1990) The current status of the *Salmonella enteritidis* control programme in the United Kingdom. In: *Proceedings of the 94th Annual* Meeting *of the United States Animal Health Association*. Carter Printing, Richmond, Virginia, pp. 450–462.

McIlroy, S.G., McCracken, R.M., Neill, S.D. and O'Brien, J.J. (1989) Control, prevention and eradication of *Salmonella enteritidis* infection in broiler and broiler breeder flocks. *Veterinary Record* 125, 545–548.

McLeod, S. and Barrow, P.A. (1992). LPS-specific IgG in egg yolk from two chicken flocks infected with *Salmonella enteritidis*. *Letters in Applied Microbiology* 13, 294–297.

Medeiros, M.A., Oliveira, D.C., Rodrigues Ddos P. and Freitas, D.R. (2011) Prevalence and antimicrobial resistance of *Salmonella* in chicken carcasses at retail in 15 Brazilian cities. *Revista Panamericana de Salud Publica (Pan American Journal of Public Health)* 30, 555–560.

Mellor, G.E., Duffy, L.L., Dykes, G.A. and Fegan, N. (2010) Relative prevalence of *Salmonella* Sofia on broiler chickens pre- and postprocessing in Australia. *Poultry Science* 89, 1544–1548.

Methner, U., Rabsch, W., Reissbrodt, R. and Williams, P.H. (2008) Effect of norepinephrine on colonisation and systemic spread of *Salmonella enterica* in infected animals: role of catecholate siderophore precursors and degradation products. *International Journal of Medical Microbiology* 298, 429–439.

M'ikanatha, N.M., Sandt, C.H., Localio, A.R., Tewari, D., Rankin, S.C., Whichard, J.M., Altekruse, S.F., Lautenbach, E., Folster, J.P., Russo, A., Chiller, T.M., Reynolds, S.M. and McDermott, P.F. (2010) Multidrug-resistant *Salmonella* isolates from retail chicken meat compared with human clinical isolates. *Foodborne Pathogens and Disease* 7, 929–934.

Mizumoto, N., Sasai, K., Tani, H. and Baba, E. (2005) Specific adhesion and invasion of *Salmonella* Enteritidis in the vagina of laying hens. *Veterinary Microbiology* 111, 99–105.

Moore, E.N. (1946) The *Occurrence of Fowl Typhoid.* Circular No. 19, University of Delaware, Newark, Delaware, pp. 1–20.

Morgan, E., Campbell, J.D., Rowe, S.C., Bispham, J., Stevens, M.P., Bowen, A., Barrow, P.A., Maskell D.J. and Wallis, T.S. (2004) Identification of host-specific colonization factors of *Salmonella enterica* serovar Typhimurium. *Molecular Microbiology* 54, 994 1010.

Morningstar-Shaw, B.R., Barker, D.A., Mackie, T.A., Muonz, M.I., Palmer, E.A., Kane, M.A., Cook, L.K. and Erdman, M.M. (2012) *Salmonella* serotypes isolated from animals in the United States: January 1 to December 31, 2010. *Proceedings 115th Annual Meeting US Animal Health Association*, 397–407.

Morris, G.K., McMurray, B.L., Galton, M.M. and Wells, J.G. (1969) A study of the dissemination of salmonellosis in a commercial broiler chicken operation. *American Journal of Veterinary Research* 30, 1413–1421.

Morse, E.V. (1978) Salmonellosis and pet animals. In: *Proceedings of the National Salmonellosis Seminar.* United States Animal Health Association and other co-sponsors, Washington, DC, 6 pp.

Nagaraja, K.V. and Halvorson, D.A. (1993) Best management practices for *Salmonella* risk reduction in turkeys. In: *Proceedings of the 97th Annual Meeting of the United States Animal Health Association.* Carter Printing, Richmond, Virginia, pp. 505–523.

Nakamura, M., Nagamine, N., Takahashi, T., Suzuki, S., Kijima, M., Tamura, Y. and Sato, S. (1994) Horizontal transmission of *Salmonella enteritidis* and effect of stress on shedding in laying hens. *Avian Diseases* 38, 282–288.

Neill, M.A., Opal, S.M., Heelan, J., Giusti, R., Cassidy, J.E., White, R. and Mayer, K.H. (1991) Failure of ciprofloxacin to eradicate convalescent faecal excretion after acute salmonellosis: experience during an outbreak in health care workers. *Annals of Internal Medicine* 114, 195–199.

Noda, I., Murakami, K., Ishiguro, Y. and Asai, T. (2010) Chicken meat is an infection source of *Salmonella* serovar Infantis for humans in Japan. *Foodborne Pathogens and Disease* 7, 727–735.

Nurmi, E. and Rantala, M. (1973) New aspects of *Salmonella* infection in broiler production. *Nature* 214, 210–211.

O'Brien, J.D.P. (1988) *Salmonella ententidis* infection in broiler chickens. *Veterinary Record* 122, 214.

Olesiuk, O.M., Carlson, V.L., Snoeyenbos, G.H. and Smyser, C.F. (1969) Experimental *Salmonella typhimurium* infection in two chicken flocks. *Avian Diseases* 13, 500–508.

Oosterom, J. (1991) Epidemiological studies and proposed preventive measures in the fight against human salmonellosis. *International Journal of Food Microbiology* 12, 41–52.

Opara, O.O., Carr, L.E., Rusek-Cohen, E., Tate, C.R., Mallinson, E.T., Miller, R.G., Stewart, L.E., Johnston, R.W. and Joseph, S.W. (1992) Correlation of water activity and other environmental conditions with repeated detection of *Salmonella* contamination on poultry farms. *Avian Diseases* 36, 664–671.

Padron, M.N. (1990) *Salmonella typhimurium* outbreak in broiler chicken flocks in Mexico. *Avian Diseases* 34, 221–223.

Paul, J. and Batchelor, B. (1988) *Salmonella enteritidis* phage type 4 and hens' eggs. *Lancet* ii, 1421.

Perales, I. and Audicana, A. (1988) *Salmonella enteritidis* and eggs. *Lancet* ii, 1133.

Petter, J.G. (1993) Detection of two smooth colony phenotypes in a *Salmonella* enteritidis isolate which vary in their ability to contaminate eggs. *Applied and Environmental Microbiology* 59, 2884–2890.

Philbrook, F.R., MacCready, R.A., Van Roekel, H., Anderson, E.S., Smyser, C.F., Sanen, F.J. and Groton, W.M. (1960) Salmonellosis spread by a dietary supplement of avian source. *New England Journal of Medicine* 263, 713–718.

Plummer, R.A.S., Blissett, S.J. and Dodd, C.E.R. (1995) *Salmonella* contamination of retail chicken products sold in the UK. *Journal of Food Protection* 58, 843–846.

Pomeroy, B.S. (1984) Fowl typhoid. In: Hofstad, M.S., Barnes, H.J., Calnek, B.W., Reid, W.M. and Yoder, H.W. (eds) *Diseases of Poultry*, 8th edn. Iowa State University Press, Ames, Iowa, pp. 79–91.

Poppe, C. and Gyles, C. (1987) Relation of plasmids to virulence and other properties of salmonellae from avian sources. *Avian Diseases* 31, 844–854.

Poppe, C., Irwin, R.J., Forsberg, C.M., Clarke, R.C. and Oggel, J. (1991a) The prevalence of *Salmonella enteritidis* and other *Salmonella* spp. among Canadian registered commercial layer flocks. *Epidemiology and Infection* 106, 259–270.

Poppe, C., Irwin, R.J., Messier, S., Finley, G.G. and Oggel, J. (1991b) The prevalence of *Salmonella enteritidis* and other *Salmonella* spp. among Canadian registered commercial chicken broiler flocks. *Epidemiology and Infection* 107, 201–211.

Poppe, C., McFadden, K.A., Brouwer, A.M. and Demczuk, W. (1993a) Characterization of *Salmonella enteritidis* strains. *Canadian Journal of Veterinary Research* 57, 176–184.

Poppe, C., Demczuk, W., McFadden, K. and Johnson, R.P. (1993b) Virulence of *Salmonella enteritidis* phage types 4, 8, and 13 and other *Salmonella* spp. for day-old chicks, hens and mice. *Canadian Journal of Veterinary Research* 57, 281–287.

Rampling, A., Anderson, J.R., Upson, R., Peters, E., Ward, L.R. and Rowe, B. (1989) *Salmonella enteritidis* phage type 4 infection of broiler chickens - a hazard to public health. *Lancet* ii, 436–438.

Read, D.H., Kinde, H. and Daft, B.M. (1994) Pathology of *Salmonella enteritidis* phage type 4 infection in commercial layer chickens in southern California. In: *Proceedings of the 44th Meeting of the Western Poultry Disease Conference,* Sacramento, California, 5–7 March 1995, pp. 76–78.

Reilly, W.J., Forbes, G.I., Sharp, J.C.M., Oboegbulem, S.I., Collier, P.W. and Paterson, G.M. (1988) Poultry-borne salmonellosis in Scotland. *Epidemiology and Infection* 101, 115–122.

Renwick, S.A., Irwin, R.J., Clarke, R.C., McNab, W.B., Poppe, C. and McEwen, S.A. (1992) Epidemiological associations between characteristics of registered broiler chicken flocks in Canada and the *Salmonella* culture status of floor litter and drinking water. *Canadian Veterinary Journal* 33, 449–458.

Rettger, L.F. (1900) Fatal septicaemia among young chicks. *New York Medical Journal* 71, 803–805.

Rettger, L.F. (1909) Further studies on fatal septicaemia in young chickens, or 'white diarrhoea'. *Journal of Medical Research* 21, 115–123.

Revolledo, L., Ferreira, C.S. and Ferreira, A.J. (2009) Prevention of *Salmonella* Typhimurium colonization and organ invasion by combination treatment in broiler chicks. *Poultry Science* 88, 734–743.

Rigby, C.E. and Pettit, J.R. (1979) Some factors affecting *Salmonella typhimurium* infection and shedding in chickens raised on litter. *Avian Diseases* 23, 442–455.

Rivoal, K., Protais, J., Quéguiner, S., Boscher, E., Chidaine, B., Rose, V., Gautier, M., Baron, F., Grosset, N., Ermel, G. and Salvat, G. (2009) Use of pulsed-field gel electrophoresis to characterize the heterogeneity and clonality of *Salmonella* serotype Enteritidis, Typhimurium and Infantis isolates obtained from whole liquid eggs. *International Journal of Food Microbiology* 129, 180–186.

Roberts, D. (1991) *Salmonella* in chilled and frozen chicken. *Lancet* 337, 984–985.

Rodrigue, D.C., Tauxe, R.V. and Rowe, B. (1990) International increase in *Salmonella* enteritidis: a new pandemic? *Epidemiology and Infection* 105, 21–27.

Sadler, W.W., Brownell, J.R. and Fanelli, M.J. (1969) Influence of age and inoculum level on shed pattern of *Salmonella typhimurium* in chickens. *Avian Diseases* 13, 793–803.

Saeed, A.M. (1999) Salmonella enterica *Serovar enteritidis* in *Humans and Animals: Epidemiology, Pathogenesis and Control.* Iowa State University Press, Ames, Iowa.

Saeed, A.M. and Koons, C.W. (1993) Growth and heat resistance of *Salmonella enteritidis* in refrigerated and abused eggs. *Journal of Food Protection* 56, 927–931.

Salem, M., Odor, E.M. and Pope, C. (1992) Pullorum disease in Delaware roasters. *Avian Diseases* 36, 1076–1080.

Sasaki, Y., Murakam, M., Maruyama, N., Tsujiyama, Y., Kusukawa, M., Asai, T. and Yamada, Y. (2012) Risk factors for *Salmonella* prevalence in laying-hen farms in Japan. *Epidemiology and Infection* 140, 982–990.

Schaaf, J. (1936) Die Salmonellose (infektiöse Enteritis, Paratyphose) des Geflügels, ihre Bedeutung und Bekämpfung. *Zeitschrift für Infektionskrankheiten, Parasitäre Krankheiten und Hygiene der Haustiere* 49, 322–332.

Schaffer, J.M., MacDonald, A.D., Hall, W.J. and Bunyea, H. (1931) A stained antigen for the rapid whole blood test for pullorum disease. *Journal of the American Veterinary Medical Association* 79, 236–240.

Seeliger, H.P.R. and Maya, A.E. (1964) Epidemiologie der Salmonellosen in Europa 1950-1960. In: van Oye, E. (ed.) *The World Problem of Salmonellosis.* W. Junk Publishers, The Hague, pp. 245–294.

Setta, A.M., Barrow, P.A., Kaiser, P. and Jones, M.A. (2012a) Early immune dynamics following infection with *Salmonella enterica* serovars Enteritidis, Infantis, Pullorum and Gallinarum: Cytokine and chemokine gene expression profile and cellular changes of chicken cecal tonsils. *Comparative Immunology Microbiology and Infectious Diseases* 35, 397–410.

Setta, A., Barrow, P.A., Kaiser, P. and Jones, M.A. (2012b) Immune dynamics following infection of avian macrophages and epithelial cells with typhoidal and non-typhoidal *Salmonella enterica* serovars; bacterial invasion and persistence, nitric oxide and oxygen production, differential host gene expression, NF-κB signalling and cell cytotoxicity. *Veterinary Immunology and Immunopathology* 146, 212–224.

Seuna, E., Nagaraja, K.V. and Pomeroy, B.S. (1985) Gentamicin and bacteria culture (Nurmi culture) treatments either alone or in combination against experimental *Salmonella hadar* infection in turkey poults. *Avian Diseases* 29, 617–629.

Shah, D.H., Lee, M.J., Park, J.H., Lee, J.H., Eo, S.K., Kwon, J.T. and Chae, J.S. (2005) Identification of *Salmonella gallinarum* virulence genes in a chicken infection model using PCR-based signature-tagged mutagenesis. *Microbiology* 151, 3957–3968.

Shivaprasad, H.L. (2000) Fowl Typhoid and Pullorum Disease. *Scientific and Technical Review of the Office International des Epizooties* 19, 405–424.

Shivaprasad, H.L. (2008) Arizonosis. In: Saif, Y.M. *et al.* (eds) *Diseases of Poultry*, 12th edn. Blackwell Publishing, Ames, Iowa, pp. 665–674.

Shivaprasad, H.L. and Barrow, P.A. (2008) Pullorum Disease and Fowl Typhoid. In: Saif, Y.M. *et al.* (eds) *Diseases of Poultry*, 12th edn. Blackwell Publishing, Ames, Iowa, pp. 620–636.

Shivaprasad, H.L., Cortes, P. and Crespo, R. (2006) Otitis interna (Labyrinthitis) associated with *Salmonella enterica arizonae* in turkey poults. *Avian Diseases* 50, 135–138.

Silva, E.M., Snoeyenbos, G.H., Wienack, O.M. and Smyser, C.F. (1981) Studies on the use of 9R strain of *Salmonella gallinarum* as a vaccine in chickens. *Avian Diseases* 25, 38–52.

Singh, P., Foley, S.L., Nayak, R. and Kwon, Y.M. (2012) Multilocus sequence typing of *Salmonella* strains by high-throughput sequencing of selectively amplified target genes. *Journal of Microbiological Methods* 88, 127–133.

Smith, H.W. and Tucker, J.F. (1975) The effect of antibiotic therapy on the faecal excretion of *Salmonella typhimurium* by experimentally infected chickens. *Journal of Hygiene (London)* 75, 275–292.

Smith, H.W. and Tucker, J.F. (1980) The virulence of *Salmonella* strains for chickens; their excretion by infected chicken. *Journal of Hygiene, Cambridge* 84, 479–488.

Snoeyenbos, G.H. (1984) Pullorum disease. In: Hofstad, M.S., Barnes, H.J., Calnek, B.W., Reid, W.M. and Yoder, H.W. (eds) *Diseases of Poultry*, 8th edn. Iowa State University Press, Ames, Iowa, pp. 66–79.

Snoeyenbos, G.H., Carlson, V.L., Smyser, C.F. and Olesiuk, O.M. (1969) Dynamics of *Salmonella* infection in chicks reared on litter. *Avian Diseases* 13, 72–83.

Sojka, W.J., Wray, C., Hudson, E.B. and Benson, J.A. (1975) Incidence of *Salmonella* infection in animals in England and Wales, 1968-73. *Veterinary Record* 96, 280–287.

Steinert, L., Virgil, D., Bellemore, E., Williamson, B., Dinda, E., Harris, D., Scheider, D., Fanella, L., Bogacki, V., Liska, F., Birkhead, G.S., Guzewich, J.J., Fudala, J.K., Kondracki, S.F., Shayegani, M., Morse, D.L., Dennis, D.T., Healey, B., Tavris, D.R., Duffy, M. and Drinnen, K. (1990) Update: *Salmonella enteritidis* infections and grade A shell eggs - United States, 1989. *Morbidity and Mortality Weekly Report* 38, 877–880.

Stevens, A., Joseph, C., Bruce, H., Fenton, D., O'Mahony, M., Cunningham, D., O'Connor, B. and Rowe, B. (1989) A large outbreak of *Salmonella enteritidis* phage type 4 associated with eggs from overseas. *Epidemiology and Infection* 103, 425–433.

St Louis, M.E., Morse, D.L., Potter, M.E., DeMelfi, T.M., Guzewich, J.J., Tauxe, R.V., Blake, P.A and the *Salmonella enteritidis* Working Group (1988) The emergence of grade A eggs as a major source of *Salmonella enteritidis* infections. *Journal of the American Medical Association* 259, 2103–2107.

Tannock, G.W. and Smith, J.M.B. (1971) Studies on the survival of *Salmonella typhimurium* and *Salmonella bovis- morbificans* on pasture and in water. *Australian Veterinary Journal* 47, 557–559.

Taylor, M., Leslie, M., Ritson, M., Stone, J., Cox, W., Hoang, L. and Galanis, E. (2012) Investigation of the Concurrent Emergence of *Salmonella enteritidis* in Humans and Poultry in British Columbia, Canada, 2008-2010. *Zoonoses and Public Health* 10.1111.

Telzak, E.E., Budnick, L.D., Zweig Greenberg, M.S., Blum, S., Shayegani, M., Benson, C.E. and Schultz, S. (1990) A nosocomial outbreak of *Salmonella enteritidis* infection due to the consumption of raw eggs. *New England Journal of Medicine* 323, 394–397.

Thain, J.A. and Blandford, T.B. (1981) A long-term serological study of a flock of chickens naturally infected with *Salmonella pullorum*. *Veterinary Record* 109, 136–138.

Thiagarajan, D., Saeed, A.M. and Asem, E.K. (1994) Mechanism of transovarian transmission of *Salmonella enteritidis* in laying hens. *Poultry Science* 73, 89–98.

Thiagarajan, D., Saeed, M., Turek, J. and Asem, E. (1996) *In vitro* attachment and invasion of chicken ovarian granulosa cells by *Salmonella enteritidis* phage type 8. *Infection and Immunity* 64, 5015–5021.

Tietjen, M. and Fung, D.Y.C (1995) Salmonellae and food safety. *Critical Reviews in Microbiology* 21, 53–83.

Timms, L.M., Marshall, R.N. and Breslin, M.F. (1990) Laboratory assessment of protection given by an experimental *Salmonella enteritidis* PT4 inactivated, adjuvant vaccine. *Veterinary Record* 127, 611–614.

Timoney, J.F., Shivaprasad, H.L., Baker, R.C. and Rowe, B. (1989) Egg transmission after infection of hens with *Salmonella enteritidis* phage type 4. *Veterinary Record* 125, 600–601.

Truscott, R.B. (1981) Oral *Salmonella* antigens for the control of *Salmonella* in chicks. *Avian Diseases* 25, 810–820.

Tucker, J.F. (1967) Survival of salmonellae in built-up litter for housing of rearing and laying fowls. *British Veterinary Journal* 123, 92–103.

Turnbull, P.C.B. and Snoeyenbos, G.H. (1973) Experimental salmonellosis in the chicken I. Fate and host response in alimentary canal, liver, and spleen. *Avian Diseases* 18, 153–177.

Turner, A.K., Lovell, M.A., Hulme, S.D., Zhang-Barber, L. and Barrow, P.A. (1998) Identification of *Salmonella typhimurium* genes required for colonization of the alimentary tract and for virulence in newly hatched chickens. *Infection and Immunity* 66, 2099–2106.

van de Giessen, A.W., Peters, R., Berkers, P.A.T.A., Jansen, W.H. and Notermans, S.H.W. (1991) *Salmonella* contamination of poultry flocks in The Netherlands. *Veterinary Quarterly* 13, 41–46.

van de Giessen, A.W., Dufrenne, J.B., Ritmeester, W.S., Berkers, P.A.T.A., van Leeuwen, W.J. and Notermans, S.H.W. (1992) The identification of *Salmonella enteritidis*-infected poultry flocks associated with an outbreak of human salmonellosis. *Epidemiology and Infection* 109, 405–411.

Wales, A.D. and Davies, R.H. (2011) A critical review of *Salmonella* Typhimurium infectivity in laying hens. *Avian Pathology* 40, 429–436.

Wallis, T.S. and Galyov, E.E. (2000) Molecular basis of *Salmonella*-induced enteritis. *Molecular Microbiology* 36, 997–1005.

Wierup, M., Wold-Troell, M., Nurmi, E. and Hakkinen, M. (1987) Epidemiological evaluation of the *Salmonella* controlling effect of a nationwide use of a ‘competitive exclusion’ culture in poultry. In: *Proceedings of an International Workshop on Competitive Exclusion of Salmonellas from Poultry*, Bristol Laboratory, Langford, UK, p. 7.

Wigley, P., Hulme, S.D., Powers, C., Beal, R.K., Berchieri, A. Jr, Smith, A. and Barrow, P. (2005) Infection of the reproductive tract and eggs with *Salmonella enterica* serovar pullorum in the chicken is associated with suppression of cellular immunity at sexual maturity. *Infection and Immunity* 73, 2986–2990.

Williams, J.E. (1981) Salmonellas in poultry feeds – a worldwide review. Methods in isolation and identification. *World's Poultry Science Journal* 37, 19–25.

Williams, J.E., Dillard, L.H. and Hall, G.O. (1968) The penetration patterns of *Salmonella typhimurium* through the outer structures of chicken eggs. *Avian Diseases* 12, 445–466.

Withanage, G.S., Sasai, K., Fukata, T., Miyamoto, T., Lillehoj, H.S. and Baba, E. (2003) Increased lymphocyte subpopulations and macrophages in the ovaries and oviducts of laying hens infected with *Salmonella enterica* serovar Enteritidis. *Avian Pathology* 32, 583–590.

Withanage, G.S.K., Kaiser, P., Wigley, P., Powers, C., Mastroeni, P., Brooks, H., Barrow, P.A., Smith, A., Maskell, D.J. and McConnell, I. (2004) Rapid expression of chemokines and pro-inflammatory cytokines in newly hatched chickens infected with *Salmonella enterica* serovar Typhimurium. *Infection and Immunity* 72, 2152–2159.

Wray, C. (1985) Is salmonellosis still a serious problem in veterinary practice? *Veterinary Record* 116, 485–489.

Xu, Y.M., Pearson, G.R. and Hinton, M. (1988) The colonization of the alimentary tract and visceral organs of chicks with salmonellas following challenge via the feed – bacteriological findings. *British Veterinary Journal* 144, 403–404.

Yang, B., Qu, D., Zhang, X., Shen, J., Cui, S., Shi, Y., Xi, M., Sheng, M., Zhi, S. and Meng, J. (2010) Prevalence and characterization of *Salmonella* serovars in retail meats of marketplace in Shaanxi, China. *International Journal of Food Microbiology* 141, 63–72.

10 *Salmonella* Infections in Turkeys

Hafez Mohamed Hafez*
Free University of Berlin, Department of Veterinary Medicine, Institute of Poultry Diseases, Germany

Introduction

Salmonellosis and *Salmonella* infections in turkey are distributed worldwide and result in severe economic losses when no effort is made to control them. The large economic losses are caused by high poult mortality during the first weeks of age, high medication costs, reductions in egg production in breeder flocks, poor poult quality and high costs for eradication and control measures. The most important aspect, however, is the continuing effect of *Salmonella*-contaminated turkey meat and meat-products on public health.

The economic costs of salmonellosis in humans as well as for the poultry industry are enormous. This includes absence from work and medical treatment in humans as well as the expense of investigations, control measures, disposal of contaminated material, lost leisure-time spending and other costs in poultry.

In turkeys as well as in chickens a distinction is usually made between infections caused by the two non-motile host-adapted serovars of *Salmonella* (*S.*) Pullorum (pullorum disease) and *S.* Gallinarum (fowl typhoid), and the remainder of the motile *Salmonella* (paratyphoid infection) including the *S.* subsp. *arizonae* subgenera (arizonosis).

Historical Perspective

The first case of paratyphoid infection in domestic poultry was reported by Moore (1895), who described an outbreak of infectious enteritis in pigeons due to a bacillus of the hog cholera group. The first occurrence of paratyphoid infections (PT) in turkey poults was reported by Pfaff (1921) in the USA. Pomeroy and Fenstermacher (1939) observed the infection in Minnesota turkeys in 1932. Paratyphoid infections cause major losses predominantly in young poults and Hinshaw and McNeil (1940) found that *S.* Typhimurium accounted for approximately 50% of the PT outbreaks in turkeys which they investigated.

The causative agent of pullorum disease was first isolated by Rettger in 1899. In 1909 he named it *Bacterium pullorum* (Rettger, 1909) and later changed it to *S.* Pullorum. Pullorum disease in turkey was first described in 1928 by Hewitt. According to Hinshaw and McNeil (1940), the infection appeared to be introduced

* Author, e-mail: hafez@zedat.fu-berlin.de

© CAB International 2013. *Salmonella in Domestic Animals, 2nd Edition* (eds P.A. Barrow and U. Methner)

into turkeys by contact with infected chickens in hatcheries and/or by brooding chicks and poults together. Likewise contact with chickens or yards used by chickens is an important factor in the spread of fowl typhoid to turkeys. Pfeiler and Roepke (1917) and other authors reported the disease in turkeys reared on farms where it was also prevalent in chickens.

The first description of an organism now classified as *S.* Arizonae was by Caldwell and Ryerson (1939) in which attention was drawn to a bacterium isolated from diseased chuckwallas, horned lizards and gila monsters. The first reports of *S.* Arizonae in turkeys were by Peluffo *et al.* (1942) and Edwards *et al.* (1943). Later Hinshaw and McNeil (1946) isolated Arizona serotype 7:1,7,8 now classified as O18:$_{Z4:Z32}$ and O18:$_{Z4:Z23}$ from a number of outbreaks in poults and showed that all infections were traceable to eggs produced in a defined area in California.

In poultry the genus *Salmonella* of the family *Enterobacteriaceae*, which includes more than 2500 serovars, can roughly be classified into three categories or groups:

1. **Group 1.** Highly host-adapted and invasive serovars: this group includes species restricted and invasive *Salmonella* such as *S.* Pullorum, *S.* Gallinarum in poultry and *S.* Typhi in humans.
2. **Group 2.** Non-host-adapted and invasive serovars: this group consists of approximately 10–20 serovars that are able to cause an invasive infection in poultry and may be capable of infecting humans. Currently, the most important serovars are *S.* Enteritidis, *S.* Typhimurium, *S.* Hadar, *S.* Heidelberg, *S.* Saintpaul and *S.* Infantis.
3. **Group 3.** Non-host-adapted and non-invasive serovars: most serovars of the genus *Salmonella* belong to this group and may cause disease in humans and other animals.

Aetiology

Salmonella belong to the family *Enterobacteriaceae* and all members are gram-negative, non-sporing rods that do not have capsules. According to the latest nomenclature, which reflects recent advances in *Salmonella* taxonomy, the genus *Salmonella* consists of two species: *Salmonella bongori and S. enterica*. *Salmonella enterica* is divided into the following six subspecies: *S. enterica* subsp. *enterica*, *S. enterica* subsp. *salamae*, *S. enterica* subsp. *arizonae*, *S. enterica* subsp. *diarizonae*, *S. enterica* subsp. *houtenae* and *S. enterica* subsp. *indica*. There are also regular changes to serovar classifications as new evidence on genetic relatedness becomes available, e.g. *S.* Pullorum is now classified as *S.* Gallinarum biovar Pullorum and *S.* Thomasville is designated as an antigenic variant of *S.* Orion (Le Minor and Popoff, 1987; Grimont and Weill, 2007) (see Chapter 1, this volume). Beside the conventional phenotyping several modern molecular biological tests for genotyping of *Salmonella* have been developed (Brunner *et al.*, 1983; Eisenstein, 1990; Bailey, 1998; Eyigor and Carli, 2003; Fratamico, 2003).

Epidemiology

Many different *Salmonella* serovars have been isolated from turkeys; however, their exact number is difficult to estimate. Some serovars may be predominant for a number of years in a region or countries and then disappear to be replaced by another serovar. For example, *Salmonella* surveillance in commercial turkey flocks in Germany was carried out between 1993 and 1995 by Hafez *et al.* (1997), whose results showed that the most frequently isolated serovars were *S.* Newport (34.6%) and *S.* Reading (30.3%) followed by *S. Bredeney* (10.6%). *Salmonella* Enteritidis phage type 8 was detected only for a short period (5 weeks) in one flock. *Salmonella* shedding was of intermittent duration and varied between 1 and 20 weeks. In eight out of 24 monitored meat turkey flocks *Salmonella* could not be detected during the entire rearing period. Seven flocks (29.2%) appeared to be infected with only one serovar and in another three flocks (12.5%) two different serovars were isolated during the rearing period, in some cases concurrently. More than two serovars could be detected in the remaining six flocks (25.0%).

Recently, Hafez (2011) monitored 10,243 fattening turkey flocks in Germany for *Salmonella* between 2001 and 2009. Two boot swab samples were collected from each monitored flock 3 weeks prior to slaughtering and examined bacteriologically. The results obtained showed a continuous reduction in the prevalence of all *Salmonella* serovars during that time. From 2002 to 2004 a strong reduction was observed from 18.1% positive flocks to 5%. Between 2007 and 2009 the number of positive tested flocks varied from 3.2% to 5.0%. The prevalence of *S.* Typhimurium showed a similar reduction. *Salmonella* Enteritidis could not be detected in any samples examined since 2006. Papadopoulou *et al.* (2009) summarized data from the scanning surveillance of turkey flocks in Great Britain for *Salmonella* from 1995 to 2006 and compared them with trends in other livestock and animal feed. *Salmonella* Typhimurium was the predominant serovar. The peak of this serovar in turkeys in the late 1990s occurred in parallel with the *S.* Typhimurium DT104 epidemic in other livestock species, especially cattle and pigs. *Salmonella* Enteritidis reports peaked in the mid- to late 1990s, but decreased considerably after 2000. This decrease was also seen in flocks of domestic fowl. On the other hand they reported an increase in *S.* Kottbus and *S.* Kedougou incidence during the last 3–5 years of the investigation period.

In the EU and Norway the most frequently isolated serovars in fattening turkey flocks between 2006 and 2007 were *S.* Bredeney (16.5%), *S.* Hadar (12.9%), *S.* Saintpaul (10.9%), *S.* Derby 9.8%), *S.* Kottbus (7.5%), *S.* Typhimurium (7.1%), *S.* Ohio (6.0%), *S.* Infantis (5.3%) and *S.* Enteritidis (3.1%) (EFSA, 2008).

Transmission

Transmission and spread of *Salmonella* occurs by vertical and/or horizontal routes. The true-vertical transmission occurs primarily by ovarian transmission, by passage through the oviduct or by contact with infected peritoneum or air sacs (Cherrington *et al.*, 1937). Pseudo vertical transmission happens by contamination of the egg content as a result of faecal contamination of the eggshell from cloaca and/or contaminated nests, floor or incubators, with subsequent penetration into the eggs (Pomeroy and Fenstermacher, 1941; Stokes *et al.*, 1956); this pseudo-vertical transmission has similar outcomes to true-vertical transmission.

True-vertical transmission is the most important route of infection in turkey for *S. Gallinarum*, *S.* Pullorum (Snoeyenbos, 1991), *S.* Arizonae, *S.* Senftenberg (Kumar *et al.*, 1971), *S.* Typhimurium (Lee *et al.*, 1936), *S.* Enteritis and *S.* Hadar (Mayer *et al.*, 1984). Williams and Dillard (1968) found that unpigmented turkey eggs were more frequently penetrated by *S.* Typhimurium than normal pigmented eggs. Such unpigmented eggs have thinner shells and larger pores. Within the above mentioned invasive *Salmonella* serovars a significant variation between the strains and among the same serovars exists (Saeed *et al.*, 2006). In addition, Iaffaldano *et al.* (2010) reported about the possibility of transmission of *Salmonella* spp. to breeder flocks by use of contaminated cryopreserved semen artificially contaminated with *S.* Liverpool, *S.* Montevideo and *S.* Braenderup. Donoghue *et al.* (2004) evaluated the efficacy of semen extenders to reduce or eliminate pathogens; pooled ejaculates were contaminated with *Campylobacter* or *Salmonella* and treated with commercial poultry extenders containing various concentrations of antibiotics or an antibiotic combination previously demonstrated to remove *Campylobacter* from mammalian semen. The results obtained revealed that commercial turkey semen may contain *Campylobacter* or *Salmonella*, and the semen extenders tested either did not reduce the bacteria or resulted in a reduction but not elimination of these bacteria from semen.

Hatcheries are one of the major sources for early horizontal transmission. Horizontal spread of *Salmonella* occurring during hatching was shown in chickens, when contaminated and *Salmonella*-free eggs were incubated together (Jodas, 1992; Cason *et al.*, 1994). Hatched birds may become infected by aerosols containing *Salmonella* (Baskerville *et al.*, 1992; Agabou, 2009). *Salmonella* can also spread through the hatchery by means of contamination of ventilation ducting, belt slots or door seals within hatchers, but may also result from infection and contamination that continuously recycles between hatchers, hatched birds, dust and crate-washing equipment (Davies and Wray 1994; Davies and Bedford, 2001). *Salmonella* spp. can persist for many years within the hatchery (Friend and Franson, 1999). Hoover *et al.* (1997) examined poult-box liners and poults at day 0 on the arrival to the commercial farm and revealed positive *Salmonella* results. They concluded that *Salmonella* contamination may have been acquired from the breeder flocks or the hatchery. Jodas and Hafez (2002) reported on the isolation of *S.* Enteritidis PT4 in a turkey hatchery in 7 out of 231 examined meconium samples. In addition, *S.* Enteritidis was detected in 10 out of 112 tested fluff samples, 2 out of 70 investigated eggs and in 6 out of 306 tested day-old poults. From 146 environmental swabs collected at the hatchery *S.* Enteritidis could not be isolated. Immediately after the first *S.* Enteritidis isolation in the hatchery all turkey breeder flocks, which belonged to the hatchery owner, were intensively bacteriologically examined. From two out of three examined breeder flocks (52–53 weeks of age) and from one brooding flock (6 weeks old) *S.* Enteritidis was isolated.

During rearing the infection is transmitted horizontally by direct contact between infected and uninfected turkeys, and by indirect contact with contaminated environments through ingestion or inhalation of *Salmonella* organisms. Subsequently, there are many possibilities for lateral spread of the organisms through live and dead vectors. Transmission frequently occurs via faecal contamination of feed, water, equipment, environment and dust in which *Salmonella* can survive for long periods. Failure to clean and disinfect properly after an infected flock has left the site can result in infection of the next batch of birds. *Salmonella* have been reported to survive in turkey litter for up to 9 months after removal of an infected flock. *Salmonella* colonization of turkey flocks and the spread of *Salmonella* within the environment were extensive once initial contamination of the production house occurred. Drinkers, feeders, litter and air were critical sources of horizontal transmission within each pen as well as between pens (Hoover *et al.*, 1997).

Significant reservoirs for *Salmonella* are human, farm animals, water fowl and wild birds. Rodents, pet's insects and litter beetles are also potential reservoirs and transmit the infection to birds and between houses. The organisms are often localized in the gut of these carriers, which shed *Salmonella* intermittently in their faeces thus contaminating the poultry environment. Rodents constitute a persistent reservoir of *Salmonella* infection from which poultry houses and stored feeding stuffs must be protected as far as possible (Kumar *et al.*, 1971; McCapes *et al.*, 1991; Henzler and Opitz, 1992; Skov *et al.*, 2004; Wales *et al.*, 2010).

Probably one of the most common sources for lateral spread of the organisms is feed. Nearly every ingredient ever used in the manufacture of poultry feedstuffs has been shown at one time or another to contain *Salmonella*. The organism occurs most frequently in protein from animal products such as meat and bone meal, blood meal, poultry offal, feather meal and fish meal. Protein of vegetable origin has also been shown to be contaminated with *Salmonella*. Turkey feed samples have been investigated by Bryan *et al.* (1968), Willinger *et al.* (1986) and Hafez *et al.* (1997), who detected *Salmonella* contamination rates between 3% and 9%. Studies in Canada have shown that *Salmonella* are widespread in the environment of turkey farms and Irwin *et al.* (1994) recovered *Salmonella* from 9.8% of feed samples, 79.6% of litter samples and 80.4% of dust samples. Recently, Dutta *et al.* (2010) reported that turkey feed contaminated with *S.* Enteritidis was responsible for a severe outbreak of gastroenteritis in turkeys with a mortality rate of 34.38%.

Factors Influencing the Course of Infection

The course of the infection and the prevalence of salmonellosis in turkeys depend on different factors, such as the *Salmonella* serovar, age of birds, infectious dose and route of infection. Further stress-producing circumstances such as bad management, poor ventilation, high stocking density or concurrent diseases may also contribute to the development of a systemic infection with possible heavy losses among young poults. Koinarski *et al.* (2006) estimated the effect of *Eimeria adenoeides* challenge upon the course of *S.* Enteritidis infection in turkey poults under experimental condition. The highest mortality rate as well as the most frequent and most prolonged isolation of *Salmonella* from parenchymal organs was observed in the group where the *Eimeria* infection preceded the *Salmonella* infection. Generally, after recovery, birds continue to excrete *Salmonella* in their faeces, and such birds must be considered as a potential vector of the microorganisms.

Pullorum Disease

Pullorum disease is an acute systemic disease of young poults, characterized by sudden death and high mortality. The disease is mostly egg transmitted. In adult turkeys the disease is often localized and can cause lifelong latent infections and lead to a decrease in egg production and fertility, as well as hatchability.

Clinical signs

The incubation period is 3 to 5 days. Morbidity and mortality are highly variable from less than 10% to as high as 100%. The first indication of disease by vertical transmission is usually an increase in the number of dead-in-shell poults. Infected hatched poults appear moribund and sudden death without clinical symptoms may occur. Mortality begins to increase around the fourth or fifth day of age with a peak mostly between the second and third week.

The symptoms are not characteristic and are similar to those of paratyphoid infection. Laboured breathing due to pneumonia is commonly observed. Some poults show white diarrhoea with a pasting of feathers round the vent ('pasty vent'). Conjunctivitis, swelling of joints and synovial sheaths as well as lameness may also be observed. In rare instances nervous symptoms have been observed. Survivors are often irregular in size, stunted or poorly feathered and many remain carriers and disseminate the causative agent. Adult turkeys usually show no clinical signs, though some appear unthrifty. Variable degrees of decreased egg production, fertility and hatchability have been observed (Shivaprasad and Barrow, 2008).

Lesions

Salmonella Pullorum may cause severe systemic lesions although their severity is highly variable. Lesions are limited in young poults that die suddenly in the early stages. The liver may be enlarged, congested or discoloured and may be streaked with haemorrhages. Changes are commonly accompanied with small white focal necrosis. Necrotic foci or greyish white nodules are also seen in heart, lungs, gizzard muscle and the caeca. The intestine usually lacks tone and contains an excessive mucous discharge. The caeca may contain a caseous core and sometimes are filled with blood. Peritonitis is frequently manifested and pericarditis may be observed. The yolk sac and its contents reveal slight or no alteration. In more protracted cases the absorption of the yolk sac may be poor and the contents may be of creamy or of pasty consistency. The spleen may be enlarged, the kidneys congested and the ureters may be distended with urates. In septicaemia forms, hyperaemia may also be found in other organs.

In adult birds, the lesions most frequently found in chronic carrier hens are misshapen, pedunculated, discoloured cystic ova, which usually contain oily and caseous material enclosed in a thickened capsule. The ovary may be haemorrhaged with atrophic discoloured follicles. Ovarian and oviduct dysfunction may lead to abdominal ovulation or impassable oviduct, which might lead to extensive peritonitis and adhesions of the abdominal viscera. In male birds, the testes may be atrophied with thickening of tunica albuginea and multiple abscesses. Occasional myocarditis with pericarditis and ascites may also occur in both sexes.

Fowl Typhoid

Fowl typhoid is a septicaemic disease caused by *S.* Gallinarum; the mortality and course of the disease are variable, depending on the virulence of the strain involved.

Clinical signs

The incubation period is about 5 days and the losses may extend over 2–3 weeks with a tendency for recurrence. The initial outbreak is mostly accompanied by high mortality rates of up to 26.5% (Hinshaw, 1930) followed by intermittent recurrence with less severe losses. The clinical symptoms of fowl typhoid in turkeys are similar to those described in pullorum disease and are not characteristic. However, some infected poults show green to greenish yellow diarrhoea with pasting of feathers around the vent, increased thirst, anorexia, somnolence, retarded growth and respiratory distress. In growing and mature turkeys increased thirst, listlessness and a tendency to separate from healthy birds have been observed. Body temperatures increase several degrees to as high as 44°C–45°C just before death.

Lesions

In young poults the lesions resemble those observed in pullorum disease. In peracute cases, post-mortem lesions may be absent and in acute cases subcutaneous blood vessels are injected. The skeletal muscles are congested, dark in colour and often appear as if partially cooked. The heart is swollen and small greyish necrotic foci are seen in the myocardium. The liver is enlarged, friable with necrotic foci and a bronze coloration. The spleen and kidneys are enlarged. The lungs are congested and have small grey areas of focal necrosis. Haemorrhagic enteritis especially in the duodenum and ulceration of the intestine are more or less consistent lesions in turkeys. Usually an increased percentage of large retained yolk sacs are present.In adult carriers there is a predilection for the reproductive organs, and lesions are similar to those described in pullorum disease (Shivaprasad and Barrow, 2008).

Paratyphoid Infection

Infection of avian species with motile *Salmonella*, with the exception of *S.* Arizonae, are designated as paratyphoid (PT) infections and, generally, such infections are more prevalent in turkey than any other avian species. Moran (1959) reported that serovar *S.* Typhimurium was encountered four times more frequently in turkeys than in chickens. This group of infections is one of the most important bacterial diseases in the turkey breeder sector and results in high losses among turkey poults during the first month after hatching with maximum loss occurring in the first 10 days. Among valuable breeder flocks, infections are generally accompanied by severe economic losses because of its chronic nature and the difficulty of eradication. In many cases the infection seriously impairs fertility, hatchability and egg production.

Clinical signs

Incubation periods range from 2 to 5 days. Mortality in young poults varies from negligible to 10–20% and in severe outbreaks may reach 80% or more. The severity of an outbreak in young poults depends on the serovar involved, virulence, degree of exposure, the age of birds (Bierer, 1960), environmental conditions and presence of concurrent infections. The age at which the disease is first observed in poults will depend on whether the poults are infected in the incubator or after being placed in the brooder. In poults infected orally at day 1 of age with 10^8 colony-forming units (cfu) per bird with either *S.* Typhimurium, *S.* Anatum, *S.* Thompson, *S.* Meleagridis or *S.* Chester losses started at

2 days and stopped 8 days post-exposure. The mortality rate ranged between 70 and 90% (Shahata *et al.*, 1984). Similar results were obtained by Mitrovic (1956) and Bierer (1960). On the other hand, neither mortality nor clinical signs were observed after experimental oral infection of 3-day-old poults with either 10^6 cfu per bird *S.* Enteritidis phage type 8 or 4 (Hafez and Stadler, 1997). Poults may be infected from a few days after hatching to maturity. Clinical signs may be absent even if infection occurs in the incubator or a few days after hatching. If infection was egg transmitted or occurred in the incubator there are a lot of unpipped and pipped eggs with dead embryos. Symptoms usually seen in young poults are somnolence, weakness, drooping wings, ruffled feathers and huddling together near heat sources. Many poults that survive for several days will become emaciated, and the feathers around the vent will be matted with faecal material. However, in young poults diarrhoea is not a constant symptom. Lameness caused by arthritis may also be present.

Adult birds usually show little or no evidence of the infection and serve mostly as intestinal or internal organ carriers over long periods. Experimental PT infection has resulted in an acute disease of short duration when the birds showed inappetence, increased water consumption, diarrhoea, dehydration and general listlessness. Also Chaplin and Hamilton (1957) reported synovitis in turkeys infected intravenously with *S.* Thompson. Leg weakness in mature birds is not uncommon. Higgins *et al.* (1944) encountered a flock of 24-week-old turkeys infected with PT in which 10% of the birds were so severely affected with an arthritic condition that they were unsuitable for marketing.

Lesions

Lesions may be entirely absent in extremely severe outbreaks. Birds that die in an acute phase of the disease show a persistent yolk sac, catarrhal and haemorrhagic enteritis, necrotic foci in liver, spleen and heart muscle. Furthermore, congestion of the liver, kidney, gall bladder and heart muscle are the most constant post-mortem findings (Gast, 2008). The pericardial sac is often filled with a straw-coloured fluid. Another common finding is a caseous caecal core, which is sometimes filled with blood. Lung and heart lesions are rare but air-sac involvement is common (Hinshaw, 1959).

In adult turkeys, marked inflammation of the intestine with occasional necrotic ulcers has been observed and in these cases the liver and spleen is usually swollen and congested.

Arizonosis

Arizonosis caused by serovars O18:$_{Z4:Z32}$ and O18:$_{Z4:Z23}$ (formerly 7,1,7,8) is a serious problem in the turkey industry due to high mortality and reduced production and hatchability. The turkey appears to be the primary poultry host for these particular serovars, although the host range for other serovars of *S.* Arizonae is unlimited. The infection is egg transmitted and most of the outbreaks occur in young turkeys during the first 3 weeks of age. The infection can be masked in day-old poults by antibiotic treatment. Crespo *et al.* (2004) investigated the possible relationships between *S.* Arizonae isolated from breeder flocks, hatching eggs and fattening flocks belonging to a single turkey integrator. The presence of common pulsed-field patterns between isolates from breeder flocks, eggs and fattening flocks suggested that *S.* Arizonae was being transmitted vertically from the breeder flock.

Clinical signs

The incubation period ranges between 5 and 10 days. Mortality varies greatly; 3.5–15% is common, although losses up to 90% have been reported. Mortality is generally highest during the first 3 weeks after hatching and may continue through 5 weeks after hatch (Greenfield *et al.*, 1971). In turkeys *S.* Arizonae infection is indistinguishable from other forms of salmonellosis. Young poults appear in poor condition, listless, shivering, huddling near heat sources and sit on their hocks. In addition, diarrhoea with pasting in the vent area, uni- or bilateral blindness as well as nervous disorders like uncoordinated gaits, convulsions, twisted neck and torticollis have been observed in birds with brain lesions (Kowalski and Stephans, 1968). Poor growth and moderate to marked uneven growth in the flock is often seen after the clinical disease has ended.

Shivaprasad *et al.* (2006) reported on inflammation of internal ears (otitis interna) in turkey poults associated with *S. enterica* arizonae. The following clinical signs were observed: paralysis, opisthotonus, torticollis and blindness accompanied with increased mortality. *Salmonella* arizonae was isolated from the brains, eyes, intestines, yolk sacs and livers. They assumed that the *S.* Arizonae infection spread from the brain to the internal ears through the vestibulocochlear nerve.

Clinical signs are rarely found in mature turkeys and they seldom die from the infection (Sato and Adler, 1966). They remain, however, latent carriers and shed the organisms. Infected parent stocks may show decreased egg production, fertility and hatchability (Shivaprasad, 2008).

Lesions

In poults that die with septicaemia, lesions may be absent. Frequently, however, there is an enlarged, congested, mottled, yellow liver with pin-point necrotic foci, distended gall bladder and retained yolk sac. Marked congestion and erosion of the gastrointestinal tract and caseous casts filling the caecal lumen are common findings. Other lesions include accumulation of caseous exudate in air sacs and the abdominal or thoracic cavities.

A small but significant number of poults have eye lesions. The eye usually has a normal cornea but an opaque lens and a cheesy exudate covers the retina. This lesion is not pathognomonic, because it also occurs with PT, aspergillosis or colibacillosis, although it occurs more frequently with arizonosis. Purulent exudate in the meninges, lateral ventricles of the brain, or in the middle and inner ear is seen in birds with central nervous system signs. In adult birds small caseous mesenteric lesions and cystic ovules have been described by Hinshaw and McNeil (1946).

Diagnosis of *Salmonella* Infections in Turkeys

Clinical signs and lesions are of little value in diagnosis, because in many cases the infection is not accompanied with clinical disease or lesions. Accurate diagnosis must be substantiated by isolation, identification of the causative bacteria and/or detection of antibodies using serological examination. In general, however, many factors such as governmental regulation, goal of examinations, cost benefit analysis, equipment facilities, availability of reagents and experiences of the staff are influenced and to some extent limit the choice of the laboratory methods (Hafez, 2001). Currently, isolation of the organism is mostly laid down in legislation. Voluntary control schemes may, however, use serology or other techniques to detect infected flocks

Isolation and Identification

Usually the organism can be detected in hatching eggs, dead-in-shell embryos, heart blood, liver, spleen, kidney, crop, intestinal content, unabsorbed yolk, faeces and environmental samples such as drag swabs, floor litter, nest litter and dust.

Yamamota *et al.* (1961) found *S.* Typhimurium in higher number in caecal faeces than in intestinal faeces after experimental inoculation of bacteria into crop of adult turkey. Faddoul and Fellows (1966) found that in 70% of the positive turkey consignments, *Salmonella* could be isolated only from intestinal tracts, where they have a predilection to establish a chronic infection in the caeca. Hafez and Stadler (1997) inoculated 3-day-old poults orally with 10^6 cfu per bird of *S.* Enteritidis (one group with phage type 8 and the other with phage type 4). Samples of heart, liver, lung, spleen, crop, proventriculus, duodenum, caeca, bursa of Fabricius and bone marrow were collected at 21 days of age and cultured separately for the presence of *Salmonella*. The highest detection rates were obtained by culturing the spleen and caeca. Culturing caseous material covering the retina is useful for the detection of *S.* Arizonae in infected birds (Kowalski and Stephans, 1968).

Method of isolation

A large number of studies on *Salmonella* isolation from poultry flocks and poultry products have been published, however, there is no optimal universal technique and each laboratory is advised to use the methods with which it is familiar. Since the experimental designs concerning the kind of specimens, the *Salmonella* serovars involved and culture procedures have varied widely, it is difficult to compare the results. In addition there is no single, ideal scheme for isolation of all serotypes. According to Fricker (1987):

> It is a foolish person who suggests the use of a single procedure for the isolation of all salmonellas from all types of samples. One must decide upon which medium or media to use in the light of knowledge of the type of sample being studied and the types of *Salmonella* likely to be present.

The type and the amount of sample, and the culture techniques (media, amount of inoculum, temperature and time of incubation) can influence the isolation. The type of sample reflects the degree of contamination with other competing microbes and may indirectly provide some knowledge about the type and number of *Salmonella* in a sample (Hafez, 2001):

- Faeces: highly contaminated with other competing microorganisms;
- Eggs: generally a very small number of *Salmonella* are expected;
- Fresh poultry meat and egg products: the degree of contamination varies widely;
- Frozen products: contain sub-lethally injured *Salmonella*;
- Poultry feed: small number of *Salmonella*, which are unevenly distributed in the sample;
- Environmental samples: contain usually low numbers of *Salmonella*.

In most publications, pre-enrichment followed by selective enrichment and streaking on selective agar is accepted to provide the most satisfactory results.

The World Health Organization (WHO) provided guidelines on detection and monitoring of *Salmonella*-infected poultry flocks with particular reference to *S.* Enteritidis (Wray and Davies, 1994). They recommend the use of buffered peptone water as non-selective pre-enrichment followed by selective enrichment in Rappaport Vassiliadis medium and streaking on xylose lysine desoxycholate and brilliant green agar. In addition, bismuth sulfite agar is an excellent plating medium for isolation of *S.* Arizonae (Mallinson and Snoeyenbos, 1989). Hafez *et al.* (1993) carried out a study in turkey flocks to determine the best technique for isolation of *Salmonella* from turkey faeces using different selective enrichment media. The results revealed that using semi-solid Rappaport-Vassiliadis (Diasalm agar) as selective enrichment gives the best results. Since 2008 samples taken for obligatory monitoring of turkey flocks in the EU should be prepared and tested in accordance with the requirements of the Annex in Commission Regulation (EC) No 584/2008 (EC, 2008) using the method recommended by the Community Reference Laboratory for *Salmonella* in Bilthoven, the Netherlands. The method is described in Annex D of ISO 6579 (2002). This includes a non-selective pre-enrichment stage to revitalize *Salmonella* that may be in a stressed condition and to increase the number of organisms before transfer of an inoculum (0.1 ml after 16–20 h incubation at 37°C) to modified semi-solid Rappaport-Vassiliadis medium (MSRV), supplemented by novobiocin to reduce gram-positive competing organisms, which is incubated at 41.5°C for 48 h. A loop of this growth is streaked on to two selective indicator agars, xylose lysine decarboxylase agar and a second media of choice, although the value of the second media is often debatable (Carrique-Mas *et al.*, 2009) and greater detection could normally be achieved by testing more samples with a single plate method (Carrique-Mas and Davies, 2008). Suspect colonies are confirmed biochemically and/or by slide agglutination tests and isolates can then be submitted for serotyping and further characterization.

Conventional cultural procedures for hatching eggs using egg yolk, albumen or shell samples have generally resulted in low isolation rates. Other sample and culture techniques such as the 'egg moulding method' described by Baxter-Jones and Wilding (1982) have shown increased isolation rates of *Salmonella* in turkey hatching eggs in comparison with conventional culture methods. Hafez *et al.* (1986) described a further modification using enrichment media in empty egg shells. The re-isolation rate of *S.* Senftenberg using this method was always higher than examination of yolk and/or albumen alone from artificially contaminated broiler chicken, turkey and quail hatching eggs. Investigation on isolation of *S.* Enteritidis from experimentally contaminated chicken hatching eggs (layer type) using pre-enrichment of empty egg shell samples led to significantly higher detection rates in comparison to the same samples cultured without pre-enrichment after contamination with 10^2 cfu ml^{-1} *S.* Enteritidis (Hafez and Jodas, 1992).

Serological examination

Invasive host-adapted *Salmonella* are generally able to stimulate the production of circulating antibodies and different serological techniques may be used to detect the infection. The advantage of the serological tests over bacteriological examination is that antibodies in serum of infected birds persist for a longer time and the bacteria shedding in faeces of infected birds are intermittent. On the other hand, some poultry with a positive serological response may not be infected with *Salmonella* organisms and poultry in the early stages of infection may be serologically negative.

Several serological tests have been developed for the diagnosis of *Salmonella* infections in turkeys. The rapid whole blood test (WBT), first used in the 1920s by Runnells *et al.* (1927), progressed into a stained antigen slide agglutination test (Schaffer *et al.*, 1931). WBT was shown to be undependable in detecting either pullorum or fowl typhoid in turkeys (Hinshaw and McNeil, 1940; Winter *et al.*, 1952). However, the serum agglutination test (SAT) has been shown to be effective for testing turkey flocks for antibodies against *S.* Typhimurium and *S.* Arizonae infections (Timms, 1971; Kumar *et al.*, 1974). The standard tube agglutination test is used to test turkey serum for pullorum-typhoid, *S.* Typhimurium and *S.* Arizonae infection (DeLay *et al.*, 1954; Mallinson and Snoeyenbos, 1989). Further methods such as microagglutination/microantiglobulin have been used with varying degrees of success (Williams and Whittemore, 1971; Kumar *et al.*, 1977).

In addition, enzyme-linked immunosorbent assay (ELISA) using a variety of antigens, including somatic lipopolysaccharide, flagella, SEF14 fimbriae, outer membrane proteins and crude antigen preparations, has been used especially for detection of *S.* Enteritidis and *S.* Typhimurium carriers in chicken but there is no available literature on the use of these methods in turkey flocks. In general, ELISA provided a satisfactory tool for serological examination of serum as well as egg yolk for antibodies to *S.* Typhimurium, *S.* Enteritidis, *S.* Gallinarum and *S.* Pullorum (Barrow *et al.*, 1996).

Nagaraja *et al.* (1984, 1986) successfully used the outer membrane protein as ELISA antigen for detection of antibodies against *S.* Arizonae infection in turkey breeder flocks. Antigens and macroserological tests for detection of antibodies against *Salmonella* in poultry have been described and discussed elsewhere.

Differential Diagnosis

Young birds with generalized salmonellosis and arizonosis infections may show signs and lesions identical to any acute septicaemia caused by a wide variety of bacteria, including *Escherichia coli*. In severe outbreaks of salmonellosis, liver and heart lesions may be very similar to those seen with secondary invaders in avian mycoplasmosis. Lesions in the caecum may be similar to those caused by *Histomonas meleagridis*; nervous symptoms may resemble those of Newcastle disease, avian influenza, *Ornithobacterium rhinotracheale*, aspergillosis (Hafez and Jodas, 1997) or other diseases affecting the central nervous system. The heavy yellowish white cheesy exudate covering the retina is, as indicated previously, not pathognomic of turkey poults with arizonosis.

Treatment

Generally, the use of antimicrobials will tend to promote the development of antibiotic resistance in bacteria. In addition, according to Commission Regulation (EC) No 1177/2006 (EC, 2006) antimicrobials shall not be used as a specific method to control *Salmonella* in poultry. In some cases, however, the use of antimicrobial can be permitted.

Sensitivity testing of the involved *Salmonella* isolates should be done concurrently with the commencement of medication, because the results of resistance tests in different regions are not comparable and the sensitivity of *Salmonella* varies from time to time. Treatment of salmonellosis in turkeys with antimicrobial drugs is highly effective in reducing mortality and clinical signs, but not for elimination of the infection, if the treatment is administered early in the outbreak. Administration of tetracyclines, neomycin, amoxycillin, trimethoprim/sulfonamide, polymixin B, fluoroquinolones and gentamicin in drinking water, in feed or by injection have been shown to be very effective. However, the majority of survivors become carriers. So far no drug or combination of drugs has been found to be able to eliminate the infection and treat symptomless carriers from treated flocks. Hafez *et al.* (1997) found that the treatment of turkey flocks with different antimicrobials to combat respiratory disease conditions or coccidiosis did not reduce the shedding of *Salmonella* in the faeces of naturally infected flocks. On the other hand, Guillot and Milleman (1990) reported that the use of enrofloxacin appears to be very effective in reducing the intestinal carrier of *S.* Typhimurium after experimental infection. Ekperigin *et al.* (1983) controlled severe outbreaks of disease in flocks of poults caused by a gentamicin-resistant *S.* Arizonae strain by the use of oral and parenteral administration of tetracyclines.

Control of *Salmonella* Infections in Turkeys

In countries with intensive poultry production it has been determined that under current conditions it would be very difficult to eliminate *Salmonella* contamination in poultry production. However, the possibility to eliminate host-specific serovars and to reduce non-host-specific invasive serovars (PT) is realistic (Hafez, 1999, 2005).

In November 2003, the European Parliament Council Regulation 2160/2003/EC (EC, 2003a) on the control of *Salmonella* and other specified food-borne zoonotic agents was passed. This regulation covers the adoption of targets for the reduction of the prevalence of specified zoonoses in animal populations at the level of primary production, including meat turkey. After the relevant control programme has been approved, food business operators must have samples taken and analysed for the zoonoses and zoonotic agents. The flocks should be sampled also by the competent authority.

In June 2008 Commission Regulation (EC) No 584/2008 of implementing Regulation (EC) No 2160/2003 of the European Parliament and of the Council as regards a Community target for the reduction of the prevalence of *S.* Enteritidis and *S.* Typhimurium in turkeys was put into force (EC, 2008). The Community target is the reduction of both *Salmonella* serovars to the maximum percentage of fattening and breeder flocks remaining positive to 1% or less by 31 December 2012. The testing scheme necessary to verify progress in the achievement of the Community target is set out in the Annex of this regulation and should apply from 1 January 2010. All flocks of fattening and breeding turkeys should be investigated on the initiative of the food business operator within 3 weeks before the birds are moved to the slaughterhouse. In fattening turkeys at least two pairs of boot/sock swabs shall be taken. For free-range flocks of turkeys, samples shall only be collected in the area inside the house. All boot/sock swabs must be pooled into one sample.

In addition, flocks of breeding turkeys should be investigated during the rearing at day-old, at 4 weeks of age and 2 weeks before moving to the laying phase: during the laying period they are to be investigated at least every third week at the holding or at the hatchery.

Sampling by the competent authority in a breeding turkey flock with at least 250 birds should be carried out as follows:

- Once a year, all flocks or 10% of holdings with at least 250 adult breeding turkeys between 30 and 45 weeks of age but including in any case all holdings where *S.* Enteritidis or *S.* Typhimurium was detected during the previous 12 months and all holdings with elite, great grandparents and grandparent breeding turkeys; this sampling may also take place at the hatchery;
- All flocks on holdings in case of detection of *S.* Enteritidis or *S.* Typhimurium from samples taken at the hatchery by food business operators or within the frame of official controls, to investigate the origin of infection;
- Each time the competent authority considers it necessary.

Sampling by the competent authority in holdings with at least 500 fattening turkeys should be carried out as mentioned for breeding flocks

Specific requirement concerning fresh poultry meat

Starting from 12 December 2010 fresh poultry meat may not be placed on the market for human consumption when *Salmonella* was detected. The criterion laid down does not apply to fresh poultry meat destined for industrial heat treatment or another treatment to eliminate *Salmonella* in accordance with Community legislation on food hygiene (EC, 2003a).

In general, the main strategy for control of *Salmonella* in turkey should include: cleaning the production pyramid from the top by culling infected breeder flocks infected with invasive serovars, hatching egg sanitation and limiting introduction and spread at the farm level and hatchery through good animal husbandry practices (GAHPs). To achieve GAHPs, effective hygiene measures should be applied to poultry houses, their environment and the feed. In addition, reducing *Salmonella* colonization by using feed additives, competitive exclusion or vaccines are further possibilities. All these measures should be considered in the specific governmental legislations as well as legislations related to global trade with live turkeys, hatching eggs and turkey meat.

Clean the production chain from the top

The major strategy to control *Salmonella* in poultry should now be directed to clean the production chain from the top to prevent the vertical transmission of *Salmonella*. The success or failure of any *Salmonella* reduction programme begins at the primary breeder level, which supplies seed stock to most of the world's turkey industry. Breeders must be committed to reduce and eliminate *Salmonella* in their stock and also in grandparent stocks.

Pullorum disease and fowl typhoid have been nearly or totally eradicated from most countries with a modern turkey industry through consequent testing and eradication of the infected breeding flocks. Similar development appears to have been achieved with *S.* Arizonae, *S.* Typhimurium and *S.* Enteritidis in turkey breeding stocks.

In addition, control measures to prevent the introduction and spread of *Salmonella* infection in breeder flocks should concentrate on high standards of animal management with bacteriological and serological monitoring of breeding birds. These measures must be coupled with meticulous attention to all stages of hatching egg production.

All eggs should be collected not less than three times daily and the shells should be disinfected soon after collection on the farm, since the penetration of the shell by microorganisms is particularly rapid. If the bacteria penetrate the shell before the egg reaches the hatchery, it is difficult to find an effective method to counteract such contamination (Clayton *et al.*, 1985). Generally, two methods are used to disinfect turkey hatching eggs under field conditions, namely fumigation or dipping in a solution of detergent or disinfectant.

Fumigation is best done with formaldehyde gas for at least 20 min with a concentration of 35 ml formalin mixed with 17.5 g potassium permanganate and 20 ml water m^{-3} space. Temperature during fumigation must be maintained at a minimum of 20–24°C and relative humidity at 70%. The eggs should be placed in trays that will permit the fumigant to contact as much of the shell surface as possible. After fumigation, hygienic measures should be followed to preclude recontamination. Because of the unpleasant nature of formaldehyde gas and its possible health hazards to the operator, some owners elect to use wet treatments. Different sanitizing solutions are used and most of them are based on chlorine, glutaraldehyde or quaternary ammonium compounds. Weand and Horsting (1978) reported that chlorine, quaternary ammonium compounds and formalin are the most effective and practical disinfectants for sanitizing hatching eggs.

Egg dipping in detergents or in disinfectants is highly effective in greatly reducing or eliminating the bacteria from the shell when performed correctly. However, there is little or no effect on those bacteria that have already penetrated the shell (Baxter-Jones and Wilding, 1981). Manufacturer's instructions for the chemicals used should be followed, particularly those concerning the number of eggs that may be dipped per litre of solution and how often fresh solution has to be provided. Attention also must be directed to the temperature of the detergent, which must be higher than the egg temperature.

Eggs sent to the hatchery should not be dry cleaned as damage to the cuticle increases the risk of subsequent microbial penetration.

Hatcheries must be designed to permit only a one-way flow of traffic from the egg entry room through egg trays, incubation, hatching and holding rooms to the van loading area. The ventilation system must prevent recirculation of contaminated air. Trays used for hatchery should be thoroughly cleaned and disinfected before eggs are placed on them. Fumigation and disinfection programmes should not be used to replace cleanliness but to support it. All eggs should be sanitized on arrival at the hatchery (presetting treatment) using fumigation. Additionally fumigation can be carried out after setting. This provides a final disinfection following handling, transport and various environmental contaminations during storage of hatching eggs. Further fumigations are mostly carried out immediately after the transfer of hatching eggs from setter to the hatch.

Dipping turkey hatching eggs in disinfectant and/or antibiotics using temperature differential dipping (TDD) or pressure differential dipping (PDD) to control egg-transmitted *Salmonella* and other bacterial pathogens has been widely investigated and is of great value. Baxter-Jones and Wilding (1981) pointed out that egg treatment methods to reduce egg-borne *Salmonella* should be: non-antibiotics in order to avoid resistance problems; effective for at least 48 h; neither affect hatchability, nor poult quality, inexpensive, easy to use and safe for the staff. Use of disinfectants in TDD on turkey hatching eggs artificially infected with *S.* Typhimurium resulted in elimination of the infection. Similar results have been obtained by treatment of broiler chicken hatching eggs experimentally infected with *S.* Senftenberg (Mandel *et al.*, 1987). However, application of the TDD and PDD methods using different disinfectants on hatching eggs from layer birds artificially infected with *S.* Enteritidis did not significantly reduce the *S.* Enteritidis re-isolation rate of newly hatched chicks (Jodas, 1992). Lucas *et al.* (1970) dipped infected turkey hatching eggs in kanamycin, neomycin and spectinomycin. The first two were able to significantly reduce *S.* Saintpaul but not *S.* Typhimurium. Investigation by Saif *et al.* (1971) revealed that *S.* Arizonae could be eliminated from artificially infected turkey hatching eggs using the TDD method with gentamicin sulfate. In addition, Saif and Shelly (1973) were able to reduce the re-isolation rate significantly using the TDD method and 1000 ppm gentamicin sulfate on turkey hatching eggs artificially infected with 25 different *Salmonella* strains. To control the egg transmission of *S.* Arizonae, Ghazikhanian *et al.* (1984) dipped preheated turkey hatching eggs for 2–3 min into 400 ppm gentamicin sulfate and 300 ppm quaternary ammonium compound. The eggs were then injected via the small end with 0.6 mg of gentamicin per egg. Results indicated that the proper application of the dual hatching egg treatment with effective antibiotic would totally remove *S.* Arizonae contamination distributed in different segments of hatching eggs.

Techniques and equipment for dipping turkey hatching eggs using PDD in solutions of antibiotics are now commercially available. These methods are largely used for eradication of mycoplasma infection in turkeys and still used to combat other egg-borne infections including *Salmonella*.

Some turkey hatcheries in Germany wash the hatching eggs after delivery with disinfectants, water and then dry them with hot air followed by subsequently dipping in 1000 ppm gentamicin and/or 500 ppm enrofloxacin under reduced pressure of 500 mbar for 5 min. The partial vacuum is then released and the eggs allowed soaking in the antibiotics at atmospheric pressure for a further 10 min. After removal from the dip, eggs are allowed to drain and dry before setting in the incubator.

In a 2-year investigation of parent turkey flocks and the hatchery, different *Salmonella* serovars (Montevideo, Mbandaka, Braenderup and Hadar) were isolated from hatching eggs delivered to the hatchery from four out of six parent flocks examined. Bacteriological examinations of 485 samples collected from the hatchery (dead-in-shell, hatchery debris, meconium, day-old chicks, transport cartons) at 18 different hatching days, failed to isolate *Salmonella*. The possibility of hatching eggshell contamination with isolated *Salmonella* serovars and vertical transmission to hatched poults could not be demonstrated, since all hatching eggs were sanitized by fumigation on the farm and PPD using enrofloxacin at the hatchery (Hafez *et al.*, 1997).

Precautions should be followed, since dipping solutions can become excessively contaminated with resistant microorganisms such as pseudomonads and organic material. To prevent bacterial contamination of the solution, filtering with subsequent cool storage and/or addition of disinfectants is the most effective method. Thorough and continuous bacteriological monitoring of dip solution is also required. The concentration of the antibiotics must be examined regularly and renewed routinely. By using enrofloxacin the pH-value of the dipping solution can be corrected during storage. According to Froyman (1994) the use of egg dipping in antimicrobials should be critically evaluated, because of the irregular uptake of dip solution, uneven distribution of active substance in the egg compartments and lack of standardization in dipping technique.

Additionally, it is known that different disinfectants used for washing can influence negatively the antibiotic uptake of hatching eggs. Therefore, it is recommended that the compatibility of different disinfectants used for egg washing and/or used in dipping solution has to be examined before application (Bickford *et al.*, 1973).

As the uptake of active agent by the hatching egg can be very irregular during dipping, individual egg injection with accurate delivery of the proper dose is preferred in elite and grandparent stock breeding. Automated systems for *in ovo* drug disposition before hatch is being developed and in use in some countries.

Hygienic measures

The biosecurity of farms for *Salmonella* control has to be upgraded to a much higher level than that for disease control. The level of biosecurity should be high, but it is difficult and expensive to maintain a high level of biosecurity at all times and at all production levels. An all-in, all-out principle should be adopted wherever possible. Multiple ages of birds on a farm constitute a serious disease risk, in particular if multiple-age birds are closely associated.

It is important to maintain a very high level of biosecurity at breeder flocks. In general, other animal species such as cattle or pigs must never be present on the farm. Employees should not have or work with other domestic animal species at home. Dogs and cats should not be present in the barns, and no other kinds of poultry should be permitted. Turkey houses should be kept locked and unwanted visitors should have no access to the poultry buildings. Vehicles (feed trucks) could be permitted if the wheels and underside are sprayed with disinfectant (Gazdzinski, 2004). Further precautions related to staff should be taken, by regular bacteriological examination to identify the carriers and to prevent transmission and cross-contamination on the farm.

Cleaning, disinfection and vector control must be integrated in a comprehensive *Salmonella* control programme. When a turkey house is depopulated, all droppings and litter should be removed from the house prior to cleaning. The procedure should be tailored to meet the particular needs. The cleaning and disinfection programme should include time schedule, type of disinfectant and concentration, desired level as well as check and microbiological monitoring of the procedures. Mueller-Doblies *et al.* (2010) compared the efficacy of different disinfection methods in eliminating *Salmonella* contamination from turkey houses. Fifty depopulated turkey houses that had all housed *Salmonella*-positive flocks were visited after cleaning and disinfection. Houses were grouped according to the disinfectant that had been used and the efficacy of the different groups of disinfectants was compared. Of these houses, 68% tested positive for *Salmonella* after cleaning and disinfection. There was no significant difference in the level of residual contamination between breeding, rearing and finishing houses. Products containing a mixture of formaldehyde, glutaraldehyde and quaternary ammonium compounds performed significantly better than products containing hydrogen peroxide and peracetic acid. Cleaning and disinfection was least effective in nest boxes and anterooms. Single disinfection is not sufficient to kill *Salmonella* in the barn environment. It is more effective to use two or three different kinds of disinfectants on different days (chlorine, phenol and formaldehyde). Barn disinfection is not complete if disinfection of water lines and feed lines is not performed. Water lines can be effectively sanitized with 2000 ppm of sodium hypochloride overnight. Feed lines can be disinfected with special feed flush containing 2% propionic acid. Such feed flush should be left for at least 8 h in the feed lines in order to be effective for *Salmonella* disinfection. Effectiveness of disinfection has to be checked by collecting drag swabs from critical 'hot spots' in a barn.

Rodents, especially rats and mice, are particularly important sources of *Salmonella* contamination of poultry houses. An intensive and sustained rodent control is essential and needs to be well planned and routinely performed and its effectiveness should be monitored. Rodent killing by routine baiting and trapping, both inside and outside of the houses, is standard on-farm practice. All baits have to be applied in pipes or plastic boxes. Random placement of baits around the barn is rarely very effective. There are many products on the market, of which the single-dose anticoagulants seem to be the most effective. Traps placed inside the entrance to a barn and in feed rooms play a very important role in the rodent control programme. Monitoring and recording rodent activity and bait consumption is an important part of a rodent control programme (Gazdzinski, 2004).

Wild birds can be carriers of different serovars of *Salmonella*, and so their presence inside barns is not acceptable. Houses should be constructed in a manner that makes it difficult for wild birds to enter. They have to be kept in good repair to prevent entry and nesting. In addition, darkling beetles are important carriers of *Salmonella* and other pathogens of turkeys (Hazeleger *et al.*, 2008). Control of darkling beetles relies on applying insecticides as soon as the birds are moved out of the barn. After cleaning and disinfection leave the house empty for 2–4 weeks before a new flock is placed (Gazdzinski, 2004). Restocking of day-old poults from a known *Salmonella*-free source is important.

Litter to use should be of good quality. Storage of litter, either straw or shavings, must be done in barns with good rodent, wild bird and animal control. Contamination of litter during storage can be a major *Salmonella* source in the turkey industry. Precautions should be taken especially with straw, which can be contaminated in the field. Therefore, at least a 3-month quarantine of straw is recommended instead of using fresh straw. Litter moisture is directly related to *Salmonella* contamination in turkeys. It has been found that low litter surface humidity can lead to low litter surface *Salmonella* contamination and this can lead to low contamination of carcasses. To effectively control *Salmonella* in the litter the following measures are recommended: maintain proper barn ventilation to keep litter at proper moisture level, prevent splashing/leakage from drinkers and use products acidifying litter, particularly around and under drinkers (Gazdzinski, 2004). Vicente *et al.* (2007) suggested that the administration of selected probiotic candidate bacteria in combination with a commercial organic acid may reduce environmental *Salmonella* in turkey houses. Recently, Featherstone *et al.* (2010) investigated the risk factors for *Salmonella* on fattening-turkey farms. The results obtained revealed that a decreased risk of *Salmonella* spp. infection was associated with a history of intestinal illness in the sampled flock, the use of wood shavings as litter, use of disinfectant in the cleaning process, incineration of dead birds on farm and seasonal production.

Feed hygiene

Contaminated feed has long been recognized as the most common source of new *Salmonella* serovars for poultry flocks. Investigations in different countries have shown that many poultry feed ingredients are contaminated with *Salmonella*. The level of contamination frequently varies between the time of feed manufacture and its delivery, which indicates the highly important role of transport in the recontamination of both raw materials and finished feed (McIllroy, 1996). Different approaches have been utilized to reduce the *Salmonella* contamination of feed ingredients as well as finished feed (see Chapter 19, this volume). Häggblom (1993) and Renggli (1996) reviewed the different methods used and the level of decontamination achieved. A review of practical *Salmonella* control measures in animal feed was recently published by Jones (2011). It is important to point out that feeding mush and feed processed in sub-optimal temperatures contributes to higher incidence of *Salmonella* in turkeys. There are different opinions regarding the temperature that is required to kill *Salmonella* in contaminated feed ingredients (Jones, 2011). Contaminated feed ingredients are an important source of *Salmonella* and they can be effectively decontaminated by the pelleting process. However, dust accumulation around the pellet mill can negatively influence this process. Usually the pellet cooler is a major area for recontamination (Gazdzinski, 2004). Therefore, dust control in feed mills is a very critical control point. Preventing recontamination of feed with *Salmonella* is currently the biggest challenge in feed mills. Control of *Salmonella* in the feed using organic acid, formaldehyde or a combination can address the problem of recontamination (Jones, 2011).

Feed additives

Short chain organic acids

Chemical methods have been established to prevent the recontamination of finished feed. Short chain organic acids (formic acid, propionic acid) have been used recently as feed additives. There are two fundamentally different applications: (i) for the decontamination very high acidification is needed (6% propionic acid); and (ii) for the prevention of (re-)contamination lower doses (0.5–0.7%) are required and have been shown to reduce *Salmonella* colonization in birds consuming the treated feed (Cherrington *et al.*, 1991). The antimicrobial effect of the organic acids decontaminates infected feed on contact and, as a further effect, its residual activity prevents subsequent re-infection (Hinton, 1996). The acids do not eliminate *Salmonella* from dry feed but they kill the organisms in the crop of the birds when the feed has been moistened after consumption by the combined effects of the acids, higher water activity and temperature. Berchieri and Barrow (1996) showed that formic and propionic acid in feed was able to reduce significantly the transmission of *S.* Gallinarum strain 9R between birds after experimental infection. Also the morbidity and mortality in 1-week-old birds were significantly lower (33.3%) in a group receiving acid-treated feed compared with 75.6% in a group receiving untreated feed. The results suggest that some protection could be possible against other invasive *Salmonella*, such as *S.* Pullorum, *S.* Enteritidis and *S.* Arizonae and that the treatment might be used to reduce the extent of vertical transmission by these pathogens. Treatment of feed with organic acids must be considered as an important support to good hygiene and husbandry on all production chains.

Carbohydrates

Other feed additives such as carbohydrates (lactose, mannose, galactose, saccharose), which are able to influence the caecal environment by increasing the amount of acid produced by bacterial fermentation thus decreasing the pH, have been found to reduce *Salmonella* colonization (Oyofo *et al.*, 1989; DeLoach *et al.*, 1990). Corrier *et al.* (1991) found that the addition of lactose to the diet of turkey poults decreased the caecal pH and when it was combined with volatile fatty acids (VFA) producing anaerobic caecal microflora markedly increased the concentration of undissociated VFA thus preventing *Salmonella* colonization. Other sugars within more complex carbohydrates have been successful (Bailey *et al.*, 1991). On the other hand, Valancony *et al.* (2001) examined different feed additives (avilamycin, a manno-oligosaccharide prebiotic, a mixture of essential oils and spices, and a mixture of organic acids) for their influence on weight gain and on the caecal colonization of *S.* Typhimurium in turkey poults but did not find any efficacy.

Antimicrobials

For decades it has been generally known that supplementation of poultry feed with antibiotic growth promoters (AGPs) improves performance of livestock. The effect of AGP on the gut flora results in a more stable balance of the microbial population, an improvement of digestion and better absorption of nutrients. As a consequence this is accompanied with reduced intestinal disorders. The antibiotics not only affect *Salmonella* but also several types of gut flora that are inhibitory for *Salmonella*. Few antimicrobials are effective in reducing faecal shedding and they may prolong excretion. However, AGP can also increase the prevalence of drug-resistant bacteria. Due to concerns about increased prevalence of drug-resistant bacteria, the EU decided to ban the use of AGPs in feed of food-producing animals completely by January 2006 (EC, 2003b).

Probiotics

Probiotics are products that are able to proliferate in the intestinal tract and beneficially affect the host animal by improving its intestinal microbial balance and consequently enhance the growth, production and the health of farm animals. The word probiotic is derived from the Greek meaning 'for life' (Fuller, 1992). These products are mainly composed of lactobacilli, streptococci, bifidobacteria, bacilli and yeasts. These microorganisms are able to inhibit growth of potentially pathogenic microorganisms by lowering the pH through production of lactate, lactic acid and VFA (Mulder, 1996). The use of probiotics in chickens was reviewed by Barrow (1992).

In turkey, the *in ovo* inoculation at the time of transfer of embryonated eggs from the setter to the hatcher or spray application of *Lactobacillus reuteri* have beneficial effects in promoting greater viability associated with enhanced colonization of the caecum with *L. reuteri* and more rapid shedding of *Salmonella* when the birds were challenged with either *S.* Typhimurium or *S.* Senftenberg at hatch or 1 day after hatch (Edens *et al.*, 1991).

Casas *et al.* (1993) reported the use of *L. reuteri* in turkey under field conditions. Three applications using spray formulation in hatchery, the first at 15% pipping (26 days on incubation), the second at 40–60% pipping and the third at 12 h before taking the poults out of the hatcher, resulted in good protection against in-hatcher contamination with *S.* Typhimurium. Feed application to meat turkey resulted in improved viability, body weight and feed conversion. Similar results have been found by Damron *et al.* (1981). Improvement of body weight and feed intake was reported in male turkeys at 20 weeks of age (Jirophocaked *et al.*, 1990) after using dried *Bacillus subtilis* culture. Vicente *et al.* (2007) studied the efficacy of two probiotic culture candidates to reduce environmental *Salmonella* in commercial turkey flocks 2 weeks prior to processing, with or without the use of a commercial organic acid. The results obtained revealed that the administration of selected probiotic candidate bacteria in combination with organic acid may reduce environmental *Salmonella* contamination in turkey houses. Wolfenden *et al.* (2011) evaluated the efficacy of two *Bacillus* isolates as probiotics (*Bacillus laterosporus* and *Bacillus subtilis*) using turkey poults raised under commercial conditions. These isolates were shown to significantly increase body weight gain and decrease the level of colonization of *Salmonella* organisms. On the other hand, Johannsen *et al.* (2004) did not find any colonization-inhibition effect of *Lactobacillus acidophilus* against *S.* Typhimurium in domestic turkey.

Competitive exclusion

Competitive exclusion (CE), also named 'Nurmi concept' or exclusion flora, in combination with conventional hygienic measures has been shown to be very effective as a preventive measure against *Salmonella* infection in poultry. CE is a culture from an undefined mixture of microorganisms from the crop and intestinal tract contents of adult birds (Nurmi and Rantala, 1973) or from defined cultures (Impey *et al.*, 1984; Stavric, 1992). Schneitz (2005) presented an excellent review on CE with special reference to history, development, safety, administration in chickens and turkeys, benefits and mechanism of function.

CE should be applied to newly hatched chicks or turkey poults as soon as possible at the hatchery or farm. Administration can be carried out by spray in the hatchery. The droplet size should be at least 1 mm in diameter (Pivnick and Nurmi, 1982). According to Mulder (1996), the administration of the flora in the hatchery, however, causes some opposition, because it is very illogical to spray a large number of microorganisms in an environment that has by all possible means to be kept more or less sterile to prevent contamination. An alternative is to apply the CE preparation via drinking water, when chicks or poults are delivered to the farm (Schneitz and Nuotio, 1992; Wierup *et al.*, 1992). Spray application in hatchery followed by drinking water administration on the farm has also been found to be effective in controlling *Salmonella* in commercial broiler chickens (Blankenship *et al.*, 1993). Further applications in older birds after antibiotic treatment to regenerate the intestinal microflora have shown satisfactory results. The results of Corrier *et al.* (1991) indicate that intracloacal inoculation of newly hatched poults with intestinal flora from adult chickens or addition of lactose to the feed both significantly decreased caecal colonization by *S.* Senftenberg. Inoculation of turkeys with intestinal extracts has also been demonstrated to increase resistance to *Salmonella* colonization (Lloyd *et al.*, 1977). Furthermore, combined treatment with intestinal flora and provision of dietary lactose resulted in generally lower levels of *Salmonella* colonization than did either of the two treatments alone. According to Fowler and Mead (1990), combination of antibiotic therapy and CE was able to reduce the *Salmonella* infection rate in broiler breeder flocks and the vertical transmission to the end-product. On the other hand, according to Anderson *et al.* (1984), use of caecal cultures may also be limited by the interference of antibiotics for the control of *Salmonella* in turkeys.

Turkey poults are fully protected with CE prepared from chickens or turkeys (Impey *et al.*, 1984; Reid and Barnum, 1984; Seuna *et al.*, 1984; Schneitz and Nuotio, 1992). Hollister *et al.* (1999) studied the effects of chicken-derived, CE culture of caecal bacteria on the reduction of *S.* Typhimurium caecal colonization in growing turkey poults. The results indicated that treatment of turkey poults with the characterized chicken-derived culture effectively decreased *Salmonella* caecal colonization. On the other hand, Hofacre *et al.* (2000) investigated the efficacy of two commercial CE products, a chicken-origin lyophilized culture (Aviguard, Bayer Animal Health) and a probiotic culture (Avian Pac Soluble Plus) containing only *Lactobacillus acidophilus*, with that of fresh and 24-h-old adult turkey caecal material against *Salmonella* colonization. The results showed that Aviguard was protective, but fresh turkey caecal material was significantly more protective in three of the four trials.

Many authors reported that treatment must precede exposure to *Salmonella* to be protective (Anderson *et al.*, 1984). However, evidence exists that CE treatment given after *Salmonella* challenge reduces the number of *Salmonella* in the chicken caeca and the number of infected birds in a flock (Schneitz, 2005).

Vaccination

Vaccines may be useful in controlling clinical salmonellosis caused by host-adapted or invasive serovars. However, the application of vaccines to control colonization with non-invasive *Salmonella* is unlikely to be effective since humoral or cell-mediated immunity will have little influence on events in the lumen of the gastrointestinal tract (Barrow, 1991). In addition, there is evidence that highly invasive strains are likely to stimulate a stronger immune response and be eliminated earlier than would occur with less invasive strains (Barrow *et al.*, 1988).

Live and inactivated vaccines are used to control *Salmonella* in poultry, although there appears to be no report of the use of live vaccines in turkeys. Recently Krüger *et al.* (2008) investigated the efficacy of a commercially available *S.* Enteritidis live vaccine in fattening turkey flocks. The birds were vaccinated at day 1 of age via spray boostered at 6 and 11 weeks of age via drinking water. Two challenge trials with *S.* Enteritidis PT4 at dose level of 1×10^8 cfu per bird were carried out at the age of 7 weeks and at 16 weeks of age. The birds were observed during 11 days for clinical signs, abnormal reactions, mortality and *Salmonella* shedding. At the end of the challenge the turkeys were necropsied and examined for post-mortal lesions. Caecum with content, liver and spleen were chosen for bacteriological examination. No post-vaccinal reactions in all immunized turkeys could be detected. After challenge there was no reduction in shedding as well as of the colonization of internal organs. They concluded that application of this live *Salmonella* vaccine alone seems to be not suitable for the control of *S.* Enteritidis infections in turkeys.

McCapes *et al.* (1967) studied the use of a *Salmonella* bacterin in turkey breeders, particularly to determine whether any parental resistance would be passed to their poults. Poults originated from *S.* Typhimurium-vaccinated hens exhibited resistance to yolk sac challenge with both the B group *S.* Typhimurium and *S.* Schwarzengrund but not with the E group *S.* Anatum. According to Thain *et al.* (1984), administration of an inactivated *S.* Hadar vaccine to turkey breeding stock may be of value in limiting the spread of this serotype in young poults. They found that the use of this vaccine produced high levels of IgG antibodies, which were passed on through the egg to the poults. Successful vaccination of turkey breeders for the control of *Salmonella* with autogenous mineral oil adjuvant vaccines prepared from the serovars *S.* Sandiego and *S.* Arizonae were applied by Nagaraja *et al.* (1988). Their results suggested that outer membrane proteins of the organism give better protection than formalin-killed whole cell bacterin. In a study by Charles *et al.* (1993), the use of the subunit vaccines prepared from outer membrane proteins (OMP) from *S.* Heidelberg incorporating them into lipid-conjugated immunostimulating complexes for protection against homologous and heterologous *Salmonella* challenge in turkeys was investigated. The re-isolation rate of *Salmonella* from internal organs after challenge with *S.* Heidelberg, *S.* Reading or *S.* Enteritidis in turkeys was completely negative for the homologous serotype and significantly lower for the heterologous serotype in vaccinated turkeys. The results also indicate that fewer turkeys shed *Salmonella* after vaccination with ISCOM preparations than after vaccination with OMP alone.

Tenk *et al.* (2000) studied the efficacy of an inactivated *S.* Enteritidis commercial vaccine (Salenvac®) on *Salmonella* shedding in two breeding turkey flocks. Flock 'A' was vaccinated twice intramuscularly on weeks 20 and 27, whereas flock 'B' received the vaccine three times at weeks 8, 20 and 27. The ELISA test on week 54 from flock 'A' indicated low serum antibody titres. Following vaccination *Salmonella*-associated losses and condemnations were reduced to one-third of the level observed prior to vaccination. After vaccination the hatching performance improved, the quality of the day-old poults was better and performance figures were higher. Recurrences of excretion and egg contamination may occur during periods of stress such as the onset of lay, overheating or the final stages of lay.

Jodas and Hafez (2002) carried out an investigation to evaluate the efficacy of a commercial *S.* Enteritidis inactivated vaccine under field conditions in a turkey breeder farm with *S.* Enteritidis history. *Salmonella* shedding in vaccinated flocks was investigated by intensive bacteriological examination from faecal samples, cloacal swabs, hatching eggs, meconium, hatchery fluff and 1-day-old poults collected at several intervals. In addition, the serological response was determined using a commercial available *S.* Enteritidis ELISA test. After introducing the vaccine at the farm *Salmonella* spp. could not be isolated from faecal samples of turkey breeder flocks or from samples collected at the hatchery. The results indicate that the application of an inactivated vaccine together with improvement in the production hygiene has been remarkably successful in controlling *S.* Enteritidis infection.

Ghazikhanian *et al.* (1984) showed that using autogenous oil emulsion *S.* Arizonae bacterin resulted in a significant reduction of the overall egg transmission rate in vaccinated challenged hens compared with non-vaccinated challenged turkeys.

Education programmes

Since the success of any disease control programme depends on the farm and personal sanitation, it is essential to incorporate education programmes about microorganisms, modes of transmission as well as awareness of the reasons behind such control programmes by people involved in poultry production. In addition, effective education programmes must be implemented to increase public awareness of the necessary measures to be taken for protection against *Salmonella* in food products from turkeys. Finally, research must continue to find additional control and preventive means.

Public Health Aspects

In spite of significant improvement in technology and hygienic practices at all stages of food production accompanied with advanced improvement in public sanitation, salmonellosis and *Salmonella* infections remain a persistent threat to human and animal health (Newell *et al.*, 2010). Recent investigations estimate 80.3 million annual cases of food-borne disease related to *Salmonella* worldwide (Majowicz *et al.*, 2010).

Scallan *et al.* (2011) estimated food-borne illness using data from active and passive surveillance and other sources. They found out that each year 31 major pathogens acquired in the USA caused 9.4 million episodes of food-borne illness, 55,961 hospitalizations and 1351 deaths. Most (58%) illnesses were caused by norovirus, followed by non-typhoidal *Salmonella* spp. (11%), *Clostridium perfringens* (10%) and *Campylobacter* spp. (9%). Leading causes of hospitalization were non-typhoidal *Salmonella* spp. (35%), norovirus (26%), *Campylobacter* spp. (15%) and

Toxoplasma gondii (8%). Leading causes of death were non-typhoidal *Salmonella* spp. (28%), *T. gondii* (24%), *Listeria monocytogenes* (19%) and norovirus (11%).

In 2009 a total of 5550 food-borne outbreaks were reported in the European Union, causing 48,964 human cases, 4356 hospitalizations and 46 deaths. Most of the reported outbreaks were caused by *Salmonella*, viruses and bacterial toxins. The most important food sources were eggs and egg products, mixed or buffet meals and pig meat and products thereof. In addition, 15 water-borne outbreaks were reported in 2009 related to the contamination of private or public water sources. The number of salmonellosis cases in humans decreased by 17.4%, compared to 2008. In total 108,614 confirmed human cases were reported in 2009 and, in particular, human cases caused by *S*. Enteritidis decreased markedly. The case fatality rate was 0.08%. It is assumed that the observed reduction of salmonellosis cases is mainly attributed to successful implementation of national *Salmonella* control programmes in fowl populations; but other control measures along the food chain may also have contributed to the reduction. In foodstuffs, *Salmonella* was most often detected in fresh broiler, turkey and pig meat, on average at levels of 5.4%, 8.7% and 0.7%, respectively (EFSA, 2011).

In view of the high prevalence and contamination rate of turkey meat and products with *Salmonella* it is not surprising that turkey products should be considered as a source of human *Salmonella* infection. In the turkey industry the practice of further processing turkey carcasses for sale as portion, sausage or burgers etc. has increased worldwide. The contaminated products cause food-borne illness as a result of inadequate cooking or cross-contamination of working surfaces in the kitchen environment. Large outbreaks are mostly associated with the food prepared in food service establishments such as hotels, restaurants and institutions and by catered foods.

The most recently (2010/2011) reported human multistate outbreaks of human *S*. Hadar and *S*. Heidelberg infections in the USA were proved to be linked to turkey burgers and ground turkey, respectively. In both outbreaks the isolated strains were resistant to numerous commonly prescribed antibiotics, which could increase the risk of hospitalization or possible treatment failure in infected individuals (CDC, 2011).

The deficiency of the human population to apply hygienically acceptable food handling and cooking practice, and the fact that the processing plants are not able to reduce the level of pathogenic bacteria in poultry products, means that every effort must be made to reduce the *Salmonella* contamination of the live birds before despatch to processing plants (Hafez, 1999).

New approaches to the problem of contamination must be adopted and the discussion on the decontamination of the end-product must be re-evaluated carefully and without emotion.

References

Agabou, A. (2009) Air-borne bacterial contaminations in two broiler hatcheries in the North-East of Algeria. *Veterinary World*, 2, 48–49.

Anderson, W.R., Mitchell, W.R., Barnum, D.A. and Julian, R.J. (1984) Practical Aspects of Competitive Exclusion for the Control of *Salmonella* in Turkeys. *Avian Diseases* 28, 1071–1078.

Bailey, J.S. (1998) Detection of *Salmonella* cells within 24 to 26 hours in poultry samples with the polymerase chain reaction BAX system. *Journal of Food Protection* 61(7), 792–795.

Bailey, J.S., Blankenship, L.C. and Cox, N.A. (1991) Effect of fructo-oligosaccaharide on *Salmonella* colonisation of the chicken intestine. *Poultry Science* 70, 2433–2438.

Barrow, P.A. (1991) Immunological control of *Salmonella* in poultry. In: Blankenship, L.C. (ed.) *Colonization Control of Human Bacterial Enteropathogens in Poultry*. Academic Press, San Diego, pp. 199–217.

Barrow, P.A. (1992) Probiotics for chickens. In: Fuller, R. (ed.) *Probiotics*. Chapman Hall, London, pp. 1–8.

Barrow, P.A., Simpson, J.M. and Lovell, M.A. (1988) Intestinal colonization in the chicken by food-poisoning *Salmonella* serotypes; microbial characteristics associated with faecal excretion. *Avian Pathology* 17, 571–588.

Barrow, P.A., Desmidt, M., Ducatelle, R., Guittet, M., van der Heijden, H.M.J.F., Holt, P.S., Huis in't Velt, J.H.J., McDonough, P., Nagaraja, K.V., Porter, R.E., Proux, K., Sisak, F., Staak, C., Steinbach, G., Thorns, C.J., Wray, C. and van Zijderveld, F. (1996) World Health Organisation – supervised interlaboratory comparison of ELISAs for the serological detection of *Salmonella enterica* serovar Enteritidis in chickens. *Epidemiology and Infection* 117, 69–77.

Baskerville, A., Humphrey, T.J., Fitzgeorge, R.B., Cook, R.W., Chart, H., Rowe, B. and Whitehead, A. (1992) Airborne infection of laying hens with *Salmonella enteritidis* phage type 4. *Veterinary Record* 130, 395–398.

Baxter-Jones, C. and Wilding, G.P. (1981) *Salmonella* contamination of turkeys: recent progress towards improved control. *Hohenheimer Arbeiten* 116, 21–30.

Baxter-Jones, C. and Wilding, G.P. (1982) Controlling egg-borne pathogens. *Poultry International* 6, 12–22.

Berchieri, A. and Barrow, P.A. (1996) Reduction in Incidence of Experimental Fowl Typhoid by Incorporation of a Commercial Formic-Acid Preparation (Bio-Add[ä]) into Poultry Feed. *Poultry Science* 75, 339–341.

Bickford, S.M., Soy, J.I. and Barnes, L.E. (1973) Gentamycin concentrations in turkey eggs and in tissues of progeny following egg dipping. *Avian Disease* 17, 301–307.

Bierer, W.B. (1960) Effect of age factor on mortality in *Salmonella typhimurium* infection in turkey poults. *Journal of American Veterinary Medicine Association* 137, 657–658.

Blankenship, L.C., Bailey, J.S., Cox, N.A., Stern, N.J., Brewer, R. and Williams, O. (1993) Two-step mucosal competitive exclusion flora treatment to diminish *salmonella*e in commercial broiler chickens. *Poultry Science* 72, 1667–1672.

Brunner, F., Margadant, A., Peduzzi, R. and Piffaretti, J.C. (1983) The plasmid pattern as an epidemiological tool for *Salmonella* typhimurium epidemics: comparison with the lysotype. *Journal of Infectious Diseases* 148, 7–11.

Bryan, F.T., Ayres, J.C. and Kraft, A.A. (1968) Contributory sources of Salmonellae on turkey products. *American Journal of Epidemiology* 87, 578–591.

Caldwell, M.E. and Ryerson, D.L. (1939) Salmonellosis in certain reptiles. *Journal of Infectious Disease* 65, 242–245 (cit. Greenfield *et al.*, 1971).

Carrique-Mas, J.J. and Davies, R.H. (2008) Sampling and bacteriological detection of *Salmonella* in poultry and poultry premises: a review. *OIE Scientific and Technical Review* 27, 66.

Carrique-Mas, J.J., Barnes, S., Mclaren, I. and Davies, R. (2009) Comparison of three plating media for the isolation of *Salmonella* from poultry environmental samples in Great Britain using ISO 6579:2002 (Annex D). *Journal of Applied Microbiology,* 107(6), 1976–1983.

Casas, I.A., Edens, F.W., Dobrogosz, W.J. and Parkhurst, C.R. (1993) Performance of GAIAfeed and GAIAspray: *Lactobacillus reuteri*-based probiotic for poultry. In: Jenson, J.F., Hinton, M.H. and Mulder, R.W.A.W. (eds) *Proceeding of 'Prevention and control of potentially pathogenic microorganisms in poultry and poultry meat processing' 12. Probiotics and pathogenicity.* 'Het Spelderholt' Agriculture Research Department DLO-NL, Beekbergen, the Netherlands, meeting held at Vedbaek, Denmark, pp. 63–72.

Cason, J.A., Cox, N.A. and Bailey, J.S. (1994) Transmission of *Salmonella typhimurium* during hatching of broiler chicks. *Avian Diseases* 38, 583–588.

CDC (2011) Investigation Update: Multistate Outbreak of Human *Salmonella* Heidelberg Infections Linked to Ground Turkey. Available at: http://www.cdc.gov/Salmonella/heidelberg/111011/index.html (accessed February 2013).

Chaplin, W.C. and Hamilton, C.M. (1957) A synovitis in turkeys produced by *Salmonella* thompson. *Poultry Science* 36, 1380–1381.

Charles, S.D., Nagaraja, K.V. and Sivanandan, V. (1993) A Lipid-Conjugated Immunostimulating Complex Subunit Vaccine against *Salmonella* Infection in Turkeys. *Avian Diseases* 37, 477–484.

Cherrington, C.A., Hinton, M., Mead, G.C. and Chopra, I. (1991) Organic Acids: Chemistry, Antibacterial Activity and Practical Applications. *Advances in Microbial Physiology* 32, 87–108.

Cherrington, V.A., Gildow, E.M. and Moore, P. (1937) Paratyphoid in turkeys. *Poultry Science* 16, 226–231.

Clayton, G.A., Lade, R.E., Nixey, C., Jones, D.R., Charles, D.R., Hopkins, J.R., Binstead, J.A. and Prickett, R. (1985) *Turkey Production. Breeding and Husbandry*. MAFF. Her Majesty's Stationery Office, London.

Corrier, D.E., Hinton, A., Kubena, L.F., Zirpin, R.L. and DeLoach, J.R. (1991) Decreased *Salmonella* colonisation in turkey poults inoculated with anaerobic caecal microflora and provided dietary lactose. *Poultry Science* 70, 1345–1350.

Crespo, R., Jeffrey, J.S., Chin, R.R., Senties-Cue, G. and Shivaprasad, H.L. (2004) Phenotypic and genotypic characterization of *Salmonella* arizonae from an integrated turkey operation. *Avian Diseases* 48, 344–350.

Damron, B.L., Wilson, H.R., Voitle, R.A. and Harms, R.H. (1981) A mixed Lactobacillus culture in the diet of Broad Breasted Large White turkey hens. *Poultry Science* 60, 1350–1351.

Davies, R.H. and Bedford, S. (2001) Observations on *Salmonella* contamination in five turkey hatcheries. In: *Proceedings of the 'Current Topics in Veterinary Science' 55th Annual Conference*, Scarborough, 9–12 April. *Research in Veterinary Science*, 22.

Davies, R.H. and Wray, C. (1994) *Salmonella* pollution in poultry units and associated enterprises. In: Dewi, A., Axford, R. and Marai, F.M. (eds) *Pollution in Livestock Production Systems*. CAB International, Wallingford, UK, pp. 137–165.

DeLay, P.D., Jackson, T.W., Jones, E.E. and Stover, D.E. (1954) A testing service for the control of *Salmonella* typhimurium infection in turkeys. *American Journal of Veterinary Research* 15, 122–129.

DeLoach, J.R., Oyofo, B.A., Corrier, D.E., Kubena, R.L., Zirpin, R.L. and Mollenhauer, H.H. (1990) Reduction of *Salmonella* typhimurium concentration in broiler chickens by milk or whey. *Avian Diseases* 34, 389–392.

Donoghue, A.M., Blore, P.J., Cole, K., Loskutoff, N.M. and Donoghue, D.J. (2004) Detection of *Campylobacter* or *Salmonella* in turkey semen and the ability of poultry semen extenders to reduce their concentrations. *Poultry Science* 83, 1728–1733.

Dutta, T.K., Roychoudhury, P. and Bandypadhyay, S. (2010) Molecular epidemiology and virulence properties of *Salmonella* Enteritidis isolated from an outbreak of gastroenteritis in turkeys. *Indian Journal of Animal Sciences* 80, 391–397.

EC (2003a) Regulation (EC) No 2160/2003 of the European Parliament and of the Council of 17 November 2003 on the control of *Salmonella* and other specified foodborne pathogens. *Official Journal of the European Commission* L 325, 1–15.

EC (2003b) Regulation (EC) No 1831/2003 of the European Parliament and of the Council of 22 September 2003 on additives for use in animal nutrition. *Official Journal of the European Commission* L 268, 29–43.

EC (2006) Regulation (EC) No 1177/2006 of 1 August 2006 implementing Regulation (EC) No 2160/2003 of the European Parliament and of the Council as regards requirements for the use of specific control methods in the framework of the national programmes for the control of *Salmonella* in poultry. *Official Journal of the European Commission* L 212, 3–5.

EC (2008) Regulation (EC) No 584/2008 of 20 June 2008 implementing Regulation (EC) No 2160/2003 of the European Parliament and of the Council as regards a Community target for the reduction of the prevalence of *Salmonella enteritidis* and *Salmonella typhimurium* in turkeys. *Official Journal of the European Commission* L 162, 3–8.

Edens, F.W., Parkhurst, C.R. and Casas, I.A. (1991) *Lactobacillus reuteri* and whey reduce *Salmonella* colonization in the ceca of turkey poults. *Poultry Science* 70 (Suppl.1), 158.

Edwards, P.R., Cherry, W.B. and Bruner, D.W. (1943) Further studies on coliform bacteria serologically related to the genus *Salmonella*. *Journal of Infectious Disease* 73, 229–238.

EFSA (2008) Report of the Task Force on Zoonoses Data Collection on the Analysis of the baseline survey on the prevalence of Salmonella in turkey flocks, in the EU, 2006-2007. *The EFSA Journal* 134, 1–91.

EFSA (2011) The European Union Summary Report on Trends and Sources of Zoonoses, Zoonotic Agents and Food-borne Outbreaks in 2009. *The EFSA Journal* 9, 2090. Available at: http://www.efsa.europa.eu/en/efsajournal/pub/2090.htm (accessed 27 March 2011).

Eisenstein, B.I. (1990) New molecular techniques for microbial epidemiology and the diagnosis of infectious diseases. *Journal of Infectious Disease* 161, 595–602.

Ekperigin, H.E., Jang, S. and McCapes, R.H. (1983) Effective control of a gentamicin-resistant Salmonella arizonae infection in turkey poults. *Avian Diseases* 27, 822–829.

Eyigor, A. and Carli, K.T. (2003) Rapid detection of *Salmonella* from poultry by real-time polymerase chain reaction with fluorescent hybridization probes. *Avian Diseases* 47, 380–386.

Faddoul, G.P. and Fellows, G.W. (1966) A five-year survey of the incidence of Salmonellae in avian species. *Avian Diseases* 10, 296–304.

Featherstone, C.A., Reichel, R., Snow, L.C., Davies, R.H., Christiansen, K.H., Carrique-Mas, J.J. and Evans, S.J. (2010) Investigation of risk factors for *Salmonella* on fattening-turkey farms. *Epidemiology and Infection* 138, 1427–1438.

Fowler, N.G. and Mead, G.C. (1990) Competitive exclusion and *Salmonella* enteritidis. *Veterinary Record* 126, 489.

Fratamico, P.M. (2003) Comparison of culture, polymerase chain reaction (PCR), TaqMan Salmonella, and Transia Card Salmonella assays for detection of *Salmonella* spp. in naturally-contaminated ground chicken, ground turkey, and ground beef. *Molecular and Cellular Probes* 17, 215–221.

Fricker, C.R. (1987) The isolation of Salmonellas and Campylobacters. *Journal of Applied Bacteriology* 63, 99–116.

Friend, M. and Franson, J.C. (1999) *Salmonellosis, Field Manual of Wildlife Diseases*. General Field Procedures and Diseases of Birds, Edition, USGS, pp. 99–109.

Froyman, R. (1994) The potential use of enrofloxacin (Baytril[ä]), either alone of combined with competitive exclusion flora, in *Salmonella* sanitation programs for poultry. World Health Organisation. Unpublished report of the WHO-FEDESA-FEP workshop on competitive Exclusion, vaccination and antibiotics in *Salmonella* control in poultry, WHS/CDS/VOPH/94. 134 (WHO, Geneva).

Fuller, R. (1992) History and development of probiotics. In: Fuller, R. (ed.) *Probiotics*. Chapman Hall, London, pp. 1–8.

Gast, R.K. (2008) Paratyphoid infections. In: Saif, Y.M., Fadly, A.M., Glisson, J.R., McDougald, L.R., Nalon, L.K. and Swayne, D.E. (eds) *Diseases of Poultry*, 12th edn. Iowa State Press, Ames, Iowa, pp. 637–665.

Gazdzinski, P. (2004) *Salmonella* control in turkeys at farm level. In: Hafez, H.M. (ed.) *Proceedings of the 5th International Symposium on Turkey Diseases Berlin*. DVG-Service-GmbH, Giessen, pp. 57–63.

Ghazikhanian, G.Y., Kelly, B.J. and Dungan, W.M. (1984) *Salmonella* orizonae control program. In: Snoeyenbos, G.H. (ed.) *Proceedings of the International Symposium on Salmonella*. American Association of Avian Pathologists Inc., Kennett Square, Pennsylvania. Meeting held at New Orleans, Louisiana, pp. 142–149.

Greenfield, J., Bigland, C.H. and Dukes, T.W. (1971) The genus *Arizona* with special reference to Arizona disease in turkeys. *Veterinary Bulletin* 41, 605–612.

Grimont, P.A.D. and Weill, F.-X. (2007) *Antigenic Formulae of the* Salmonella *Serovars*, 9th edn. World Health Organization Collaborating Centre for Reference and Research on *Salmonella*. Institut Pasteur, Paris, France.

Guillot, J.F. and Milleman, Y. (1990) Intestinal colonization of chickens and turkeys by *Salmonella* and antibiotic decontamination. In: Mulder, R.W.A.W. (ed.) *Proceeding of Prevention and Control of Potentially Pathogenic Microorganisms in Poultry and Poultry Meat Processing. 1. Colonisation Control*. Meeting held at Ploufragan, France. 'Het Spelderholt' Agricultural Research Service (DLO-NL), Beekbergen, the Netherlands, pp. 31–44.

Hafez, H.M. (1999) Poultry meat and food safety: pre- and post-harvest approaches to reduce food borne pathogens. *World's Poultry Science Journal* 55, 269–280.

Hafez, H.M. (2001) *Salmonella* infections in poultry: diagnosis and control. *Periodicum Biologorum* 103, 103–113.

Hafez, H.M. (2005) Governmental regulations and concept behind eradication and control of some important poultry diseases. *World's Poultry Science Journal* 61, 569–582.

Hafez, H.M. (2011) *Salmonella* of turkeys: Update. In: Hafez, H.M. (ed.) *Turkey production and Health: An Update. Proceedings of the 6th International Symposium on Turkey Production*, Meeting of the Working Group 10 (Turkey) of WPSA, Berlin. Mensch & Buch Verlag, Berlin, pp. 250–255.

Hafez, H.M. and Jodas, S. (1992) Effect of sample selection from hatching eggs on *Salmonella enteritidis* detection rate. *Deutsche Tieraerztliche Wochenschrift* 99, 489–490.

Hafez, H.M. and Jodas, S. (1997) *Putenkrankheiten*. Ferdinand Enke Verlag, Stuttgart.

Hafez, H.M. and Stadler, A. (1997) *Salmonella enteritidis* colonization in turkey poults. *Deutsche Tieraerztliche Wochenschrift* 104, 118–120.

Hafez, H.M., Mandl, J. and Woernle, H. (1986) Einfache und empfindliche Methode zum Nachweis von Salmonellen in Eiern. 2. Mitteilung: Dekontamination mit Sysovet-PA und Schlupfergebnisse. *Deutsche Tieraerztliche Wochenschrift*. 93, 37–38.

Hafez, H.M., Stadler, A. and Jodas, S. (1993) *Salmonella* isolation in poultry and factors influencing: Review. In: Fanchini, A. and Mulder, R.W.A.W. (eds) *Proceedings of Prevention and Control of Potentially Pathogenic Microorganisms in Poultry and Poultry Meat Processing. 13. Consequences of the Zoonosis Order: Monitoring, methodology and data registration*. Meeting held at Bologna, Italy. 'Het Spelderholt' Agricultural Research Service (DLO-NL), Beekbergen, the Netherlands, pp. 65–72.

Hafez, H.M., Stadler, A. and Kösters, J. (1997) Surveillance on *Salmonella* in turkey flocks and processing plants. *Deutsche Tieraerztliche Wochenschrift* 104, 33–35.

Häggblom, P. (1993) Monitoring and control of *Salmonella* in animal feed. In: Bengtson S.O. (ed) *Proceedings of International Course on Salmonella Control in Animal Production and Products*. A presentation of the Swedish Salmonella Programme. WHO, pp. 127–137.
Hazeleger, W.C., Bolder, N.M.. Beumer, R.R. and Jacobs-Reitsma, W.F. (2008) Darkling beetles (*Alphitobius diaperinus*) and their larvae as potential vectors for the transfer of *Campylobacter jejuni* and *Salmonella enterica* serovar Paratyphi B variant Java between successive broiler flocks. *Applied and Environmental Microbiology* 74, 6887–6891.
Henzler, D.J. and Opitz, H.M. (1992) The role of mice in the epizootiology of *Salmonella enteritidis* infection on chicken layer farms. *Avian Diseases* 36, 625–631.
Hewitt, E.A. (1928) Bacillary white diarrhea in baby turkeys. *Cornell Veterinarian* 18, 272–276 (cit. Hinshaw, 1959).
Higgins, W.A., Christiansen, J.B. and Schroeder, C.H. (1944) A *Salmonella enteritidis* infection associated with leg deformity in turkeys. *Poultry Science* 23, 340–341.
Hinshaw, W.R. (1930) Fowl typhoid of turkeys. *Veterinary Medicine* 25, 514–517.
Hinshaw, W.R. (1959) Diseases of the turkeys. In: Biester, H.E. and Schwarte, L.H. (eds) *Diseases of Poultry*, 4th edn. Iowa State University Press, Ames, Iowa, pp. 974–1076.
Hinshaw, W.R. and McNeil, E. (1940) Eradication of pullorum disease from turkey flocks. In: *Proceeding of 44th Annual Meeting United States Livestock Sanitation Association*, pp.178–194 (cit. Snoeyenbos, 1991).
Hinshaw, W.R. and McNeil, E. (1946) The occurrence of type 10 paracolon in turkeys. *Journal of Bacteriology* 53, 281–280.
Hinton, M. (1996) Organic acids for control of *Salmonella*. *Misset World Poultry Salmonella Special* 33–34.
Hofacre, C.L., Primm, N.D., Vance, K., Vance, K., Goodwin, M.A. and Brown, J. (2000) Comparison of a lyophilized chicken-origin competitive exclusion culture, a lyophilized probiotic, and fresh turkey cecal material against *Salmonella* colonization. *Journal of Applied Poultry Research* 9, 195–203.
Hollister, A.G., Corrier, D.E., Nisbet, D.J. and Deloach, J.R. (1999) Effects of chicken-derived cecal microorganisms maintained in continuous culture on cecal colonization by *Salmonella typhimurium* in turkey poults. *Poultry Science* 78, 546–549.
Hoover, N.J., Kenney, P.B., Amick, J.D. and Hypes, W.A. (1997) Preharvest sources of *Salmonella* colonization in turkey production. *Poultry Science* 76, 1232–1238.
Iaffaldano, N., Reale, A., Sorrentino, E., Coppola, R., Di Iorio, M. and Rosato, M.P. (2010) Risk of *Salmonella* transmission via cryopreserved semen in turkey flocks. *Poultry Science* 89, 1975–1980.
Impey, C.S., Mead, G.C. and George, S.M. (1984) Evaluation of treatment with defined and undefined mixtures of gut microorganisms for preventing *Salmonella* colonization in chicks and turkey poults. *Food Microbiology* 1, 143–147.
Irwin, R.J., Poppe, C., Menier, S., Finley, G.G. and Oggel, J. (1994) A national survey to estimate the prevalence of *Salmonella* species among Canadian registered commercial turkey flocks. *Canadian Journal of Veterinary Research* 58, 263–267.
Jirophocaked, S., Sullivan, T.W. and Shahani, K.M. (1990) Influence of a dried *Bacillus subtilis* culture and antibiotics on performance and intestinal microflora in turkeys. *Poultry Science* 69, 1966–1973.
Jodas, S. (1992) Behandlungsverfahren zur Bekämpfung von Salmonella enteritidis bei künstlich infizierten Bruteiern (Legehybriden). Vet. Med. Diss., München (Dr. med. vet. Thesis Munich University, Germany).
Jodas, S. and Hafez, H.M. (2002) Field investigations on the efficacy of inactivated *Salmonella enteritidis* vaccine (Salenvac®) in turkey breeder flocks. In: Hafez, H.M. (ed.) *Proceedings of the 4th International Symposium on Turkey Diseases, Berlin*. ISBN 3-936815-58-5, pp. 259–270.
Johannsen, S.A., Griffith, R.W., Wesley, I.V. and Scanes, C.G. (2004) *Salmonella enterica* serovar typhimurium colonization of the crop in the domestic turkey: influence of probiotic and prebiotic treatment (*Lactobacillus acidophilus* and lactose). *Avian Diseases* 48, 279–286.
Jones, F.T. (2011) A review of practical *Salmonella* control measures in animal feed. *Journal of Applied Poultry Research* 20, 102–113.
Koinarski, V., Lyutskanov, M. and Urumova, V. (2006) Effect of *Eimeria adenoeides* challenge upon the course of an experimental *Salmonella* enteritidis infection in turkey poults. *Turkish Journal of Veterinary and Animal Sciences* 30, 489–495.
Kowalski, L.M. and Stephans, J.F. (1968) Arizona 7:1,7,8 Infection in young turkeys. *Avian Diseases* 12, 317–329.
Krüger, A., Redmann, T. and Krajewski, V. (2008) Field investigations on the efficacy of a live vaccine of *Salmonella* Enteritidis in meat turkeys. In: Hafez, H.M. (ed.) *Proceedings of the 7th International Symposium on Turkey Diseases*, Berlin. Verlag der DVG Service GmbH - ISBN 978-3-939902-96-6, pp. 300–311.

Kumar, M.C., York, M.D., McDowell, J.R. and Pomeroy, B.S. (1971) Dynamics of *Salmonella* infection in fryer roaster turkeys. *Avian Diseases* 15, 221–232.

Kumar, M.C., Nivas, S.C., Bahl, A.K., York, M.D. and Pomeroy, B.S. (1974) Studies on natural infection and egg transmission of *Arizona hinshawii* 7:1,7,8 in turkeys. *Avian Diseases* 18, 416–426.

Kumar, M.C., York, M.D. and Pomeroy, B.S. (1977) Development of microagglutination test for detecting *Arizona hinshawii* 7:1,7,8 in turkeys. *American Journal of Veterinary Research* 38, 255–257.

Le Minor, L. and Popoff, M.Y. (1987) Request for an opinion. Designation of *Salmonella enterica* sp. nov. norm. rev. as the type and only species of the genus *Salmonella*. *International Journal of Systematic Bacteriology* 37, 465–468.

Lee, C.D., Holm, G. and Murray, C. (1936) Paratyphoid infection in turkeys. *Journal of American Veterinary Medical Association* 89, 65–76.

Lloyd, A.B., Cumming, R.B. and Kent, R.D. (1977) Prevention of *Salmonella typhimurium* infection in poultry by pretreatment of chickens and poults with intestinal extracts. *Australian Veterinary Journal* 53, 82–87.

Lucas, T.E., Kumar, M.C., Kleven, S.H. and Pomeroy, B.S. (1970) Antibiotic treatment of turkey hatching eggs preinfected with Salmonellae. *Avian Diseases* 14, 455–462.

Majowicz, S.E., Musto, J., Scallan, E., Angulo, F.J., Kirk, M., O'Brien, S.J., Jones, T.F., Fazil, A. and Hoekstra, R.M. (2010) The global burden of nontyphoidal *Salmonella gastroenteritidis*. *Clinical Infectious Diseases* 50, 882–889.

Mallinson, E.T. and Snoeyenbos, G.H. (1989) Salmonellosis. In: Purchase, H.G., Arp, L.H., Domermuth, C.H. and Pearson, J.E. (eds) *Isolation and Identification of Avian Pathogens*, 3rd edn. Kendall/Hunt Publishing Company, Dubuque, Iowa, pp. 3–11.

Mandel, J., Hafez, H.M., Woernle, H. and Kösters, J. (1987) Wirksamkeit unterschiedlicher Methoden zur Desinfektion *Salmonella*-kontaminierter Huehnerbruteier (Mastrasse) 2. Mitteilung: Dekontamination mit Lysovet-PA und Schlufpergebnisse. *Archiv für Geflügelkunde* 51, 141–144.

Mayer, H., Geßler, K., Weiss, H.-E., Hetkamp, D. and Verhalen, K.-H. (1984) Infektketten und Infektionszyklen der Salmonellen in der Broiler -und Putenproduktion. *Tierärztliche Umschau* 39, 538–548.

McCapes, R.H., Coffland, R.T. and Christie, L.E. (1967) Challenge of turkey poults originating from hens vaccinated with *Salmonella typhimurium* bacteria. *Avian Diseases* 11, 15–24.

McCapes, R.H., Osburn, B.I. and Riemann, H. (1991) Safety of foods of animal origin: model for elimination of *Salmonella* contamination of turkey meat. *Journal of American Veterinary Medicine Association* 199, 875–880.

McIlIroy, S.G. (1996) How did birds become infected by a *Salmonella* serotype. *World Poultry Misset Salmonella Special*, May, pp. 15–17.

Mitrovic, M. (1956) First report of paratyphoid infection in turkey poults due to *Salmonella* reading. *Poultry Science* 35, 171–174.

Moore, V.A. (1895) On a pathogenic bacillus of the hog-cholera group associated with a fatal disease in pigeons. *USDA BAI Bull* 8, pp. 71–76 (cit. Nagaraja *et al.*, 1991a).

Moran, A.B. (1959) *Salmonella* in animals: a report for 1957. *Avian Diseases* 3, 85–88.

Mueller-Doblies, D., Carrique-Mas, J.J., Sayers, A.R. and Davies, R.H. (2010) A comparison of the efficacy of different disinfection methods in eliminating *Salmonella* contamination from turkey houses. *Journal of Applied Microbiology* 109, 471–479.

Mulder, R.W.A.W. (1996) Probiotics and competitive exclusion microflora against *Salmonella*. *World Poultry Misset Salmonella Special*, May, pp. 30–32.

Nagaraja, K.V., Emery, D.A., Newman, J.A. and Pomeroy, B.S. (1984) Detection of *Salmonella arizonae* in turkey flocks by ELISA. In: *Proceeding of the 27th Annual Meeting of American Association Vet. Lab Diag.*, pp. 185–204.

Nagaraja, K.V., Ausherman, L.T., Emery, D.A. and Pomeroy, B.S. (1986) Update on enzyme linked immunosorbent assay for its field application in the detection of *Salmonella arizonae* infection in breeder flocks of turkeys. In: *Proceeding of the 29th Annual Meeting of American Association Vet. Lab Diag.*, pp. 347–356.

Nagaraja, K.V., Kim, C.J. and Pomeroy, B.S. (1988) Prophylactic vaccines for the control and reduction of *Salmonella* in turkeys. In: *Proceedings of 92nd Annual Meeting US Animal Health Association*, pp. 347–348.

Newell, D.G., Koopmans, M., Verhoef, L., Duizer, E., Aidara-Kane, A., Sprong, H., Opsteegh, M., Langelaar, M., Threfall, J., Scheutz, F., van der Giessen, J.V. and Kruse, H. (2010) Food-borne diseases – The challenges of 20 years ago still persist while new ones continue to emerge. *International Journal of Food Microbiology* 139(Suppl. 1), 3–15.

Nurmi, E. and Rantala, M. (1973) New aspects of *Salmonella* infections in broiler production. *Nature, London* 241, 210–211.

Oyofo, B.A., De Loach, J.R., Corrier, D.E., Norman, J.O., Zirpin, R.L. and Mollenhauer, H.H. (1989) Effect of carbohydrates on *Salmonella typhimurium* colonization in broiler chickens. *Avian Diseases* 33, 531–534.

Papadopoulou, C., Davies, R.H., Carrique-Mas, J.J. and Evans, S.J. (2009) *Salmonella* serovars and their antimicrobial resistance in British turkey flocks in 1995 to 2006. *Avian Pathology* 38, 349–357.

Peluffo, C.A., Edwards, P.R. and Brunner, D.W. (1942) A Group of Coliform Bacilli Serologically Related to the Genus *Sallvionella*. *Journal of Infectious Disease* 70, 185–192 (cit. Geenfield *et al.*, 1971).

Pfaff, F. (1921) Eine Truthühnerseuche mit Paratyphus-Befund. *Zentralblatt für Infektionskrankheite der Haustiere* 22, 285–292.

Pfeiler, W. and Roepke, W. (1917) Zweite Mitteilung über das Auftreten des Huehnertyphus und die Eigenschaften seines Erregers. *Zentralblatt für Bakteriologie I. Original* 79, 125 (cit. Hinshaw, 1959).

Pivnick, H. and Nurmi, E. (1982) The Nurmi Concept and its role in the control of *Salmonella* in poultry. In: Davies, R. (ed.) *Developments in Food Microbiology - 1*. Applied Science Publishers, Barking, England, pp. 41–70.

Pomeroy, B.S. and Fenstermacher, R. (1939) Paratyphoid infections in turkeys. *Journal of American Veterinary Medicine Association* 94, 90–97.

Pomeroy, B.S. and Fenstermacher, R. (1941) Paratyphoid infection in turkeys. American *Journal of Veterinary Research* 2, 285–291.

Reid, C.R. and Barnum, D.A. (1984) The effects of treatments of cecal contents on their protective properties against *Salmonella* in poults. *Avian Diseases* 29, 1–11.

Renggli, F. (1996) *Salmonella* contamination of poultry products is an important problem, and could be prevented though the routine practice of feed decontamination and proper feed handling. Different methods of decontamination exist and some of them can even be combined to enhance efficiency. *World Poultry Misset Salmonella Special*, May, pp. 34–35.

Rettger, L.F. (1909) Further studies on fatal septicaemia in young chickens, or 'white diarrhoea'. *Journal of Medical Research* 21, 115–123.

Runnells, R.A., Coon, C.J., Farley, H. and Thorp, F. (1927) An application of the rapid-method agglutination test to the diagnosis of bacillary white diarrhea infection. *Journal of American Veterinary Medicine Association* 70, 660–662.

Saeed, A.M., Walk, S.T., Mokhtar Arshad, M. and Whittam, T.S. (2006) Clonal structure and variation in virulence of *Salmonella* Enteritidis isolated from mice, chickens, and humans. *Journal of AOAC International* 89, 504–511.

Saif, Y.M. and Shelly, S.M. (1973) Effect of gentamycin sulfate dip on *Salmonella* organisms in experimentally infected turkey eggs. *Avian Diseases* 17, 574–581.

Saif, Y.M., Ferguson, L.C. and Nestor, K.E. (1971) Treatment of turkey hatching eggs for control of Arizona infection. *Avian Diseases* 15, 446–461.

Sato, G. and Adler, H.E. (1966) Experimental infection of adult turkeys with arizona group organisms. *Avian Diseases* 10, 329–336.

Scallan, E., Hoekstra, R.M., Angulo, F.J., Tauxe, R.V., Widdowson, M.-A., Roy, S.L., Jeffery, L.J. and Griffin, P.M. (2011) Foodborne Illness Acquired in the United States – Major Pathogens. *Emerging Infectious Diseases* 17, 16–22.

Schaffer, J.M., McDonald, A.D., Hall, W.J. and Bunyea, H. (1931) A stained antigen for the rapid whole blood test for pullorum disease. *Journal of American Veterinary Medicine Association* 79, 236–240.

Schneitz, C. (2005) Competitive exclusion in poultry – 30 years of research. *Food Control* 16, 657–667.

Schneitz, C. and Nuotio, L. (1992) Efficacy of different microbial preparations for controlling *Salmonella* colonisation in chicks and turkey poults by competitive exclusion. *British Poultry Science* 33, 207–211.

Seuna, E., Nagaraja, K.V. and Pomeroy, B.S. (1984) Gentamicin and bacterial culture (Nurmi culture) treatments either alone or in combination against experimental *Salmonella* hadar infection in turkey poults. *Avian Diseases* 29, 617–629.

Shahata, M.A., El-Timawy, A.A.M. and El-Dimerdash, M.Z. (1984) Some studies on Salmonellosis of turkeys. *Assuit Veterinary Medicine Journal* 11, 203–208.

Shivaprasad, H.L. (2008) Arizonosis. In: Saif, Y.M., Fadly, A.M., Glisson, J.R., McDougald, L.R., Nalon, L.K. and Swayne, D.E. (eds) *Diseases of Poultry*, 12th edn. Iowa State Press, Ames, Iowa, pp. 665–674.

Shivaprasad, H.L. and Barrow, P.A. (2008) Pullorum disease and fowl typhoid infections. In: Saif, Y.M., Fadly, A.M., Glisson, J.R., McDougald, L.R., Nalon, L.K. and Swayne, D.E. (eds) *Diseases of Poultry*, 12th edn. Iowa State Press, Ames, Iowa, pp. 620–636.

Shivaprasad, H.L., Cortes, P. and Crespo, R. (2006) Otitis interna (labyrinthitis) associated with *Salmonella enterica* arizonae in turkey poults. *Avian Diseases* 50, 135–138.

Skov, M.N., Spencer, A.G., Hald, B., Petersen, L., Nauerby, B., Carstensen, B. and Madsen, M. (2004) The role of litter beetles as potential reservoir for *Salmonella enterica* and thermophilic *Campylobacter* spp. between broiler flocks. *Avian Diseases* 48, 9–18.

Snoeyenbos, G.H. (1991) Pullorum Disease. In: Calnek, B.W., Barnes, H.J., Reid, W.M. and Yoder, H.W. Jr (eds) *Diseases of Poultry*, 9th edn. Iowa State University Press, Ames, Iowa, pp. 73–86.

Stavric, S. (1992) Defined cultures and prospects. *International Journal of Food Microbiology* 15, 245–263.

Stokes, J.L., Osborne, W.W. and Bayne, H.G. (1956) Penetration and growth of *Salmonella* in shell eggs. *Food Research* 2, 510–518.

Tenk, I., Gyorvary, I., Erdei, P., Szabo, Z., Kostyak, A. and Matray, D. (2000) Effect on *Salmonella* shedding in breeding turkey flocks of vaccine (Salenvac) against *Salmonella* Enteritidis. *Magyar Allatorvosok Lapja* 122, 737–741.

Thain, J.A., Baxter-Jones, C., Wilding, G.P. and Cullen, G.A. (1984) Serological response of turkey hens to vaccination with *Salmonella* hadar and its effect on their subsequently challenged embryos and poults. *Research in Veterinary Science* 36, 320–325.

Timms, L. (1971) Arizona infection in turkeys in Great Britain. *Journal of Medical Laboratory Technology* 28, 150–156.

Valancony, H., Humbert, F., Rukelibuga, J., Bougon, M., Balaine, L. and Lalande, F. (2001) Comparison of some substitutes for antibiotic additives in diets for turkey poults. Effects on production and on resistance to *Salmonella* colonization. *Sciences & Techniques Avicoles* 35, 25–34.

Vicente, J., Higgins, S., Bielke, L., Tellez, G., Donoghue, D., Donoghue, A. and Hargis, B. (2007) Effect of probiotic culture candidates on *Salmonella* prevalence in commercial turkey houses. *Journal of Applied Poultry Research* 16, 471–476.

Wales, A.D., Allen, V.M. and Davies, R.H. (2010) Chemical treatment of animal feed and water for the control of *Salmonella*. *Foodborne Pathogens and Disease* 7, 3–15.

Weand, D.C. and Horsting, A.G. (1978) Sanitation of hatching eggs. *Proceedings of 16th World Poultry Congress*, pp. 797–808 (cit. Nagaraja *et al.*, 1991b).

Wierup, M., Wahlstroem, H. and Engstroem, B. (1992) Experience of a 10-year use of competitive exclusion treatment as part of the *Salmonella* control programme in Sweden. *International Journal of Food Microbiology* 15, 287–291.

Williams, J.E. and Dillard, L.H. (1968) *Salmonella* penetration of fertile and infertile chicken eggs at progressive stages of incubation. *Avian Diseases* 12, 629–635.

Williams, J.E. and Whittemore, A.D. (1971) Serological diagnosis of pullorum disease with the microagglutination system. *Applied Microbiology* 21, 394–399.

Willinger, H., Flatscher, J., Dreier, F. and Wildner, T. (1986) Epidemiologische Untersuchungen zum Vorkommen von Salmonellen in Gefluegelhaltungen. *Wiener Tieraerztliche Monatsschrift* 73, 141–148.

Winter, A.R., Burkhart, B. and Widley, H. (1952) Further studies on the whole blood and tube methods of testing turkeys for *Salmonella* pullorum infection. *Poultry Science* 31, 399–404.

Wolfenden, R.E., Pumford, N.R., Morgan, M.J., Shivaramaiah, S., Wolfenden, A.D., Pixley, C.M., Green, J., Tellez, G. and Hargis, B.M. (2011) Evaluation of selected direct-fed microbial candidates on live performance and *Salmonella* reduction in commercial turkey brooding houses. *Poultry Science* 90, 2627–2631.

Wray, C. and Davies, R.H. (1994) Guidelines on detection and monitoring of *Salmonella* infected poultry flocks with particular reference to *Salmonella enteritidis*. World Health Organization Veterinary Public Health Unit, WHO/Zoon 94.173, Geneva.

Yamamota, R., Adler, H.E., Sadler, W.W. and Stewart, G.F. (1961) A study of *Salmonella typhimurium* infection in market-age turkeys. *American Journal of Veterinary Research* 22, 382–387.

11 *Salmonella* Infections in Ducks

H.L. Shivaprasad[1]* and Paul A. Barrow[2]

[1]California Animal Health and Food Safety Laboratory System, University of California, USA; [2]School of Veterinary Medicine and Science, University of Nottingham, UK

Introduction

Farming ducks for meat and eggs has been practised for several millennia and is currently most common in countries of central Asia and South-east Asia. China alone is home to 75% of the world's duck population. However, their numbers are increasing in many countries including USA and in Europe as an alternative form of agriculture and to meet the demands of consumers for duck meat and eggs. There has long been an association between ducks and *Salmonella*, largely through the consumption of duck eggs, which historically was associated with a high probability of 'food poisoning'. The concept of '*Salmonella* food poisoning' is of relatively recent origin and the present increased interest even more recent, being a side-effect of urbanization and intensive farming, combined with mass catering.

In contrast to food poisoning as a result of eating duck eggs *Salmonella* food poisoning from duck meat is very rare. This is probably due largely to the culinary methods and eating habits of the relatively small proportion of the population that eats duck meat, rather than to any great difference between duck farming and other poultry farming methods.

In spite of the long history of the association between *Salmonella* and duck, the literature on the subject is scanty and is largely confined to reports of serovars isolated from routine monitoring of post-mortem specimens either targeting poultry in general or as part of a more general *Salmonella* prevalence survey. This lack of information may simply reflect the view that the source of infection, epidemiology, diagnosis and treatments reported for the other avian species apply equally to the duck. This is, of course, largely true, but there are some differences, which may be relevant when considering monitoring procedures or treatment regimes.

The following commentary reflects mainly experiences in the UK, with references where applicable to work from other countries. All references relate to the Pekin/mallard type of duck (*Anas platyrhynchos*), unless otherwise stated.

Clinical Disease

The usual signs of clinical disease following infection are more common in the very young duckling, and generally commence in the immediate post-hatch period. The recent

* Corresponding author, e-mail: hlshivaprasad@ucdavid.edu

© CAB International 2013. *Salmonella in Domestic Animals, 2nd Edition* (eds P.A. Barrow and U. Methner)

experience with *S.* Enteritidis PT 4 was that, although immediate post-hatch infections are seen, in birds of about 3 weeks of age or more, disease also occurred under those circumstances that normally give rise to *Escherichia coli* septicaemia.

The signs of clinical salmonellosis are similar to most bacterial infections: general listlessness, hunched appearance, diarrhoea, dehydration (as evidenced by semi-closed eyes with possibly some 'gumming' of the eyelids), reduced food and water intake, possibly some signs of nervous incoordination and eventual coma and death. The progress through the various stages may take only a few hours (hence the American term 'keel disease', because 'the birds just keel over and die'). Perhaps more commonly, the clinical condition runs a course of 4–5 days. Convalescent birds may show some degree of unthriftiness, which, in some cases, can be associated with a hock or foot arthritis or synovitis. Infected adult birds generally show neither gross clinical signs nor a drop in egg production. It has, however, been reported that, following experimental challenge, there is a change in eggshell structure, which is consistent with the presence of stress within the flock (S. Solomon, unpublished data, 1997). Changes from negative to positive *Salmonella* status of a flock have no apparent effect on fertility or hatchability even though egg transmission may occur. Whether this results from the slow spread of infection through an flock or whether it reflects the resistance of the duck is not clear.

Post-mortem Findings

On post-mortem examination of birds that have died or are showing clinical signs of *Salmonella* infection, the pathological findings are similar to those in the fowl with, to varying degrees, carcass congestion, pericarditis, perihepatitis, hepatic necrotic foci, typhlitis and the emaciation, dehydration and nephrosis/nephritis that probably reflect more the general malaise of the bird than any specific effect caused by the *Salmonella*. In this context, it should be noted that nephritis, particularly when accompanied by visceral urate deposits (gout), is, in the duck, pathognomonic for lack of water intake, irrespective of the cause. Although small pale spots on the liver may result from *Salmonella* infection, streptococcal infections have a similar effect in birds of between 1 and 2 weeks of age.

Zhakov and Prudnikov (1987) reported changes in the bursa of Fabricius and thymus in ducks immunized with live *S.* Typhimurium vaccine and challenged subsequently. Bursal follicular depletion was observed, with enlargement of the medulla of the thymus and reduction in the size of the cortex. These findings may have significance with regard to the immune mechanisms being activated, but bursal changes, at least, are not specifically associated with salmonellosis and bursal regression in ducks has also been associated with reovirus infection (Smyth and McNulty, 1994). Arthritis in ducks due to salmonellosis has also been reported (Bisgaard *et al.*, 1981).

Pathogenesis

Although the prevalence of *Salmonella* in the duck population (both farmed and feral) is well recognized internationally, the degree to which the duck population itself suffers as a consequence appears to be minimal. It may be that the gregarious habits of the species in its natural habitat and the fact that it tends to swim, feed and drink in what can only be regarded as its own effluent has, over the millennia, generated increased resistance to the potentially pathogenic organisms residing in the gut to which this behaviour pattern exposes it. Whatever the reason, the duck is not uncommonly infected with *Salmonella* but is only very rarely diseased, so far as can be determined by clinical observation. This hypothesis was supported in one study where four serotypes of *Salmonella*, *S.* Typhimurium, *S.* Enteritidis, *S.* Heidelberg and *S.* Gallinarum, given orally to 1-day-old ducks failed to cause systemic infection but colonized the intestine and were excreted for at least 6 weeks (Barrow *et al.*, 1999). But in two other studies where a highly virulent *S.* Enteritidis phage type (PT4) was inoculated either intra-nasally to day-old ducklings or subcutaneously to 14-day-old ducklings bacterial genomic DNA and the antigen was demonstrated in cells of various tissues in addition to mild pathology in various organs (Deng *et al.*, 2009a, b). Age is an important feature in the extent of infection and colonization (Yu *et al.*, 2008). As far as is known, wound infection/insect bites in the duck are not a significant factor in the spread of salmonellosis, although injection of *S.* Virchow has been reported to result in faecal excretion and vertical transmission (Gosh *et al.*, 1990).

Septicaemia due to *Salmonella* may occasionally arise but can usually be traced to some form of environmental or managemental stress. Such infections are most common in very young ducklings that have been exposed to chilling stress or where lack of good hatchery hygiene has permitted massive challenge.

Public Health Significance

Due to the popularity of ducks either for hobby or as a small enterprise, sold by the hatcheries or also by feed stores, the number of human salmonellosis cases is increasing in the USA due to *Salmonella* Hadar (CDC, 1992), *S.* Infantis (CDC, 2000), *S.* Altona and *S.* Johannesburg (CDC, 2012), due to *S.* Enteritidis PT4 in Italy (Nastasi *et al.*, 1998), due to *S.* Shubra and *S.* Saintpaul in Egypt (Osman *et al.*, 2010) and due to S. Typhimurium DT8 in England and Northern Ireland (Noble *et al.*, 2012). In the England and Northern Ireland outbreak there was a strong correlation between salmonellosis in humans who had consumed duck eggs contaminated with *S.* Typhimurium DT8. In the USA most of the outbreaks were due to ducklings being sold as mail-order by hatcheries. Infection mainly affected children and resulted from handling of ducklings. Some of these outbreaks involved as many as 28 states out of 50.

Sources of Infection

Salmonella infections can be spread both horizontally and vertically.

Horizontal transmission

A comparison of raw feed-material isolates and duck isolates suggests that horizontal transmission accounts for most of the changes in serovar prevalence that occur on farms. This can also include litter material contamination, residual environmental contamination and feral vectors. The latter two may account for the recrudescence of infections considered to have been eliminated from the farm.

Feed

Although heat treatment of duck feed and the incorporation of organic acids into the feed have significantly reduced the prevalence of feed-borne *Salmonella* it will not prevent the contamination of feed during the latter stages of manufacture, storage and transport. This situation is improving but until such time as raw materials are free of *Salmonella* contamination it is likely to be a major source of infection.

Environment and feral vectors

The role of fomites and possibly even human vectors in horizontal transmission tends to be forgotten, but lapses in biosecurity from these sources are probable. In flocks that conform to the requirements of the UK Poultry Health Scheme, horizontal transmission from these sources is under good control. In the UK, a dramatic change has taken place over the last 20 years and *Salmonella*-negative breeder flocks are now becoming more common.

Salmonella-negative grower flocks are less common, mainly because economic factors give rise to multi-age sites, where satisfactory inter-crop clean-down may be compromised by the proximity of other livestock with a safe haven for vermin. There is, however, a significant move towards resolving the situation.

Litter

One of the main differences between the management practices of duck growing and broiler or turkey growing is the need to replenish the duck litter material on a daily basis. In the UK, the litter can be either of wood by-products origin (shavings or sawdust) or straw (usually barley or wheat straw).

Salmonella-free litter sources are far from common. Contamination of straw occurs both in the field and, more probably, in the stack, which, unless preventive steps are taken, becomes home to rats/mice and wild birds, and home/hunting-ground to cats, all of which are potential carriers and disseminators of *Salmonella*. The situation with regard to wood shavings or sawdust is similar. Although the faecal material that might carry the contamination is relatively easier to identify in wood shavings there is little that can be done to remove any such contamination. Ducks sift through the fresh litter provided, for nutritious material. Straw, shavings, litter and almost anything else are likely to be swallowed. Proper storage of the bulk material at source before delivery to the distributor and proper packaging of the final product prior to farm delivery are essential if *Salmonella* contamination from these sources is to be avoided.

Vertical transmission

True egg transmission occurs when the egg is infected before laying. The alternative route of vertical transmission, egg contamination, may occur in conjunction with or independently of egg transmission. The duck egg usually has a very thick cuticle, which may help to prevent invasion of the egg by *Salmonella* via eggshell pores, but cuticle cover can vary considerably. Additionally, partial cuticle removal may be seen as a result of the surface of the egg being scraped by the parent or another duck while the cuticle is still soft after laying. Ducks have a habit of defecating in the nesting-boxes provided and duck faeces are of a fluid consistency. Baker *et al.* (1985) observed that good egg hygiene is helpful in minimizing hatchery contamination. Under normal circumstances, true egg transmission of *Salmonella* in the duck is very largely confined to transmission of *S.* Typhimurium. The successful use of neomycin to control faecal excretion and the continued appearance of *S.* Enteritidis-infected day-old ducklings suggests vertical transmission via an infected reproductive tract (R.R. Henry, personal observation).

Vertical transmission has been identified in mature layers as soon as 8 days after challenge following artificial infection through the drinking water with *S.* Typhimurium, supplied at the rate of 10^3 cfu per bird in their water.

Egg transmission of *S.* Hadar has been noted in the Muscovy (Barbary) duck (*Cairina moschata*). This type of bird is, in many ways, more goose-like than duck-like in many of its attributes. Gosh *et al.* (1990) reported the vertical transmission of *S.* Virchow following both oral and intraperitoneal challenge of adult birds.

Hatchery transmission

Whether *Salmonella* egg infection takes place by true egg transmission, shell penetration or external shell contamination, the end result is contamination of: (i) the hatchlings and hatcher in which the eggs are hatched; (ii) ducklings of the same and other parentage in the same hatcher; and, (iii) the general hatchery environment, from which further duckling infection may take place at a later date.

Salmonella Serovars

The Salmonella serovars that may infect ducks and give rise to general infection and/or gut carrier status appear to differ little from those that would be expected to behave similarly in the fowl or turkey, except that the fowl-adapted *S.* Pullorum/Gallinarum does not appear to be a particular duck pathogen (Buchholz and Fairbrother, 1992), although its presence has been recorded on occasions (Chute and Gershman, 1963; Anderson *et al.*, 2006).

More information is available now on the prevalence of *Salmonella* in ducks including eggs, faeces, internal organs etc. Information from European Union countries from 2003 to 2004 (EFSA, 2006) indicates levels of flock infections between 4.8 and 57.2% with some countries such as Denmark having high levels of infection (57.2%), Germany having less (10.7%) and Norway having none at all. The figure for duck-breeder flocks in Poland was 7.9%. Ireland found 18.6% of duck meat to be contaminated.

Prevalence studies of *Salmonella* in Vietnam have ranged from 8.8% in adult ducks to 24.7% in ducklings (Hanh, 1998). Similarly the prevalence in internal organs has ranged from 6.3% to 14.3% in different regions of Vietnam whereas the incidence ranged from 3.2% to 31.7% in dead duck embryos (Hanh, 1998; Hanh *et al.*, 2006). In another study from the Mekong Delta 14 different serovars were isolated from the faeces or intestinal contents of ducks with *S.* Typhimurium being the most common (Tran *et al.*, 2004).

In extensive testing of *Salmonella* from cloacal swabs in 2000 ducks from 100 duck farms in Taiwan an overall prevalence rate of 4.6% was found (Tsai and Hsiang, 2005). A total of 12 serotypes were identified in this study out of which *S.* Potsdam was the most frequently (31.9%) isolated serotype. In a study in Chinese duck and goose hatcheries, 110 *Salmonella* isolates were identified (Su *et al.*, 2011). These isolates were serotyped by four multiplex PCR methods and it was found that 97.3% of the isolates were of *S.* Potsdam serotype suggesting that this serotype is the predominant one in duck farms in China and Taiwan. In Thailand isolation of *Salmonella* from 564 eggshells and egg contents resulted in 133 isolates from which 23 serotypes were identified (Saitanu *et al.*, 1994). The four most common serotypes identified were *S.* Typhimurium (5.5%), *S.* Cerro (4.1%), *S.* Tennessee (2.8%) and *S.* Amsterdam (2.1%).

In Belgium a recent study of the prevalence of *Salmonella* serotypes in male mule ducks over a period of 32 months in 100 flocks resulted in the isolation of 95 strains of *Salmonella* belonging to 11 serotypes (Flament *et al.*, 2012). *Salmonella* Indiana (42.1%) and *S.* Regent (36.8%) were the two most common serotypes, whereas *S.* Typhimurium and *S.* Enteritidis were found only once (1.1%). In another study on trends in phage types of *S.* Enteritidis in ducks between 2001 and 2005 in England it was found that PTs 6, 6a, 9b and 14b increased during the period (Carrique-Mas *et al.*, 2008). *Salmonella* Enteritidis has also been identified on the eggshells from ducks in the USA (Baker *et al.*, 1985). A survey in the USA by Price *et al.* (1962) on 7029 post-mortem occasions carried out over 10 years isolated 491 *Salmonella*. Of these, 457 (93%) isolates were *S.* Typhimurium and there were fewer than ten each of the other serovars (Table 11.1). These organisms were isolates

Table 11.1. *Salmonella* serovars isolated from ducks.

Serovar	Author	Serovar	Author	Serovar	Author
S. Agona	2, 2*, 3	*S.* Hadar	2, 2*, 3	*S.* Nagoya	3
S. Amsterdam	4	*S.* Heidelberg	2, 2*, 3	*S.* Newport	1, 2*, 3
S. Anatum	1, 2*, 3	*S.* Indiana	3, 5	*S.* Oregon	1
S. Bareilly	2, 2*	*S.* Infantis	3	*S.* Orion	3
S. Binza	3	*S.* Kedougou	3	*S.* Panama	1, 2*
S. Braenderup	3	*S.* Lille	2*	S. Potsdam	4
S. Bredeny	2*, 3	*S.* Livingstone	3	*S.* Regent	3, 5
S. Cerro	4	*S.* London	2	*S.* Saintpaul	1
S. Choleraesuis	2*	*S.* Manchester	1	*S.* Senftenberg	1, 3
S. Derby	3	*S.* Manhattan	1	S. Tennessee	4
S. Enteritidis	1, 2*, 3	*S.* Mbandaka	3	*S.* Thomasville	3
S. Fresno	3	*S.* Meleagridis	2	*S.* Typhimurium	1, 2, 2*, 3
S. Gallinarum/Pullorum	2	*S.* Montevideo	2	*S.* Virchow	2
S. Give	1, 3			*S.* Wangata	3

Authors: 1, Price *et al.*, 1962; 2, Simko, 1988: ducks; 2*, Simko, 1988: geese; 3, MAFF (1997); 4, Saitanu *et al.*, 1994; Flament *et al.*, 2012.

from ducklings considered to be clinically affected with 'keel disease', but in retrospect the role of some of the isolates as the primary cause of disease may be doubtful. A similar survey in Slovakia by Simko (1988) reported on 679 *Salmonella* isolations, of which 61% were *S.* Typhimurium, 22% *S.* Anatum, 4% *S.* Meleagridis and other serovars (Table 11.1) were less than 1%. He also reported 706 isolations from goose farms, of which 41% were *S.* Enteritidis, 17% *S.* Typhimurium, 16% *S.* Anatum and 11% *S.* Newport and other serovars listed in Table 11.1.

Because of changes in both EU legislation and public attitudes, considerable attention has been paid to the presence of *Salmonella* in the gut of many species, including ducks. Routine surveillance has shown carrier status of the serovars listed in Table 11.1, both in healthy ducks and, rarely, associated with clinical infections of ducklings in the first few days of life. In recent years in the UK, *S.* Typhimurium and *S.* Enteritidis have been associated with septicaemia in young ducklings, but as a primary cause of disease they did not and do not figure strongly.

Many isolates from ducks have usually been seen as transient gut infections and occasionally as short-term hatchery or farm residents. *Salmonella* Typhimurium is almost certainly the predominant serovar in many countries because, in addition to horizontal transmission, it is the subject of vertical transmission by more than one route.

The mainly feed-material contamination will result in broadly similar serovars being isolated around the world and across species at risk, following the common economic pressures for cheap feed ingredients as raw material.

Diagnosis

There are, in general, two situations in which diagnosis of *Salmonella* infections is required: the first of these is where clinical signs of disease are present, with, and occasionally without, gross pathological changes to be found in dead or sacrificed birds, while the second is the more challenging requirement for accurate but economically sustainable monitoring of layer/breeder flocks for *Salmonella* infection/colonization and transmission to the egg.

For the purpose of diagnosis of clinical disease, it is usual to culture affected organs on blood agar and MacConkey agar media, with subsequent aerobic incubation at 37°C for 18–24 h. Almost pure growth of *Salmonella* can be expected from cases of acute salmonellosis if the specimens are reasonably fresh. Although multiple-serovar carrier status is not uncommon, clinical salmonellosis appears to be due mainly to single serovars.

Salmonella can also be recovered with reasonable certainty from the brains of ducks that have died or have shown either nervous signs or general malaise. Contaminants will be less prevalent in the brain than, for instance, in liver or spleen. Recovery of *Salmonella* from the brain of birds that merely show presumptive *Salmonella*-associated malaise is less common, possibly because the level of malaise at which culls may be taken varies considerably, or possibly because the assumed association is false, despite the fact that the bird may be a *Salmonella* carrier.

Serovar-specific real-time polymerase chain reaction (RT-PCR) or fluorescence-based quantitative PCR (FQ-PCR) can detect genomic DNA of *S.* Enteritidis for diagnosis (Deng *et al.*, 2008a, 2009b). By these methods the organisms could be detected in blood, liver, spleen, heart, kidney, pancreas, gall bladder, thymus, bursa of Fabricius, Harderian gland in acute infection and the organisms could be detected in the spleen up to 9 to 14 days post-infection. (Deng *et al.*, 2008a, b).

Isolation of *Salmonella*

The culture of *Salmonella* from material of duck origin may be carried out with almost any of the recognized pre-enrichment, enrichment and selective media in common use. Although the growth characteristics of *Salmonella* on selective media are well documented, the different media are usually designed to be optimal under specific conditions, which may not include unforeseen types of background flora such as occur in ducks. In the case of under-investigated species, such as ducks, *ad hoc* investigations of new media are recommended, in view of the findings of Mann and McNabb (1984), who investigated the prevalence of *Salmonella* in geese. An unpublished trial using neck-flap or sliced giblets by R. Henry indicated that Rappaport-Vassiliadis broth (RV), lysine desoxycholate (XLD) agar and brilliant green agar (BGA) were all effective.

The procedure for the examination of egg material may follow any of the procedures outlined above, but similar findings involving 15,000 eggs suggest that, if egg-shells are suitably disinfected, the pre-enrichment incubation of whole, macerated 10-day-incubated dead-embryo or clear eggs at 37°C overnight, followed by direct plating to BGA and XLD with novobiocin, is a more cost-effective procedure for detecting contaminated eggs. Should results prove equivocal, pre-enrichment broth can still be subjected to selective enrichment at 48 h post-inoculation.

It has been noted that XLD (with or without 10 ppm novobiocin) has the unexplained and unmatched property of showing duck-associated *S.* Typhimurium as a noticeably smaller colony than other sources. This property is retained even after the *Salmonella* has been sub-cultured on non-selective media four times. The colony size, which is also independent of the H_2S production characteristics of the isolate, is a useful marker in the laboratory, enhancing the ability to 'pick off' multiple isolates and saving on time spent on identification of the selected small colony.

Monitoring Programmes

The diagnosis of carrier status/egg-transmitter status is more complex, mainly because of the limitations imposed by costs and practicalities. The wide range of programmes designed for monitoring flocks for the presence of *Salmonella* demonstrates the unsuitability of any one of them for all situations.

In considering the sustainability of a programme for any given set of circumstances the following factors should be considered.

1. Egg transmission can occur without clinical signs in either parent or offspring.
2. Infection results in faecal shedding of the organism for a greater or lesser length of time, irrespective of when the first infection occurred.
3. In any flock, egg transmission of one *Salmonella* serovar may take place with faecal shedding of a different serovar.
4. Seroconversion in the parent always appears to accompany egg transmission.

Sampling strategy

The strategy for monitoring parent flocks for *Salmonella* status starts with the assumption that any infection that may be present has, at some time or other, entered via the oro-pharynx and will have, shortly thereafter, appeared at the cloaca, where it will be present for a variable length of time. The optimum strategy with respect to monitoring parent flocks for potential to spread *Salmonella* to their offspring involves sufficiently frequent faecal sampling from 1 day old onwards, together with possible serological investigations.

Sampling tactics

In the UK, the Poultry Breeding Flocks and Hatcheries Order (HMSO, 1993) does not apply to duck breeders, but conformation with its requirements appears to be a sound basis for *Salmonella* monitoring. Similarly, EU legislation (Directives 92/117 and 2003/99) (Directive, 1992, 2003) introduced to begin a process of monitoring and control of food-borne pathogens in livestock has laid the main emphasis so far on fowl and pigs, reflecting the relatively small place that ducks play in meat consumption.

Although currently ducks are not subject to legislation in the EU, it is likely to happen in the medium to long term. The EU National Control Plans (NCP) for chickens and turkeys set fairly modest 'flock size' numbers and are fairly 'relaxed' as to the definition of commercial production, e.g. permitting 'local' sale (turkeys), or use in bed and breakfasts (eggs). Hence, an NCP for ducks may only 'catch' flocks of several hundred birds (or more), and may not apply to some apparently 'commercial' use of meat or eggs. Therefore, it would seem logical for small scale production (e.g. 100–200 birds), including pets/backyard egg production and also game ducks, to be considered in due course.

The UK Poultry Breeding Flocks and Hatcheries Order lays down requirements, *inter alia*, to take box liners and 'dead on arrival' from newly placed parent flocks, followed by all birds that die or are culled in the first 4 days. These examinations are useful for monitoring infection of parent or hatchery origin, provided that an adequate number of samples are taken. Although the prevalence of infection emanating from a contaminated hatchery may be high, this is not necessarily so, and equally the tendency for *Salmonella* infection to spread amongst day-old ducklings is high, but this may also not necessarily occur. There are further requirements in this Order to take composite faeces samples at 4 weeks of age and 2 weeks before 'entering the laying phase'. This frequency of monitoring may be inadequate to identify an infected flock early enough for some remedial action to be taken.

Experience has shown that the use of cloacal swabs to determine faecal excretion of *Salmonella* is less efficacious than the use of litter samples. A high percentage of the birds may not be excreting at any one time. Examination of litter samples is capable of revealing levels of excretion that may be missed by cloacal swabbing unless a very high percentage of the birds is examined. Perhaps because of the nature of duck litter management, it appears that examination of litter is more effective and more practical than the examination of drag swabs. Examination of water from drinking troughs is also a sample source for monitoring, but the number of recovered organisms (per gram of material) is not as high as from litter. Samples taken at fortnightly or monthly intervals are an appropriate compromise between cost/work load and effective surveillance. There are situations in which examination of litter samples or other sources of faecal material are not appropriate – for instance, during medication for other conditions.

Depending on the past history and age of the birds, reliance may have to be placed on serology or, if appropriate, bacteriological examination of egg material. For examination of egg material to be an effective monitoring procedure, selection of an appropriate number of eggs is essential. The binomial expansion can be used to determine the minimum number of samples to be taken based on the expected level of infection to have 95% or 99% confidence in finding a positive sample. If the *Salmonella* status of a potential breeder flock is in doubt due to lack of testing it is optimal to screen those eggs produced at the onset of lay that are not considered suitable for the production of commercially viable offspring. Almost by definition, the egg numbers will be low and infertility high, but, since examination of live eggs is not optimal for *Salmonella* recovery, this is not a problem. In the early stages of lay, it may be necessary to examine all available eggs to obtain reliable data. These eggs should be incubated for at least 10 days prior to bacteriological examination. The examination of fresh eggs is not an effective monitoring procedure.

For eggs being taken on to hatch, the eggs discarded at candling after 10 days' incubation is the most practical and productive material for *Salmonella* detection. Early dead embryos are preferred to 'clears' (i.e. infertile eggs), although *Salmonella* may not be the cause of early embryo death. However, culture of such eggs usually produces a *Salmonella* monoculture, if it is present, with a bacterial count of the order of 10^6 colony-forming units (cfu) g^{-1}.

Apart from identifying positive parent flocks with complete accuracy (and reasonable sensitivity), the technique has the advantage that it leaves time for the eggs to be hatched in isolation or diverted to another hatchery, should such options be available, thus preventing spread to other hatchlings. Given a moderate degree of care, it is possible and, in some parts of the world, commonplace to move duck eggs at about 23 days of incubation over considerable distances, for the final stages of hatching.

The examination of meconium or hatch debris/dead-in-shell, as required by the Poultry Health Scheme in the UK, is clearly too late for much useful action to be taken and, unless the hatcher contains the offspring of only one parent flock, it is considerably less accurate with regard to the identity of the parent source of any isolate(s).

Serology

Infected ducks will mount cell-mediated and humoral immune responses. The humoral response produced by the duck differs from that of the domestic fowl in the detail of the immunoglobulin G produced and in the amount and nature of the IgM (Higgins and Warr, 1993). Indeed the whole immune system of the duck is considerably less evolved than that of the fowl (see Davison *et al.*, 2008 for review).

Serological tests that depend on secondary effects such as agglutination, complement fixation, passive haemagglutination and agar gel precipitation tend to be insensitive. Experience has shown that, when using the rapid slide agglutination test against 'pullorum antigen', a 10% false-positive reaction may be expected and the significance of the results has to be considered in relation to the sensitivity of the test.

Enzyme-linked immunosorbent assays (ELISA) are currently the most useful for examining the humoral response of the duck to a wide variety of antigens, including the flagellar and lipopolysaccharide (LPS) antigens. Unfortunately, there is no common agreed protocol and workers in this field either use their own standards or utilize commercial kits, where these are available. The disadvantages are that: (i) the assay depends on the existence of a good quality standard serum; (ii) optical densities (ODs) obtained are diagnostically only useful 'in house' and therefore comparison of results with other laboratories is difficult and relies on comparing interpreted results, rather than actual titre values, or exchanging control sera; and (iii) the relatively high serum dilution used (1/500, 1/1000 or even greater dilutions are usual) may render the test 'oversensitive'. Examination of sera from the Muscovy duck can be carried out using the same methodology. Within limited experience, it would appear that this type of bird reacts, serologically, rather more vigorously that the Pekin bird, as judged by the ODs obtained under similar conditions of husbandry and challenge and in spite of using the second antibody designed for the Pekin duck.

To judge that, given a set of positive reactions, the birds have encountered the particular *Salmonella* from which the antigen was prepared (either LPS or flagellar) is an over-optimistic view of the test system. There is a tendency to regard serological reactions as a specific response to the organism providing the test antigen (e.g. *S.* Pullorum- or *S.* Enteritidis-positive), whereas the only valid inference from the test is that the serum is showing a reaction to one or more epitopes on the antigen.

Antibiotic Sensitivity

Salmonella isolates in the UK show good *in vitro* sensitivity to amoxicillin, apramycin, chloramphenicol, colistin, cotrimoxazone, enrofloxacin, framycetin, neomycin, spectinomycin, streptomycin, the tetracyclines and trimethoprim. Wasniewski and Galazka (1991) reported from Poland that, of 41 *S.* Typhimurium and 74 *S.* Enteritidis isolates, 95% and 92%, respectively, were enrofloxacin-sensitive and fewer were sensitive to streptomycin, oxytetracycline, neomycin and chloramphenicol. It will be interesting to investigate levels of resistance in countries in the Far East where levels of resistance in *Salmonella* strains isolated from fowl are much higher than in the UK and other EU countries. Certainly the few surveys that have been carried out indicate higher levels of resistance (Adzitey *et al.*, 2012).

Treatment

Treatment of ducks for clinical salmonellosis is rarely necessary. Since the disease usually follows some form of stress – frequently chilling – the primary action is to remedy the predisposing cause. Control is recommended to involve a flock-based management system and not involve drug use. There is increasing interest in nest hygiene, egg dipping and cuticle scrubbing/cleaning of eggs as a part of this. Should veterinary advice indicate that antibiotic therapy is required, the only antibiotic licensed in the UK for water administration is amoxicillin. For in-feed medication, chlortetracycline is licensed. Neither of these are necessarily the drugs one would choose for chemotherapy. The evidence that either of these is likely to be of clinical benefit for the control of salmonellosis is scanty. The clinically-affected birds tend not to eat or drink and hence do not benefit from the medication provided. Antibiotics may help to reduce the weight of challenge to the in-contact birds but neither of those mentioned above appears to prevent the carrier state. For both the above licensed medications, the withdrawal time is 7 days. Lincomycin-spectinomycin are licensed in the UK non-specifically for poultry as is enrofloxacin in the water.

Treatment of faecal excretors of *Salmonella* to limit environmental contamination is possible using neomycin in the feed at a standard rate of 320 g activity t^{-1}. The feed supply rate should be taken into account when calculating the appropriate medication rate. If birds are not fed ad libitum, there may be considerable intake of litter, with resulting medicament dilution. The use of neomycin in the food prior to moving birds from rearing to laying premises has also coincided with the disappearance of faecal shedding of some *Salmonella* serovars.

Treatment of layers to eliminate *S.* Enteritidis PT4 has been shown to be possible by the use of enrofloxacin medication, following the manufacturer's recommended regime. However, the successful eradication of *S.* Typhimurium from a positive laying flock has not been achieved so far. Prevention of egg transmission of other *Salmonella* is presumably possible by the same means, although faecal transmission may well cease spontaneously without treatment and without the appearance of egg transmission. Egg transmission of the organism has been very significantly reduced but, in a flock of only 100 layers, a low level of transmission eventually reappeared following enrofloxacin treatment. Tenk *et al.* (1994) report treatment of a flock of geese with a 31% excretion rate using enrofloxacin. *Salmonella* excretion was suspended for a period of 42 days, at which time a 4% excretion rate was observed. That this followed plucking stress is probably significant. However, for this product withdrawal periods are only specifically stated in the UK for broiler chickens, turkeys and pullets. Ducks are not specifically listed, so a 28 day meat withdrawal should be employed. Also, due to withdrawal liabilities, enrofloxacin should not be used for hens laying eggs for human consumption; therefore its use should not be recommended for ducks doing the same.

Prevention

There is increasing interest in the use of gut flora preparations and vaccination as a component of a flock-based system for controlling infection in breeders.

Although the use of anaerobic cultures of adult bowel flora to colonize the intestinal tract of the fowl has proved a useful technique in limiting the *Salmonella* carrier status (Nurmi and Rantala, 1973), the technique has not, as yet, proved useful for the duck. Ducklings infected with a *Salmonella* at 1 day old or shortly after, whether given a strictly anaerobically grown culture of adult bowel flora or not, will become carriers for a variable length of time, which may last until point of lay. Further investigation of this effect is required since the *Salmonella* carrier status may disappear spontaneously from a flock coming into lay. Efficacious commercial vaccination of day-old ducklings to prevent either *S.* Enteritidis or *S.* Typhimurium infections has been shown (Windhorst *et al.*, unpublished results) and there is experimental evidence that infection with *S.* Enteritidis resulted in a measurable protective immunity against an isogenic mutant (Barrow *et al.*, 1999). Immunization of older birds with either Bovivac (MSD Animal

Health) for its *S.* Typhimurium content or the *S.* Enteritidis vaccine (Salenvac^{TM}) failed to prevent egg transmission of these *Salmonella*. However, the prevalence of egg transmission was reduced and these vaccines may prove a useful adjunct to medication in an eradication scheme. Live vaccination (AviPro^{R} Salmonella Duo, Lohmann) of newly hatched ducklings produced significant reduction in invasion to the liver and spleen following challenge 22 or 36 days later.

In one study chicken egg-derived antibody for *S.* Enteritidis when given alone or in combination with probiotics orally to ducklings and challenged with the same serovar at day 1 or day 5 showed fewer ducks infected than the positive control birds (Fulton *et al.*, 2002).

References

Adzitey, F., Huda, N. and Rahmat Ali, G.R. (2012) Prevalence and antibiotic resistance of Campylobacter, *Salmonella*, and *L. monocytogenes* in ducks: a review. *Foodborne Pathogens and Disease* 9, 498-505.

Anderson, L.A., Miller, D.A. and Trampel, D.W. (2006) Epidemiological investigation, cleanup, and eradication of pullorum disease in adult chickens and ducks in two small-farm flocks. *Avian Diseases* 50, 142–147.

Baker, R.C., Qureshi, R.A., Sandhu, T.S. and Timoney, J.F. (1985) The frequency of salmonellae on duck eggs. *Poultry Science* 64, 646–652.

Barrow, P.A., Lovell, M.A., Murphy, C.K. and Page, K. (1999) *Salmonella* infection in a commercial line of ducks; experimental studies on virulence, intestinal colonization and immune protection. *Epidemiology and Infection* 123, 121–132.

Bisgaard, M., Folkersen, J.C. and Høg, C. (1981) Arthritis in ducks. II. Condemnation rate, economic significance and possible preventive measures. *Avian Pathology* 10, 321–327.

Buchholz, R.S. and Fairbrother, A. (1992) Pathogenicity of *Salmonella* pullorum in northern bobwhite quail and mallard ducks. *Avian Diseases* 36, 304–312.

Carrique-Mas, J.J., Papadopoulou, C., Evans, S.J., Wales, A., Teale, C.J. and Davies, R.H. (2008) Trends in phage types and antimicrobial resistance of *Salmonella enterica* serovar Enteritidis isolated from animals in Great Britain from 1990 to 2005. *Veterinary Record* 162, 541–546.

CDC (Centers for Disease Control) (1992) Salmonella hadar associated with pet ducklings – Connecticut, Maryland, and Pennsylvania, 1991 *Journal of the American Medical Association* 267, 2011.

CDC (Centers for Disease Control and Prevention) (2000) Salmonellosis associated with chicks and ducklings – Michigan and Missouri, spring 1999. *Journal of the American Medical Association* 283, 2229–2230.

CDC (Centers for Disease Control and Prevention) (2012) Notes from the field: multistate outbreak of *Salmonella* Altona and Johannesburg infections linked to chicks and ducklings from a mail-order hatchery – United States, February-October 2011. *Morbidity and Mortality Weekly Report* 61, 195.

Chute, H.L. and Gershman, M. (1963) Case Report – *Salmonella* Pullorum in a Muscovy duck (*Cairina moschata*) duck. *Avian Diseases* 7, 168–169.

Davison, T.F., Kaspers, B. and Schat, K.A. (eds) (2008) *Avian Immunology*. Elsevier Academic Press, London.

Deng, S.X., Cheng, A.C., Wang, M.S., Yan, B., Yin, N.C., Cao, S.Y., Zhang, Z.H. and Cao, P. (2008a) The pathogenesis of *Salmonella* enteritidis in experimentally infected ducks: a quantitative time-course study using taqman polymerase chain reaction. *Poultry Science* 87, 1768–1772.

Deng, S.X., Cheng, A.C., Wang, M.S., Yan, B., Yin, N.C., Cao, S.Y., Zhang, Z.H. and Cao, P. (2008b) A study of the distribution patterns and levels of *Salmonella* enteritidis in the immune organs of ducklings after oral challenge by serovar-specific real-time PCR. *Avian Diseases* 52, 507–512.

Deng, S.X., Cheng, A.C., Wang, M.S., Li, X.R. and Yan, B. (2009a) Replication kinetics of *Salmonella* enteritidis in internal organs of ducklings after oral challenge: a quantitative time-course study using real-time PCR. *Veterinary Research Communications* 33, 273–280.

Deng, S.X., Cheng, A.C., Wang, M.S. and Ye, L.G. (2009b) Quantitative analysis of *Salmonella* Enteritidis loads in ducklings after nasal inoculation. *Poultry Science* 88, 1888–1892.

Directive (1992) Concerning measures for protection against specified zoonoses and specified zoonotic agents in animals and products of animal origin in order to prevent outbreaks of food-borne infections and intoxications. *EU Directive* 92/117.

Directive (2003) On the monitoring of zoonoses and zoonotic agents amending Council Decision 90/424 and repealing Council Directive 92/117. *Official Journal of the European Union* L 325/31.

EFSA (2006) Trends and sources of zoonoses, zoonotic agents and antimicrobial resistance in the European Union in 2004. European Food Safety Authority. *The EFSA Journal* 2005, 310.

Flament, A., Soubbotina, A., Mainil, J. and Marlier, D. (2012) Prevalence of *Salmonella* serotypes in male mule ducks in Belgium. *Veterinary Record* 170, 311.

Fulton, R.M., Nersessian, B.N. and Reed, W.M. (2002) Prevention of *Salmonella enteritidis* infection in commercial ducklings by oral chicken egg-derived antibody alone or in combination with probiotics. *Poultry Science* 81, 34–40.

Gosh, S.S., Roy, A.K.B. and Nanda, S.K. (1990) Transmission of *S. virchow* in fowls and Khaki Campbell ducks. *Indian Veterinary Journal* 671, 84–85.

Hanh, T.X. (1998) Preliminary results of duck salmonellosis studies in vicinity of Ho Chi Minh city. *Veterinary Science and Technology* 5, 61–67.

Hanh, T., Nguyen, T.T., Hoang, Q.T., Le, T.T., Lam, M.T. and Nguyen, T.H. (2006) Prevalence of *Salmonella* spp. in poultry in Vietnam. *Annals of the New York Academy of Sciences* 1081, 266–268.

Higgins, D.A. and Warr, G.W. (1993) Duck immunoglobulins, structure, functions and molecular genetics. *Avian Pathology* 22, 211–236.

HMSO (1993) The Poultry Breeding Flocks and Hatcheries Order 1993. Statutory Instrument 1994 No. 1898.

MAFF (1997) *Salmonella* in Livestock Production. Veterinary Laboratories Agency, New Haw, Addlestone, UK.

Mann, E. and McNabb, C.D. (1984) Prevalence *of Salmonella* contamination in market-ready geese in Manitoba. *Avian Disease* 284, 978–983.

Nastasi, A., Mammina, C., Piersante, G.P., Robertazzo, M. and Caruso, P. (1998) A foodborne outbreak of *Salmonella enteritidis* vehicled by duck and hen eggs in southern Italy. *New Microbiologica* 21, 93–96.

Noble, D.J., Lane, C., Little, C.L., Davies, R., De Pinna, E., Larkin, L. and Morgan, D. (2012) Revival of an old problem: an increase in *Salmonella enterica* serovar Typhimurium definitive phage type 8 infections in 2010 in England and Northern Ireland linked to duck eggs. *Epidemiology and Infection* 140, 146–149.

Nurmi, E. and Rantala, M. (1973) New aspects of *Salmonella* infection in broiler production. *Nature* 241, 210–211.

Osman, K.M., Yousef, A.M., Aly, M.M. and Radwan, M.I. (2010) *Salmonella* spp. infection in imported 1-day-old chicks, ducklings, and turkey poults: a public health risk. *Foodborne Pathogens and Disease* 7, 383–390.

Price, J.I., Dougherty, E. 3rd and Bruner, D.J.W. (1962) *Salmonella* infections in white pekin duck – a short summary of the years 1950-60. *Avian Diseases* 6, 145–147.

Saitanu, K., Jerngklinchan, J. and Koowatananukul, C. (1994) Incidence of salmonellae in duck eggs in Thailand. *Southeast Asian Journal of Tropical Medicine and Public Health* 25, 328–331.

Simko, S. (1988) Salmonellae in ducks and geese on farms with latent infections and in centres of salmonellosis. *Immunoprophylaxia* 1–2, 92–101.

Smyth, J.A. and McNulty, M.S. (1994) A transmissible disease of the bursa of Fabricius of the duck. *Avian Pathology* 23, 447–460.

Su, Y.C., Yu, C.Y., Lin, J.L., Lai, J.M., Chen, S.W., Tu, P.C. and Chu, C. (2011) Emergence of *Salmonella enterica* serovar Potsdam as a major serovar in waterfowl hatcheries and chicken eggs. *Avian Diseases* 55, 217–222.

Tenk, I., Kovacs, Z. and Matray, D. (1994) Effect of enrofloxacin on the *Salmonella* excretion of plucked geese. *Magyar Allatorvosok Lapja* 498, 501–503.

Tran, T.P., Ly, T.L., Nguyen, T.T., Akiba, M., Ogasawara, N., Shinoda, D., Okatani, T.A. and Hayashidani, H. (2004) Prevalence of *Salmonella* spp. in pigs, chickens and ducks in the Mekong Delta, Vietnam. *Journal of the Veterinary Medical Science* 66, 1011–1014.

Tsai, H.J. and Hsiang, P.H. (2005) The prevalence and antimicrobial susceptibilities of *Salmonella* and *Campylobacter* in ducks in Taiwan. *Journal of the Veterinary Medical Science* 67, 7–12.

Wasniewski, A. and Galazka, V. (1991) Baytril Bayer – a preparation for treatment for salmonellosis in poultry. *Zeszty Naukowe Akademii Rolmczej we Wrocawiu, Weterynana* 49, 109–114.

Yu, C.Y., Chu, C., Chou, S.J., Chao, M.R., Yeh, C.M., Lo, D.Y., Su, Y.C., Horng, Y.M., Weng, B.C., Tsay, J. and Huang, K.C. (2008) Comparison of the association of age with the infection of *Salmonella* and *Salmonella enterica* Serovar Typhimurium in Pekin ducks and Roman geese. *Poultry Science* 87, 1544–1549.

Zhakov, M. and Prudnikov, V.S. (1987) Morphological changes in the central immune-reactive organs of ducks after oral immunisation against salmonellosis. *Veterinamaya Nauka Ponzvostvu* 25, 56–58.

12 *Salmonella* Infections in Cattle

Roberto La Ragione,[1,3]* Hannah J. Metcalfe,[2] Bernardo Villarreal-Ramos[3] and Dirk Werling[2]

[1]*Department of Microbial and Cellular Sciences, University of Surrey, UK;*
[2]*Department of Pathology and Infectious Diseases, Royal Veterinary College, UK;*
[3]*Animal Health and Veterinary Laboratories Agency (Weybridge), UK*

Introduction

Salmonella infections are an important cause of mortality and morbidity in cattle and subclinically infected cattle are frequently found. Cattle thus constitute an important reservoir for human infections. There have been numerous reviews over the years (see Mohler *et al.*, 2009), increasingly reporting about multi-drug resistant strains (Alexander *et al.*, 2009) as well as the importance of *Salmonella* for the food industry (Thorns, 2000). Interestingly, despite decades of research into salmonellosis, the disease and its public health consequences are not really resolved. This chapter extends the chapter written by C. Wray and R.H. Davies for the first edition, and aims to update our current knowledge about bovine salmonellosis.

Historical Perspective

The early history of the disease is confused as the genus *Salmonella* was initially inadequately characterized. A few of the serovars were clearly defined; however, these were often confused with members of other genera. The causative agent of *Typhus abdominalis* in humans was discovered in 1880 by Egbert and Koch, and cultivated in a pure culture in 1884 by Gaffky. However, prior to this, calf paratyphoid was recorded in Europe in the middle of the 19th century, when a specific form of calf diarrhoea ('*Kälberruhr*') attracted considerable attention in the Netherlands, Germany and Denmark. In 1865, Obich was the first to consider the disease to be caused by an infectious agent. However, it was not investigated bacteriologically until Jensen (1891) isolated a coliform bacillus from the viscera of affected calves in Denmark. This bacillus was subsequently named *Bacillus paracoli*. Thomassen (1897) isolated an organism, which he named 'pseudotyphoid bacillus', thus indicating a relationship with the recently isolated 'typhoid bacillus'. Further *Salmonella* isolations from calves were made by a number of workers; some of these appeared to be similar to *Bacillus enteritidis*, which was isolated by Gärtner in 1880 from an outbreak of food poisoning in humans (today *Salmonella* (*S.*) Enteritidis). Further confusion was also caused by the isolation of 'Breslau-bacillus' (today *S.* Typhimurium) from mice by Löffler in 1889 (Löffler, 1892). The subsequent isolation of this bacillus by Kaensche during an outbreak of food poisoning in Breslau in 1893 was linked to the sale of condemned meat from an emergency-slaughtered cow.

* Corresponding author, e-mail: r.laragione@ahvla.defra.gsi.gov.uk; r.laragione@surrey.ac.uk

© Crown copyright 2013. Reproduced with the permission of the Controller of Her Majesty's Stationery Office/Queen's Printer for Scotland and Animal Health and Veterinary Laboratories Agency

Salmonella infection was subsequently reported in adult cattle by Mohler and Buckley (1902), during a disease outbreak in the USA caused by an organism resembling *S.* Enteritidis. Many of these earlier infections of *S.* Enteritidis were subsequently shown by serology to be erroneous and are now recognized as caused by *S.* Dublin. Similar confusion existed between *S.* Paratyphi B and *S.* Typhimurium, and it was not accepted until the 1920s that these two serovars were distinct. When the genus *Salmonella* was more clearly defined, it became apparent that the serovar most commonly associated with bovine salmonellosis in those parts of Europe where the disease was endemic was *S.* Dublin, and *S.* Typhimurium was next in order of frequency.

Epidemiology

Incidence of salmonellosis in cattle

Although salmonellosis in cattle is caused by a number of different serovars, *S.* Typhimurium and *S.* Dublin are by far the most common. The disease caused by both serovars in cattle is clinically indistinguishable, but they differ epidemiologically. The host preferences and the ability of the two serovars to establish carriers in animals following initial infection also differ. Furthermore, the distribution of these two serovars may differ between countries.

On 1 March 1989 the Zoonoses Order 1975 was revoked in the UK and replaced by the Zoonoses Order 1989. Prior to this new legislation, estimates of the prevalence of salmonellosis were based on the number of cases diagnosed by the Ministry of Agriculture's laboratories. During the 1960s and early 1970s, *S.* Dublin was the predominant serovar, and the number of cases increased from 115 in 1958 to a peak of 4012 cases in 1969 (Wray and Sojka, 1977). Its prevalence has subsequently declined, with *S.* Typhimurium now being more frequent (MAFF, 1988), but in general, salmonellosis caused by both serovars are in decline (see http://vla.defra.gov.uk/reports/rep_salm_rep09.htm). With the introduction of the Zoonoses Order 1989, isolations of *Salmonella* from horses, deer and pigeons became reportable. In contrast to *Salmonella* in humans, many isolations of *Salmonella* from livestock are not associated with clinical disease, or occur on farm premises where *Salmonella* has been isolated from a group of animals rather than an individual. Since 1993 reports of *Salmonella* from livestock have been separated into 'isolations' and 'incidents'. 'Isolations' comprise individual reports of *Salmonella* made from samples and reported to Officers of the Minister. 'Incidents' afford a truer picture of the amount of *Salmonella* in the animal population as they do not include repeat isolations of a serovar that may result from a number of samplings during the course of an investigation, or monitoring activities on a particular premises. Isolates, isolations and incidents are defined as follows. An isolate is a single culture of a particular *Salmonella*, and results from a single sample. An isolation is defined as the report of the first isolate of a given *Salmonella* (defined by serovar and/or phage type, if available) from the same group of animals on a given occasion. If two submissions from the same group of animals on different dates give the same serovar, this is reported as two isolations. An incident comprises the first isolation and all subsequent isolations of the same serovar or serovar and phage/definitive type combination of a particular *Salmonella* from an animal, group of animals or their environment on a single premises, within a defined time period (usually 30 days) (for further changes in the legislation, see http://vla.defra.gov.uk/reports/rep_salm_rep09.htm).

There is no routine *Salmonella* monitoring of cattle in Great Britain, therefore the majority of isolates come from cattle with clinical disease. In the UK, *S.* Dublin remains the most common serovar isolated from cattle (68.6% of incidents), followed by *S.* Typhimurium (8.4% of incidents), *S.* Mbandaka (8.1% of incidents), *S.* Montevideo (3.7% of incidents) and *S.* Anatum (2.7% of incidents). There were three reported incidents involving *S.* Enteritidis in 2009. Infection of cattle with *S.* Dublin is more frequent than with *S.* Typhimurium in Denmark and Sweden, while the converse is the case in France and

Germany (Methner, 2005). In the Netherlands, the prevalence of *S.* Dublin appears to be increasing (Visser *et al.*, 1993). Although *S.* Dublin has been isolated from humans in New Zealand, it has not been detected in farm animals (Sanson and Thornton, 1997). *Salmonella* Dublin infection was formerly more frequent in cattle in Australia than *S.* Typhimurium, but since 1990 the latter is more common. Since 1980, *S.* Dublin has spread eastward from California to other states and northwards into Canada, where it had not been detected previously (Robinson *et al.*, 1984). Its prevalence now appears to be declining, although it was detected in 26 states during 1995/96 (Ferris and Miller, 1996).

A study of allelic variation in *S.* Dublin by Selander *et al.* (1992) identified three electrophoretic types, making three closely related clones, one of which (Du1) was globally distributed. Non-motile variants are common in the USA, comprising 24% of the *S.* Dublin isolates (Ferris and Miller, 1996). The non-motile variants recovered from the USA belonged to Du1. Strains possessing the Vi antigen were confined to clone Du3, which is apparently limited to France and Great Britain (although in our experience British isolates do not express this antigen). Studies by Ferris *et al.* (1992) of 100 clinical isolates of *S.* Dublin identified 26 groups by phage typing, but 52% belonged to one group. Seven plasmid profile groups were identified, of which 90 isolates belonged to three groups.

Many different phage types of *S.* Typhimurium have been isolated from cattle and in the UK one particular type appears to become dominant until it is replaced by another phage type. During the 1960s, multiple-resistant *S.* Typhimurium phage type 29 became widespread in calves (Anderson, 1968). This then declined and, in 1977, multiple-resistant *S.* Typhimurium phage types 204 and 193 became frequent, and the variant DT204c was the predominant type in calves (Wray *et al.*, 1987b).

Although the prevalence of DT204c decreased during the early 1990s, a subsequent increase in the prevalence of multiply resistant DT104 in both adult cattle and calves has occurred (MAFF, anonymous report, 1996; Wray and Davies, 1996). In the UK, one or two phage types usually predominate, although some 20–30 different phage types are detected annually at a much lower incidence. Surveillance in the Netherlands has shown a similar progression of multiply resistant phage types. In 1972, PT201 (Dutch typing system) was detected in calves; this was replaced by PF193 in 1977, in 1979 PT202 (corresponding to DT204c) was detected and currently PT206-DT104 is occurring (van Leeuwen *et al.*, 1984; W.J. van Leeuwen, RIVM, Bilthoven, the Netherlands, personal communication, 1998).

2009 saw a number of 'firsts' for isolations of phage types of *S.* Typhimurium: *S.* Typhimurium DT66A, DT101 and U320 were never before reported in any UK species and DT80, which was never reported in cattle or livestock before 2009. Many of these apparently 'new strains' may result from extension of phage typing schemes rather than emergence of new clonal groups of *Salmonella*. In addition, a number of irregularly occurring serovars was identified in the UK, and these seem to be mainly associated with contaminated feed ingredients.

Many *Salmonella* serovars other than *S.* Dublin and *S.* Typhimurium have been isolated from cattle (Kelterborn, 1967). During the period 1968–1974, Sojka *et al.* (1977) recorded the isolation of 101 different *Salmonella* serovars, usually at a low prevalence, detected annually in cattle (MAFF, anonymous report, 1996). In the USA, 48% of the 730 *Salmonella*, other than *S.* Dublin and *S.* Typhimurium, isolated from cattle were represented by seven serovars (Ferris and Miller, 1996). In the UK in 2009 there were ten *Salmonella* reports of non-GB origin reported from cattle, these included *S.* Typhimurium DT104, *S.* Mbandaka, *S.* Anatum and *S.* Dublin, clearly showing that importation of new strains remains a constant risk. Interestingly, the number of incidents of *S.* Newport decreased in 2009 in the UK, and these isolates continue to be monitored for multiple drug resistance (MDR) following the emergence of MDR *S.* Newport in the USA where some strains have shown resistance to at least nine antimicrobials, particularly cephalosporins. Monophasic *Salmonella* serovars have also recently been isolated from cattle (Yeruham *et al.*, 2005; Ido *et al.*, 2011).

Antimicrobial Resistance

More detailed information regarding this topic can be found in Chapter 7, this volume. Antimicrobial resistance has been monitored in *Salmonella* isolated from cattle in England and Wales since 1971. Over the years, some clones of *S.* Dublin have developed resistance to some antimicrobial drugs. Fluctuations in the prevalence of resistance are probably related to the clonal spread of particular strains as a result of husbandry and animal movement factors, in addition to the variation in the selective pressure exerted by antimicrobial usage. Similar situations occur in Scandinavia, some other European countries and Australia (Cherubin, 1981; Wilhelm *et al.*, 2009). Likewise, in France, multiply resistant *S.* Dublin has been isolated from calves but not from adult cattle (Lailler *et al.*, 2005).

Multiple antibiotic resistance in the UK is usually associated with a small number of phage types of *S.* Typhimurium, e.g. PT29 (Anderson, 1968), DT204c (Wray *et al.*, 1987b) and more recently DT104 (Hollinger *et al.*, 1998). In the Netherlands, multiply resistant phage types were 201, 193, 202, and more recently, 206 (van Duijkeren *et al.*, 2003). However, in the USA, most *S.* Typhimurium from cattle are multiply resistant, and a recent update on the situation of MDR strains/serovars for the USA can be found in Alexander *et al.* (2009). Other serovars may also acquire antimicrobial resistance (Martel *et al.*, 1995; Wray, 1997) and an account of the epidemiology of multiply resistant *S.* Newport was given by Holmberg *et al.* (1984).

Route of Infection

Infection with *Salmonella* normally occurs via the oral-faecal route. Numerous experiments have shown that oral doses ranging from 10^6 to 10^{11} colony-forming units (cfu) for *S.* Dublin and 10^4 to 10^{11} cfu for *S.* Typhimurium are necessary to cause disease in healthy cattle (Wray and Sojka, 1977). With the higher doses, the results of experimental infections are more consistent and the symptoms are more acute. These doses are likely to be higher than those encountered under natural conditions, where concurrent disease and environmental stress contribute due to immunosuppression. Nazer and Osborne (1977) found that intra-duodenal inoculation of 10^4 *S.* Dublin produced disease.

In addition to the oral route, aerosol transmission may also contribute to *Salmonella* spread. Furthermore, conjunctival infection of calves has been achieved experimentally, although De Jong and Ekdahl (1965) and Nazer and Osborne (1977) found that large doses injected supra-conjunctively were required to produce disease. More recently, experimental infection of calves by aerosol (Wathes *et al.*, 1988) as well as intra-uterine infection of calves have been reported (Counter and Gibson, 1980).

Transmission of Infection

Most infection is introduced into *Salmonella*-free herds by the purchase of infected animals, either as calves for intensive rearing or adult cattle for replacements. Purchased animals may have acquired infection on their home-farm premises, in transit or on dealers' premises (Wray *et al.*, 1990, 1991).

Adult cattle

A case-control study of *S.* Typhimurium DT104 infection in cattle showed that the introduction of newly purchased cattle to a farm increased the risk of disease and that the period of highest risk was the first 4 weeks after purchase. Purchase through dealers was associated with a four-fold increase in risk, compared with purchasing cattle directly from other farms (Evans and Davies, 1996). As indicated previously, *S.* Dublin has become widespread in some countries after being localized in an area for many years. Clonal spread within a country is also a common feature of the epidemiology of *S.* Typhimurium in cattle herds (Aarestrup *et al.*, 1997).

Some adult cattle that recover from *Salmonella* infection, especially in the case of *S.* Dublin, may become active carriers and excrete the organism continuously or intermittently in their faeces for years, if not for life. Sojka *et al.* (1974) investigated two active *S.* Dublin carriers and found that continuous excretion of the organism occurred, the number of organisms ranging from 10^2 to $10^4 g^{-1}$ faeces. In contrast, animals recovering from *S.* Typhimurium infection may continue to excrete the organism in their faeces, but this period is usually limited to a few weeks or months after recovery (Gibson, 1965). However, Evans and Davies (1996) in their investigation of *S.* Typhimurium DT104 infection commented that, while the disease outbreak was of short duration, subclinical infection in the herd could persist for up to 18 months and that recurrence of infection may occur in some herds 2–3 years after the original infection (Davies, 1997). During a study of disease caused by serovars other than *S.* Dublin and *S.* Typhimurium, Richardson (1975a) found that some cows excreted *Salmonella* for up to 11 months after the disease outbreak.

Ingestion of *Salmonella* does not necessarily lead to infection or disease, and Richardson (1975b) considered that *S.* Dublin organisms, and presumably other serovars, may be ingested by adult cattle and pass through the alimentary tract with little or no invasion on the lymph nodes. Grazing contacts of active carriers often yield positive rectal swabs, but when removed from pasture and stalled they cease shedding *Salmonella* in about 2 weeks. Likewise, during an outbreak of *S.* Newport, Clegg *et al.* (1983) frequently isolated the organism from rectal swabs from a number of animals, but when the two longest excreters were housed in clean premises, the organism was isolated neither from rectal swabs nor at post-mortem examination.

Some animals in a herd may harbour localized infection in lymph nodes or tonsils, especially following *S.* Dublin infection, without excreting the organism in their faeces. Such animals may be termed latent carriers, which are of importance in the epidemiology of *S.* Dublin infection and the persistence of the organism on farms. Watson *et al.* (1971) pointed out that no investigation had been made into cattle that had negative faeces in herds in which *S.* Dublin infection was present. During their investigation, they found that 14 of 59 cows with negative rectal swabs were infected at post-mortem examination. Latent *S.* Dublin carriers may become active carriers or even clinical cases during stress, especially during pregnancy, when abortion may occur and the organism may be excreted in the genital discharges, urine and milk.

Smith *et al.* (1994) found that some cattle in California had chronic *Salmonella* infection of the udder, and some of these cattle shed the organism in both faeces and milk. Experimental studies (Spier *et al.*, 1991) included infection by inoculation of low numbers of organisms (ca. 5000) into the teat canal, and the resulting milk contained 10^2–10^5 cfu ml^{-1} milk. Such milk may be a source of infection for calves. House *et al.* (1993) found that three heifers that were infected with *S.* Dublin as calves had infected supramammary lymph nodes when slaughtered at 13 months of age. It is likely that *S.* Dublin septicaemia may result in lymph node infections and consequent shedding during lactation. In contrast with California, where chronic *S.* Dublin infection of the udder is not uncommon, European studies indicate that mammary-gland infection with *Salmonella* is uncommon, although epidemiologically important. Giles *et al.* (1989) described an outbreak of *S.* Typhimurium in a dairy herd in which a cow excreted the organism intermittently in its milk for 2.5 years. More recently, Sharp and Rawson (1992) described possible mammary-gland infection with *S.* Typhimurium DT104 and Wood *et al.* (1991) the persistence of *S.* Enteritidis in the udder.

A number of studies have shown that *Salmonella* infection may be present on farms in the absence of clinical disease. Thus, Heard *et al.* (1972) studied patterns of *Salmonella* infection on four farms and found that, on a well-run farm, although the incidence of *Salmonella* infection was high, there was little disease. A 3-year study of a farm on which *S.* Dublin was present detected the organism in cattle and their environment in the absence of clinical disease (Wray *et al.*, 1989). Morisse *et al.* (1992) isolated *Salmonella* from 6.9% of 145 cows in 17 herds without a history of *Salmonella*. Interestingly, Smith *et al.* (1994) found 75% prevalence of *Salmonella*-infected dairy herds by serological testing. Thus, failure to recognize that the introduction of infection may sometimes precede the development of clinical disease by several months or years may lead investigators to attribute infection to somewhat unlikely sources. A sudden change in her resistance, due to concurrent disease, nutritional stress or severe weather can result in clinical disease.

Calves

The mixing of young susceptible calves and their subsequent transport is an effective means for the rapid dissemination of *Salmonella*, especially *S.* Typhimurium. Gronstol *et al.* (1974) studied the effect of transport experimentally and found that cross-infection occurred and the stress activated latent infection in calves whose faeces had been negative for 5 weeks. Indeed, it is likely that DT204c was introduced into the Netherlands by the import of British calves (Rowe *et al.*, 1979). A number of studies have shown that few calves are infected on arrival at the rearing farm (Rankin *et al.*, 1969; Osborne *et al.*, 1974; Wray *et al.*, 1987a), but infection then spreads rapidly, often in the absence of clinical disease. Wray *et al.* (1987a) showed that the infection rate for *S.* Typhimurium increases during the first week to reach a peak at 14–21 days, although the spread of *S.* Dublin appears to be slower, with a peak at 4–5 weeks. On all of the farms studies there was little clinical disease. During an analysis of the spatial and temporal patterns of *Salmonella* excretion by individually penned calves, it was observed that non-contagious or indirect routes were more important than direct contagious routes in disease spread (Hardman *et al.*, 1991). These authors suggested that the avoidance of aerosol production and the effective cleaning and disinfection of utensils between feeding and of building between batches were likely to be of great importance in the control of salmonellosis in calves.

Both active and latent carriers of *S.* Dublin may produce congenitally infected calves and, though most of these calves are often stillborn, some may survive to infect in-contact animals or to become a carrier. Calves may also be infected by drinking milk from cows with *Salmonella* infection in the udder or associated lymph nodes (Smith *et al.*, 1989).

Additional Factors in the Aetiology of Disease

Many factors, conveniently labelled as 'stress', may either exacerbate the disease or increase the susceptibility of cattle to *Salmonella* infections. Frik (1969) suggested that the persistent carrier state in adult cattle follows concurrent *S.* Dublin and *Fasciola hepactica* infection, and Richardson and Watson (1971) reported that salmonellosis in adult cattle was more prevalent on fluke-infested farms, although Taylor and Kilpatrick (1975) suggested that the two infections were independent of each other but were influenced by similar external conditions. However, in experimental studies, Aitken *et al.* (1976) found that fascioliasis increased the susceptibility to *S.* Dublin infection.

Similarly, in calves, combined *Salmonella* and bovine viral diarrhoea virus (BVDV) infection was more severe than *Salmonella* infection alone (Wray and Roeder, 1987), and severe disease was observed in a group of pregnant dairy heifers that had natural BVDV and *S.* Typhimurium DT104 infection (Penny *et al.*, 1996). Morisse and Cotte (1994), on the other hand, could find no association between BVDV and *F. hepatica* and *Salmonella* infections, because both agents had an identical prevalence in infected and control herds. They suggested, however, that metabolic and hepatic changes observed during the peripartum period could result in disturbances in the intestinal ecosystem and in the emergence of *Salmonella* populations.

In a case-control study of *S.* Typhimurium DT104 in cattle, Evans (1996) found that the feeding of purchased maize or root crops was associated with a reduced risk of disease. It is known that normal flora of the alimentary tract is inhibitory to colonization by *Salmonella* (Chambers and Lysons, 1979). The inhibitory effect is probably most dependent on the volatile fatty acid content and pH of rumen fluid, and a change in feed or an inadequate level of feeding can alter the balance of the intestinal flora to favour the multiplication of *Salmonella* (Frost *et al.*, 1988; Morisse and Cotte, 1994). Thus, it is possible that the susceptibility of an animal to *Salmonella* may be modulated by feeding changes that affect the intestinal flora balance.

Environmental Aspects

Persistence in buildings

An important aspect of the epidemiology of *Salmonella* infection in cattle is the persistence of the organism in animal accommodation after depopulation. *Salmonella* were isolated from the environment of six of nine calf units investigated after cleansing and disinfection (Wray *et al.*, 1987b). Similar results were found in markets (Wray *et al.*, 1991) and on calf dealers' premises, when the organism was detected in the environment of 10 of the 12 premises investigated (Wray *et al.*, 1990). The cleaning and disinfection routines were often ineffective and *Salmonella* were isolated from 7.6% and 5.3% of the wall and fall samples, respectively, before disinfection and 6.8% and 7.6% afterwards. Eight different *Salmonella* serovars were detected, of which the commonest was *S.* Typhimurium. On one of the premises, the *Salmonella* isolation rates increased after cleansing and disinfection, and it is possible that the use of pressure hoses may spread *Salmonella* by aerosols to other parts of the building or that vigorous cleansing may have washed *Salmonella* out from previously untouched areas. *Salmonella* Typhimurium DT204c has been shown by plasmid-profile analysis to persist in calf units for periods ranging from 4 months to 2 years (mean 14 months) (McLaren and Wray, 1991). A case-controlled study of *S.* Typhimurium DT104 indicated an increased risk of disease when cattle were housed, possibly indicating that contaminated buildings may be a source of infection or that close confinement or stress when housed increases the risk of clinical disease (Evans and Davies, 1996). In laboratory experiments, *S.* Dublin survived for almost 6 years in faeces on different building materials (Plym-Forshell and Ekesbo, 1996).

Animal wastes

Modern, intensive, cattle production systems produce large amounts of slurry, which has highlighted the risk of pasture contamination because of the disposal problems. The subject was reviewed comprehensively by Jones (1992), although many of the studies were performed in the laboratory rather than on the farm. Jones and Matthews (1975) isolated small numbers of *Salmonella*, fewer than 100 g^{-1} from 20 of 187 different samples of cattle slurry. In Sweden, Thunegard (1975) found that 35% of cattle slurry samples contained *Salmonella*, compared with on 6% of solid manure samples. Multiplication of *Salmonella* has been reported during storage of slurry (Blum, 1968, Findlay, 1973), however, in general, their numbers are reduced by storage. *Salmonella* have been shown to survive for up to 286 days in slurry, but this is a function of the initial number of organisms, storage temperatures below 10°C and in slurries containing more than 5% solids. Although *Salmonella* die rapidly in slurry during storage, there are occasions when disinfection may be necessary, and various chemicals, such as lime, formalin or chlorine, have been recommended (Jones, 1992). Aeration of slurry is also an effective method of reducing *Salmonella*; Munch *et al.* (1987) found a 90% reduction within 2 days.

Pasture contamination

Salmonella may survive for long periods in infected faeces, where their survival is dependent on a number of factors, especially climatic conditions. Field (1948) reported that *S.* Dublin survived for at least 72 days in faeces on pasture in winter and 119 days in summer. In moist, unheaped faeces, survival up to 3–4 months has been reported, although properly composted faeces heat up rapidly and *Salmonella* reduction is much quicker. Findlay (1972) found that *S.* Dublin survived for 13–24 weeks when spread in slurry on pasture, although Taylor (1973), using a small inoculum, did not isolate *S.* Dublin from soil or pasture for more than 76 days. Taylor and Burrows (1971) found that *S.* Dublin applied in slurry could be recovered from the bottom 3 inches (7.5 cm) of grass for 19 days, although it could not be recovered from the upper levels for more than 10 days. When the grass was cropped, no survival was reported beyond 7 days. From their experiments, they concluded that the disease risk was not great after 7 days and that to infect calves it was necessary to use slurry containing 10^6 *S.* Dublin g^{-1}. A similar experiment by Kelly and Collins (1978), in which cattle were allowed to graze pasture 10 days after it had been treated with slurry from a dairy herd, did not result in any animal becoming infected. However, outbreaks of disease in cattle have been described following the grazing of cattle on slurry-contaminated pasture (Rasch and Richter, 1956; Jack and Hepper, 1969), when unstored slurry has been spread or waste allowed to enter into watercourses.

Salmonella survival has been estimated to be from less than 30 days to 1 year in soil, from 200 to 259 days in soil contaminated with animal faeces, from 57 to 300 days in soil contaminated with cattle slurry and from 11 days to 9 months in soil containing sewage sludge (Jones, 1992). Davies and Wray (1996) found that, when calf carcasses contaminated with *S.* Typhimurium were placed in either a decomposition pit or a deep burial pit, *Salmonella* were isolated from the soil around the pit for 27 weeks and for 15 weeks around the burial site. *Salmonella* reappeared in soil samples during the cold weather after an apparent 9-week absence. Spread to a nearby drainage ditch occurred and wild birds became contaminated from eating *Salmonella*-infected maggots.

Sewage sludge

Sewage sludge is used as a fertilizer, and examination of 882 samples of settled sewage, sewage sludges and final effluent from eight sewage-treatment works found that 68% of the samples were positive for *Salmonella* (Jones *et al.*, 1980). An investigation of 26 outbreaks of salmonellosis in animals found that the attributed sources of infection were sewage effluent (ten incidents), septic-tank effluent (eight), sewage sludge (three), seagulls (three) and abattoir effluent (two) (Reilly *et al.*, 1981). Because sewage sludge is used as a fertilizer, guidelines on the agricultural use of sewage sludge have been produced to minimize possible risks (HMSO, 1977); these have subsequently been incorporated into UK legislation through the Sludge (Use in Agriculture) Regulation 1989, which implements the EC Directive 86/278. In the UK, there is little evidence of risk to animals when known contaminated sludge is spread on pasture, provided that the guidelines are followed (Linklater *et al.*, 1985).

In contrast, on the continent, there have been a number of reports of outbreaks that were associated with grazing cattle on pasture contaminated with sludge (Jones, 1992). Consequently, in Germany, the agricultural disposal of sewage sludge is not allowed if it is not considered hygienically safe.

Water-borne infection

There are many reports on the isolation of *Salmonella* from rivers and streams and, once a water-supply is contaminated, rapid spread of infection may occur. In Europe as well as Africa, a number of cases of *S.* Dublin infection have been associated with watercourses contaminated by grazing animals and farm effluents (Williams, 1975; Akinyemi *et al.*, 2010) Polluted water may also contaminate pasture whenever flooding occurs, and evidence indicates that many clinical outbreaks in cattle arise from grazing recently flooded pasture. Biological treatment of sewage removes most of the suspended and dissolved organic matter but it does not necessarily remove pathogenic bacteria. Consequently, surface watercourses may be heavily contaminated from this source (Harbourne *et al.*, 1978). In the Netherlands, many rivers, canals and lakes are contaminated, although the likely numbers of *Salmonella* are small (<10 *Salmonella* l^{-1}). In the USA, Gay and Hunsaker (1993) found that recycled water that had been used to flush out the accommodation and was then being pumped into the stalls was contaminated with *Salmonella* and responsible for the continued presence of *Salmonella* on the farm.

The role of wild animals

There is no routine monitoring of *Salmonella* in wild birds or wild mammals. Therefore, all isolates are usually from clinical cases or occasionally from small-scale surveys. *Salmonella* is not necessarily the primary cause of disease when identified in wild birds (Reed *et al.*, 2003). For most species of wildlife *Salmonella* is voluntarily reportable, unless the species is covered by the Zoonoses Order (see above). Infection may be introduced on to farms by free-living animals and birds. Rats and mice may acquire *S.* Dublin infection (Tablante and Lane, 1989), but available evidence suggests that they do not play a major role in the spread of infection (Gibson, 1965). Infected mice and rats may prolong the persistence of *Salmonella* on farms, but it is probably of limited duration. Evans and Davies (1996) found that wild birds and cats were possible vectors of *S.* Typhimurium DT104, particularly if they had access to feed stores. A high population density of cats around the farm and evidence of access to feed stores by wild birds were both associated with an increased risk of disease. Cats have also been shown to be infected with *S.* Typhimurium DT104 (Wall *et al.*, 1995a, 1996). Furthermore, the *S.* Typhimurium DT40 and 56 variants, which are associated with wild birds, have been isolated from cattle. In areas with a high badger density, such as Wales, south-west England and the Midlands of the UK, outbreaks of *S.* Agama have been reported in cattle.

Feedstuff

In general, the isolation rate of *Salmonella* in both official and private samples of domestic processed animal protein has risen between 2006 and 2009. This is of concern as although most of this material is not used in rations for food animals, there appear to be increasing problems with either the standard of heat treatment or prevention of recontamination, which could be relevant to treatment of specified risk material (SRM).

As the role of animal feedstuffs in epidemiology of *Salmonella* is the subject of Chapter 19, this volume, this section serves only to emphasize the more important aspects. The importation into Europe of contaminated products has often been followed by the appearance of *Salmonella* serovars previously unknown in Europe. Although *S.* Dublin and *S.* Typhimurium are the commonest serovars, the increasing prevalence in the UK of other serovars in cattle during the 1970s was associated with imported animal protein, e.g. meat and bone-meal and fish-meal. Finished feeds have also been found to be contaminated with *Salmonella*, as have vegetable proteins such as soya, rape-seed meal and cottonseed. Likewise, waste from the food industry, such as biscuit-meal, is often contaminated.

The introduction of contaminated ingredients into compound-feed mills that prepare mixed animal feedstuffs may lead to contamination of cooling systems, storage bins and other equipment, from which, in turn, other products may be contaminated. Although many of the protein ingredients are treated with heat at temperatures high enough to ensure the destruction of *Salmonella*, faulty processing and contamination during and after processing may often lead to heavy contamination of supposedly sterilized products. Various methods have been used to reduce *Salmonella* contamination of animal feeds, such as direct injection of steam, expansion, pelletization and treatment with organic acids, such as propionic and formic acid. In recent years, many farmers in the UK have been mixing their own feeds, and as Evans and Davies (1996) pointed out, poor storage conditions on the farm may allow

Salmonella contamination by animals and birds.

Clinical Findings

Adult cattle

Adult cattle generally contract either acute or subacute enteric salmonellosis, and pregnant animals may abort. As specified before, there are no significant differences between infections caused by the different *Salmonella* serovars.

During the early stages of the acute enteric disease, severely affected animals show fever, dullness, loss of appetite and depressed milk yield; Kahrs *et al.* (1972) recorded that milk production dropped from 5000 to 1000 lb day^{-1} during an outbreak of *S.* Typhimurium infection in a herd of 111 cows. These signs are followed by severe diarrhoea, which may vary from watery green-brown to fetid watery faeces containing blood, mucus and shreds or casts of necrotic bowel lining, and is foul-smelling. The acute disease lasts for about 1 week. Death occurs most frequently 4–7 days from the onset of clinical signs. In untreated cases, the case fatality rate may reach 75%, although this may be reduced to 10% by treatment. In all cases, the animals show signs of toxaemia, dehydration and associated weight loss, with the faeces remaining liquid for 10–14 days, and complete recovery may take up to 2 months.

Similar, but less severe, signs are present in animals suffering from subacute enteric salmonellosis. Fever varies or is absent and the other symptoms are less severe. The prognosis, even without treatment, is quite good, although complete recovery may take several months. In some instances, variations in the clinical disease arise from the fact that illness is not due to recently acquired infection, but to activation by some other disease or the stress of a latent infection or infection cycling through a herd (Gibson, 1965). Such cases may show a wide gradation in the severity of clinical signs, and it may be difficult to determine whether disease is caused primarily by *Salmonella* or weather *Salmonella* are playing a secondary role (Hughes *et al.*, 1971).

As mentioned earlier, sick, pregnant cows may abort. However, it has become apparent that cows may abort from *S.* Dublin infection without showing clinical signs. Indeed, *S.* Dublin in particular, but also other serovars, may cause abortion in cows at any stage of pregnancy. Abortion may either precede the onset of dysentery or follow it within 2–4 weeks. Field observations (Henner and Lugmayr, 1972) and experimental studies (Hall and Jones, 1977) have suggested that abortion is preceded by a period of pyrexia, when the organism is multiplying in the placenta. Aborted fetuses generally show signs of decomposition (Hall and Jones, 1976). In the UK, *S.* Dublin is the second most commonly diagnosed bacterial cause of abortion. Hinton (1971, 1974) studied the clinical aspects of *S.* Dublin abortion and, in 86 of 111 cases, abortion was the only clinical sign. There was no evidence of congenital infection of the calf when abortion cases that were not faecal excreters calved again. On the other hand, when constant faecal excreters were examined, congenital infection of the calf and/or transient vaginal excretion could be demonstrated.

Calves

Calves may be infected with a diverse array of *Salmonella* serovars within hours of birth (Anderson *et al.*, 2001). The subsequent manifestation of disease depends on the host immunity/ability to mount an immune response, pathogen dose and virulence of the serovars. Neonatal disease outbreaks are frequently observed in calves between 4 and 28 days of age (Anderson *et al.*, 2001), and the severity is further influenced by housing and management conditions. In calves, the clinical disease is more common after the first week of life and clinical signs are often seen at 2–6 weeks of age. The clinical picture in calves is subject to wide variation, including pulmonary infections, but the enteric form of the disease predominates. The typical clinical case is characterized by fever, loss of appetite, followed by a brown scour, with fluid, offensive faeces, which often contain blood or mucus. Affected calves quickly lose condition and become dehydrated, weak and emaciated. With *S.* Dublin, bacteraemia and respiratory signs often predominate; the calves often tend to be older than those affected with other serovars (Wray *et al.*, 1987a).

Few clinical signs of disease may be observed in calves that suffer from peracute *Salmonella* infection, with animals simply found dead. Affected animals may have been noted to suffer from profound depression, dullness, prostration, high fever (40.5–42°C), with death occurring within 24–48 h. As this form of salmonellosis shows such a ferocious progression, no further signs may be observed. Laboratory findings may include leukopenia, neutropenia, haemoconcentration associated with dehydration, metabolic acidosis, and increased blood urea nitrogen.

Inappetence and depressed mentation are typically the first clinical signs observed in acute infections. Dehydration, combined with acid–base and electrolyte derangements, contribute to weakness and depressed mentation in acutely infected calves. Pyrexia and diarrhoea follow 48 to 72 h post-infection. Fevers may persist for up to 7 days post-infection. The absence of a fever should not rule out the presence of *Salmonella* as the febrile response is transient and calves succumbing to infection are often hypothermic for 12 to 24 h before death. Faecal consistency ranges from watery, voluminous and profuse to mucofibrinous and haemorrhagic. In some cases, pneumonia may be present, as can be jaundice and nervous signs of encephalomeningitis. Calves surviving the acute phase of the disease often go through a cachectic period during recovery.

Differences are observed between infections with different serovars and potentially between different strains of the same serovar. This is a result of differences in virulence factors that can occur between infecting strains (Mohler *et al.*, 2006, 2008). *Salmonella* Typhimurium is commonly incriminated in outbreaks of enteric disease in calves less than 2 months of age (Wray *et al.*, 1987a, b; Tsolis *et al.*, 1999). In contrast, *S.* Dublin seems to be associated with disease of similar frequencies in young and adult cattle. In a longitudinal surveillance of *Salmonella* shedding by calves, both high and low mortality associated with high-prevalence *Salmonella* faecal shedding were observed (House *et al.*, 2001). In this study, the increase in mortality corresponded to a shift from isolating a mixture of different *Salmonella* serovars to a predominance of *S.* Typhimurium.

Salmonella Dublin is more invasive than *S.* Typhimurium, and invasive manifestations of disease include meningoencephalitis, septic arthritis and septic physitis. These may be observed with or without signs of enteric disease. *Salmonella* Dublin also has a propensity to cause respiratory disease in older calves around the time of weaning. Polyarthritis and osteitis have also been described occasionally, and a sequel to some cases of enteric salmonellosis is the development of dry gangrene of the extremities, including ear tips, tail tip and the limbs from the fetlock down (O'Connor *et al.*, 1972). An immune-mediated process, known as cold agglutination, has been proposed as the main cause of dry gangrene (Loeb *et al.*, 2006). A small proportion of calves infected with *S.* Dublin fail to clear the infection and remain chronically infected. These 'carrier' animals usually appear normal and go on to shed *Salmonella* in faeces and milk, thus maintaining a source of infection in the herd. Calves born from dams infected with *S.* Dublin may be stillborn, non-viable or sickly from birth.

The severity and duration of clinical disease in calves is related to virulence of the strain, challenge dose, calf age, efficiency of passive immunity, nutrition, and degree of environmental stress. The severity and duration of clinical signs are often related to the standard of husbandry and hygiene. On poorly run farms, 80% or more calves may develop clinical signs, with mortality rates of 10–50%. Contributory factors are important in determining the occurrence and severity of clinical disease. Concurrent viral diseases, such as BVDV infection, have been shown to be of importance.

Haematological and Biochemical Aspects

The haematological changes during bovine salmonellosis have not been studied in depth and their interpretation is rendered difficult, but such factors include the age of the animal, state of hydration and possible effects of endotoxaemia.

In calves that die from salmonellosis, Smith *et al.* (1979) and Endresen (1970) found that a leucopenia and associated neutropenia preceded death, whereas in experimentally infected calves, Wray (1980) observed that a terminal leucocytosis followed the leucopenia. In calves that survive salmonellosis, a leucocytosis, with an increase in immature neutrophils, occurs (Smith *et al.*, 1979; Wray, 1980; Rings, 1985).

Elevated erythrocyte counts, haemoglobin content and packed-cell volumes have been observed in cattle during the terminal phase of salmonellosis (Hall *et al.*, 1980; Wray, 1980), and in some anaemia may occur, which is masked by the haemoconcentration. In calves that survive, erythrocyte counts remain within normal values.

Alterations in the blood biochemical levels occurred terminally in some of the calves that died, blood urea levels increased markedly and alterations in sodium and potassium levels indicated the severity of dehydration (Fisher, 1971; Wray, 1980). In diarrhoeic calves that died of salmonellosis, Fisher and Martinez (1975) found that faecal solids increased, and this, coupled with a reduction in fluid intake, resulted in considerable extravascular loss of water.

Blood urea analysis, clinical chemistry and leucocyte examination may be of value in the prognosis of *Salmonella* infections of cattle and provide guidance for therapy, although care must be exercised in their interpretation because of the variability.

The Pathogenesis of *Salmonella* Infection

Within recent years, the pathogenesis of *Salmonella* infection has been heavily investigated due to the discovery of innate immune receptors, such as Toll-like receptors (TLRs) being involved in the uptake of *Salmonella*. As this is discussed in detail in a different chapter within this book (Chapter 8, this volume), we will provide here on a short summary of our current understanding. *Salmonella* must be ingested in sufficient numbers for colonization of the distal small intestine and colon to occur. Factors interfering with and disrupting the normal intestinal flora may enhance colonization and temporary overgrowth by *Salmonella*. Under these conditions, *Salmonella* may not only be able to invade via M cells, the specialized antigen-sampling cells of the mucosal immune system, but may potentially also invade underlying tissue via opened-up tight junctions, leading to colonization of Peyer's patches (Jepson and Clark, 2001). Once reaching the basal side of the epithelium, *Salmonella* is internalized, either by induced cell membrane ruffling (Hanisch *et al.*, 2010) or by phagocytosis, into macrophages, dendritic cells and neutrophils. The outcome of the interaction between *Salmonella* serovars and dendritic cells or neutrophils is detrimental to the pathogen. In some host species *Salmonella* serovars find a safe haven from humoral defences and neutrophils within macrophages, and replication within this niche appears to be a prerequisite for the development of a systemic infection. In other host species, macrophages can control bacterial growth and the infection remains localized to the intestine and mesenteric lymph nodes (for review, see Santos and Baumler, 2004). However, prior to invasion of any cell type, *Salmonella* must attach to the cellular surface, and the molecular mechanisms of this have been extensively investigated (for review, see Darwin and Miller, 1999). One of the cellular receptors used to attach is the innate immune receptor TLR5. For this receptor, the molecular interaction between FliC and TLR5 has been intensively studied (Yoon *et al.*, 2012). Interestingly, TLR5 seems to be expressed only on the basolateral side of polarized intestinal epithelial cells (Gewirtz *et al.*, 2001). This interaction results in internalization of the bacteria (Eaves-Pyles *et al.*, 2011) as well as the initial stimulation of the innate and subsequently adaptive immune response to *Salmonella*. In this respect, flagellin expression not only enhances *Salmonella* accumulation in TLR5-positive cells (Metcalfe *et al.*, 2010), but the flagellin-TLR5 interaction may also induce tolerance to subsequent exposure (Sun *et al.*, 2007). This may be counteracted by the host through a second flagellin receptor, Ipaf, which recognizes flagellin delivered into the cytosol via the SPI-1 type III and the Dot/Icm type IV secretion system (Zhou and Galan, 2001; Miao *et al.*, 2007). Thus, TLR5 responds more generally to flagellated bacteria (in their invasive form), while Ipaf responds to bacteria that express both flagellin and virulence factors. Activation of both receptor systems subsequently leads to the clinical signs of salmonellosis.

Calves

As indicated previously, the intestine does not appear to be the sole portal of entry for *Salmonella*, and infection of oesophagoectomized calves with *S.* Typhimurium resulted in haematogenous spread via the tonsil to the intestine (De Jong and Ekdahl, 1965). Most experimental studies have been made with oral challenge, where the organism gains entry to the tissues by an invasive process, mainly in the lower intestine. Here the bacteria are able to invade the intestinal mucosa via both M cells, which overlie the lymphoid follicles, and the enterocytes. The bacterial infection results in distinct pathological changes; the villi become oedematous and shortened and there is an abnormal extrusion of enterocytes. Using specific staining techniques, Segall and Lindberg (1991) showed that *S.* Dublin had a special affinity for the columnar enterocytes of the terminal jejunum and ileum, the follicle-associated epithelium over the Peyer's patches and glandular tissues in the duodenum, tonsilar area and lungs. Using ligated bovine intestinal loops, Watson *et al.* (1995) found no difference in the ability of the *S.* Typhimurium and *S.* Dublin to invade the intestinal mucosa. When isogenic mutants were used, mutations in the *sly*A (a gene postulated to regulate the expression of virulence factors) had only a small effect on invasiveness, whereas mutations in *inv*H (a gene involved in secretion of proteins from *Salmonella*) caused a significant reproduction of epithelial invasion.

The mechanisms involved in the induction of diarrhoea are poorly understood; the involvement of bacterial toxins has long been speculated upon but, to date, there is little evidence to support a role for toxins. There are numerous reports of cytotonic, cytotoxic and enterotoxic activities *in vitro*, but these reports are often contradictory (Lax *et al.*, 1994). A putative *Salmonella* enterotoxin gene (*Stn*) has been cloned (Chopra *et al.*, 1987). The effect of mutations in the *inv*H, *sly*A and *Stn* genes on the enteropathogenicity of *S.* Typhimurium and *S.* Dublin was studied in bovine ligated intestinal loops by Watson *et al.* (1997). They found that the *inv*H mutation markedly affected the secretory and inflammatory response, implicating secreted effector molecules and enteropathogenicity. Surprisingly, the *sly*A mutation had no effect on enteropathogenicity. There appeared to be a direct correlation between the inflammatory response and the secretory response, although it could not be concluded that one occurred as a consequence of the other or vice versa. A role for secreted effector molecules in *Salmonella*-induced fluid secretion has recently been confirmed. Disruption of SopB (a 60 kDa secreted protein of *S.* Dublin) does not affect intestinal invasion but abolishes secretory and inflammatory responses in bovine ileal loops (Galyov *et al.*, 1997). Pullinger *et al.* (2008) undertook a systematic analysis of virulence factors in *S.* Dublin in cattle and found Dublin-specific sequences associated with colonization in cattle.

Many *Salmonella* serovars harbour large plasmids that are associated with virulence (virulence plasmids), and a common nomenclature (*Salmonella* plasmid virulence (SPV)) has been agreed for the operon. The *S.* Dublin virulence plasmid mediates systemic infection but not the enteric phase of the disease in cattle (Wallis *et al.*, 1995), although Libby *et al.* (1997) in their studies observed diarrhoea and enhanced intracellular proliferation in intestinal tissue associated with the presence of the *spv* genes. The *S.* Dublin virulence plasmid also appears to be involved in the lysis of macrophages, although the *spv* genes do not appear to be involved (Guilloteau *et al.*, 1996). However, *sly*A and *inv*H mutations have also been shown to affect macrophage lysis (Watson *et al.*, 1997), again implicating secreted effector molecules in this process.

Many of the systemic pathological effects of salmonellosis leading to shock are believed to be caused by the release of endotoxins (cell-wall polysaccharides). Peel *et al.* (1990) did not detect increased blood levels of tumour necrosis factor in experimentally infected calves and consequently postulated that local release of endotoxin may be responsible for the pathological changes in the intestine.

Adult cattle

While there have been numerous studies of experimental *Salmonella* infections in calves, these have been very much less frequent in adult cattle. In cows that had been starved and re-fed, Brownlie and Grau (1967) observed multiplication of *S.* Dublin in the rumen. However, Hall *et al.* (1978) failed to detect multiplication of *S.* Dublin after intraruminal inoculation of animals that had not been starved. Similarly, Chambers and Lysons (1979) found that rumen fluid was inhibitory to *S.* Typhimurium. When nine pregnant heifers were dosed orally with 10^{10}–10^{11} *S.* Dublin, the response was variable: two became severally ill, three developed mild illness and four remained healthy (Hall and Jones, 1979). One of the mildly ill animals aborted. In earlier experiments (Hall and Jones, 1977), using intravenous challenge, they found that *S.* Dublin multiplied rapidly in the connective tissue of the cotyledons just before abortion, which resulted in placental destruction and hormonal changes, which initiated the abortion.

Spier *et al.* (1991) produced intramammary infection in five post-parturient cows with low numbers of *S.* Dublin and, while excretion of *S.* Dublin was intermittent, none of the cows showed clinical signs, even though persistently infected. However, following the administration of dexamethasone, one cow became acutely ill and chronic mastitis was demonstrated in the others.

Post-mortem findings

Adult cattle

Although pathologists associate salmonellosis with enteric lesions, such as diphtheritic membranes, peracute infections often have few pathologic findings. Lesions observed with peracute salmonellosis include pulmonary congestion and submucosal and subserosal petechial haemorrhages of multiple organs, including the intestines and heart. Acute salmonellosis is typically characterized by diffuse catarrhal haemorrhagic enteritis with diffuse fibrinonecrotic ileotyphlocolitis. The intestinal contents are watery, malodorous, and may contain mucus or whole blood. Inflammation of the gall bladder is common, and histopathological evidence of fibrinous cholecystitis is considered pathognomonic for acute enteric salmonellosis in calves. Enlargement, oedema and haemorrhage are commonly observed in the mesenteric lymph nodes. Abomasal mucosal erosions may be observed, particularly with *S.* Dublin infection. Chronic salmonellosis may result in thickening of the intestinal wall with a yellow-grey necrotic material overlying a red mucosal surface. These lesions, however, are insufficient to form a firm diagnosis, and bacteriological confirmation is necessary.

Calves

Animals dying of acute septicaemia show extensive submucosal and subserosal petechial haemorrhages. More prolonged cases are characterized by poor bodily condition, usually with evidence of fetid diarrhoea. The small intestine typically shows a diffuse mucoid or muco-haemorrhagic enteritis and the mesenteric lymph nodes are oedematous, congested and greatly enlarged. A severe haemorrhagic and diphtheritic enteritis has been seen in some cases of *S.* Typhimurium infection. The liver commonly shows jaundice, with thick turbid bile, and many reports refer to the presence of necrotic foci in the liver and kidneys. Gibson (1965) commented that, although such liver lesions were commonly reported in mainland Europe, they were uncommon in his experience. Sharply defined areas of pneumonia may be present in the anterior lobes of the lungs. When joints are affected, the joint cavities and adjacent tendon sheaths contain a gelatinous or serofibrinous fluid. Skeletal lesions of epiphyseal separation, osteoperiostitis and rarefying osteomyelitis of the distal limb bones were described in calves suffering from chronic *S.* Dublin infection (Gitter *et al.*, 1978).

Laboratory Diagnosis of *Salmonella* Infections

Bacteriological examination

Outbreaks of neonatal calf diarrhoea often involve multiple pathogens. During an outbreak of salmonellosis, it is not uncommon to find from 70% to 80% of calves to be shedding the bacteria. However, in experimental challenge and field studies, differences have been observed in the propensity for and persistence of faecal shedding between different *Salmonella* serovars, with *S.* Dublin having a propensity to shed intermittently despite tissue colonization. A high prevalence of *Salmonella* shedding supports a diagnosis of salmonellosis. Culture techniques are initially preferable to ELISA and PCR detection methods as isolation of the organism provides an opportunity for serotyping and antimicrobial susceptibility testing. *Salmonella* Typhimurium and *S.* Dublin are commonly associated with disease, so the serovar isolated can provide further indication regarding the likelihood of causal association. Interpretation in this regard may require some local knowledge. For example, in Australia *S.* Bovismorbificans is commonly associated with disease in livestock. However, this same serovar is uncommon in North America. Calves dying of salmonellosis are often bacteriaemic. Therefore, isolation of *Salmonella* from systemic sites at necropsy provides robust evidence of causality as well as an isolate relevant for antimicrobial susceptibility testing. If animals are euthanized for necropsy during a herd investigation, it is best to sample calves during the acute stage of the disease. The likelihood of isolating *Salmonella* from cachectic calves recovering from salmonellosis is low because survival is associated with clearance of the organism from tissues. Isolation of *Salmonella* from gut contents or mesenteric lymph nodes without demonstrating compatible histological lesions does not necessarily establish causality.

In the live animal, confirmation of clinical salmonellosis is performed by culture of rectal swabs or, preferably, freshly voided faeces. In adult cattle with clinical salmonellosis, the organism is excreted continuously and in large numbers and isolation of the organism presents no difficulties. Faecal culture, however, may give negative results in the early stages of the disease before the onset of acute diarrhoea. In the febrile stages of the disease, especially *S.* Dublin infection, the organism may be isolated by blood culture and, sometimes, from the milk. There are numerous methods of detecting *Salmonella* and, at the herd level, it is not difficult to detect or isolate the organism. The diagnostic question more specifically relates to the association between the presence of the organism and the observed disease process. This question arises from the observation that *Salmonella* may be recovered from the faeces of clinically normal calves. During a suspected outbreak of salmonellosis, ten calves in the affected age group should be sampled to determine the proportion of calves infected with *Salmonella*. While direct culture of faeces provides for rapid detection of *Salmonella*, this method of detection is insensitive because of the large number of gram-negative organisms present in faeces, which often hinder the isolation of *Salmonella* colonies. Diagnostic laboratories use enrichment media to promote the growth of *Salmonella* and inhibit other faecal flora. Enriched samples are subsequently plated on *Salmonella*-selective media and suspect colonies are tested using a series of biochemical tests and *Salmonella* antisera. Serotyping is generally conducted by reference laboratories.

In the case of active carriers, usually *S.* Dublin but occasionally other serovars, faecal cultures carried out on three occasions at 7–14 day intervals are recommended to confirm diagnosis. Latent carriers of S. Dublin may best be detected at parturition, when vaginal swabs, faeces and milk may be positive (Richardson, 1973). During an investigation of S. Dublin abortion, Hinton (1974) found that excretion of the organism in milk and the vaginal mucus did not persist beyond 4–5 weeks and faecal excretion was usually transient. When abortions occur, it is usually possible to isolate *Salmonella* from fetal stomach contents of placenta. In some cases, these materials may be culture-negative, because abortion was caused by endotoxaemia, release of endogenous prostaglandin $F_{2\alpha}$ ($PGF_{2\alpha}$) and lysis of the corpus luteum.

Faeces or rectal swabs may be used for calves, but swabs from up to 50% of the infected calves may be negative on culture, because of intermittent excretion, and samples should therefore be taken from a number of calves. The salivary excretion of S. Dublin has been described (Richardson and Fawcett, 1973), but a number of workers found that faeces were more reliable than mouth swabs.

At necropsy, the isolation of *Salmonella* from tissues and intestinal contents usually presents few problems, but care must be taken in the interpretation of the findings, especially when small numbers of the organism are isolated from a few tissues or in cases where other pathogens are present. The isolation of *Salmonella* should be correlated with clinical signs and pathological lesions in order to determine the significance of the isolation.

To identify infected herds or to monitor persistence of infection, slurry or environmental samples collected with swabs may be cultured. Likewise, milk filters, when available, may also be used to monitor dairy herds.

Culture media

Although many different media have been described, it should be remembered that S. Dublin is inhibited by brilliant green and care should be exercised in the use of media containing brilliant green. Likewise, S. Dublin may be inhibited by the incubation of enrichment broths at 43°C, e.g. Mueller-Kauffman tetrathionate (Gitter *et al.*, 1978) or Rappaport-Vassiliadis broth (Peterz *et al.*, 1989).

For cattle faeces and rectal swabs, enrichment in selenite broth and plating on brilliant green agars or deoxycholate-citrate agar are usually used in the UK. In the USA, many use xylose-lysine-Tergitol 4 (XLT4) after enrichment in selenite and tetrathionate. Our recent studies obtained better results by using pre-enrichment in buffered peptone water, subculture (1:100 dilution) into semi-solid Rappaport-Vassiliadis and plating on Rambach agar. The last method is also suitable for slurry and milk.

Serological diagnosis

Serum samples from cattle may be tested by the serum agglutination test (SAT) (Wray *et al.*, 1977), when flagellar titres of 1:320 or higher and somatic titres of 1:40 or higher are considered indicative of infection. In the cases of calves less than 4 months of age, a good flagellar response is produced, but there is little or no production of somatic agglutinins. When a calf is 3–4 months old, it is capable of producing high titre agglutinins. The SAT has been used mostly for S. Dublin but, when Lawson *et al.* (1974) evaluated the test in a known infected herd, many serologically positive animals were found not to be infected at slaughter. Other serological tests that have been used include the complement fixation test, the indirect haemagglutination test and the anti-globulin test (see Wray and Sojka, 1977), but the results have been no better than the SAT.

Rapid-detection diagnostic methods include antigen capture ELISA and PCRs. Preliminary enrichment culture is often employed with both techniques to enhance the sensitivity of detection. ELISAs have a reported sensitivity of 59% and specificity of 97.6% on enrichment cultures. Smith *et al.* (1989) used ELISA to predict the carrier status of cows in a herd where animals had mammary and intestinal infections with S. Dublin. They found that, with eight ELISA-positive cows, only 3.4% of 985 faeces and 2.5% of

756 milk samples were culture-positive (Smith *et al.*, 1992). In calves, 17.3% of 643 faeces were culture-positive. They considered that ELISAs were a better guide than culture for identified carrier status. Nielsen and Vestergaard (1992) found a sensitivity of 92% and specificity of 91% when an ELISA, read at an end-point titre of 800, was used to detect *S.* Dublin carriers. A comparison of persisting anti-lipopolysaccharide (LPS) antibodies and post-mortem culture of animals from *Salmonella*-infected herds showed that only half (14/31) *S.* Dublin-seropositive adult cattle were culture-positive, although 6/13 calves were positive. However, none of the cattle seropositive for *S.* Typhimurium was culture-positive at post-mortem. They concluded that serology was useful to identify infected herds but insufficient for the identification of persistently infected animals. Because of cross-agglutination between the *Salmonella* groups B- and D-LPS in the ELISA, Konrad *et al.* (1994) oxidized the LPS with sodium periodate to produce pure O9 antigen and so eliminate these cross-reactions.

Hoorfar *et al.* (1996) evaluated a fimbrial (SEF14) antigen to differentiate *S.* Dublin- and *S.* Typhimurium-infected herds and, while there was no complete agreement in an ELISA using a somatic antigen, they considered that the high specificity of the SEF14 antigen may increase the predictive value of the test in areas with a low prevalence of *Salmonella*.

Conventional and real-time PCR assays have also been developed to detect the presence of *Salmonella* in faeces. PCR is reported to reduce the detection limits and time compared with conventional faecal culture techniques.

The use of milk assays for *Salmonella* antibodies

A number of earlier assays based on the milk-ring test were not reliable and false-positive results were not uncommon (see Wray and Sojka, 1977). Although Hinton (1973) considered the whey agglutination test to be nearly comparable to the SAT, it was only practical to examine whey for flagellar agglutinins. However, ELISAs have been used to test milk for *Salmonella* antibodies with promising results. ELISA was used by Smith *et al.* (1989) to detect *S.* Dublin antibodies in milk; they found a good correlation between serum and milk titres and concluded that ELISAs were a useful test for detection of cattle with chronic *S.* Dublin infection of the intestine and mammary gland. All of the cattle shed *S.* Dublin in the milk and faeces; 46% of 1733 milk samples and 4% of 1733 faeces were culture-positive. Antibody titres remained elevated for long periods and there was a significant difference in milk ELISA titres between the infected group and the uninfected control group. Likewise, Hoorfar *et al.* (1994) as well as Hoorfar and Wedderkopp (1995) used the ELISA to screen milk samples for *S.* Dublin and *S.* Typhimurium antibodies; they found a good correlation between the serum and milk antibody titres, but considered that further modifications were necessary before the assay could be used for bulk milk samples.

Treatment

The choice of drugs to be used depends on tests to determine the antibacterial sensitivity of the isolate, which may depend on the geographic region. Furthermore, some *Salmonella* isolates may be multiply resistant, though early treatment based on a likely successful regimen must be used before these results are available. Dehydration, electrolyte imbalances, endotoxaemia and bacteraemia are common clinical features of *Salmonella* infections in calves. Treatment of salmonellosis in calves is directed at replacing fluid and electrolyte losses, limiting inflammatory cascades through use of non-steroidal anti-inflammatory drugs (NSAIDs), and the judicious use of antimicrobials. Parenteral fluid therapy will increase the survival rate when administered intravenously. Oral fluids will also help animals to survive the period of acute dehydration and toxaemia. Intravenous hypertonic saline ($4\,mg\,kg^{-1}$ of 7% NaCl), combined with oral rehydration with water or hypotonic sodium-contaminating fluid via a stomach tube, has proved particularly useful. Provision of a clean, dry, thermo-neutral environment and nutritional support improves outcome.

There are differences of opinion amongst veterinarians about the rationale and wisdom of treating cases of salmonellosis with antimicrobials (Whitlock, 1984), because of their efficacy and the likelihood of producing carriers. The general view of most practitioners is that prompt treatment with broad-spectrum antibiotics is beneficial. Aggressive treatment early in the course of the disease, especially in calves, where infection may become septicaemic, is required. Parenteral antimicrobial therapy has been shown to be more beneficial than oral treatment and, indeed, antimicrobial drugs have been shown to be effective in preventing the development of bacteraemia or septicaemia in animals suffering from enteric disease (Osborne *et al.*, 1978).

A number of experiments have shown that some antimicrobials may prolong *Salmonella* shedding, but the importance under farm conditions is uncertain, especially as studies of calves on farms have shown that, during outbreaks of salmonellosis, there is concomitantly a high prevalence of subclinical infection in untreated animals.

Vaccination

Vaccination is based on the induction of memory responses that contribute to control of the pathogen upon infection. It has been shown that *S. enterica* induces both humoral and cellular immune responses in cattle (Lindberg and Andersson, 1983; Roden *et al.*, 1992; Villarreal-Ramos *et al.*, 1998) and that both cellular and humoral immune responses are required for protection (Mastroeni *et al.*, 1993). Vaccines against salmonellosis in cattle can be divided into two major groups: inactivated and live attenuated bacteria.

Within the first group, there are whole-cell inactivated bacteria, such as Bovivac S, a mixture of killed *S.* Typhimurium and *S.* Dublin (http://www.msd-animal-health.co.uk/products_public/bovivac_s/090_product_datasheet.aspx) currently marketed by MSD, and subunit vaccines, such as the siderophore receptors and porins (SRP®) as used in the *S.* Newport bacterial extract (Agrilabs, St Joseph, Missouri, USA). Both these preparations are recommended for therapeutic treatment of ongoing infections and are aimed at reducing the shedding of bacteria during clinical infection (see http://www.agrilabs.com/documents/BHW %20 Dairy %20v3 %20n1 %202007 %20SPRING.pdf). Reduction of *Salmonella* shedding is regarded as one of the major contributions of these vaccines to the clearing of infection. However, there are reports with different outcomes on the use of these vaccines. Heider *et al.* (2008) reported no differences in the level of *Salmonella* shedding between vaccinated and non-vaccinated cattle in a dairy herd with subclinical infection. Similarly, Dodd *et al.* (2011) and colleagues reported no difference in the faecal prevalence of *Salmonella* bacteria or cattle health performance in feedlot cattle. On the other hand, Hermesch *et al.* (2008) reported that vaccination of healthy dairy cattle with an SRP vaccine prior to parturition increased milk production even in cattle without detectable shedding of *S.* Newport or clinical signs of salmonellosis. The mechanisms to explain this observation remain to be explored.

Live attenuated vaccines have been considered to induce better protection than killed vaccines due to their ability to stimulate both cellular and humoral immune responses (Villarreal-Ramos *et al.*, 1998). These vaccines are generated mainly through targeted gene deletion of genes that have been shown to be necessary for the pathogen in the host. *Aro*$^-$ mutants of *S.* Dublin and *S.* Typhimurium have been shown experimentally to confer protection against homologous challenge in experimental conditions (Smith *et al.*, 1984a, b, 1993; Villarreal-Ramos *et al.*, 1998). An *aro*$^-$ *S.* Dublin is licensed as vaccine in the USA for use in cattle older than 2 weeks of age. The vaccine was initially used as a parenteral vaccine in a clinical setting in 1995 (Selim *et al.*, 1995). More recently, the vaccine was used to determine whether the level of protection the vaccine would confer through the oral route, in extra label conditions, in a clinical setting

(Habing *et al.*, 2011). The authors found no difference in the morbidity and/or mortality rate between vaccinated and non-vaccinated animals. The reason for this, the authors propose, could be that having suffered an outbreak of salmonellosis, conditions in the farm were such that the incidence of *Salmonella* was at a low level due to management and herd immunity changes. There is a need to further test currently available vaccines in clinical settings to determine their ability to confer protection under natural conditions.

Control and Prevention of Bovine Salmonellosis

In general, measures for the control of bovine salmonellosis are equally applicable to all serovars, despite the differences in some aspects of their epidemiology. Three principal variables determine the outcome of host-*Salmonella* interactions: host immunity, pathogen dose and pathogen virulence. Environmental conditions have the potential to influence outcomes by impacting each of these variables. The approach to infectious disease control described by Radostits and Acres (1980) over three decades ago includes: (i) removing the source of infection from the calf's environment; (ii) removing the calf from the contaminated environment; (iii) increasing the non-specific immunity of the calf; (iv) increasing the specific immunity of the calf; and (v) reducing stress. These approaches are still applicable today and represent the core of *Salmonella* control programmes. These principles have been adapted in current production animal systems through the uptake of hazard analysis and critical control point programmes.

Measures aimed at protecting cattle

In general, strategies to mitigate the potential adverse consequences of introduced and endemic *Salmonella* come back to good feed management and implementation of good husbandry practices that avoid compromised herd immunity.

If possible, a closed-herd policy should be maintained. Improving the resistance of high-risk groups by immunization is important, as is correct feeding to maintain the intestinal flora in a balanced state. If stock are purchased or returned to the farm from markets etc., they should be: (i) kept in isolation for 4 weeks, as many disease outbreaks occur within 2–3 weeks of arrival and the quarantine period allows the infection to be contained and reduces spread to the resident stock; or (ii) bought from direct sources rather than dealers/markets. Visitors who have been on to other farms and in contact with animals should be provided with clean protective clothing and disinfected boots. Foot-baths with active disinfectants should be provided at the entry to all livestock farms. The quarantine buildings should be located as far away as possible from the resident herd, with the flow of sewage being controlled in such a way that the flow from the quarantine building does not reach healthy animals, and good hygiene (separate boots, overalls and equipment) and disinfection procedures observed. As mentioned before, waterways and pasture may be contaminated during the application of slurry and sewage sludge; therefore, surface water should be fenced off and pastures rested for 4–5 weeks after the application of slurry and sludge. Effective rodent and bird control should be carried out, because these animals have been shown to contaminate stored feed.

Animals should be inspected daily for signs of diarrhoea or other illness and, after about 3 weeks, faeces may be cultured for the presence of *Salmonella*, or checked using ELISA. These measures are likely to have the greatest impact on the reduction of salmonellosis, including diseases caused by MRD DT104 serovars (Aarestrup *et al.*, 1997). In the case of adults, a positive serological test for *S.* Dublin or *S.* Typhimurium will indicate that the animal should be kept in isolation and its faeces cultured.

Calf-rearing units

Calves have numerous opportunities to become infected with *Salmonella*. On dairy farms experiencing problems with neonatal salmonellosis, it is not uncommon to find evidence of disease and a high prevalence of *Salmonella* faecal shedding in postpartum cows. Here, calves may become infected through faecal material from the dam during birth-process, or when calves contact the underside of the cow during suckling. Similar as with risk-herds, salmonellae may also proliferate in organic bedding material used in calving pens. The presence of moisture in the environment favours *Salmonella* proliferation and can result in environmental loads of 10^7 salmonellae g^{-1}. It is important to appreciate that significant pathogen exposure can occur during the first hours of life. However, as before, these points can be easily controlled through good husbandry and appropriate management. A very good review summarizing the most important aspects of preventing calves from contracting salmonellosis can be found in Mohler *et al.* (2009).

Control measures on farms rearing purchased calves from different sources should be planned on the probability that *Salmonella* infection will be introduced sooner or later. Sick calves or calves from known infected cows should not be introduced into an already occupied calf house or unit. One infected calf can give rise to widespread infection in a calf house, irrespective of whether the calves are single penned or group-housed. The risk of introducing *Salmonella* is especially high with purchased calves coming from different resources.

Disease is not, however, inevitable and its prevention depends on two main factors:

1. Minimizing the number of *Salmonella* to which the calves are exposed.
2. Maintaining maximum resistance by optimal nutrition and management practices.

An all-in, all-out system should be adopted and buildings thoroughly cleaned and disinfected, allowing at least 2 weeks between batches to minimize carry-over of infections. Ideally, calves should be bought in age-matched groups directly from local farms, using the purchaser's own transport; if this is not possible, calves should be bought from as few sources as possible, using reputable dealers or reliable buying groups. Markets should be avoided if possible. Body weight, condition and adequate colostral antibody status are useful guides. Journey times should be as short as possible, using suitable vehicles and complying with appropriate regulations. Housing, i.e. the general layout of the site and construction of the calf house, should take account of drainage to minimize cross-infection. All fittings, utensils and surfaces should lend themselves to effective cleansing and disinfection. A strict hygiene routine for buckets and teats should be maintained. Each calf should have its own bucket and automatic feeders should be dismantled, cleaned and disinfected daily. Concurrent infection, especially respiratory diseases or BVDV, may precipitate clinical disease and sick calves should be nursed in isolation facilities. The use of vaccines has been questioned on the grounds that calves may be infected on arrival, but their use is preferable to the prophylactic use of antibiotics.

Control measures during outbreaks

Sick calves can shed 10^9 salmonellae g^{-1} faeces, thus amplifying bacterial load in the environment, increasing the risk of contamination for personnel and equipment. Once salmonellosis has occurred, the priority is to stop it spreading to other animals and people. Thus, it is of outmost importance that the calf attendant needs to follow a strict regime of disinfection on entering and leaving the house and, if possible, should not deal with healthy calves in another house, or should care for healthy calves first.

Clinically affected animals should be kept in isolation, such as sick pens, or segregated, to reduce the large weight of environmental contamination. However, it has to be kept in mind that once an infected calf has been identified, the other calves in the group have already been exposed. Thus, movement of calves may be contraindicated to prevent spreading the infection. Animals that have recovered may still excrete the organism and should remain in isolation until *Salmonella* excretion ceases (usually 2–12 weeks). In many *Salmonella* outbreaks, infection will be found to be widespread, with healthy animals excreting *Salmonella* in their faeces. Stressful events, such as parturition, nutritional stress, anorexia, other disease etc., may trigger clinical disease and, because newly calved cows are susceptible, disease often occurs in calving boxes or stalls. These should not be used for other animals until they have been thoroughly cleaned and disinfected.

Salmonella spreads around the farm environment on boots, tractors, other equipment, surface water, effluent from animal accommodation, birds, rodents, domestic animals etc., and every effort should be made to attain a very high standard of cleanliness and discipline at all times. All manure and effluent should be contained for disposal or treated in such a way as to minimize environmental contamination. Slurry should be stored for at least 3 months and bedding from the isolation areas is best burned. Manure and slurry are best spread on arable land.

Public Health Aspects

Although *Salmonella* are an important cause of food poisoning, it should not be forgotten that humans may be infected by direct contact with infected cattle. Skin lesions caused by *S.* Dublin and other serovars have been described in veterinarians following obstetrical manipulations (Williams, 1980; Visser, 1991). It was reported by Evans and Davies (1996) that, on 20% of the cattle farms where *S.* Typhimurium DT104 infection was present, possible or confirmed associated human illness occurred in farm workers or their families. A study of human cases of salmonellosis found that 30% were associated with contact with infected cattle (Fone and Barker, 1994) and, in a case-control study, 10% of the cases originated on farms (Wall *et al.*, 1994, 1995b).

Milk-borne *Salmonella* infection

Contamination of milk may occur by a variety of routes. Cattle may occasionally, during the febrile stages of salmonellosis, excrete the organism in their milk (Gibson, 1965; Maclachlan, 1974) or, more commonly, infected faeces from either a clinical case or a healthy carrier may contaminate milk during the milking process (McEwen *et al.*, 1988). In western Europe, udder infection with *Salmonella* appears infrequent, although the excretion of *S.* Typhimurium has been reported (Ogilvie, 1986; Giles and King, 1987). In herds that had experienced acute outbreaks of salmonellosis, Morisse *et al.* (1984) detected *Salmonella* in 10–60% of aseptically drawn milk samples. During a herd investigation by Giles *et al.* (1989), a cow was detected that excreted *S.* Typhimurium intermittently from the udder for 2.5 years. In California, udder infections with *S.* Dublin do not appear to be uncommon (Smith *et al.*, 1989; Spier *et al.*, 1991) and *S.* Dublin infection of humans from drinking raw milk has been documented (Werner *et al.*, 1979, 1984). Milk may also be contaminated by the use of polluted water (Gay and Hunsaker, 1993) or dirty equipment. Indirect contamination may also occur when the udders, flanks etc., of cattle become contaminated when they wade into polluted streams and the *Salmonella* enter the milk during milking (George *et al.*, 1972).

Many outbreaks of human salmonellosis have been associated with the drinking of raw milk (Sharp *et al.*, 1980; Potter *et al.*, 1984) and in Scotland an outbreak of human illness caused by *S.* Dublin involved at least 700 people (Small and Sharp, 1979). During the period 1992–1996, Djuretic *et al.* (1997) described 11 general outbreaks associated with milk and dairy products, such as cheese. Some of these outbreaks involved pasteurized milk and, although the heat treatment used during pasteurization is adequate to destroy *Salmonella* in milk, pasteurization-plant failure and post-pasteurization contamination can occur. Ryan *et al.* (1987) reported one such outbreak when over 16,000 culture-confirmed cases of human *S.* Typhimurium infection occurred after drinking pasteurized milk from a plant where post-processing contamination occurred. Milk products, such as cheese (Rampling, 1996), ice-cream (Djuretic *et al.*, 1997), dried milk powder (Rowe *et al.*, 1987) and others (Becker and Terplan, 1986), have frequently been associated with human salmonellosis.

Meat and meat products

The most serious hazard to public health is that arising from the sick or casualty animal; in such animals, latent *Salmonella* infection may become generalized and so infect other animals in the lairage or during transit. Although there have been many surveys of the incidence of *Salmonella* in healthy cattle at abattoirs, there has been no uniformity of the material examined or the sampling techniques, and consequently the results are not comparable. Surveys in various countries have shown that in adult cattle the incidence of *Salmonella* varied from 0.3 to 11.6% and in calves from 4.3 to 14.3% (see Wray and Sojka, 1977).

The transfer of *Salmonella* from animals carrying the organisms both externally and internally can be limited only by cleanliness of the lairage and strict adherence to hygienic procedures during slaughter and dressing. The presence of even small numbers of *Salmonella* in carcass meat and edible offal may lead to heavy contamination of minced meat and sausage. In 1971, Edel and Kampelmacher (1971) found 33.7% minced meat samples, 20% tartar, 16.7% beef burgers and 16.9% raw sausages to be contaminated with *Salmonella*. Roberts *et al.* (1975) found the prevalence of *Salmonella* in sausages and sausage meat from several different producers to range from about 2 to 60%. A more recent survey found 17% of 786 samples of raw sausage to be contaminated with *Salmonella*, which included *S.* Typhimurium DT104 (Nichols and de Louvois, 1995). Improperly cooked and stored beef was associated with an outbreak of *S.* Typhimurium DT104 (Davies *et al.*, 1996) and a study of food in Manchester (UK) found 0.5% of cooked meat and 3.2% of tripe and udder to be contaminated with *Salmonella* (Barrell, 1987). Such contaminated meat and meat products may either cause direct infection or indirect contamination through cross-contamination in the kitchen.

References

Aarestrup, F.M., Jensen, N.E. and Beggensen, D.L. (1997) Clonal spreads of tetracycline resistant *Salmonella* Typhimurium in Danish dairy herds. *Veterinary Record* 140, 313–314.

Aitken, M.M., Jones, P.W., Hall, G.A. and Hughes, D.L. (1976) The effect of fascioliasis on susceptibility of cattle to *Salmonella* Dublin. *British Veterinary Journal* 132, 119–120.

Akinyemi, K.O., Philipp, W., Beyer, W. and Bohm, R. (2010) Application of phage typing and pulsed-field gel electrophoresis to analyse *Salmonella* enterica isolates from a suspected outbreak in Lagos, Nigeria. *Journal of Infection in Developing Countries* 4, 828–833.

Alexander, K.A., Warnick, L.D. and Wiedmann, M. (2009) Antimicrobial resistant *Salmonella* in dairy cattle in the United States. *Veterinary Research Communications* 33, 191–209.

Anderson, E.S. (1968) Drug resistance in *Salmonella* Typhimurium and its implications. *British Medical Journal* 3, 333–339.

Anderson, R.J., House, J.K., Smith, B.P., Kinde, H., Walker, R.L., Vande Steeg, B.J. and Breitmeyer, R.E. (2001) Epidemiologic and biological characteristics of salmonellosis in three dairy herds. *Journal of the American Veterinary Medical Association* 219, 310–322.

Barrell, R.A. (1987) isolations of salmonellas from humans and foods in the Manchester area: 1981–1985. *Epidemiology and Infection* 98, 277–284.

Becker, H. and Terplan, G. (1986) *Salmonella* in milk and milk products. *Zentralblatt für Veterinärmedizin B* 33, 1–25.

Blum, J. (1968) Studies on the occurrence, tenacity, growth and disinfection of salmonellas in waste waters of agricultural enterprises. *Schweizer Archiv Tierheilkunde* 110, 243–261.

Brownlie, L.E. and Grau, F.H. (1967) The effect of food intake on growth and survival of salmonellas and *E. coli* in the bovine rumen. *Journal of General Microbiology* 46, 125–134.

Chambers, P.G. and Lysons, R.J. (1979) The inhibitory effect of bovine rumen fluid on *Salmonella* Typhimurium. *Research in Veterinary Science* 26, 273–276.

Cherubin, C.E. (1981) Antibiotic resistance of *Salmonella* in Europe and the United States. *Reviews of Infectious Diseases* 3, 1105–1126.

Chopra, A.K., Houston, C.W., Peterson, J.W., Prasad, R. and Mekalanos, J.J. (1987) Cloning and expression of the *Salmonella* enterotoxin gene. *Journal of Bacteriology* 169, 5095–5100.

Clegg, F.G., Chiejina, S.N., Duncan, A.L., Kay, R.N. and Wray, C. (1983) Outbreaks of *Salmonella* Newport infection in dairy herds and their relationship to management and contamination of the environment. *Veterinary Record* 112, 580–584.

Counter, D.E. and Gibson, E.A. (1980) *Salmonella* Dublin infection in self contained dairy herds in East Anglia: excretion at calving. *Veterinary Record* 107, 191–193.

Darwin, K.H. and Miller, V.L. (1999) Molecular basis of the interaction of *Salmonella* with the intestinal mucosa. *Clinical Microbiology Reviews* 12, 405–428.

Davies, A., O'Neil, P., Towers, L. and Cooke, M. (1996) An outbreak of *Salmonella* Typhimurium DT104 food poisoning associated with eating beef. *PHLS Communicable Disease Report* 6, R159–R162.

Davies, R.H. (1997) A two year study of *Salmonella* Typhimurium DT104 infection and contamination on cattle farms. *Cattle Practice* 5, 189–194.

Davies, R.H. and Wray, C. (1996) Seasonal variations in the isolation of *Salmonella* Typhimurium, *Salmonella* Enteritidis, *Bacillus cereus* and *Clostridium perfingens* from environmental samples. *Journal of Veterinary Medicine B* 43, 119–127.

De Jong, H. and Ekdahl, M.O. (1965) Salmonellosis in calves – the effect of dose rate and other factors on transmission. *New Zealand Veterinary Journal* 13, 59–64.

Djuretic, T., Wall, P.G. and Nicholls, G. (1997) General outbreaks of infectious intestinal disease associated with milk and dairy products in England and Wales: 1992-1996. *PHLS Communicable Disease Report* 7, R41–R45.

Dodd, C.C., Renter, D.G., Thomson, D.U. and Nagaraja, T.G. (2011) Evaluation of the effects of a commercially available *Salmonella* Newport siderophore receptor and porin protein vaccine on fecal shedding of *Salmonella* bacteria and health and performance of feedlot cattle. *American Journal of Veterinary Research* 72, 239–247.

Eaves-Pyles, T., Bu, H.F., Tan, X.D., Cong, Y., Patel, J., Davey, R.A. and Strasser, J.E. (2011) Luminal-applied flagellin is internalized by polarized intestinal epithelial cells and elicits immune responses via the TLR5 dependent mechanism. *PloS ONE* 6, e24869.

Edel, W. and Kampelmacher, E.H. (1971) *Salmonella* infection in fattening calves at the farm. *Zentralblatt für Veterinärmedizin (B)* 18, 617–621.

Endresen, H.A. (1970) Evaluation of leucopenia in cattle. *Journal of the American Veterinary Medicine Association* 156, 858–866.

Evans, S.J. (1996) *A Case Control Study of Multiple-resistant* S. *Typhimurium DT104 Infection of Cattle in Great Britain*. Report AHVG, MAFF, Tolworth, Surrey.

Evans, S.J. and Davies, R.H. (1996) Case control of multiple-resistant *Salmonella* Typhimurium DT104 infection in cattle in Great Britain. *Veterinary Record* 139, 557–558.

Ferris, K.E. and Miller, D.A. (1996) *Salmonella* serovars from animals and related sources reported during July 1995-June 1996. *Proceedings of the US Animal Health Association* 100, 505–526.

Ferris, K.E., Andrews, R.E., Thoen, C.O. and Blackburn, B.O. (1992) Plasmid profile analysis phage typing and antibiotic sensitivity of *Salmonella* Dublin from clinical isolates in the United States. *Veterinary Microbiology* 32, 51–62.

Field, H.I. (1948) A survey of bovine salmonellosis in Mid and West Wales. *Veterinary Journal* 104, 294–302.

Findlay, C.R. (1972) The persistence of *Salmonella* Dublin in slurry in tanks and on pasture. *Veterinary Record* 91, 233–235.

Findlay, C.R. (1973) Salmonellae in sewage sludge: multiplication. *Veterinary Record* 93, 102–103.

Fisher, E.W. (1971) Hydrogen ion and electrolyte disturbances in neonatal calf diarrhoea. *Annals of the New York Academy of Sciences* 176, 223–230.

Fisher, E.W. and Martinez, A.A. (1975) Studies of neonatal calf diarrhoea III. Water balance studies in neonatal salmonellosis. *British Veterinary Journal* 131, 643–651.

Fone, D.L. and Barker, R.M. (1994) Association between human and farm animal infection with *Salmonella* Typhimurium DT104 in Herefordshire. *Communicable Disease Report* 4, 136–140.

Frik, J.F. (1969) *Salmonella* Dublin infectis bij runderen in Nederland. Thesis, University of Utrecht.

Frost, A.J., O'Boyle, D. and Samual, J.L. (1988) The isolation of *Salmonella* spp. from feed lot cattle managed under different conditions before slaughter. *Australian Veterinary Journal* 65, 224–225.

Galyov, E.E., Wood, M.W., Rosqvist, R., Mullan, P.B., Watson, P.R., Hedges, S. and Wallis, T.S. (1997) A secreted effector protein of *Salmonella* Dublin is translocated into eukaryotic cells and mediates inflammation and fluid secretion in infected ileal mucosa. *Molecular Microbiology* 25, 903–912.

Gay, J.M. and Hunsaker, M.E. (1993) Isolation of multiple *Salmonella* serovars from a dairy two years after a clinical salmonellosis outbreak. *Journal of the American Veterinary Medicine Association* 203, 1314–1320.

George, J.T.A., Wallace, J.G., Morrison, H.R. and Harbourne, J.F. (1972) Paratyphoid in man and cattle. *British Medical Journal* iii, 208–211.

Gewirtz, A.T., Navas, T.A., Lyons, S., Godowski, P.J. and Madara, J.L. (2001) Cutting edge: bacterial flagellin activates basolaterally expressed TLR5 to induce epithelial proinflammatory gene expression. *Journal of Immunology* 167, 1882–1885.

Gibson, E.A. (1965) Reviews of the progress of dairy science *Salmonella* infection in cattle. *Journal of Dairy Research* 32, 97–134.

Giles, N. and King, S.C. (1987) Excretion of *S.* Typhimurium from a cow's udder. *Veterinary Record* 120, 23.

Giles, N., Hopper, S.A. and Wray, C. (1989) Persistence of *S.* Typhimurium in a large dairy herd. *Epidemiology and Infection* 103, 235–241.

Gitter, M., Wray, C., Richardson, C. and Pepper, R.T. (1978) Chronic *Salmonella* Dublin infection in calves. *British Veterinary Journal* 134, 113–121.

Gronstol, H., Osbourne, A.D. and Pethiyagoda, S. (1974) Experimental *Salmonella* infection in calves. (1) The effect of stress factors on the carrier state. *Journal of Hygiene, Cambridge* 72, 155–162.

Guilloteau, L.A., Wallis, T.S., Gautier, A.V., MacIntyre, S., Platt, D.J. and Lax, A.J. (1996) The *Salmonella* virulence plasmid enhances *Salmonella*-induced lysis of macrophages and influences inflammatory responses. *Infection and Immunity* 64, 3385–3393.

Habing, G.G., Neuder, L.M., Raphael, W., Piper-Youngs, H. and Kaneene, J.B. (2011) Efficacy of oral administration of a modified-live *Salmonella* Dublin vaccine in calves. *Journal of the American Veterinary Medicine Association* 238, 1184–1190.

Hall, G.A. and Jones, P.W. (1976) An experimental study of *Salmonella* Dublin abortion in cattle. *British Veterinary Journal* 132, 60–65.

Hall, G.A. and Jones, P.W. (1977) A study of the pathogenesis of experimental *Salmonella* Dublin abortion in cattle. *Journal of Comparative Pathology* 87, 53–65.

Hall, G.A. and Jones, P.W. (1979) Experimental oral infection of pregnant heifers with *Salmonella* Dublin. *British Veterinary Journal* 135, 75–82.

Hall, G.A., Jones, P.W. and Aitken, M.M. (1978) The pathogenesis of experimental intra-ruminal infection of cows with *Salmonella* Dublin. *Journal of Comparative Pathology* 88, 409–417.

Hall, G.A., Jones, P.W., Parsons, K.R., Young, E.R. and Aitken, M. (1980) The haematology of experimental *Salmonella* Dublin infections in pregnant heifers. *British Veterinary Journal* 136, 182–189.

Hanisch, J., Ehinger, J., Ladwein, M., Rohde, M., Derivery, E., Bosse, T., Steffen, A., Bumann, D., Misselwitz, B., Hardt, W.D., Gautreau, A., Stradal, T.E. and Rottner, K. (2010) Molecular dissection of *Salmonella*-induced membrane ruffling versus invasion. *Cellular Microbiology* 12, 84–98.

Harbourne, J.F., Thomas, G.W. and Luery, K.W. (1978) *Salmonella* in effluent waters and river sites in North Yorkshire. *British Veterinary Journal* 134, 350–357.

Hardman, P.M., Wathes, C.M. and Wray, C. (1991) Transmission of salmonellae among calves penned individually. *Veterinary Record* 129, 327–329.

Heard, T.W., Jennet, N.E. and Linton, A.H. (1972) Changing patterns of *Salmonella* excretion in various cattle populations. *Veterinary Record* 90, 359–364.

Heider, L.C., Meiring, R.W., Hoet, A.E., Gebreyes, W.A., Funk, J.A. and Wittum, T.E. (2008) Evaluation of vaccination with a commercial subunit vaccine on shedding of *Salmonella* enterica in subclinically infected dairy cows. *Journal of the American Veterinary Medical Association* 233, 466–469.

Henner, S. and Lugmayr, D. (1972) Enzootisches Verwerfen bei Rindern verursacht durch Salmonellen. [Enzootic abortion in cattle caused by salmonellae.] *Tierärztliche Umschau* 27, 271–272.

Hermesch, D.R., Thomson, D.U., Loneragan, G.H., Renter, D.R. and White, B.J. (2008) Effects of a commercially available vaccine against *Salmonella* enterica serotype Newport on milk production, somatic cell count, and shedding of *Salmonella* organisms in female dairy cattle with no clinical signs of salmonellosis. *American Journal of Veterinary Research* 69, 1229–1234.

Hinton, M.H. (1971) *Salmonella* abortion in cattle. *Veterinary Bulletin* 41, 973–980.

Hinton, M.H. (1973) *Salmonella* Dublin abortion in cattle. II. Observations on the whey agglutination tests and the milk ring test. *Journal of Hygiene, Cambridge* 71, 471–479.

Hinton, M.H. (1974) *Salmonella* Dublin abortion in cattle: studies on the clinical aspects of the condition. *British Veterinary Journal* 130, 556–563.

HMSO (1977) *Report of the Working party on the disposal of Sewage Sludge to Land.* Report No. 5, Department of the Environment Standing Technical Committee, London.

Hollinger, K., Wray, C., Evans, S., Pascoe, S., Chappell, S. and Jones, Y. (1998) *Salmonella* Typhimurium DT104 in cattle in Great Britain. *Journal of the American Veterinary Medical Association* 213, 1732–1733.

Holmberg, S.D., Osterholm, M.T., Senger, K.A. and Cohen, M.L. (1984) Drug-resistant *Salmonella* from animals fed antimicrobials. *New England Journal of Medicine* 311, 617–622.

Hoorfar, J. and Wedderkopp, A. (1995) Enzyme-linked immunosorbent assay for screening of milk samples for *Salmonella* Typhimurium in dairy herds. *American Journal of Veterinary Research* 56, 1549–1554.

Hoorfar, J., Lind, P. and Bitsch, V. (1994) Evaluation of an O-antigen enzyme-linked immunosorbent assay for screening of milk samples for *Salmonella* Dublin infection in dairy herds. *Canadian Journal of Veterinary Research* 59, 142–148.

Hoorfar, J., Lind, P., Bell, M.M. and Thorns, C.J. (1996) Seroreactivity of *Salmonella*-infected cattle herds against a fibrial antigen in comparison with lipopolysaccharide antigens. *Journal of Veterinary Medicine B* 43, 461–467.

House, J.K., Smith, B.P., Dilling, G.W. and Rosden, L.D. (1993) Enzyme-linked immunosorbent assay for serological detection of *Salmonella* Dublin carriers on a large dairy. *American Journal of Veterinary Research* 54, 1391–1399.

House, J.K., Ontiveros, M.M., Blackmer, N.M., Dueger, E.L., Fitchhorn, J.B., McArthur, G.R. and Smith, B.P. (2001) Evaluation of an autogenous *Salmonella* bacterin and a modified live *Salmonella* serotype Choleraesuis vaccine on a commercial dairy farm. *American Journal of Veterinary Research* 62, 1897–1902.

Hughes, L.E., Gibson, E.A., Roberts, H.E., Davies, E.T., Davies, G. and Sojka, W.J. (1971) Bovine salmonellosis in England and Wales. *British Veterinary Journal* 127, 225–238.

Ido, N., Kudo, T., Sasaki, K., Motokawa, M., Iwabuchi, K., Matsudate, H., Seimiya, Y.M. and Akiba, M. (2011) Molecular and phenotypic characteristics of *Salmonella enterica* serovar 4,5,12:i:- isolated from cattle and humans in Iwate Prefecture, Japan. *Journal of Veterinary Medical Science* 73, 241–244.

Jack, E.J. and Hepper, P.T. (1969) An outbreak of *Salmonella* Typhimurium infection associated with the spreading of slurry. *Veterinary Record* 84, 196–198.

Jensen, C.O. (1891) Om den infektiose Kalvediarrhoe og dens Aarsag. *Maanedsskr Dyrlaeger* 4, 140–162.

Jepson, M.A. and Clark, M.A. (2001) The role of M cells in *Salmonella* infection. *Microbes and infection/ Institut Pasteur* 3, 1183–1190.

Jones, P.W. (1992) Salmonellas in animal wastes and hazards for other animals and humans from handling animal wastes. In: Salmonella *and Salmonellosis*, 15-17 September 1992, Ploufragen/St Brieuc, France, pp. 280-294. (Obtainable from ~ISPAIA, BPT, 22440 Ploufragen, France, 450FF + postage).

Jones, P.W. and Matthews, P.R.J. (1975) Examination of slurry from cattle for pathogenic bacteria. *Journal of Hygiene, Cambridge* 74, 57–64.

Jones, P.W., Rennison, L.M., Lewin, V.H. and Redhead, D.L. (1980) The occurrence and significance to animal health of salmonellas in sewage and sewage sludge. *Journal of Hygiene, Cambridge* 84, 47–62.

Kahrs, F.R., Bentink-Smith, J., Bjorck, G.R., Bruner, D.W., King, J.M. and Lewis, N.F. (1972) Epidemiological investigation of an outbreak of fatal enteritis and abortion associated with dietary change and *Salmonella* Typhimurium infection in a dairy herd, a case report. *Cornell Veterinarian* 62, 175–191.

Kelly, W.R. and Collins, J.D. (1978) The potential health significance of antibiotic-resistant *E. coli* and other infectious agents present in farm effluent. In: *Animals and Human Health*, CEC Eur. 6009 EN, pp. 172–188.

Kelterborn, E. (1967) Salmonella *Species: First Isolation, Names and Occurrence*. W. Junk, The Hague.

Konrad, J., Smith, B.P., Dilling, G.W. and House, J.K. (1994) Production of *Salmonella* serogroup D (O9)-specific enzyme-linked immunosorbent assay antigen. *American Journal of Veterinary Research* 55, 1647–1651.

Lailler, R., Sanaa, M., Chadoeuf, J., Fontez, B., Brisabois, A., Colmin, C. and Millemann, Y. (2005) Prevalence of multidrug resistant (MDR) *Salmonella* in bovine dairy herds in western France. *Preventive Veterinary Medicine* 70, 177–189.

Lawson, G.H.K., McPherson, E.A. and Wooding, P. (1974) The epidemiology of *Salmonella* Dublin infection in a dairy herd. II. Serology. *Journal of Hygiene, Cambridge* 72, 329–337.

Lax, A.J., Barrow, P.A., Jones, P.W. and Wallis, T.S. (1994) Current perspectives in salmonellosis. *British Veterinary Journal* 151, 351–377.

Libby, S.J., Adams, L.G., Ficht, T.A., Allen, C., Whitford, H.A., Buchmeier, N.A., Bossie, S. and Guiney, D.G. (1997) The *spv* genes on the *Salmonella* Dublin virulence plasmid are required for severe enteritis and systemic infection in the natural host. *Infection and Immunity* 65, 1768–1792.

Lindberg, A.A. and Andersson, J.A. (1983) *Salmonella* Typhimurium infection in calves: cell-mediated and humoral immune reactions before and after challenge with live virulent bacteria in calves given live or inactivated vaccines. *Infection and Immunity* 41, 751–757.

Linklater, K.A., Graham, M.M. and Sharp, J.C.M. (1985) Salmonellae in sewage sludge and abattoir effluent in south-east Scotland. *Journal of Hygiene, Cambridge* 94, 301–307.

Loeb, E., Toussaint, M.J., Rutten, V.P. and Koeman, J.P. (2006) Dry gangrene of the extremities in calves associated with *Salmonella* Dublin infection; a possible immune-mediated reaction. *Journal of Comparative Pathology* 134, 366–369.

Löffler, F. (1892) Über Epidemien unter den im hygienischen Institute zu Greifswald gehaltenen Mäusen und über Bekämpfung der Feldmaus plage. *Zentralblatt für Bakteriologie* 11, 129–141.

Maclachlan, J. (1974) Salmonellosis in Midlothian and Peebleshire. *Public Health, London* 88, 79–87.

MAFF (1988) Salmonella *in Livestock Production*. Veterinary Laboratories Agency (Weybridge), Addlestone, UK.

Martel, J.L., Chaslus-Dancla, E., Coudert, M., Poumarat, F. and Lafont, J.P. (1995) Survey of antimicrobial resistance in bacterial isolates from diseased cattle in France. *Microbial Drug Resistance* 1, 273–283.

Mastroeni, P., Villarreal-Ramos, B. and Hormaeche, C.E. (1993) Adoptive transfer of immunity to oral challenge with virulent salmonellae in innately susceptible BALB/c mice requires both immune serum and T-cells. *Infection and Immunity* 61, 3981–3984.

McEwen, S.A., Martin, W.S., Clarke, R.C., Tamblyn, S.E. and McDermott, J.J. (1988) The prevalence, incidence, geographical distribution, antimicrobial sensitivity patterns and plasmid profiles of milk filter *Salmonella* isolates from Ontario dairy farms. *Canadian Journal of Veterinary Research* 52, 18–22.

McLaren, I.M. and Wray, C. (1991) Epidemiology of *Salmonella* Typhimurium infection in calves: persistence of salmonellae in calf units. *Veterinary Record* 129, 461–462.

Metcalfe, H.J., Best, A., Kanellos, T., La Ragione, R.M. and Werling, D. (2010) Flagellin expression enhances *Salmonella* accumulation in TLR5-positive macrophages. *Developmental & Comparative Immunology* 34, 797–804.

Methner, U. (2005) Situation of bovine salmonellosis in Germany from 1995-2003 according to the data from the National Animal Disease Reporting System. *Berl Munch Tierarztl Wochenschr.* 118(11–12), 449–455.

Miao, E.A., Andersen-Nissen, E., Warren, S.E. and Aderem, A. (2007). TLR5 and Ipaf: dual sensors of bacterial flagellin in the innate immune system. *Seminars in Immunopathology* 29, 275–288.

Mohler, J.R. and Buckley, J.S. (1902) *19th Report*. US Bureau Animal Industry, p. 297.

Mohler, V.L., Heithoff, D.M., Mahan, M.J., Walker, K.H., Hornitzky, M.A., McConnell, C.S., Shum, L.W. and House, J.K. (2006) Cross-protective immunity in calves conferred by a DNA adenine methylase deficient *Salmonella* enterica serovar Typhimurium vaccine. *Vaccine* 24, 1339–1345.

Mohler, V.L., Heithoff, D.M., Mahan, M.J., Walker, K.H., Hornitzky, M.A., Shum, L.W., Makin, K.J. and House, J.K. (2008) Cross-protective immunity conferred by a DNA adenine methylase deficient *Salmonella* enterica serovar Typhimurium vaccine in calves challenged with *Salmonella* serovar Newport. *Vaccine* 26, 1751–1758.

Mohler, V.L., Izzo, M.M. and House, J.K. (2009) *Salmonella* in calves. The Veterinary clinics of North America. *Food Animal Practice* 25, 37–54, vi.

Morisse, J.P. and Cotte, J.P. (1994) Evaluation of some risk factors in bovine salmonellosis. *Veterinary Research* 25, 185–191.

Morise, J.P., Cotte, J.P. and Huonnic, D. (1984) Dissemination of salmonellae by chronically infected dairy cows. *Point Vétérinaire* 15, 55–59.

Morisse, J.P., Cotte, J.P., Argente, G. and Daniel, L. (1992) Approche épidémiologique de l'exrétion de salmonelles dans un réseau de 50 exploitations bovine laitiers avec et sans antecedents cliniques. *Annals de Médicine Vétérinaire* 136, 403–409.

Munch, B., Errebo Larsen, H. and Aalbaek, B. (1987) ii. Experimental studies on the survival of pathogenic and indicator bacteria in aerated and non-aerated cattle and pig slurry. *Biological Wastes* 22, 49–65.

Nazer, A.H.K. and Osborne, A.D. (1977) Experimental *Salmonella* Dublin infection in calves. *British Veterinary Journal* 133, 388–398.

Nichols, G.L. and de Louvois, J. (1995) The microbiological quality of raw sausages sold in the UK. *PHLS Microbiology Digest* 12, 236–242.

Nielsen, B.B. and Vestergaard, E.M. (1992) Use of ELISA in the eradication of *Salmonella* Dublin infection. In: *Proceedings International* Salmonella *and Salmonellosis*. ISPAIA, Ploufragen, France, pp. 220–224.

Obich (1865) Woschenschrift für Thierheilkunde und Viezucht. Cited by Jensen, C.O. (1893) Ueber die Külberruhr und deren Aetiologie. Monatschefte für Praktishe Thierheilkundel, Band 597–124. Reprinted in Jensen, C.O. (1948) *Selected Papers 1886-1908*, vol. 1. Einar Munksgaard, Copenhagen, p. 180.

O'Connor, P.J., Rogers, P.A.M., Collins, J.D. and McErlean, B.A. (1972) On the association between salmonellosis and the occurrence of osteomyelitis and terminal dry gangrene in calves. *Veterinary Record* 90, 459–460.

Ogilvie, T.H. (1986) The persistent isolation of *Salmonella* Typhimurium from the mammary gland of a dairy cow. *Canadian Veterinary Journal* 27, 329–331.

Osborne, A.D., Linton, A.H. and Pethiyagoda, S. (1974) Epidemiology of *Salmonella* infection in calves. (2) Detailed study in a large beef rearing unit. *Veterinary Record* 94, 604–610.

Osborne, A.D., Nazer, A.H. and Shimeld, C. (1978) Treatment of experimental calf salmonellosis with amoxycillin. *Veterinary Record* 103, 233–237.

Peel, J.M., Viorol, M.J., Kolly, C., Gobert, D. and Martinod, S. (1990) Induction of circulating tumour necrosis factor cannot be demonstrated during septicaemic salmonellosis in calves. *Infection and Immunity* 58, 439–442.

Penny, C.D., Low, J.C., Nettleton, P.F., Scott, P.R., Sargison, N.D., Strachan, W.D. and Honeyman, P.C. (1996) Concurrent bovine viral diarrhoea virus and *Salmonella* Typhimurium DT104 infection in a group of pregnant dairy heifers. *Veterinary Record* 138, 485–489.

Peterz, M., Wiberg, C. and Norberg, P. (1989) The effect of incubation temperature and magnesium chloride concentration on growth of *Salmonella* in home-made and in commercially available dehydrated Rappaport-Vassiliadis broths. *Journal of Applied Bacteriology* 66, 523–528.

Plym-Forshell, L. and Ekesbo, I. (1996) Survival of salmonellas in urine and dry-faeces from cattle – an experimental study. *Acta Veterinaria Scandinavica* 37, 127–131.

Potter, M.E., Kaufmann, A.F., Blake, P.A. and Feldman, R.A. (1984) Unpasteurised milk: the hazards of a health fetish. *Journal of the American Medical Association* 252, 2048–2052.

Pullinger, G.D., Dziva, F., Charleston, B., Wallis, T.S. and Stevens, M.P. (2008) Identification of *Salmonella enterica* serovar Dublin specific sequences by subtractive hybridization and analysis of their role in intestinal colonization and systemic translocation in cattle. *Infection and Immunity* 76, 5310–5321.

Radostits, O.M. and Acres, S.D. (1980) The prevention and control of epidemics of acute indifferentiated diarrhea of beef calves in Western Canada. *Canadian Veterinary Journal* 21(9), 243–249.

Rampling, A. (1996) Raw milk, cheeses and *Salmonella*. *British Medical Journal* 312, 67–68.

Rankin, J.D., Taylor, R.J. and Burrows, M.R. (1969) *Salmonella* infection in young calves. *Veterinary Record* 85, 582.

Rasch, K. and Richter, J. (1956) Endemiologisches um einen bovine Dauerausscheider von Salmonella Heidelberg. *Berliner und Münchener Tierarztliche Wochenschrift* 69, 211–214.

Reed, K.D., Meece, J.K., Henkel, J.S. and Shukla, S.K. (2003) Birds, migration and emerging zoonoses: west nile virus, lyme disease, influenza A and enteropathogens. *Clinical Medicine & Research* 1, 5–12.

Reilly, W.J., Forbes, G.I., Paterson, G.M. and Sharp, J.C.M. (1981) Human and animal salmonellosis in Scotland associated with environmental contamination. *Veterinary Record* 108, 553–555.

Richardson, A. (1973) The transmission of *Salmonella* Dublin to calves from adult carrier cows. *Veterinary Record* 92, 112–115.

Richardson, A. (1975a) Outbreaks of a bovine salmonellosis caused by serovars other than *S*. Dublin and *S*. Typhimurium. *Journal of Hygiene, Cambridge* 74, 195–203.

Richardson, A. (1975b) Salmonellosis in cattle [review]. *Veterinary Record* 96, 329–331.

Richardson, A. and Fawcett, A.R. (1973) *Salmonella* Dublin infection in calves: the value of rectal swabs in diagnosis and epidemiological studies. *British Veterinary Journal* 129, 151–156.

Richardson, A. and Watson, W.A. (1971) A contribution to the epidemiology of *Salmonella* Dublin infection in cattle. *British Veterinary Journal* 127, 172–183.

Rings, D.M. (1985) Salmonellosis in calves. *Veterinary Clinics North America Food Animal Practitioners* 1, 529–530.

Roberts, D., Boag, K., Hall, M.L. and Shipp, C.R. (1975) The isolation of salmonellas from British pork sausages and sausage-meat. *Journal of Hygiene, Cambridge* 75, 173–184.

Robinson, R.A., Blackburn, B.O., Murphy, C.D., Morse, E.V. and Potter, M.E. (1984) Epidemiology of *Salmonella* Dublin in the USA. In: *Proceedings of the International Symposium on* Salmonella, *New Orleans*

1984. Avian Association of Avian Pathologists, New Bolton Center, Kennet Square, Pennsylvania, pp. 182–193.

Roden, L.D., Smith, B.P., Spier, S.J. and Dillings, G.W. (1992) Effect of calf age and *Salmonella* bacterin type on ability to produce immunoglobulins directed against *Salmonella* whole cells or lipopolysacharide. *American Journal of Veterinary Research* 53, 1895–1899.

Rowe, B., Threlfall, E.J., Ward, L.R. and Ashley, A.S. (1979) International spread of multi-resistant strains of *Salmonella* Typhimurium phage types 204 and 193 from Britain to Europe. *Veterinary Record* 105, 468–469.

Rowe, B., Begg, N.T., Hutchinson, D.N., Dawkins, H.C., Gilbert, R.J., Jacob, M., Hales, B.H., Rae, F.A. and Jepson, M. (1987) *Salmonella* Ealing infections associated with consumption of infant dried milk. *Lancet* ii, 900–903.

Ryan, C.A., Nickels, M.K., Hargett-Bean, N.T., Potter, M.E., Endo, T., Mayer, L., Langkop, C.W., Gibson, C., McDonald, R.C., Kenney, R.T., Buhr, N.D., McDonnell, P.J., Cohen, M.L. and Blake, P.A. (1987) Massive outbreak of antimicrobial-resistant salmonellosis traced to pasteurised milk. *Journal of American Medical Association* 258, 3269–3274.

Sanson, R.L. and Thornton, R.N. (1997) A modelling approach to the quantification of the benefits of a national surveillance programme. *Preventive Veterinary Medicine* 30, 37–47.

Santos, R.L. and Baumler, A.J. (2004) Cell tropism of *Salmonella* enterica. *International Journal of Medical Microbiology: IJMM* 294, 225–233.

Segall, T. and Lindberg, A.A. (1991) Experimental oral *Salmonella* Dublin infection in calves: a bacteriological and pathological study. *Journal of Veterinary Medicine B* 38, 169–185.

Selander, R.K., Smith, N.H., Li, J., Beltran, P., Ferris, K.E., Kopecko, D.J. and Rubin, F.A. (1992) Molecular evolutionary genetics of the cattle-adapted serovar *Salmonella* Dublin. *Journal of Bacteriology* 174, 2587–3592.

Selim, S.A., Cullor, J.S., Smith, B.P., Blanchard, P., Farver, T.B., Hoffman, R., Dilling, G., Roden, L.D. and Wilgenburg, B. (1995) The effect of *Escherichia coli* J5 and modified live *Salmonella* Dublin vaccines in artificially reared neonatal calves. *Vaccine* 13, 381–390.

Sharp, J.C.M., Paterson, G.M. and Forbes, G.I. (1980) Milk-borne salmonellosis in Scotland. *Journal of Infection* 2, 333–340.

Sharp, M.W. and Rawson, B.C. (1992) Persistent *Salmonella* Typhimurium DT104 in a dairy herd. *Veterinary Record* 131, 375–376.

Small, R.G. and Sharp, J.C.M. (1979) A milk-borne outbreak due to *Salmonella* Dublin. *Journal of Hygiene, Cambridge* 82, 95–100.

Smith, B.P., Habasha, F., Reina-Guerra, M. and Hardy, A.J. (1979) Bovine salmonellosis: experimental production and characterisation of the disease in calves, using oral challenge with *Salmonella* Typhimurium. *American Journal of Veterinary Research* 40, 1511–1513.

Smith, B.P., Reina-Guerra, M., Hoiseth, S.K., Stocker, B.A.D., Habasha, F., Johnson, E. and Merrit, F. (1984a) Aromatic-dependent *Salmonella* Typhimurium as modified live vaccines for calves. *American Journal of Veterinary Research* 45, 59–66.

Smith, B.P., Reina-Guerra, M., Stocker, B.A., Hoiseth, S.K. and Johnson, E. (1984b) Aromatic-dependent *Salmonella* Dublin as a parenteral modified live vaccine for calves. *American Journal of Veterinary Research* 45, 2231–2235.

Smith, B.P., Oliver, D.G. and Singh, P. (1989) Detection of *Salmonella* Dublin mammary gland infection in carrier cows using enzyme linked immunosorbent assay for antibody in milk and serum. *American Journal of Veterinary Research* 50, 1352–1260.

Smith, B.P., House, J.K., Dilling, G.W., Roden, L.D. and Spier, S.J. (1992) Identification of *Salmonella* Dublin infected in cattle. In: *Proceedings of* Salmonella *and Salmonellosis*. Ploufragen, France, pp. 225–230.

Smith, B.P., Dillings, G.W., Roden, L.D. and Stocker, B.A.D. (1993) Vaccination of calves with orally administered aromatic-dependent *Salmonella* Dublin. *American Journal of Veterinary Research* 54, 1249–1255.

Smith, B.P., Roden, L.D., Tharmond, M.C., Dilling, G.W., Konrad, H., Pelton, J.A. and Picanso, J.R. (1994) Prevalence of salmonellae in cattle and in the environment on California dairies. *Journal of American Veterinary Medicine Association* 205, 467–471.

Sojka, W.J., Thomson, P.D. and Hudson, E.B. (1974) Excretion of *Salmonella* Dublin by adult bovine carriers. *British Veterinary Journal* 130, 482–488.

Sojka, W.J., Wray, C., Shreeve, J. and Benson, J.A. (1977) Incidence of *Salmonella* infections in animals in England and Wales, 1968-74. *Journal of Hygiene, Cambridge* 78, 43–56.

Spier, S.J., Smith, B.P., Cullor, J.S., Olander, H.J., Roden, L.D. and Dilling, G.W. (1991) persistent experimental *Salmonella* Dublin intramammary infection in dairy cows. *Journal of Veterinary Internal Medicine* 5, 341–350.

Sun, J., Fegan, P.E., Desai, A.S., Madara, J.L. and Hobert, M.E. (2007) Flagellin-induced tolerance of the Toll-like receptor 5 signaling pathway in polarized intestinal epithelial cells. American journal of physiology. *Gastrointestinal and Liver Physiology* 292, G767–778.

Tablante, N. and Lane, V.M. (1989) Wild mice as potential reservoirs of *Salmonella* Dublin in a closed dairy herd. *Canadian Veterinary Journal* 30, 590–592.

Taylor, R.J. (1973) ii. A further assessment of the potential hazard in calves allowed to graze pasture contaminated with *Salmonella* Dublin in slurry. *British Veterinary Journal* 129, 354–358.

Taylor, R.J. and Burrows, M.R. (1971) The survival of *Escherichia coli* and *Salmonella* Dublin in slurry on pastures and the infectivity of *S.* Dublin for grazing calves. *British Veterinary Journal* 127, 536–643.

Taylor, S.M. and Kilpatrick, D. (1975) The relationship between concurrent live fluke infection and salmonellosis in cattle. *Veterinary Record* 96, 342–343.

Thomassen, M. (1897) Une nouvelle septicémie des baux avec néphrite et urocystite (bactériurie) consecutives. *Annales de l'Institut Pasteur* 11, 523, 540.

Thorns, C.J. (2000) Bacterial food-borne zoonoses. *Revue Scientifique et Technique* 19, 226–239.

Thunegard, E. (1975) On the persistence of bacteria in manure: a field and experimental study with special reference to *Salmonella* in liquid manure. *Acta Veterinarie Scandinavica* 16 (Suppl. 56), 86 pp.

Tsolis, R.M., Adams, L.G., Ficht, T.A. and Baumler, A.J. (1999) Contribution of *Salmonella* Typhimurium virulence factors to diarrheal diease in calves. *Infection and Immunity* 67, 4879–4885.

van Duijkeren, E., Wannet, W.J., Houwers, D.J. and van Pelt, W. (2003) Antimicrobial susceptibilities of *Salmonella* strains isolated from humans, cattle, pigs, and chickens in the Netherlands from 1984 to 2001. *Journal of Clinical Microbiology* 41, 3574–3578.

van Leeuwen, W.J., Voogd, C.E. and Guinee, P.A.M. (1984) Antibiotic resistance in *Salmonella* in the Netherlands. In: Pohl and Leunen, J. (eds) *Resistance and Pathogenic Plasmids*. CEC Seminar, Brussels, p. 1.

Villarreal-Ramos, B., Manser, J., Collins, R.A., Dougan, G., Chatfield, S.N. and Howard, C. (1998) Immune responses in calves immunised orally or subcutaneously with a live *Salmonella* Typhimurium aro vaccine. *Vaccine* 16, 45–54.

Visser, I.J.R. (1991) Cutaneous salmonellosis in veterinarians. *Veterinary Record* 129, 364.

Visser, I.J.R., Veen, M., vander Giessen, J.W.B., Peterse, D.J. and Wouda, W. (1993) *Salmonella* Dublin in dairy herds in north Netherlands. *Tijdschrift voor Diergeneeskunde* 118, 84–87.

Wall, P.G., Morgan, D., Lamden, K., Ryan, M., Giffin, M., Threlfall, E.J., Ward, L.R. and Rowe, B. (1994) A case control study of infection with an epidemic strain of multi-resistant *Salmonella* Typhimurium DT104 in England and Wales. *Communicable Disease Review* 4, R130.

Wall, P.G., Davis, S., Threlfall, E.J., Ward, L.R. and Ewbank, A.J. (1995a) Chronic carriage of multidrug resistant *Salmonella* Typhimurium in a cat. *Journal of Small Animal Practice* 36, 279–281.

Wall, P.G., Morgan, D., Lamden, K., Griffin, M., Threlfall, E.J., Ward, L.T. and Rowe, B. (1995b) Transmission of multi-resistant strains of *Salmonella* Typhimurium from cattle to man. *Veterinary Record* 136, 591–592.

Wall, P.G., Threlfall, E.J., Ward, L.R. and Rowe, B. (1996) Multi-resistant *Salmonella* Typhimurium DT104 in cats: a public health risk. *Lancet* 348, 471.

Wallis, T.S., Paulin, S.M., Plested, J.S., Watson, P.R. and Jones, P.W. (1995) The *Salmonella* Dublin virulence plasmid mediates systemic but not enteric phases of salmonellosis in cattle. *Infection and Immunity* 63, 2755–2761.

Wathes, C.M., Zaidan, W.A.R., Pearson, G.R., Hinton, M. and Todd, N. (1988) Aerosol infection of calves and mince with *Salmonella* Typhimurium. *Veterinary Record* 123, 590–594.

Watson, P.R., Paulin, S.M., Bland, A.P., Jones, P.W. and Wallis, T.S. (1995) Characterisation of intestinal invasion by *Salmonella* Typhimurium and *Salmonella* Dublin and effect of a mutation in the inv H gene. *Infection and Immunity* 63, 2743–2754.

Watson, P.R., Paulin, S.M., Jones, P.W. and Wallis, T.S. (1997) Role of stn, sly A and inv H in *Salmonella* induced enteritis in cattle. In: *Proceedings* Salmonella *and Salmonellosis*. ISPAIA, Ploufragen, pp. 53–156.

Watson, W.A., Wood, B. and Richardson, A. (1971) *Salmonella* Dublin infection in a beef herd. *British Veterinary Journal* 127, 294–298.

Werner, S.B., Humphrey, G.L. and Kamei, I. (1979) Association between raw milk and human *Salmonella* Dublin infection. *British Medical Journal* 2, 238–241.

Werner, S.B., Morrison, F.R. and Humphrey, G.L. (1984) *Salmonella* Dublin and raw milk consumption. *Journal of the American Medical Association* 251, 2195–2199.
Whitlock, R.H. (1984) Therapeutic strategies involving antimicrobial treatment of the gastrointestinal tract in large animals. *Journal of the American Veterinary Medical Association* 185, 1210–1213.
Wilhelm, B., Rajic, A., Waddell, L., Parker, S., Harris, J., Roberts, K.C., Kydd, R., Greig, J. and Baynton, A. (2009) Prevalence of zoonotic or potentially zoonotic bacteria, antimicrobial resistance, and somatic cell counts in organic dairy production: current knowledge and research gaps. *Foodborne Pathogens and Disease* 6, 525–539.
Williams, B.M. (1975) Environmental considerations in salmonellosis. *Veterinary Record* 96, 318–321.
Williams, E. (1980) Veterinary surgeons as vectors of *Salmonella* Dublin. *British Medical Journal* 22, 815–818.
Wood, J.D., Chalmers, G.A., Fenton, R.A., Pritchard, J., Schoonderwoerd, M. and Lichtenberger, W.L. (1991) The persistent shedding of *Salmonella* Enteritidis from the udder of a cow. *Canadian Veterinary Journal* 32, 738–741.
Wray, C. (1980) Some haematological and blood biochemical findings during experimental *Salmonella* Typhimurium infection in calves. *Zentralblatt für Veterinärmedizin B* 27, 365–373.
Wray, C. (1997) Development of antibiotic resistance: a vet's tale. *Journal of Medical Microbiology* 46, 26–28.
Wray, C. and Davies, R.H. (1996) *Salmonella* in animals – a veterinary viewpoint. *PHLS Microbiology Digest* 13, 44–48.
Wray, C. and Roeder, P.L. (1987) Effect of bovine virus-diarrhoea-mucosal disease infection on *Salmonella* infections in calves. *Research in Veterinary Science* 42, 213–218.
Wray, C. and Sojka, W.J. (1977) Reviews of the progress of dairy science: bovine salmonellosis. *Journal of Dairy Research* 44, 383–425.
Wray, C., Todd, N. and Hinton, M.H. (1987a) The epidemiology of *Salmonella* Typhimurium infection in calves: excretion of *S.* Typhimurium in faeces of calves in different management systems. *Veterinary Record* 121, 293–296.
Wray, C., McLaren, I., Parkinson, N.M. and Beedell, Y. (1987b) Differentiation of *Salmonella* Typhimurium DT204c by plasmid profile and biotyping. *Veterinary Record* 121, 514–516.
Wray, C., Wadsworth, Q.C., Richards, D.W. and Morgan, J.H. (1989) A three-year study of *Salmonella* Dublin in a closed dairy herd. *Veterinary Record* 124, 532–535.
Wray, C., Todd, M., McLaren, I.M., Breedall, Y.E. and Rowe, B. (1990) The epidemiology of *Salmonella* infection in calves: the role of dealers. *Epidemiology and Infection* 105, 295–305.
Wray, C., Sojka, W.J. and Callow, R.J. (1977) The serological response in cattle to salmonella infection. *British Veterinary Journal* 133(1), 25–32.
Wray, C., Todd, M., McLaren, I.M. and Beedell, Y.E. (1991) The epidemiology of *Salmonella* in calves: the role of markets and vehicles. *Epidemiology and Infection* 107, 521–525.
Yeruham, I., Elad, D., Mechani, M. and Lublin, A. (2005) Outbreak of salmonellosis in calves in a dairy herd caused by monophasic *Salmonella* serovar 9,12:l,v:-. *Veterinary Record* 157, 778–779.
Yoon, S.I., Kurnasov, O., Natarajan, V., Hong, M., Gudkov, A.V., Osterman, A.L. and Wilson, I.A. (2012) Structural basis of TLR5-flagellin recognition and signaling. *Science* 335, 859–864.
Zhou, D. and Galan, J. (2001) *Salmonella* entry into host cells: the work in concert of type III secreted effector proteins. *Microbes and Infection/Institut Pasteur* 3, 1293–1298.

13 *Salmonella* Infections in Pigs

Mark P. Stevens[1]* and Jeffrey T. Gray[2]
[1]*The Roslin Institute and Royal (Dick) School of Veterinary Studies, University of Edinburgh, UK;* [2]*Office of the Vice President for Research, Des Moines University, USA*

Historical Perspectives

The organism now known as *Salmonella enterica* serovar Choleraesuis was first isolated from pigs by Salmon and Smith (1886), when they considered it to be the cause of swine fever (hog cholera). The importance of the organism as a cause of porcine disease was neglected when the viral aetiology of swine fever was discovered, and a number of years elapsed before *S.* Choleraesuis was recognized as a primary pathogen capable of causing several disease syndromes in pigs. It was later recognized that a variety of antigenically distinct *S. enterica* serovars can be isolated from pigs, some of which are of public health importance as they transmit through the food chain and farm environment to humans, where they typically cause acute but self-limiting gastroenteritis (Buxton, 1957). Though such serovars may cause transient disease in pigs, they are often persistently shed in a subacute carrier state, and therefore pose a significant challenge to those involved in production and processing of pigs. *Salmonella* are a major cause of economic loss in pig production, resulting in millions of dollars in lost income to the pork industry (Griffith *et al.*, 2006).

Epidemiology

Members of the genus *Salmonella* are extremely widespread in nature. They are recovered from nearly all vertebrates, as well as insects, and are often referred to as universal pathogens (Taylor and McCoy, 1969; Falkow and Mekalanos, 1990). Selected serovars of *S. enterica* have varied reservoir hosts and can move readily between host species. Others appear adapted to cause disease in specific hosts, or a narrow range of hosts. They are shed efficiently in faeces, persist within the environment and are spread readily between food-producing animals in the farm environment. Though diseased animals shed high numbers of *Salmonella*, asymptomatic carriers can shed *Salmonella* in faeces continuously or intermittently in the absence of overt pathology, further spreading the organism (Wood *et al.*, 1991). Shedding of the organism can be exacerbated by a long list of stressors, all of which are prevalent at the end of the production cycle, including mixing, transportation and food deprivation. In turn, such stressors can be expected to enhance entry of *Salmonella* into the human food chain.

* Corresponding author, e-mail: Mark.Stevens@roslin.ed.ac.uk

© CAB International 2013. *Salmonella in Domestic Animals, 2nd Edition* (eds P.A. Barrow and U. Methner)

It is convenient to consider porcine *Salmonella* as consisting of two groups separated by host range and clinical presentation. The first group consists of the host-adapted serovar *S.* Choleraesuis, which tends to elicit systemic disease. The second group consists of all other serovars, which have a broader host range and tend to elicit transient enteritis, such as *S.* Typhimurium. Such broad host range serovars are associated with food-borne non-typhoidal salmonellosis in humans worldwide (Falkow and Mekalanos, 1990). This classification is imperfect as *S.* Typhimurium can cause severe systemic disease in neonatal and immunocompromised pigs and host-adapted *S.* Choleraesuis has been reported to cause systemic disease in humans with high mortality (Cherubin, 1980). Global demand for pork is accelerating fast, driven largely by demand in Asia owing to population growth, urbanization and rising affluence. In turn, the impact of *S. enterica* serovars that affect pig and human health is increasing with no single intervention appearing to be effective in control of the problem.

Prevalent Serovars and Phage Types

In the UK, *S.* Choleraesuis was the predominant serovar in pigs during the 1950s and 1960s and, in 1958 and 1968, it constituted 90% and 74.2%, respectively, of all *Salmonella* isolates from pigs (Sojka *et al.*, 1977). Subsequently its prevalence has declined in the UK to the point where it is infrequently reported, or not seen from year-to-year. The same trend has been reported in a number of other European countries (Laval *et al.*, 1992; Baggesen and Christensen, 1997; Helmuth *et al.*, 1997). The last decade has also seen a decrease in isolations and disease from *S.* Choleraesuis in North America, likely as a consequence of improvements in swine management and the advent of efficacious live-attenuated vaccines. Regional variation in salmonellosis incidence is loosely correlated to pig density, husbandry practices and co-mingling of pigs.

A year-long survey during 2006–2007 detected *Salmonella* in the ileocaecal lymph node of 21.2% of pigs at slaughter in the UK, with *S.* Typhimurium by far the most prevalent serovar (EFSA, 2008). This compared to an average across Member States of the European Union of 10.3% (EFSA, 2008). In the UK in the same year as the survey there were over 13,000 laboratory-confirmed cases of human salmonellosis, though it was estimated that four times as many human cases were not captured by national surveillance and the proportion of cases attributable to pig products was unknown (DEFRA, 2007). European Community-wide it is estimated that 10–20% of human non-typhoidal salmonellosis may be linked to pigs (EFSA, 2010). This is consistent with evidence of entry of the pathogen into the food chain from pigs. For example, *Salmonella* was isolated from 5.3% of UK pig carcass swabs during 1999–2000, at a time when 23.0% of caecal contents were positive at slaughter (Davies *et al.*, 2004). Quantitative microbiological risk assessments have predicted that the incidence of human infections due to pig products would fall in proportion to *Salmonella* prevalence in pigs (EFSA, 2010). Toward this aim, proposed legislation (European Union, 2003) will require Member States to act to control porcine salmonellosis to reduce zoonosis and enhance pig health. *Salmonella* Derby is frequently the second most prevalent serovar in pigs and can be detected on carcass swabs (Davies *et al.*, 2004), yet this serovar rarely appears in humans. The reasons for this are unclear and analysis of the genome sequence of serovar Derby strains, and the nature of infection in pigs, may help to explain differences in the zoonotic potential of pig-associated serovars. Consideration of such trends is necessary when considering whether control strategies are required to control all *Salmonella* serovars found in pigs, or those posing the greatest threat of zoonosis. The reader is referred to annual European Food Standards Agency reports for data on prevalence of serovars in each Member State of Europe, though in most cases serovars Typhimurium and Derby are isolated most frequently.

In the USA, the most common serovars isolated from pigs during the National Animal Health Monitoring Survey in both 2000 and 2006 were Typhimurium, Derby, Agona, Typhimurium-Copenhagen and Heidelberg, three of which were also in the top five serotypes isolated from humans in the same period (Haley *et al.*, 2012). The recovery of a serovar varies by source, as well as geographical location (Currier *et al.*, 1986; Davies *et al.*, 1997). The number of reports of some other serovars has increased during the last 20 years, but it is not known whether this is the result of better monitoring or whether it indicates increased disease or environmental prevalence. It is evident that the problem of *Salmonella* in pigs is not restricted geographically, and this is significant considering the scale of global trade in pork as individual countries are no longer isolated from world events. For example, a recent study in Brazil indicated that the prevalence in swine facilities ranged between 26% on finishing pen floors to 90% on slaughter holding pens, and 46% in swine lymph nodes with the final post-chilled carcass surfaces at 24% (Kich *et al.*, 2011).

Of the different phage types of *S.* Typhimurium, the most frequent in pigs in the UK are DT104, DT193 and DT208, all of which are resistant to a number of antibiotics (Wray *et al.*, 1997; Davies *et al.*, 2004). In 1997, only 15.8% of the *Salmonella* isolates from predominantly diseased pigs were fully susceptible to the antibiotics used for monitoring; tetracycline resistance was the most frequent. In the USA in 1997, 19% of the diagnostic and 44.2% of the slaughter isolates were fully susceptible to all antimicrobials. Multiple resistance to five or more antimicrobials was observed in 23.3% of diagnostic and 16.8% of slaughter isolates (NARMS-EB, 1997). However, in a survey covering healthy swine performed in 2000 and again in 2006 the proportion of *Salmonella* isolates that were susceptible to all antimicrobials (pan-susceptible) was 38.1% in 2000 and 20.4% in 2006. The proportion of *Salmonella* isolates that were resistant to three or more antimicrobials (multi-drug resistant) was similar in 2000 and in 2006 (52.8 and 57.7%, respectively) (Haley *et al.*, 2012). While direct comparison between these years and studies is not possible, the trend in these results seems to indicate an increase in multi-drug resistance over the past decade.

Since the mid-1990s a monophasic variant of *S.* Typhimurium with the serotype 4,[5],12:i:- began to be isolated in Spain (Echeita *et al.*, 1999). Molecular characterization (sequencing the *fliA-fliB* intergenic region, phage sensitivity and tRNA sequencing) indicated that this was a true variant of *S.* Typhimurium in which the phase 2 flagella antigen was missing as a result of a deletion in the *fljB* gene. Other deletions were also present. This variant has since spread to many other countries in Europe and elsewhere and monophasic variants of the multi-antibiotic-resistant ST193 have begun to emerge in Germany, which have also spread to other countries. It has since become one of the most frequently isolated serovars worldwide (CDC, 2005). These are thought to represent multiple clones emerging through independent deletions (Switt *et al.*, 2009). It represents a human health risk and can be isolated from pork meat (Hauser *et al.*, 2010).

Transmission

Transmission of *Salmonella* between hosts is thought to occur via the faecal–oral route of exposure. Since *Salmonella* are often shed in large numbers in the faeces, it is plausible that this is a major route for transmission of the organism. A number of studies have reproduced experimental infection by the oral route and, during acute disease, pigs will shed up to 10^6 colony-forming units (CFU) of *S.* Choleraesuis (Smith and Jones, 1967) or 10^7 CFU *S.* Typhimurium (Gutzmann *et al.*, 1976) per gram of faeces. Generally, high doses have to be used and disease is frequently difficult to reproduce. Neutralization of stomach pH by use of antacids can improve reproducibility. Dawe and Troutt (1976) produced moderate disease following oral inoculation of 10^6 CFU, but most authors report successful induction of disease with doses of 10^8–10^9 *Salmonella* (Gray *et al.*, 1995, 1996a, b). During a study on two farms, Williams *et al.* (1981) were unable to reach any firm conclusions as to the natural route of transmission of *S.* Choleraesuis and they suggested that cannibalism of piglets may be important in the spread of the organism.

As early as 1965, De Jong and Ekdahl (1965), after oesophagectomizing calves and giving an oral challenge, proposed that both haematogenous and lymphatogenous routes of infection are important in the dissemination of *Salmonella*, particularly *S.* Typhimurium. Hardman *et al.* (1991) further demonstrated that calves penned individually were susceptible to infection with *Salmonella*. Aerosol experiments in chickens and mice have shown that infections with *Salmonella* can be achieved more regularly via the lungs than by oral inoculation (Clemmer *et al.*, 1960; Darlow *et al.*, 1961). This gave support to the role that aerosols may also play in the transmission and dissemination of *Salmonella*. Further studies in pigs using oesophagotomy indicated that the upper respiratory tract may be equally important in transmission (Fedorka-Cray *et al.*, 1995b) and that the tonsils and lungs may be important sites for the invasion and dissemination of *Salmonella*. Pneumonia associated with experimental *S.* Choleraesuis infection has been previously described (Baskerville and Dow, 1973) and *S.* Choleraesuis-associated pneumonia is not infrequent in the field (Turk *et al.*, 1992). It is unclear whether this predilection for the lung is due solely to the pathogen, poor ventilation in large confinement buildings or some combination of these and other factors. Experimental infection models have not provided good answers, because positive lung samples have been regarded as an artefact of intranasal or per oesophageal inoculation. However, in addition to the oesophagotomy work by Fedorka-Cray *et al.* (1995b), Gray *et al.* (1996b) also demonstrated that the lung is colonized in pigs that are naturally exposed to pigs infected with *S.* Choleraesuis, indicating that lung colonization is not an artefact of experimental inoculation. Collectively, these studies indicate that while the traditional paradigm of faecal-oral transmission predominates, other routes, such as aerosol or dust-borne transmission, are also relevant.

The presence of *Salmonella* in herds of swine is typically endemic and largely asymptomatic. Dutch studies suggest that about 25% of herds are never infected, 24% are constantly infected and 50% are infected intermittently much of the time. Infection tends to occur in naïve animals in the first weeks after arrival or co-mingling and can reach 80–100% prevalence within 2–3 weeks. In such circumstances, about 30% of the pigs are still excreting salmonellae at the end of the finishing period. The National Animal Health Monitoring Service (NAHMS) reported 53% of US herds were infected with at least one serovar of *Salmonella*, with prevalence being highest in herds marketing greater than 10,000 pigs annually (Haley *et al.*, 2012). Transmission at the end of the finishing period occurs significantly between pigs during market transport and lairage at abattoirs, with infection rates proportional to time spent in transport and lairage (Griffith *et al.*, 2006). It is likely that physiological changes associated with stress result in release of immune-modulators and stress-related catecholamines, decreased gastric acid production and increased intestinal motility, though the impact of such changes on *Salmonella* remain ill-defined.

Environmental Considerations

Although transmission of *Salmonella* typically occurs through faecal–oral or aerogenous transmission, other vectors may mediate dissemination of the organism. In pigs, observed sources of contamination include wild animals and feedstuffs (Clarke and Gyles, 1993; McChesney *et al.*, 1995). Mouse faecal pellets have been shown to contain up to 10^5 CFU of *Salmonella* (Henzler and Opitz, 1992). During an investigation of *Salmonella* contamination, which involved 23 pig farms, Davies and Wray (1997) found a wide range of wild animals, including rats, mice and cats associated with contamination of feed and grain stores, and rodents were involved in the perpetuation of infection in specific buildings on the farm. Infected foxes were most common on outdoor breeding farms. Flies and dust can also act as mechanical vectors that spread *Salmonella* throughout the facility or environment (Edel *et al.*, 1967, 1970). It is well known that animal feeds frequently contain *Salmonella* and that animals fed contaminated feed often become infected (Linton and Jennet, 1970). The rate of contamination of animal protein delivered to a large feed-mill in the south-eastern part of the USA was reported over a 10-month period (Williams *et al.*, 1969). Of 311 pig feed samples, 68% contained one or more of the 68 *Salmonella* serovars identified in the study. Samples were found to be contaminated in 86% of the meat-meal and 18% of the fish-meal. In another study to determine the prevalence of *Salmonella* in pig feeds, 2.8% of the feeds and feed ingredients taken from farm environments were positive for *Salmonella* (Harris *et al.*, 1997). Feed trucks have also been implicated as a source for feed and feedstuff contamination (Fedorka-Cray *et al.*, 1997a). A large study conducted in Brazil indicated that 29% of swine feeds were positive for *Salmonella*, indicating that the problem exists widely (Kich *et al.*, 2011). There have been reports that feed consistency is associated with prevalence of *Salmonella* in herds. However, a recent review of available data indicated there is no strong evidence regarding associations between presence of *Salmonella* and the other feed characteristics (O'Connor *et al.*, 2008).

The role of interactions between *Salmonella* and other microbes in the environment in promoting transmission is open to question. It was reported that passage of *S.* Typhimurium or *S.* Choleraesuis in the free-living protozoan *Acanthamoeba castellanii* enhances virulence in pigs compared to passage in Hep-2 cells (Xiong *et al.*, 2010). Selected virulence-associated genes are up-regulated and required for survival during *S.* Typhimurium infection of *Acanthamoeba polyphaga* (Bleasdale *et al.*, 2009), and it is plausible that amoebic passage in the environment primes *Salmonella* gene expression required for infection of the porcine host.

Salmonella may persist in the pig production environment for long periods and Linton *et al.* (1970) considered such persistence an important risk factor. Berends *et al.* (1996) suggested that contamination of finishing sites was the predominant source of infection of finished pigs, rather than infection originating from breeding farms or other sources, though the latter is more important when pigs from various sources are mixed on finishing farms. Baggesen *et al.* (1997) isolated *Salmonella* from faeces, pens, dust, equipment, ventilation equipment and slurry during their studies on pig farms. Gray and Fedorka-Cray (1995) showed that *S.* Choleraesuis survives in dry faeces for at least 13 months post-shedding, demonstrating the importance of cleaning organic matter from the environment. Davies and Wray (1997) found a high level of *Salmonella* persisting in pig pens even after disinfection.

Disease in Pigs

Clinical porcine salmonellosis can be broadly separated into two syndromes: septicaemia associated with *S.* Choleraesuis and entercolitis associated with *S.* Typhimurium or other serovars. In the USA and UK, salmonellosis in pigs is most frequently due to infection with *S.* Typhimurium and is often associated with predisposing factors such as intercurrent illnesses, conditions of poor hygiene that allow exposure to high doses of the organism, or neonatal or immunologically naïve pigs. The latter situation appears to be more frequently encountered with modern production systems utilizing age-segregated production. Clinical disease has also been associated with *S.* Typhisuis. This serovar is difficult to isolate and, as a consequence, may be responsible for more outbreaks than is attributed by culture (Wilcock and Schwartz, 1992). In addition, there have been reports of both *S.* Dublin (Lawson and Dow, 1966) and *S.* Enteritidis (Reynolds *et al.*, 1967) causing disease in pigs. The vast majority of *S.* Choleraesuis outbreaks in pigs are due to the H_2S-producing variant Kunzendorf (Wilcock and Schwartz, 1992). However, the non-H_2S-producing *S.* Choleraesuis has been as high as number two in the top ten commonest *Salmonella* isolates from pigs in a given year (Ferris and Thomas, 1993).

The frequency of entry of pigs into a subacute carrier state after clinical salmonellosis, and the sites of bacterial persistence, have been studied following experimental infection. After oral dosing of 7- to 8-week-old piglets with 10^{10} CFU *S.* Typhimurium, faecal excretion was observed in all pigs for at least 22 weeks but with more variation between individuals from 8 weeks post-inoculation and long after resolution of clinical symptoms (Wood *et al.*, 1989). In this study, and an independent study using a similar oral dose of *S.* Typhimurium (Wood and Rose, 1992), post-mortem analysis revealed persistence of *Salmonella* in the tonsils and selected lymph nodes and intestinal sites even at 28 weeks post-infection. However, another study using 8-week-old pigs and 10^{10} CFU of a different *S.* Typhimurium strain revealed uniform faecal excretion for just 3 weeks post-inoculation, with more variable isolation thereafter (Fedorka-Cray *et al.*, 1994). A similarly rapid decline in excretion was also observed in c. 20 kg pigs in the grower phase inoculated with 10^8 CFU *S.* Typhimurium (Nielsen *et al.*, 1995). Oral inoculation of 7-week-old pigs with a *S.* Newport strain by Wood and colleagues (Wood *et al.*, 1991) yielded similar patterns of excretion and persistence in tissues to that observed by the same workers with *S.* Typhimurium (Wood *et al.*, 1989; Wood and Rose, 1992); however, other studies have reported differences in the kinetics and sites of persistence of other serovars, and in pigs inoculated directly with *Salmonella* compared to those exposed to excreting pigs (Anderson *et al.*, 1998). Faecal-oral cycling of *Salmonella* is likely to play a role in perpetuating *Salmonella* in pig herds but the host, bacterial and production factors influencing entry into the carrier state, and reactivation from it, require further study.

Populations affected

Intensively reared, weaned pigs are most often affected by *Salmonella* infection. In general, *S.* Typhimurium tends to cause disease in young pigs from 6 to 12 weeks of age. Alternatively, disease from *S.* Choleraesuis occurs among a wider range of ages. Mortality tends to be higher in younger than in older pigs, while morbidity is often equal regardless of age. Disease from *S.* Choleraesuis in the adult is rare, however, if a susceptible population is exposed the animals will be significantly affected (Wilcock and Schwartz, 1992). It is not known how common subclinical infection is in the adult. Normally, only moribund suspect cases are cultured for *S.* Choleraesuis. The occurrence of salmonellosis in suckling pigs is rare, presumably because of maternal transfer of antibody, but infection is not uncommon (Gooch and Haddock, 1969; Wilcock *et al.*, 1976). However, neonatal pigs are susceptible to oral challenge with *Salmonella* and develop a disease similar to that observed in weaned pigs (Wilcock and Olander, 1978).

Septicaemia

The septicaemic form of porcine salmonellosis is usually caused by *S.* Choleraesuis. Affected pigs are inappetent, lethargic and febrile, with temperatures of up to 107°F (41.7°C). Respiratory signs may consist of a shallow, moist cough and diaphragmatic breathing. Clinical signs first appear after 24–36 h of infection (Reed *et al.*, 1986). Often, producers will find the first evidence of disease as dead pigs with cyanotic extremities and abdomens. In most outbreaks, mortality is high and morbidity is variable but generally less than 10% (Reed *et al.*, 1986; Wilcock and Schwartz, 1992). Diarrhoea is normally not a feature of *S.* Choleraesuis infection until at least the fourth or fifth day of infection. It may last from 5 to 7 days after onset in the absence of chronic re-infection. Gross lesions include colitis, infarction of gastric mucosa, swollen mesenteric lymph nodes, splenomegaly, hepatomegaly and lung congestion. Random white foci of necrosis are often observed on the liver (Reed *et al.*, 1986; Wilcock and Schwartz, 1992). The microscopic lesion that is most often associated with *S.* Choleraesuis in pigs is the paratyphoid nodule. This lesion can be viewed in the liver as clusters of histiocytes amid foci of acute coagulative hepatocellular necrosis and corresponds to the white foci seen grossly (Lawson and Dow, 1966). Other lesions may include fibrinoid thrombi in venules of gastric mucosa and cyanotic skin and glomerular capillaries. Swelling of histiocytes and epithelial cells, typical of Gram-negative sepsis, as well as hyperplasia of reticular cells of the spleen and lymph nodes, is often observed (Wilcock *et al.*, 1976).

Enterocolitis

Enterocolitis in pigs is typically associated with *S.* Typhimurium infection. In contrast to the septicaemic disease, the initial sign of infection is often watery, yellow diarrhoea. Infected pigs are inappetent, febrile and lethargic. Mortality is usually low, however morbidity can be high within a few days of infection (Wilcock and Schwartz, 1992). The major gross lesion at necropsy is focal or diffuse necrotic colitis and typhlitis. Mesenteric lymph nodes are often greatly enlarged. Intestinal lesions develop as red, rough mucosal surfaces, which may also have grey-yellow debris. Colon and caecal contents are bile-stained and scant, often with black or sand-like gritty material on the surface. Intestinal necrosis may be seen as sharply delineated button ulcers, often associated with resolving lesions (Wilcock and Olander, 1978; Wilcock and Schwartz, 1992; Wood and Rose, 1992). In cases of *S.* Typhimurium enterocolitis, the liver and spleen are not enlarged except by terminal congestion (Wilcock and Schwartz, 1992). Necrotic ileitis in swine has historically been attributed to several agents, including *Salmonella*. However, when necrotic enteritis is seen on necropsy the pathology may actually be secondary to porcine proliferative enteropathy (PPE) and *Salmonella* may or may not be present (Griffith *et al.*, 2006).

Histopathological examination of enteric lesions will typically contain necrotic crypt and surface enterocytes that can be both focal and/or diffuse in appearance. Macrophages and lymphocytes appear in the lamina propria and submucosa whereas neutrophils are observed only in the very early lesions. The necrosis frequently extends to involve muscularis mucosa, submucosa and lymphoid follicles (Griffith *et al.*, 2006). It is not uncommon to see lymphoid atrophy or regenerative hyperplasia associated with this disease (Wilcock *et al.*, 1976; Jubb *et al.*, 1985; Reed *et al.*, 1986).

Pathogenesis

In general, experimental models reproduce the differential virulence of serovars and disease presentation seen in naturally-infected pigs. In age-matched weaned piglets, oral dosing with c. 10^8 CFU of *S.* Typhimurium 4/74 rapidly induced fever, diarrhoea and vomiting; however, by 2–3 days post-inoculation clinical signs were normal (Watson *et al.*, 2000). In contrast, symptoms were more severe and prolonged following inoculation with *S.* Choleraesuis 14/74, with severe pyrexia, intermittent diarrhoea, depression and lethargy for the duration of the experiment. In the same study, a *S.* Dublin isolate that causes bovine typhoid was cleared by pigs in the absence of overt pathology. Bacterial recoveries from intestinal sites were far higher with *S.* Choleraesuis than for any other serovar, and only *S.* Choleraesuis was recovered from systemic sites in quantifiable numbers 7 days post-infection (Watson *et al.*, 2000). Comparative studies in 4-week-old piglets have also been reported, with *S.* Typhimurium causing transient enterocolitis but *S.* Choleraesuis frequently producing necrotic and ulcerative lesions in the colonic mucosa, septicaemia, interstitial pneumonia and multifocal hepatic necrosis (Reed *et al.*, 1986).

Studies in experimentally infected swine have indicated that *S.* Choleraesuis exhibits a preferential tropism for ileal M cells while *S.* Typhimurium has a low tendency to invade the ileal mucosa (Pospischil *et al.*, 1990). In contrast, in porcine ligated ileal loops, strains of serovars Choleraesuis and Typhimurium enter both M cells and enterocytes directly, with no evidence of preferential association with Peyer's patch mucosa (Reed *et al.*, 1986; Bolton *et al.*, 1999). Such studies confirm earlier reports that *Salmonella* can enter cells that are not normally phagocytic (Finlay *et al.*, 1988). In porcine ileal loops, recoveries of gentamicin-protected (intracellular) *S.* Choleraesuis A50 were lower than those of *S.* Typhimurium 4/74 3 h post-inoculation (Paulin *et al.*, 2007), suggesting that the magnitude of initial invasion may not be associated with the systemic virulence of the strains. Fluid secretion and recruitment of ^{111}In-labeled neutrophils was markedly higher in loops inoculated with *S.* Typhimurium relative to *S.* Choleraesuis, consistent with the elevated induction of TNFα, IL-8 and IL-18 mRNA in ileal mucosa by the former 24 h after oral dosing (Paulin *et al.*, 2007). Analysis of the partitioning of a temperature-sensitive plasmid in the two strains indicated that *S.* Typhimurium 4/74 replicates faster than *S.* Choleraesuis A50 in the intestinal mucosa; therefore the higher levels of inflammation observed with the former may partly reflect the elevated bacterial load (Paulin *et al.*, 2007). Recently it was reported that *Salmonella*-induced enteritis releases tetrathionate as an electron acceptor for bacterial respiration in the murine intestines and calf ileal loops (Winter *et al.*, 2010). It was subsequently reported that this promotes anaerobic respiration of ethanolamine as a carbon source (Thiennimitr *et al.*, 2011), enabling the bacteria to compete with the indigenous microflora. It is therefore plausible that growth of *S. enterica* serovars in the porcine intestines follows inflammation rather than vice versa. *Salmonella* Choleraesuis A50 was found to persist better than *S.* Typhimurium 4/74 in mesenteric lymph nodes serving the ileum and colon (Paulin *et al.*, 2007), and the tissue- and cell-interactions that dictate the outcome of infection require further study.

The mechanisms underlying the induction of enteritis and systemic translocation of *Salmonella* in pigs are ill-defined. Most studies on these topics have relied on murine and bovine models of enteritis and typhoid (reviewed in Tsolis *et al.*, 2011), and data supporting the role of host and bacterial factors in the outcome of *Salmonella* infection in pigs are comparatively scarce. Analysis of transcriptional responses of pigs challenged repeatedly by the oral route with *S.* Typhimurium or *S.* Choleraesuis has identified differences in the timing, location and magnitude of expression of genes related to immunity (Burkey *et al.*, 2007; Uthe *et al.*, 2007; Wang *et al.*, 2007, 2008). It has been suggested that the failure of *S.* Choleraesuis to elicit responses that control *Salmonella* at the mucosal surface may lead to dissemination by 'stealth'. For example, neutrophils play a role in control of *Salmonella* in the porcine intestines (Foster *et al.*, 2003, 2005) and heritable resistance of pigs to systemic salmonellosis (van Diemen *et al.*, 2002), yet *S.* Choleraesuis attracts lower numbers of neutrophils in a manner that may be associated with weaker pro-inflammatory cytokine responses in the ileal mucosa relative to *S.* Typhimurium (Paulin *et al.*, 2007). A lack of strong dendritic cell-mediated antigen presentation in *S.* Choleraesuis-infected mesenteric lymph nodes has also been proposed to aid dissemination (Wang *et al.*, 2008). After rapid induction of pro-inflammatory responses it has been reported that *Salmonella* suppresses the NF-kB pathway (Wang *et al.*, 2007) and it is plausible this aids persistence and entry into the carrier state. Evasion of innate immune recognition is a common strategy among pathogens causing enteric fever (reviewed in Tsolis *et al.*, 2008), and further studies are required to unravel how host immune responses relate to the pathology observed with different serovars.

As indicated above, the upper respiratory tract may be a portal of entry of *Salmonella* (Fedorka-Cray *et al.*, 1995b; Gray *et al.*, 1995) and *Salmonella* often persist within the palatine tonsils (Wood *et al.*, 1989). It is unclear how *Salmonella* spreads from the tonsils and lungs, or what factors mediate persistence at such sites. Macrophages are often cited to play a role in the translocation of *Salmonella* from subepithelial spaces such as the lamina propria to visceral organs. *Salmonella* Choleraesuis has been reported to be phagocytosed by macrophages and polymorphonuclear cells in lung tissue (Baskerville *et al.*, 1972, 1973), but the role of such cells in the control or pathogenesis of porcine salmonellosis is unclear. Survival of *Salmonella* in porcine peripheral blood monocytes has been reported to be associated with suppression of production of reactive oxygen species (Roof and Kramer, 1989; Donné *et al.*, 2005); however, it is noteworthy that serovar Typhimurium and Dublin strains persist within, and produce damage to, primary porcine alveolar macrophages at a greater level than strains of serovar Choleraesuis (Watson *et al.*, 2000). This indicates that the systemic virulence of *S.* Choleraesuis cannot be attributed to intra-macrophage survival *per se*, although one cannot exclude the possibility that *Salmonella* may interact differently with macrophages from other sites.

The basis of the persistent subacute carrier state is ill-defined, however it has been suggested that *Salmonella* may modulate its growth rate *in vivo* to evade detection (reviewed in Tierrez and García-del Portillo, 2005) and that it may actively suppress the local induction of inflammatory responses. As indicated above, stress caused by transportation has been associated with reactivation of subacute *S.* Typhimurium infections in pigs (Isaacson *et al.*, 1999; Larsen *et al.*, 2003), and social stress due to mixing increases faecal excretion and invasion of *S.* Typhimurium in early-weaned pigs (Callaway *et al.*, 2006). A partial explanation for such events arises from the recent finding that *Salmonella* are able to sense and respond to host stress-related catecholamines (Freestone *et al.*, 2008). A key response of the enteric nervous system to stress is the release of norepinephrine (NE). NE augments *Salmonella* virulence in bovine, avian and murine models (Williams *et al.*, 2006; McCuddin *et al.*, 2008; Methner *et al.*, 2008; Pullinger *et al.*, 2010a) and studies in pigs have indicated that the release of endogenous NE upon administration of the selective neurotoxin 6-hydroxydopamine transiently reactivates faecal excretion of *S.* Typhimurium (Pullinger *et al.*, 2010b). Culture of *S.* Typhimurium in the presence of NE has been reported to alter the tissue distribution of *Salmonella* in pigs (Toscano *et al.*, 2007), however, this effect was likely due to use of distinct media as such effects were not apparent in subsequent studies using NE in the same medium (Pullinger *et al.*, 2010b). It has been proposed that *Salmonella* senses and responds to NE via the putative bacterial adrenergic receptor QseC (Rasko *et al.*, 2008). QseC contributes to intestinal colonization of swine (Bearson and Bearson, 2008; Bearson *et al.*, 2010). However, it remains unclear if its role in colonization reflects the sensing of NE or other cues. In calves, NE augments *Salmonella*-induced enteritis in a manner associated with increased net replication and independent of QseC (Pullinger *et al.*, 2010a). This is consistent with the finding that NE can promote *Salmonella* growth, both from a viable non-culturable state (Reissbrodt *et al.*, 2002) and in iron-restricted serum-rich media in a manner that requires specific iron-uptake systems (Bearson and Bearson, 2008; Methner *et al.*, 2008). It remains unclear whether the concentrations of stress-related catecholamines released by pigs subject to stress are sufficient to augment *Salmonella* pathogenesis.

It is becoming clear that the intestinal microflora influences the ability of *Salmonella* to colonize the intestines, induce enteritis and transmit between hosts. Thus in mice, antibiotic-mediated depletion of the flora enables *S.* Typhimurium to produce enterocolitis (Barthel *et al.*, 2003) and influences shedding and clearance dynamics (Lawley *et al.*, 2008; Endt *et al.*, 2010). Germ-free piglets lacking indigenous microflora are exquisitely sensitive to *Salmonella* infection, but the relative importance of the flora in competitive exclusion of *Salmonella* as opposed to maturation of mucosal immunity remains ill-defined. The impact of treatments for porcine salmonellosis such as antibiotics and flora preparations for competitive exclusion (as discussed below) may not therefore be easy to predict.

Virulence Factors

Comparative analysis of the genome sequences of strains of serovar Choleraesuis and Typhimurium has identified an elevated number of pseudogenes in serovar Choleraesuis (Chiu *et al.*, 2005; Richardson *et al.*, 2011). In common with other host-restricted or host-specific serovars, such gene decay may provide a partial explanation for the narrowing of host tropism relative to serovars with a generally broad host range. Phylogenetic analysis has indicated that *S.* Choleraesuis and human-adapted *S.* Paratyphi C may have evolved from a common ancestor (Porwollik *et al.*, 2004; Liu *et al.*, 2009). As the sequences of further swine-associated serovars become available, it will be of interest to determine whether patterns exist in the conservation, or attrition, of genes or pathways within serovars associated with swine enterocolitis or septicaemia. The sequenced *S.* Choleraesuis strain SC-B67 contains two plasmids: a 138 kb self-transmissible plasmid that confers resistance to multiple antibiotics used to treat systemic salmonellosis (Ye *et al.*, 2011); and a 50 kb plasmid that exhibits homology to the *spv*-encoding virulence plasmids of other serovars (Yu *et al.*, 2006). Loss of the 50 kb plasmid attenuates *S.* Choleraeusis in mice (Kawahara *et al.*, 1988) and pigs (Danbara *et al.*, 1992), and some plasmid-cured derivatives have been evaluated as live-attenuated vaccines (Kennedy *et al.*, 1999; Chu *et al.*, 2007). The contribution of individual plasmid-encoded genes to the pathogenesis of swine typhoid remains unclear. Though the literature describes the production of at least three cytotoxins in *Salmonella* (Reitmeyer *et al.*, 1986; Ashkenazi *et al.*, 1988; Libby *et al.*, 1990; Prasad *et al.*, 1990, 1992), the advent of complete genome sequences for several *S. enterica* serovars has indicated an absence of classical enterotoxins (akin to cholera toxin or *Escherichia coli* heat-labile or heat-stable toxins) that could mediate the induction of enteritis in isolation of other factors.

Genes associated with the virulence of *Salmonella* in pigs have been sought by signature-tagged mutagenesis (STM). This method relies on the assembly of pools of random bacterial transposon mutants, each harbouring a unique oligonucleotide sequence that can be detected by polymerase chain reaction and hybridization. Mutants that are negatively-selected *in vivo* are inferred to have insertions in virulence-associated loci, which can then be identified by subcloning and sequencing. Screening of a library of 960 signature-tagged mutants of *S.* Choleraesuis by intranasal inoculation of pigs identified 33 attenuating mutations (Ku *et al.*, 2005). Among the genes required for virulence in this model were those encoded by *Salmonella* pathogenicity island (SPI)-1 and -2, which respectively encode Type III secretion systems (T3SS)-1 and -2. These systems act in a manner akin to molecular syringes and inject a set of bacterial proteins into host cells, which then subvert cellular processes to the benefit of the pathogen. T3SS-1 is believed to promote bacterial uptake by epithelial cells via the injection of effectors that rearrange the subcortical actin cytoskeleton leading to membrane 'ruffling', whereas T3SS-2 promotes net intracellular replication of the bacteria (reviewed in Stevens *et al.*, 2009). Evidence exists that T3SS-1 promotes invasion of porcine ileal mucosa by *S.* Typhimurium (Paulin *et al.*, 2007), and by analogy with events in calves and streptomycin-pretreated mice it is inferred that this system may also be important in the induction of enteritis (Stevens *et al.*, 2009). Ku *et al.* (2005) detected other attenuating mutations in *S.* Choleraesuis affecting lipopolysaccharide (LPS) biosynthesis, transport of small molecules, regulators and bacteriophage-encoded genes. Two such mutants (with defects in SPI-2 or the Gifsy-1 prophage) were considered superior to a live-attenuated vaccine strain available at the time in terms of safety and protective efficacy (Ku *et al.*, 2005). The role of LPS is supported by earlier studies that suggested a role in invasion of cultured cells (Finlay *et al.*, 1988), and resistance to phagocytosis and complement-mediated killing (Saxen *et al.*, 1987; Robbins *et al.*, 1992). LPS also plays a key role in activation of innate immunity and endotoxic reactions during septicaemia, but the relative potency of LPS from different serovars in pigs is unclear.

STM has also been used to identify *S.* Typhimurium genes mediating intestinal colonization of pigs (Carnell *et al.*, 2007), as well as those promoting survival in swine gastric contents *ex vivo* (Bearson *et al.*, 2006). Some attenuating mutations were common to both screens. Carnell *et al.* (2007) screened 1045 random mutants in pigs and reported the phenotype of 227 mutants. As with the screen by Ku *et al.* (2005), the authors identified attenuating mutations in SPI-1 and -2, cell envelope and transport-associated genes as well as regulators and prophage elements. This screen also identified attenuating mutations in other SPIs (3 to 6), fimbriae and flagella, central metabolism and numerous genes of unknown function. The same library was previously screened following oral inoculation of calves and chicks (Morgan *et al.*, 2004) and comparison of the datasets indicates that *Salmonella* may deploy conserved- and host-specific factors during intestinal colonization.

Though powerful, STM is labour- and time-intensive and the identity of the majority of mutants screened remains unknown. It also relies on highly subjective visual assessment of the intensity of hybridization signals between input and output pools and between co-screened mutants. Massively-parallel sequencing of transposon-flanking regions can be used to simultaneously describe the location and relative abundance of mutations in complex pools. Transposon-directed insertion-site sequencing (TraDIS; Langridge *et al.*, 2009) has recently assigned phenotypes to 7701 *S.* Typhimurium mutants during intestinal colonization of pigs, calves and chickens, providing data on the role of 2715 different genes (Chaudhuri *et al.*, 2013). This has confirmed the role of the *Salmonella* pathogenicity islands specified above, but also assigned roles to hundreds of *S.* Typhimurium genes of previously unknown function in pigs, providing key data for the rational design of control strategies.

Whilst screening of mutant libraries has provided valuable insights, such studies provide only a snapshot of the infection process and do not reveal the spatial or temporal role of genes. For example, it has been reported that the SPI-1 regulator HilA plays a role in intestinal colonization of pigs by *S.* Choleraesuis after oral infection, but not intraperitoneal challenge (Lichtensteiger and Vimr, 2003). Similarly, a mutant lacking the SPI-2 regulatory system SsrAB was defective for colonization of visceral organs after intravenous infection of pigs, but did not exhibit a significant defect in intestinal persistence (Boyen *et al.*, 2008). The limited role for T3SS-2 in colonization of the porcine intestines is supported by observations with a *S.* Typhimurium DT104 *sseD* mutant (Brumme *et al.*, 2007). Tissue-specific phenotypes may also exist. For example after oral dosing of pigs, T3SS-1 mediates invasion of intestinal mucosa but not the tonsils (Boyen *et al.*, 2006b). This finding was supported by gentamicin treatment and immunocytochemical analysis of single-cell suspensions of porcine tonsils, which suggest that most bacteria reside outside cells at this site (van Parys *et al.*, 2010). One must also consider that studies with random or defined mutants are conducted with a small number of prototype strains that may not be representative of the wider serovar. It is becoming clear that subtle variation in the repertoire, sequence or expression of genes may lead to differences in virulence. Indeed, between serovar Typhimurium and Choleraesuis strains it is noteworthy that variation exists in the sequence and transcription of components of T3SS-1 and -2, as well as the repertoire of secreted effectors, which may partially explain the differential virulence of the organisms (Paulin *et al.*, 2007; Eswarappa *et al.*, 2008).

Competition between mutants screened in complex pools has the potential to exaggerate fitness defects and transposon insertions may have polar effects. A need therefore exists to confirm the role of specific genes via analysis of defined mutant and repaired or complemented strains. Few such studies have been reported for *Salmonella* in pigs to date. In addition to those described above with SPI-1 and -2 mutants, the regulators RpoS and PhoP, which are important for survival of *S.* Typhimurium in swine gastric fluid *ex vivo* (Bearson *et al.*, 2006), were found to contribute to intestinal colonization of pigs by *S.* Choleraesuis (Domínguez-Bernal *et al.*, 2008). Type I fimbriae mediate adherence of *S.* Typhimurium to porcine enterocytes and influence intestinal colonization (Althouse *et al.*, 2003). Saf fimbriae were also implicated in the carriage of *S.* Typhimurium in pigs, albeit that the defect in shedding did not attain statistical significance relative to the parent (Carnell *et al.*, 2007). Mutation of the *S.* Typhimurium regulators *cpxR* and *lon* has been reported to be attenuating in pregnant sows and to confer protection in suckling pigs (Hur and Lee, 2010). Moreover, a plasmid-cured catabolite repression (*crp*) mutant of *S.* Choleraesuis is attenuated in pigs (Chu *et al.*, 2007), supporting earlier findings with *cya crp* derivatives (Kennedy *et al.*, 1999). An adenine histidine auxotroph of *S.* Typhimurium is also attenuated in pigs (Selke *et al.*, 2007) as are mutants with defects affecting aromatic amino acid biosynthesis (Barrow *et al.*, 2001; Trebichavsky *et al.*, 2006; Paulin *et al.*, 2007). A predicted class-II aminoacyl-tRNA synthetase (PoxA), required for survival in swine gastric contents *ex vivo* (Bearson *et al.*, 2006), has been confirmed to be required for tonsillar and intestinal colonization of pigs (Bearson *et al.*, 2011), however its mode of action remains unclear.

As discussed in detail elsewhere (Bearson and Bearson, 2011), factors influencing *Salmonella* virulence in rodent models occasionally play no role in swine, as reported for the fibronectin-binding Type V secreted adhesin ShdA, which influences long-term persistence in mice (Kingsley *et al.*, 2000) but not pigs (Boyen *et al.*, 2006a). Similarly, combined mutation of the *fepA*, *iroN* and *cirA* genes involved in iron acquisition attenuates *S*. Typhimurium in mice (Williams *et al.*, 2006) but not swine (Bearson *et al.*, 2008). Taken together with observations on the phenotype of random transposon mutants screened in multiple hosts, such data support the notion that *Salmonella* deploys host-specific virulence factors in pigs and reinforces the need for research in target hosts where feasible.

An alternative approach to identify genes influencing *Salmonella* pathogenesis in pigs has been to identify *in vivo*-induced genes. A recombinase-based promoter-trap screen was used to identify 55 clones containing promoters that were induced during intestinal colonization of pigs but not during growth in laboratory medium (Huang *et al.*, 2007). Among the 31 unique genes located downstream of the promoters in such clones were genes for synthesis of Bcf fimbriae (*bcfA*), LPS (*rffG*), a two-component sensory system related to zinc tolerance (*hydH*), and genes involved in the degradation of aromatic compounds (*hpaBR*), heat-shock response (*hscA*) and virulence in mice (*yciR, metL*) (Huang *et al.*, 2007). Of the 55 clones, 19 were isolated from both the tonsils and the intestine, while 23 were identified only in the intestine and 13 only in tonsils, consistent with the requirement for different *Salmonella* genes in distinct anatomical niches. The existence of tissue-specific patterns of transcription is supported by an independent promoter-trap screen reliant on rescue from purine auxotrophy (van Parys *et al.*, 2011). These authors identified 37 *S*. Typhimurium genes induced 3 weeks post-oral inoculation in the tonsils, ileum and ileocaecal lymph nodes of pigs. Several genes were expressed in all three organs analysed, while others were only expressed in one or two organs. For examples, *efp* and *rpoZ*, which encode elongation factor P and the omega subunit of RNA polymerase respectively, were specifically expressed in the ileocaecal lymph nodes (van Parys *et al.*, 2011). One of the *S*. Typhimurium genes predicted to be expressed in the tonsils and ileum (STM4067, encoding a putative ADP-ribosylglycohydrolase) was subsequently shown to play a role in intestinal colonization in pigs, while another *in vivo*-induced gene encoding the SPI-2 effector SifB did not affect persistence (van Parys *et al.*, 2011).

Treatment

Various antibiotics have been used to treat severe *Salmonella* infections in pigs, but actual controlled trials to judge their efficacy are few. Wilcock and Schwartz (1992) mention a number of trials, but the general conclusion was that therapy was equivocal or of little merit. Antimicrobials have also been used to reduce, but not eliminate, the shedding of *Salmonella* by sick or recovered pigs (Holcomb and Fedorka-Cray, 1997). However, anecdotal information from practitioners suggests that severe *Salmonella* infections will respond to appropriate antimicrobial therapy. Ancillary therapy, such as the use of fluids to replace lost electrolytes and to prevent dehydration, will assist recovery.

Detection of *Salmonella*

Culture

Interest has grown in the animal-production and food-processing industries to develop and evaluate methods to detect, either directly or indirectly, the presence of *Salmonella*. Traditional culture methods may take 3–5 days to complete and much effort has been directed towards finding more rapid methods. However, the culture of *Salmonella* is the standard by which all other methods are measured. Recovery of the organism is the only means by which classification into serotypes and phage types can be achieved, and is thus key to epidemiological investigations.

Most of the original methods were developed for the diagnosis of clinical salmonellosis in humans and other animals. In pigs, clinical salmonellosis is uncommon. The sensitivity of the culture method may also be affected by the phase of the infection. In acute salmonellosis, large numbers of *Salmonella* are shed in the faeces, whereas a chronically infected pig or a carrier may excrete only low numbers of *Salmonella* intermittently. Thus, for clinical samples, direct culture may suffice, whereas samples from chronically infected pigs or from the environment will almost certainly require pre-enrichment and selective enrichment or a different approach altogether.

Many different culture media and methods have been developed and used for *Salmonella* detection. For the isolation of *S.* Choleraesuis, Smith (1952) found it absolutely necessary to utilize media other than tetrathionate broth and selenite F broth, both of which have been reported to be toxic for the organism. It has been suggested that this may explain the infrequent isolation of *S.* Choleraesuis in pigs during epidemiological surveys (Ewing, 1986). During a study on the prevalence of *Salmonella* in finishing pigs, Davies *et al.* (1997) failed to isolate *S.* Choleraesuis on xylose-lysine-Tergitol 4 (XLT4) medium, though the organism grew on modified brilliant green agar. When possible, a combination of enrichment media should be employed and may include Gram-negative (GN)-Hajna broth and tetrathionate broth (Ewing, 1986; Fedorka-Cray *et al.*, 1995a). Many plating media have been devised for the isolation and differentiation of *Salmonella* (see OIE, 2010) and the choice of the media will be governed by the operators' experience and requirements. It should also be remembered that the classical *S.* Choleraesuis does not produce H_2S and may be missed on media, such as xylose lysine desoxycholate (XLD), which incorporate an H_2S indicator. When considering swine, in all cases, pooled faecal samples are preferred over rectal swabs for the detection of *Salmonella* carrier pigs (McCall *et al.*, 1966).

Enzyme-linked immunosorbent assays

Enzyme-linked immunosorbent assays (ELISA) can be used to detect either the organism or a humoral immune response to the organism. Antigen-capture ELISA to detect microorganisms in food and feedstuffs are gaining widespread use in the industry. Whereas culture may take 3–7 days to identify the organism, ELISA can detect the organism in a much shorter period of time, usually 1 day or less. However, the reliability of some of these assays is questionable. In general, the cleaner the sample, the better the assay will perform. Usually faeces or faeces-contaminated samples do not test as well as food and feedstuffs. Feng (1992) listed and described several commercial rapid-screening assays. Several antigen-capture immunoassays have been utilized to detect *Salmonella* in pig faeces (Araj and Chugh, 1987; Lambiri *et al.*, 1990; van Poucke, 1990). They have the same disadvantage as many ELISA tests in that they require 10^4–10^5 CFU *Salmonella* ml^{-1} to detect the organism (Dziezak, 1987). In order to achieve these numbers, a time-consuming and expensive concentration protocol or a lengthy pre-enrichment step must be employed. Some investigators have had success in utilizing rapid-enrichment protocols to detect *Salmonella* in pig faeces (Cherrington and Huis in't Veld, 1993). The second use of ELISA is to detect animals that have been, or are currently, infected with *Salmonella*. The detection of antibodies to the O antigen of *Salmonella* has been used successfully in pigs (Nielsen *et al.*, 1994). The mixed ELISA utilizes LPS produced from both *S.* Typhimurium and *S.* Choleraesuis. The majority of pig-related *Salmonella* serovars produce high titres to the O-antigens that are present. Although the test can be utilized at the herd level, it is not suitable as an individual pig test (Nielsen *et al.*, 1995). The mixed ELISA has been used for routine screening of breeding, multiplying and slaughter pig herds in Denmark since 1993. The screening of breeding and multiplying herds is performed on serum samples, whereas meat juice is used for slaughter pigs. The meat juice is obtained by freezing a 10 g sample of muscle tissue at −20°C overnight and then allowing it to thaw, thereby releasing antibody-containing tissue fluid. On the basis of the ELISA results, further farm investigations may be undertaken, using culture methods. Unfortunately, experimentally and naturally-infected pigs have been shown to have a titre to LPS for at least 12 weeks after exposure to *S.* Choleraesuis, even after clearing the bacteria (Gray *et al.*, 1996b). This may result in a number of ELISA-positive pigs that are no longer infected. It is unclear what effect licensed or candidate vaccines have on the outcome of this assay. However, data indicate that pigs vaccinated with a commercially available, modified, live, plasmid-free *S.* Choleraesuis vaccine do not initiate a humoral immune response to *S.* Choleraesuis antigens (Schwarz *et al.*, 2011). This would suggest that pigs vaccinated with this strain would appear as non-infected pigs in a diagnostic test.

Another ELISA has been used to detect antibodies in *Salmonella*-infected pigs, employing a heat-extracted antigen (Kramer *et al.*, 1994). The results from this study indicate that most pigs infected with *S.* Typhimurium or *S.* Choleraesuis have an antibody response to this antigen. This assay shows a correlation between prevalence and severity of infection and the magnitude of the antibody response. ELISA tests have been shown to be useful for the detection of farms that are regularly contaminated with *Salmonella*; however, such tests cannot give information on the infectious status of a single animal or a group at the point of slaughter (Nowak *et al.*, 2007). ELISA is best used in combination with management measures to prevent the spread of infections by trade and transport (Nowak *et al.*, 2007).

Polymerase chain reaction

The extraordinary ability of the polymerase chain reaction (PCR) to exponentially replicate a target DNA sequence has made it a very powerful tool in the armoury of the diagnostician, epidemiologist and molecular biologist. This assay is based on the ability of target (organism)-specific primers, through complementary DNA base-pairing, to anneal only to the target sequence. Thermostable DNA polymerase recognizes the template primer complex as a substrate, which results in the simultaneous copying of both strands of the segment of DNA between the two annealed primers. The denaturation, annealing and elongation steps take place in a cyclical fashion, relying on the thermostability of the polymerase, until the target sequence is amplified to detectable amounts (Ehrlich and Sirko, 1994). The PCR assay has been used to identify *Salmonella* in food and clinical samples (Araj and Chugh, 1987; Rahn *et al.*, 1992; Cohen *et al.*, 1993). However, obstacles in the detection of organisms include the presence of substances inhibitory to PCR (Wilde *et al.*, 1990; Rossen *et al.*, 1992) and the inability to detect $<10^3$ CFU g^{-1} of sample without pre-enrichment (Ehrlich and Sirko, 1994). Investigators have improved detection methods in PCR assays by combining it with immunomagnetic separation (Widjojoatmodjo *et al.*, 1991, 1992) or by enrichment culture (Stone *et al.*, 1994). Analytical approaches for pork quality control programmes now recommend combining ELISA tests with PCR to increase sensitivity and increase ease of sample handling (Nowak *et al.*, 2007).

Considerable progress has been made utilizing PCR and/or immunoassays to detect *Salmonella* in foods of swine origin. Hoerner *et al.* (2011) have shown immunoassay to have sensitivity of 99% and specificity of 100%, demonstrating that post-harvest monitoring can be valuable. Additionally, several options exist for post-harvest monitoring of swine origin foodstuffs with multiplex PCR detecting multiple pathogens including *Salmonella*. Suo *et al.* (2010) reported that enrichment combined with PCR appears to be a viable post-harvest approach to detect a range of pathogens. Recent studies by Wilkins *et al.* (2011) compared culture, PCR and ELISA in detecting *Salmonella* status in herds. With a Bayesian model specifying dependence between the two tests, the sensitivity of culture and real-time PCR (RT-PCR) was 79% to 86%, depending on the cut-off value for the ELISA. When culture specificity was assumed to be 100%, RT-PCR had a specificity of 94%.

Vaccination

A systematic review of literature from 1979 to 2007 relating to the efficacy of vaccines for control of *Salmonella* in pigs may be found elsewhere (Denagamage *et al.*, 2007). Of the trials surveyed, just five were considered to provide robust evidence that vaccination reduces *Salmonella* prevalence in pigs. The authors make clear the requirement for careful study design and sampling of pigs at slaughter age if conclusions on the impact of vaccination on control of zoonosis are to be justified. Though many promising candidates have been reported in murine models, this section deals only with those vaccines tested for immunogenicity or protective efficacy in pigs.

It is generally accepted that live, attenuated, orally administered *Salmonella* vaccines provide the best protection against *Salmonella* infection. The superior protection achieved in comparison with inactivated bacterins and subunit vaccines is generally attributed to the ability of live vaccines to stimulate a more effective cell-mediated immune response capable of targeting intracellular *Salmonella*. Oral administration allows the attenuated mutant to utilize natural routes of infection, which facilitates the crucial step of antigen presentation to lymphocytes in the gut-associated lymphoid tissue. These events induce the production of secretory immunoglobulin A (IgA) on mucosal surfaces (Clarke and Gyles, 1993). To some extent, live-attenuated vaccines may also protect in the short term by competitive exclusion (Lovell and Barrow, 1999; Foster *et al.*, 2003).

In many countries inactivated vaccines are available and their efficacy is equivocal. Linton *et al.* (1970) considered that immunization with a killed vaccine conferred only weak protection against *Salmonella* infection in general. Davies and Wray (1997) showed that vaccination of breeding stock on a farm with an inactivated *S.* Typhimurium/*S.* Dublin vaccine was associated with a reduction of *Salmonella* from 67% to 12% in weaned pigs and from 52% to 5% in the adults. In Denmark, Dahl *et al.* (1997) demonstrated that the use of killed vaccines reduced the clinical impact of *S.* Typhimurium infection in pigs but did not reduce subclinical infection. It may be feasible to rationally improve bacterins by culture of the bacteria under conditions that mimic the *in vivo* environment, thereby enhancing expression of factors required for persistence in the host.

Several strategies have been used to construct live-attenuated *Salmonella* vaccines, including for expression of heterologous antigens, via the introduction of stable and specific mutations (Chatfield *et al.*, 1992). A mutation in the *galE* region in *S.* Typhi results in a deficiency in UDP-glucose-4-epimerase, the enzyme that converts UDP-glucose to UDP-galactose, an essential component of *Salmonella* smooth LPS (Levine *et al.*, 1989). In several trials in humans, this mutant has appeared to be efficacious, therefore *galE* mutations have been employed in other *Salmonella* serovars, including *S.* Typhimurium (Nnalue and Lindberg, 1990). However, a *galE* mutation in *S.* Choleraesuis does not reduce virulence in pigs. This may be due to the fact that galactose is missing from the oligosaccharide repeating unit of the O-antigen side-chain of *S.* Choleraesuis (Nnalue and Stocker, 1986). The somatic antigens of *Salmonella* serogroups facilitate survival in the gastrointestinal tract and entry into deeper tissues (Nnalue and Lindberg, 1990; Ku *et al.*, 2005; Carnell *et al.*, 2007; Chaudhuri *et al.*, 2013). Other LPS mutants have therefore been evaluated, some of which are effective in mice and may be suitable for differentiating vaccinated from naturally-infected pigs (Leyman *et al.*, 2011)

An alternative strategy for attenuation involves the creation of auxotrophs that require metabolites not available in animal tissues. Mutations in the aromatic amino acid biosynthetic pathway impose a requirement for aromatic metabolites, such as p-aminobenzoate and 2,3-dihydroxybenzoate. Oral vaccination with *aroA*, *aroD* mutants in mice and calves has been effective in reducing disease and has been shown to be safe (Robertsson *et al.*, 1983; Smith *et al.*, 1984; Hook, 1990). Experiments using an *aroA* mutant of *S.* Typhimurium indicated that vaccinated pigs shed *Salmonella* significantly less frequently than non-vaccinated pigs (Lumsden *et al.*, 1991). An auxotrophic mutant derived by chemical mutagenesis with requirements for adenine and histidine has also been reported to be effective in control of *S.* Typhimurium in pigs (Selke *et al.*, 2007). This vaccine, which is licensed as Salmoporc in some European countries, has been further improved by the inclusion of an *ompD* mutation, which permits the differentiation of vaccinated and naturally-infected animals (Selke *et al.*, 2007). An adenine-deficient strain of *S.* Choleraesuis has also been used for immunization of pigs in Germany (Meyer *et al.*, 1993).

Mutations in global regulatory pathways have also been a popular means of attenuation. Several studies have utilized strains with deletions in the genes for adenylate cyclase (*cya*) and for cAMP-receptor protein (*crp*). Cyclic AMP and cAMP-receptor protein regulate at least 200 genes, many of which are required for the breakdown of catabolites. *Salmonella* with deletion mutations in the *cya*, *crp* genes have been shown to be safe and effective in eliciting protective immunity in mice, chickens and pigs (Curtiss and Kelly 1987; Stabel *et al.*, 1990, 1991; Coe and Wood, 1992; Kelly *et al.*, 1992; Kennedy *et al.*, 1999) but retain virulence for germ-free pigs (Barrow *et al.*, 2001).

An attenuated strain of *S.* Choleraesuis var. Kunzendorf that has been cured of the 50 kb virulence plasmid (SC-54) has been shown to be safe and efficacious in pigs (Kramer *et al.*, 1992). It also reduces seroprevalence and isolation of *Salmonella* at slaughter after vaccination on the first day of life (Schwarz *et al.*, 2011). The non-specific mutation was obtained by repeated passage through porcine neutrophils. The plasmid-free variant lacks the ability to invade Vero cell monolayers and porcine neutrophils, as well as having increased resistance to killing by hydrogen peroxide (H_2O_2) and phagocytic killing by porcine neutrophils (Roof *et al.*, 1992).

Another approach has been to target the function of key *Salmonella* virulence factors. For example, it is known that *S.* Typhimurium requires Type III secretion systems and other secreted virulence factors to colonize the porcine intestines, therefore an inert vaccine comprising the secreted fraction of *S.* Typhimurium was evaluated (Carnell *et al.*, 2007). Vaccines comprising of factors precipitated from culture supernatants reduce the prevalence of enterohaemorrhagic *E. coli* O157 in cattle, however only a modest reduction in faecal excretion of *S.* Typhimurium was observed on a single day post-challenge of vaccinated pigs relative to controls (Carnell *et al.*, 2007). The weak protective effect was independent of T3SS-1-secreted proteins as it was also observed when the secreted fraction of a *prgH* mutant was used (Carnell *et al.*, 2007), and it is likely that other secreted proteins or LPS may be responsible for the effects observed.

The use of vaccines should be considered as part of an overall strategy to control *Salmonella* on the farm and their use should be in conjunction with other measures (EFSA, 2006). Where protection is required in early life, vaccination of sows to prime maternal transfer of antibody may be more useful than delivering vaccines to immunologically naïve neonates. For the same reason, feeding of *Salmonella*-specific antibodies purified from the yolk of eggs from immunized chickens may offer some protection. Reviews on the efficacy of vaccination in swine populations indicate desirable impact; however, the available data do not include, or translate into, large-scale impact studies. The majority of vaccine challenge studies also do not report the necessary data to completely evaluate vaccine efficacy (Denagamage *et al.*, 2007). It is desirable that future studies follow the recommended guidelines for reporting described by O'Connor *et al.* (2010).

Competitive Exclusion

Competitive exclusion has been used successfully in poultry for control of *Salmonella* and relies on the ability of harmless exogenous microbes to persist in the intestines and outcompete or eliminate incoming or resident pathogens (Bailey, 1987; Bailey *et al.*, 1992; Blankenship *et al.*, 1993). A mucosal competitive-exclusion culture from swine (MCES) was developed by Fedorka-Cray *et al.* (1999). Following application in suckling pigs and subsequent challenge with *S.* Choleraesuis, 28% of the gut tissues from the MCES-treated pigs were positive versus 79% positive tissues from the control pigs. A 2 to 5 $\log_{10}$ CFU/g reduction of *Salmonella* in the caecal contents or ileocolic junction was observed in the MCES-treated pigs when compared with the controls. Competitive exclusion also appeared to be effective when used in neonatal and weaned piglets (Genovese *et al.*, 2003). A mixture of five lactic acid bacteria (two strains of *Lactobacillus murinus* and one strain each of *Lactobacillus salivarius* subsp. *salivarius*, *Lactobacillus pentosus*, and *Pediococcus pentosaceous*), has been reported to reduce shedding of *S.* Typhimurium and alleviate disease symptoms in challenged piglets (Casey *et al.*, 2007). However, the challenge of finding single microorganisms capable of excluding *Salmonella* is emphasised by independent reports suggesting that *Enterococcus faecium* NCIMB 10415 confers no protective effect against *S.* Typhiumurium DT104 challenge in weaned or weaning pigs, and may even enhance the course of *Salmonella* infection (Szabó *et al.*, 2009; Kreuzer *et al.*, 2012). Continuous delivery of *E. faecium* as a mix with two *Bacillus* strains in drinking water also offered no protection against *S.* Typhimurium infection (Walsh *et al.*, 2012). The challenge of finding species or mixtures that persistently colonize the porcine intestines and effectively exclude a range of *Salmonella* serovars, as well as being safe and cheap to manufacture in a reproducible manner, has hindered development of competitive exclusion approaches for pigs. However, probiotics continue to be developed to prevent or treat human gastrointestinal syndromes and it is likely that further candidates will be explored in swine. It is evident that some serovars (e.g. *S.* Infantis) and attenuated *Salmonella* (e.g. Δ*aroA* mutants) protect gnotobiotic piglets against otherwise lethal challenge with *S.* Typhimurium in a manner associated with neutrophil recruitment to the intestines (Foster *et al.*, 2003). Use of such strains would interfere with current immunoassays for *Salmonella* contamination and, as with live-attenuated vaccines, a need would exist for marked strains that could permit the differentiation of treated and naturally-infected animals and which would not persist to the point of entry of pigs into the food chain.

Other Control Measures

During the last decade, the structure of the pig industry has changed markedly, with the introduction of large integrated systems and breeding pyramids, akin to those of the poultry industry. The introduction of outdoor 'welfare-friendly' systems in some developed countries also poses new challenges. In the absence of vaccines or treatments that can eliminate *Salmonella*, control measures are of increasing importance owing to rising demand and consumer concerns about food safety. Epidemiological studies in recent years suggest that *Salmonella* infection of suckling piglets is much lower than that of older animals, because of lactogenic immunity, and that, by the application of integrated quality control systems agreed upon by all staff, the prevalence of *Salmonella* on pig farms can be reduced. Application of these systems requires some knowledge of the *Salmonella* prevalence on an individual farm and this can be monitored, as indicated earlier, by either serology or culture.

In recognition of the major role that pigs play in transmission of food-poisoning *Salmonella* serovars to man via the food chain, the European Union introduced legislation (European Union, 2003) requiring control measures to be introduced in each Member State for the control of *Salmonella* serovars of public health significance in poultry and pigs and which includes breeding pigs. Vaccination was regarded as a method to control infection which might be considered as a valid component of this overall scheme.

The main components of an integrated quality control system are as follows.

Biosecurity

As indicated previously there are many routes by which *Salmonella* can be introduced on to a farm and the organism is often disseminated widely on farms. Control measures include changes of clothing and boots for visitors, bird and rodent control, footbaths containing active disinfectant outside houses, limiting access to the site by visitors and lorries, etc. Farm size, stocking densities and pig density within a region all have a negative effect on the *Salmonella* status of a farm, perhaps by predisposing to *Salmonella* spread within and between farms.

All-in, all-out systems

Effective cleaning and disinfection are important aspects of disease control. It is generally accepted that farms should operate an all-in, all-out policy, with adequate cleaning and disinfection after the pen is empty. Linton *et al.* (1970) found that uninfected animals, which remained in disinfected pens, usually stayed free of *Salmonella*, but, as the number of pigs per pen increased, a higher prevalence of infection was found. Tielen *et al.* (1997) found that *Salmonella*-negative piglets placed in clean accommodation remained free, despite serological evidence of *Salmonella* in the sows. Fedorka-Cray *et al.* (1997b) weaned pigs at 14–21 days and removed them to clean accommodation, where the piglets remained free of *Salmonella*. Improved disinfection of weaner and grower pens on several farms produced a significant reduction in the incidence of positive batches (from 80% to 11% on one farm) (Davies and Wray, 1997).

A word of caution should be introduced, however, as other investigators have shown no reduction in the prevalence of *Salmonella* using all-in, all-out management of finishing pigs, compared with conventional farrow-to-finish systems, in North Carolina, USA (Davies *et al.*, 1997).

Feeding systems

Many batches of animal feed are contaminated with *Salmonella* (see Chapter 19, this volume). In the Netherlands, it was found that the prevalence of *Salmonella* infection was ten times lower in pigs fed a porridge than those fed dry feed (Tielen *et al.*, 1997). A study of 40 fattening farms in the Netherlands isolated *Salmonella* from 19.4% of the samples from farms using whey, compared with 64.4% of farms using water (Van Schie and Overgoor, 1987). Field studies in Denmark found a lower prevalence of *Salmonella* on farms mixing their own feed and feeding liquid feed (Bager, 1994). It is possible that the size of the feed particles can influence the intestinal flora or the distribution of organic acids, which have been shown to be inhibitory (Prohaszka *et al.*, 1990). Naturally fermented feed is now being recommended for reduction of *Salmonella* infection in Denmark. Likewise, the use of acidified feed may improve the response to treatment and reduce the spread of disease, though no protective effect of delivery of organic acids in drinking water was observed in a recent study (Walsh *et al.*, 2012). One may caution that use of acidified water or diets may lead to excretion of acid-tolerant *Salmonella* that may be better adapted to transit through the acid barrier of the stomach to initiate infection. Supplementation of drinking water with chlorate preparations has been reported to reduce *Salmonella* levels in both weaned and finisher pigs (Anderson *et al.*, 2004, 2006). The impact of a range of feed characteristics, including feed formulation, was reviewed in 2008 (O'Connor *et al.*, 2008). The ultimate conclusion of this review was that there is, as yet, no strong association between the presence of *Salmonella* in market weight finishers and feed characteristics that could form the basis of science-led changes to diet to control *Salmonella*.

It is important that control is based on a detailed knowledge of the epidemiology of infection and a specific control programme for each enterprise. While a range of interventions have been trialled to reduce *Salmonella* in swine, including vaccination, competitive exclusion, treatments of feed and water, antibiotic administration, disinfection of animals and segregated weaning into clean facilities, it continues to be the segregated weaning approaches that yield the most consistent results (reviewed by Wales *et al.*, 2011). No control measure in isolation has been successful on its own, but improved hygiene and disease security, combined with vaccination and/or strategic medication, are methods that have been used successfully in other sectors of the livestock industry. Implementation of the hazard analysis critical control point

(HACCP) principles on the farm and at slaughter, to identify risk factors and target control strategies, is an important ongoing step. In most cases methods useful for pre-harvest *Salmonella* reduction in swine populations such as HACCP are related to sound management practices that also improve the overall health of a swine operation (Griffith *et al.*, 2006).

Public Health Aspects

Pigs are an important reservoir of human non-typhoidal salmonellosis and there have been many reports on the isolation of the organism from pork and pork products (Buxton, 1957; Bryan, 1980). Salmonellosis continues to be one of the most common food-borne illnesses in humans in the developed world. There is considerable public awareness of microbiological hazards of food and improved monitoring. Although *Salmonella* contamination of poultry and beef products exceeds that of pork in some countries, *Salmonella* control programmes in swine continue to be a key focus of food safety initiatives. The majority of swine herds in the USA are positive for *Salmonella* (Haley *et al.*, 2012). In Europe continued concern over pork products and *Salmonella* infection in humans are borne out of recent outbreaks due to products such as pork sausage (Gossner *et al.*, 2012).

In the period 1992–1999, in England and Wales, 73 (32%) of 228 meat-related outbreaks of food-borne diseases were associated with pig meat. Of these, 35 (15%) were caused by *Salmonella*. The most important serovars involved were *S.* Typhimurium (13), *S.* Enteritidis (13) and other *Salmonella* serovars (9), indicating the importance of pigs and pig meat as a vehicle for *Salmonella* (Smerdon *et al.*, 2001). Similarly, in the Netherlands 22% of human salmonellosis cases were associated with consumption of pork (reported in European Food Safety Authority, 2006).

Reports indicate that a wide range of *Salmonella* may be present in fresh pork (Bozzano *et al.*, 1993; Fernandez-Escartin *et al.*, 1995). In Greece, 28% of pork pig carcasses were found to be contaminated with *Salmonella* (Epling *et al.*, 1993). Carcass contamination was 17.5% in Canada (Lammerding *et al.*, 1998), 21% in the Netherlands (Oosterom *et al.*, 1985), 6.5% in the USA (FSIS, 1999) and 27% in Belgium (Korsak *et al.*, 1998). Pig meat products, such as hot vacuum-packaged pork (Van Laack *et al.*, 1993), especially those incorporating low-grade material, such as mechanically recovered meat (Banks and Board, 1983), are frequently contaminated with *Salmonella*. In many countries, the relationship between human illness and *Salmonella* contamination of pig meat is unclear.

The problem persists with continuing reports from many countries and variable levels of antibiotic resistance, which reflect the levels of usage in each country. Levels of contamination varied from 1.6% in Canada (Bohaychuk *et al.*, 2011) to 31% in China (Yang *et al.*, 2010). The prevalence of contamination is also increasing in some countries with levels from between 1% and 1.8% in 2002 increasing to 4.2% to 8.6% in 2006 in Denmark (Hansen *et al.*, 2010).

The prevalence of *Salmonella* in the intestine of individual pigs from different sources is extremely variable (Gray *et al.*, 1995, 1996a, b). Individual animals may remain as carriers for up to 36 weeks (Wood and Rose, 1992). In Denmark, 6.2% of caecal samples were found positive, usually with one serovar or phage type predominating from each farm source (Baggesen *et al.*, 1996). Sampling methods are important in these surveys, because it has been shown that rectal swabs provide an underestimate of the level of infection, as may carcass swabs. Davies *et al.* (1999) investigated *Salmonella* contamination at a large abattoir and isolated *Salmonella* from 7.0% of 2211 carcass swabs and 11.6% of 2205 samples of large-intestinal contents. Many of the isolates were resistant to antibiotics. It is commonly supposed that lairage of pigs will increase the chance of cross-infection and contamination of pigs (Morgan *et al.*, 1987). *Salmonella* shedding may be increased by any stress factor, including transport (Scheepens *et al.*, 1994; Berends *et al.*, 1996), but stress levels, and possibly *Salmonella* excretion, are reduced by overnight lairage (Warriss *et al.*, 1998). There appears to be little difference in the magnitude of this effect in relation to the distance travelled (Rajkowski *et al.*, 1998). Davies *et al.* (1999) found a reduced rate of intestinal carriage of *Salmonella* and carcass contamination in pigs that had been held overnight in lairage, as compared with pigs slaughtered within 2–3 h of arrival.

The slaughter process in a well-run pig abattoir is capable of reducing the level of surface contamination of carcasses, because of the scalding and singeing stages, but any *Salmonella* that survive these stages can be spread between carcasses by the de-hairing equipment (Gill and Bryant, 1993). Most of the contamination, however, results from escape of intestinal contents during evisceration (Saide-Albornoz *et al.*, 1995). The studies of Davies *et al.* (1999) indicated that there was little increase in carcass contamination after evisceration, although further increases caused by trimming and meat inspection have been described (Mousing *et al.*, 1997). HACCP-style procedures have been widely adopted in abattoirs, but the level of microbial monitoring to verify the critical control points and the correct application of procedures is often insufficient (von Langer, 1995). Employment of HACCP principles in the abattoir appear to have decreased the recovery of *Salmonella* from pig carcasses in the USA (FSIS, 1999). It is clear that biosecurity and hygiene precautions to control *Salmonella* should be taken throughout the pig meat production and distribution chain, from nucleus breeders to hot-dog stalls (Simonsen *et al.*, 1987).

Future Perspectives

Global demand for pork is fast accelerating owing to population growth, urbanization and rising affluence. With the implementation of effective vaccines and biosecurity measures for control of *Salmonella* in poultry, attention is increasingly focusing toward pigs as a reservoir of human non-typhoidal salmonellosis. In some countries swine typhoid continues to adversely impair the welfare of farmed pigs and it is noteworthy that the evolution of *S. enterica* has been punctuated by the emergence of epidemic and drug-resistant variants with the potential to spread worldwide via trade and travel. The basis of the differential virulence and host tropism of serovars found in pigs, and of the emergence and decline of epidemic variants over time, has eluded researchers for decades. The advent of rapid whole-genome sequencing, and of methods to simultaneously assign the role of hundreds of *Salmonella* genes *in vivo*, offers scope to unravel why some serovars pose threats to porcine and/or public health. Though information on the repertoire, sequence and function of genes will be valuable, it is likely that variation will also exist at the levels of transcription and translation, and quantification of bacterial gene expression *in vivo* poses significant technical challenges. 'Systems' approaches that integrate such disparate variables may help to distil testable hypotheses relating to virulence and host specificity. As our knowledge of the role and immunogenicity of factors deployed by *Salmonella* in pigs increases, so too will scope for inclusion of such factors into subunit vaccines and development of specific inhibitors. Some consider that cell-mediated immunity induced by live-attenuated vaccines will be required for clearance of *Salmonella* from intracellular niches; however, predicting which mutations will provide the desired balance of cross-serovar protection versus safety and persistence remains difficult. Vaccine design will benefit from studies on the immunological basis of resistance conferred by vaccination and challenge, and require investment to develop reagents to study porcine innate and adaptive responses at levels currently only feasible in mice and humans. Use of novel adjuvants and immunomodulatory substances to potentiate responses to existing vaccines or stimulate clearance prior to slaughter also merits study. In the long term, marker-assisted selection for pigs with improved heritable resistance to *Salmonella* and understanding of the role of indigenous microbiota in exclusion may also offer solutions, though care will be needed to ensure that such resistance is not to the detriment of other production traits or disease resistances. Any such interventions will need to be considered as part of a holistic plan that also considers the impact of biosecurity, diet, management practices and stressors.

References

Althouse, C., Patterson, S., Fedorka-Cray, P. and Isaacson, R.E. (2003) Type 1 fimbriae of *Salmonella enterica* serovar Typhimurium bind to enterocytes and contribute to colonization of swine in vivo. *Infection and Immunity* 71, 6446–6452.

Anderson, R.C., Nisbet, D.J., Buckley, S.A., Genovese, K.J., Harvey, R.B., Deloach, J.R., Keith, N.K. and Stanker, L.H. (1998) Experimental and natural infection of early weaned pigs with *Salmonella* cholerae-suis. *Research in Veterinary Science* 64, 261–262.

Anderson, R.C., Hume, M.E., Genovese, K.J., Callaway, T.R., Jung, Y.S., Edrington, T.S., Poole, T.L., Harvey, R.B., Bischoff, K.M. and Nisbet, D.J. (2004) Effect of drinking-water administration of experimental chlorate ion preparations on *Salmonella enterica* serovar Typhimurium colonization in weaned and finished pigs. *Veterinary Research Communications* 28, 179–189.

Anderson, R.C., Jung, Y.S., Genovese, K.J., McReynolds, J.L., Callaway, T.R., Edrington, T.S., Harvey, R.B. and Nisbet, D.J. (2006) Low level nitrate or nitroethane preconditioning enhances the bactericidal effect of suboptimal experimental chlorate treatment against *Escherichia coli* and *Salmonella* Typhimurium but not *Campylobacter* in swine. *Foodborne Pathogens and Disease* 3, 461–465.

Araj, G. and Chugh, T.D. (1987) Detection of *Salmonella* spp. in clinical specimens by capture enzyme-linked immunosorbent assay. *Journal of Clinical Microbiology* 25, 2150–2153.

Ashkenazi, S., Cleary, T.G., Murray, B.C., Wagner, A. and Pickering, L.K. (1988) Quantitative analysis and partial characterisation of cytotoxin production by *Salmonella* strains. *Infection and Immunity* 56, 3089–3094.

Bager, F. (1994) *Salmonella* in Danish pig herds: risk factors and sources of infection. In: *Proceedings of the XVII Nordic Veterinary Congress*. Reykjavik, pp. 79–82.

Baggesen, D.L. and Christensen, J. (1997) Distribution of *Salmonella enterica* serovars and phage types in Danish pig herds. In: *Proceedings of the 2nd International Symposium on Epidemiology and Control of* Salmonella *in Pork*, Copenhagen, Denmark, 20–22 August 1997, pp. 107–109.

Baggesen, D.L., Wegener, H.C., Bager, F., Stege, H. and Christensen, J. (1996) Herd prevalence of *Salmonella enterica* infections in Danish slaughter pigs determined by microbiological testing. *Preventive Veterinary Medicine* 26, 201–213.

Baggesen, D.L., Dahl, J., Wingstrand, A. and Nielsen, B. (1997) Detection of *Salmonella enterica* in different materials from the environment of pig farms. In: *Proceedings of the 2nd International Symposium on Epidemiology and Control of* Salmonella *in Pork*, Copenhagen, Denmark, 20–22 August 1997, pp. 173–175. (Obtainable from Federation of Danish Pig Producers and Slaughterhouses, Axelborg, Axeltorv 3, 1609 Copenhagen V, Denmark. Price DK 350 + postage).

Bailey, J.S. (1987) Factors affecting microbial competitive exclusion in poultry. *Food Technology* 47, 88–92.

Bailey, J.S., Cox, N.A., Blankenship, L.C. and Stern, N.J. (1992) Effect of competitive exclusion microflora on the distribution of *Salmonella* serovars in an integrated poultry operation. *Poultry Science* 71 (Suppl. 1).

Banks, J.G. and Board, R.G. (1983) Incidence and level of contamination of British pork sausages and ingredients with salmonellas. *Journal of Hygiene (Cambridge)* 90, 213–224.

Barrow, P.A., Page, K. and Lovell, M.A. (2001) The virulence for gnotobiotic pigs of live attenuated vaccine strains of *Salmonella enterica* serovars Typhimurium and Enteritidis. *Vaccine* 19, 3432–3436.

Barthel, M., Hapfelmeier, S., Quintanilla-Martínez, L., Kremer, M., Rohde, M., Hogardt, M., Pfeffer, K., Rüssmann, H. and Hardt, W.D. (2003) Pretreatment of mice with streptomycin provides a *Salmonella enterica* serovar Typhimurium colitis model that allows analysis of both pathogen and host. *Infection and Immunity* 71, 2839–2858.

Baskerville, A. and Dow, C. (1973) Pathology of experimental pneumonia in pigs produced by *Salmonella choleraesuis*. *Journal of Comparative Pathology* 83, 207–215.

Baskerville, A., Dow, C., Curran, W.L. and Hanna, J. (1972) Ultrastructure of phagocytosis of *Salmonella choleraesuis* by pulmonary macrophages *in vivo*. *British Journal of Experimental Pathology* 53, 641–647.

Baskerville, A., Dow, C., Curran, W.L. and Hanna, J. (1973) Further studies on experimental bacterial pneumonia: ultrastructure changes produced in the lungs by *Salmonella choleraesuis*. *British Journal of Experimental Pathology* 54, 90–98.

Bearson, B.L. and Bearson, S.M. (2008) The role of the QseC quorum-sensing sensor kinase in colonization and norepinephrine-enhanced motility of *Salmonella enterica* serovar Typhimurium. *Microbial Pathogenesis* 44, 271–278.

Bearson, B.L. and Bearson, S.M. (2011) Host specific differences alter the requirement for certain *Salmonella* genes during swine colonization. *Veterinary Microbiology* 150, 215–219.

Bearson, B.L., Bearson, S.M., Uthe, J.J., Dowd, S.E., Houghton, J.O., Lee, I., Toscano, M.J. and Lay, D.C. Jr (2008) Iron regulated genes of *Salmonella enterica* serovar Typhimurium in response to norepinephrine and the requirement of *fepDGC* for norepinephrine-enhanced growth. *Microbes and Infection* 10, 807–816.

Bearson, B.L., Bearson, S.M., Lee, I.S. and Brunelle, B.W. (2010) The *Salmonella enterica* serovar Typhimurium QseB response regulator negatively regulates bacterial motility and swine colonization in the absence of the QseC sensor kinase. *Microbial Pathogenesis* 48, 214–219.

Bearson, S.M., Bearson, B.L. and Rasmussen, M.A. (2006) Identification of *Salmonella enterica* serovar Typhimurium genes important for survival in the swine gastric environment. *Applied and Environmental Microbiology* 72, 2829–2836.

Bearson, S.M., Bearson, B.L., Brunelle, B.W., Sharma, V.K. and Lee, I.S. (2011) A mutation in the *poxA* gene of *Salmonella enterica* serovar Typhimurium alters protein production, elevates susceptibility to environmental challenges, and decreases swine colonization. *Foodborne Pathogens and Disease* 8, 725–732.

Berends, B.R., Urlings, H.A.P., Snijders, J.M.A. and Van Knapen, F. (1996) Identification and quantification of risk factors in animal management and transport regarding *Salmonella* spp in pigs. *International Journal of Food Microbiology* 30, 37–53.

Blankenship, L.C., Bailey, J.S., Cox, N.A., Stern, N.J., Brewer, R. and Williams, O. (1993) Two-step mucosal competitive exclusion flora treatment to diminish *Salmonella* in commercial broiler chickens. *Poultry Science* 72, 1667–1672.

Bleasdale, B., Lott, P.J., Jagannathan, A., Stevens, M.P., Birtles, R.J. and Wigley, P. (2009) The *Salmonella* pathogenicity island 2-encoded type III secretion system is essential for the survival of *Salmonella enterica* serovar Typhimurium in free-living amoebae. *Applied and Environmental Microbiology* 75, 1793–1795.

Bohaychuk, V.M., Gensler, G.E. and Barrios, P.R. (2011) Microbiological baseline study of beef and pork carcasses from provincially inspected abattoirs in Alberta, Canada. *Canadian Veterinary Journal* 52, 1095–100.

Bolton, A.J., Osborne, M.P., Wallis, T.S. and Stephen, J. (1999) Interaction of *Salmonella* Choleraesuis, *Salmonella* Dublin and *Salmonella* Typhimurium with porcine and bovine terminal ileum *in vivo*. *Microbiology* 145, 2431–2441.

Boyen, F., Pasmans, F., Donné, E., Van Immerseel, F., Morgan, E., Adriaensen, C., Hernalsteens, J.P., Wallis, T.S., Ducatelle, R. and Haesebrouck, F. (2006a) The fibronectin binding protein ShdA is not a prerequisite for long term faecal shedding of *Salmonella typhimurium* in pigs. *Veterinary Microbiology* 115, 284–290.

Boyen, F., Pasmans, F., Van Immerseel, F., Morgan, E., Adriaensen, C., Hernalsteens, J.P., Decostere, A., Ducatelle, R. and Haesebrouck, F. (2006b) *Salmonella* Typhimurium SPI-1 genes promote intestinal but not tonsillar colonization in pigs. *Microbes and Infection* 8, 2899–2907.

Boyen, F., Pasmans, F., Van Immerseel, F., Morgan, E., Botteldoorn, N., Heyndrickx, M., Volf, J., Favoreel, H., Hernalsteens, J.P., Ducatelle, R. and Haesebrouck, F. (2008) A limited role for SsrA/B in persistent *Salmonella* Typhimurium infections in pigs. *Veterinary Microbiology* 128, 364–373.

Bozzano, A.I., Diguerdos, G., Saccares, S., Bilet, S., Zottola, T., Brozzi, A.M., Panfilli, G. and Fontanelli, G. (1993) Occurrence of *Salmonella* in pork meat and processed pork products in the Latium region, central Italy from 1980–1989. *Italian Journal of Food Science* 5, 167–172.

Brumme, S., Arnold, T., Sigmarsson, H., Lehmann, J., Scholz, H.C., Hardt, W.D., Hensel, A., Truyen, U. and Roesler, U. (2007) Impact of *Salmonella* Typhimurium DT104 virulence factors *invC* and *sseD* on the onset, clinical course, colonization patterns and immune response of porcine salmonellosis. *Veterinary Microbiology* 124, 274–285.

Bryan, F.L. (1980) Foodborne diseases in the United States associated with meat and poultry. *Journal of Food Protection* 43, 140–150.

Burkey, T.E., Skjolaas, K.A., Dritz, S.S. and Minton, J.E. (2007) Expression of Toll-like receptors, interleukin 8, macrophage migration inhibitory factor, and osteopontin in tissues from pigs challenged with *Salmonella enterica* serovar Typhimurium or serovar Choleraesuis. *Veterinary Immunology and Immunopathology* 115, 309–319.

Buxton, A. (1957) Public health aspects of salmonellosis in animals. *Veterinary Record* 69, 105–109.

Callaway, T.R., Morrow, J.L., Edrington, T.S., Genovese, K.J., Dowd, S., Carroll, J., Dailey, J.W., Harvey, R.B., Poole, T.L., Anderson, R.C. and Nisbet, D.J. (2006) Social stress increases fecal shedding of *Salmonella typhimurium* by early weaned piglets. *Current Issues in Intestinal Microbiology* 7, 65–71.

Carnell, S.C., Bowen, A., Morgan, E., Maskell, D.J., Wallis, T.S. and Stevens, M.P. (2007) Role in virulence and protective efficacy in pigs of *Salmonella enterica* serovar Typhimurium secreted components identified by signature-tagged mutagenesis. *Microbiology* 153, 1940–1952.

Casey, P.G., Gardiner, G.E., Casey, G., Bradshaw, B., Lawlor, P.G., Lynch, P.B., Leonard, F.C., Stanton, C., Ross, R.P., Fitzgerald, G.F. and Hill, C. (2007) A five-strain probiotic combination reduces pathogen shedding and alleviates disease signs in pigs challenged with *Salmonella enterica* serovar Typhimurium. *Applied and Environmental Microbiology* 73, 1858–1863.

Centers for Disease Control Prevention (CDC) (2005) Salmonella*: Annual Summary, 2005*. CDC, Division of Foodborne, Bacterial and Mycotic Diseases, Atlanta, Georgia.

Chatfield, S., Li, L.J.L., Sydenham, M., Douce, G. and Dougan, G. (1992) *Salmonella* genetics and vaccine development. In: Hoermache, C.E., Penn, C.W. and Smyth, C.J. (eds) *Molecular Biology of Bacterial Infections: Current Status and Future Perspectives*. Cambridge University Press, Cambridge, pp. 299–312.

Chaudhuri, R.R., Morgan, E., Peters, S.E., Pleasance, S.J., Hudson, D.L., Davies, H.M., Wang, J., van Diemen, P.M., Buckley, A.M., Bowen, A.J., Pullinger, G.D., Turner, D.J., Langridge, G.C., Turner, A.K., Parkhill, J., Charles, I.G., Maskell, D.J. and Stevens, M.P. (2013) Comprehensive assignment of roles for *Salmonella* Typhimurium genes in intestinal colonization of food-producing animals. *PLoS Genetics* 9, e1003456.

Cherrington, C.A. and Huis in't Veld, J.H.J. (1993) Development of a 24 h screen to detect viable Salmonellas in faeces. *Journal of Applied Bacteriology* 75, 58–64.

Cherubin, C.E. (1980) Epidemiologic assessment of antibiotic resistance in *Salmonella*. In: *CRC Handbook on Zoonosis*. CRC Press, Boca Raton, Florida, pp. 173–200.

Chiu, C.H., Tang, P., Chu, C., Hu, S., Bao, Q., Yu, J., Chou, Y.Y., Wang, H.S. and Lee, Y.S. (2005) The genome sequence of *Salmonella enterica* serovar Choleraesuis, a highly invasive and resistant zoonotic pathogen. *Nucleic Acids Research* 33, 1690–1698.

Chu, C.Y., Wang, S.Y., Chen, Z.W., Chien, M.S., Huang, J.P., Chen, J.J., Hong, L.S., Shiau, A.L., Tsai, J.L. and Wu, C.L. (2007) Heterologous protection in pigs induced by a plasmid-cured and *crp* gene-deleted *Salmonella choleraesuis* live vaccine. *Vaccine* 25, 7031–7040.

Clarke, R.C. and Gyles, C.L. (1993) *Salmonella*. In: Gyles, C.L. and Thoen, C.O. (eds) *Pathogenesis of Bacterial Infections in Animals*, 2nd edn. Iowa State University Press, Ames, Iowa, pp. 133–153.

Clemmer, D.I., Hickey, J.L.S., Bridges, J.F., Schlossmann, D.J. and Shaffer, M.F. (1960) Bacteriologic studies of experimental air-borne salmonellosis in chicks. *Journal of Infectious Disease* 106, 197–210.

Coe, N. and Wood, R.L. (1992) The effect of exposure to a *cya/crp* mutant of *Salmonella typhimurium* on the subsequent colonization of swine by the wild-type parent strain. *Veterinary Microbiology* 31, 207–220.

Cohen, N.D., Neibergs, H.L., McGruder, E.D., Whitford, H.W., Behle, R.W., Ray, P.M. and Hargis, B.M. (1993) Genus-specific detection of salmonellae using the polymerase chain reaction (PCR). *Journal of Veterinary Diagnostic Investigation* 5, 368–371.

Currier, M., Singleton, M., Lee, J. and Lee, D.R. (1986) *Salmonella* in swine at slaughter: incidence and serovar distribution at different seasons. *Journal of Food Protection* 49, 366–368.

Curtiss, R. III and Kelly, S.M. (1987) *Salmonella typhimurium* deletion mutants lacking adenylate cyclase and cyclic AMP receptor protein are avirulent and immunogenic. *Infection and Immunity* 55, 3035–3043.

Dahl, J., Wingstrand, A., Baggesen, D.L. and Nielsen, B. (1997) Strategies for elimination of *Salmonella typhimurium* In: *Proceedings of the 2nd International Symposium on Epidemiology and Control of* Salmonella *in Pork*, Copenhagen, Denmark, 20–22 August 1997, pp. 153–156.

Danbara, H., Moriguchi, R., Suzuki, S., Tamura, Y., Kijima, M., Oishi, K., Matsui, H., Abe, A. and Nakamura, M. (1992) Effect of 50 kilobase-plasmid, pKDSC50, of *Salmonella choleraesuis* RF-1 strain on pig septicemia. *Journal of Veterinary Medical Science* 54, 1175–1178.

Darlow, H.M., Bale, W.R. and Carter, G.B. (1961) Infection of mice by the respiratory route with *Salmonella* Typhimurium. *Journal of Hygiene (Cambridge)* 59, 303–308.

Davies, P.R., Morrow, W.E.M., Jones, E.T., Deen, J., Fedorka-Cray, P.J. and Harris, I.T. (1997) Prevalence of *Salmonella* in finishing swine raised in different production systems in North Carolina, USA. *Epidemiology and Infection* 119, 237–244.

Davies, R.H. and Wray, C. (1997) Distribution of *Salmonella* on 23 pig farms in the UK. In: *Proceedings of the 2nd International Symposium on Epidemiology and Control of* Salmonella *in Pork*, Copenhagen, Denmark, 20–22 August 1997, pp. 137–141.

Davies, R.H., McLaren, I.M. and Bedford, S. (1999) Observations on the distribution of *Salmonella* in a pig abattoir. *Veterinary Record* 145, 655–661.

Davies, R.H., Dalziel, R., Gibbens, J.C., Wilesmith, J.W., Ryan, J.M., Evans, S.J., Byrne, C., Paiba, G.A., Pascoe, S.J. and Teale, C.J. (2004) National survey for *Salmonella* in pigs, cattle and sheep at slaughter in Great Britain (1999–2000). *Journal of Applied Microbiology* 96, 750–760.

Dawe, D.L. and Troutt, H.F. (1976) Treatment of experimentally induced salmonellosis in weanling pigs with trimethoprim and sulfadiazine. In: *Proceedings of the 4th International Pig Veterinary Association*, Ames, Iowa, p. M4.

De Jong, H. and Ekdahl, M.O. (1965) Salmonellosis in calves – the effect of dose rate and other factors on transmission. *New Zealand Veterinary Journal* 13, 59–64.

DEFRA (Department for the Environment, Food and Rural Affairs, UK) (2007) Zoonoses report. Available at: http://archive.defra.gov.uk/foodfarm/farmanimal/diseases/atoz/zoonoses/documents/reports/zoonoses2007.pdf (accessed 4 March 2013).

Denagamage, T.N., O'Connor, A.M., Sargeant, J.M., Rajić, A. and McKean, J.D. (2007) Efficacy of vaccination to reduce *Salmonella* prevalence in live and slaughtered swine: a systematic review of literature from 1979 to 2007. *Foodborne Pathogens and Disease* 4, 539–549.

Domínguez-Bernal, G., Tierrez, A., Bartolomé, A., Martínez-Pulgarín, S., Salguero, F.J., Antonio Orden, J. and de la Fuente, R. (2008) *Salmonella enterica* serovar Choleraesuis derivatives harbouring deletions in *rpoS* and *phoP* regulatory genes are attenuated in pigs, and survive and multiply in porcine intestinal macrophages and fibroblasts, respectively. *Veterinary Microbiology* 130, 298–311.

Donné, E., Pasmans, F., Boyen, F., Van Immerseel, F., Adriaensen, C., Hernalsteens, J.P., Ducatelle, R. and Haesebrouck, F. (2005) Survival of *Salmonella* serovar Typhimurium inside porcine monocytes is associated with complement binding and suppression of the production of reactive oxygen species. *Veterinary Microbiology* 107, 205–214.

Dziezak, J.D. (1987) Rapid methods for microbiological analysis of food. *Food Technology* 41, 56–73.

Edel, W., Guinee, P.A.M., van Schothorst, M. and Kampelmacher, E.H. (1967) *Salmonella* infection in pigs fattened with pellets and unpelleted meal. *Zentralblatt fur Veterinarmedizin* 14, 393–401.

Edel, W., van Schothorst, M., Guinee, P.A.M. and Kampelmacher, E.H. (1970) Effect of feeding pellets on the prevention and sanitation of *Salmonella* infections in fattening pigs. *Zentralblatt fur Veterinarmedizin* 17, 730–738.

EFSA (European Food Safety Authority) (2006) Risk assessment and mitigation options of *Salmonella* in pig production. *EFSA Journal* 341, 1–131.

EFSA (European Food Safety Agency) (2008) Report of the task force on zoonoses data: collection on the analysis of the baseline survey on the prevalence of *Salmonella* in slaughter pigs in the EU, 2005–2007, Part A. *EFSA Journal* 135, 1–111.

EFSA (European Food Safety Agency) (2010) Scientific opinion on a quantitative microbiological risk assessment of *Salmonella* in slaughter and breeder pigs. *EFSA Journal* 8, 1547.

Ehrlich, G.D. and Sirko, D.A. (1994) PCR and its role in clinical diagnostics. In: Ehrlich, G.D. and Greenberg, S.J. (eds) *PCR-based Diagnostics in Infectious Disease*. Blackwell Scientific Publications, Boston, Massachusetts, pp. 1.1–1.3.

Eicheta, M.A., Aladuena, A., Cruchaga, S. and Usera, M.A. (1999) Emergence and spread of an atypical *Salmonella enterica* subsp. enterica serotype 4,5,12:i:- strain in Spain. *Journal Clinical Microbiology* 37, 3425.

Endt, K., Stecher, B., Chaffron, S., Slack, E., Tchitchek, N., Benecke, A., Van Maele, L., Sirard, J.C., Mueller, A.J., Heikenwalder, M., Macpherson, A.J., Strugnell, R., von Mering, C. and Hardt, W.D. (2010) The microbiota mediates pathogen clearance from the gut lumen after non-typhoidal *Salmonella* diarrhea. *PLoS Pathogens* 6, e1001097.

Epling, L.K., Carpenter, J.A. and Blankenship, L.C. (1993) Prevalence of *Campylobacter* and *Salmonella* spp. on pork carcasses and the reduction effected by spraying with lactic acid. *Journal of Food Protection* 53, 536–537.

Eswarappa, S.M., Janice, J., Nagarajan, A.G., Balasundaram, S.V., Karnam, G., Dixit, N.M. and Chakravortty, D. (2008) Differentially evolved genes of *Salmonella* pathogenicity islands, insights into the mechanism of host specificity in *Salmonella*. *PLoS One* 3, e3829.

European Union (2003) Regulation (EC) No 2160/2003 of the European Parliament and of the council of 17 November 2003 on the control of *Salmonella* and other specified food-borne zoonotic agents 12.12.2003. *Official Journal of the European Union* L 325/1.

Ewing, W.H. (1986) Isolation and preliminary identification. In: Edwards, P.R. and Ewing, W.H. (eds) *Identification of* Enterobacteriaceae, 4th edn. Elsevier Science Publishing, New York, pp. 27–45.

Falkow, S. and Mekalanos, J. (1990) The enteric bacilli and vibrios. In: Davis, B., Dulbecco, R., Eisen, H. and Ginsberg, H. (eds) *Microbiology*, 4th edn. J.B. Lippincott, Philadelphia, pp. 576–579.

Fedorka-Cray, P.J., Whipp, S.C., Isaacson, R.E., Nord, N. and Lager, K. (1994) Transmission of *Salmonella typhimurium* to swine. *Veterinary Microbiology* 41, 333–344.

Fedorka-Cray, P.J., Gray, J.T. and Thomas, L.A. (1995a) Comparison of culture media for the isolation of *Salmonella* species. In: *Symposium Diagnosis of* Salmonella *Infections, Proceedings of the US Animal Health Association*, Reno, Nevada, pp. 116–123.

Fedorka-Cray, P.J., Kelley, L.C., Stabel, T.J., Gray, J.T. and Laufer, J.A. (1995b) Alternate routes of invasion may affect pathogenesis of *Salmonella typhimunum* in swine. *Infection and Immunity* 63, 2658–2664.

Fedorka-Cray, P.J., Hogg, A., Gray, J.T., Lorenzen, K., Velasquez, J. and von Behren, P. (1997a) Feed and feed trucks as sources of *Salmonella* contamination in swine. *Swine Health and Production* 5, 189–193.

Fedorka-Cray, P.J., Harris, D.L. and Whipp, S.C. (1997b) Using isolated weaning to raise *Salmonella*-free swine. *Veterinary Medicine*, April, 375–382.

Fedorka-Cray, P.J., Bailey, J.S., Stern, N. and Cox, N.A. (1999) Mucosal competitive exclusion to reduce *Salmonella* in swine. *Journal of Food Protection* 62, 1376–1380.

Feng, P. (1992) Rapid methods for detecting food-borne pathogens. In: *FDA Bacteriological Analytical Manual*, 7th edn. Appendix 1.

Fernandez-Escartin, F., Saldana Lozano, J., Rodriguez, D., Marnnez-Gonzales, N. and Torres, J.A. (1995) Incidence and level of *Salmonella* serovars in raw pork obtained from Mexican butcher shops. *Food Microbiology* 12, 435–439.

Ferris, K. and Thomas, L.A. (1993) *Salmonella* serovars from animals and related sources during July 1992–June 1993. In: *Proceedings 97th Annual Meeting US Animal Health Association*. Cummings Corporation and Carter Printing, Richmond, Virginia, pp. 538.

Finlay, B.B., Starnbach, M.N., Francis, C.L., Stocker, B.A.D., Chatfield, S., Dougan, G. and Falkow, S. (1988) Identification and characterization of Tn*phoA* mutants of *Salmonella* that are unable to pass through a polarized MDCK epithelial cell monolayer. *Molecular Microbiology* 6, 757–766.

Foster, N., Lovell, M.A., Marston, K.L., Hulme, S.D., Frost, A.J., Bland, P. and Barrow, P.A. (2003) Rapid protection of gnotobiotic pigs against experimental salmonellosis following induction of polymorphonuclear leukocytes by avirulent *Salmonella enterica*. *Infection and Immunity* 71, 2182–2191.

Foster, N., Hulme, S., Lovell, M., Reed, K. and Barrow, P. (2005) Stimulation of gp91 phagocytic oxidase and reactive oxygen species in neutrophils by an avirulent *Salmonella enterica* serovar infantis strain protects gnotobiotic piglets from lethal challenge with serovar Typhimurium strain F98 without inducing intestinal pathology. *Infection and Immunity* 73, 4539–4547.

Freestone, P.P., Sandrini, S.M., Haigh, R.D. and Lyte, M. (2008) Microbial endocrinology, how stress influences susceptibility to infection. *Trends in Microbiology* 16, 55–64.

FSIS (Food Safety and Inspection Service) (1999) HACCP Implementation – First Year: *Salmonella*. Available at: http://www.fsis.usda.gov/ophs/salmdata.htm (accessed 4 March 2013).

Genovese, K.J., Anderson, R.C., Harvey, R.B., Callaway, T.R., Poole, T.L., Edrington, T.S., Fedorka-Cray, P.J. and Nisbet, D.J. (2003) Competitive exclusion of *Salmonella* from the gut of neonatal and weaned pigs. *Journal of Food Protection* 66, 1353–1359.

Gill, C.O. and Bryant, J. (1993) The presence of *Escherichia coli*, *Salmonella* and *Campylobacter* in pig carcasses dehairing equipment. *Food Microbiology* 10, 337–344.

Gooch, J.M. and Haddock, R.L. (1969) Swine salmonellosis in a Hawaiian piggery. *Journal of the American Veterinary Medical Association* 154, 1051–1054.

Gossner, C.M., van Cauteren, D., Le Hello, S., Weill, F.X., Terrien, E., Tessier, S., Janin, C., Brisabois, A., Dusch, V., Vaillant, V. and Jourdan-da Silva, N. (2012) Nationwide outbreak of *Salmonella enterica* serotype 4,[5],12:i:- infection associated with consumption of dried pork sausage, France, November to December 2011. *Euro Surveillance* 17, 20071.

Gray, J.T. and Fedorka-Cray, P.J. (1995) Survival and infectivity of *Salmonella choleraesuis* in swine feces. In: *76th Conference on Research Workers in Animal Disease*, pp. 94.

Gray, J.T., Fedorka-Cray, P.J., Stabel, T.J. and Ackermann, M.R. (1995) Influence of inoculation route on the carrier state of *Salmonella choleraesuis* in swine. *Veterinary Microbiology* 47, 43–59.

Gray, J.T., Stabel, T.J. and Fedorka-Cray, P.J. (1996a) Effect of dose on the immune response and persistence of *Salmonella choleraesuis* infection in swine. *American Journal of Veterinary Research* 57, 313–319.

Gray, J.T., Fedorka-Cray, P.J., Stabel, T.J. and Kramer, T.T. (1996b) Natural transmission of *Salmonella choleraesuis* in swine. *Applied and Environmental Microbiology* 62, 141–146.

Griffith, R.W., Schwartz, K.J. and Meyerholz, D.K. (2006) Salmonellosis. In: Straw, B.E., Zimmerman, J.J., D'Allaire, S. and Taylor, D.J. (eds) *Diseases of Swine*, 9th edn. Blackwell Publishing, Oxford, UK, pp. 739–754.

Gutzmann, F., Layton, H., Simiins, K. and Jarolman, H. (1976) Influence of antibiotic-supplemented feed on the occurrence and persistence of *S. typhimunum* in experimentally infected swine. *American Journal of Veterinary Research* 37, 649–655.

Haley, C.A., Dargatz, D.A., Bush, E.J., Erdman, M.M. and Fedorka-Cray, P.J. (2012) *Salmonella* prevalence and antimicrobial susceptibility from the National Animal Health Monitoring System Swine 2000 and 2006 studies. *Journal of Food Protection* 75, 428–436.

Hansen, T.B., Christensen, B.B. and Aabo, S. (2010) *Salmonella* in pork cuttings in supermarkets and butchers' shops in Denmark in 2002 and 2006. *Zoonoses and Public Health* 57(Suppl. 1), 23–29.

Hardman, P.M., Wathes, C.M. and Wray, C. (1991) Transmission of Salmonellae among calves penned individually. *Veterinary Record* 129, 327–329.

Harris, I.T., Fedorka-Cray, P.J., Gray, J.T., Thomas, L.A. and Ferris, K. (1997) Prevalence of *Salmonella* organisms in swine feed. *Journal of the American Veterinary Medicinal Association* 210, 382–385.

Hauser, E., Tietze, E., Helmuth, R., Junker, E., Blank, K., Prager, R., Rabsch, W., Appel, B., Fruth, A. and Malorny, B. (2010) Pork contaminated with *Salmonella enterica* serovar 4,[5],12:i:-, an emerging health risk for humans. *Applied Environmental Microbiology* 76, 4601–4610.

Helmuth, R., Kasbohrer, A., Geue, L., Rabsch, W. and Protz, D. (1997) Pilot study on the prevalence of *Salmonella* in slaughter pigs in Germany: III Detection of *Salmonella* by PCR, serovar distribution and population analysis of isolates. In: *Proceedings of the 2nd International Symposium on Epidemiology and Control of* Salmonella *in Pork*, Copenhagen, Denmark, 20–22 August 1997, pp. 103–106.

Henzler, D.J. and Opitz, H.M. (1992) The role of mice in the epizootiology of *Salmonella enteritidis* infection on chicken layer farms. *Avian Diseases* 336, 625–631.

Hoerner, R., Feldpausch, J., Gray, R.L., Curry, S., Islam, Z., Goldy, T., Klein, F., Tadese, T., Rice, J. and Mozola, M. (2011) Reveal *Salmonella* 2.0 test for detection of *Salmonella* spp. in foods and environmental samples. Performance Tested Method 960801. *The Journal of AOAC International* 94, 1467–1580.

Holcomb, H.L. and Fedorka-Cray, P.J. (1997) Effect of Naxel and Baytril on persistence of *Salmonella heidelberg* in swine. In: *Abstracts of the Annual Meeting of the American Society for Microbiology*. ASM, Washington, DC, pp. 445.

Hook, E.W. (1990) *Salmonella* species (including typhoid fever). In: Mandell, G.L., Douglas, R.G. and Bennet, J.E. (eds) *Principles and Practices of Infectious Disease*. Churchill Livingstone, New York, pp. 1700–1722.

Huang, Y., Leming, C.L., Suyemoto, M. and Altier, C. (2007) Genome-wide screen of *Salmonella* genes expressed during infection in pigs, using *in vivo* expression technology. *Applied and Environmental Microbiology* 73, 7522–7530.

Hur, J. and Lee, J.H. (2010) Immunization of pregnant sows with a novel virulence gene deleted live *Salmonella* vaccine and protection of their suckling piglets against salmonellosis. *Veterinary Microbiology* 143, 270–276.

Isaacson, R.E., Firkins, L.D., Weigel, R.M., Zuckermann, F.A. and DiPietro, J.A. (1999) Effect of transportation and feed withdrawal on shedding of *Salmonella typhimurium* among experimentally infected pigs. *American Journal of Veterinary Research* 60, 1155–1158.

Jubb, K.V., Kennedy, P.C. and Palmer, N.C. (1985) Infectious and parasitic diseases. In: Jubb, K.V., Kennedy, P.C. and Palmer, N. (eds) *Pathology of Domestic Animals*, 3rd edn. Academic Press, New York, pp. 135–143.

Kawahara, K., Haraguchi, Y., Tsuchimoto, M., Terakado, N. and Danbara, H. (1988) Evidence of correlation between 50-kilobase plasmid of *Salmonella choleraesuis* and its virulence. *Microbial Pathogenesis* 4, 155–163.

Kelly, S.M., Bosecker, B.A. and Curtiss, R. III (1992) Characterization and protective properties of attenuated mutants of *Salmonella choleraesuis*. *Infection and Immunity* 60, 4881–4890.

Kennedy, M.J., Yancey, R.J. Jr, Sanchez, M.S., Rzepkowski, R.A., Kelly, S.M. and Curtiss, R. 3rd. (1999) Attenuation and immunogenicity of Δ*cya* Δ*crp* derivatives of *Salmonella choleraesuis* in pigs. *Infection and Immunity* 67, 4628–4636.

Kich, J.D., Coldebella, A., Morés, N., Nogueira, M.G., Cardoso, M., Fratamico, P.M., Call, J.E., Fedorka-Cray, P. and Luchansky, J.B. (2011) Prevalence, distribution, and molecular characterization of *Salmonella* recovered from swine finishing herds and a slaughter facility in Santa Catarina, Brazil. *International Journal of Food Microbiology* 151, 307–313.

Kingsley, R.A., van Amsterdam, K., Kramer, N. and Bäumler, A.J. (2000) The *shdA* gene is restricted to serotypes of *Salmonella enterica* subspecies I and contributes to efficient and prolonged fecal shedding. *Infection and Immunity* 68, 2720–2727.

Korsak, N., Daube, G., Ghafir, Y., Chahed, A., Jolly, S. and Vindevogel, H. (1998) An efficient sampling technique used to detect for food-borne pathogens on pork and beef carcasses in nine Belgian abattoirs. *Journal of Food Protection* 61, 535–541.

Kramer, T.T., Roof, M.B. and Matheson, R.R. (1992) Safety and efficacy of an attenuated strain of *Salmonella choleraesuis* for vaccination of swine. *American Journal of Veterinary Research* 53, 444–448.

Kramer, T.T., Rhiner, J., Gray, J.T. and Fedorka-Cray, P.J. (1994) Comparison of IgG ELISA and bacteriologic diagnosis in experimental swine salmonellosis. In: *Proceedings of the 75th Annual Conference Research Workers in Animal Disease*, Chicago, Illinois.

Kreuzer, S., Janczyk, P., Aßmus, J., Schmidt, M.F., Brockmann, G.A. and Nöckler, K. (2012) No beneficial effects evident for *Enterococcus faecium* NCIMB 10415 in weaned pigs infected with *Salmonella enterica* serovar Typhimurium DT104. *Applied and Environmental Microbiology* 78, 4816–4825.

Ku, Y.W., McDonough, S.P., Palaniappan, R.U., Chang, C.F. and Chang, Y.F. (2005) Novel attenuated *Salmonella enterica* serovar Choleraesuis strains as live vaccine candidates generated by signature-tagged mutagenesis. *Infection and Immunity* 73, 8194–8203.

Lambiri, M., Mavridou, A., Richardson, S.C. and Papadakis, J.A. (1990) Comparison of the TECRA *Salmonella* immunoassay with the conventional culture method. *Letters in Applied Microbiology* 11, 182–184.

Lammerding, A.M., Garcia, M.M., Mann, E.D., Robinson, Y., Dorward, W.J., Truscott, R. and Tittinger, F. (1998) Prevalence of *Salmonella* and thermophyllic *Campylobacter* in fresh pork. *Journal of Food Protection* 51, 47–52.

Langridge, G.C., Phan, M.D., Turner, D.J., Perkins, T.T., Parts, L., Haase, J., Charles, I., Maskell, D.J., Peters, S.E., Dougan, G., Wain, J., Parkhill, J. and Turner, A.K. (2009) Simultaneous assay of every *Salmonella* Typhi gene using one million transposon mutants. *Genome Research* 19, 2308–2316.

Larsen, S.T., McKean, J.D., Hurd, H.S., Rostagno, M.H., Griffith, R.W. and Wesley, I.V. (2003) Impact of commercial preharvest transportation and holding on the prevalence of *Salmonella enterica* in cull sows. *Journal of Food Protection* 66, 1134–1138.

Laval, A., Morvan, H., Despez, G. and Corbion, B. (1992) Salmonellosis in swine. In: *Reports and Communications,* Salmonella *and Salmonellosis,* 15-17 September, 1993 Ploufragan/St Brieuc, France, pp. 164–175.

Lawley, T.D., Bouley, D.M., Hoy, Y.E., Gerke, C., Relman, D.A. and Monack, D.M. (2008) Host transmission of *Salmonella enterica* serovar Typhimurium is controlled by virulence factors and indigenous intestinal microbiota. *Infection and Immunity* 76, 403–416.

Lawson, G. and Dow, C. (1966) Porcine salmonellosis. *Journal of Comparative Pathology* 76, 363–371.

Levine, M.M., Ferreccio, C., Black, R.E., Tacket, C.O. and Germanier, R. (1989) Progress in vaccines against typhoid fever. *Review of Infectious Disease* 11, S552–S567.

Leyman, B., Boyen, F., Van Parys, A., Verbrugghe, E., Haesebrouck, F. and Pasmans, F. (2011) *Salmonella* Typhimurium LPS mutations for use in vaccines allowing differentiation of infected and vaccinated pigs. *Vaccine* 29, 3679–3685.

Libby, S.J., Goebel, W., Muir, S., Songer, G. and Heffron, F. (1990) Cloning and characterization of a cytotoxin gene from *Salmonella typhimurium*. *Research in Microbiology* 141, 775–783.

Lichtensteiger, C.A. and Vimr, E.R. (2003) Systemic and enteric colonization of pigs by a *hilA* signature-tagged mutant of *Salmonella choleraesuis*. *Microbial Pathogenesis* 34, 149–154.

Linton, A.H. and Jennet, N.E. (1970) Multiplication of *Salmonella* in liquid feed and its influence on the duration of excretion in pigs. *Research in Veterinary Science* 11, 452–457.

Linton, A.H., Heard, T.W., Grimshaw, J.J. and Pollaed, P. (1970) Computer-based analysis of epidemiological data arising from salmonellosis in pigs. *Research in Veterinary Science* 11, 523–532.

Liu, W.Q., Feng, Y., Wang, Y., Zou, Q.H., Chen, F., Guo, J.T., Peng, Y.H., Jin, Y., Li, Y.G., Hu, S.N., Johnston, R.N., Liu, G.R. and Liu, S.L. (2009) *Salmonella paratyphi* C, genetic divergence from *Salmonella choleraesuis* and pathogenic convergence with *Salmonella typhi*. *PLoS One* 4, e4510.

Lovell, M.A. and Barrow, P.A. (1999) Intestinal colonisation of gnotobiotic pigs by *Salmonella* organisms: interaction between isogenic and unrelated strains. *Journal of Medical Microbiology* 48, 907–916.

Lumsden, J.S., Wilkie, B.N. and Clarke, R.C. (1991) Resistance to faecal shedding in pigs and chickens vaccinated with an aromatic dependent mutant of *Salmonella typhimunum*. *Amencan Journal of Veterinary Research* 52, 1784–1787.

McCall, C.E., Martin, W.T. and Boring, J.R. (1966) Efficiency of cultures of rectal swabs and faecal specimens in detecting salmonellae carriers: correlation with numbers of salmonellas excreted. *Journal of Hygiene (Cambridge)* 64, 261–269.

McChesney, D.G., Kaplan, G. and Gardner, P. (1995) FDA survey determines *Salmonella* contamination. *Feedstuffs* 7, 20–23.

McCuddin, Z.P., Carlson, S.A. and Sharma, V.K. (2008) Experimental reproduction of bovine *Salmonella* encephalopathy using a norepinephrine-based stress model. *Veterinary Journal* 175, 82–88.

Methner, U., Rabsch, W., Reissbrodt, R. and Williams, P.H. (2008) Effect of norepinephrine on colonisation and systemic spread of *Salmonella enterica* in infected animals, role of catecholate siderophore precursors and degradation products. *International Journal of Medical Microbiology* 298, 429–439.

Meyer, H., Koch, H., Methner, U. and Steinbach, G. (1993) Vaccines in salmonellosis control in animals. *Zentralblatt fur Bakteriologie* 278, 407–415.

Morgan, E., Campbell, J.D., Rowe, S.C., Bispham, J., Stevens, M.P., Bowen, A.J., Barrow, P.A., Maskell, D.J. and Wallis, T.S. (2004) Identification of host-specific colonization factors of *Salmonella enterica* serovar Typhimurium. *Molecular Microbiology* 54, 994–1010.

Morgan, I.R., Krautil, F.L. and Craven, J.A. (1987) Effect of lairage on caecal and *Salmonella* carcass contamination of slaughter pigs. *Epidemiology and Infection* 98, 323–330.

Mousing, J., Kyrrval, J., Jensen, T.K., Aalbaek, B., Buttenschon, J., Svensmark, B. and Willeberg, P. (1997) Meat safety consequences of implementing visual post-mortem meat inspection procedures in Danish slaughter pigs. *Veterinary Record* 140, 472–477.

NARMS-EB (1997) *Annual Report*. FDA, USDA-ARS, USDA-APHIS, USDA-FSIS, Athens, Georgia.

Nielsen, B., Baggesen, D., Bager, F. and Lind, P. (1994) Serological diagnosis of *Salmonella* infections in swine by ELISA. In: *Proceedings of the 13th International Pig Veterinary Science Congress*, Bangkok, Thailand, 26–30 June.

Nielsen, B., Baggesen, D., Bager, F., Haugegaard, J. and Lind, P. (1995) The serological response to *Salmonella* serovars Typhimurium and Infantis in experimentally infected pigs. The time course followed with an indirect anti-LPS ELISA and bacteriological examinations. *Veterinary Microbiology* 47, 205–218.

Nnalue, N.A. and Lindberg, A.A. (1990) *Salmonella choleraesuis* strains deficient in O antigen remain fully virulent for mice by parenteral inoculation but are avirulent by oral administration. *Infection and Immunity* 58, 2493–2501.

Nnalue, N.A. and Stocker, B.A.D. (1986) Some *galE* mutants of *Salmonella choleraesuis* retain virulence. *Infection and Immunity* 54, 635–640.

Nowak, B., von Müffling, T., Chaunchom, S. and Hartung, J. (2007) *Salmonella* contamination in pigs at slaughter and on the farm: a field study using an antibody ELISA test and a PCR technique. *International Journal of Food Microbiology* 115, 259–267.

O'Connor, A.M., Denagamage, T., Sargeant, J.M., Rajić, A. and McKean, J. (2008) Feeding management practices and feed characteristics associated with *Salmonella* prevalence in live and slaughtered market-weight finisher swine: a systematic review and summation of evidence from 1950 to 2005. *Preventative Veterinary Medicine* 87, 213–228.

O'Connor, A.M., Sargeant, J.M., Gardner, I.A., Dickson, J.S., Torrence, M.E., Dewey, C.E., Dohoo, I.R., Evans, R.B., Gray, J.T., Greiner, M., Keefe, G., Lefebvre, S.L., Morley, P.S., Ramirez, A., Sischo, W., Smith, D.R., Snedeker, K., Sofos, J., Ward, M.P. and Wills, R. (2010) The REFLECT statement: Methods and processes of creating reporting guidelines for randomized control trials for livestock and food safety (LFS) by modifying the CONSORT statement. *Journal of Food Protection* 73, 132–139.

OIE (2010) *Manual of Diagnostic Tests and Vaccines for Terrestrial Animals*. CAB International, Wallingford, UK.

Oosterom, J., Dekker, R., Dewilde, G.J.A., Van Kempende, T.F. and Engels, G.B. (1985) Prevalence of *Campylobacter jejuni* and *Salmonella* during pig slaughtering. *Veterinary Quarterly* 7, 31–34.

Paulin, S.M., Jagannathan, A., Campbell, J., Wallis, T.S. and Stevens, M.P. (2007) Net replication of *Salmonella enterica* serovars Typhimurium and Choleraesuis in porcine intestinal mucosa and nodes is associated with their differential virulence. *Infection and Immunity* 75, 3950–3960.

Porwollik, S., Boyd, E.F., Choy, C., Cheng, P., Florea, L., Proctor, E. and McClelland, M. (2004) Characterization of *Salmonella enterica* subspecies I genovars by use of microarrays. *Journal of Bacteriology* 186, 5883–5898.

Pospischil, A., Wood, R.L. and Anderson, T.D. (1990) Peroxidase-antiperoxidase and immunogold labeling of *Salmonella typhimurium* and *Salmonella choleraesuis var kunzendorf* in tissues of experimentally infected swine. *American Journal of Veterinary Research* 51, 619–624.

Prasad, R., Chopra, A.K., Peterson, J.W. and Pericas, R. (1990) Biological and immunological characterization of a cloned cholera toxin-like enterotoxin from *Salmonella typhimurium Microbial Pathogenesis* 9, 315–329.

Prasad, R., Chopra, A.K., Charry, P. and Peterson, J.W. (1992) Expression and characterization of the cloned *Salmonella typhimurium* enterotoxin. *Microbial Pathogenesis* 13, 109–121.

Prohaszka, L., Jayarao, B.M., Fabian, A. and Kovacs, S. (1990) The role of intestinal volatile fatty acids in the *Salmonella* shedding of pigs. *Journal of Veterinary Medicine B* 37, 570–574.

Pullinger, G.D., Carnell, S.C., Sharaff, F.F., van Diemen, P.M., Dziva, F., Morgan, E., Lyte, M., Freestone, P.P. and Stevens, M.P. (2010a) Norepinephrine augments *Salmonella enterica*-induced enteritis in a manner associated with increased net replication but independent of the putative adrenergic sensor kinases QseC and QseE. *Infection and Immunity* 78, 372–380.

Pullinger, G.D., van Diemen, P.M., Carnell, S.C., Davies, H., Lyte, M. and Stevens, M.P. (2010b) 6-hydroxydopamine-mediated release of norepinephrine increases faecal excretion of *Salmonella enterica* serovar Typhimurium in pigs. *Veterinary Research* 41, 68.

Rahn, K., De Grandis, S.A., Clarke, R.C., McEwen, S.A., Galan, J.E., Ginocchio, R., Curtiss, R. III and Gyles, C.L. (1992) Amplification of an *invA* gene sequence of *Salmonella typhimunum* by polymerase chain reaction as a specific method of detection of *Salmonella*. *Molecular and Cellular Probes* 6, 271–279.

Rajkowski, K.T., Eblen, S. and Laubauch, C. (1998) Efficiency of washing and sanitising trailers used for swine transport in reduction of *Salmonella* and *Escherichia coli*. *Journal of Food Protection* 61, 35–37.

Rasko, D.A., Moreira, C.G., Li, de R., Reading, N.C., Ritchie, J.M., Waldor, M.K., Williams, N., Taussig, R., Wei, S., Roth, M., Hughes, D.T., Huntley, J.F., Fina, M.W., Falck, J.R. and Sperandio, V. (2008) Targeting QseC signaling and virulence for antibiotic development. *Science* 321, 1078–1080.

Reed, W.M., Olander, H.J. and Thacker, H.L. (1986) Studies on the pathogenesis of *Salmonella typhimurium* and *Salmonella choleraesuis* var *kunzendorf* infection in weanling pigs. *American Journal of Veterinary Research* 47, 75–83.

Reissbrodt, R., Rienaecker, I., Romanova, J.M., Freestone, P.P., Haigh, R.D., Lyte, M., Tschäpe, H. and Williams, P.H. (2002) Resuscitation of *Salmonella enterica* serovar Typhimurium and enterohemorrhagic *Escherichia coli* from the viable but nonculturable state by heat-stable enterobacterial autoinducer. *Applied and Environmental Microbiology* 68, 4788–4794.

Reitmeyer, J.C., Peterson, J.W. and Wilson, K.J. (1986) *Salmonella* cytotoxin: a component of the bacterial outer membrane. *Microbial Pathogenesis* 1, 503–510.

Reynolds, I.M., Miner, P.W. and Smith, R.E. (1967) *Salmonella enteritidis* from porcine meningitis – a case report. *Cornell Veterinarian* 50, 100–105.

Richardson, E.J., Limaye, B., Inamdar, H., Datta, A., Manjari, K.S., Pullinger, G.D., Thomson, N.R., Joshi, R.R., Watson, M. and Stevens, M.P. (2011) Genome sequences of *Salmonella enterica* serovar Typhimurium, Choleraesuis, Dublin and Gallinarum strains of well-defined virulence in food-producing animals. *Journal of Bacteriology* 193, 3162–3163.

Robbins, J.B., Chu, C. and Sneerson, R. (1992) Hypothesis for vaccine development: protective immunity to enteric diseases caused by nontyphoidal salmonellae and shigellae may be conferred by serum IgG antibodies to the O-specific polysaccharide of their lipopolysaccharides. *Clinical Infectious Diseases* 15, 346–361.

Robertsson, J.A., Lindberg, A.A., Hoiseth, S. and Stocker, B.A.D. (1983) *Salmonella typhimunum* infection in calves- protection and survival of virulent challenge bacteria after immunization with live or inactivated vaccines. *Infection and Immunity* 41, 742–750.

Roof, M.B. and Kramer, T.T. (1989) Porcine neutrophils function in the presence of virulent and avirulent *Salmonella choleraesuis*. *Veterinary Immunology and Immunopathology* 23, 365–376.

Roof, M.B., Kramer, T.T., Roth, J.A. and Minion, F.C. (1992) Characterization of a *Salmonella choleraesuis* isolate after repeated neutrophil exposure. *American Journal of Veterinary Research* 53, 1328–1332.

Rossen, L., Norskov, K., Holmstrom, K. and Rasmussen, O.F. (1992) Inhibition of PCR by components of food samples, microbial diagnostic assays and DNA-extraction solutions. *International Journal of Food Microbiology* 17, 37–45.

Saide-Albornoz, J.J., Knipe, C.L., Murano, E.A. and Beran, G.W. (1995) Contamination of carcasses during slaughter, fabrication and chilled storage. *Journal of Food Protection* 58, 993–997.

Salmon, D.E. and Smith, T. (1886) The bacterium of swine plague. *American Monthly Microbiology Journal* 7, 204.

Saxen, H., Reima, I. and Makela, P.H. (1987) Alternative complement pathway activation by *Salmonella* O polysaccharide as a virulence determinant in the mouse. *Microbial Pathogenesis* 2, 15–28.

Scheepens, C.J.M., Hessing, M.J.C., Hensen, E.J. and Hendricks, P.A.J. (1994) Effect of climatic stress on the immunological reactivity of weaned pigs. *Veterinary Quarterly* 16, 137–143.

Schwarz, P., Kich, J.D., Kolb, J. and Cardoso, M. (2011) Use of an avirulent live *Salmonella* Choleraesuis vaccine to reduce the prevalence of *Salmonella* carrier pigs at slaughter. *Veterinary Record* 169, 553.

Selke, M., Meens, J., Springer, S., Frank, R. and Gerlach, G.F. (2007) Immunization of pigs to prevent disease in humans, construction and protective efficacy of a *Salmonella enterica* serovar Typhimurium live negative-marker vaccine. *Infection and Immunity* 75, 2476–2483.

Simonsen, B., Bryan, F.L., Christian, J.H.B., Roberts, T.A., Tomkins, R.B. and Silliker, J.H. (1987) Prevention and control of food-borne salmonellosis through application of hazard analysis critical control (HACCP). *International Journal of Food Microbiology* 4, 227–247.

Smerdon, W.J., Adak, G.K., O'Brien, S.J, Gillespie, I.A. and Reacher, M. (2001) General outbreaks of infectious intestinal disease linked with red meat, England and Wales, 1992-1999. *Communicable Disease and Public Health* 4, 259–267.

Smith, B.P., Reina-Guerra, M., Hoiseth, S.K., Stocker, B.A.D., Habasha, F., Johnson, E. and Merritt, F. (1984) Aromatic-dependent *Salmonella typhimunum* as modified live vaccines for calves. *American Journal of Veterinary Research* 45, 59–66.

Smith, H.W. (1952) The evaluation of culture media for the isolation of *Salmonella* from faeces. *Journal of Hygiene (Cambridge)* 50, 21–36.

Smith, H.W. and Jones, J.E.T. (1967) Observations on experimental oral infections with *S. dublin* in calves and *S. choleraesuis* in pigs. *Journal of Pathology and Bacteriology* 93, 141–156.

Sojka, W.J., Wray, C., Shreeve, J. and Benson, A.J. (1977) Incidence of *Salmonella* infections in animals in England and Wales, 1968-1974. *Journal of Hygiene (Cambridge)* 78, 43–56.

Stabel, T.J., Mayfield, J.E., Tabatabai, L.B. and Wannemuehler, M.J. (1990) Oral immunization of mice with attenuated *Salmonella typhimurium* containing a recombinant plasmid which codes for production of a 31-kilodalton protein of *Brucella abortus*. *Infection and Immunity* 58, 2048–2055.

Stabel, T.J., Mayfield, J.E., Tabatabai, L.B. and Wannemuehler, M.J. (1991) Swine immunity to an attenuated *Salmonella typhimurium* mutant containing a recombinant plasmid which codes for production of a 31-kilodalton protein of *Brucella abortus*. *Infection and Immunity* 59, 2941–2947.

Stevens, M.P., Humphrey, T.J. and Maskell, D.J. (2009) Molecular insights into farm animal and zoonotic *Salmonella* infections. *Philosophical Transactions of the Royal Society of London (B) Biological Sciences* 364, 2709–2723.

Stone, G.G., Oberst, R.D., Hays, M.P., McVey, S. and Chengappa, M.M. (1994) Detection of *Salmonella* serovars from clinical samples by enrichment broth cultivation-PCR procedure. *Journal of Clinical Microbiology* 32, 1742–1749.

Suo, B., He, Y., Tu, S.I. and Shi, X. (2010) A multiplex real-time polymerase chain reaction for simultaneous detection of *Salmonella* spp., *Escherichia coli* O157, and *Listeria monocytogenes* in meat products. *Foodborne Pathogens and Disease* 7, 619–628.

Switt, A.I., Soyer, Y., Watnick, L.D. and Wiedmann, M. (2009) Emergence, distribution, and molecular and phenotypic characteristics of *Salmonella enterica* serotype 4,5,12:i:–. *Foodborne Pathogens and Disease* 6, 407–415.

Szabó, I., Wieler, L.H., Tedin, K., Scharek-Tedin, L., Taras, D., Hensel, A., Appel, B. and Nöckler, K. (2009) Influence of a probiotic strain of *Enterococcus faecium* on *Salmonella enterica* serovar Typhimurium DT104 infection in a porcine animal infection model. *Applied and Environmental Microbiology* 75, 2621–2628.

Taylor, J. and McCoy, J.H. (1969) *Salmonella* and Arizona infections and intoxications. In: Riemann, H. (ed.) *Foodborne Infections and Intoxications*. Academic Press, New York, pp. 3–71.

Thiennimitr, P., Winter, S.E., Winter, M.G., Xavier, M.N., Tolstikov, V., Huseby, D.L., Sterzenbach, T., Tsolis, R.M., Roth, J.R. and Bäumler, A.J. (2011) Intestinal inflammation allows *Salmonella* to use ethanolamine to compete with the microbiota. *Proceedings of the National Academy of Science USA* 108, 17480–17485.

Tielen, M.J.M., van Schie, F.W., van der Wolf, P.J., Elbers, A.R.W., Koppens, J.M.C.C. and Wolbers, W.B. (1997) Risk factors and control measures for subclinical infection in pig herds. In: *Proceedings of the 2nd International Symposium on Epidemiology and Control of* Salmonella *in Pork*, Copenhagen, Denmark, 20–22 August 1997, pp. 32–35.

Tierrez, A. and García-del Portillo, F. (2005) New concepts in *Salmonella* virulence, the importance of reducing the intracellular growth rate in the host. *Cellular Microbiology* 7, 901–909.

Toscano, M.J., Stabel, T.J., Bearson, S.M.D., Bearson, B.L. and Lay, D.C. (2007) Cultivation of *Salmonella enterica* serovar Typhimurium in a norepinephrine-containing medium alters *in vivo* tissue prevalence in swine. *Journal of Experimental Animal Science* 43, 329–338.

Trebichavsky, I., Splichalova, A., Rychlik, I., Hojna, H., Muneta, Y., Mori, Y. and Splichal, I. (2006) Attenuated *aroA Salmonella enterica* serovar Typhimurium does not induce inflammatory response and early protection of gnotobiotic pigs against parental virulent LT2 strain. *Vaccine* 24, 4285–4289.

Tsolis, R.M., Young, G.M., Solnick, J.V. and Bäumler, A.J. (2008) From bench to bedside, stealth of enteroinvasive pathogens. *Nature Reviews Microbiology* 6, 883–892.

Tsolis, R.M., Xavier, M.N., Santos, R.L. and Bäumler, A.J. (2011) How to become a top model, impact of animal experimentation on human *Salmonella* disease research. *Infection and Immunity* 79, 1806–1814.

Turk, J.R., Fales, W.H., Maddox, C., Miller, M., Pace, L., Fischer, J., Kreeger, J., Johnson, G., Turnquist, S., Ramos, J.A. and Gosser, H.S. (1992) Pneumonia associated with *Salmonella choleraesuis* infection in swine: 99 cases (1987-1990). *Journal of the American Veterinary Medical Association* 201, 1615–1616.

Uthe, J.J., Royaee, A., Lunney, J.K., Stabel, T.J., Zhao, S.H., Tuggle, C.K. and Bearson, S.M. (2007) Porcine differential gene expression in response to *Salmonella enterica* serovars Choleraesuis and Typhimurium. *Molecular Immunology* 44, 2900–2914.

van Diemen, P.M., Kreukniet, M.B., Galina, L., Bumstead, N. and Wallis, T.S. (2002) Characterisation of a resource population of pigs screened for resistance to salmonellosis. *Veterinary Immunology and Immunopathology* 88, 183–196.

Van Laack, R.L.J.M., Johnson, J.L., van der Palen, C.J.N.M., Smulders, F.J.M. and Snijders, J.M.A. (1993) Survival of pathogenic bacteria on pork loins as influenced by hot processing and packaging. *Journal of Food Protection* 56, 847–851.

van Parys, A., Boyen, F., Volf, J., Verbrugghe, E., Leyman, B., Rychlik, I., Haesebrouck, F. and Pasmans, F. (2010) *Salmonella* Typhimurium resides largely as an extracellular pathogen in porcine tonsils, independently of biofilm-associated genes *csgA*, *csgD* and *adrA*. *Veterinary Microbiology* 144, 93–99.

Van Parys, A., Boyen, F., Leyman, B., Verbrugghe, E., Haesebrouck, F. and Pasmans, F. (2011) Tissue-specific *Salmonella* Typhimurium gene expression during persistence in pigs. *PLoS One* 6, e24120.

van Poucke, L.S.G. (1990) *Salmonella*-TEK, a rapid screening method for *Salmonella* species in food. *Applied and Environmental Microbiology* 56, 924–927.

Van Schie, F.W. and Overgoor, G.H.A. (1987) An analysis of the possible effects of different feed upon the excretion of *Salmonella* bacteria in clinically normal groups of fattening pigs. *Veterinary Quarterly* 9, 185–188.

von Langer, L. (1995) The need for microbiological examination to improve the standards of fresh meat hygiene. *Tierarztiches Umshau* 50, 47–52.

Wales, A.D., Cook, A.J. and Davies, R.H. (2011) Producing *Salmonella*-free pigs: a review focusing on interventions at weaning. *Veterinary Record* 168, 267–276.

Walsh, M.C., Rostagno, M.H., Gardiner, G.E., Sutton, A.L., Richert, B.T. and Radcliffe, J.S. (2012) Controlling *Salmonella* infection in weanling pigs through water delivery of direct-fed microbials or organic acids. Part I: effects on growth performance, microbial populations, and immune status. *Journal of Animal Science* 90, 261–271.

Wang, Y., Qu, L., Uthe, J.J., Bearson, S.M., Kuhar, D., Lunney, J.K., Couture, O.P., Nettleton, D., Dekkers, J.C. and Tuggle, C.K. (2007) Global transcriptional response of porcine mesenteric lymph nodes to *Salmonella enterica* serovar Typhimurium. *Genomics* 90, 72–84.

Wang, Y., Couture, O.P., Qu, L., Uthe, J.J., Bearson, S.M., Kuhar, D., Lunney, J.K., Nettleton, D., Dekkers, J.C. and Tuggle, C.K. (2008) Analysis of porcine transcriptional response to *Salmonella enterica* serovar Choleraesuis suggests novel targets of NFkappaB are activated in the mesenteric lymph node. *BMC Genomics* 9, 437.

Warriss, P.D., Brown, S.N., Edwards, J.E. and Knowles, T.G. (1998) Effect of lairage time on levels of stress and meat quality in pigs. *Animal Science* 66, 255–261.

Watson, P.R., Paulin, S.M., Jones, P.W. and Wallis, T.S. (2000) Interaction of *Salmonella* serotypes with porcine macrophages *in vitro* does not correlate with virulence. *Microbiology* 146, 1639–1649.

Widjojoatmodjo, M.N., Fluit, A.C., Torensma, R., Keller, B.H.I. and Verhoef, J. (1991) Evaluation of the magnetic immune-PCR assay for the rapid detection of *Salmonella*. *European Journal of Clinical Microbiology and Infectious Disease* 10, 935–938.

Widjojoatmodjo, M.N., Fluit, A.C., Torensma, R., Verdonk, G.P.H.T. and Verhoef, J. (1992) The magnetic immuno-polymerase chain reaction assay for direct detection of salmonellae in fecal samples. *Journal of Clinical Microbiology* 30, 3195–3199.

Wilcock, B. and Olander, H. (1978) Influence of oral antibiotic feeding on the duration and severity of clinical disease, growth performance and pattern of shedding in swine inoculated with *Salmonella typhimurium*. *Journal of the American Veterinary Medical Association* 172, 472–477.

Wilcock, B.P. and Schwartz, K. (1992) Salmonellosis. In: Leman, A.D., Straw, B.E., Mengeling, W.E., D'Allaire, S. and Taylor, D.J. (eds) *Diseases of Swine*, 7th edn. Iowa State University Press, Ames, Iowa, pp. 570–583.

Wilcock, B., Armstrong, C. and Olander, H. (1976) The significance of the serovar in the clinical and pathologic features of naturally occurring porcine salmonellosis. *Canadian Journal of Comparative Medicine* 40, 80–88.

Wilde, J., Eiden, J. and Yolken, R. (1990) Removal of inhibitory substances from human fecal specimens for detection of group A rotavirus by reverse transcriptase and polymerase chain reaction. *Journal of Clinical Microbiology* 28, 1300–1307.

Wilkins, W., Waldner, C., Rajić, A., McFall, M., Chow, E. and Muckle, A. (2011) Comparison of bacterial culture, polymerase chain reaction, and a mix-enzyme-linked immunosorbent assay for the detection of *Salmonella* status in grow-to-finish pigs in western Canada with a Bayesian approach. *Canadian Journal of Veterinary Research* 75, 308–311.

Williams, D.R., Hunter, D., Binder, J. and Hough, E. (1981) Observations on the occurrence of *Salmonella choleraesuis* and other salmonellas in two herds of feeder pigs. *Journal of Hygiene (Cambridge)* 86, 369–377.

Williams, L.P., Vaughn, J.P., Scott, A. and Blanton, V. (1969) A ten-month study on *Salmonella* contamination in animal protein meals. *Journal of the American Veterinary Medical Association* 155, 167–174.

Williams, P.H., Rabsch, W., Methner, U., Voigt, W., Tschäpe, H. and Reissbrodt, R. (2006) Catecholate receptor proteins in *Salmonella enterica*, role in virulence and implications for vaccine development. *Vaccine* 24, 3840–3844.

Winter, S.E., Thiennimitr, P., Winter, M.G., Butler, B.P., Huseby, D.L., Crawford, R.W., Russell, J.M., Bevins, C.L., Adams, L.G., Tsolis, R.M., Roth, J.R. and Bäumler, A.J. (2010) Gut inflammation provides a respiratory electron acceptor for *Salmonella*. *Nature* 467, 426–429.

Wood, R.L. and Rose, R. (1992) Populations of *Salmonella typhimurium* in internal organs of experimentally infected carrier swine. *American Journal of Veterinary Research* 53, 653–657.

Wood, R.L., Pospischil, A. and Rose, R. (1989) Distribution of persistent *Salmonella typhimurium* infection in internal organs of swine. *American Journal of Veterinary Research* 50, 1015–1021.

Wood, R.L., Rose, R., Coe, N.E. and Ferris, K.E. (1991) Experimental establishment of persistent infection in swine with a zoonotic strain of *Salmonella newport*. *American Journal of Veterinary Research* 52, 813–819.

Wray, C., Davies, R.H., Jones, Y.E. and Chappell, S. (1997) Antibiotic resistance and *Salmonella* infections in pigs. In: *Proceedings of the 2nd International Symposium on Epidemiology and Control of* Salmonella *in Pork*, Copenhagen, Denmark, 20–22 August 1997, pp. 247–250.

Xiong, N., Brewer, M.T., Day, T.A., Kimber, M.J., Barnhill, A.E. and Carlson, S.A. (2010) Evaluation of the pathogenicity and virulence of three strains of *Salmonella* organisms in calves and pigs. *American Journal of Veterinary Research* 71, 1170–1177.

Yang, B., Qu, D., Zhang, X., Shen, J., Cui, S., Shi, Y., Xi, M., Sheng, M., Zhi, S. and Meng, J. (2010) Prevalence and characterization of *Salmonella* serovars in retail meats of marketplace in Shaanxi, China. *International Journal of Food Microbiology* 141, 63–72.

Ye, J., Su, L.H., Chen, C.L., Hu, S., Wang, J., Yu, J. and Chiu, C.H. (2011) Analysis of pSC138, the multidrug resistance plasmid of *Salmonella enterica* serotype Choleraesuis SC-B67. *Plasmid* 65, 132–140.

Yu, H., Wang, J., Ye, J., Tang, P., Chu, C., Hu, S. and Chiu, C.H. (2006) Complete nucleotide sequence of pSCV50, the virulence plasmid of *Salmonella enterica* serovar Choleraesuis SC-B67. *Plasmid* 55, 145–151.

14 *Salmonella* Infections in Sheep

Sergio Uzzau*
Dipartimento di Scienze Biomediche, Centre for Biotechnology Development and Biodiversity Research, Università di Sassari, Italy

Introduction – Historical

Sheep and goats were the first livestock species to be domesticated when the Neolithic agricultural revolution developed over 10,000 years BP in Southwest Asia. Initially, sheep were domesticated mainly for meat and, later, for secondary products such as wool and milk (Ryder, 1983). Since then, sheep lifestyle imposed by domestication has certainly had an impact on the evolutive adaptation of sheep bacterial pathogens, including serovars of *Salmonella enterica*. From Asia, domesticated sheep moved to Europe and North Africa together with the nomadic herders and the new sedentary farmers. Sheep have been constantly exposed to contact with other individuals of the same community (flock) and, frequently, with other feral or domesticated animal species. Over many thousands of years, therefore, strains of *S. enterica* serovars have been circulating within the ovine species and evolved toward a host-restricted pathogenic lifestyle, while other serovars were responsible for disease in sheep and other warm-blooded animals, including humans and their domesticated animals (i.e. pigs, dogs and cattle).

Epidemiology

In most countries of the world with a large sheep population, including the UK, Australia, New Zealand and the USA, sheep salmonellosis is apparently rare and does not represent a relevant economic issue. In these countries, sheep infections occur with a wide range of *S. enterica* serovars that are non-restricted to ovine (i.e. serovars Typhimurium, Indiana, Arizonae, Derby, Dublin, Brandenburg and Montevideo; Walton, 1972; Findlay, 1973; Sojka *et al.*, 1977; Linklater, 1983; Pritchard, 1990; Hjartardóttir *et al.*, 2002; Clark *et al.*, 2004; Oloya *et al.*, 2007; Luque *et al.*, 2009; Kidanemariam *et al.*, 2010). These serovars do not establish an endemic pattern and their occurrence appears to be related to pastures contaminated by wild bird faeces, in which *Salmonella* can survive for more than 2 years (Hjartardóttir *et al.*, 2002; Lillehaug *et al.*, 2005; Pennycott *et al.*, 2006; Luque *et al.*, 2009). Disease distribution and prevalence of infections due to ubiquitous serovars is typically seasonal and associated with animal movement and shipping (Gardiner and Craig, 1970; Linklater, 1983; Richards *et al.*, 1989; Higgs *et al.*, 1993). Exposition to prolonged environmental stress,

* Author, e-mail: uzzau@uniss.it

© CAB International 2013. *Salmonella in Domestic Animals, 2nd Edition* (eds P.A. Barrow and U. Methner)

including cold, poor nutrition and concurrent diseases, might be important to activate latent infection and *Salmonella* shedding in faeces (Higgs *et al.*, 1993).

Epidemiological studies have assessed a clear linkage between the occurrence of human salmonellosis outbreaks and contact with live infected animals or consumption of contaminated animal food. Examination of slaughter-age healthy sheep and identification of *Salmonella* species have been often reported in the past few years, due to public health concerns of these serovars entering the human food chain (Hjartardóttir *et al.*, 2002; Molla *et al.*, 2006; Vanselow *et al.*, 2007). Ovine salmonellosis might be an important zoonotic reservoir for human infection and a number of studies have reported food-borne transmission to humans (Evans *et al.*, 1999; Baker *et al.*, 2007; Hess *et al.*, 2008).

A different epidemiology pattern occurs when infection is due to the *S.* Abortusovis, which is entirely host-specific to sheep, as it could be isolated only from sheep under natural conditions. In the case of this serovar, outbreaks are reported with a cyclic rhythm in the frequency of abortion. In endemic areas, abortion occurs in 30–50% of sheep in a flock, generally during the first pregnancy and mainly during the last period of gestation (Jack, 1968; Pardon *et al.*, 1988; Uzzau *et al.*, 2000). Prevalence of *S.* Abortusovis infection is high in Italy, Spain, France, Greece, Switzerland, Russia, the Middle East and northern Africa, and losses, due uniquely to abortion, might have serious economic consequences in these countries. Epidemiological studies have been performed by means of pulsed field gel electrophoresis (PFGE), IS200 fingerprinting, ribotyping and plasmid profiling, to trace the spread of different *S.* Abortusovis genotypes and to identify the predominant clones (Colombo *et al.*, 1992; Nikbakht *et al.*, 2002; Dionisi *et al.*, 2006; Schiaffino *et al.*, 1996; Valdezate *et al.*, 2007; Belloy *et al.*, 2009). Taken together, these studies suggest that a wide number of specific clones disseminate within the same endemic areas and present evidence of co-isolation of different genotypes within the same affected flock. Preliminary data obtained with IS*1414* element as molecular epidemiology marker provide evidence of the existence of two different clusters of *S.* Abortusovis strains. The former, to which belong isolates carrying a high copy number of IS*1414* genomic insertion, is widespread in European countries. In the other cluster are found isolates that do not possess IS*1414* and are predominant in Asian countries (Bacciu *et al.*, 2004).

Transmission

Serovar Abortusovis strains, being host-restricted to ovines, are expected to be introduced into a flock by an infected sheep and transmitted by the faecal–oral route (Mura and Contini, 1954; Jack, 1968). There is no convincing evidence of bacterial spread by feed, water, or other host's faeces. Hence, caution has to be taken when moving animals from a flock with history of infection into non-infected ones. In particular, while many authors have reported faecal shedding of culturable infectious bacteria up to 3 months following abortion (Uzzau *et al.*, 2000), *S.* Abortusovis DNA has also been detected in faeces up to 12 months from abortion (Belloy *et al.*, 2009), suggesting that sheep may be long-term asymptomatic carriers. Experimental infection studies have demonstrated that sheep may become infected by the conjunctival and vaginal routes (Jack, 1968; Sanchis *et al.*, 1986, 1991; Uzzau *et al.*, 2000), but their importance in natural transmission has not been assessed. Since serovars Abortusovis, Dublin and others cause pneumonia in young lambs, infection of grazing animals through the nasal route might also be possible and respiratory secretion may spread the infection to other individuals. High bacterial load in aborted fetuses and expelled placenta, excretion of bacteria with vaginal discharges following abortion and by scouring lambs are the main source of transmission throughout a flock during the lambing season (Jack, 1968; Belloy *et al.*, 2009).

As noted above, ubiquitous *Salmonella* serovars are transmitted to ovine flocks by faecal contamination of feed and water due to other animal species, including wild birds (Hjartardóttir *et al.*, 2002; Luque *et al.*, 2009).

Clinical Features

Signs and symptoms of ovine salmonellosis vary depending on the serovar involved and the animal age, but usually an outbreak is manifested by epidemic abortion in ewes at the last third of pregnancy, stillbirths, and premature and non-viable lambs. In addition to abortion, ewes may exhibit a vaginal discharge around the time of abortion and transient fever, but otherwise appear healthy. For these reasons, *Salmonella* infection often goes undetected in sheep flocks until it is too late to adopt effective measures during the lambing period. Infected ewes that do not abort may deliver weak lambs that generally develop bacteraemia and die within a few days. Lambs may also be born strong and become infected and die within the first 2 weeks after birth. Less frequently, the ewes die of septicaemia, acute metritis and peritonitis resulting from placental retention. In non-pregnant ewes and rams, infection might be totally asymptomatic. Instead, lambs infected during the first month show signs of pneumonia, enteritis (diarrhoea), or polyarthritis. These clinical manifestations typically occur in ovine salmonellosis associated with the sheep-restricted *S.* Abortusovis but also with other serovars, including Montevideo and Indiana, that are more frequently responsible for salmonellosis in other animal species including humans (Jack, 1968; Linklater, 1983; Sharp *et al.*, 1983; Uzzau *et al.*, 2000; Luque *et al.*, 2009). While the death of the ewe is not common, abortion occurs in 30–50% of sheep in a flock, generally during the first pregnancy.

Of all serovars isolated from ovine salmonellosis, few determine gastroenteritis, pneumonia and death in adult animals, including serovars Brandenburg, Arizonae and Typhimurium. Affected animals might have both systemic and enteric signs of infection, with malaise, pyrexia, profuse diarrhoea, and die because of dehydration and septicaemia (Saunders *et al.*, 1966; Baker *et al.*, 1971; Hunter *et al.*, 1976; Long *et al.*, 1978; Richards *et al.*, 1993; Clark *et al.*, 2007). Serovar Dublin causes both enteritis and abortion in adult sheep and the disease is often associated with metritis, anorexia and loss of wool (Ekdahl and Allan, 1966; McCaughey *et al.*, 1971).

Diagnosis

The definitive diagnosis of *Salmonella* abortion in ewes depends upon the isolation of the bacteria from the aborted fetus tissues, vaginal discharges or faecal samples. Specimens are evaluated by direct culture on selective agars, such as MacConkey agar, XLD, *Salmonella-Shigella* agar. Samples taken from fetus tissues and vaginal discharges, in the first few days following salmonellosis abortion, show high bacterial load of non-lactose-fermenting bacteria and should not require enrichment media or further serological analysis to confirm animal infection. The examination of bacterial colonies and serological and biochemical testing allow rapid identification of the *Salmonella* serovar involved. Serovar Abortusovis grows slowly and forms small colonies, posing special difficulties in direct isolation from specimens with other overgrowing bacteria (i.e. faeces). Typically, colonies reach a size of 1–2 mm after 48–72 h of growth. To obtain pure cultures, bacteria must be re-inoculated in rich media since *S.* Abortusovis carries several auxotrophies (Uzzau *et al.*, 2000). This serovar can be distinguished by other *Salmonella* members by biochemical kits or serology testing. It is also possible to rely on PCR amplification of a serovar-specific 900 bp fragment, corresponding to a selected IS*200* chromosomal copy (Schiaffino *et al.*, 1996; Beuzón *et al.*, 1997; Habrun *et al.*, 2006; Masala *et al.*, 2007).

The retrospective identification of *Salmonella* infection in ewes is challenging as excretion of the causative agent is transient and the serum antibodies fall to low titres soon after the abortion (Uzzau *et al.*, 2000, 2005; Belloy *et al.*, 2009). A number of serum agglutination and microagglutination tests have been developed (Sojka *et al.*, 1977; Ivanov *et al.*, 1982; Pardon *et al.*, 1990a; Giannati *et al.*, 1999). ELISA tests based on *S.* Abortusovis antigens proved to be more sensitive than agglutination and may allow distinction between the early IgM response and later IgG response (Sting *et al.*, 1997; Uzzau *et al.*, 2005; Wirz-Dittus *et al.*, 2010a, b). Furthermore, ELISA can detect positive antibody levels for up to 10 months after abortion, suggesting that this test can be used for flock surveillance testing (Wirz-Dittus *et al.*, 2010a). An indirect ELISA test has been developed also for IgG antibodies specific for *S.* Brandenburg salmonellosis in sheep (Perera and Murray, 2009).

Detection of *S.* Abortusovis-specific DNA, both in faeces and vaginal excretions, up to 12 months following abortion, suggests that *S.* Abortusovis might be shed in culture negative samples and that it is possible to diagnose infection in asymptomatic carriers (Habrun *et al.*, 2006).

Pathology

On post-mortem examination of ewes and lambs that have died of salmonellosis, the pathological findings cover a wide range of reactions, reflecting the particular disease provoked by *Salmonella* serovars. Sheep that experienced systemic infection by *S.* Typhimurium or die following abortion due to other serovars manifest congested organs, with splenic enlargement, liver focal necrosis and intravasal coagulation. Clinical evidence of anorexia and scour are normally associated with swollen liver, abomasitis, enteritis and enlarged lymph nodes (Richards *et al.*, 1993). Intestinal fluid content might be high and associated to haemorrhagic necrotic lesions. Aborted fetuses are generally fresh and placentae appear slightly damaged and inflamed. Sometime fetuses are rotten when abortion occurs in the latest days of pregnancy. Placenta lesions are not specific. Histological examination reveals areas of necrosis with leucocyte infiltration and thrombosis within the caruncle's blood vessels.

Morphological changes induced in infected ileal mucosa have been recorded in an experimental ewe model of infection (Uzzau *et al.*, 2001). In this study, microscopic analysis confirmed the induction of intense inflammatory reaction as defined by villous atrophy, extrusion of enterocytes, and infiltration of inflammatory cells into the submucosa and epithelium, by enteritis-causing serovars Typhimurium and Dublin. The architecture of mucosa infected with *S.* Abortusovis was not affected and appeared indistinguishable from that of the uninfected control. These finding correlates well with the absence of enteritis in *S.* Abortusovis-infected ewes (Uzzau *et al.*, 2001).

Pathogenesis

The capability of *Salmonella* to colonize the host mucosal barrier and disseminate to deeper tissues and organs depends heavily on its interplay with the lymphoid submucosal tissue. Here, bacteria survive and replicate within professional phagocytic cells, inducing the release of inflammatory cytokines. In this respect, as for other animal hosts, the initial site of *Salmonella* invasion in sheep mainly occurs within the intestinal mucosa following the oral route of natural infection. In addition to this gut-associated lymphoid tissue (GALT), sheep are among the *Salmonella* host species where the bronchus-associated lymphoid tissue (BALT) is rather abundant. These follicle-like aggregations with lymphocytes infiltrating the epithelium show specialized epithelial cells and a structure similar to that seen in the small intestine. According to these anatomic features, together with the occurrence of pneumonia among the clinical outcomes of *Salmonella* infection in both lambs and ewes, the nasal route of infection (i.e. faecal-nasal), in addition to the oral one, cannot be ruled out. In this case, the primary site of infection may be represented by non-intestinal tissues, such as the tonsil and the lung as hypothesized in case of serovars Choleraesuis and Typhimurium infection in swine and in cattle, respectively (De Jong and Ekdahl, 1965; Gray *et al.*, 1995). Other routes of infection have been experimentally investigated, and successful reproduction of sheep salmonellosis has been obtained by intra-vaginal and intra-conjunctival infections (Pardon *et al.*, 1990a), while the significance of these routes in natural epidemic dissemination are unclear.

Pathogenesis of abortion has been clearly demonstrated to be affected by the timing of infection along the gestation period. In experimental infections with serovars Abortusovis and Montevideo, abortion occurred 2–3 weeks after infection of ewes at their 90–110 days of gestation, while almost all pregnant ewes infected during earlier stages of gestation did not abort (Linklater, 1983; Sanchis and Pardon, 1984). Since aborted fetuses are usually well developed and do not have gross anatomical abnormalities, placentitis appears to be a key element in pathogenesis. In sheep, macrophages accumulate in the uterine endometrium during pregnancy (Tekin and Hansen, 2004), where they may be needed to guarantee an effective immune surveillance. In addition, regulatory (gamma-delta) T cells also accumulate in the uterus during pregnancy (Lee *et al.*, 1992; Majewski *et al.*, 2001), with the probable task to balance immunological responses and avoid immunological causes of pregnancy losses. Taking into account that *Salmonella*-infected pregnant ewes usually abort without other signs of infection and appear healthy even during abortion, placentitis might be a consequence of local alterations in maternal immunity during pregnancy.

As noted in previous paragraphs, the majority of *Salmonella* serovars isolated from sheep are associated with enteric disease, as occur in other animal species. Pathogenesis of inflammatory diarrhoea might be essentially dependent on the activity of several effectors secreted by the SPI-1 encoded type 3 secretion system (TTSS-1), and the innate response triggered by the wide assortment of TLR ligands produced by *Salmonella*. Host-specific *S.* Abortusovis, on the other hand, shows different pathogenic traits. Sheep experimental infections with *S.* Abortusovis showed that this serovar invades the intestinal mucosa in relatively low numbers and fails to elicit enteritis (Uzzau *et al.*, 2001). Since Abortusovis reaches significantly lower counts in this tissue compared to enteritogenic *S.* Dublin, the absence of enteritis in *S.* Abortusovis-infected ewes might depend on poor induction of the innate immune response. Deletion of SPI-1 encoded gene *invH* has been shown to further decrease *S.* Abortusovis bacterial load in the intestine, while virulence plasmid encoded genes do not influence intestinal invasion (Uzzau *et al.*, 2001). Molecular analysis of SPI-1 encoded effectors in *S.* Abortusovis has shown that SipA, SopA, SopB, SopD and SopE are expressed to a lesser extent by intracellular bacteria and that *sopD* is a pseudogene. Further, AvrA, a deubiquitinase effector that might dampen inflammatory response, is maintained at a level over ten-fold higher than *S.* Typhimurium (Collier-Hyams *et al.*, 2002; Uzzau, 2003). While the acute intestinal inflammatory response may act to control colonization by the majority of *Salmonella* serovars that cause sheep salmonellosis, the avoidance of a strong inflammation by highly host-restricted serovars like Abortusovis may facilitate their systemic spread and promote the establishment of a chronic carrier lifestyle.

Genomics

Strains isolated from ovine salmonellosis all belong to subspecies I, in which a high frequency of recombination has been reported (Falush *et al.*, 2006; Octavia and Lan, 2006). However, most of these strains have not been subjected to detailed genetic analysis and their population structure at serovar level is not available. Therefore, to date, it is not known whether the ovine salmonellosis isolates, belonging to different serovars, have acquired similar pathogenic traits by means of recombination within the subspecies I, or they have adapted themselves to the ovine host independently by convergent evolutionary processes. Comparison of genomes corresponding to different serovar strains isolated from ovine salmonellosis will provide models to identify possible bias toward ovine infection.

Most of the current knowledge on the genetic structure of *Salmonella* isolates from sheep salmonellosis is given by epidemiology reports that made use of molecular techniques to assess strains genetic relatedness. In particular, PFGE has been applied to strains isolated from an outbreak of sheep salmonellosis by *S.* Indiana (Luque *et al.*, 2009), where isolates were found to be highly clonal and related to wild birds isolates. On the contrary, recent studies on *S.* Abortusovis epidemic populations in Europe demonstrated an important heterogeneity of genotypes circulating over the years and/or within the same outbreak (Dionisi *et al.*, 2006; Valdezate *et al.*, 2007; Belloy *et al.*, 2009). In addition to their relevance for epidemiology purposes, these findings highlighted the existence of a heterogeneous genomic structure in *S.* Abortusovis.

Genomes of *S.* Abortusovis clinical isolates appear to accumulate high numbers of recombination events also according to genomic insertion profiles of IS*1414*, a genetic element that is peculiar to this serovar (Bacciu *et al.*, 2004). As observed for other host-restricted *Salmonella* serovars (Parkhill *et al.*, 2001; Thomson *et al.*, 2008), analysis by micro-array technology suggested that Abortusovis appeared to have been subjected to extensive genome reduction (McClelland *et al.*, 2004; Porwollik *et al.*, 2004).

Vaccination

Control of epidemic ovine salmonellosis is a major concern for countries in which sheep herding is of great importance. Efforts to prevent the disease are frequently made by administration of inactivated vaccines. This is particularly true for salmonellosis with an endemic pattern and a well-known trend of reduced abortions in the year following an outbreak, suggesting that the animals develop resistance to the disease. With *S.* Abortusovis, strong protective immunity and successful reproduction in subsequent seasons provide compelling evidence of a protective, adaptive immune response in ewes that have aborted. To elicit this protective state against *S.* Abortusovis, a number of inactivated and live attenuated vaccines have been developed (Pardon *et al.*, 1990a, b, c; Sanchis *et al.*, 1995; Giannati-Stefanou *et al.*, 1999; Uzzau *et al.*, 2005; Estevan *et al.*, 2006). A live attenuated vaccine, strain Rv6, was selected as a non-dependent reverse mutant from a streptomycin-dependent strain and, to date, it has been tested as safe in field conditions and widely administered subcutaneously to pregnant ewes in France and other European countries (Pardon *et al.*, 1990a, c). Significant protection has been achieved also with a live attenuated strain of *S.* Typhimurium obtained by means of 'metabolic drift' mutation (Linde *et al.*, 1992). This strain has been administered subcutaneously in two large field studies in Kirgiziya. The study included 178,000 pregnant ewes, and reported that immunization with the attenuated vaccine induced a strong protection from Abortusovis infection, compared to animals vaccinated with a killed strain and to unvaccinated controls. Derivative strains of *S.* Typhimurium have been obtained also by *aroA* gene deletion and used as sheep salmonellosis vaccine (Mukkur *et al.*, 1987, 1995; Begg *et al.*, 1990; Mukkur and Walker, 1992). These vaccine were found more effective when administered parenterally rather than orally and protection against challenge with wild-type parental strains persisted for up to 6 months. Live vaccine candidates of *S.* Abortusovis have also been developed by deleting *aroA* or *cya crp cdt* genes, or by curing parental strain from the virulence plasmid (Uzzau *et al.*, 2005). Immunization efficacies were evaluated in terms of inducing serum antibodies and protecting against abortion after challenge with wild-type parental strain in pregnant ewes. Pregnancy failure of vaccinated ewes was reduced compared to that of non-immunized controls. All three vaccine candidates appear to be safe for use in pregnant ewes. The protection efficacy was paralleled by the values of vaccine-induced specific IgM and IgG antibodies at the time of challenge, with the plasmid-cured strain inducing the highest level of immunogenicity.

In addition, a special need for sheep salmonellosis control occurs for those zoonotic diseases directly transmitted to humans with an occupational contact with live animals or carcasses (Baker *et al.*, 2007; Hess *et al.*, 2008). In this direction, efforts have been made by evaluating the protection efficacy of a *S.* Typhimurium-attenuated mutant and a subunit formulate of Brandenburg antigens against *S.* Brandenburg salmonellosis, but significant protection has yet to be achieved (Li *et al.*, 2005).

References

Bacciu, D., Falchi, G., Spazziani, A., Bossi, L., Marogna, G., Leori, G.S., Rubino, S. and Uzzau, S. (2004) Transposition of the heat-stable toxin *astA* gene into a gifsy-2-related prophage of *Salmonella enterica* serovar Abortusovis. *Journal of Bacteriology* 186, 4568–4574.

Baker, J.R., Faull, W.B. and Rankin, J.E. (1971) An outbreak of salmonellosis in sheep. *Veterinary Record* 88, 270–277.

Baker, M.G., Thornley, C.N., Lopez, L.D., Garrett, N.K. and Nicol, C.M. (2007) A recurring salmonellosis epidemic in New Zealand linked to contact with sheep. *Epidemiology and Infection* 135, 76–83.

Begg, A.P., Walker, K.H., Love, D.N. and Mukkur, T.K. (1990) Evaluation of protection against experimental salmonellosis in sheep immunised with 1 or 2 doses of live aromatic-dependent *Salmonella* typhimurium. *Australian Veterinary Journal* 67, 294–298.

Belloy, L., Decrausaz, L., Boujon, P., Hächler, H. and Waldvogel, A.S. (2009) Diagnosis by culture and PCR of *Salmonella* abortusovis infection under clinical conditions in aborting sheep in Switzerland. *Veterinary Microbiology* 138, 373–377.

Beuzón, C.R., Schiaffino, A., Leori, G., Cappuccinelli, P., Rubino, S. and Casadesús, J. (1997) Identification of *Salmonella* abortusovis by PCR amplification of a serovar-specific IS200 element. *Applied and Environmental Microbiology* 63, 2082–2085.

Clark, R.G., Fenwick, S.G., Nicol, C.M., Marchant, R.M., Swanney, S., Gill, J.M., Holmes, J.D., Leyland, M. and Davies, P.R. (2004) *Salmonella* Brandenburg – emergence of a new strain affecting stock and humans in the South Island of New Zealand. *New Zealand Veterinary Journal* 52, 26–36.

Clark, R.G., Gill, J.M., Fairley, R.A. and Smart, J.A. (2007) Abortions in sheep caused by *Salmonella* Brandenburg: pathological findings. *New Zealand Veterinary Journal* 55, 356–357.

Collier-Hyams, L.S., Zeng, H., Sun, J., Tomlinson, A.D., Bao, Z.Q., Chen, H., Madara, J.L., Orth, K. and Neish, A.S. (2002) Cutting edge: *Salmonella* AvrA effector inhibits the key proinflammatory, anti-apoptotic NF-kappa B pathway. *The Journal of Immunology* 169, 2846–2850.

Colombo, M.M., Leori, G., Rubino, S., Barbato, A. and Cappuccinelli, P. (1992) Phenotypic features and molecular characterization of plasmids in *Salmonella* abortusovis. *Journal of General Microbiology* 138, 725–731.

de Jong, H. and Ekdahl, M.O. (1965) Salmonellosis in calves – the effect of dose rate and other factors on transmission. *New Zealand Veterinary Journal* 13, 59–64.

Dionisi, A.M., Carattoli, A., Luzzi, I., Magistrali, C. and Pezzotti, G. (2006) Molecular genotyping of *Salmonella enterica* Abortusovis by pulsed field gel electrophoresis. *Veterinary Microbiology* 116, 217–223.

Ekdahl, M.O. and Allan, C.M. (1966) Isolation of *Salmonella* Dublin from a sheep in New Zealand. *New Zealand Veterinary Journal* 14, 93.

Estevan, M., Irache, J.M., Grilló, M.J., Blasco, J.M. and Gamazo, C. (2006) Encapsulation of antigenic extracts of *Salmonella enterica* serovar. Abortusovis into polymeric systems and efficacy as vaccines in mice. *Veterinary Microbiology* 118, 124–132.

Evans, M.R., Salmon, R.L., Nehaul, L., Mably, S., Wafford, L., Nolan-Farrell, M.Z., Gardner, D. and Ribeiro, C.D. (1999) An outbreak of *Salmonella* typhimurium DT170 associated with kebab meat and yogurt relish. *Epidemiology and Infection* 122, 377–383.

Falush, D., Torpdahl, M., Didelot, X., Conrad, D.F., Wilson, D.J. and Achtman, M. (2006) Mismatch induced speciation in *Salmonella*: model and data. *Philosophical Transactions of the Royal Society B: Biological Science* 361(1475), 2045–2053.

Findlay, C.R. (1973) Abortion in ewes caused by *Salmonella* derby. *Veterinary Record* 93, 81.

Gardiner, M.R. and Craig, J. (1970) Factors affecting survival in the transportation of sheep by sea in the tropics and subtropics. *Australian Veterinary Journal* 46, 65–69.

Giannati, A., Koptopoulos, G., Hatzopoulou, E. and Sarris, K. (1999) Preparation of a high titre *Salmonella* abortusovis H-antigen and antiserum and improvement of the microagglutination test. *Journal of Microbiological Methods* 35, 219–223.

Giannati-Stefanou, A., Koptopoulos, G., Hatzopoulou, E. and Sarris, K. (1999) A *Salmonella* abortusovis inactivated vaccine protects mice from abortion after challenge. *Veterinary Microbiology* 66, 285–290.

Gray, J.T., Fedorka-Cray, P.J., Stabel, T.J. and Ackermann, M.R. (1995) Influence of inoculation route on the carrier state of *Salmonella* choleraesuis in swine. *Veterinary Microbiology* 47, 43–59.

Habrun, B., Listes, E., Spicic, S., Cvetnic, Z., Lukacevic, D., Jemersic, L., Lojkic, M. and Kompes, G. (2006) An outbreak of *Salmonella* Abortusovis abortions in sheep in south Croatia. *Journal of Veterinary Medicine, Series B* 53, 286–290.

Hess, I.M., Neville, L.M., McCarthy, R., Shadbolt, C.T. and McAnulty, J.M. (2008) A *Salmonella* Typhimurium 197 outbreak linked to the consumption of lambs' liver in Sydney, NSW. *Epidemiology and Infection* 136, 461–467.

Higgs, A.R., Norris, R.T. and Richards, R.B. (1993) Epidemiology of salmonellosis in the live sheep export industry. *Australian Veterinary Journal* 70, 330–335.

Hjartardóttir, S., Gunnarsson, E. and Sigvaldadóttir, J. (2002) *Salmonella* in sheep in Iceland. *Acta Veterinaria Scandinavica* 43, 43–48.

Hunter, A.G., Mathieson, A.O., Scott, J.A. and Corrigall, W. (1976) An outbreak of *S.* typhimurium in sheep and its consequences. *Veterinary Record* 98, 126–130.

Ivanov, I.N., Draganov, M. and Masalski, N. (1982) Active immunoprophylaxis of *Salmonella* abortion in sheep. *Veterinarno-meditsinski nauki* 19, 22–29.

Jack, E.J. (1968) *Salmonella* abortusovis: an atypical *Salmonella*. *Veterinary Record* 82, 558–561.

Kidanemariam, A., Engelbrecht, M. and Picard, J. (2010) Retrospective study on the incidence of *Salmonella* isolations in animals in South Africa, 1996 to 2006. *Journal of the South African Veterinary Association* 81, 37–44.

Lee, C.S., Meeusen, E., Gogolin-Ewens, K. and Brandon, M.R. (1992) Quantitative and qualitative changes in the intraepithelial lymphocyte population in the uterus of nonpregnant and pregnant sheep. *American Journal of Reproductive Immunology* 28, 90–96.

Li, H., McFarlane, R.G. and Wagner, J. (2005) Vaccination of pregnant ewes against infection with *Salmonella* Brandenburg. *New Zealand Veterinary Journal* 53, 416–422.

Lillehaug, A., Monceyron Jonassen, C., Bergsjø, B., Hofshagen, M., Tharaldsen, J., Nesse, L.L. and Handeland, K. (2005) Screening of feral pigeon (*Colomba livia*), mallard (*Anas platyrhynchos*) and graylag goose (*Anser anser*) populations for *Campylobacter* spp., *Salmonella* spp., avian influenza virus and avian paramyxovirus. *Acta Veterinaria Scandinavica* 46, 193–202.

Linde, K., Bondarenko, V. and Sviridenko, V. (1992) Prophylaxis of *Salmonella* abortus ovis-induced abortion of sheep by a *Salmonella* typhimurium live vaccine. *Vaccine* 10, 337–340.

Linklater, K.A. (1983) Abortion in sheep associated with *Salmonella* montevideo infection. *Veterinary Record* 112, 372–374.

Long, J.R., Finley, G.G., Clark, M.H. and Rehmtulla, A.J. (1978) Ovine fetal infection due to *Salmonella arizonae*. *Canadian Veterinary Journal* 19, 260–263.

Luque, I., Echeita, A., León, J., Herrera-León, S., Tarradas, C., González-Sanz, R., Huerta, B. and Astorga, R.J. (2009) *Salmonella* Indiana as a cause of abortion in ewes: genetic diversity and resistance patterns. *Veterinary Microbiology* 134, 396–399.

Majewski, A.C., Tekin, S. and Hansen, P.J. (2001) Local versus systemic control of numbers of endometrial T cells during pregnancy in sheep. *Immunology* 102, 317–322.

Masala, G., Porcu, R., Daga, C., Denti, S., Canu, G., Patta, C. and Tola, S. (2007) Detection of pathogens in ovine and caprine abortion samples from Sardinia, Italy, by PCR. *Journal of Veterinary Diagnostic Investigation* 19, 96–98.

McCaughey, W.J., Kavanagh, P.J. and McClelland, T.G. (1971) Experimental *Salmonella* Dublin infection in sheep. *British Veterinary Journal* 127, 557–566.

McClelland, M., Sanderson, K.E., Clifton, S.W., Latreille, P., Porwollik, S., Sabo, A., Meyer, R., Bieri, T., Ozersky, P., McLellan, M., Harkins, C.R., Wang, C., Nguyen, C., Berghoff, A., Elliott, G., Kohlberg, S., Strong, C., Du, F., Carter, J., Kremizki, C., Layman, D., Leonard, S., Sun, H., Fulton, L., Nash, W., Miner, T., Minx, P., Delehaunty, K., Fronick, C., Magrini, V., Nhan, M., Warren, W., Florea, L., Spieth, J. and Wilson, R.K. (2004) Comparison of genome degradation in Paratyphi A and Typhi, human-restricted serovars of *Salmonella enterica* that cause typhoid. *Nature Genetics* 36, 1268–1274.

Molla, W., Molla, B., Alemayehu, D., Muckle, A., Cole, L. and Wilkie, E. (2006) Occurrence and antimicrobial resistance of *Salmonella* serovars in apparently healthy slaughtered sheep and goats of central Ethiopia. *Tropical Animal Health and Production* 38, 455–462.

Mukkur, T.K. and Walker, K.H. (1992) Development and duration of protection against salmonellosis in mice and sheep immunised with live aromatic-dependent *Salmonella* typhimurium. *Research of Veterinary Science* 52, 147–153.

Mukkur, T.K., McDowell, G.H., Stocker, B.A. and Lascelles, A.K. (1987) Protection against experimental salmonellosis in mice and sheep by immunisation with aromatic-dependent *Salmonella* typhimurium. *Journal of Medical Microbiology* 24, 11–19.

Mukkur, T.K., Walker, K.H., Baker, P. and Jones, D. (1995) Systemic and mucosal intestinal antibody response of sheep immunized with aromatic-dependent live or killed *Salmonella* typhimurium. *Comparative Immunology, Microbiology and Infectious Diseases* 18, 27–39.

Mura, D. and Contini, A. (1954) Sorgenti e vie di trasmissione dell'infezione abortovine e caprino da *Salmonella*: importanza del maschio reproduttore. *Veterinaria Italiana* 5, 788–802.

Nikbakht, G.H., Raffatellu, M., Uzzau, S., Tadjbakhsh, H. and Rubino, S. (2002) IS200 fingerprinting of *Salmonella enterica* serotype Abortusovis strains isolated in Iran. *Epidemiology and Infection* 128, 333–336.

Octavia, S. and Lan, R. (2006) Frequent recombination and low level of clonality within *Salmonella enterica* subspecies I. *Microbiology* 152, 1099–1108.

Oloya, J., Theis, M., Doetkott, D., Dyer, N., Gibbs, P. and Khaitsa, M.L. (2007) Evaluation of *Salmonella* occurrence in domestic animals and humans in North Dakota (2000-2005). *Foodborne Pathogens and Disease* 4, 551–563.

Pardon, P., Sanchis, R., Marly, J., Lantier, F., Pépin, M. and Popoff, M. (1988) [Ovine salmonellosis caused by *Salmonella* abortus ovis]. *Annales de Recherches Vétérinaires* 19, 221–235.

Pardon, P., Sanchis, R., Marly, J., Lantier, F., Guilloteau, L., Buzoni-Gatel, D., Oswald, I.P., Pépin, M., Kaeffer, B., Berthon, P. *et al.* (1990a) Experimental ovine salmonellosis (*Salmonella* abortusovis): pathogenesis and vaccination. *Research in Microbiology* 141, 945–953.

Pardon, P., Marly, J., Lantier, F. and Sanchis, R. (1990b) Vaccinal properties of *Salmonella* abortusovis mutants for streptomycin: screening with an ovine model. *Annales de Recherches Vétérinaires* 21, 57–67.

Pardon, P., Sanchis, R., Molenat, G., Marly, J. and Renard, D. (1990c) Serological and allergic reactions of ewes after simultaneous vaccinations with two living attenuated strains of Brucella and *Salmonella*. *Annales de Recherches Vétérinaires* 21, 153–160.

Parkhill, J., Dougan, G., James, K.D., Thomson, N.R., Pickard, D., Wain, J., Churcher, C., Mungall, K.L., Bentley, S.D., Holden, M.T., Sebaihia, M., Baker, S., Basham, D., Brooks, K., Chillingworth, T., Connerton, P., Cronin, A., Davis, P., Davies, R.M., Dowd, L., White, N., Farrar, J., Feltwell, T., Hamlin, N., Haque, A., Hien, T.T., Holroyd, S., Jagels, K., Krogh, A., Larsen, T.S., Leather, S., Moule, S., O'Gaora, P., Parry, C., Quail, M., Rutherford, K., Simmonds, M., Skelton, J., Stevens, K., Whitehead, S. and Barrell, B.G. (2001) Complete genome sequence of a multiple drug resistant *Salmonella enterica* serovar Typhi CT18. *Nature* 413(6858), 848–852.

Pennycott, T.W., Park, A. and Mather, H.A. (2006) Isolation of different serovars of *Salmonella enterica* from wild birds in Great Britain between 1995 and 2003. *Veterinary Record* 158, 817–820.

Perera, K. and Murray, A. (2009) Development of an indirect ELISA for the detection of serum IgG antibodies against region IV of phase 1 flagellin of *Salmonella enterica* serovar Brandenburg in sheep. *Journal of Medical Microbiology* 58, 1576–1581.

Porwollik, S., Boyd, E.F., Choy, C., Cheng, P., Florea, L., Proctor, E. and McClelland, M. (2004) Characterization of *Salmonella enterica* subspecies I genovars by use of microarrays. *Journal of Bacteriology* 186, 5883–5898.

Pritchard, J.A. (1990) *Salmonella* arizonae in sheep. *Canadian Veterinary Journal* 31, 42.

Richards, R.B., Norris, R.T., Dunlop, R.H. and McQuade, N.C. (1989) Causes of death in sheep exported live by sea. *Australian Veterinary Journal* 66, 33–38.

Richards, R.B., Norris, R.T. and Higgs, A.R. (1993) Distribution of lesions in ovine salmonellosis. *Australian Veterinary Journal* 70, 326–330.

Ryder, M.L. (1983) *Sheep and Man.* Duckworth, London.

Sanchis, R. and Pardon, P. (1984) Experimental infection of sheep with *Salmonella* abortus ovis: effect of the gestational stage. *Annales de Recherches Vétérinaires* 15, 97–103.

Sanchis, R., Pardon, P., Abadie, G., Marly, J. and Polveroni, G. (1986) Experimental infection with *Salmonella* abortus ovis in rams. *Annales de Recherches Vétérinaires* 17, 387–393.

Sanchis, R., Pardon, P. and Abadie, G. (1991) Abortion and serological reaction of ewes after conjunctival instillation of *Salmonella enterica* subsp *enterica* ser abortusovis. *Annales de Recherches Vétérinaires* 22, 59–64.

Sanchis, R., Abadie, G. and Pardon, P. (1995) Subcutaneous and conjunctival vaccination with a live attenuated strain of *Salmonella* Abortusovis: effect of gestation on serological response of ewes. *Veterinary Research* 26, 110–115.

Saunders, C.N., Kinch, D.A. and Martin, R.D. (1966) An outbreak of *Salmonella* Typhimurium infection in sheep. *Veterinary Record* 79, 554–556.

Schiaffino, A., Beuzón, C.R., Uzzau, S., Leori, G., Cappuccinelli, P., Casadesús, J. and Rubino, S. (1996) Strain typing with IS200 fingerprints in *Salmonella* abortusovis. *Applied and Environmental Microbiology* 62, 2375–2380.

Sharp, J.C., Reilly, W.J., Linklater, K.A., Inglis, D.M., Johnston, W.S. and Miller, J.K. (1983) *Salmonella* montevideo infection in sheep and cattle in Scotland, 1970-81. *Journal of Hygiene (London)* 90, 225–232.

Sojka, W.J., Wray, C., Shreeve, J. and Benson, A.J. (1977) Incidence of *Salmonella* infection in animals in England and Wales 1968–1974. *Journal of Hygiene (London)* 78, 43–56.

Sting, R., Nagel, C. and Steng, G. (1997) Detection methods for *Salmonella* abortus ovis and examinations in sheep flocks in northern Baden-Württemberg. *Zentralblatt für Veterinärmedizin, Reihe B* 44, 87–98.

Tekin, S. and Hansen, P.J. (2004) Regulation of numbers of macrophages in the endometrium of the sheep by systemic effects of pregnancy, local presence of the conceptus, and progesterone. *American Journal of Reproductive Immunology* 51, 56–62.

Thomson, N.R., Clayton, D.J., Windhorst, D., Vernikos, G., Davidson, S., Churcher, C., Quail, M.A., Stevens, M., Jones, M.A., Watson, M., Barron, A., Layton, A., Pickard, D., Kingsley, R.A., Bignell, A., Clark, L., Harris, B., Ormond, D., Abdellah, Z., Brooks, K., Cherevach, I., Chillingworth, T., Woodward, J., Norberczak, H., Lord, A., Arrowsmith, C., Jagels, K., Moule, S., Mungall, K., Sanders, M., Whitehead, S., Chabalgoity, J.A., Maskell, D., Humphrey, T., Roberts, M., Barrow, P.A., Dougan, G. and Parkhill, J. (2008) Comparative genome analysis of *Salmonella* Enteritidis PT4 and *Salmonella* Gallinarum 287/91 provides insights into evolutionary and host adaptation pathways. *Genome Research* 18, 1624–1637.

Uzzau, S. (2003) *ASM Conference on* Salmonella: *Pathogenesis, Epidemiology, and Vaccine Development*, 20–24 September, Alghero, Italy.

Uzzau, S., Brown, D.J., Wallis, T., Rubino, S., Leori, G., Bernard, S., Casadesús, J., Platt, D.J. and Olsen, J.E. (2000) Host adapted serotypes of *Salmonella enterica*. *Epidemiology and Infection* 125, 229–255.

Uzzau, S., Leori, G.S., Petruzzi, V., Watson, P.R., Schianchi, G., Bacciu, D., Mazzarello, V., Wallis, T.S. and Rubino, S. (2001) *Salmonella enterica* serovar-host specificity does not correlate with the magnitude of intestinal invasion in sheep. *Infection and Immunity* 69, 3092–3099.

Uzzau, S., Marogna, G., Leori, G.S., Curtiss, R. 3rd, Schianchi, G., Stocker, B.A. and Rubino, S. (2005) Virulence attenuation and live vaccine potential of aroA, crp cdt cya, and plasmid-cured mutants of *Salmonella enterica* serovar Abortusovis in mice and sheep. *Infection and Immunity* 73, 4302–4308.

Valdezate, S., Astorga, R., Herrera-León, S., Perea, A., Usera, M.A., Huerta, B. and Echeita, A. (2007) Epidemiological tracing of *Salmonella enterica* serotype Abortusovis from Spanish ovine flocks by PFGE fingerprinting. *Epidemiology and Infection* 135, 695–702.Vanselow, B.A., Hornitzky, M.A., Walker, K.H., Eamens, G.J., Bailey, G.D., Gill, P.A., Coates, K., Corney, B., Cronin, J.P. and Renilson, S. (2007) *Salmonella* and on-farm risk factors in healthy slaughter-age cattle and sheep in eastern Australia. *Australian Veterinary Journal* 85, 498–502.

Walton, J.R. (1972) Bacteriological, biochemical and virulence studies on *Salmonella* dublin from abortion and enteric disease in cattle and sheep. *Veterinary Record* 90, 236–240.

Wirz-Dittus, S., Belloy, L., Doherr, M.G., Hüssy, D., Sting, R., Gabioud, P. and Waldvogel, A.S. (2010a) Use of an indirect enzyme-linked immunosorbent assay for detection of antibodies in sheep naturally infected with *Salmonella* Abortusovis. *Journal of Veterinary Diagnostic Investigation* 22, 531–536.

Wirz-Dittus, S., Belloy, L., Hüssy, D., Waldvogel, A.S. and Doherr, M.G. (2010b) Seroprevalence survey for *Salmonella* Abortusovis infection in Swiss sheep flocks. *Preventive Veterinary Medicine* 97, 126–130.

15 *Salmonella* Infections in Horses

John Timoney*
Gluck Equine Research Centre, University of Kentucky, USA

Historical Perspective

The earliest available records of *Salmonella* infection in horses date to 1893 when Kilborne (1893) and Smith (1893) independently described *Salmonella enterica* serovar Abortusequi-induced abortion in mares in North America. By the 1950s, this host-adapted *Salmonella* sp. had disappeared from the USA following widespread use of bacterin and other control measures. The non-host-adapted serovar *S.* Typhimurium was first recognized as a cause of colitis in 1919 (Graham *et al.*, 1919) and has since dominated globally as a cause of equine salmonellosis. The initial report linked outbreaks of disease with the stress of cross-country rail transportation. A voluminous body of literature has since appeared describing risk factors associated with outbreaks of salmonellosis on breeding farms and in veterinary hospitals. Nosocomial infections involving antibiotic-resistant strains of *S.* Typhimurium and a few other serovars have been a recurring problem over the past 40 years and a serious cause of mortality and source of economic loss (Baker, 1969; van Duijkeren *et al.*, 1994; Ekiri *et al.*, 2010). Antibiotic usage in combination with stressors associated with hospitalization have proved to be potent influences in increasing susceptibility of the horse to invasion by *Salmonella* spp. and in selection of resistant strains. Colitis frequently followed by bacteraemia is the most common clinical manifestation of salmonellosis in adult horses. Bacteraemia/septicaemia, with or without colitis, is commonly seen in foals.

Epidemiology

Salmonella infections occur by ingestion of food or water contaminated by faeces and so transmission is often termed 'faecal–oral'. However, the organism can survive and replicate for long periods in moist environments and so the original faecal source may be remote in time. It should also be mentioned that host-adapted *S.* Abortusequi, now absent from many parts of the world, may attain large numbers in fetal membranes and fluids, which then may be a source for pregnant mares or foals in that herd.

Salmonellosis is most commonly observed on breeding farms and in veterinary hospitals. Foals and young horses on breeding farms are more likely to be affected than adults. Hospitalization and its associated surgical and medical interferences greatly increase susceptibility of horses of all ages to

* Author, e-mail: jtimoney@uky.edu

© CAB International 2013. *Salmonella in Domestic Animals, 2nd Edition*
(eds P.A. Barrow and U. Methner)

Salmonella strains that persist in the hospital environment and/or are cycled through patients during their confinement (Morse *et al.*, 1976b; Kikuchi *et al.*, 1982; Hird *et al.*, 1984, 1986; van Duijkeren *et al.*, 1994; Tillotson *et al.*, 1997; House *et al.*, 1999; Schett *et al.*, 2001; Ekiri *et al.*, 2010). In addition to the stress that predisposes to nosocomial infection in hospitals, transportation, food/water deprivation, anthelminthic administration, poor sanitation, overcrowding, parasite burden, harsh weather, parturition, antimicrobial therapy and gastrointestinal surgery have been associated with onset of clinical salmonellosis (Cordy and Davis, 1946; Owen *et al.*, 1983; McClintock and Begg, 1990).

The protective effect of the gut flora is in part mediated by the inhibitory effects of volatile fatty acids (VFAs) and the low oxidation and reduction potentials they produce in the gut (Meynell, 1963).

Anorexia, antimicrobial administration, intestinal surgery and marked changes in diet increase the susceptibility of horses to *Salmonella* challenge (Hird *et al.*, 1984, 1986; Carter *et al.*, 1986; Traub-Dargatz *et al.*, 1990). Changes in the quality of substrate ingested have profound effects on bacterial and protozoal populations in the large bowel (Argenzio, 1975; Clarke *et al.*, 1990). Concentrate (grain) feeding is associated with an increase in bacterial counts and a reduction in the protozoal counts and pH in the caecum (Goodson *et al.*, 1988). Acetic, propionic and butyric acids are the predominant end-products of carbohydrate digestion, with less lactic and succinic acid present. Increasing concentrations of lactic acid are found when there is an excess of rapidly fermentable carbohydrate (Argenzio *et al.*, 1974; Argenzio, 1975). Reduction of motility favours the growth of anaerobes, such as *Clostridium* spp., and facultative anaerobes, including *S. enterica* (Linerode and Goode, 1970). Feeding following a period of fasting is associated with an increased proportion of soluble carbohydrate delivered to the caecum, thus promoting rapid fermentation and lactate production (Breukink, 1974).

Surveys based on culture of faeces and mesenteric lymph nodes of healthy horses and of animals euthanized for reasons other than enteric disease have revealed a wide range (0–70%) in frequency of positive animals (Smith *et al.*, 1978; Roberts and O'Boyle, 1981; McCain and Powell, 1990). PCR data suggest much higher rates of faecal shedding than are revealed by culture (Cohen *et al.*, 1996; Amavisit *et al.*, 2001; Ward *et al.*, 2005a). This disparity may in part be due to residual DNA, similar DNA sequence from a different intestinal bacterium, or less than optimal enrichment/plating conditions since fewer than 100 organisms g^{-1} faeces are seldom detected by culture. Results of PCR may therefore be misleading and so the gold standard is demonstration of live *Salmonella* in samples from one or more animals in the herd.

Carrier horses are a common source of *Salmonella* spp. for other horses (Bryans *et al.*, 1961; Baker, 1969; Binde *et al.*, 1983; Begg *et al.*, 1988; McCain and Powell, 1990). Bryans *et al.* (1961) showed that foals shed *S.* Typhimurium for many months following recovery from clinical disease. However, the risk that infections acquired from carriers will cause clinical disease in the presence of predisposing environmental or host factors is determined by the virulence and antimicrobial resistance of the *Salmonella* spp. involved.

Transportation and antimicrobial therapy exacerbated the severity of physical disease and shedding in ponies experimentally infected with *S.* Typhimurium (Owen *et al.*, 1983). In another study extending over 5 years on 1931 horses in an extensive-care facility, the stress of hospitalization did not convert healthy carriers of *S.* Typhimurium or *S.* Krefeld into clinical cases although the risk of mortality was greater for horses shedding *S.* Typhimurium (Mainar-Jaime *et al.*, 1998). Nosocomial *Salmonella* infections, although shown to be more frequent in compromised hospitalized horses (House *et al.*, 1999), did not significantly impact the mortality rate of the infected horses.

Horses with colic that undergo abdominal surgery experience different degrees of ileus associated with evacuation of lavage of the large colon or caecum, withholding of feed and anaesthesia. These events result in a patient that is extremely susceptible when exposed to even very small numbers of virulent organisms. In particular, horses with large colon impactions appear to be at greater risk of acquiring nosocomial *Salmonella* infections in a veterinary-hospital environment (House *et al.*, 1999). The frequency of *Salmonella* outbreaks and shedding by asymptomatic horses tends to increase in hot weather (Smith *et al.*, 1978; Carter *et al.*, 1986). In another study, high ambient temperature was a risk factor for nosocomial *Salmonella* infections in hospitalized horses (House *et al.*, 1999). Presumably heat stress impairs host immunity, while at the same time reduction in bacterial generation time increases the environmental challenge dose. A survey conducted in the USA in 1998 showed that *Salmonella* shedding by normal horses increased from 0.2% of the population in winter to 1.1% in summer (NAHMS, 2001). Also, the prevalence of shedding was seven times higher in horses in the northern USA compared to the warmer south.

Although foals born to mares that are shedding *Salmonella* in their faeces are often infected and may become clinically ill shortly after birth, there are no reports of *Salmonella* shedding in the colostrum and milk of these mares. *Salmonella* exposure may result from faecal contamination at birth, coprophagia or during the immediate peripartum period as the foal searches for the udder. Mares shedding at and following parturition are usually asymptomatic (Kikuchi *et al.*, 1982; Binde *et al.*, 1983; Walker *et al.*, 1991). The greater susceptibility of neonates is explained by their incompletely developed immune system and relative lack of competitive gut flora.

Salmonella Abortusequi, the cause of equine paratyphoid, is the sole *Salmonella* host adapted for equids. Once a common infection throughout the world, the organism is now limited to specific locations in Japan, India, Argentina, China and some Balkan and African countries. Infection is acquired by food and water contaminated by infected fetal fluids and membranes. Many of the infections are clinically inapparent and eliminated in a few months by immune responses in healthy animals maintained under good sanitary conditions. Pregnant mares may develop placentitis and abort in the later stages of pregnancy. Immunity developed during these infections is protective and so later pregnancies proceed normally. Host adaptation in combination with effective protective immunity generated by exposure or by use of bacterins seem to have been valuable in eradication of *S.* Abortusequi from the USA, Canada and many other areas of the world over the past 60 years. Studies in Japan have shown that isolates from Japan, Mongolia and Croatia form distinct genetic clusters, reflecting their evolution in isolated geographic areas (Akiba *et al.*, 2003).

A notable feature of the epidemiology of equine salmonellosis in the USA has been the rise and fall in incidence of infection by specific serovars (Fig. 15.1). This may reflect

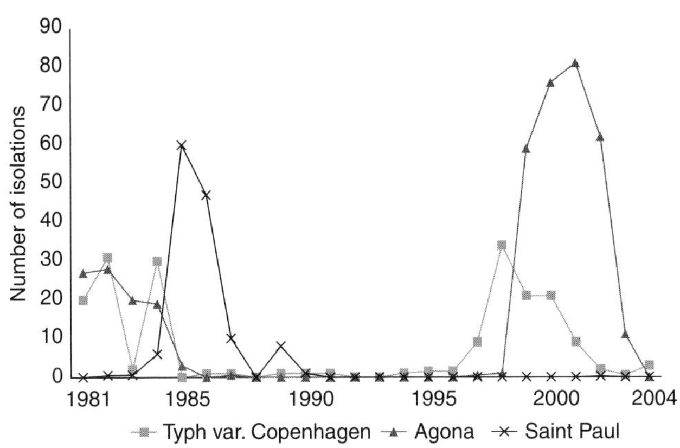

Fig. 15.1. Serovars of *Salmonella enterica* isolated from equine specimens submitted to the Livestock Animal Disease Diagnostic Laboratory, Lexington, Kentucky, USA from 1981 to 2004 (courtesy J. Michael Donahue).

development of herd immunity and/or loss of virulence of the specific serovar. The latter may be driven by the selection pressure of antibody as herd immunity progresses. Local spikes in the frequency of isolation of specific serovars is often correlated with nosocomial outbreaks in local veterinary hospitals wherein there is enhanced transmission. Control measures including closure of affected facilities will reduce the number of new cases ultimately contributing to disappearance of the epidemic serovar.

Although *Salmonella* isolated during nosocomial outbreaks in hospitalized horses are often resistant to antimicrobial drugs, equine isolates in general show lower frequencies of resistance than isolates from swine, poultry or cattle (Timoney, 1978; Vo *et al.*, 2007; Zhao *et al.*, 2007; Veterinary Laboratories Agency, 2008). This reflects the fact that horses are not subject to antibiotic selection pressure via feed and are not usually maintained under conditions of intensive housing that favour transfer of R factors in the local microbial flora.

Nevertheless, isolates in veterinary hospitals frequently contain R plasmids (Sato *et al.*, 1984; Ikeda and Hirsh, 1985; Donahue, 1986; Hartmann and West, 1995; Vo *et al.*, 2007). Some reports, e.g. Vo *et al.* (2007) and van Duijkeren *et al.* (2002), indicate a higher frequency of antibiotic resistance in *S.* Typhimurium than in other serovars from horses. *Salmonella* Typhimurium is usually more virulent for horses than other serovars and so is more likely to be exposed to therapeutic antibiotic selection pressure. The Dutch research also indicates that equine isolates of *S.* Typhimurium have the capability to acquire a variety of integrin-based resistance genes presumably acquired from a range of different microbial sources (van Duijkeren *et al.*, 2002). *Salmonella* Typhimurium DT104 with multiple antibiotic resistance represented 37% of all isolates of this serovar from horses in the UK in 1996.

In the hospital environment, R-factor-based antimicrobial resistance may be passed between *Salmonella* serovars and also between isolates of the same serovar (Ikeda and Hirsh, 1985). Since different resistance genes are usually linked on the same R-factor plasmid, resistance to antimicrobials never used in the clinic may be selected.

Clinical Features

Salmonella infections in the horse produce a wide spectrum of effect ranging from asymptomatic carrier states to invasive septicaemic disease with high mortality. Disease severity is related to the serovar involved, age and immune status and presence of stresses such as anthelmintic administration, hospitalization, high ambient temperature and transportation. Acute severe diarrhoea is the most common manifestation of infection by *S.* Typhimurium, although in young foals, bacteraemia is often present in the early stages of the disease. Low serum IgG is an important risk factor.

Diarrhoea is due to colitis and typhlitis that result in massive rapid fluid and electrolyte losses. There may be cramping and fluid distension of the bowel and signs of colic, which may be evident before onset of diarrhoea. Therefore, horses with colic that are febrile and have a reddened rectal mucosa should be regarded as suspect *Salmonella* cases and checked for neutropenia (Dorn *et al.*, 1975; Smith *et al.*, 1979). Faecal colour may be brown or blood coloured with liquid consistency and foul odour. Protein and fibrin are present as a result of loss of mucosal integrity, which also may predispose to absorption of endotoxin. The resulting endotoxaemia then induces depression, anorexia, poor capillary refill, rapid heart rate, weak pulse and neutropenia. Fluid electrolyte and protein losses lead to dehydration, electrolyte imbalances, acid–base abnormalities and renal shutdown. Foals less than 2 months of age infected with *Salmonella* Typhimurium are likely to become bacteraemic and to exhibit a rapid, weak pulse, and they may either die acutely from endotoxic shock or develop focal organ, bone and joint infections, in addition to experiencing dehydration and electrolyte imbalances, associated with diarrhoea. Focal infections are most common in growth plates (physes) and joints, resulting in arthritis (Morgan *et al.*,

1974; Goedegebuure *et al.*, 1980; Poyade-Alvarado and Marcoux, 1993). Pneumonia, bacterial endocarditis, septic renal infarcts and meningo-encephalitis may also occur (Stuart *et al.*, 1973). Growth plate infections are caused by lodgement of *Salmonella* in metaphyseal vessel loops. Transphyseal vessels connecting the metaphyseal and epiphyseal vessel loops close at 7 to 10 days and so bacterial lodgement is more likely in older foals (Clase *et al.*, 2010).

Horses surviving the acute phase of the disease may progress to a chronic form in which diarrhoea persists for months. The faeces may have a 'cow pie' consistency (Morse *et al.*, 1976b). Some of these chronic cases steadily lose condition until unable to rise. Others may develop colic months after apparent recovery – a result of abdominal adhesions and intestinal scarring (Bryans *et al.*, 1961).

Infection (equine paratyphoid) caused by the host-adapted *S.* Abortusequi is often inapparent until a day or two before the mare aborts. Premonitory signs include slight fever, inappetance and diarrhoea. Abortion most often occurs toward the end of pregnancy. Fetal membranes are oedematous, haemorrhagic and with areas of necrosis. The heart, lungs and spleen may have petechial haemorrhages and fluid may have accumulated in the pericardium and peritoneum. Foals born alive have pneumonia and enteritis. In addition to abortion, *S.* Abortusequi has occasionally been associated with bronchopneumonia, arthritis, bursitis and orchitis. Most often, infection of non-pregnant animals is asymptomatic and cleared in a few months by adaptive protective immune responses.

Clinical Pathology

The most dramatic clinical pathologic changes are neutropenia and/or a toxic left shift, loss of plasma proteins and increase in red blood cell packed volume (PCV). Neutropenia is often quite profound (<1000 neutrophils μl^{-1}) and neutrophils may be vacuolated. Decrease in neutrophils is explained by margination in the splanchnic vasculature, invasion of villous cores and loss into the intestinal lumen. These effects are closely related to the endotoxic activity of the lipid A component of *Salmonella* cell wall lipopolysaccharide (LPS) to which equids are extremely sensitive. Damage to the intestinal mucosa also facilitates entry of bacterial components into the portal bloodstream. Hepatocytes may be irreversibly damaged resulting in marked elevations of serum levels of enzymes, e.g. sorbitol dehydrogenase (SDM) and aspartate transaminase (AST). Dehydration is associated with altered electrolyte levels, blood pH and a pre-renal azotaemia, indicated by elevated blood urea nitrogen and serum creatinine. The prognosis is poor when plasma-protein values decline, PCV increases or a high PCV persists in a patient receiving fluid therapy.

Immune Responses

Resistance to *Salmonella* infection in the immunologically naïve horse is largely dependent on intact innate immunity and a normal intestinal flora. It is unclear how stress adversely affects these defences in the horse.

Serum antibody responses to *Salmonella* infection were first measured by the agglutination and complement fixation tests (Good and Corbett, 1913). These authors showed that serum agglutinins in mares that had aborted due to *S.* Abortusequi infection were elevated 3- to 20-fold compared to levels in normal horses. Complement-fixing antibodies were also significantly elevated. Soon after this time, a vaccine consisting of heat-killed cells of *S.* Abortusequi was shown to be effective in immunizing mares on endemic farms against abortion (Good and Dimock, 1927). Bruner *et al.* (1948) showed that *S.* Abortusequi agglutinins in vaccinated mares were passed in colostrum and that these antibodies persisted for at least 1 month in the foal's serum. Serum agglutinins specific for *S.* Enteritidis and *S.* Typhimurium similar to those induced following infection are induced by immunization with heat killed, formalinized bacterins (Bryans *et al.*, 1961). The relatively insensitive agglutination reaction has been replaced by ELISAs utilizing *Salmonella* sonicates and purified LPS (Sheoran *et al.*, 2001; Gall *et al.*, 2006). Bacterins are effective in stimulating serum antibodies to both O (LPS) and H (flagellar) antigens.

Bacterin-type vaccines have been less effective against disease caused by non-host-adapted serovars, in part because they fail to stimulate cell-mediated immunity and mucosal IgA as generated by infection with live organisms (Mestecky, 1987). To circumvent this problem, a *Salmonella* mutant attenuated by deletion of essential genes *cya* and *crp* has been applied mucosally to induce both cell-mediated and serum and mucosal antibody responses in the horse (Sheoran *et al.*, 2001). Following intranasal administration, a Δ *cya* Δ *crp-pabA* deletion mutant MGN-707 of equine isolate of *S.* Typhimurium UK1 stimulated specific serum IgG and mucosal IgA responses in ponies within 25 days (Tables 15.1 and 15.2).

These antibodies declined slowly over the following 2–3 months but were rapidly recalled to levels higher than originally stimulated following a second intranasal inoculation at 140 days. The isotype profile (elevated IgGa (G1), IgGb (G4), low IgG (T) (G3, 5)) of the antibodies produced indicated the response of the ponies was Th1 biased as expected following infection with live *Salmonella*. Ponies were not challenged with virulent *S.* Typhimurium so protective efficacy of the intranasal vaccine is unknown. Interestingly, a strong response to the second vaccination was not blocked by residual mucosal IgA. The intranasal immunogenicity of MGN-707 is probably accounted for by the presence of M cells in the nasopharyngeal tonsillar epithelium (Kumar *et al.*, 2001). These cells in the intestinal Peyer's patches are well established as preferred sites of entry of *Salmonellae* through the intestinal epithelial barrier with subsequent priming of specific B cells in adjacent lymphoid tissue (Kraehenbuhl and Neutra, 1992). The intranasal vaccine also stimulated *Salmonella*-specific IgA, IgGb (G4) and IgGa (G1) and IgA and IgGb in jejunal and vaginal secretions, respectively, an indication of stimulation of a common mucosal system as well as the possibility of local stimulation of the intestinal mucosal compartment by vaccine organisms swallowed following intranasal administration. The efficacy of a MGN-707 attenuated *Salmonella* expressing SzP of *Streptococcus zooepidemicus* in stimulating remote *Salmonella* and SzP-specific IgA and IgG in the equine uterus has been demonstrated (Causey *et al.*, 2010). No adverse reactions have been recorded in ponies and horses inoculated with MGN-707 and there is no detectable faecal shedding or contact transmission.

The efficacy of attenuated *Salmonella* strains or bacterins other than *S.* Abortusequi in protecting against natural and nosocomial exposure is unknown. Bryans *et al.* (1961) concluded that an autogenous bacterin composed of *S.* Typhimurium and *S.* Enteritidis is effective in stimulating antibody that controlled

Table 15.1. Serum antibody responses to *Salmonella* sonicate of six ponies inoculated intranasally with attenuated *S.* Typhimurium MGN-707 Δcya Δcrp-pab A. Median and ranges of reciprocal ELISA titres are shown (Sheoran *et al.*, 2001).

Day	IgGa (G1)	IgGb (G4)	IgG(T)	IgA
0[a]	0[b]	0[b]	0[b]	0[b]
25	12,800[c,d] (6,400–51,200)	25,600[c,d] (12,800–102,400)	800[c,d] (0–3,200)	6,400[c] (1600–25,600)
69	3,200[d,e] (1,600–6,400)	12,800[d,e] (6,400–25,600)	400[b,d] (0–400)	400[c,e] (400–1,600)
83	3,200[d,f] (1,600–6,400)	6,400[d,f] (6,400– 25,600)	400[b,d] (0–800)	400[d,e] (0–1,600)
140[a]	400[b,e,f] (0–1,600)	3,200[e,f] (3,200–6,400)	0[b] (0–200)	200[b,e] (0–800)
151	102,400[c] (6,400–102,400)	102,400[c] (12,800–204,800)	3,200[c] (0–3,200)	25,600[c] (6,400–51,200)

Values within a column with different superscripts (b–f) are significantly (P <0.05) different.
[a] Days inoculated.

Table 15.2. Nasal mucosal antibody responses to *Salmonella* sonicate of five ponies inoculated intranasally with attenuated *S.* Typhimurium MGN-707 Δcya Δcrp-pab A. Median and ranges of reciprocal ELISA titres are shown (Sheoran *et al.*, 2001).

Day	IgGa (G1)	IgGb (G4)	IgA
0[a]	0[b]	0[b]	0[b]
25	80 (20–320)[c]	160 (40–640)[c,d]	1,280 (0–5,120)[c,d]
69	0 (0–40)[b]	80 (0–160)[b,d]	320 (0–1,280)[b,d]
83	0[b]	0 (0–80)[b]	0 (0–320)[b]
140[a]	0[b]	0[b]	0 (0–160)[b]
151	320 (0–640)[c]	320 (20–640)[d]	1,280 (1,280–10,240)[c]

Values within a column with different superscripts (b–d) are significantly ($P < 0.05$) different.
[a] Days inoculated.

salmonellosis on Kentucky, USA, farms. Nevertheless, given the importance of cell-mediated responses in resistance to *Salmonella*, an effective vaccine should stimulate these responses with the caveat that stress may adversely affect cell-mediated immunity.

Diagnosis

Definitive diagnosis of salmonellosis requires culture of the organism from faeces, blood or tissue by direct plating on selective/differential media and by enrichment and selenite or tetrathionate (10% faeces by volume) followed by direct plating. Suspicious colonies may be checked by slide agglutination with antisera against the O antigens of serovars commonly encountered from equine sources, i.e. Typhimurium, Newport, Enteritidis, St Paul, Agona, Anatum and Heidelberg. Knowledge of serovar(s) circulating in the geographic area will guide choice of O grouping sera for screening unknown isolates. *Salmonella*-like colonies on differential/selective media may also be confirmed using commercially available antibody-based lateral flow platform technology or by DNA hybridization (Reveal 2.0; GeneQuence, Neogen Corporation, Michigan). Culture of faeces from cases of salmonellosis in adult horses is often ineffective for reasons unknown and repeated culturing may be necessary to confirm a diagnosis. Shedding is much more likely to be detected by culture in animals less than 1 year old. Foals are more likely to be positive following culture of blood since bacteraemia is a frequent sequela of intestinal infection. PCR applied to faeces is often 3–5 times more sensitive than culture and has the advantage of providing results within hours of sample submission. Ekiri *et al.* (2010) have provided an excellent evaluation of PCR as a tool in diagnosis and hospital surveillance. Depending on the gene targeted in the PCR, sensitivity ranged from 80 to 100% with a specificity of 86 to 96%. Gene targets have included *spaQ*, *inv*-A, *hisJ* and *invA* (Gentry-Weeks *et al.*, 2002; Kurowski *et al.*, 2002; Ward *et al.*, 2005a; Bohaychuk *et al.*, 2007; Pusterla *et al.*, 2010). However, although PCR appears to be sensitive and specific in experiments incorporating equine faeces samples spiked with known numbers of *S.* Typhimurium, its application in field and hospital surveys has indicated a high percentage of false positives among equine patients with no clinical signs of salmonellosis (Ward *et al.*, 2005b). These workers found that one or more samples from 87 (75%) hospitalized horses were PCR positive yet only 11 (9.5%) of these yielded *Salmonella* spp. on culture. This suggests specificity is in question assuming absence of laboratory contamination. A possible source of error is contamination of reagents with DNA sequences of *Escherichia coli*, since the latter is the usual vector for production of enzymes used in the PCR. It is possible but unlikely that DNA of the target gene persists much longer in the intestine than live *Salmonella* spp. The sensitivity of PCR may be increased by pre-enrichment of the sample before amplification (Pusterla *et al.*, 2010). Development of real-time PCR protocols should be helpful in resolving some of the problems associated with conventional PCR since they would allow an approach targeting more than one gene target and would have reduced risk of laboratory contamination. Finally, it should not be forgotten that direct microscopic examination of stained faecal smears from acute cases of enteric salmonellosis often reveals large numbers of neutrophils.

Therapy

Horses with diarrhoea require aggressive intravenous fluid electrolyte and plasma replacement. These replacement regimes are adjusted based on acid–base and electrolyte data and are complemented by use of anti-inflammatory drugs to mitigate inflammatory cascades initiated by endotoxin and to help prevent laminitis. Endotoxaemia is associated with inadequate perfusion of vital tissues, multi-system organ dysfunction and rapid margination of neutrophils and resulting leucopenia. These effects are seen following systemic invasion of the young foal by *Salmonella* spp. and require prompt administration of antimicrobials based on available information of antimicrobial sensitivity patterns of local isolates. Native *Salmonella* spp. are sensitive to amikacin, gentamicin, third-generation cephalosporins including ceftiofur, chloramphenicol, fluoroquinolones and trimethoprim-sulfonamide. However, multi-resistant strains are frequent in hospital environments and so sensitivity testing must be constantly performed to aid in selection of appropriate antimicrobials. Antimicrobials are strongly indicated in treatment of foals at risk of bacteraemia but are contraindicated in older equids with non-bacteraemic enterocolitis because they seldom alter the course of the disease or reduce faecal shedding and because they may exacerbate the clinical condition should an infectious *Salmonella* spp. have acquired resistance to the antibiotic (Morse *et al.*, 1976a; van Duijkeren *et al.*, 1994). Antimicrobial disruption of the normal defensive intestinal flora is a well-established precursor to *Salmonella* colonization of the intestine and may convert asymptomatic infection to clinical disease.

Pathologic Findings

Salmonella invasion of the intestine results in a fibronecrotic typhlocolitis. Necrosis and ulceration of the mucosa and lamina propria, with severe oedema and congestion of the mucosal and submucosal blood-vessels, may be observed in the small and large colons and caecum. The submucosal lymphoid patches are the most severely affected. The mucosa usually appears congested and covered with a thin film of fibrin. The mesenteric and colonic lymph nodes are often oedematous and congested. Periportal cholangiohepatitis may be present, secondary to the necrotizing process in the gastrointestinal tract. Generalized petechiae and ecchymoses are associated with septicaemia and disseminated intravascular coagulation.

Prevention and Control

The widespread distribution of *Salmonella* spp. in wild and domestic animals and their environment is a significant obstacle to the maintenance of a *Salmonella*-free horse population on a farm or following admission to a veterinary hospital. The origin of infection is often not known in the early stages of an outbreak and so initial control efforts must be focused on strict isolation of clinically suspicious animals with diarrhoea or colic or those known to be shedding *Salmonella* spp. Control measures on farms differ in some important respects from what are required in a hospital environment.

Outbreaks of salmonellosis on horse farms most frequently occur in the summer months, a reflection both of availability of a susceptible population of foals but also of greater activity and numbers of wildlife that may serve as sources of infection. As an example, pigeons are a common source of *S.* Typhimurium var. Copenhagen and so equine cases infected with this variant may have been directly or indirectly infected from this source. Other wild birds and rodents as well as domestic livestock are also possible sources of *S.* Typhimurium and other serovars. Recurrence of outbreaks on the same farm indicates inter-epizootic maintenance in healthy carrier animals. Recovered foals have shed *S.* Typhimurium for up to 14 months (Bryans *et al.*, 1961). Ideally, control of *Salmonella* infections depends on separation of healthy non-infected animals from direct or indirect contact with the organism. Acute cases may shed up to 10^9 cfu g^{-1} faeces and so not only will the organism quickly contaminate the immediate environment but also be widely dispersed on footwear and equipment and by water droplets from hosed surfaces (Hird *et al.*, 1986). Thus, an important element in sanitation of stalls and passages is avoidance of high-pressure water hoses. Compounding the problem is the ability of *Salmonella* spp. to persist for extended periods on moist surfaces.

Identification and isolation of shedder animals is also critical with the caveat that some of these animals are unlikely to be discovered by culture of faeces. Manure from diagnosed and suspect cases should be removed in designated labelled garbage containers and ensiled for at least 6 months to decompose. *Salmonella* spp. are sensitive to 56°C for 5–10 min and so populations on surfaces may be greatly reduced or eliminated by application of steam or hot water (70°C). It should also be mentioned that multiplication in moist environments will occur at warmer ambient temperatures in summer but will be absent at temperatures of 5°C or lower.

During an outbreak, caretakers must wear separate outer distinctive clothing/ boots that are stored at the isolation facility. Disinfectant foot baths and hand-washing facilities must be available at the entrance to the facility.

An extensive literature is available on salmonellosis control and prevention in hospitalized horses (Baker, 1969; Hird *et al.*, 1984; van Duijkeren *et al.*, 1994; House *et al.*, 1999; Dunowska *et al.*, 2007; Ekiri *et al.*, 2009, 2010). Salmonellosis may develop following nosocomial infection acquired in the hospital or by activation of a pre-existing asymptomatic carrier state. Nosocomial infections usually are manifest following hospitalization for 72 h or longer. The causative *Salmonella* spp. is identical (antibiotic resistance phenotype and 'O' antigens) to the clone currently circulating in the hospital. Ideally, all horses should be screened by culture/PCR of faeces at admission to guide discussions about subsequent segregation and need for aggressive environmental decontamination. Animals admitted with clinical signs of salmonellosis (diarrhoea, fever, leucopenia) should be isolated pending laboratory confirmation of diagnosis. The very large numbers of organisms potentially found in the many litres of liquid faeces of horses/foals with enteric salmonellosis make containment efforts exceedingly difficult. Access of rodents/flies will compound the problem. Oral administration of antimicrobials should be avoided where feasible because of the well-established association of antimicrobial therapy and increased risk of nosocomial salmonellosis (Hird *et al.*, 1986). Oral use of the antibiotic to which a *Salmonella* species is resistant has the potential to convert a localized infection into a life-threatening bacteraemia because of its destructive effect on the protective normal flora.

Personnel training is also an important aspect of control. Caretakers and nursing technicians must have an understanding of the ease by which *Salmonella* spp. may be spread in a facility including its zoonotic potential and the measures including change of outer protective clothing and boots, hand washing, avoidance of aerosols, use of dedicated equipment restricted to the facility that are required to prevent escape of the organism or personal contamination. They must be cognizant of the risk of splashes to the face and the need to avoid duty in the isolation facility at times when they are receiving antibiotic treatment.

Autogenous bacterins have been used to aid in control of *S.* Typhimurium and other selected serovars and have been shown to be potent in elicitation of serum antibody to their polysaccharide and protein antigens (Bryans *et al.*, 1961; Bailey *et al.*, 2010). No adverse effects of vaccination have been recorded by these authors other than slight swelling at injection sites in some horses. Vaccination of pregnant mares was effective in elevating colostrum and post-suckling serum antibody levels in their foals (Bailey *et al.*, 2010). It should therefore have value to control of neonatal salmonellosis, since affected foals are often bacteraemic.

Future research must address the efficacy of bacterins and live attenuated vaccines in prevention of *Salmonella* infection on horse farms and in veterinary hospitals. These vaccines have been shown to be safe and potent. Controlled clinical trials that evaluate protective efficacy are potentially more feasible, informative and cost effective than vaccination-challenge experiments that require expensive isolation facilities and study limitations imposed by animal welfare considerations.

References

Akiba, M., Uchida, I., Nishimori, K., Tanaka, K., Anzai, T., Kumoto, Y., Wada, R., Ohya, T. and Ito, H. (2003) Comparison of *Salmonella enterica* serovar Abortusequi isolates of equine origin by pulsed-field gel electrophoresis and fluorescent amplified-fragment length polymorphism fingerprinting. *Veterinary Microbiology* 92, 379–388.

Amavisit, P., Browning, G.F., Lightfoot, D., Church, S., Anderson, G.A., Whitaker, K.G. and Markham, P.F. (2001) Rapid PCR detection of *Salmonella* in horse faecal samples. *Veterinary Microbiology* 79, 63–74.

Argenzio, R.A. (1975) Functions of the equine large intestine and their interrelationship in disease. *Cornell Veterinarian* 65, 303–330.

Argenzio, R.A., Southworth, M. and Stevens, C.E. (1974) Sites of organic acid production and absorption in the equine gastrointestinal tract. *American Journal of Physiology* 226, 1043–1050.

Baker, J.R. (1969) An outbreak of salmonellosis involving veterinary hospital patients. *Veterinary Record* S5, S-IQ.

Bailey, C.S., Fallon, L., Wang, W., Borst, L. and Timoney, J. (2010) Use of a bacterin in pregnant mares to neonatal salmonellosis. *Animal Reproduction Science* 121, 367–368.

Begg, A.P., Johnston, K.G., Hutchins, D.R. and Edwards, D.J. (1988) Some aspects of the epidemiology of equine salmonellosis. *Australian Veterinary Journal* 65, 221–223.

Binde, M., Gronstol, H. and Berg, C. (1983) Outbreak of salmonellosis in horses. *Norsk Veterinaertidsskrift* 95, 627–631.

Bohaychuk, V.M., Gensler, G.E., McFall, M.E., King, R.K. and Renter, D.G. (2007) A real-time PCR for the detection of *Salmonella* in a wide variety of food and food-animal matrices. *Journal of Food Protection* 5, 1080–1087.

Breukink, H.J. (1974) Oral mono- and disaccharide tolerance tests in ponies. *American Journal of Veterinary Research* 35, 1523–1527.

Bruner, D.W., Edwards, P.R. and Doll, E.R. (1948) Passive immunity in the newborn foal. *Cornell Veterinarian* 38, 363–366.

Bryans, J.T., Fallon, H. and Shephard, B.P. (1961) Equine salmonellosis. *Cornell Veterinarian* 51, 467–477.

Carter, J.D., Hird, D.W., Farver, T.B. and Hjerpe, C.A. (1986) Salmonellosis in hospitalized horses: seasonality and case fatality rates. *Journal of the American Veterinary Medical Association* 188, 163–167.

Causey, R.C., Artiushin, S.C., Crowley, I.F., Weber, J.A., Homola, A.D., Kelley, A., Stephenson, L.A., Opitz, H.M., Guilmain, S. and Timoney, J.F. (2010) Immunisation of the equine uterus against *Streptococcus equi* subspecies *zooepidemicus* using an intranasal *Salmonella* vector. *Veterinary Journal* 184, 156–161.

Clarke, L.L., Roberts, M.C. and Argenzio, R.A. (1990) Feeding and digestive problems in horses: physiologic responses to a concentrated meal. *Veterinary Clinics of North America Equine Practice* 6, 433–450.

Clase, K., Gerard, M., Davidson, G. and Schramme, M. (2010) Successful treatment of infectious (*Salmonella* type III:44) polyarthritis and osteomyelitis in a 4-week-old foal. *Equine Veterinary Education* doi:10.1111/j.2042-3292.2010.00152x.

Cohen, N.D., Martin, L.J., Simpson, R.B., Wallis, D.E. and Neibergs, H.L. (1996) Comparison of polymerase chain reaction and microbiological culture for detection of Salmonellae in equine faeces and environmental samples. *American Journal of Veterinary Research* 57, 780–786.

Cordy, D.R. and Davis, R.W. (1946) An outbreak of salmonellosis in horses and mules. *Journal of the American Veterinary Medical Association* 108, 20–24.

Donahue, J.M. (1986) Emergence of antibiotic-resistant *Salmonella* agona in horses in Kentucky. *Journal of the American Veterinary Medical Association* 188, 592–594.

Dorn, C.R., Coffman, J.R., Schmidt, D.A., Gamer, H.E., Addison, J.B. and McCune, E.L. (1975) Neutropenia and salmonellosis in hospitalized horses. *Journal of the American Veterinary Medical Association* 166, 65–67.

Dunowska, M., Morley, P.S., Traub-Dargatz, J.L., Davis, M.A., Patterson, G., Frye, J.G., Hyatt, D.R. and Dargatz, D.A. (2007) Comparison of *Salmonella enterica* serotype Infantis isolates from a veterinary teaching hospital. *Journal of Applied Microbiology* 102, 1527–1536.

Ekiri, A.B., MacKay, R.J., Gaskin, J.M., Freeman, D.E., House, A.M., Giguere, S., Troedsson, M.R., Schuman, C.D., van Charnier, M.M., Henry, K.M. and Hernandez, J.A. (2009) Epidemiologic analysis of nosocomial salmonella infections in hospitalized horses. *Journal of the American Veterinary Medical Association* 234, 108–119.

Ekiri, A.B., Morton, A.J., Long, M.T., MacKay, R.J. and Hernandez, J.A. (2010) Review of the epidemiology and infection control aspects of nosocomial *Salmonella* infections in hospitalized horses. *Equine Veterinary Education* 22, 631–641.

Gall, D., Nielsen, K., Bermudez, R.M., Munoz del Real, M.C., Halbert, G., Groulx, R., Moreno, F., Chow, E.Y. and Checkley, S.L. (2006) Development of an indirect enzyme-linked immunosorbent assay for detecting equine serum antibodies to the lipopolysaccharide of *Salmonella abortusequi*. *Research in Veterinary Science* 81, 215–217.

Gentry-Weeks, C., Hutcheson, H.J., Kim, L.M., Bolte, D., Traub-Dargatz, J., Morley, P., Powers, B. and Jassen, M. (2002) Identification of the two phylogenetically related organisms from feces by PCR for detection of *Salmonella* spp. *Journal of Clinical Microbiology* 4, 1487–1492.

Goedegebuure, S.A., Dik, K.J., Firth, E.G. and Merkens, H.W. (1980) Polyarthritis and polyosteomyelitis in foals. *Veterinary Pathology* 17, 651.

Good, E.S. and Corbett, L.S. (1913) Investigation of the etiology of infectious abortion of mares and jennets in Kentucky. *Journal of Infectious Diseases* 13, 53–68.

Good, E.S. and Dimock, W.W. (1927) Studies on abortion in mares, II. The results of vaccination against contagious abortion in mares. *Journal of the Veterinary Medical Association* 71, 31–34.

Goodson, J., Tyznik, W.J., Cline, J.H. and Dehority, B.A. (1988) Effects of an abrupt diet change from hay to concentrate on microbial numbers and physical environment in the caecum of the pony. *Applied Environmental Microbiology* 54, 1946–1950.

Graham, R., Francois, V.C. and Reynolds, H.K. (1919) Bacteriologic studies of a peracute disease of horses and mules. *Journal of the American Veterinary Medical Association* 56, 378–393.

Hartmann, F.A. and West, S.E. (1995) Antimicrobial susceptibility profiles of multidrug-resistant *Salmonella* anaturn isolated from horses. *Journal of Veterinary Diagnostic Investigation* 7, 159–161.

Hird, D.W., Pappaioanou, M. and Smith, B.P. (1984) Case-control study of risk factors associated with isolation of *Salmonella saintpaul* in hospitalized horses. *American Journal of Epidemiology* 120, 852–864.

Hird, D.W., Casebolt, D.B., Carter, J.D., Pappaioanou, M. and Hjerpe, C.A. (1986) Risk factors for salmonellosis in hospitalized horses. *Journal of the American Veterinary Medical Association* 188, 173–177.

House, J.K., Mainar-Jaime, R.G., Smith, B.P., House, A. and Kamiya, D.Y. (1999) Case-control study of risk factors for nosocomial *Salmonella* infection among hospitalized horses. *Journal of the American Veterinary Medical Association* 214, 1511–1516.

Ikeda, J.S. and Hirsh, D.C. (1985) Common plasmid encoding resistance to ampicillin, chloramphenicol, gentamicin, and trimethoprim-sulfadiazine in two serovars of *Salmonella*, isolated during an outbreak of equine salmonellosis. *American Journal of Veterinary Research* 46, 769–773.

Kikuchi, N., Kawakami, Y., Murase, N., Ohishi, H., Tomioka, Y., Iwata, K., Fujimura, M. and Sakazaki, R. (1982) Isolation of *Salmonella typhimurium* from foals with pyrexia and diarrhoea. *Bulletin of Equine Research Institute, Japan* 19, 43–50.

Kilborne, F.S. (1893) *Bulletin of the Bureau of Animal Industry United States Department of Agriculture* 3, 49.

Kraebenbuhl, J.P. and Neutra, M.R. (1992) Molecular and cellular basis of immune protection of mucosal surfaces. *Physiology Review* 72, 853–879.

Kumar, P., Timoney, J.F. and Sheoran, A.S. (2001) M cells and associated lymphoid tissue of the equine nasopharyngeal tonsil. *Equine Veterinary Journal* 33, 324–330.

Kurowski, P.B., Traub-Dargatz, J.L., Morley, P.S. and Gentry-Weeks, C.R. (2002) Detection of *Salmonella* spp in fecal specimens by use of real-time polymerase chain reaction assay. *American Journal of Veterinary Research* 6, 1265–1268.

Linerode, P.A. and Goode, R.L. (1970) The effects of colic on the microbial activity of the equine large intestine. In: *Proceedings 16th Convention American Association of Equine Practitioners*, Montreal, pp. 321–341.

Mainar-Jaime, R.C., House, J.K., Smith, B.P., Hird, D.W., House, A.M. and Kamiya, D.Y. (1998) Influence of fecal shedding of *Salmonella* organisms on mortality in hospitalized horses. *Journal of the American Veterinary Medical Association* 213, 1162–1166.

McCain, C.S. and Powell, K.C. (1990) Asymptomatic salmonellosis in healthy adult horses. *Journal of Veterinary Diagnostic Investigation* 2, 236–237.

McClintock, S.A. and Begg, A.P. (1990) Suspected salmonellosis in seven broodmares after transportation. *Australian Veterinary Journal* 67, 265–267.

Mestecky, J. (1987) The common mucosal immune system and current strategies for induction of immune response in external secretions. *Journal of Clinical Immunology* 7, 265–276.

Meynell, G.G. (1963) Antibacterial mechanisms of the mouse gut II: the role of EH and volatile fatty acids in the normal gut. British *Journal of Experimental Pathology* 44, 209–219.

Morgan, J.P., van der Watering, C. and Kersjes, A.W. (1974) *Salmonella* bone infection in colts and calves: its radiographic diagnosis. *Journal of the American Veterinary Radiology Society* 15, 66–76.

Morse, E.V., Duncan, A.M., Fessler, J.F. and Page, E.A. (1976a) The treatment of salmonellosis in Equidae. *Modern Veterinary Practice* 57, 47–51.

Morse, E.V., Duncan, M.A., Page, E.A. and Fessler, J.F. (1976b) Salmonellosis in Equidae: a study of 23 cases. *Cornell Veterinarian* 66, 198–213.

NAHMS (2001) USDA National Animal Health Monitoring System. *Salmonella* and the US horse population. Information Sheet, Center for Epidemiology and Animal Health Veterinary Services, USDA–APHIS.

Owen, R.A., Fullerton, J. and Barnum, D.A. (1983) Effects of transportation, surgery, and antibiotic therapy in ponies infected with *Salmonella*. *American Journal of Veterinary Research* 44, 46–50.

Poyade-Alvarado, A. and Marcoux, M. (1993) Haematogenous septic arthritis and osteomyelitis in foals: 39 cases (1985-1989). *Pratique Veterinaire Equine* 25, 275–280.

Pusterla, N., Byrne, B.A., Hodzic, E., Mapes, S. and Jang, S. (2010) Use of quantitative real-time PCR for the detection of *Salmonella* spp in fecal samples from horses at a veterinary teaching hospital. *The Veterinary Journal* 186, 252–255.

Roberts, M.C. and O'Boyle, D.A. (1981) The prevalence and epizootiology of salmonellosis among groups of horses in south east Queensland. *Australian Veterinary Journal* 57, 27–35.

Sato, G., Nakaoka, Y., Ishiguro, N., Ohishi, H., Senba, H., Kato, H., Honma, S. and Nagase, N. (1984) Plasmid profiles of *Salmonella typhimurium* var. Copenhagen strains isolated from horses. *Bulletin of Equine Research Institute* 21, 105–109.

Schett, H.C., Ewart, S.L., Walker, R.D., Dwyer, R.M., Dietrich, S., Eberhart, S.W., Kusey, J., Stick, J.A. and Derksen, F.J. (2001) An outbreak of salmonellosis among horses at a veterinary teaching hospital. *Journal of the American Veterinary Medical Association* 218, 1151–1159.

Sheoran, A.S., Timoney, J.F., Tinge, S.A., Sundaram, P. and Curtiss III, R. (2001) Intranasal immunogenicity of a Δ *cya* Δ *crp-pabA* mutant of *Salmonella enterica* serotype *Typhimurium* for the horse. *Vaccine* 19, 3787–3795.

Smith, B.P., Reina-Guerra, M. and Hardy, A.J. (1978) Prevalence and epizootiology of equine salmonellosis. *Journal of the American Veterinary Medical Association* 172, 353–356.

Smith, B.P., Reina-Guerra, M., Hardy, A.J. and Habasha, F. (1979) Equine salmonellosis: experimental production of four syndromes. *American Journal of Veterinary Research* 40, 1072–1077.

Smith, T. (1893) *Bulletin of the Bureau of Animal Industry, United States Department of Agriculture* 3, 53.

Stuart, B.P., Martin, B.R., Williams, L.P., Jr and Byern, H.V. (1973) *Salmonella*-induced meningoencephalitis in a foal. *Journal of the American Veterinary Medical Association* 162, 211–213.

Tillotson, K., Savage, C.J., Salmon, M.D., Gentry-Weeks, C.R., Rice, D., Fedorka-Cray, P.J., Hendrickson, D.A., Jones, R.L., Nelson, W. and Traub-Dargatz, J.L. (1997) Outbreak of *Salmonella infantis* infection in a large animal veterinary teaching hospital. *Journal of the American Veterinary Medical Association* 211, 1554–1557.

Timoney, J.F. (1978) The epidemiology and genetics of antibiotic resistance of *Salmonella typhimurium* isolated from diseased animals in New York State. *Journal of Infectious Diseases* 137, 67–73.

Traub-Dargatz, J.L., Salman, M.D. and Jones, R.L. (1990) Epidemiologic study of Salmonellae shedding in the faeces of horses and potential risk factors for development of the infection in hospitalized horses. *Journal of the American Veterinary Medical Association* 196, 1617–1622.

van Duijkeren, E., Sloet-van Oldruitenborgh-Oosterbaan, M.M., Houwers, D.J., van Leeuwen, W.J. and Kalsbeek, H.C. (1994) Equine salmonellosis in a Dutch veterinary teaching hospital. *Veterinary Record* 135, 248–250.

van Duijkeren, E., Wannet, W.J.B. and Heck, M.E.O.C. (2002) Sero types, phage types and antibiotic susceptibilities of *Salmonella* strains isolated from horses in The Netherlands from 1993 to 2000. *Veterinary Microbiology* 86, 203–213.

Veterinary Laboratories Agency (2008) Chapter 2.4. In: *Reports of* Salmonella *in Deer, Horses and Rabbits*. Department for Environment, Food and Rural Affairs of the United Kingdom.

Vo, A.T., van Duijkeren, E., Fluit, A.C. and Gaastra, W. (2007) A novel *Salmonella* genomic island and rare integron types in *Salmonella typhimurium* isolates from horses in The Netherlands. *Journal of Antimicrobial Chemotherapy* 59, 594–599.

Walker, R.L., Madigan, J.E., Hird, D.W., Case, J.T., Villanueva, M.R. and Bogenrief, D.S. (1991) An outbreak of equine neonatal salmonellosis. *Journal of Veterinary Diagnostic Investigation* 3, 223–227.

Ward, M.P., Alinovi, C.A., Couetil, L.L. and Wu, C.C. (2005a) Evaluation of a PCR to detect *Salmonella* in fecal samples of horses admitted to a veterinary teaching hospital. *Journal of Veterinary Diagnostic Investigation* 17, 118–123.

Ward, M.P., Brady, T.H., Couetil, L.L., Liljebjelke, K., Maurer, J.J. and Wu, C.C. (2005b) Investigation and control of an outbreak of *Salmonella typhimurium* in a population of hospitalized horses. *Veterinary Microbiology* 107, 233–240.

Zhao, S., McDermott, P.F., White, D.G., Qaiyumi, S., Friedman, S.L., Abbott, J.W., Glenn, A., Ayers, S.O.L., Post, K.W., Fales, W.H., Wilson, R.B., Reggiardo, C. and Walker, R.D. (2007) Characterization of multidrug resistant *Salmonella* recovered from diseased animals. *Veterinary Microbiology* 123, 122–132.

16 *Salmonella* Infections in Dogs and Cats

Malcolm A. Cobb* and Jenny Stavisky
School of Veterinary Medicine and Science, University of Nottingham, UK

Introduction

Salmonella enterica subsp. *enterica* serovars are found worldwide in companion animal populations. Infection is of twofold importance, as they may cause disease in the host species and also have the potential for zoonotic transfer (Wall *et al*., 1996). In cats and dogs this is particularly important given that they often live in close proximity to humans; for example, in a study in the UK, 14% of dog owners reported that their dogs slept on their beds and 11% sometimes or often licked their owners' faces (Westgarth *et al*., 2008).

Carriage of *Salmonella* in dogs and cats may be asymptomatic, with intermittent shedding. Disease occurs intermittently, and ranges from mild to severe gastroenteritis, with occasional occurrence of abortion, systemic spread or septicaemia (Caldow and Graham, 1998; Tauni and Österlund, 2000; Durgut *et al*., 2003; Stiver *et al*., 2003). Infection can also occur in combination with other pathogens, such as endoparasites and feline panleukopenia virus (Fox and Beaucage, 1979). Recovered animals may shed *Salmonella* for several weeks, and chronic carriage with periods of recrudescence is possible. Immunosuppression, for example with chemotherapeutic drugs, has also been associated with shedding of *Salmonella* (Calvert and Leifer, 1982).

A consensus opinion on the diagnosis, epidemiology, treatment and control of the primary enteropathogenic bacteria, including *Salmonella*, in dogs and cats has been published recently (Marks *et al*., 2011). This statement recognizes the challenges associated with making a diagnosis of bacterial-associated diarrhoea in the absence of objective recommendations for faecal testing and the fact that similar isolation rates have been established for putative bacterial enteropathogens in some populations of animals with and without diarrhoea (Sokolow *et al*., 2005; Ojo and Adetosoye, 2009; Stavisky *et al*., 2011).

Serovars and Sources of Infection

All known *Salmonella* are currently thought to belong to one of two species, with a number of subspecies and a wide variety of serological variants or serovars within these. Some serovars have adaptations leading them to favour particular host species, for example *Salmonella* serovar Dublin in cattle; others, such as *S*. Typhimurium, are less selective (van Duijkeren *et al*., 2002). Both selective and

* Corresponding author, e-mail: malcom.cobb@nottingham.ac.uk

© CAB International 2013. *Salmonella in Domestic Animals, 2nd Edition* (eds P.A. Barrow and U. Methner)

non-selective serovars have potential for zoonotic spread, and may also be important in the emergence of antimicrobial resistance in the bacterial population (Lynne *et al.*, 2009).

Serovars may be further subcategorized in several different ways. Phenotypes may be differentiated by antimicrobial sensitivity panels, which may be useful in clinical situations. Phage typing is also commonly used, and relies on using a panel of bacteriophages to lyse bacterial isolates. However, phage typing results may vary between laboratories, and it seems likely that in the future molecular methods will overtake phage typing in the characterization of epidemic strains (Baggesen *et al.*, 2010).

Prevalence, Routes of Infection and Transmission in Dogs

Infection usually occurs orally, via food, water or fomites (Schotte *et al.*, 2007; Finley *et al.*, 2008). Leonard *et al.* (2011) found that contact with livestock, receiving a probiotic in the previous 30 days, feeding a commercial or homemade raw food diet, feeding raw meat and eggs, feeding a homemade cooked diet and having more than one dog in the household were all risk factors for dogs testing positive for the presence of *Salmonella*.

Salmonella can be a cause of enteritis and diarrhoea in dogs, but can also be isolated from the faeces of clinically normal dogs, making the interpretation of the significance of *Salmonella* isolation difficult. Several studies have investigated the prevalence of *Salmonella* shedding in normal, asymptomatic dogs and identified a prevalence typically of between 1% and 4% (Galton *et al.*, 1952; Stucker *et al.*, 1952; Nastasi *et al.*, 1986; Kwaga *et al.*, 1989; Weber *et al.*, 1995; Seepersadsingh *et al.*, 2004; Tsai *et al.*, 2007; Murphy *et al.*, 2009). In animals living outside of the typical 'pet' environment, the prevalence of *Salmonella* spp. shedding may be substantially higher. In a study of dogs in Taiwan, 6.3% (33/491) of stray and shelter-housed dogs were shedding, as compared to 2.1% (9/437) of household pet dogs (Tsai *et al.*, 2007). In a study of stray dogs in Turkey, 11% (9/82) were shedding *Salmonella* in their faeces (Kocabiyik *et al.*, 2006).

A prevalence of 68–79% has been noted in healthy racing sled dogs, and it has been suggested that this is due to the diet these dogs consume, which is based principally on raw meat (Cantor *et al.*, 1997; McKenzie *et al.*, 2010). Similarly, 61% of non-diarrhoeic faecal samples from greyhounds fed raw meat were found to contain *Salmonella* spp. (Stone *et al.*, 1993). It is not known in these circumstances whether the dogs were truly infected and possessed a degree of immunity, or whether the *Salmonella* spp. simply transited through the dogs' gastrointestinal tracts.

The results of a number of more recent studies of the prevalence of *Salmonella* spp. shedding by normal dogs and dogs with diarrhoea are summarized in Table 16.1.

Prevalence in kennelled dogs

Dogs kennelled in military, research or veterinary facilities are generally more likely to be colonized with *Salmonella*. Burgess *et al.* (2004) took environmental samples from locations within a veterinary teaching hospital. From 452 cultured environmental samples 54 *S. enterica* isolates (11.9%) were recovered. Of the environmental isolates, 41 of 54 (75.9%) could be matched to phenotypes of isolates obtained from animal submissions in the month prior to collection of environmental samples. In a similar study, rectal swabs from 100 dogs that were admitted to a veterinary clinic and from 100 randomly selected dogs from one kennel were examined for the presence of *Salmonella* (Bagcigil *et al.*, 2007). *Salmonella* Enteritidis was isolated from a household dog and *S.* Typhimurium was isolated from a dog from the kennel. Wright *et al.* (2005) reported four outbreaks of gastrointestinal illness due to *S.* Typhimurium in employees, clients and client animals from three companion animal veterinary clinics and one animal shelter. More than 45 people and companion animals became ill. In studies of greyhounds in Florida, 3072 cultures yielded 1390 positive specimens and 1741 isolations of *Salmonella*. In addition, the proportion of animals that tested positive increased with the number of examinations, reaching 98% in those cultured five or more

Table 16.1 The results of recent studies of the prevalence of faecal *Salmonella* shedding by clinically healthy dogs and dogs with diarrhoea.

Study	Country	Sample	(*n*)	Proportion positive for *Salmonella* spp.	Method of detection (if described)	Serovars recovered
Holt (1980)	UK	Healthy dogs' faeces	100	1 (1%)		Poona
		Dogs with diarrhoea	100	0		
Nastasi *et al*., 1986	Italy	Dog faeces	212	5 (2.4%)		
Adesiyun *et al*., 1997	Trinidad	Healthy dogs' faeces	65	2 (3.1%)	Culture	Rubislaw
		Dogs with diarrhoea	65	4 (6.2%)		Javiana Virchow Jaminara Rubislaw
Caldow and Graham, 1998	UK	Dog rectal swabs	61	50 (85%)	Culture	Montevideo
Kallo and Hasso, 2001	Iraq	Rectal swabs normal and diarrhoeic dogs	150	17 (11.3%)		Typhimurium Give Enteritidis
Fukata *et al*., 2002	Japan	Healthy dogs' faeces	1013 faeces samples	1/1013 (0.1%)	Culture	Typhimurium
Souza *et al*., 2002	Italy	Rectal swabs normal and diarrhoeic dogs	193	3 (1.6%)		Saintpaul
Kozak *et al*., 2003	Slovakia	Dogs with 'digestive disorder' – diarrhoea not specified	187	1 (0.5%)	Culture	Dublin
Hackett and Lappin, 2003	USA	Normal dogs' faeces	59	1/59 (1.7%)	Culture	Group E
		Diarrhoea	71	2/71 (2.8%)		Group C-1 (1) Unidentified (1)
Maciel *et al*., 2004	Brazil	Dog faecal samples	190	18 (9.5%)	Culture	Gafsa Rubislaw Carrau Houtenae

Seepersadsingh *et al.*, 2004	Trinidad	Healthy dogs' faeces	1391	50 (3.6%)	Culture	28 serotypes: Javiana (12) Newport (6) Arechavaleta (5) Heidelberg (5)
Sokolow *et al.*, 2005	USA	Non-diarrhoeic shelter dogs	60	0	Culture	
		Diarrhoeic shelter dogs	60	0		
Kocabiyik *et al.*, 2006	Turkey	Stray dogs' faeces: healthy	49	6 (12.2%)	Culture	Corvallis
		Stray dogs' faeces: diarrhoeic	33	3 (9.1%)		Corvalis
Bagcigil *et al.*, 2007	Turkey	Faeces from non-diarrhoeic vet-visiting dogs (82)	82	1 (1.2%)	Culture	Enteritidis
		Faeces from diarrhoeic vet-visiting dogs	12	0		Typhimurium
		Faeces from diarrhoeic kennelled dogs	100	1 (1%)		
Verma *et al.*, 2007	India	Rectal swabs	250	1 (0.4%) 6 (2.4%)	Culture PCR	Weltevreden
Tsai *et al.*, 2007	Taiwan	Healthy household dogs	424	8/424 (1.9%)	Culture	Duesseldorf and many others
		Diarrhoeic household dogs	13	1 (7.7%)		Not specified
		Stray dogs (not stated whether diarrhoeic)	491	33 (6.7%)		Dusseldorf and Enteritidis most common
Ojo and Adetosoye, 2009	Nigeria	Non-diarrhoeic dogs	332	17 (3.7%)	Culture	Typhimurium
		Diarrhoeic dogs	126	5 (4%)		

(*Continued*)

Table 16.1 (Continued)

Study	Country	Sample	(*n*)	Proportion positive for *Salmonella* spp.	Method of detection (if described)	Serovars recovered
Tarsitano *et al.*, 2010	Italy	Faecal samples found in public places	152	0	PCR	
Parungao *et al.*, 2010	Philippines	Rectal swabs – normal dogs	62	1 (1.6%) 26 (42%)	Culture PCR	Not specified
Leonard *et al.*, 2011	Canada	Pet dogs' faeces – number with diarrhoea unclear but 'not significantly associated with *Salmonella* carriage.'	138 dogs from 84 households	32/138 (23.2%) (dogs) gave 39 isolates 21/84 (25%) of the households had at least one dog shedding *Salmonella*	Culture	Typhimurium (13/39) Kentucky (6/39) Brandenburg (6/39) Heidelberg (5/39).
Adley *et al.*, 2011	Ireland	Dog rectal swabs	86	0	Culture and PCR	Not applicable
Stavisky *et al.*, 2011	UK	Faecal samples from non-diarrhoeic vet-visiting dogs	147	0	Culture	Not specified
		Faecal samples from diarrhoeic vet-visiting dogs	80	1 (1.3%)		

times (Stucker *et al.*, 1952). Stone *et al.* (1993) reported *Salmonella* in faeces from 11% of asymptomatic greyhounds and 61% of diarrhoeic greyhounds. The same researchers also identified a high prevalence in raw meat from rendering plants, which formed the typical diet for these dogs (Chengappa *et al.*, 1993).

Cantor *et al.* (1997) found a high prevalence of shedding of *Salmonella* in Alaskan sled dogs. Faecal samples from 26 clinically normal dogs were obtained prior to a race and samples from 30 diarrhoeic dogs and 23 non-diarrhoeic dogs were obtained during the race and were tested for a panel of enteropathogens, including *Salmonella*. During the race, 30 dogs with diarrhoea were sampled and 19 of these were positive for *Salmonella* (63%). Of these isolates, ten were *S.* Typhimurium or *S.* Typhimurium var. Copenhagen. Of the non-diarrhoeic dogs, 13/23 (57%) were *Salmonella*-positive (all *S.* Typhimurium or *S.* Typhimurium var. Copenhagen). In a similar study, McKenzie *et al.* (2010) collected freshly voided faeces from 55 dogs before racing and from 80 dogs after 400 miles of racing. Samples were visually scored for diarrhoea, mucus, blood and melaena and cultured for a number of potentially pathogenic bacteria. Diarrhoea occurred in 36% of dogs during racing, and haematochezia, faecal mucus or melaena, or all three occurred in 57.5% of dogs. *Salmonella* was isolated from 78.2% of dogs before racing and from 71.3% of dogs during racing; no significant correlation was found between the presence of diarrhoea and a positive *Salmonella* culture. Finally, Caldow and Graham (1998) investigating an outbreak of abortions in foxhounds, found 50 of 61 faecal samples taken from the affected kennel's samples were positive for *S.* Montevideo.

Dietary sources of *Salmonella* in dogs

Feeding raw meat appears to be a common source of *Salmonella* infection in different populations of dogs (Chengappa *et al.*, 1993). Faecal samples from 200 healthy therapy dogs were collected from each dog every 2 months for 1 year, along with a log of places visited, antimicrobial use within the home, dog health status and diet (Lefebvre *et al.*, 2008). Specimens were cultured for a variety of potentially zoonotic organisms including *Salmonella*. Of the dogs, 40 (20%) were reported to have been fed raw meat at some point during the year. The incidence rate of *Salmonella* shedding in the raw meat-fed dogs was significantly higher than in dogs that were not fed raw meat. Dogs that consumed raw meat were significantly more likely to test positive for *Salmonella* at least once during the year than dogs that did not eat raw meat. Specific *Salmonella* serovars were more common among dogs that consumed raw meat versus those that did not and included *S.* Typhimurium, *S.* Heidelberg and *S.* Kentucky.

Similarly, Lenz *et al.* (2009) explored the impact of feeding raw meat to dogs on the faecal prevalence of several enteric bacterial zoonotic pathogens. Responses to a questionnaire suggested that dog owners were aware of or refused to acknowledge the risks associated with raw meat-feeding. *Salmonella enterica* was isolated from 2/40 (5%) of the raw meat feeds, 6/42 (14%) raw meat-fed dog faeces (but from none of the dogs that did not receive raw meat), 4/38 (10.5%) of the vacuum cleaner waste samples from households where raw meat was fed, and 2/44 (4.5%) of vacuum cleaner waste samples from households where raw meat was not fed to dogs. A study by Joffe and Schlesinger (2002) examined bones and raw food (BARF) diets and faecal samples of dogs consuming them and isolated *Salmonella* from 80% of the BARF diet samples and from 30% of the faecal samples from dogs fed the diet. All food and faecal samples from control dogs fed a variety of commercial dry dog foods were culture-negative.

In kennelled or working dogs, large outbreaks of salmonellosis may occur as the dogs share a common food source and potentially contaminated environment. Schotte *et al.* (2007) reported an outbreak of canine salmonellosis in military dogs due to *S.* Montevideo. *Salmonella* was isolated from faecal samples in 51 out of 80 exposed dogs (63.8%) from four kennels. Most of the infections were clinically silent, but mild diarrhoea without fever developed in only nine dogs from one kennel. Two commercial dehydrated dog feeds were identified as suspected infectious sources and *S.* Montevideo and *S.* Give with similar plasmid profiles and PFGE-restriction patterns were isolated from the suspected dog feeds and faecal samples.

A cross-sectional study examined 138 adult and juvenile greyhound dogs and made observations regarding the environment and took faecal, food and environmental specimens for culture (Morley *et al.*, 2006). *Salmonella enterica* was recovered from 88 of 133 (66%) samples of all types and from 57 of 61 (93%) faecal samples. Of the isolates, 83 (94.3%) were *S.* Newport, 77 (87.5%) of which had identical antibiotic resistance phenotypes. Genetic evaluations suggested that several strains of *S. enterica* existed at the facility, but there was a high degree of relatedness among many of the Newport isolates. Multiple strains of *S.* Newport were recovered from raw meat fed on one day. Finally, Selmi *et al.* (2011) describe an outbreak of canine salmonellosis in a municipal kennel in Tuscany. During the outbreak, 174 samples of 'diarrhetic' (sic) and 'normal' faeces and two batches of commercial dehydrated dog food were cultured for pathogenic bacteria. Of a total of 41 dogs, 25 (60.9%) had at least one faecal sample positive for *Salmonella* while nine of ten samples of dehydrated food were positive. Ten totally different serotypes were isolated from dry food and faeces: the results of the pulsed-field gel electrophoresis (PFGE) referred to similarity between the *S.* Montevideo, *S.* Muenster and *S.* Worthington isolates recovered from both the food and canine faecal samples.

A study by Urban and Broce (1998) set out to determine whether enteric pathogens such as *Salmonella* could be spread to pups through contaminated flies. Flies were trapped or were net-collected from ten dog breeding kennels, identified and counted to determine population numbers, and netted flies were cultured in tetrathionate broth and streaked to medium selecting for *Salmonella* and other lactose-negative Gram-negative bacteria. The most common enteric bacteria found were *Proteus* spp., followed by *Providencia* spp., *Pseudomonas* spp. and *Salmonella* spp., and it was suggested that infection was largely mediated by the flies' access to dog faeces. The apparent high incidence of contamination of flies with enteric bacteria clearly implicates them as vectors of these diseases in kennels.

More recent studies have shown dogs fed raw meat diets can go on to shed the organism in the faeces for a variable period of time. Twenty-eight research dogs were enrolled to determine the prevalence of *Salmonella* shedding after consumption of a *Salmonella*-contaminated commercial raw food diet meal (Finley *et al.*, 2007). Sixteen dogs were exposed to *Salmonella*-contaminated commercial raw food diets and 12 to *Salmonella*-free commercial raw food diets. Seven of the exposed dogs shed *Salmonella* spp. for 1–7 days after consumption of *Salmonella*-contaminated raw food diets. None of the dogs fed *Salmonella*-free diets shed *Salmonella*. No clinical signs were observed in either group. Five of the seven dogs shed the same serovars as those recovered from food samples used for feeding. Dogs fed *Salmonella*-contaminated raw food diets can shed *Salmonella* and may, therefore, be a source of environmental contamination potentially leading to human or animal illness. Previous studies have shown *Salmonella* contamination of commercial meat sold as fit for consumption for humans and dogs. Finley *et al.* (2008) took a total of 166 commercial frozen raw food diet samples purchased from randomly selected local pet stores in three Canadian cities for a period of 8 months. All samples were evaluated for the presence of *Salmonella*, serotyped and tested for antimicrobial susceptibility. The *Salmonella* prevalence was 21% in all samples; chicken was an ingredient for 67% of the *Salmonella*-positive diets. Eighteen different *Salmonella* serovars were recovered, and resistance was observed to 12 of the 16 antimicrobials tested. In contrast, Herrera *et al.* (2009) found no *Salmonella* in 30 samples of commercially available packed dog pellets.

Weber *et al.* (2002) isolated *Salmonella* from 40 (12.3%) of 324 samples of dried dog food made using a variety of bovine and porcine raw materials. In a later study, a total of 240 samples from 20 raw meat diets for dogs, 24 samples from two dry dog foods and 24 samples from two canned dog foods, all purchased commercially on four dates approximately 2 months apart, were evaluated for the presence of a variety of bacteria and protozoal organisms, including *Salmonella* spp. (Strohmeyer *et al.*, 2006). *Salmonella enterica* was recovered from 17 (5.9%) samples, all of which were raw meat products. Similarly, *Salmonella* spp. were detected in five of 25 (20%) commercial raw diets for dogs and cats which were evaluated bacteriologically (one each of beef-, lamb-, quail-, chicken- and ostrich-based diets) (Weese *et al.*, 2005).

Samples of dog chews imported into the UK from Thailand, China, India and Sri Lanka were collected and examined according to the PHLS standard method for the detection of *Salmonella* species by Willis (2001). A total of 2369 dog chew samples were examined over a period of 2 years (1998/2000). Twenty-nine *Salmonella* serovars were detected in 184 samples (7.8%). The most common serovars were Havana and Binza, accounting for 39.7 and 12.5% of isolates, respectively. The contaminant was observed in 26 samples from Thailand, 16 from India, six from China and one from Sri Lanka.

A total of 158 dog treats derived from pig ears and other animal parts were collected and assayed for the presence of *Salmonella* (White *et al.*, 2003). Of these samples, 41% (65/158) were positive for *Salmonella*, and 84 isolates, comprising 24 serovars, were recovered from the 65 positive samples. Fourteen samples were contaminated with more than one *Salmonella* serovar. The majority of *Salmonella* isolates were susceptible to the antimicrobials tested; however, ten (13%) isolates displayed resistance to four or more antimicrobials. Two isolates were identified as *S.* Typhimurium DT104 with the characteristic penta-resistance phenotype (ampicillin, chloramphenicol, streptomycin, sulfamethoxazole and tetracycline). One *S.* Brandenburg isolate was resistant to eight antimicrobials.

Wong *et al.* (2007) examined 300 samples of imported and domestic pet chews bacteriologically and isolated *Salmonella* from 16 (5.3%) of the imported and 20 (6.7%) of the domestic pet chews. *Salmonella* Borreze, which had never been recorded in New Zealand prior to this study, was detected from Australian rawhide. Finally, Adley *et al.* (2011) examined 102 pig ear pet treats in Ireland, and 24.5% of samples were positive for *Salmonella* on culture.

Given the risk of contamination of diets as a consequence of the use of infected raw materials and the time taken typically to culture the organism, several groups have attempted to develop rapid methods of assessing diets for the presence of *Salmonella* spp. Stone *et al.* (1998) developed a PCR-oligonucleotide ligation assay for detecting *Salmonellae* in processed pet food and Maciorowski *et al.* (2000, 2005, 2006) used methods including PCR.

Prevalence, Routes of Infection and Transmission in Cats

Cats have also been shown to carry *Salmonella*. Studies of the prevalence of *Salmonella* shedding in normal, asymptomatic cats have identified a prevalence typically of between 0.8–2.1% in cats (Gow *et al.*, 2009; Nadir *et al.*, 2005; Spain *et al.*, 2001). As discussed above the prevalence of *Salmonella* shedding in cats living outside the typical 'pet' environment may be higher; in one study of laboratory cats sourced from dealers, 15/142 (10.6%) were found to be shedding *Salmonella* spp. (Fox and Beaucage, 1979). The epidemiology, prevalence, clinical signs, diagnosis and pathological findings and sources of salmonellosis in 100 cats in Scotland and England during 1955–2007 were reported by Philbey *et al.* (2009). The most frequent serovars isolated were *S.* Typhimurium, Heidelberg, Dublin, Enteritidis, Choleraesuis, Agona, Arechavelata, Copenhagen, Hessarek, Paratyphi and Newport. Isolates were obtained from the faeces, liver, small intestine, mesenteric lymph node, lungs and spleen. Of the 49 isolates, 28 (57%) were from kittens less than 6 months of age. Shimi and Barin (1977) examined rectal swabs from 301 cats in Tehran, Iran, from two sources. First, a colony of 160 apparently healthy cats from which 15 *Salmonella* spp. (9.4%), mostly *S.* Typhimurium, were isolated. The second source comprised a total of 141 pet cats of which 26 (18.4%) yielded *Salmonella* of 16 different serotypes. In this latter group, 32 cats had gastroenteritis and the rest were apparently healthy. Similarly, Hill *et al.* (2000) assessed the prevalence of enteric zoonotic organisms in cats in north-central Colorado. Serum and faecal samples were obtained from 87 cats with diarrhoea, 106 cats without diarrhoea and 12 cats for which faecal consistency was unknown. Using bacterial culture, *S.* Typhimurium was detected in 1.0% of the samples. A similar prevalence study of several enteric zoonotic bacterial and parasitic infections was conducted in 263 faecal samples from cats that were between 1 and 12 months old, of which 149 were in humane shelters and 114 were presented to primary-care veterinarians (Spain *et al.*, 2001). Of these samples, two (0.8%) were positive for *Salmonella* spp. Van Immerseel *et al.* (2004) evaluated rectal-swab specimens from cats and found that 18 (51.4%) of 35 group-housed cats, five (8.6%) of 58 diseased cats (5/58), and one (0.36%) of 278 healthy house cats excreted *Salmonella* spp.; the most frequently isolated serovars were *S.* Typhimurium, Enteritidis and Bovismorbificans. Gow *et al.* (2009) collected faecal samples from 57 clinically healthy kittens presented for initial vaccination in the UK. Routine bacteriological examination identified *Salmonella* species in only one sample. Seepersadsingh *et al.* (2005) sampled 94 non-diarrhoeic cats in Trinidad and found two (2.1%) were positive for *Salmonella* with two serovars identified, *S.* Johannesburg and a serovar belonging to Group C. In most of these cases, the feeding of a contaminated diet did not result in clinical disease, but the practice of feeding raw meat-based diets to two co-habiting domestic cats has resulted in clinical gastro-enteric salmonellosis and septicaemia (Stiver *et al.*, 2003). Both cats were fed a home-prepared, raw meat-based diet and *S.* Newport was isolated from multiple organs in both cats and from samples of the diet.In terms of their role in the transmission of salmonellosis, cats were found to be the most abundant ecological compartment (125 of all samples positive) in a 2-year survey of the distribution of *Salmonella* on 12 pig production units in the USA (Barber *et al.*, 2002). In addition, the presence of cats on the farm was identified as a significant risk factor for outbreaks of clinical salmonellosis on Dutch dairy farms (Veling *et al.*, 2002).

Tauni and Österlund (2000) described an outbreak of *S.* Typhimurium in cats and humans associated with infection in wild birds in Sweden in 1999. A total of 62 sick cats were examined. All were anorectic and lethargic, 57% were vomiting and 31% had diarrhoea. It was considered likely that salmonellosis was transmitted from cats to humans, but there were only a few such cases. Similarly, Hauser *et al.* (2009) isolated similar strains of *Salmonella* from humans, birds and cats and suggested cats could play a role in transmitting the organisms from wild birds to humans. Philbey *et al.* (2008) isolated wild bird strains of *S.* Typhimurium from nine cats with enteric disease, all of which had a history of hunting birds. Finally, Taylor and Philbey (2010) confirmed that cats can be infected with *S.* Typhimurium DT40 by catching and eating garden birds, and suggested that both cats and the garden environment are a potential source of infection for human beings.

Gastroenteritis caused by a multidrug-resistant *S.* Typhimurium was diagnosed in a 12-week-old kitten (Wall *et al.*, 1995), which recovered from the acute episode but continued to shed the organism in its faeces for a further 12 weeks. Carriage was finally cleared by administering a 14-day course of treatment with parenteral enrofloxacin.

These studies suggest that *Salmonella* shedding is relatively rare in cats and that clinical signs such as diarrhoea are not reliable predictors of whether a cat is actively shedding enteric organisms. However, when infection does occur, cats may play an important role in the transmission of the organism.

Pathogenesis

As discussed above, the prevalence of *Salmonella* spp. in healthy dogs and cats is very similar to the prevalence in diarrhoeic dogs and cats while the prevalence in stray or kennelled dogs and cats is often higher. In addition, the prevalence of *Salmonella* has also been shown to be much higher in dogs that are fed raw food diets; however, in most cases following exposure to *Salmonella*, the organism is eventually cleared by the host's defences. Infection in dogs and cats therefore is generally subclinical, but in a small proportion of cases the organism may survive leading to the establishment of a carrier state (Tanaka *et al.*, 1976; Sugiyama *et al.*, 1993; van Duijkeren and Houwers, 2002). A range of predisposing causes can then precipitate clinical salmonellosis in a carrier animal. The likelihood of an infected host developing disease is determined by the balance between the host's innate defence and capacity to mount an immune response clinical disease has been particularly reported in hospitalized patients, particularly when stressed (Burnie *et al.*, 1983), young (Barrs *et al.*, 1999; Perkins *et al.*, 2004) or immunosuppressed (Foley *et al.*, 1999; Bhaiyat *et al.*, 2009) and the virulence of the organism, which in turn is determined by the particular strain involved, the infectious dose and the presence or absence of virulence genes.

Clinical Signs

Clinical salmonellosis is rare in healthy, adult dogs and cats; most infections do not result in the development of clinical signs. *Salmonella* gastroenteritis is uncommon in dogs, generally accounting for <3% of cases of canine diarrhoea (Cave *et al.*, 2002; Hackett and Lappin, 2003; Marks and Kather, 2003). Descriptions of clinical signs associated with *Salmonella* infection in dogs and cats are limited to individual case reports and case series (Wall *et al.*, 1995; Sato and Kuwamoto, 1999; Philbey *et al.*, 2009) and occasional reports of outbreaks in kennelled populations of dogs (Wright *et al.*, 2005; Schotte *et al.*, 2007; Selmi *et al.*, 2011) or cats or veterinary facilities (Tauni and Österlund, 2000).

Clinical signs reported in affected individuals are variable but include acute onset pyrexia, anorexia, abdominal pain, diarrhoea, which is often haemorrhagic, and vomiting, individuals may become systemically ill as a consequence of septicaemia and endotoxaemia. Individual cases describing the isolation of *Salmonella* spp. infection include conjunctivitis, osteomyelitis and meningitis (Fox *et al.*, 1984; Perkins *et al.*, 2004), pneumonia (Foster *et al.*, 2004), pyothorax (Barrs *et al.*, 2005), pyelonephritis, cholangiohepatitis (Brain *et al.*, 2006), orchitis (Fukuyama *et al.*, 1999) and reproductive failure (Caldow and Graham, 1998).

Recovery normally occurs over days or weeks, depending on the severity of clinical signs. Recovered animals may shed *Salmonella* spp. for several weeks, and chronic carriage with recrudescence during stress can be a feature of salmonellosis in some host species such as the horse (Feary and Hassel, 2006); it has been suggested that this may also occur in dogs (German, 2005).

Diagnosis

Diagnosis is usually made based on growth and identification of the causative organism from a faecal or rectal swab or from a faecal sample or other appropriate sample initially grown in enrichment broth followed by subculture on to a selective agar. Serovars are identified by serotyping and by using a panel of biochemical tests. Submission of faecal samples from dogs and cats with acute and chronic diarrhoea for culture to identify potentially enteropathogenic bacteria is common in small animal practice. In suspected cases of salmonellosis, multiple or pooled samples may be submitted to improve the likelihood of recovering the causative organism. Of 6589 faecal samples from diarrhoeic dogs examined in one veterinary laboratory only 69 (1%) yielded *Salmonella* (van Duijkeren and Houwers, 2002). As discussed, the isolation of *Salmonella* from faecal samples from dogs with gastrointestinal disease does not necessarily mean the organism is responsible for the clinical signs, as *Salmonella* are occasionally isolated from the faeces of apparently healthy dogs. Nevertheless, culture may be useful in procuring isolates for the application of molecular techniques for detection of specific virulence genes or molecular typing of isolated strains to establish clonality in suspected outbreaks.

The diagnostic value of running a faecal panel that assesses a faecal sample or samples from dogs or cats with diarrhoea for a variety of enteropathogenic bacteria appears to very low (Cave *et al.*, 2002). Given the poor sensitivity and the time taken to get a test result using conventional culture methods there has been significant interest in the utility of more sensitive and rapid molecular methods that have been developed within the last few years such as variable number of tandem repeats (VNTR), real-time PCR and PFGE (Ward *et al.*, 2005; Bohaychuk *et al.*, 2007; Baggesen *et al.*, 2010).

Treatment

The use of antimicrobials is not generally advised in uncomplicated episodes of *Salmonella* infection. Instead, supportive therapy based around correction and maintenance of fluid and electrolyte balance is recommended. Antimicrobials may be indicated in animals that are systemically ill or immunocompromised, and ideally antimicrobial selection should be based on susceptibility testing of isolated organisms; however, empirically, a combination of ampicillin and enrofloxacin is often advised.

Resistance of *Salmonella* isolated from dogs and cats to some classes of antimicrobial has been shown to be comparatively high in some studies. Among 54 *Salmonella* isolates recovered from wildlife including stray dogs, 50 (92.6%) were resistant to tetracycline and streptomycin, 47 (87.0%) to nalidixic acid, 35 (64.8%) to kanamycin and 26 (48.1%) to neomycin (Adesiyun, 1999). Kallo and Hasso (2001) tested 17 isolates from 150 normal and diarrhoeic dogs and found them all to be sensitive to gentamicin and 97.1% of isolates were sensitive to chloramphenicol. Ojo and Adetosoye (2009) demonstrated a similarly high susceptibility to chloramphenicol (89.2%) and ciprofloxacin (100%) in *S.* Typhimurium isolates, but all isolates were resistant to erythromycin and cloxacillin; resistance was also exhibited to tetracycline (70.6%), ampicillin (47.1%), cefuroxime (52.9%), amoxicillin (35.3%), cotrimoxazole (76.5%), augmentin (52.9%), gentamicin (35.3%) and streptomycin (35.3%).

Six of the seven *S.* Typhimurium DT56V isolates from cats in the study by Philbey *et al.* (2008) were sensitive to ampicillin, cefotaxime, chloramphenicol, ciprofloxacin, furazolidone, gentamicin, kanamycin, nalidixic acid, netilmicin, spectinomycin, streptomycin, sulfonamide, tetracycline and trimethoprim.

Prevention

Studies have been performed to assess the ability of prebiotics and probiotics to prevent the development of clinical salmonellosis in treated individuals. Apanavicius *et al.* (2007) showed that fructan supplementation appeared to attenuate some of the negative responses associated with *Salmonella* challenge and may provide protection against infection in weanling puppies. Food intake decreased and body temperature increased in puppies experimentally infected with *S.* Typhimurium DT104. However, the decrease in food intake and the severity of enterocyte sloughing was less severe in the treated puppies than in those fed the control diet. Another study, however, demonstrated that while an 18-day application of the probiotic *Enterococcus faecium* product did indeed induce changes in the gastrointestinal microflora in all treated dogs, *Salmonella* spp. and *Campylobacter* spp. counts were higher in most dogs post-treatment than they were before the application (Vahjen and Manner, 2003).

It has been suggested that isolation and screening of Lactobacilli and Bifidobacteria adherent to healthy canine gastrointestinal tissue might yield strains with commensal activity in dog. To this end canine-derived bacterial strains with commensal traits have been isolated and *Bifidobacterium animalis* AHC7 has been shown to have significant potential for improving canine gastrointestinal health, having been shown to adhere to epithelial cells, transit the gastrointestinal tract in high numbers and significantly lead to reduced *S.* Typhimurium translocation in an experimental mouse model (O'Mahony *et al.*, 2009). However, its clinical application in the dog remains to be assessed.

The chi4127-attenuated strain of *S.* Typhimurium has demonstrated potential for use as a vaccine for canine salmonellosis. In oral challenge experiments, morbidity in the dogs challenged with wild-type *S.* Typhimurium was 8.3% in immunized dogs but 100% in the non-vaccinated controls. Of the 12 control dogs, nine developed both gastrointestinal and respiratory tract signs with pyrexia that persisted through 5 days after challenge. Serum IgG response against *S.* Typhimurium lipopolysaccharide significantly increased in vaccinated dogs and in non-vaccinated dogs after challenge and the non-vaccinated dogs had 3 to 4 logs higher numbers of *S.* Typhimurium in splenic and hepatic tissue than did the vaccinated dogs (McVey *et al.*, 2002).

Human Health Implications

Human salmonellosis occurs mainly as a result of handling or consuming contaminated food products. A small percentage of cases are related to other, less well-defined exposures, such as contact with companion animals. Transmission of *Salmonella* from pets (chicken, dog, cat, rabbit, rodent, ferret, turtle, iguana and other reptiles) is reported to account for 15–20% of total cases of *Salmonella* spp. infection in humans (Plaut *et al.*, 1996) and it is estimated that 1% of the number of cases of salmonellosis reported annually in the USA are associated with contact with companion animals (Stehr-Green and Schantz, 1987). Infection can be transmitted by direct or indirect contact (e.g. with water in which pets swim or which they drink) and a number of pet-associated cases are in children aged 1–9 years (Sato *et al.*, 2000). Birnbaum *et al.* (1980) published a case report describing a facial infection due to *S.* Typhimurium, caused by bites from the family's pet dog. Westgarth *et al.* (2008) investigated the nature and frequency of the contacts that occur between dogs, and between dogs and people, by means of a questionnaire survey of 260 dog-owning households in a community in Cheshire, UK. The contacts were highly variable and were affected by the size, sex and age of the dog, individual dog behaviours, human behaviours and human preferences in the management of the dog. A number of situations were identified that may be important in relation to zoonoses, including sleeping areas, playing behaviours, greeting behaviours, food sources, walking, disposal of faeces, veterinary preventive treatment and general hygiene.

Behravesh *et al.* (2010) investigated an outbreak of *S.* Schwarzengrund primarily affecting young children. Affected households were significantly more likely than control households to report dog contact and to have recently purchased a particular brand of dry pet food. Illness among infant case-patients was significantly associated with feeding pets in the kitchen and the outbreak strain was isolated from opened bags of dry dog food and faecal samples from dogs that ate it. In 2004–2005, contact with *Salmonella*-contaminated pet treats of beef and seafood origin resulted in nine cases of human *S.* Thompson infections in the USA and in western Canada (Brisdon *et al.*, 2006). The increasing popularity of raw food diets and natural pet treats for companion animals is another potential pet-associated source of *Salmonella* organisms; however, pets that consume contaminated pet treats and raw food diets can be colonized with the organism without exhibiting clinical signs, making them a possible hidden source of contamination in the household (Finley *et al.*, 2006, 2007). Bacterial contamination, including *Salmonella*, is common in commercially available raw meat diets (Strohmeyer *et al.*, 2006).

Another 2001 study investigating a dramatic rise in the incidence of *S.* Infantis infections in humans in Alberta, Canada, established that the outbreak was associated with pet treats for dogs produced from processed pig ears (Clark *et al.*, 2001). Laboratory investigations using phage typing and PFGE established that isolates from the ear treats and humans exposed to the treats comprised a well-defined subset of all isolates analysed. Of the 53 subtypes of *S.* Infantis obtained around the time of the outbreak as defined by PFGE and phage typing, only six subtypes were associated with both human infection and isolation from pig ears. During the course of this outbreak, several other *Salmonella* serovars were also isolated from pet treats, suggesting these products may be an important source of enteric infection in both humans and dogs.

Subsequently, Pitout *et al.* (2003) described human infections with a multidrug-resistant strain of *S.* Newport phage type 14 related to the handling of pet treats containing dried beef. These strains were isolated from five patients in Canada during 2002 and were compared to a strain cultured from a commercial pet treat present at the property of one of the patients. All strains were shown to express the plasmid-encoded AmpC β-lactamase, CMY-2. PFGE showed the human and pet treat *Salmonella* strains to be highly related.

Pet-assisted therapy (PAT) is becoming increasingly common in hospitals and care homes, but the risks to patient health associated with this activity, particularly among those patients who are immunocompromised, has received relatively little attention. One cross-sectional study evaluated the prevalence of zoonotic agents in a group of 102 PAT dogs from a variety of sources (Lefebvre *et al.*, 2006). Owners were interviewed using a questionnaire while dogs underwent a physical examination. A specimen of faeces, hair-coat brushings and one rectal, aural, nasal, oral and pharyngeal swab were collected from each dog and tested for 18 specific pathogens. All dogs were judged to be in good health clinically. Zoonotic agents were isolated from 80 out of 102 (80%) dogs. The primary pathogen was *Clostridium difficile*, which was isolated from 58 (58%) faecal specimens, but organisms of the genus *Salmonella* were isolated from three (3%) dogs. Two hundred healthy PAT dogs were enrolled in a Canadian study (Lefebvre *et al.*, 2008); faecal samples were collected from each dog every 2 months for 1 year, and a record kept of places visited, antimicrobial use within the home, dog health status and diet. Specimens were cultured for a variety of potential zoonotic pathogens including *Salmonella*. Of the dogs, 40 (20%) were reported to have been fed raw meat at some point during the year. The incidence rate of *Salmonella* shedding was significantly greater in the raw meat-fed dogs than in dogs that were not fed raw meat. Dogs that consumed raw meat were significantly more likely to test positive for *Salmonella* at least once during the year than dogs that did not eat raw meat. It has been suggested therefore that dogs fed raw meat should not be entered into PAT programmes, particularly when the programmes involve interaction with humans at high risk of infection, and also that the feeding of raw meat to pets should perhaps be avoided in homes in which immunocompromised people live.

In 1999 and 2000, three US state health departments reported four outbreaks of gastrointestinal illness due to *S.* Typhimurium in employees, clients and client-owned animals from three companion animal veterinary clinics and one animal shelter (Wright *et al.*, 2005). Forty-seven people and several companion animals became ill. Four independent investigations resulted in the testing of 19 human samples and over 200 animal samples; 18 persons and 36 animals were culture-positive for *S.* Typhimurium. One outbreak was due to multidrug-resistant *S.* Typhimurium R-type ACKSSuT, while the other three were due to multidrug-resistant *S.* Typhimurium R-type ACSSuT DT104. This report documents nosocomial transmission of *S.* Typhimurium and demonstrates that companion animal facilities may serve as foci of transmission for *Salmonella* between animals and humans if adequate precautions are not followed. Similarly, Cherry *et al.* (2004) reported an outbreak of disease associated with *S.* Typhimurium in a veterinary clinic in the USA where seven people (two technicians, four people associated with clinic patients and a nurse not linked to the clinic) in addition to a cat were all affected. Murphy *et al.* (2010) found that 2% of environmental swabs submitted for culture for a range of zoonotic organisms from 101 community veterinary hospitals were positive for *Salmonella*, suggesting the presence of an environmental reservoir of pathogens in veterinary hospitals. Maha and Lotfy (2009) confirmed the presence of *Salmonella* in 20% of kennel attendants, 33.3% of puppies and 41.67% of dogs in one kennel, again confirming that captive dogs can act as a potential source of zoonotic pathogen. As indicated above, contact with livestock, receiving a probiotic in the previous 30 days, feeding a commercial or homemade raw food diet, feeding raw meat and eggs, feeding a homemade cooked diet, and having more than one dog in the household have all been shown to be management factors associated with the presence of *Salmonella* spp. in the faeces of household dogs (Leonard *et al.*, 2011). Finally, a total of 123 children with laboratory-confirmed *Salmonella* infections were shown by multivariable analysis matched on age group to have contact with reptiles and cats more commonly than 139 age-matched control children who had not experienced symptoms of gastrointestinal illness (Younus *et al.*, 2010).

Conclusion

In summary, the prevalence of *Salmonella* infection in healthy dogs and cats is very similar to the prevalence in diarrhoeic dogs, and in most populations is likely to be under 4%. The prevalence of *Salmonella* infection in stray or kennelled dogs and cats is often higher. Most cases of salmonellosis in dogs and cats are sub-clinical. Following exposure to *Salmonella*, the organism is generally cleared by the host's defences. However, in a small proportion of cases the organism may survive leading to the establishment of a carrier state.

Salmonella infection is a rare cause of clinical signs in healthy, adult dogs and cats. When clinical signs do occur, signs of gastroenteritis, including vomiting, diarrhoea, inappetance and lethargy may occur. However, infection may occur in almost any body system, and CNS, ocular and urogenital infections have been reported.

Salmonella have been isolated from a high proportion of raw meat-based diets and pet treats of animal origin, and the prevalence of *Salmonella* infection has been shown to be much higher in dogs that are fed raw food diets.

A small percentage of cases of human salmonellosis are related to contact with infected dogs and cats. These usually occur as a result of closely sharing an environment with an infected animal or its contaminated food, and therefore owners of infected dogs and animal health professionals are likely to be at the highest risk of zoonotic transfer.

References

Adesiyun, A.A. (1999) Antibiograms of thermophilic *Campylobacter* and *Salmonella* species isolated from stray and pet animals and wildlife on Trinidad. *Veterinarski Arhiv* 69, 229–237.

Adesiyun, A.A., Campbell, M. and Kaminjolo, J.S. (1997) Prevalence of bacterial enteropathogens in pet dogs in Trinidad. *Journal of Veterinary Medicine Series B* 44, 19–27.

Adley, C., Dillon, C., Morris, C.P., Delappe, N. and Cormican, M. (2011) Prevalence of *Salmonella* in pig ear pet treats. *Food Research International* 44, 193–197.

Apanavicius, C.J., Powell, K.L., Vester, B.M., Karr-Lilienthal, L.K., Pope, L.L., Fastinger, N.D., Wallig, M.A., Tappenden, K.A. and Swanson, K.S. (2007) Fructan supplementation and infection affect food intake, fever, and epithelial sloughing from *Salmonella* challenge in weanling puppies. *Journal of Nutrition* 137, 1923–1930.

Bagcigil, A.F., Ikiz, S., Dokuzeylu, B., Basaran, B., Or, E. and Ozgur, N.Y. (2007) Fecal shedding of *Salmonella* spp. in dogs. *The Journal of Veterinary Medical Science* 69, 775–777.

Baggesen, D.L., Sorensen, G., Nielsen, E.M. and Wegener, H.C. (2010) Phage typing of *Salmonella* Typhimurium – is it still a useful tool for surveillance and outbreak investigation? *Eurosurveillance* 15, 19471.

Barber, D.A., Bahnson, P.B., Isaacson, R., Jones, C.J. and Weigel, R.M. (2002) Distribution of *Salmonella* in swine production ecosystems. *Journal of Food Protection* 65, 1861–1868.

Barrs, V.R., Swinney, G.R., Martin, P. and Nicoll, R.G. (1999) Concurrent *Aelurostrongylus abstrusus* infection and salmonellosis in a kitten. *Australian Veterinary Journal* 77, 229–232.

Barrs, V.R., Allan, G.S., Martin, P., Beatty, J.A. and Malik, R. (2005) Feline pyothorax: a retrospective study of 27 cases in Australia. *Journal of Feline Medicine and Surgery* 7, 211–222.

Behravesh, C.B., Ferraro, A., Deasy, M.R., Dato, V., Moll, M., Sandt, C., Rea, N.K., Rickert, R., Marriott, C., Warren, K.Y., Urdaneta, V., Salehi, E., Villamil, E., Ayers, T., Hekstra, R.M., Austin, J.L., Ostroff, S. and

Williams, I.T. (2010) Human *Salmonella* infections linked to contaminated dry dog and cat food, 2006-2008. *Pediatrics* 126, 477–483.

Bhaiyat, M.I., Hariharan, H., Chikweto, A., Brathwaite-Sylvester, E., Burnett, P.J.A., Matthew, V., Oliveira, S. and Johnson, C. (2009) Concurrent lymphosarcoma and *Salmonella enteritidis* infection in a cat: a case report. *Veterinarni Medicina* 54, 451–454.

Birnbaum, M., Miller, K. and Stratigos, G.T. (1980) *Salmonella typhi* facial infection. Report of case. *Oral Surgery, Oral Medicine and Oral Pathology* 49, 219–220.

Bohaychuk, V.M., Gensler, G.E., McFall, M.E., King, R.K. and Renter, D.G. (2007) A real-time PCR assay for the detection of *Salmonella* in a wide variety of food and food-animal matricest. *Journal of Food Protection* 70, 1080–1087.

Brain, P.H., Barrs, V.R., Martin, P., Baral, R., White, J.D. and Beatty, J.A. (2006) Feline cholecystitis and acute neutrophilic cholangitis: clinical findings, bacterial isolates and response to treatment in six cases. *Journal of Feline Medicine and Surgery* 8, 91–103.

Brisdon, S., Galanis, E., Colindres, R., Crowe, L., McIntyre, L., Baer, R., MacDougall, L., Wilcott, L., Gustafson, L., Paccagnella, A., Chui, L., Everett, D., MacDonald, D., Ellis, A., Leslie, M., Keys, C.E., Ekperigin, H., Collins, M.L., Drake, A., Koepsell, J., Debolt, C., McKeirnan, S., Duchin, J., Johnson, J.M. and Farmer, D.E. (2006) An international outbreak of human salmonellosis associated with animal-derived pet treats – Canada and Washington State, 2005. *Canada Communicable Disease Report* 32, 150–155.

Burgess, B.A., Morley, P.S. and Hyatt, D.R. (2004) Environmental surveillance for *Salmonella enterica* in a veterinary teaching hospital. *Journal of the American Veterinary Medical Association* 225, 1344–1348.

Burnie, A., Simpson, J., Lindsay, D. and Miles, R. (1983) The excretion of campylobacter, salmonellae and<u>Giardia lamblia</u> in the faeces of stray dogs. *Veterinary Research Communications* 6, 133–138.

Caldow, G.L. and Graham, M.M. (1998) Abortion in foxhounds and a ewe flock associated with *Salmonella montevideo* infection. *Veterinary Record* 142, 138–139.

Calvert, C.A. and Leifer, C.E. (1982) Salmonellosis in dogs with lymphosarcoma. *Journal of the American Veterinary Medical Association* 180, 56–58.

Cantor, G.H., Nelson, S. Jr, Vanek, J.A., Evermann, J.F., Eriks, I.S., Basaraba, R.J. and Besser, T.E. (1997) *Salmonella* shedding in racing sled dogs. *Journal of Veterinary Diagnostic Investigation* 9, 447–448.

Cave, N.J., Marks, S.L., Kass, P.H., Melli, A.C. and Brophy, M.A. (2002) Evaluation of a routine diagnostic fecal panel for dogs with diarrhea. *Journal of the American Veterinary Medical Association* 221, 52–59.

Chengappa, M.M., Staats, J., Oberst, R.D., Gabbert, N.H. and McVey, S. (1993) Prevalence of *Salmonella* in raw meat used in diets of racing greyhounds. *Journal of Veterinary Diagnostic Investigation* 5, 372–377.

Cherry, B., Burns, A., Johnson, G.S., Pfeiffer, H., Dumas, N., Barrett, D., McDonough, P.L. and Eidson, M. (2004) *Salmonella* Typhimurium outbreak associated with veterinary clinic. (Zoonotic diseases). *Emerging Infectious Diseases* 10, 2249–2251.

Clark, C., Cunningham, J., Ahmed, R., Woodward, D., Fonseca, K., Isaacs, S., Ellis, A., Anand, C., Ziebell, K., Muckle, A., Sockett, P. and Rodgers, F. (2001) Characterization of *Salmonella* associated with pig ear dog treats in Canada. *Journal of Clinical Microbiology* 39, 3962–3968.

Durgut, R., Celik, S., Ozturk, S. and Pekkaya, S. (2003) Evaluation of dogs with colitis and ulcerative colitis using radiographic, electrocardiographic and laboratory findings. *Turk Veterinerlik ve Hayvanclk Dergisi* 27, 541–547.

Feary, D.J. and Hassel, D.M. (2006) Enteritis and Colitis in Horses. *Veterinary Clinics of North America: Equine Practice* 22, 437–479.

Finley, R., Raid-Smith, R. and Weese, J.S. (2006) Human health implications of *Salmonella*-contaminated natural pet treats and raw pet food. *Clinical Infectious Diseases* 42, 686–691.

Finley, R., Ribble, C., Aramini, J., Vandermeer, M., Popa, M., Litman, M. and Reid-Smith, R. (2007) The risk of salmonellae shedding by dogs fed *Salmonella*-contaminated commercial raw food diets. *Canadian Veterinary Journal* 48, 69–75.

Finley, R., Reis-Smith, R., Ribble, C., Popa, M., Vandermeer, M. and Aramini, J. (2008) The occurrence and antimicrobial susceptibility of salmonellae isolated from commercially available canine raw food diets in three Canadian cities. *Zoonoses and Public Health* 55, 462–469.

Foley, J.E., Orgad, U., Hirsh, D.C., Poland, A. and Pedersen, N.C. (1999) Outbreak of fatal salmonellosis in cats following use of a high-titer modified-live panleukopenia virus vaccine. *Journal of the American Veterinary Medical Association* 214, 67–70, 43–64.

Foster, S.F., Martin, P., Allan, G.S., Barrs, V.R. and Malik, R. (2004) Lower respiratory tract infections in cats: 21 cases (1995-2000). *Journal of Feline Medicine and Surgery* 6, 167–180.

Fox, J.G. and Beaucage, C.M. (1979) The incidence of *Salmonella* in random-source cats purchased for use in research. *Journal of Infectious Diseases* 139, 362–365.

Fox, J.G., Beaucage, C.M., Murphy, J.C. and Niemi, S.M. (1984) Experimental *Salmonella*-associated conjunctivitis in cats. *Canadian Journal of Comparative Medicine and Veterinary Science* 48, 87–91.

Fukata, T., Naito, F., Yoshida, N., Yamaguchi, T., Mizumura, Y. and Hirai, K. (2002) Incidence of *Salmonella* infection in healthy dogs in Gifu Prefecture, Japan. *Journal of Veterinary Medical Science* 64, 1079–1080.

Fukuyama, M., Hayashi, S., Hara, M., Kishikawa, S., Nakajima, H., Kawakami, S., Suzuki, Y., Sato, M., Isayama, Y. and Tabuchi, K. (1999) Isolation of *Salmonella infantis* from a dog with orchitis. *Journal of the Japan Veterinary Medical Association* 52, 32–35.

Galton, M.M., Scatterday, J.E. and Hardy, A.V. (1952) Salmonellosis in Dogs. *Journal of Infectious Diseases* 91, 1–4.

German, A.G. (2005) Diseases of the small intestine. In: Hall, E.J., Simpson, J.W. and Williams, D.A. (eds) *BSAVA Manual of Canine and Feline Gastroenterology*. BSAVA, Quedgeley, pp. 176–202.

Gow, A.G., Gow, D.J., Hall, E.J., Langton, D., Clarke, C. and Papasouliotis, K. (2009) Prevalence of potentially pathogenic enteric organisms in clinically healthy kittens in the UK. *Journal of Feline Medicine and Surgery* 11, 655–662.

Hackett, T. and Lappin, M.R. (2003) Prevalence of enteric pathogens in dogs of North-Central Colorado. *Journal of the American Animal Hospital Association* 39, 52–56.

Hauser, E., Huhn, S., Junker, E., Jaber, M., Schroeter, A., Helmuth, R., Rabsch, W., Winterhoff, N. and Malorny, B. (2009) Characterisation of a phenotypic monophasic variant belonging to *Salmonella enterica* subsp. *enterica* serovar Typhimurium from wild birds and its possible transmission to cats and humans. *Berliner und Münchener Tierärztliche Wochenschrift* 122, 169–177.

Herrera, M.M., Mena, J.E., Rojas, S.C., Rodriguez, C.E., Chaves, U.C. and Arias, E.M.L. (2009) Microbiological analysis of commercial adult dog pellets sold in Costa Rica. *Analecta Veterinaria* 29, 10–15.

Hill, S.L., Cheney, J.M., Taton-Allen, G.F., Reif, J.S., Bruns, C. and Lappin, M.R. (2000) Prevalence of enteric zoonotic organisms in cats. *Journal of the American Veterinary Medical Association* 216, 687–692.

Holt, P.E. (1980) Incidence of *Campylobacter*, *Salmonella* and *Shigella* infections in dogs in an industrial town. *Veterinary Record* 107, 254.

Joffe, D.J. and Schlesinger, D.P. (2002) Preliminary assessment of the risk of *Salmonella* infection in dogs fed raw chicken diets. *Canadian Veterinary Journal* 43, 441–442.

Kallo, O.J. and Hasso, S.A. (2001) Prevalence of salmonellosis serotypes in dogs and their sensitivity to antimicrobials. *Iraqi Journal of Veterinary Sciences* 14, 67–71.

Kocabiyik, A.L., Cetin, C. and Dedicova, D. (2006) Detection of *Salmonella* spp. in stray dogs in Bursa Province, Turkey: first isolation of *Salmonella* Corvallis from dogs. *Journal of Veterinary Medicine. Series B* 53, 194–196.

Kozak, M., Horosova, K., Lasanda, V., Bilek, J. and Kyselova, J. (2003) Do dogs and cats present a risk of transmission of salmonellosis to humans? *Bratislavske Lekarske Listy* 104, 323–328.

Kwaga, J.K.P., Adesiyun, A.A., Abdullahi, S.U. and Bello, C.S.S. (1989) Prevalence of salmonellae, shigellae and Plesiomonas shigelloides in dogs in Zaria, Nigeria. *British Veterinary Journal* 145, 174–177.

Lefebvre, S.L., Waltner-Toews, D., Peregrine, A.S., Reid-Smith, R., Hodge, L., Arroyo, L.G. and Weese, J.S. (2006) Prevalence of zoonotic agents in dogs visiting hospitalized people in Ontario: implications for infection control. *Journal of Hospital Infection* 62, 458–466.

Lefebvre, S.L., Reid-Smith, R., Boerlin, P. and Weese, J.S. (2008) Evaluation of the risks of shedding salmonellae and other potential pathogens by therapy dogs fed raw diets in Ontario and Alberta. *Zoonoses and Public Health* 55, 470–480.

Lenz, J., Joffe, D., Kauffman, M., Zhang, Y. and Lejeune, J. (2009) Perceptions, practices, and consequences associated with foodborne pathogens and the feeding of raw meat to dogs. *Canadian Veterinary Journal* 50, 637–643.

Leonard, E.K., Pearl, D.L., Finley, R.L., Janecko, N., Peregrine, A.S., Reid-Smith, R.J. and Weese, J.S. (2011) Evaluation of pet-related management factors and the risk of *Salmonella* spp. carriage in pet dogs from volunteer households in Ontario (2005-2006). *Zoonoses and Public Health* 58, 140–149.

Lynne, A.M., Dorsey, L.L., David, D.E. and Foley, S.L. (2009) Characterisation of antibiotic resistance in host-adapted *Salmonella enterica*. *International Journal of Antimicrobial Agents* 34, 169–172.

Maciel, B.M., Argolo Filho, R.C., Freitas, E.S.D., Kruschewsky, F.F., Santos, B.F., Rocha, G.D., Wetler, R.M.C. and Martins, L.A.F. (2004) Occurrence of exotic *Salmonella* serovars in asymptomatic dogs in Ilheus City/BA - Brazil. *Brazilian Journal of Veterinary Research and Animal Science* 41, 247–253.

Maciorowski, K.G., Pillai, S.D. and Ricke, S.C. (2000) Efficacy of a commercial polymerase chain reaction-based assay for detection of *Salmonella* spp. in animal feeds. *Journal of Applied Microbiology* 89, 710–718.

Maciorowski, K.G., Pillai, S.D., Jones, F.T. and Ricke, S.C. (2005) Polymerase chain reaction detection of food-borne *Salmonella* spp. in animal feeds. *Critical Reviews in Microbiology* 31, 45–53.

Maciorowski, K.G., Herrera, P., Jones, F.T., Pillai, S.D. and Ricke, S.C. (2006) Cultural and immunological detection methods for *Salmonella* spp. in animal feeds - A review. *Veterinary Research Communications* 30, 127–137.

Maha, A.S. and Lotfy, H.S. (2009) Captive dogs as reservoirs of some zoonotic pathogens. *Assiut Veterinary Medical Journal* 55, 333–349.

Marks, S.L. and Kather, E.J. (2003) Bacterial-associated diarrhea in the dog: a critical appraisal. (Gastroenterology). *Veterinary Clinics of North America, Small Animal Practice* 33, 1029–1060.

Marks, S.L., Rankin, S.C., Byrne, B.A. and Weese, J.S. (2011) Enteropathogenic bacteria in dogs and cats: diagnosis, epidemiology, treatment, and control. *Journal of Veterinary Internal Medicine* 25, 1195–1208.

McKenzie, E., Riehl, J., Banse, H., Kass, P.H., Nelson, S. Jr and Marks, S.L. (2010) Prevalence of diarrhea and enteropathogens in racing sled dogs. *Journal of Veterinary Internal Medicine* 24, 97–106.

McVey, D.S., Chengappa, M.M., Mosier, D.E., Stone, G.G., Oberst, R.D., Sylte, M.J., Gabbert, N.M., Kelly-Aehle, S.M. and Curtiss, R. (2002) Immunogenicity of chi4127 phoP- *Salmonella enterica* serovar Typhimurium in dogs. *Vaccine* 20, 1618–1623.

Morley, P.S., Strohmeyer, R.A., Tankson, J.D., Hyatt, D.R., Dargatz, D.A. and Fedorka-Cray, P.J. (2006) Evaluation of the association between feeding raw meat and *Salmonella enterica* infections at a Greyhound breeding facility. *Journal of the American Veterinary Medical Association* 228, 1524–1532.

Murphy, C., Reid-Smith, R.J., Prescott, J.F., Bonnett, B.N., Poppe, C., Boerlin, P., Weese, J.S., Janecko, N. and McEwen, S.A. (2009) Occurrence of antimicrobial resistant bacteria in healthy dogs and cats presented to private veterinary hospitals in southern Ontario: a preliminary study. *Canadian Veterinary Journal* 50, 1047–1053.

Murphy, C.P., Reid-Smith, R.J., Boerlin, P., Weese, J.S., Prescott, J.F., Janecko, N., Hassard, L. and McEwen, S.A. (2010) *Escherichia coli* and selected veterinary and zoonotic pathogens isolated from environmental sites in companion animal veterinary hospitals in southern Ontario. *Canadian Veterinary Journal* 51, 963–972.

Nadira, S., Adesiyun, A.A. and Ravi, S. (2005) Serovars and antibiotic sensitivity of *Salmonella* spp. isolated from non-diarrhoeic cats in Trinidad. *Veterinarski Arhiv* 75, 223–231.

Nastasi, A., Massenti, M.F., Scarlate, G., Mammina, C., Calco, C. and Villafrate, M.R. (1986) *Salmonella* and *Yersinia enterocolitica* in soil and dog faeces. *Bollettino dell'Istituto Sieroterapico Milanese* 65, 150–152.

O'Mahony, D., Murphy, K.B., Macsharry, J., Boileau, T., Sunvold, G., Reinhart, G., Kiely, B., Shanahan, F. and O'Mahony, L. (2009) Portrait of a canine probiotic *Bifidobacterium*-from gut to gut. *Veterinary Microbiology* 139, 106–112.

Ojo, O.E. and Adetosoye, A.I. (2009) *Salmonella* Typhimurium infection in diarrhoeic and non-diarrhoeic dogs in Ibadan, Nigeria. *Veterinarski Arhiv* 79, 371–377.

Parungao, S.P., Gordoncillo, M.J.N., Baldrias, L.R. and Ramirez, T.J. (2010) Isolation and molecular detection of *Salmonella* spp. from the feces of apparently healthy dogs. *Philippine Journal of Veterinary Medicine* 47, 73–77.

Perkins, M.C., Martin, P. and Malik, R. (2004) Successful treatment of *Salmonella* meningitis and osteomyelitis in a young maltese dog. *Australian Veterinary Practitioner* 34, 67–75.

Philbey, A.W., Mather, H.A., Taylor, D.J. and Coia, J.E. (2008) Isolation of avian strains of *Salmonella enterica* serovar Typhimurium from cats with enteric disease in the United Kingdom. *Veterinary Record* 162, 120–122.

Philbey, A.W., Brown, F.M., Mather, H.A., Coia, J.E. and Taylor, D.J. (2009) Salmonellosis in cats in the United Kingdom: 1955 to 2007. *Veterinary Record* 164, 120–122.

Pitout, J.D.D., Reisbig, M.D., Mulvey, M., Chui, L., Louie, M., Crowe, L., Church, D.L., Elsayed, S., Gregson, D., Ahmed, R., Tilley, P. and Hanson, N.D. (2003) Association between handling of pet treats and infection with *Salmonella enterica* serotype Newport expressing the AmpC β-lactamase, CMY-2. *Journal of Clinical Microbiology* 41, 4578–4582.

Plaut, M., Zimmerman, E.M. and Goldstein, R.A. (1996) Health hazards to humans associated with domestic pets. *Annual Review of Public Health* 17, 221–245.

Sato, Y., Mori, T., Koyama, T. and Nagase, H. (2000) *Salmonella* virchow infection in an infant transmitted by household dogs. *Journal of Veterinary Medical Science* 62, 767–769.

Sato, Y. and Kuwamoto, R. (1999) A case of canine salmonellosis due to *Salmonella* infantis. *Journal of Veterinary Medical Science* 61, 71–72.

Schotte, U., Borchers, D., Wulff, C. and Geue, L. (2007) *Salmonella* Montevideo outbreak in military kennel dogs caused by contaminated commercial feed, which was only recognized through monitoring. *Veterinary Microbiology* 119, 316–323.

Seepersadsingh, N., Adesiyun, A.A. and Seebaransingh, R. (2004) Prevalence and antimicrobial resistance of *Salmonella* spp. in non-diarrhoeic dogs in Trinidad. *Journal of Veterinary Medicine. Series B* 51, 337–342.

Seepersadsingh, N., Adesiyun, A.A. and Seebaransingh, R. (2005) Serovars and antibiotic sensitivity of *Salmonella* spp. isolated from non-diarrhoeic cats in Trinidad. *Veterinarski Arhiv* 75, 223–231.

Selmi, M., Stefanelli, S., Bilei, S., Tolli, R., Bertolotti, L., Marconi, P., Giurlani, S., De Lucia, P.G., Ruggeri, G. and Pagani, A. (2011) Contaminated commercial dehydrated food as source of multiple *Salmonella* serotypes outbreak in a municipal kennel in Tuscany. Mangime commerciale disidratato all'origine di un focolaio di salmonellosi sostenuto da diversi sierotipi in un Canile municipale in Toscana *Veterinaria Italiana* 47, 183-190.

Shimi, A. and Barin, A. (1977) *Salmonella* in cats. *Journal of Comparative Pathology* 87, 315–318.

Sokolow, S.H., Rand, C., Marks, S.L., Drazenovich, N.L., Kather, E.J. and Foley, J.E. (2005) Epidemiologic evaluation of diarrhea in dogs in an animal shelter. *American Journal of Veterinary Research* 66, 1018–1024.

Souza, L.C.D., Langoni, H., Franco, S.R.V.D.S., Pinheiro, E., Mota, M.D.A. and Listoni, F.J.P. (2002) Epidemiological aspects of salmonellosis in dogs in the city of Botucatu - SP. *Veterinaria e Zootecnia* 11, 133–140.

Spain, C.V., Scarlett, J.M., Wade, S.E. and McDonough, P. (2001) Prevalence of enteric zoonotic agents in cats less than 1 year old in Central New York State. *Journal of Veterinary Internal Medicine* 15, 33–38.

Stavisky, J., Radford, A.D., Gaskell, R., Dawson, S., German, A., Parsons, B., Clegg, S., Newmann, J. and Pinchbeck, G. (2011) A case-control study of pathogen and lifestyle risk factors for diarrhoea in dogs. *Preventive Veterinary Medicine* 99, 185–192.

Stehr-Green, J.K. and Schantz, P.M. (1987) The impact of zoonotic diseases transmitted by pets on human health and the economy. *Veterinary Clinics of North America - Small Animal Practice* 17, 1–15.

Stiver, S.L., Frazier, K.S., Mauel, M.J. and Styer, E.L. (2003) Septicemic salmonellosis in two cats fed a raw-meat diet. *Journal of the American Animal Hospital Association* 39, 538–542.

Stone, G.G., Chengappa, M.M., Oberst, R.D., Gabbert, N.H., McVey, S., Hennessy, K.J., Muenzenberger, M. and Staats, J. (1993) Application of polymerase chain reaction for the correlation of *Salmonella* serovars recovered from greyhound feces with their diet. *Journal of Veterinary Diagnostic Investigation* 5, 378–385.

Stone, G.G., Chengappa, M.M., Hays, M.P. and Oberst, R.D. (1998) Application of polymerase chain reaction-oligonucleotide ligation assay for the detection of salmonellae in processed meat, poultry, fish, and pet foods. *Journal of Rapid Methods and Automation in Microbiology* 6, 119–128.

Strohmeyer, R.A., Morley, P.S., Hyatt, D.R., Dargatz, D.A., Scorza, A.V. and Lappin, M.R. (2006) Evaluation of bacterial and protozoal contamination of commercially available raw meat diets for dogs. *Journal of the American Veterinary Medical Association* 228, 537–542.

Stucker, C.L., Galton, M.M., Cowdery, J. and Hardy, A.V. (1952) Salmonellosis in dogs. *Journal of Infectious Diseases* 91, 6–11.

Sugiyama, Y., Sugiyama, F. and Yagami, K.I. (1993) Isolation of *Salmonella* from impounded dogs introduced to a laboratory. *Experimental Animals* 42, 119–121.

Tanaka, Y., Katsube, Y. and Imaizumi, K. (1976) Experimental carrier in dogs produced by oral administration of *Salmonella typhimurium*. *Japanese Journal of Veterinary Science* 38, 569–578.

Tarsitano, E., Greco, G., Decaro, N., Nicasio, F., Lucente, M.S., Buonavoglia, C. and Tempesta, M. (2010) Environmental monitoring and analysis of faecal contamination in an urban setting in the city of Bari (Apulia region, Italy): health and hygiene implications. *International Journal of Environmental Research and Public Health* 7, 3972–3986.

Tauni, M.A. and Österlund, A. (2000) Outbreak of *Salmonella typhimurium* in cats and humans associated with infection in wild birds. *Journal of Small Animal Practice* 41, 339–341.

Taylor, D.J. and Philbey, A.W. (2010) *Salmonella* infections in garden birds and cats in a domestic environment. *Veterinary Record* 167, 26–28.

Tsai, H.J., Huang, H.C., Lin, C.M., Lien, Y.Y. and Chou, C.H. (2007) Salmonellae and campylobacters in household and stray dogs in Northern Taiwan. *Veterinary Research Communications* 31, 931–939.

Urban, J.E. and Broce, A. (1998) Flies and their bacterial loads in greyhound dog kennels in Kansas. *Current Microbiology* 36, 164–170.

Vahjen, W. and Manner, K. (2003) The effect of a probiotic *Enterococcus faecium* product in diets of healthy dogs on bacteriological counts of *Salmonella* spp., *Campylobacter* spp. and *Clostridium* spp. in faeces. *Archiv für Tierernahrung* 57, 229–233.

Van Duijkeren, E. and Houwers, D. (2002) *Salmonella*-enteritis bij de hond, niet relevant? [*Salmonella* enteritis in dogs, not relevant?] *Tijdschrift voor Diergeneeskunde* 127, 716–717.

Van Duijkeren, E., Wannet, W.J.B., Houwers, D.J. and Van Pelt, W. (2002) Serotype and phage type distribution of *Salmonella* strains iolated from humans, cattle, pigs, and chickens in The Netherlands from 1984 to 2001. *Journal of Clinical Microbiology* 40, 3980–3985.

Van Immerseel, F., Pasamans, F., Buck, J.D., Rychlik, I., Hradecka, H., Collard, J.M., Wildemauwe, C., Heyndrickx, M., Ducatelle, R. and Haesebrouck, F. (2004) Cats as a risk for transmission of antimicrobial drug-resistant *Salmonella*. (Zoonotic diseases). *Emerging Infectious Diseases* 10, 2169–2174.

Veling, J., Wilpshaar, H., Frankena, K., Bartels, C. and Barkema, H.W. (2002) Risk factors for clinical *Salmonella enterica* subsp. *enterica* serovar Typhimurium infection on Dutch dairy farms. *Preventive Veterinary Medicine* 54, 157–168.

Verma, A.K., Sinha, D.K. and Singh, B.R. (2007) Salmonellosis in apparently healthy dogs. *Journal of Veterinary Public Health* 5, 37–39.

Wall, P.G., Davis, S., Threllfall, E.J., Ward, L.R. and Ewbank, A.J. (1995) Chronic carriage of multidrug resistant *Salmonella typhimurium* in a cat. *Journal of Small Animal Practice* 36, 279–281.

Wall, P.G., Threllfall, E.J., Ward, L.R. and Rowe, B. (1996) Multiresistant *Salmonella typhimurium* DT104 in cats: a public health risk. *The Lancet* 348, 471–471.

Ward, M.P., Brady, T.H., Couetil, L.L., Liljebjelke, K., Maurer, J.J. and Wu, C.C. (2005) Investigation and control of an outbreak of salmonellosis caused by multidrug-resistant *Salmonella typhimurium* in a population of hospitalized horses. *Veterinary Microbiology* 107, 233–240.

Weber, A., Wachowitz, R., Weigl, U. and Schäfer-Schmidt, R. (1995) Occurrence of *Salmonella* in fecal samples of dogs and cats in northern Bavaria from 1975 to 1994. *Berliner und Münchener Tierärztliche Wochenschrift* 108, 401–404.

Weber, A., Mölle, G., Wachowitz, R., Schafer-Schmidt, R. and Stieger, E. (2002) Prevalence of *Salmonella* in dried dog feed produced from bovine ears, lungs, rumen, ox loin and pigs' ears etc. *Tierärztliche Umschau* 57, 616–618.

Weese, J.S., Rousseau, J. and Arroyo, L. (2005) Bacteriological evaluation of commercial canine and feline raw diets. *Canadian Veterinary Journal* 46, 513–516.

Westgarth, C., Pinchbeckk, G.L., Bradshaw, J.W.S., Dason, S., Gaskell, R.M. and Christley, R.M. (2008) Dog-human and dog-dog interactions of 260 dog-owning households in a community in Cheshire. *Veterinary Record* 162, 436–442.

White, D.G., Datta, A., McDermott, P., Friedmann, S., Qaiyumi, S., Ayers, S., English, L., McDermott, S., Wagner, D.D. and Zhao, S. (2003) Antimicrobial susceptibility and genetic relatedness of *Salmonella* serovars isolated from animal-derived dog treats in the USA. *Journal of Antimicrobial Chemotherapy* 52, 860–863.

Willis, C. (2001) Isolation of *Salmonella* species from imported dog chews. *Veterinary Record* 149, 426–427.

Wong, T.L., Thom, K., Nicol C., Heffernan, H. and Macdiarmid, S. (2007) *Salmonella* serotypes isolated from pet chews in New Zealand. *Journal of Applied Microbiology* 103, 803–810.

Wright, J.G., Tengelsen, L.A., Smith, K.E., Bender, J.B., Frank, R.K., Grendon, J.H., Rice, D.H., Thiessen, A.M.B., Gilbertson, C.J., Sivapalasingam, S., Barrett, T.J., Besser, T.E., Hancock, D.D. and Angulo, F.J. (2005) Multidrug-resistant *Salmonella* Typhimurium in four animal facilities. *Emerging Infectious Diseases* 11, 1235–1241.

Younus, M., Wilkins, M.J., Davies, H.D., Rahbar, M.H., Funk, J., Nguyen, C., Siddiqi, A.E., Cho, S. and Saeed, A.M. (2010) The role of exposures to animals and other risk factors in sporadic, non-typhoidal *Salmonella* infections in Michigan children. *Zoonoses and Public Health* 57, e170–e176.

17 *Salmonella* Infections in Exotic Pets

Frank Pasmans,* Filip Boyen and Freddy Haesebrouck
Laboratory of Veterinary Bacteriology and Mycology, Department of Pathology, Bacteriology and Avian Diseases, Ghent University, Belgium

Salmonella Infections in Reptiles

Reptiles are well-known carriers of *Salmonella*. Since the probable first isolation of *Salmonella* from reptiles in 1939 (Caldwell and Reyrson, 1939), numerous reports describe the high prevalence of *Salmonella* infections in reptiles (e.g. Zwart, 1960). In fact, each reptile should be considered as *Salmonella* carrier until the contrary is proven. Both *Salmonella enterica* and *Salmonella bongori*, their subspecies and serovars can be found in reptiles (e.g. Zwart *et al.*, 1970; Bäumler *et al.*, 1998; Pedersen *et al.*, 2009). Moreover, reptiles can be infected by multiple serovars at the same time. Known host-adapted and host-restricted serovars are rarely reported from reptiles, an example being a *S.* Dublin strain that was isolated from the snake *Walterinnesia aegyptia* (Greenberg and Sechter, 1992). Although there is some evidence that *Salmonella* might be transferred vertically in reptiles (Chiodini, 1982; Schröter *et al.*, 2006), the horizontal route of infection through oral-faecal contact is probably the most common one. Coprophagia, which is a natural phenomenon in many herbivorous reptiles, enables direct transfer of *Salmonella*. Freshly laid turtle eggs are frequently infected shortly after egg-laying. D'Aoust *et al.* (1990) found 21% of turtle eggs exported from the USA to be infected with *Salmonella*. Egg-laying females often moisten the nesting site with *Salmonella*-contaminated fluid from the accessory bladder. Subsequently, the bacteria penetrate the eggshell, resulting in infection of the egg contents within 1 h (Feeley and Treger, 1969).

The pathogenesis of a *Salmonella* infection in ectothermic hosts such as reptiles is poorly known. After infection, the bacterium mainly resides in the gut. Colonization of the chelonian host is restricted to the distal intestinal tract, without invasion of intestinal tissues and colonization of internal organs (Dimow, 1966; Pasmans *et al.*, 2002a). In the hindgut, chelonians can carry and excrete *Salmonella* for at least 1 year (Dimow, 1966) and even for up to 9 years (Boycott, 1962). Experimental inoculation of bearded dragons (*Pogona vitticeps*) with a *S.* Enteritidis strain did result in persistent colonization of both the intestinal tract and liver and spleen in the absence of inflammation and clinical signs (F. Pasmans, unpublished results). The mechanisms *Salmonella* uses to persistently colonize the reptilian host are poorly understood. The N-acylhomoserine lactone receptor SdiA, involved in quorum sensing, appears to become active only in the chelonian, but not in the avian or mammalian gut (Smith *et al.*, 2008). The fluctuating body temperature of the ectothermic reptiles may have a

* Corresponding author, e-mail: frank.pasmans@UGent.be

© CAB International 2013. *Salmonella in Domestic Animals, 2nd Edition* (eds P.A. Barrow and U. Methner)

pronounced effect on the host–bacterium interactions. *Salmonella* appears to be perfectly capable of surviving and even proliferating intracellularly in chelonian and saurian macrophages, which are known to play a vital role in *Salmonella* persistency in mammals (Pasmans *et al.*, 2002b, and unpublished results). Reptiles, infected orally with *Salmonella*, generally do not seroconvert, opposed to animals inoculated parenterally (Chiodini, 1982; Pasmans *et al.*, 2002a). The role of the *Salmonella* pathogenicity islands (SPI) in the reptile–*Salmonella* interaction is far from being clear yet. Recent results show that SPI1, SPI2, SPI3 and SPI4 but not SPI5 of *Salmonella* Enteritidis contribute to intestinal persistence and that SPI1, SPI2 and SPI3 but not SPI4 and SPI5 contribute to persistence in the liver of bearded dragons (unpublished results). Stress-induced re-excretion of *Salmonella* by carriers appears to exist as suggested by enhanced *Salmonella* excretion after dehydration of turtles (Du Ponte *et al.*, 1978). Overall, the available scarce knowledge concerning the pathogenesis of *Salmonella* infections in reptiles suggests a complex host–bacterium interaction.

Clinical salmonellosis is rare in reptiles but might present as salpingitis, coelomitis, dermatitis, abscessation, osteomyelitis, arthritis, septicaemia or granulomatous disease (Fig. 17.1; Onderka and Finlayson, 1985; González Candela *et al.*, 2005; Bemis *et al.*, 2007). Its role in enteric disease in reptiles is not clear but at least in chelonians and bearded dragons, no signs of enteritis can be seen after experimental inoculation. When *Salmonella* is isolated from the internal organs of chelonians showing clinical signs, other predisposing factors such as stress, heavy parasitic loads, traumata, tumours and other infectious diseases are generally associated (Cambre *et al.*, 1980). Also in lizards and snakes, viral infections (e.g. adenovirosis in lizards) or heavy intestinal parasitic infections often coincide with these *Salmonella*-associated lesions. A primary role of *Salmonella* in the development of disease in reptiles has still to be demonstrated. Even when infected intracardially, subcutaneously or intracelomically with *Salmonella*, chelonians and snakes mostly do not show any clinical signs of salmonellosis (Blanc *et al.*, 1960; Delage, 1966; Dimow, 1966, Chiodini, 1982). Nevertheless, parenterally infected chelonians are capable of mounting an antibody response towards *Salmonella* (Blanc *et al.*, 1960; Dimow, 1966; Pasmans *et al.*, 2002a). An intriguing series of cases of clinical *Salmonella* infections with the subspecies *arizonae*, causing osteomyelitis in rattle snakes has been reported (Ramsay *et al.*, 2002; Bemis *et al.*, 2007). However, until clear evidence is presented, *Salmonella* should generally be considered as facultative pathogen in reptiles, which occurs as a natural component of their intestinal microbiota.

It is now generally accepted that, with the exception of host-restricted serovars like Gallinarum, most serovars of *Salmonella* are able to cause salmonellosis in humans (Aleksic *et al.*, 1996). Indeed, reptilian *Salmonella* isolates should be considered pathogenic to humans (Pasmans *et al.*, 2005). Because a high percentage of reptiles excrete high numbers of *Salmonella* bacteria as asymptomatic carriers, they constitute a source of *Salmonella* infections to humans and homoeothermic animals. The longer reptiles stay in captivity, the higher the probability that they are infected with *Salmonella* (e.g. Pfleger *et al.*, 2003). Human salmonellosis and *Salmonella* infections in chelonians were linked for the first time in 1962 (Communicable Disease Center, 1963). Since then, an increasing number of reptile-associated salmonellosis cases have been reported. In the 1970s, between

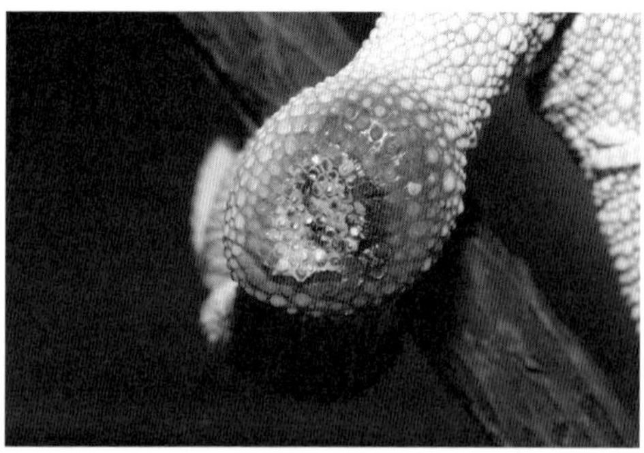

Fig. 17.1. *Salmonella* polyarthritis in a veiled chameleon (*Chamaeleo calyptratus*).

11% and 22% of all registered human salmonellosis cases were caused by chelonians (Lamm *et al.*, 1972; Cohen *et al.*, 1980). Reptile-associated *Salmonella* infections generally cause gastroenteritis in humans. However, depending on the age or immune status of the patient and the serovar involved, generalization may occur, leading to septicaemia, abortion and even death (Woodward *et al.*, 1997). In particular, immune deficiencies, for instance caused by leukaemia, systemic lupus erythematosus or HIV infections predispose for a very severe clinical course (Ackman *et al.*, 1995; Woodward *et al.*, 1997). In 1975, the sale of turtles with a carapace length less than 4 cm was prohibited, which resulted in an estimated annual reduction of 100,000 *Salmonella* infections in US children between 1 and 9 years old (Cohen *et al.*, 1980). A recent study estimates that 6% of all sporadic *Salmonella* infections in the USA can be attributed to reptiles (Mermin *et al.*, 2004). Of the top 20 increasing serovars isolated from 1987 until 1997 in the USA, seven were common reptile-associated *Salmonella* serovars (Olsen *et al.*, 2001). Turtle-associated salmonellosis was estimated to cost about 12.5m in the USA in 1987 (Stehr Green and Schantz, 1987). Sources of infection for humans are: contact with reptiles, their faeces or contaminated water and objects such as aquaria or feeding bowls (Ackman *et al.*, 1995). Consumption of undercooked reptile meat may result in human salmonellosis as well (reviewed in Magnino *et al.*, 2009). In particular, children younger than 5 years of age are at risk, probably due to the combination of their higher susceptibility to infection and limited hygienic conscience (Mermin *et al.*, 2004; Jones *et al.*, 2006; Aiken *et al.*, 2010).

Antimicrobial treatment of reptiles does not eliminate a *Salmonella* infection as demonstrated in a study of Mitchell and Shane (2001), in which prolonged administration of enrofloxacin to green iguanas did not result in complete clearance of *Salmonella*. Antibiotic treatment of infected turtles was equally unsuccessful (Weber, 1973; Koopman and Kennis, 1976). Efforts have been made to produce *Salmonella*-free turtles in farms in the USA. Treatment of pond water with copper sulfate reduced the number of *Salmonella* bacteria in the water but did not lower the number of infected turtle progeny (Kaufmann *et al.*, 1972). Decontamination of turtle eggs resulted in a significant reduction of infected turtles. Siebeling *et al.* (1975) treated eggs with tetracycline and chloramphenicol using the temperature differential egg dip method, which proved to be effective if the eggs were treated for 24 h after deposition. The pressure differential method using gentamicin was developed by Michael-Marler *et al.* (1983). *Salmonella*-free turtles were hatched from treated eggs, even if treatment was performed at 48 h after deposition. Besides antibiotic treatment, the management of the eggs has improved. Eggs are collected earlier after deposition, washed and superficially decontaminated using for instance chlorine solution. All these measures led to a decrease in the amount of infected juvenile turtles from 40% in 1980 to less than 1% in 1985 (Shane *et al.*, 1990). However, the use of antibiotics promoted the development of acquired antibiotic resistance of *Salmonella*, notably to gentamicin (D'Aoust *et al.*, 1990). This in turn caused an increase in the amount of infected juvenile turtles. A total of 21% of juvenile turtles and from 8 to 80% of turtle eggs examined by D'Aoust *et al.* (1990) were positive for *Salmonella*. Non-antibiotic treatment of eggs using a combination of hypochlorite and polyhexamethylene presents a valuable alternative (Mitchell *et al.*, 2007).

Overall, acquired antimicrobial resistance in reptilian *Salmonella* isolates varies from near absence (Pasmans *et al.*, 2005) to relatively high resistances to tetracyclines, sulfonamides, chloramphenicol and streptomycin (Maciel *et al.*, 2010). Recently, plasmid-mediated quinolone resistance determinants *qnrB19*, *qnrS1* and *aac(6')-Ib-cr* were detected in Germany in isolates from reptiles (Guerra *et al.*, 2010).

Extensive guidelines to avoid transmission of *Salmonella* from reptiles to humans have been proposed by several organizations, including the Association of Reptile and Amphibian Veterinarians and the American Veterinary Medical Association. Basically, these include hygienic measures and limiting contact between immunocompromised humans and reptiles (Warwick *et al.*, 2001).

The following guidelines are proposed regarding the handling of reptiles and strongly reduce the risk of contracting salmonellosis from reptiles: thorough washing of hands, using soap and hot water after direct or indirect contact with reptiles, separating reptile accessories from all utensils used for human food preparation, no free-roaming of reptiles in places accessible to children and, finally, keeping reptiles away from children younger than 5 years of age, pregnant women and immunodeficient persons. Raising awareness of reptile owners concerning the zoonotic risk their pet poses is an important task for any reptile veterinarian.

Salmonella Infections in Amphibians and Ornamental Fish

Ornamental fish or aquarium water have repeatedly been mentioned to contain *Salmonella* (Sanyal *et al.*, 1987; Black *et al.*, 1992; Manfrin *et al.*, 2001; Seepersadsingh and Adesiyun, 2003; Gaulin *et al.*, 2005). The presence of *Salmonella* is well documented also in amphibians, particularly in anurans (frogs and toads, Ang *et al.*, 1973; Bartlett *et al.*, 1977; Devi and Shivananda, 1983; Moreno *et al.*, 1995; Rajendran *et al.*, 1998). In urodelans (salamanders and newts), *Salmonella* infections probably only exceptionally occur. None of 100 faecal samples from captive urodelans from three different collections yielded any *Salmonella* isolates (F. Pasmans, unpublished results). Possibly, the low body temperatures of most urodelan species (<20°C and even <15°C) may limit colonization by *Salmonella*. This finding is in support of the hypothesis that ectothermic vertebrates with low body temperatures are not suitable hosts for *Salmonella* bacteria.

Although pathogenic significance has been suggested for infections with *Salmonella* Paratyphi B and *Salmonella enterica* subsp. *arizonae* in fish (Kodama *et al.*, 1987; Musto *et al.*, 2006), no clinical evidence has so far been produced to attribute clinical importance to *Salmonella* infections in amphibians and fish. Their sole significance appears to be their zoonotic potential. Indeed, keeping amphibians is considered to enhance the risk of contracting salmonellosis (Mermin *et al.*, 2004). Salmonellosis associated with amphibian contact has been described previously (e.g. Srikantiah *et al.*, 2004), one notorious outbreak, caused by *S.* Typhimurium, involving at least 85 people from 31 US states (CDC, 2010). This outbreak was linked to contact with water of aquaria containing African dwarf clawed frogs (*Hymenochirus* sp.). The consumption of contaminated frog legs also poses a public health risk (Purushothaman *et al.*, 1981; Catsaras, 1983; Rajagopalan *et al.*, 1983). Salmonellosis contracted from ornamental fish or their aquarium water has been described as well, with the notable report of multidrug-resistant *Salmonella* Paratyphi B, which caused severe disease, particularly in young children (Levings *et al.*, 2006; Musto *et al.*, 2006).

Salmonella Infections in Companion Birds

Salmonella infections in Galliformes have been described elsewhere in this book (Chapter 9, this volume). In companion birds, salmonellosis is a frequent cause of disease and mortality. The outcome of infection may vary from the development of asymptomatic carriers to disease outbreaks with high mortality. In this section, we will make a clear distinction between paratyphoid in pigeons and in other avian species. Indeed, in pigeons, the majority of clinical *Salmonella* infections are caused by host-adapted phage types of *S.* Typhimurium, resulting in a typhoid-like syndrome. In other avian species (excluding poultry), the aetiology and pathogenesis of *Salmonella* infections have been much less studied and it is at present not clear whether host-adapted *Salmonella* strains cause disease in e.g. psittacines and passerines.

Salmonellosis in passerine and psittacine birds

Although salmonellosis in passerine and psittacine birds can be caused by a wide variety of serovars, *S.* Typhimurium is possibly the most frequently isolated serovar from these birds. The *S.* Typhimurium phage types DT40, DT41, DT56 and DT160 may be adapted to passerine birds, resulting in endemic infections and context-driven epizootics (Wobeser and Finlayson, 1969; Pennycott *et al.*, 1998, 2010; Daoust *et al.*, 2000; Hughes *et al.*, 2010; Taylor and Philbey, 2010).

Sources of infection probably include direct or indirect contact with wild birds (e.g. in aviaries), the introduction of pet trade-derived *Salmonella*-infected birds (e.g. Sawa *et al.*, 1981), contaminated feed (Madadgar *et al.*, 2009), other pets (for example an iguana, Oros *et al.*, 1998), rodents etc. Since *Salmonella* is able to persist for prolonged periods in the environment, the infected avian environment constitutes a continuous source of re-infection. Vertical transmission might occur in some avian species and with more host-adapted *Salmonella* strains but has not yet been unambiguously proven at present in passerine and psittacine birds. Although asymptomatic carriers occur, it is difficult to estimate the role of these birds as a reservoir for *Salmonella. Salmonella* carriage in apparently healthy wild birds appears to be uncommon (<1%, Brittingham *et al.*, 1988; for a comprehensive review of salmonellosis in wild birds, see Daoust and Prescott, 2007). Exceptions are wild birds such as, for example, gulls, starlings and house sparrows that forage in *Salmonella*-contaminated areas, most often near human settlements (e.g. waste dumps, feeders) and farming operations (Fenlon, 1981; Davies and Wray, 1996; Craven *et al.*, 2000; Refsum *et al.*, 2003; Taylor and Philbey, 2010), which promotes infection with and subsequent spread of *Salmonella*, for example to aviaries.

Due to different methodology used, studies examining the prevalence of *Salmonella* in healthy, captive birds are difficult to compare. Studies concerning the prevalence of *Salmonella* infections yield highly variable results, largely depending on the method used: bacterial isolation (with or without the use of pre-enrichment and enrichment), serology or PCR. A large *invA*-based PCR screening of healthy psittacine birds yielded 13.2% positive birds (Allgayer *et al.*, 2008). However, neither isolates could be obtained nor could antibodies against serovars Gallinarum, Enteritidis or Typhimurium be demonstrated. Bacteriological studies generally yield a lower prevalence of approximately 1% in healthy pet birds (Scope *et al.*, 1998; Seepersadsingh and Adesiyun, 2003; Ok and Yardimci, 2010). However, asymptomatic carriers may be easily overlooked due to intermittent excretion of low numbers of *Salmonella.* Besides, care must be taken not to overlook 'atypical' (e.g. lactose positive, H_2S negative, lysine decarboxylase negative) isolates since e.g. *S. enterica* subsp. *arizonae* has been detected in psittacines. Serological examination often results in a high prevalence estimate, up to 67% (Deem *et al.*, 2005). However, care should be taken to interpret these results since the tests used have most often not been validated in the species tested and do not reflect the bacteriological status of the bird.

Clinical outbreaks of salmonellosis both in passerine and psittacine birds have been reported on numerous occasions (Harrington *et al.*, 1975; Panigrahy and Gilmore, 1983; Reinhard *et al.*, 1988; Shima and Osborn, 1989; Orosz *et al.*, 1992; Oros *et al.*, 1998; Raidal, 1998; Ward *et al.*, 2003; Allgayer *et al.*, 2009; Madadgar *et al.*, 2009; Vigo *et al.*, 2009; Piccirillo *et al.*, 2010). Species with caeca such as *Amazona* sp. or macaws may be more often infected asymptomatically (Gerlach, 1994). Indeed, contrary to galliform birds, most passerine and many psittacine birds have no or only residual caeca and concurring intestinal microbial ecosystem. Clinical signs vary from acute and massive mortality to a more chronic atypical disease with anorexia, diarrhoea, dyspnoea, lethargy, cachexia, fluffed or ruffled feathers, subcutaneous granulomas, conjunctivitis, arthritis and ocular problems such as panophthalmitis. Probably, periods of stress such as catching, transport, disturbance of social structures and concurrent disease predispose for a clinical course of infection. Indeed, outbreaks affecting a large number of animals are often noticed upon transportation of birds for the pet trade (Harrington *et al.*, 1975; Sawa *et al.*, 1981).

In acutely diseased birds, macroscopic lesions are often discrete or absent. In less acute cases, generally, hepato- and splenomegaly, lung congestion and enteritis are present. Multifocal necrotic foci are frequently present in the liver. Pennycott *et al.* (1998) and Daoust *et al.* (2000) report a high prevalence of ingluviitis and oesophagitis in passerine birds. In chronic cases, granulomas may develop. Microscopic lesions are characterized by necrosis and pronounced inflammation, involving granulocytes and macrophages. The latter are the host cells in which the *Salmonella* bacteria reside and constitute an important component of the *Salmonella* granulomas. In chronic infections, multinucleated giant cells are formed. Overall, the clinical signs, macroscopic and microscopic lesions of salmonellosis are highly similar to those caused by *Yersinia pseudotuberculosis*.

Diagnosis of salmonellosis in psittacine and passerine birds should be based on the combination of the presence of clinical signs and/or lesions and demonstration of the presence of *Salmonella*, preferably from lesions in a pure and abundant culture. Control of salmonellosis in collections of captive birds should include preventive and curative measures. Preventive measures comprise proper quarantine of any newly acquired bird. During this quarantine period, the bird should be examined for the presence of *Salmonella* using bacteriological or molecular examination of multiple faecal samples, collected over a period of several days. Vaccination is not routinely applied. Curative measures include isolation of clinically ill birds, antimicrobial treatment of all birds in the infected flocks and thorough disinfection of all fomites, cages and aviaries.

Salmonellosis in pigeons

Salmonella Typhimurium is the most important bacterial pathogen in pigeons. Pigeons are predominantly infected with pigeon-specific pathogenic *Salmonella* strains, notably *Salmonella enterica* subsp. *enterica* serovar Typhimurium (*S.* Typhimurium) variant Copenhagen phage types 2 and 99 (Pohl *et al.*, 1983; Rabsch *et al.*, 2002; Methner and Lauterbach, 2003; Pasmans *et al.*, 2004), but also infections with other serotypes, such as Enteritidis, are possible. *Salmonella* Typhimurium phage types 2 and 99 can be considered host-restricted, which is reflected by increased toxicity of these phage types to pigeon macrophages (Pasmans *et al.*, 2003). Although infections of humans with pigeon-associated *Salmonella* strains are rare, these strains are able to cause severe disease in Balb/C mice (Pasmans *et al.*, 2004) and fluid accumulation in bovine ileal loops (Andrews-Polymenis *et al.*, 2004). The phage types DT2 and DT99 are genetically highly similar to the fully sequenced *S.* Typhimurium LT2 strain (Andrews-Polymenis *et al.*, 2004).

Pigeons are infected by oral uptake of the agent from contaminated feed, drinking water, baskets, etc. Asymptomatic carriers frequently occur and maintain the infection in a flock of pigeons through intermittent faecal shedding of *Salmonella*. Vertical transmission is highly likely due to predilection of these *Salmonella* strains to the pigeons' gonads.

Salmonellosis in pigeons is characterized by enteritis and septicaemia. Symptoms include anorexia, lethargy, (slimy to bloody) diarrhoea, cachexia, polyuria, (poly-) arthritis, notably of the elbow joint, nervous symptoms, dermatitis, panophtalmitis and death (Devriese, 1986). Infertility of breeder birds, embryonic death and mortality of squabs frequently occur. Chronically infected birds develop abscesses and granulomata in multiple organs, resulting in ill condition and, finally, death (Fig. 17.2).

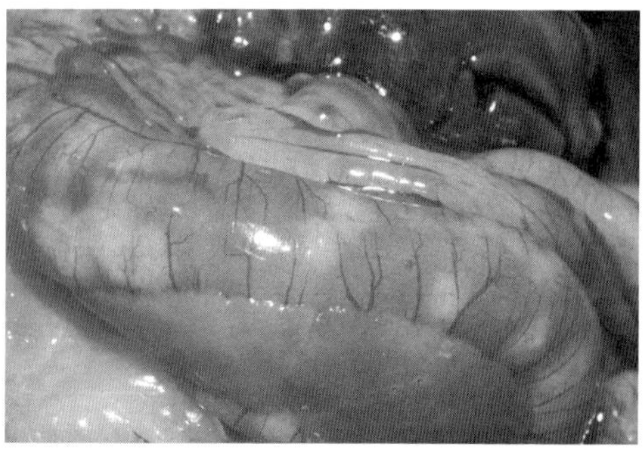

Fig. 17.2. Paratyphoid in pigeon with intestinal granuloma formation.

The diagnosis of paratyphoid in pigeons should be based on demonstration of *S.* Typhimurium, associated with the presence of clinical signs of paratyphoid in the flock. To assess the presence of *Salmonella* in a pigeon flock, pooled samples over a 5-day period are recommended, due to the intermittent excretion of the bacterium. Generally, *Salmonella* can be isolated in abundant culture from acutely diseased birds, both from the intestine and from the internal organs. In chronically infected and carrier birds, the numbers of *Salmonella* may be considerably lower, requiring multiple sampling and/or enrichment. A slide agglutination test with stained, formaldehyde inactivated bacteria can be used to detect anti-*Salmonella* antibodies (Devriese, 1986). However, false negatives frequently occur and this test mainly yields positive results in the case of clinically and acutely infected pigeons.

Controlling pigeon paratyphoid presents a challenge due to the presence of asymptomatic carriers, persistency of *Salmonella* in the environment, vertical transmission and difficulties to eliminate *Salmonella* bacteria from infected animals. Except for very valuable birds, clinically infected pigeons should be euthanized to prevent the development of chronic carriers. If treated, clinically infected birds should be quarantined. Re-introduction of these birds in the flock should only be considered after repeated bacteriological examinations of faecal samples for the presence of *Salmonella*. Since asymptomatically infected carrier birds cannot be reliably detected, all contact birds should be treated using e.g. fluoroquinolones. Interestingly, acquired antimicrobial resistance is largely absent in *Salmonella* isolates from pigeons, despite the disturbing abuse of antimicrobials by pigeon fanciers and subsequent development of acquired antimicrobial resistance in other bacteria from pigeons (Kimpe *et al.*, 2002). The use of certain antimicrobials such as florfenicol has been proven to promote the development of carriers (Pasmans *et al.*, 2008). Besides antimicrobial treatment, hygienic measures including thorough cleaning and decontamination of the pigeon loft is vital. Breeding must be interrupted, and overpopulation avoided. Preventive or therapeutic vaccination using inactivated bacterins is widely used and promotes elimination of *Salmonella*, reduces the severity of the disease, faecal shedding and mortality (Uyttebroek *et al.*, 1991; Methner and Lauterbach, 2003). The outcome of the control programme has to be assessed on the basis of regular bacteriological examinations of pooled faecal samples. Vaccination does not guarantee protection against entry of *Salmonella* into the pigeon loft.

Rodents

Many domestic and wild-living rodents can carry *Salmonella* in their intestinal tract without showing any clinical symptoms, but extensive epidemiological data are surprisingly scarce. The prevalence of *Salmonella* carriage in rodents seems to vary between 1 and 32%, depending on geographical location and vicinity to humans or other animals (Shimi *et al.*, 1979; Singh *et al.*, 1980; Kirchner *et al.*, 1982; Oboegbulem and Okoronkwo, 1990; Barber *et al.*, 2002; Hilton *et al.*, 2002; Meerburg *et al.*, 2006; Yokoyama *et al.*, 2007; Lapuz *et al.*, 2008).

Rodents are considered as possible reservoir hosts for many pathogens, including *Salmonella*. Rodent control is therefore an important aspect of the biosafety measures in the vicinity of food-producing animals. Mice and rats are often considered to be more susceptible to a *Salmonella* infection, especially to infection with *S.* Typhimurium (hence Typhimurium), mainly based on the finding that this serovar has caused massive epidemics in laboratory mice in the past (Friedman *et al.*, 1996) and that laboratory mice are used as a model for human typhoid in *Salmonella* pathogenesis research. However, only a few specific inbred mouse lines show this increased susceptibility to a *Salmonella* infection. This increased susceptibility can almost entirely be ascribed to the absence of the *slc11a1* gene (also known as *Ity* or *Nramp*). This gene is thought to play an important role in the limitation of intracellular pathogens in macrophages (Wigley, 2004). Until otherwise proven, wild-living and domesticated rodents (except for certain laboratory inbred lines) can be considered equally susceptible to *Salmonella* compared to other mammalian hosts. Especially (very) young animals, old animals, immunocompromised or stressed animals (for example hypovitaminosis C in guinea pigs) and gravid animals are susceptible for clinical infections. The relatively low susceptibility of rodents to clinical salmonellosis renders the application of *Salmonella* as rodenticide inappropriate (Painter *et al.*, 2004). The use of *Salmonella*-based rodenticides may even increase the prevalence of *Salmonella* infections in rodents.

A *Salmonella* infection in mice and hamsters generally does not lead to diarrhoea, except when these animals are pre-treated with antibiotics, such as streptomycin (Bohnhoff and Miller, 1962; Hapfelmeier and Hardt, 2005). In rats and guinea pigs, distention and ulceration of ileum and caecum and production of soft stools may develop. The systemic phase of infection, however, can be devastating in rodents, leading to septicaemia, organ localization (mainly in liver and spleen) and death, especially in *slc11a1*$^{-/-}$ animals. Symptoms often observed in rodents are anorexia, weight loss, lethargy, dull hair coat and occasionally conjunctivitis (Albert *et al.*, 1991). Post mortem, oedema, leucocyte infiltration (mainly neutrophils) and/or necrosis can be observed in the intestines, gut-associated lymphoid tissue and internal organs, such as liver and spleen. Acute infections can be self-limiting, become chronic or eventually lead to death. Nevertheless, the majority of infections in mice are subclinical and do not cause overt symptoms. Asymptomatic carrier animals can pose a threat to both animal and human health (Porcalla and Rodriguez, 2001; Anonymous, 2005; Skov *et al.*, 2008; Featherstone *et al.*, 2010; Harker *et al.*, 2010).

Rabbits

Salmonella can be isolated from wild rabbits at a high prevalence (Vieira-Pinto *et al.*, 2011), and only occasionally from modern commercially farmed rabbits or pet rabbits (Zahraei *et al.*, 2010; Borrelli *et al.*, 2011), even though *Salmonella* infections on commercial rabbitries have resulted in substantial economic losses in the past (Harwood, 1989; Agnoletti *et al.*, 1999). Nowadays, rabbit meat and rabbit pets are possible, but probably infrequent, sources for *Salmonella* infections in humans (Rodríguez-Calleja *et al.*, 2006; Zahraei *et al.*, 2010). *Salmonella* Typhimurium and *S.* Enteritidis are most frequently associated with disease in rabbits; however, other serotypes can also be present (Onyekaba, 1985; Harwood, 1989; Agnoletti *et al.*, 1999; Borrelli *et al.*, 2011; Vieira-Pinto *et al.*, 2011). Sources of infection can be other animals, cages, bedding materials, feed, water or even humans.

Salmonellosis in rabbits is not common, but can cause serious problems with both high morbidity and mortality (Harwood, 1989; Agnoletti *et al.*, 1999). As in other host species, predisposing factors, such as stress, very low or very high age, gravidity and possibly coccidiosis (Harwood, 1989), significantly increase the chance of clinical disease. Most animals, however, will not develop clinical signs and will eliminate the bacterium or will become a persistent asymptomatic carrier. Since rabbits have been used as a model for studying the pathogenesis, and more specifically the intestinal phase, of salmonellosis in the past, some information on the pathogenesis is available (Giannella *et al.*, 1973; Wallis *et al.*, 1989; Hanes *et al.*, 2001). During the intestinal phase of the infection, epithelial cell invasion, leucocyte infiltration and fluid secretion is mediated by the SPI-1 type 3 secretion system (Everest., 1999). Even though (haemorrhagic) diarrhoea is an important clinical sign, this is not always present (Harwood, 1989; Agnoletti *et al.*, 1999). If the bacterium is able to breach the intestinal barrier, the animals can develop septicaemia, resulting in anorexia, lethargy and acute death, increased neonatal losses and in (necrotic) metritis and abortion, most commonly in does in the latter stage of the pregnancy (Harwood, 1989; Agnoletti *et al.*, 1999). Considering the fact that (multiple) antimicrobial resistance has been reported in *Salmonella* strains isolated from rabbits (Borrelli *et al.*, 2011), the choice of antimicrobial agent for treatment should be based on antimicrobial susceptibility tests and on the absence of adverse reactions in rabbits (Harwood, 1989; Agnoletti *et al.*, 1999).

References

Ackman, D.M., Drabkin, P., Birkhead, G. and Cieslak, P. (1995) Reptile-associated salmonellosis in New York State. *Pediatric Infectious Disease Journal* 14, 955–959.

Agnoletti, F., Lenarduzzi, M., Ricci, A. and Marotta, A. (1999) Isolation of *Salmonella* spp. from Italian commercial rabbitries. *2nd International Conference on Rabbit Production in Hot Climates*, Zaragoza. *CIHEAM - Options Méditerranéennes* 189–193.

Aiken, A.M., Lane, C. and Adak, G.K. (2010) Risk of *Salmonella* infection with exposure to reptiles in England, 2004-2007. *Eurosurveillance* 15, 11–18.

Albert, M.J., Ansaruzzaman, M., Faruque, S.M., Haider, K., Qadri, F., Islam, M.M., Kibriya, A.K. and Tzipori, S. (1991) Outbreak of keratoconjunctivitis due to *Salmonella* Weltevreden in a guinea pig colony. *Journal of Clinical Microbiology* 29, 2002–2006.

Aleksic, S., Heinzerling, F. and Bockemuhl, J. (1996) Human infection caused by Salmonellae of subspecies II to VI in Germany, 1977-1992. *Zentralblatt für Bakteriologie* 283, 391–398.

Allgayer, M.C., Lima-Rosa, C.A.V., Weimer, T.A., Rodenbusch, C.R., Pereira, R.A., Streck, A.F., Oliveira, S.D. and Canal, C.W. (2008) Molecular diagnosis of *Salmonella* species in captive psittacine birds. *The Veterinary Record* 162, 816–819.

Allgayer, M.C., de Oliveira, S.J., Mottin, V.D., Loiko, M.R., Abilleira, F., Guedes, N.M.R., Passos, D.T. and Weimer, T.D. (2009) *Salmonella* Braenderup isolation in hyacinth macaw (*Anodorhynchus hyacinthinus*). *Ciencia Rural* 39, 2542–2545.

Andrews-Polymenis, H.L., Rabsch, W., Porwollik, S., McClelland, M., Rosetti, C., Adams, L.G. and Baumler, A.J. (2004) Host restriction of *Salmonella enterica* serotype Typhimurium pigeon isolates does not correlate with loss of discrete genes. *Journal of Bacteriology* 186, 2619–2628.

Ang, O., Ozek, O., Cetin, E.T. and Toreci, K. (1973) *Salmonella* serotypes isolated from tortoises and frogs in Istanbul. *Journal of Hygiene* 71, 85–88.

Anonymous (2005) Outbreak of multidrug-resistant *Salmonella* Typhimurium associated with rodents purchased at retail pet stores – United States, December 2003-October 2004. *Morbidity and Mortality Weekly Report* 54, 429–433.

Barber, D.A., Bahnson, P.B., Isaacson, R., Jones, C.J. and Weigel, R.M. (2002) Distribution of *Salmonella* in swine production ecosystems. *Journal of Food Protection* 65, 1861–1868.

Bartlett, K., Trust, T.J. and Lior, H. (1977) Small pet aquarium frogs as a source of *Salmonella*. *Applied and Environmental Microbiology* 33, 1026–1029.

Bäumler, A.J., Tsolis, R.M., Ficht, T.A. and Adams, L.G. (1998) Evolution of host adaptation in *Salmonella enterica*. *Infection and Immunity* 66, 4579–4587.

Bemis, D.A., Grupka, L.M., Liamthong, S., Folland, D.W., Sykes, J.M. and Ramsay, E.C. (2007) Clonal relatedness of *Salmonella* isolates associated with invasive infections in captive and wild-caught rattlesnakes. *Veterinary Microbiology* 120, 300–307.

Black, D.A., Hay, J., Mead, A.J.C. and Seal, D.V. (1992) *Salmonella* in tropical freshwater fish 'carriage water'. *Public Health* 106, 413–414.

Blanc, B., Delage, B. and Ascione, L. (1960) Comportement des salmonelles inoculées par voie sanguine à *Testudo graeca*. *Bulletin de la Société de Pathologie Exotique* 53, 131–133.

Bohnhoff, M. and Miller, C.P. (1962) Enhanced susceptibility to *Salmonella* infection in streptomycin-treated mice. *Journal of Infectious Diseases* 111, 117–127.

Borrelli, L., Fioretti, A., Ruggiero, V., Santaniello, A., Cringoli, G., Ricci, A., Barco, L., Menna, L.F. and Dipineto, L. (2011) *Salmonella* Typhimurium DT104 in farmed rabbits. *Journal of Veterinary Medical Science* 73, 385–387.

Boycott, J.A. (1962) *Salmonella* species in turtles. *Science* 137, 761.

Brittingham, M.C., Temple, S.A. and Duncan, R.M. (1988) A survey of the prevalence of selected bacteria in wild birds. *Journal of Wildlife Diseases* 24, 299–307.

Caldwell, M.E. and Reyrson, D.L. (1939) Salmonellosis in certain reptiles. *Journal of Infectious Diseases* 65, 242–245.

Cambre, R.C., Green, D.E., Smith, E.E., Montali, R.J. and Bush, M. (1980) Salmonellosis and arizonosis in the reptile collection at the National Zoological Park. *Journal of the American Veterinary Medical Association* 177, 800–803.

Catsaras, M. (1983) *Salmonella* in frog legs – hygienic considerations. *Bulletin de l'Académie Vétérinaire de France* 56, 261–270.

Centers for Disease Control and Prevention (CDC) (2010) Multistate outbreak of human *Salmonella* Typhimurium infections associated with aquatic frogs – United States, 2009. *Journal of the American Medical Association* 303, 502–504.

Chiodini, R.J. (1982) Transovarian passage, visceral distribution, and pathogenicity of *Salmonella* in snakes. *Infection and Immunity* 36, 710–713.

Cohen, M.L., Potter, M., Pollard, R. and Feldman, R.A. (1980) Turtle-associated salmonellosis in the United States: effect of Public Health Action, 1970 to 1976. *Journal of the American Medical Association* 243, 1247–1249.

Communicable Disease Center (1963) Salmonella *surveillance report 1963* 10, 22–24.

Craven, S.E., Stern, N.J., Line, E., Bailey, J.S., Cox, N.A. and Fedorka-Cray, P. (2000) Determination of the incidence of *Salmonella* spp., *Campylobacter jejuni*, and *Clostridium perfringens* in wild birds near broiler houses by sampling intestinal droppings. *Avian Diseases* 44, 715–720.

D'Aoust, J.Y., Daley, E., Crozier, M. and Sewell, A.M. (1990) Pet turtles: a continuing international threat to public health. *American Journal of Epidemiology* 132, 233–238.

Daoust, P.Y. and Prescott, J.F. (2007) Salmonellosis. In: Thomas, N.J., Hunter, D.B. and Atkinson, C.T. (eds) *Infectious Diseases of Wild Birds*. Blackwell Publishing, Oxford, UK, pp. 270–288.

Daoust, P.Y., Busby, D.G., Ferns, L., Goltz, J., McBurney, S., Poppe, C. and Whitney, H. (2000) Salmonellosis in songbirds in the Canadian Atlantic provinces during winter-summer 1997-98. *Canadian Veterinary Journal* 41, 54–59.

Davies, R.H. and Wray, C. (1996) Persistence of *Salmonella enteritidis* in poultry units and poultry food. *British Poultry Science* 37, 589–596.

Deem, S.L., Noss, A.J., Cuellar, R.L. and Karesh, W.B. (2005) Health evaluation of free-ranging and captive blue-fronted Amazon parrots (*Amazona aestiva*) in the Gran Chaco, Bolivia. *Journal of Zoo and Wildlife Medicine* 36, 598–605.

Delage, B. (1966) Survie des *Salmonella* ingérées dans le tractus digestif de quelques animaux. *Bulletin de la Société de Pathologie Exotique* 59, 943–949.

Devi, J.N.S. and Shivananda, P.G. (1983) Frogs as natural reservoirs of *Salmonella*. *Indian Journal of Medical Research* 78, 465–470.

Devriese, L. (1986) *Ziekten van Siervogels en Duiven*, 3rd edn. Rijksuniversiteit, Ghent.

Dimow, I. (1966) Versuche Landschildkröten der Arten *Testudo graeca* und *Testudo hermanni* mit *Salmonella*-bakterien zu infizieren. *Zentblatt für Bakteriologie, Parasitenkunde, Infektionskrankheiten und Hygiene, Abt. I Orig. A* 199, 181–184.

Du Ponte, M.W., Nakamura, R.M. and Chang, E.M.L. (1978) Activation of latent *Salmonella* and *Arizona* organisms by dehydration in red-eared turtles, *Pseudemys scripta elegans*. *American Journal of Veterinary Sciences* 39, 529–530.

Everest, P., Ketley, J., Hardy, S., Douce, G., Khan, S., Shea, J., Holden, D., Maskell, D. and Dougan, G. (1999) Evaluation of *Salmonella* Typhimurium mutants in a model of experimental gastroenteritis. *Infection and Immunity* 67, 2815–2821.

Featherstone, C.A., Reichel, R., Snow, L.C., Davies, R.H., Christiansen, K.H., Carrique-Mas, J.J. and Evans, S.J. (2010) Investigation of risk factors for *Salmonella* on fattening-turkey farms. *Epidemiology and Infection* 138, 1427–1438.

Feeley, B.S. and Treger, M.D. (1969) Penetration of turtle eggs by *Salmonella* braenderup. *Public Health Report USA* 84, 156–158.

Fenlon, D.R. (1981) Seagulls (*Larus* spp.) as vectors of salmonellae: an investigation into the range of serotypes and numbers of salmonellae in gull faeces. *Journal of Hygiene* 86, 195–202.

Friedman, C.R., Malcolm, G., Rigau-Pérez, J.G., Arámbulo, P. 3rd and Tauxe, R.V. (1996) Public health risk from *Salmonella*-based rodenticides. *The Lancet* 347, 1705–1706.

Gaulin, C., Vincent, C. and Ismail, J. (2005) Sporadic infections of *Salmonella* Paratyphi B var. Java associated with fish tanks. *Canadian Journal of Public Health* 96, 471–474.

Gerlach, H. (1994) Bacteria. In: Ritchie, B.W., Harrison, G.J. and Harrison, L.R. (eds) *Avian Medicine, Principles and Applications*. Wingers Publishing, Lake Worth, Florida, pp. 949–983.

Giannella, R.A., Formal, S.B., Dammin, G.J. and Collins, H. (1973) Pathogenesis of salmonellosis. Studies of fluid secretion, mucosal invasion, and morphologic reaction in the rabbit ileum. *Journal of Clinical Investigation* 52, 441–453.González Candela, M.G., Atance, P.M., Seva, J., Pallarés, F.J. and Vizcaíno, L.L. (2005) Granulomatous hepatitis caused by *Salmonella* Typhimurium in a spur-thighed tortoise (*Testudo graeca*). *The Veterinary Record* 157, 236–237.

Greenberg, Z. and Sechter, I. (1992) *Salmonella* serotypes isolated from snakes and other reptiles - Israel, 1953-1989. *Israel Journal of Veterinary Medicine* 47, 49–60.

Guerra, B., Helmuth, R., Thomas, K., Beutlich, J., Jahn, S. and Schroeter, A. (2010) Plasmid-mediated quinolone resistance determinants in *Salmonella* spp. isolates from reptiles in Germany. *Journal of Antimicrobial Chemotherapy* 65, 2043–2045.

Hanes, D.E., Robl, M.G., Schneider, C.M. and Burr, D.H. (2001) New Zealand white rabbit as a nonsurgical experimental model for *Salmonella enterica* gastroenteritis. *Infection and Immunity* 69, 6523–6526.

Hapfelmeier, S. and Hardt, W.D. (2005) A mouse model for *S.* Typhimurium-induced enterocolitis. *Trends in Microbiology* 13, 497–503.

Harker, K.S., Lane, C., De Pinna, E. and Adak, G.K. (2010) An outbreak of *Salmonella* Typhimurium DT191a associated with reptile feeder mice. *Epidemiology and Infection* 14, 1–8.

Harrington, R., Blackburn, B.O. and Cassidy, D.R. (1975) Salmonellosis in canaries. *Avian Diseases* 19, 827–829.

Harwood, D.G. (1989) *Salmonella* Typhimurium infection in a commercial rabbitry. *The Veterinary Record* 125, 554–555.

Hilton, A.C., Willis, R.J. and Hickie, S.J. (2002) Isolation of *Salmonella* from urban wild brown rats (*Rattus norvegicus*) in the West Midlands, UK. *International Journal of Environmental Health Research* 12, 163–168.

Hughes, L.A., Wigley, P., Bennett, M., Chantrey, J. and Williams, N. (2010) Multi-locus sequence typing of *Salmonella enterica* serovar Typhimurium isolates from wild birds in northern England suggests host-adapted strain. *Letters in Applied Microbiology* 51, 477–479.

Jones, T.F., Ingram, L.A., Fullerton, K.E., Marcus, R., Anderson, B.J., McCarthy, P.V., Vugia, D., Shiferaw, B., Haubert, N., Wedel, S. and Angulo, F.J. (2006) A case-control study of the epidemiology of sporadic *Salmonella* infection in infants. *Pediatrics* 118, 2380–2387.

Kaufmann, A.F., Fox, M.D., Morris, G.K., Wood, B.T., Feeley, J.C. and Frix, M.K. (1972) Turtle-associated salmonellosis. III. The effects of environmental *Salmonellae* in commercial turtle breeding ponds. *American Journal of Epidemiology* 95, 521–528.

Kimpe, A., Decostere, A., Martel, A., Haesebrouck, F. and Devriese, L.A. (2002) Prevalence of antimicrobial resistance among pigeon isolates of *Streptococcus gallolyticus, Escherichia coli* and *Salmonella enterica* serotype Typhimurium. *Avian Pathology* 31, 393–397.

Kirchner, B.K., Dixon, L.W., Lentsch, R.H. and Wagner, J.E. (1982) Recovery and pathogenicity of several *Salmonella* species isolated from mice. *Laboratory Animal Science* 32, 506–508.

Kodama, H., Nakanishi, Y., Yamamoto, F., Mikami, T., Izawah, H., Imagawa T., Hasimoto, Y. and Kudo, N. (1987) *Salmonella arizonae* isolated from a pirarucu, *Arapaima gigas* Cuvier, with septicaemia. *Journal of Fish Diseases* 10, 509–512.

Koopman, J.P. and Kennis, H.M. (1976) Occurrence and treatment of *Salmonella* carriers in tejus (*Tupinambis teguixin*) and tortoises (*Testudo hermanni*). *Tijdschrift voor Diergeneeskunde* 101, 957–961.

Lamm, S.H., Taylor, A., Gangarosa, E.J., Anderson, H.W., Young, W., Clark, M.H. and Bruce, A.R. (1972) Turtle-associated salmonellosis. An estimation of the magnitude of the problem in the United States. *American Journal of Epidemiology* 95, 511–517.

Lapuz, R., Tani, H., Sasai, K., Shirota, K., Katoh, H. and Baba, E. (2008) The role of roof rats (*Rattus rattus*) in the spread of *Salmonella* Enteritidis and *S.* Infantis contamination in layer farms in eastern Japan. *Epidemiology and Infection* 136, 1235–1243.

Levings, R.S., Lightfoot, D., Hall, R.M. and Djordjevic, S.P. (2006) Aquariums as reservoirs for multidrug-resistant *Salmonella* Paratyphi B. *Emerging Infectious Diseases* 12, 507–509.

Maciel, B.M., Argolo, R.C., Nogueira, S.S.C., Dias, J.C.T. and Rezende, R.P. (2010) High prevalence of *Salmonella* in tegu lizards (*Tupinambis merianae*), and susceptibility of the serotypes to antibiotics. *Zoonoses and Public Health* 57, e23–e36.

Madadgar, O., Salehi, T.Z., Ghafari, M.M., Tamai, I.A., Madani, S.A. and Yahyareyat, R. (2009) Study of an unusual paratyphoid epornitic in canaries (*Serinus canaria*). *Avian Pathology* 38, 437–441.

Magnino, S., Colin, P., Dei-Cas, E., Masen, M., McLauchlin, J., Nöckler, K., Maradona, M.P., Tsigarida, E., Vanopdenbosch, E. and Van Peteghem, C. (2009) Biological risks associated with consumption of reptile products. *International Journal of Food Microbiology* 134, 163–175.

Manfrin, A., Friso, S., Perin, R., Qualtieri, K. and Bovo, G. (2001) Tropical fish importation from third countries: the potential risk of introducing human and aquatic animal pathogens. In: Rodgers, C.J. (ed.) *Risk Analysis in Aquatic Animal Health. Proceedings of the OIE International Conference* held in Paris, France, 8–10 February 2000, pp. 167–170.

Meerburg, B.G., Jacobs-Reitsma, W.F., Wagenaar, J.A. and Kijlstra, A. (2006) Presence of *Salmonella* and *Campylobacter* spp. in wild small mammals on organic farms. *Applied and Environmental Microbiology* 72, 960–962.

Mermin, J., Hutwagner, L., Vugia, D., Shallow, S., Daily, P., Bender, J., Koehler, J., Marcus, R. and Angulo, F.J. (2004) Reptiles, amphibians, and human *Salmonella* infection: a population-based, case-control study. *Clinical Infectious Diseases* 38, 253–261.

Methner, U. and Lauterbach, L. (2003) Studies on the detection of *Salmonella* Typhimurium variant Copenhagen DT2 in fancy pigeons. *Deutsche Tierärztliche Wochenschrift* 110, 239–244.

Michael-Marler, S., Brown, M.L. and Siebeling, R.J. (1983) Eradication of *Arizona henshawii* from artificially infected turtle eggs. *Applied and Environmental Microbiology* 45, 748–754.

Mitchell, M.A. and Shane, S.M. (2001) *Salmonella* in reptiles. *Seminars in Avian and Exotic Pet Medicine* 10, 25–35.

Mitchell, M.A., Adamson, T.W., Singleton, C.B., Roundtree, M.K., Bauer, R.W. and Acierno, M.J. (2007) Evaluation of a combination of sodium hypochlorite and polyhexamethylene biguanide as an egg wash for red-eared slider turtles (*Trachemys scripta elegans*) to suppress or eliminate *Salmonella* organisms on egg surfaces and in hatchlings. *American Journal of Veterinary Research* 68, 158–164.

Moreno, C.M., Vargas, M.M.O., Echeita, A. and Usera, M.A. (1995) Occurrence of *Salmonella* in cold-blooded animals in Gran Canaria, Canary islands, Spain. *Antonie Van Leeuwenhoek International Journal of General and Molecular Microbiology* 68, 191–194.

Musto, J., Kirk, M., Lightfoot, D., Combs, B.G. and Mwanri, L. (2006) Multi-drug resistant *Salmonella* Java infections acquired from tropical fish aquariums, Australia, 2003-04. *Communicable Disease Intelligence* 30, 222–227.

Oboegbulem, S.I. and Okoronkwo, I. (1990) Salmonellae in the African great cane rat (*Thryonomys swinderianus*). *Journal of Wildlife Diseases* 26, 119–121.

Ok, A. and Yardimci, H. (2010) Isolation of *Salmonella* spp. in cage birds in Ankara. *Ankara Universitesi Veteriner Fakultesi Dergisi* 57, 201–203.

Olsen, S.J., Bishop, R., Brenner, F.W., Roels, T.H., Bean, N., Tauxe, R.V. and Slutsker, L. (2001) The changing epidemiology of *Salmonella*: trends in serotypes isolated from humans in the United States, 1987–1997. *Journal of Infectious Diseases* 183, 753–761.

Onderka, D.K. and Finlayson, D.C. (1985) Salmonellae and salmonellosis in captive reptiles. *Canadian Journal of Comparative Medicine* 49, 268–270.

Onyekaba, C.O. (1985) *Salmonella* Ochiogu: experimental infection of laboratory rabbits (*Oryctolagus cuniculus*). *Laboratory Animals* 19, 32–34.

Oros, J., Rodriguez, J.L., Fernandez, A., Herraez, P., de los Monteros, A.E. and Jacobson, E.R. (1998) Simultaneous occurrence of *Salmonella arizonae* in a sulfur crested cockatoo (*Cacatua galerita galerita*) and iguanas. *Avian Diseases* 42, 818–823.

Orosz, S.E., Chengappa, M.M., Oyster, R.A., Morris, P.J., Trock, S. and Altekruse, S. (1992) *Salmonella* Enteritidis infection in 2 species of psittaciformes. *Avian Diseases* 36, 766–769.

Painter, J.A., Mølbak, K., Sonne-Hansen, J., Barrett, T., Wells, J.G. and Tauxe, R.V. (2004) *Salmonella*-based rodenticides and public health. *Emerging Infectious Diseases* 10, 985–987.

Panigrahy, B. and Gilmore, W.C. (1983) Systemic salmonellosis in an African gray parrot and *Salmonella* osteomyelitis in canaries. *Journal of the American Veterinary Medical Association* 183, 699–700.

Pasmans, F., De Herdt, P. and Haesebrouck, F. (2002a) Pathogenesis of infections with *Salmonella enterica* serovar Muenchen in the turtle *Trachemys scripta scripta*. *Veterinary Microbiology* 87, 315–325.

Pasmans, F., De Herdt, P. and Haesebrouck, F. (2002b) Interactions of *Salmonella enterica* serovar Muenchen with macrophages of the turtle *Trachemys scripta scripta*. *Developmental and Comparative Immunology* 26, 295–304.

Pasmans, F., Van Immerseel, F., Heyndrickx, M., Godard, C., Wildemauwe, C., Ducatelle, R. and Haesebrouck, F. (2003) Host adaptation of pigeon isolates of *Salmonella* serovar Typhimurium var. Copenhagen PT99 is associated with macrophage cytotoxicity. *Infection and Immunity* 71, 6068–6074.

Pasmans, F., Van Immerseel, F., Hermans, K., Heyndrickx, M., Collard, J.M., Ducatelle, R. and Haesebrouck, F. (2004) Assessment of virulence of pigeon isolates of *Salmonella enterica* subsp. *enterica* serovar Typhimurium variant Copenhagen for humans. *Journal of Clinical Microbiology* 42, 2000–2002.

Pasmans, F., Martel, A., Boyen, F., Vandekerchove, D., Wybo, I., Van Immerseel, F., Heyndrickx, M., Collard, J.M., Ducatelle, R. and Haesebrouck, F. (2005) Characterization of *Salmonella* isolates from captive lizards. *Veterinary Microbiology* 110, 285–291.

Pasmans, F., Baert, K., Martel, A., Bousquet-Melou, A., Lanckriet, R., De Boever, S., Van Immerseel, F., Eeckhaut, V., de Backer, P. and Haesebrouck, F. (2008) Induction of the carrier state in pigeons infected with *Salmonella enterica* subspecies *enterica* serovar Typhimurium PT99 by treatment with florfenicol: a matter of pharmacokinetics. *Antimicrobial Agents and Chemotherapy* 52, 954–961.

Pedersen, K., Lassen-Nielsen, A.M., Nordentoft, S. and Hammer, A.S. (2009) Serovars of *Salmonella* from captive reptiles. *Zoonoses Public Health* 56, 238–242.

Pennycott, T.W., Ross, H.M., McLaren, I.M., Park, A., Hopkins, G.F. and Foster, G. (1998) Causes of death of wild birds of the family *Fringillidae* in Britain. *The Veterinary Record* 143, 155–158.

Pennycott, T.W., Mather, H.A., Bennett, G. and Foster, G. (2010) Salmonellosis in garden birds in Scotland, 1995 to 2008: geographic region, *Salmonella enterica* phage type and bird species. *The Veterinary Record* 166, 419–422.

Pfleger, S., Benyr, G., Sommer, R. and Hassl, A. (2003) Pattern of *Salmonella* excretion in amphibians and reptiles in a vivarium. *International Journal of Hygiene and Environmental Health* 206, 53–59.

Piccirillo, A., Mazzariol, S., Caliari, D. and Menandro, M.L. (2010) *Salmonella* Typhimurium phage type DT160 infection in two Moluccan cockatoos (*Cacatua moluccensis*): clinical presentation and pathology. *Avian Diseases* 54, 131–135.

Pohl, P., Lintermans, P., Vandendriessche, A. and Boutiflat, Y. (1983) Epidémiologie de *Salmonella typhimurium* variété Copenhagen. *Annales de Médecine Vétérinaire* 127, 279–287.

Porcalla, A.R. and Rodriguez, W.J. (2001) Soft tissue and cartilage infection by *Salmonella* Oranienburg in a healthy girl. *Southern Medical Journal* 94, 435–437.

Purushothaman, V., Jayaraman, M.S. and Balaprakasam, R.A. (1981) *Salmonella* contamination of frog legs and shrimps in Madras. *Cheiron* 10, 197–200.

Rabsch, W., Andrews, H.L., Kingsley, R.A., Prager, R., Tschape, H., Adams, L.G. and Baumler, A.J. (2002) *Salmonella enterica* serotype Typhimurium and its host-adapted variants. *Infection and Immunity* 70, 2249–2255.

Raidal, S.R. (1998) Salmonellosis in two canary (*Serinus canaria*) flocks. *Australian Veterinary Practitioner* 28, 58.

Rajagopalan, D., Deshpande, C.K. and Joshi, L. (1983) Lactose positive *Salmonella* – inpraw from processed frog legs. *Indian Journal of Medical Research* 78, 177–180.

Rajendran, P., Jainamboo, K.S.M. and Thyagarajan, S.P. (1998) A study on the green frog (*Rana hexadactyla*) in relation to the environmental dissemination of enteric human pathogens. *Journal of Environmental Biology* 19, 73–78.

Ramsay, E.C., Daniel, G.B., Tryon, B.W., Merryman, J.L., Morris, P.J. and Bemis, D.A. (2002) Osteomyelitis associated with *Salmonella enterica* subsp. *arizonae* in a colony of ridgenose rattlesnakes (*Crotalus willardi*). *Journal of Zoo and Wildlife Medicine* 33, 301–310.

Refsum, T., Vikoren, T., Handeland, K., Kapperud, G. and Holstad, G. (2003) Epidemiologic and pathologic aspects of *Salmonella typhimurium* infection in passerine birds in Norway. *Journal of Wildlife Diseases* 39, 64–72.

Reinhard, G.R., Harbison, M.L., Tolles, A.K. and Zaoutis, T.E. (1988) Subcutaneous *Salmonella* granulomas in canaries. *Laboratory Animal Sciences* 38, 505.

Rodríguez-Calleja, J.M., García-López, I., García-López, M.L., Santos, J.A. and Otero, A. (2006) Rabbit meat as a source of bacterial foodborne pathogens. *Journal of Food Protection* 69, 1106–1112.

Sanyal, D., Burge, S.H. and Hutchings, P.G. (1987) Enteric pathogens in tropical aquaria. *Epidemiology and Infection* 99, 635–640.

Sawa, H., Hirai, K., Kinjo, T., Shibata, I. and Shimakura, S. (1981) *Salmonella typhimurium* infection in imported passerine and psittacine birds. *Japanese Journal of Veterinary Sciences* 43, 967–969.

Schröter, M., Speicher, A., Hofmann, J. and Roggentin, P. (2006) Analysis of the transmission of *Salmonella* spp. through generations of pet snakes. *Environmental Microbiology* 8, 556–559.

Scope, A., Hofer, E. and Vosacek, L. (1998) Occurrence of pathogenic bacteria in clinically healthy psittacines. *Wiener Tierärztliche Monatsschrift* 85, 82–86.

Seepersadsingh, N. and Adesiyun, A.A. (2003) Prevalence and antimicrobial resistance of *Salmonella* spp. in pet mammals, reptiles, fish aquarium water and birds in Trinidad. *Journal of Veterinary Medicine B* 50, 488–493.

Shane, S.M., Gilbert, R. and Harrington, K.S. (1990) *Salmonella* colonization in commercial pet turtles (*Pseudemys scripta elegans*). *Epidemiology and Infection* 105, 307–316.

Shima, A.L. and Osborn, K.G. (1989) An epornitic of *Salmonella* Typhimurium in a collection of lories and lorikeets. *Journal of Zoo and Wildlife Medicine* 20, 373–376.

Shimi, A., Keyhani, M. and Hedayati, K. (1979) Studies on salmonellosis in the house mouse, *Mus musculus*. *Laboratory Animals* 13, 33–34.

Siebeling, R.J., Neal, P.M. and Granberry, W.D. (1975) Treatment of *Salmonella-Arizona*-infected turtle eggs with terramycin and chloromycetin by the temperature-differential egg dip method. *Applied Microbiology* 30, 791–799.

Singh, S.P., Sethi, M.S. and Sharma, V.D. (1980) The occurrence of salmonellae in rodent, shrew, cockroach and ant. *International Journal of Zoonoses* 7, 58–61.

Skov, M.N., Madsen, J.J., Rahbek, C., Lodal, J., Jespersen, J.B., Jørgensen, J.C., Dietz, H.H., Chriél, M. and Baggesen, D.L. (2008) Transmission of *Salmonella* between wildlife and meat-production animals in Denmark. *Journal of Applied Microbiology* 105, 1558–1568.

Smith, J.N., Dyszel, J.L., Soares, J.A., Ellermeier, C.D., Altier, C., Lawhon, S.D., Adams, L.G., Konjufca, V., Curtiss 3rd, R., Slauch, J.M. and Ahmer, B.M. (2008) SdiA, an N-acylhomoserine lactone receptor, becomes active during the transit of *Salmonella enterica* through the gastrointestinal tract of turtles. *PLoS ONE*, e2826

Srikantiah, P., Lay, J.C., Hand, S., Crump, J.A., Campbell, J., Van Duyne, M.S., Bishop, R., Middendor, R., Currier, M., Mead, P.S. and Mølbak, K. (2004) *Salmonella enterica* serotype Javiana infections associated with amphibian contact, Mississippi, 2001. *Epidemiology and Infection* 132, 273–281.

Stehr Green, J.K. and Schantz, P.M. (1987) The impact of zoonotic disease transmitted by pets on human health and the economy. *Veterinary Clinics of North America – Small Animal Practice* 17, 5–7.

Taylor, D.J. and Philbey, A.W. (2010) *Salmonella* infections in garden birds and cats in a domestic environment. *The Veterinary Record* 164, 26–28.

Uyttebroek, E., Devriese, L.A., Gevaert, D., Ducatelle, R., Nelis, J. and Haesebrouck, F. (1991) Protective effects of vaccines against experimental salmonellosis in racing pigeons. *Veterinary Record* 128, 152–153.

Vieira-Pinto, M., Morais, L., Caleja, C., Themudo, P., Torres, C., Igrejas, G., Poeta, P. and Martins, C. (2011) *Salmonella* sp. in Game (*Sus scrofa* and *Oryctolagus cuniculus*). *Foodborne Pathogens and Disease* 8(6), 739–740.

Vigo, G.B., Origlia, J., Gornatti, D., Piscopo, M., Salve, A., Caffer, M.I., Pichel, M., Binsztein, N. and Leotta, G.A. (2009) Isolation of *Salmonella* Typhimurium from dead blue and gold macaws (*Ara araurana*). *Avian Diseases* 53, 135–138.

Wallis, T.S., Hawker, R.J., Candy, D.C., Qi, G.M., Clarke, G.J., Worton, K.J., Osborne, M.P. and Stephen, J. (1989) Quantification of the leucocyte influx into rabbit ileal loops induced by strains of *Salmonella* Typhimurium of different virulence. *Journal of Medical Microbiology* 30, 149–156.

Ward, M.P., Ramer, J.C., Proudfoot, J., Garner, M.M., Juan-Salles, C. and Wu, C.C. (2003) Outbreak of salmonellosis in a zoologic collection of lorikeets and lories (*Trichoglossus, Lorius*, and *Eos* spp.). *Avian Diseases* 47, 493–498.

Warwick, C., Lambiris, A.J.L., Westwood, D. and Steedman, C. (2001) Reptile-related salmonellosis. *Journal of the Royal Society of Medicine* 94, 124–126.

Weber, A. (1973) Ueber einen Behandlungsversuch bei latent met Salmonellen infizierten Schildkröten. *Kleintier Praxis* 18, 48–50.

Wigley, P. (2004) Genetic resistance to *Salmonella* infection in domestic animals. *Research in Veterinary Science* 76, 165–169.

Wobeser, G.A. and Finlayson, M.C. (1969) *Salmonella typhimurium* infection in house sparrows. *Archives of Environmental Health* 19, 882–884.

Woodward, D.L., Khakhria, R. and Johnson, W.M. (1997) Human salmonellosis associated with exotic pets. *Journal of Clinical Microbiology* 35, 2786–2790.

Yokoyama, E., Maruyama, S., Kabeya, H., Hara, S., Sata, S., Kuroki, T. and Yamamoto, T. (2007) Prevalence and genetic properties of *Salmonella enterica* serovar Typhimurium definitive phage type 104 isolated from *Rattus norvegicus* and *Rattus rattus* house rats in Yokohama City, Japan. *Applied and Environmental Microbiology* 73, 2624–2630.

Zahraei, T., Mahzouniehand, M. and Khaksar, E. (2010) Detection of *Salmonella* serovars in zoo and pet reptiles, rabbits, and rodents in Iran by culture and PCR methods. *Comparative Clinical Pathology* 19, 199–202.

Zwart, P. (1960) *Salmonella* and *Arizona* infections in reptiles in the Netherlands. *A. Van Leeuw, Journal of Microbiology and Serology* 26, 250–254.

Zwart, P., Poelma, F.G. and Strik, W.J. (1970) The distribution of various types of salmonellae and arizonas in reptiles. *Zentralblatt für Bakteriologie, Parasitenkunde Infektionskranheiten und Hygiene Abteilung* 1, 213, 201–212.

18 Public Health Aspects of *Salmonella* Infections

Wolfgang Rabsch,[1]* Sandra Simon[1] and Tom Humphrey[2]

[1]*National Reference Centre for Salmonella and other Enteric Pathogens at the Robert Koch Institute, Germany;* [2]*National Centre for Zoonosis Research, University of Liverpool, UK*

Historical Perspective

In 1880, Karl Joseph Eberth described a bacillus that he suspected to be the cause of typhoid fever (Eberth, 1880). In 1884, the pathologist Georg Theodor August Gaffky confirmed Eberth's findings, and the organism was named Gaffky-Eberth bacillus. At that time, it was also known that bacteria similar to *Salmonella* serovar Typhi could cause enteric disease in humans and farm animals. This was proved when Salmon and Smith reported the isolation of the bacteria responsible for 'hog cholera' or 'swine fever' in 1885. The name *Salmonella* was subsequently adopted in honour of Salmon, an American veterinary surgeon.

In the early to mid-20th century there were many pioneering studies into the identification and differentiation of *Salmonella*. The schemes that were developed made use of the fact that, although *Salmonella* show considerable antigenic diversity, they elicit two principal antibody reactions in infected animals. Thus antibodies are produced against cell-surface or somatic O antigens and flagella or H antigens. In 1929, White developed a typing scheme based on this antigenic variation, which was later modified by Kauffmann. This work enabled the differentiation of *Salmonella* into serovars. In 1934, the first Kauffmann-White scheme containing 44 serovars was published by Kauffmann and the *Salmonella* Subcommittee (Kelterborn, 1967).

Later, biochemical methods were introduced into the scheme to better identify the diverse characteristics of *Salmonella* species and subspecies. In the following years, supplements describing novel serovars of different subspecies had been published by the WHO Collaborating Centre for Reference and Research on *Salmonella* under the leadership of Le Minor. In recognition of the importance of the work by Le Minor in the 1970s and 1980s, the scheme was renamed the White-Kauffmann-Le Minor scheme. Two species had been classified within the genus *Salmonella*: *S. enterica* (grouped in six subspecies) and *S. bongori* (former subsp. V, with only 23 serovars). The vast majority of serovars (1547) belong to *S. enterica* subsp. *enterica*. The last supplement (no. 47) was edited in 2010 by Weill and specifies 2610 *Salmonella* serovars. To date, the White-Kauffmann-Le Minor scheme is the benchmark for *Salmonella* typing worldwide (Guibourdenche *et al.*, 2010). Today the scientifically correct term for the bacillus that causes typhoid fever is *Salmonella enterica* subsp. *enterica* serovar Typhi or short *S.* Typhi.

* Corresponding author, e-mail: rabschw@rki.de

© CAB International 2013. *Salmonella in Domestic Animals, 2nd Edition* (eds P.A. Barrow and U. Methner)

Since some of the common serovars such as *S.* Enteritidis and *S.* Typhimurium not only cause human infections but are also major livestock colonizers, the *Salmonella* subclassification requires more discriminative methods than serotyping. During the past 50 years, phage typing became a very valuable tool for epidemiological purposes. The scheme for *S.* Typhimurium developed by Felix in 1956 (England) played a major role in many outbreak investigations and the *S.* Enteritidis scheme from Ward (Ward *et al.*, 1987) and Lalko/Laszlo (Poland and Hungary, Laszlo *et al.*, 1985) has been invaluable in the investigation of egg- and poultry-associated outbreaks that have been carried out worldwide from the 1980s to the present.

Prior to 1960, the majority of *Salmonella* isolates worldwide were fully susceptible to the available antibiotics but since 1962 drug-resistant *Salmonella* strains have dramatically increased. Today, monitoring for antimicrobial resistance is standard practice. The combined determination of serovar, phage type and resistance markers played a major role in tracking *Salmonella* outbreaks in Germany, particularly for *S.* Typhimurium belonging to the definitive phage type 9 (DT9) in the 1960s or to the multiresistant DT204 in the 1970s and DT104 in the 1990s (Callow, 1959; Anderson *et al.*, 1977; Rabsch *et al.*, 2001a). In parallel with the appearance of antibiotic resistance in *Salmonella*, plasmid-mediated transfer of drug resistance and spontaneous segregation and recombination of resistance factors were described for *S.* Typhimurium by Watanabe and Lyang in 1962. Many studies on plasmid typing followed. This method represents another helpful tool for strain differentiation but is of limited use in serovars such as *S.* Enteritidis where the majority of isolates carry one single plasmid. In numerous outbreak investigations these classical typing methods combined with molecular approaches such as pulsed-field gel electrophoresis (PFGE), ribotyping or multiple-locus variable number tandem repeat analysis (MLVA) allowed trace back the source of infection to a contaminated food product.

Human salmonellosis is one of the main causes of gastrointestinal infections worldwide and raises enormous public health problems in both developing and developed countries. In addition, the world has been getting 'smaller' during the last decades. To meet the ever-growing challenge produced by increased travelling and the dramatic growth of food import and export, surveillance networks became necessary to manage the international salmonellosis problems. Therefore, the Salm-Net surveillance network, which concentrated on standardization of *Salmonella* phage typing and the establishment of an efficient international *Salmonella* database, was funded in 1994 by the EU. In numerous outbreak investigations Salm-Net and later Enter-Net demonstrated that the timely cross-national exchange of information allows effective public health activities in Europe and outside. In October 2007, the Enter-Net network was integrated into the European Centre for Disease Prevention and Control (ECDC) Food- and Waterborne Disease unit (FWD) in Stockholm.

The European Food Safety Authority (EFSA), located in Parma, Italy, was funded by the European Community as an independent agency in 2002. It is responsible for food safety and possesses regulatory authority with the objective of consumer protection. The ECDC, an EU-agency based in Stockholm, Sweden, was established in 2005. The function of the ECDC is the enhancement of European defence strategies against infectious diseases.

Human Salmonellosis in Change of Time – a Summary for Germany

Recent salmonellosis data from Germany are presented as example for the trends in most of the EU Member States. Facilitated by improved living conditions and better hygiene and health care schemes the case numbers of typhoid salmonellosis decreased steadily during the last decades and can be assumed at present to be less than 100 per year. In contrast, the number of enteric salmonellosis cases is high with more than 25,300 infections in 2010 in industrial livestock farming and food production. The altered food consumption patterns play an important role in transfer and spread of *Salmonella* organisms. Livestock cleaning and prevention of environmental dissemination of pathogenic bacteria (e.g. by waste water) represent essential needs to break transmission routes and to eliminate reservoirs of enteric *Salmonella* (Biesold and Behrend, 1970; Heuvelink *et al.*, 2007).

Most of the infective *Salmonella* are still transmitted to humans via contaminated food containing raw eggs or undercooked meat but vegetables, including fresh produce (lettuce, sprouts etc.), are gaining more and more in importance. Now and then fairly uncommon infection sources, spices, groundnuts or even chocolate have been detected. Although the reported cases of salmonellosis have varied since the legal validity of the Federal Law on Epidemic Control (BSeuchG, 1962-2000, Infection Protection Act (IfSG)) the overall trend showed increasing infection numbers from 1962 until 1992 (Fig. 18.1). Considered retrospectively, the implementation of the recommended control measures of the council of the federal board of health (Kolpinghaus Berlin report, 1984; Votum of Bundesgesundheitsrat, 1985) were less successful, because in the following years the *Salmonella* infections caused by raw or 'undercooked' eggs increased dramatically. From the early 1990s the incidence rate dropped year by year as a consequence of numerous implemented *Salmonella* control programmes for the most common serovars (regulations on table eggs and on *Salmonella* in poultry) and the immunization strategy now applied using a safe live vaccine in poultry (Rabsch *et al.*, 2001b). The number of outbreaks decreased from 844 with total cases from 3229 in 2009 to 562 outbreaks with 2108 cases from 2009 to 2010. However, the real frequency of *Salmonella*-caused disease is hard to estimate since patients with mild diarrhoea and short illness frequently do not approach a physician. On the other hand, the rising cost pressure in the public health sector and, as a consequence, the minimized microbiological diagnostics applied to patients with diarrhoea result in the reduction of reported infections, which impedes the early recognition of pathogen transition or transformation. The number of unreported cases is assumed to be from 10- to 15-fold higher. The highest incidence is observed in children younger than 10 years with a maximum in infants.

The Most Important *Salmonella* Serovars

Enteric salmonellosis is provoked by a great variety of *Salmonella* serovars (Table 18.1), which have their primary reservoir often within livestock populations where they persist subclinically – and undetected. The bacteria are typically transmitted to humans via contaminated food and animal products (pork, poultry meat or eggs etc.). The vast

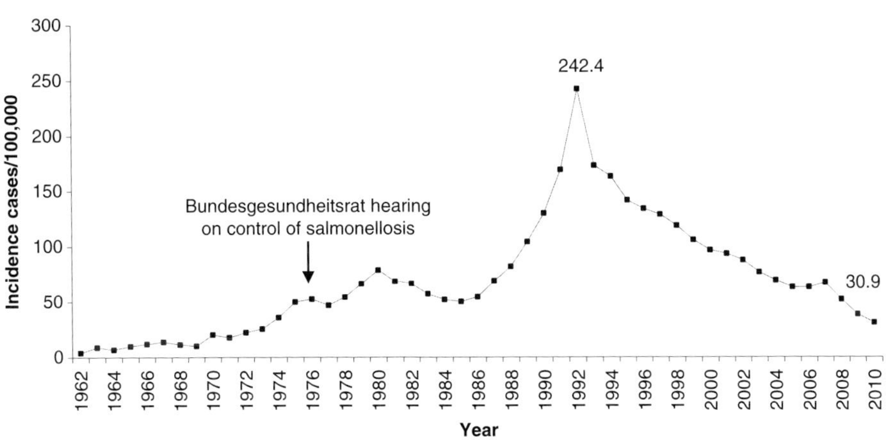

Fig. 18.1. Incidence of salmonellosis in Germany; reported cases 1962–2010.

majority of *Salmonella* isolates sent to the National Reference Centre (NRC) for subtyping belong to serovars Enteritidis and Typhimurium (~80%). While the former is mostly associated with hen eggs and chicken, the latter is commonly transmitted by pork and meat products. *Salmonella* Enteritidis had been the first-ranked serovar in Germany for several decades but recently it has been observed that *S.* Typhimurium is going to take that position since *S.* Enteritidis infections have decreased rapidly over the last few years. There were 34,679 cases in 2007 and only 9482 in 2010, while *S.* Typhimurium cases have declined much more slowly: 11,377 in 2007 compared to 8362 in 2010. An explanation for the rapid drop of reported *S.* Enteritidis cases could be the implemented *Salmonella* control measures. The serovars ranked 3 to 20 vary in their order frequently although the individual share seldom rises above 1%.

Phage typing provides a valuable epidemiological tool for further sub-differentiation of distinct serovars and is of extraordinary importance in outbreak investigations. At the NRC this method has been established for serovars Enteritidis, Typhimurium and some others. Furthermore, molecular techniques such as ribotyping (for *S.* Enteritidis) and PFGE (for *S.* Typhimurium and others) are applied to supposed outbreak isolates. The routine phage typing of *S.* Enteritidis was performed according to the typing system of Ward/Lalko and Laszlo, e.g. PT 4/6: phage type 4 according to Ward and 6 according to Lalko and Laszlo (Laszlo *et al.*, 1985; Ward *et al.*, 1987). The two most frequently reported phage types of *S.* Enteritidis were PT4/6 and PT8/7, although PT4/6 has shown a remarkable decrease during recent years. Other phage types are also involved in mainly raw egg-associated outbreaks. The ribotype differentiation is very helpful especially for

Table 18.1. The most common reported *Salmonella* serovars isolated from humans in Germany (Robert Koch-Institut, 2011a).

Serovar	Percentage						
	2004	2005	2006	2007	2008	2009	2010
S. Enteritidis	64.15	61.06	61.66	62.58	53.45	48.37	37.5
S. Typhimurium	19.78	22.12	20.83	20.53	25.58	27.39	33
S. Infantis	1.32	0.87	061	0.72	0.82	1.2	1.56
S. Goldcoast	0.57	0.25	0.08	0.12	0.3	0.23	0.11
S. Virchow	0.34	0.35	0.29	0.31	0.26	0.32	0.39
S. Give	0.27	0.05	0.04	0.03	0.03	0.02	0.05
S. Derby	0.28	0.3	0.4	0.3	0.4	0.44	0.67
S. Bovismorbificans	0.27	1.07	0.22	0.23	0.53	0.22	0.27
S. Brandenburg	0.25	0.16	0.19	0.17	0.27	0.3	0.29
S. Kentucky	0.19	0.21	0.15	0.14	0.15	0.16	0.41
S. Livingston	0.18	0.09	0.08	0.14	1.23	0.23	0.21
S. Anatum	0.17	0.27	0.07	0.08	0.13	0.05	0.06
S. Hadar	0.16	0.24	0.56	0.17	0.14	0.24	0.2
S. Agona	0.12	0.09	0.09	0.08	0.17	0.19	0.19
S. Newport	0.14	0.27	0.33	0.27	0.29	0.33	0.33
S. London	0.11	0.08	0.07	0.08	0.15	0.18	0.3
S. Stanley	0.07	0.17	0.11	0.07	0.09	0.06	0.12
S. Muenchen	0.04	0.06	0.17	0.09	0.11	0.13	0.24
S. Montevideo	0.09	0.12	0.09	0.12	0.14	0.1	0.25
S. Panama	0.07	0.06	0.1	0.13	0.21	0.18	0.28
S. Senftenberg	0.06	0.05	0.04	0.08	0.23	0.05	0.22
S. Saintpaul	0.06	0.12	0.1	0.06	0.15	0.11	0.14
S. Corvallis	0.09	0.15	0.09	0.08	0.15	0.16	0.23

S. Enteritidis where PFGE is not discriminative enough (Table 18.2).

Together, these approaches allow the clear distinction of outbreak events from each other and from single infections as well as the definite identification of the infection source.

Serological sub-differentiation of *Salmonella* isolates over decades allows the recognition of pathogen changes (quantified by means of the epidemiological dominance in humans) as well as pathogen microevolution within a defined serovar (Rabsch *et al.*, 2001a). Both events are of high epidemiological concern and therefore are explained in more detail below.

Pathogen Dynamics

The dominant serovars *S.* Typhimurium and *S.* Enteritidis in different decades

In many countries, there was a marked upsurge in the number of cases of human salmonellosis between the mid-1980s and

Table 18.2. Detected outbreaks of *S.* Enteritidis in 2006 in Germany (NRC data).

Federal state	No. of outbreaks (*n*=73)		Phage type	Ribotype
North Rhine-Westphalia	16	11	4/6	1 (5×), 7, 18, 1c (2×), 12 (2×)
		1	21c/1b	
		3	8/7	
		1	21/1b	
Bavaria	8	4	4/6	1, 3, 6, 7
		2	8/7	
		2	14b/n.c.	
Mecklenburg-Western Pomerania	7	4	4/6	3 (3×), 1
		1	1/1	
		1	21/1b	
		1	4b/6	
Baden- Württemberg	6	1	4/6	I
		1	6/6b	
		2	5/6c	
		1	8/7	
		1	1/1	
Rhineland-Platinate	7	3	8/7	
		1	21/1b	
		3	4/6	1c (2×), 3
Brandenburg	2	2	4/6	1, 6
Hamburg	1	1	21c/1b	
Hesse	3	2	4/6	1, 9
		1	1/1	
Lower Saxony	7	6	4/6	1, 3 (2×), 5, 9, 1c
		1	5c/n.c.	
Saxony	6	2	4/6	1, 7
		2	2/1b	
		1	8/7	
		1	28/7	
Saxony-Anhalt	5	3	4/6	1 (2×), 16
		2	21/1b	
Thuringia	4	2	4/6	1, 3
		1	8/7	
		1	21/1b	
Schleswig-Holstein	1	1	4/6	1

mid-1990s. Much of this has been associated with *S.* Enteritidis, and the worldwide increase in human infection has been referred to as a pandemic (Rodrigue *et al.*, 1990; Wall and Ward, 1999; Cogan and Humphrey, 2003). During this *S.* Enteritidis pandemic, the majority of outbreaks in Europe and the Americas were traced back to foods containing raw or undercooked chicken eggs or contaminated chicken meat (St Louis *et al.*, 1988; Henzler *et al.*, 1994). In the USA *S.* Enteritidis steadily increased in frequency from being the sixth most common serovar in 1963 to becoming the most frequently reported serovar in 1990 (Aserkoff *et al.*, 1970; Mishu *et al.*, 1994). Since its peak in 1995 the number of human cases has declined in the USA, which resulted in *S.* Enteritidis becoming again replaced by *S.* Typhimurium as the most common serovar in 1997 (CDC, 1998). In Germany, since the 1930s, *S.* Typhimurium and *S.* Enteritidis have been reported as the most common serovars (Table 18.3). Apparently these serovars circulate among livestock, environment and humans and therefore are dominant over a long period. Epidemiological studies from the 20th century are summarized in Table 18.3. After the Second World War, both serovars were almost equally distributed (Table 18.3).With the excessive import of feeding stuff and egg products from overseas during the 1950s a variety of 'exotic' *Salmonella* serovars emerged and resulted in a remarkable percentage decrease of *S.* Typhimurium and Enteritidis isolates. During this period other serovars like *S.* Bareilly caused outbreaks (June 1953 with 10,000 cases) and were frequently isolated (Winkle and Rohde, 1979). The *Salmonella* epidemiology changed fundamentally when developing countries entered the international trade markets and exported feeding stuff, which, due to less stringent controls, was already contaminated either in the countries of origin or on intercontinental transport. In the 1960s and 1970s *S.* Typhimurium had been the most important serovar in humans in both German states. During the mid-1980s it had been replaced from this top position by *S.* Enteritidis, but it remained second (Table 18.3; Tschäpe *et al.*, 1999). The decreasing percentage of *S.* Enteritidis and the increasing percentage of *S.* Typhimurium in the 21st century is shown in Table 18.1.

Pathogen changes within a serovar (microevolution within a serovar)

Pathogen transformation in terms of *Salmonella* describes alterations within a serovar. Like other enterobacterial species, *Salmonella* easily exchanges genetic material via horizontal gene transfer. The acquisition or loss of plasmids, prophages and other genetic elements might result in changes of phage type, resistance pattern or virulence properties (Rabsch *et al.*, 2011). Deletions of flagella-related genes are responsible for the inability to express the phase two flagellar antigen e.g. in monophasic variants of *S.* Typhimurium.

Table 18.3. Percentage of *S.* Typhimurium and *S.* Enteritidis in reported human cases in different decades of the 20th century in Germany.

Period	*S.* Typhimurium	*S.* Enteritidis	Studies and reports
1931–1935	63.0	31.0	R. Meyer, German Empire
1946–1948	49.5	42.8	Trüb, Reploh, North Rhine-Westphalia
1948–1950	22.3	27.0	Markuse, Berlin
1953–1955	12.3	10.0	Seeliger, Federal Republic of Germany
1956–1961	37.2	5.0	Seeliger, Federal Republic of Germany
1957–1971	40.3	11.9	Kiesewalter, German Democratic Republic
1972–1983	41.5	7.6	Kiesewalter, German Democratic Republic
1973–1982	48.4	6.1	Pöhn, Federal Republic of Germany
1986–1998	20.1	57.3	GDR, Berlin and new federal states

Alterations within *S.* Typhimurium have been reported regularly since the 1960s. Under selective pressure caused by the intensive use of antibiotics in veterinary medicine and livestock farming multidrug-resistant strains emerged and spread rapidly. Notably, the dominant phage type of *S.* Typhimurium seems to change periodically about every 15 years, when a new type arises and the previous dominant type almost disappears (Fig. 18.2). Sensitive strains of phage type DT9 were most important until 1972, then sulphonamide- and tetracycline-resistant (later multiresistant) strains of DT204 emerged and were dominant until the late 1980s when they were replaced by multiresistant DT104 (Rabsch *et al.*, 2001a). Phage type DT104 strains with an additional nalidixic acid (Nx) resistance were responsible for the increase in 2010 (Fig. 18.2). Since 2006 a monophasic variant of *S.* Typhimurium has been disseminating rapidly in Germany and the vast majority of these strains belong to phage type DT193. Thus besides the novel molecular approaches, phage typing is still a powerful epidemiological tool, especially for outbreak investigation but also for retrospective or long-term studies.

An emerging monophasic variant of *S.* Typhimurium

Since 2006, monophasic *S. enterica* 1,4,[5],12:i:- phage type DT193 strains have been emerging in Germany, causing numerous large diffuse outbreaks and many sporadic infections. Most isolates of DT193 exhibit the ASSuT resistance type. A remarkable increase in the prevalence of serovar 1,4,[5],12:i:- (resistance-type ASSuT) had been noted in food-borne infections and in pigs/pig meat in several European countries between 2006 and 2009 (Mossong *et al*, 2007; EFSA report, 2010; Hauser *et al.*, 2010). Recent inquiries to the ECDC Extranet EPIS refer to an increase of serovar 1,4,5,12:i:- DT193 human infections in Ireland in 2009 and in the UK and France in 2011.

An EFSA-Panel found that it is currently difficult to monitor trends in the proliferation of monophasic strains because of the inconsistent way in which they are reported by different organisations within and between EU member states and also internationally. To ensure complete consistency of reporting, all isolates of putative *Salmonella* should ideally be fully serotyped in accordance with the White-Kauffman-Le Minor scheme, and the full antigenic formula should be reported, as

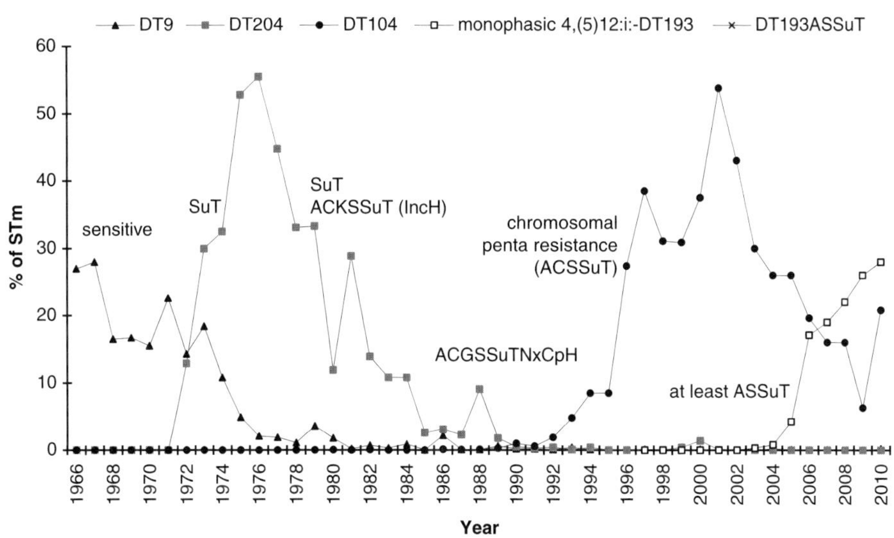

Fig. 18.2. Dominance of *S.* Typhimurium phage types DT9, DT204, DT104 and monophasic DT193 from humans (Germany; 1966–2010, NRC data).

recommended by the WHO Collaborating Centre for Reference and Research on *Salmonella*. If the full antigenic formula is not available but a phage type that is consistent with *S.* Typhimurium lacking phase two flagellar antigens has been confirmed, and the lack of the second phase flagellar antigen has been verified by PCR, then the term 'monophasic *S.* Typhimurium' is recommended for reporting purposes in the current situation (Rabsch, 2009; Torpdahl *et al.*, 2009; EFSA, 2010).

Salmonellosis in Europe Based on ECDC and EFSA Data

The ECDC annual epidemiological report on communicable diseases in Europe and the community summary report of the EFSA from 2010 give an overview of the situation of salmonellosis in Europe (EFSA/ECDC, 2010).

In 2008, a total of ~131,000 confirmed cases of human salmonellosis (notification rate 26.4 per 100,000 of population) were reported from 27 countries. As in Germany, the total number of reported human salmonellosis cases in the EU decreased steadily by several thousand cases annually from 2004, from ~196,000 cases in 2004 to ~131,000 cases in 2008. Ten out of 27 member states reported a decrease in the notification rates compared to the previous year. This might be partly explained by the obligation of the member states to implement *Salmonella* control programmes for the most common serovars reported in human cases in poultry flocks. Seven countries still show a significantly increasing trend.

In 2007 and 2008, despite 17 member states reporting an increase in the number of confirmed cases, the total number reported decreased by ~20,000 cases within 1 year, mainly due to the strong decrease in reported cases in Germany and the Czech Republic. Nine member states and Iceland experienced an increase of more than 30% confirmed cases. One of the most affected countries was Denmark, where the number of confirmed cases more than doubled from 1600 in 2007 to 3700 in 2008. This might be explained by the national *S.* Typhimurium outbreak in 2008. Germany, the UK and the Czech Republic accounted for half of the confirmed cases (49.5%) in 2008 (EFSA/ECDC, 2010). The proportion of *Salmonella* cases that were reported as domestically acquired in member states remained approximately the same in 2008 as in 2007 (63.6% versus 65.1%). The same observation was made for the proportion of imported cases or those acquired while travelling abroad, which in 2008 was 7.8% compared to 7.9% in 2007. While many member states report a clear dominance of domestically acquired *Salmonella* infections, three of the four Nordic countries, Sweden, Finland and Norway, reported the highest proportions of imported cases of salmonellosis (82.1%, 83.2% and 83.6%, respectively; EFSA/ECDC, 2010.

Information on human serovars was provided by 26 member states. As in the previous years, the two most frequently reported *Salmonella* serovars in 2008 were *S.* Enteritidis and *S.* Typhimurium, representing 58.0% and 21.9% of all reported serovars in confirmed human infections ($n = 120{,}760$), respectively. Reported *S.* Enteritidis serovars decreased by 14.0% in the EU while, in contrast, reported *S.* Typhimurium serovars increased by 27.1%. The *S.* Enteritidis notification rate in the EU decreased from 19.4 per 100,000 in 2007 to 14.6 per 100,000 in 2008. In parallel, the *S.* Typhimurium notification rate increased from 4.9 to 5.5 cases per 100,000, based on the TESSy data; 16 member states showed a decline in the reported number of *S.* Enteritidis cases. The remaining eight of the top ten serovars reported in the EU were only slightly different from 2007. *Salmonella* Bovismorbificans was a new entry on the list with an increase from 281 in 2007 to 501 in 2008. *Salmonella* Agona cases increased by 64.3% from 387 in 2007 to 636 in 2008. The two most frequently reported phage types Ward of *S.* Enteritidis in 2008 were PT4 (21.9%) and PT8 (19.3%), although PT4 showed a remarkable decrease of 39.4% during the previous year. The top seven most common phage types remained the same between 2007 and 2008, though PT21 surpassed PT1 in 2008 due to a marked decrease of PT1 by 41.5%. The European-wide emergence of *S.* Typhimurium monophasic DT193 and DT120 strains of R-type ASSuT since the late 1990s in pigs, humans, cattle and to a lesser extent in poultry and companion animals, have been described (Rabsch, 2009; Torpdahl *et al.*, 2009; Hauser *et al.*, 2010; Hopkins *et al.*, 2010). Monophasic *S.* Typhimurium isolates have also been observed overseas (Switt *et al.*, 2009; EFSA, 2010).

Salmonella in Pork and Pork Products

Pork and pork products are progressively recognized as important sources of human salmonellosis. The increasing antimicrobial resistance associated with pork-related serovars such as *S.* Typhimurium (including its monophasic variant) and *S.* Derby may become a serious human health hazard in the near future (Boyen *et al.*, 2008).

From 2001 to 2005, five large outbreaks were reported in Germany with pork being the probable vehicle of infection (Jansen *et al.*, 2007). Two of them had been caused by *S.* Goldcoast and the others by *S.* Muenchen, *S.* Give and *S.* Bovismorbificans. In the latter outbreak, 525 cases were reported within 3 months, one of them with a fatal outcome. The larger *S.* Goldcoast outbreak affected more than 250 people, two of whom died. Infections caused by *S.* Give led to hospitalization of more than half of the 115 patients. In all three events, case-control studies suspected raw minced pork as the infection origin, which was confirmed by the detection of outbreak strains in isolates from both patients and pork using PFGE and – for *S.* Bovismorbificans – phage typing (Gilsdorf *et al.*, 2005).

All outbreaks showed disperse spatial distribution, affecting multiple federal states. In two of them, cross-national pig trading seemed to play a role. To prevent further human infections from contaminated pork products, an integrated programme for the reduction of *Salmonella* in all stages of pork production is warranted. In addition, the collaboration between epidemiologists and microbiologists from both sides, the human and the veterinarian, should be strengthened in the future.

Because of the high prevalence of serovars Typhimurium (monophasic) and Derby in pigs in Europe clonal investigation was initiated in Germany. Two major clonal lineages of the monophasic *S.* Typhimurium variant were detected, which can be differentiated by phage typing (DT193 70% and DT120 19%) and PFGE (Hauser *et al.*, 2010). For *S.* Derby four major clonal groups were identified based on PFGE, and sequence data of the virulence genes *sopA*, *sopB* and *sopD* (Hauser *et al.*, 2011).

Is *Salmonella* Infantis the Next European *Salmonella* Problem?

The results of an EFSA study demonstrate that *S.* Enteritidis und *S.* Typhimurium cause the major problems in laying hens in most European countries (EFSA/ECDC, 2010). In several countries immunization using both live and inactivated vaccines against both serovars has been established in the recent years. Immunization against the dominant serovars might offer an ecological niche for other *Salmonella* serotypes from different O-groups to enter and persist within an animal population. Quite possibly, the worldwide decade-long–and finally successful–fight against serovar *S.* Gallinarum enabled *S.* Enteritidis to invade the poultry flocks (Rabsch *et al.*, 2000) and recent data suggest that *S.* Infantis seems to take advantage of the constant repression of *S.* Enteritidis. In Germany, *S.* Infantis has been the third most frequent serovar in human *Salmonella* infections for several years (Table 18.2) and multiple outbreaks have been described worldwide (Wegener and Baggesen, 1996; Pessoa-Silva *et al.*, 2002). According to an EFSA study (EFSA/ECDC, 2010), *S.* Infantis was the most frequently reported serovar on broiler meat in the EU in 2008 with 40.1%. In Hungary this serovar is dominant with 95.7% in broiler meat. The percentage of *S.* Infantis isolates from broiler meat is also high in other EU member states: Slovenia 53.8%, Austria 28.9%, Poland 22.43%, Czech Republic 20.8% and Slovakia 10%. With nearly 1300 reported cases in humans in 2007 and 2008, this serovar plays an EU-wide epidemiological role (EFSA/ECDC, 2010).

To meet the increasing public health need, a phage typing system for *S.* Infantis was developed at the Robert Koch Institute that allows outbreak investigation and subdifferentiation of *S.* Infantis isolates for epidemiological purposes. Several outbreak investigations revealed the dominant phage type 29. In combination with PFGE, the most frequently observed clone PT 29/*Xba*I 27 was detected in broiler and human outbreaks. Furthermore, it was demonstrated that PT 29/*Xba*I 27, PT 4/*Xba*I 4 and PT 29/*Xba*I 5 were frequently isolated from broilers. The strains of PT 29/*Xba*I 5 were associated with imported broilers from Hungary (Miller, 2009).

Salmonella Outbreaks Caused by Fresh Produce, Herbs, Spices and Sweets

Salmonella outbreaks linked to consumption of fresh agricultural products increased remarkably during the last decades (Hanning *et al.*, 2009). Bean and Griffin (1990) reported that fruits and vegetables had been the cause of 2% of the food-borne outbreaks in the USA between 1973 and 1987. In the 1990s, this fraction rose to 6% of all reported food-borne outbreaks, affecting more than 16,000 people in the USA (Sivapalasingam *et al.*, 2004). Recent data indicate that 13% of the outbreaks in the USA have been related to contaminated agricultural products (Doyle and Erickson, 2008). *Salmonella enterica* outbreaks linked to fresh fruits and fruit juices are also reported worldwide and the diversity of contaminated fruits (mango, cantaloupe, water melon, grapes, tomatoes, peppers etc.) is as wide as the variety of *Salmonella* serovars involved (e.g. *S.* Newport, *S.* Poona, *S.* Senftenberg, *S.* Saintpaul, *S.* Braenderup, *S.* Strathcona). In September/October 2011 a *Salmonella* outbreak caused by the rare serovar *S.* Strathcona was observed in Denmark, Germany, Austria and. Italy. Small tomatoes of the type datterino have been found to be the source of the infections (S. Ethelberg and K. Molbak, pers. comm.). In the case of fruit juices, mainly unpasteurised orange juice (contaminated with *S.* Typhimurium, *S.* Muenchen, *S.* Anatum etc.) has been identified as source of numerous, quite severe outbreaks, with hundreds of people affected (Raybaudi-Massilia *et al.*, 2009). *Salmonella* Saintpaul, *S.* Rubislaw and *S.* Javiana spread by paprika and paprika-powdered potato chips caused outbreaks with more than 1000 infected people, primarily children younger than 14 years (Lehmacher *et al.*, 1995). A large outbreak caused by multiresistant *S.* Typhimurium DT204b (resistance pattern ACGNeKSSuTTmNxCpL) and affecting around 400 people mainly in the UK, Germany and the Netherlands was traced back to imported lettuce (Crook *et al.*, 2003). European outbreaks of *S.* Stanley and *S.* Newport have occurred where imported groundnuts were the infection vehicle (Kirk *et al.*, 2004). *Salmonella* Senftenberg caused an outbreak of infection associated with pre-packed basil in the UK, Denmark and the Netherlands (Pezzoli *et al.*, 2008). There were also outbreaks of *S.* Thompson infection in Scandinavia and the UK linked to consumption of rocket leaves (Nygård *et al.*, 2008) and *S.* Anatum associated with imported basil caused an outbreak in Denmark (Pakalniskiene *et al.*, 2009). These are further examples for the growing significance of contaminated agricultural products in human *Salmonella* infections. These data emphasize the challenges for the agro-industrial sector as well as for the public health authorities worldwide. Of important interest in this context are very recent data, showing that *Salmonella* is capable of penetrating the epidermis of iceberg lettuce leaves via open stomata in a process that involves flagella motility and chemotaxis (Kroupitski *et al.*, 2009). Not only fresh produce causes *Salmonella* infections in humans; (dried) herbs and spices are also of increasing importance. A rapid cross-national increase of *S.* Oranienburg infections was registered in 2001/2002. Multi-state matched case-control studies revealed the consumption of chocolate as probable infection source (Werber *et al.*, 2005). In 2001, several countries reported an increase of salmonellosis cases due to *S.* Typhimurium DT104. Mainly young patients with a migration background characterized the cases.

Here helva (a sweet-like dessert made from sesame paste) and tahini (sesame paste) from a Turkish factory were found to be contaminated and the consumption of these products was statistically associated with infection. In this context, 117 ready-to-eat sesame seed products were examined. *Salmonella* spp. were isolated from 11 samples (9.4%), including *S*. Typhimurium in helva from different countries and manufacturers and *S*. Offa, *S*. Tennessee and *S*. Poona from sesame paste (tahini) and sesame seed, which was sold for raw consumption in cereals (Brockmann *et al*., 2004).

From October 2002 to July 2003, a total of 42 *S*. Agona cases in infants younger than 13 months were reported compared with three infections in this age group during the same period in the previous year. To understand the recent spread and to trace back the route of infection, phage typing and PFGE were applied and proved to be very helpful tools for epidemiological subtyping of *S*. Agona isolates. The clonal identity between *S*. Agona isolates from infantile gastroenteritis and herbal tea containing anise, fennel and caraway seeds could be confirmed. Subsequently, a batch of imported aniseed from Turkey was determined as the contaminated source (Koch *et al*., 2005; Rabsch *et al*., 2005).

Herbs and spices usually show a high level of bacterial contamination. This is due to their natural microflora and partly to post-harvesting factors. Microbial tests of herbs and spices reveal that *Salmonella* spp. was regularly found within a variety of other *Enterobacteriaceae*. Detailed analyses of 5754 samples collected from 1994 to 2005 show that about 4% of them were contaminated with *Salmonella* species and examples include chamomile, melissa, onion, laurel leaves, dill, rosemary, cumin, peppermint, thyme, basil sage, ginger, marjoram, tarragon, oregano, chilli, common horse tail calendula, mugwort, senna leaves, parsley and cilantro (Hartwig *et al*., 2006). Because of the high contamination rate and the extensive consumption, herbs and spices should be part of a continuous microbiological monitoring. It is known that *Salmonella* bacteria on plant surfaces form large microcolonies (biofilm) with other bacteria (Römling *et al*., 2007). *Salmonella* Thompson showed biofilm formation on the plant surface with the indigenous bacterial flora and when *Pantoea agglomerans*, a cilantro plant isolate, was co-incubated with *Salmonella* (Brandl and Mandrell, 2002).

Phage Typing or Multiplex PCR – Tools to Conclude on the Origin of Certain Serovars

Examples shown are for *S*. Typhimurium, *S*. Enteritidis and *S*. Paratyphi B.

Salmonella Typhimurium variants

The question of how bacteria overcome species barriers and adapt to new hosts is essential for the understanding of both the origin of infectious diseases and the emergence of new pathogens. Phage typing is one approach to differentiate, e.g. serovar Typhimurium isolates for epidemiological purposes. The sensitivity and reproducibility of phage typing make it a very attractive method for determining the spread of different, yet very closely related, *S*. Typhimurium clones over time (Fig. 18.2). Several studies show that DT2 and DT99 represent the phage types predominantly isolated from pigeons in Europe and other continents but very seldom from other species (Rabsch *et al*., 2002). This observation illustrates that these *S*. Typhimurium variants have a narrow host range. Conversely, pigeons are hardly ever infected with phage types other than DT2 and DT99, indicating that other *S*. Typhimurium isolates are not well adapted to this host species. It is therefore reasonable to conclude that phage types DT2 and DT99 represent a pigeon-adapted variant of *S*. Typhimurium.

In 2008/2009, the National Reference Laboratory for *Salmonella* (NRL-Salm) received an increasing number of *Salmonella* strains with the antigenic formula 4,12:-:1,2 isolated from perished wild birds, particularly siskins. The flagellar antigen of the first phase was phenotypically not detectable in these isolates. By PCR, a gene fragment coding for the H:i flagellar antigen could be amplified. Consequently, these strains represent a phenotypically monophasic variant of S. Typhimurium var. Copenhagen (antigenic formula 4,12:i:1,2). Phage typing revealed that most of the isolates belonged to phage type DT40, the most common phage type associated with S. Typhimurium infections in wild birds. Genotypically identical DT40 strains had been isolated from wild birds, humans, particularly infants, and cats. This refers to a direct or indirect transmission of the pathogen from wild birds to humans. By coming in contact with contaminated birds, domestic cats could play an important role as vehicle between birds and humans (Hauser *et al.*, 2009). Phage type DT40 has been reported to be responsible for annual spring incidents of wild bird (mainly songbirds and finches) mortality in England (Pennycott *et al.*, 1998). Phage type DT40 was responsible for an epizootic of salmonellosis in feeder birds (mainly northern flocking songbirds) in north-eastern America in the winter of 1997/1998, and this phage type was noted to be very rarely isolated from other species (Daoust *et al.*, 2000). These data suggest that phage type DT40 represents an avian-adapted S. Typhimurium variant with a narrow host range and wide geographic distribution (Rabsch *et al.*, 2002).

In the past, DT8 and DT46 were associated with a small number of human S. Typhimurium infections traced back to the consumption of raw or undercooked duck eggs, but were hardly ever connected with other sources. Investigations of geese and ducks confirmed a narrow host range by phage-typing analysis (Rabsch *et al.*, 2002). In 2010 a salmonellosis outbreak in Ireland of S. Typhimurium DT8 associated with duck eggs confirmed this association (Noble *et al.*, 2012).

Salmonella Enteritidis variants

Since 1984, S. Enteritidis has been the predominant serovar in Germany in humans, and phage types (PT) 4/6 have been the most important while chicken meat and table eggs have been demonstrated to be the main infection sources (Tschäpe *et al.*, 1999). However, S. Enteritidis PT11/n.c. (Ward/Lalko and Laszlo schemes) and PT9a/n.c. belong to the uncommon phage types causing disease in humans (Laszlo *et al.*, 1985; Ward *et al.*, 1987). Within the years 1996–2006, PT11/n.c. and PT9a/n.c. were isolated from hedgehogs in different German Federal states. The strains were isolated from organs and faeces. In the same period, 38 human cases of PT11/n.c. and two cases of PT9a/n.c. were detected. In 2008, a 2-year-old boy became ill and S. Enteritidis PT9a/n.c. was isolated. A telephone interview with the mother identified that the boy ate unwashed windfall fruit in an area where hedgehogs were present. In Great Britain, 13 of 74 hedgehogs were reported to be infected with S. Enteritidis PT11 (Keymer *et al.*, 1991). In Denmark, the association of both these phage types with hedgehogs has also been confirmed. Interestingly, both phage types are indistinguishable by PFGE *Xba*I analysis and *Hin*dIII RFLP plasmid analysis (Nauerby *et al.*, 2000).

Salmonella Paratyphi B variants

Serovar Paratyphi B can be classified into one systemic and one enteric pathovar according to its capability to ferment *d*-tartrate. While *d*-tartrate-nonfermenting (dT^-) strains exhibit an enhanced human pathogenicity causing typhoid-like disease, *d*-tartrate-fermenting strains (dT^+, former variant Java) provoke a less severe gastroenteric disease. Molecular approaches support this classification into pathovars (Prager *et al.*, 2003). Sequence analysis revealed a single nucleotide exchange within the start codon of gene *STM3356* in the *d*-tartrate-nonfermenting strains of the systemic pathovar (Malorny *et al.*, 2003) that allows a clear discrimination by PCR. Together with the *sopE* and *avrA* gene amplification, the enteric pathovar (EPV) can be further subdivided into variants 1 to 4 (Fig. 18.3). In Germany, EPV3 ($sopE^-$, $avrA^+$) is the dominant one. So in outbreak investigations a combination of phage typing and pathovar discrimination can be helpful. Evidence for a possible vehicle in a multinational outbreak of *S.* Paratyphi B var. Java PT3b var 9 is based on a case-control study conducted in Sweden. The cases were strongly associated with the consumption of imported baby spinach (Denny *et al.*, 2007). Such strains of PT3b var9 (dT^+, former variant Java) belonging to EVP1 were also observed in 2011 in Germany. The poultry-associated *S.* Paratyphi B strains that are described in the Netherlands (van Pelt *et al.*, 2003) and also observed in Germany often belong to EVP3. It is proposed that the PCR technique for testing for the presence of the virulence genes *sopE1* and *avrA* could be used as a diagnostic tool for identifying both pathovars of *S. enterica* serovar Paratyphi B (Prager *et al.*, 2003). This will be of great public health importance, since strains of *S.* Paratyphi B have recently re-emerged worldwide. The revision of the reporting scheme to take the subdivision of *S.* Paratyphi B into account would be reasonable, since the enteric pathovar is frequently found in poultry (EFSA/ECDC 2010) and from there might be transferred to humans. The systemic *S.* Paratyphi B pathovar SPV1 is mainly acquired by travelling, e.g. to Turkey (Prager *et al.*, 2003).

Reptile Exotic Pet-Associated Salmonellosis

Although the main focus of this chapter is on food-borne *Salmonella* infections, it should not be forgotten that man to man transmission is common during outbreaks, especially in institutions like hospitals, nursing homes, playschools etc.

Each year infections are also acquired through direct or indirect animal contact in homes, veterinary clinics, zoological gardens, farm environments or other public,

lane	strain no.	sopE	d-tartrate	avrA
1 SPV	08-7067	+	–	–
2 EPV1	04-4960	–	+	–
3 EPV2	05-3498	+	+	–
4 EPV3	08-7086	–	+	+
5 EPV4	07-109	+	+	+

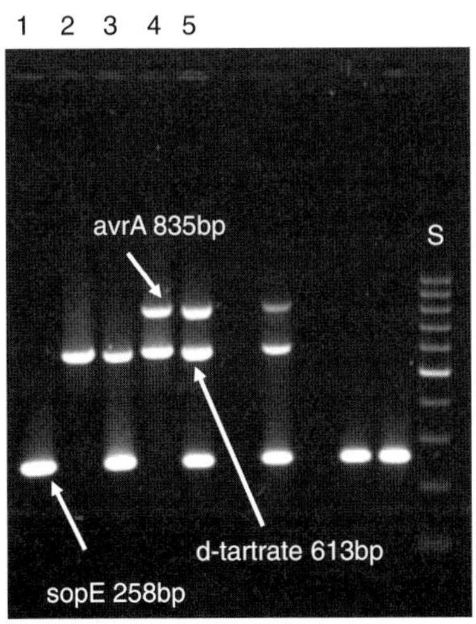

Fig. 18.3. *Salmonella* Paratyphi B multiplex PCR for pathovar differentiation SPV and EPV (S = 500 bp ladder).

professional or private settings. Clinically affected animals may exhibit a higher prevalence of shedding than apparently healthy animals, but both can shed *Salmonella* over long periods of time. In addition, environmental contamination and indirect transmission through contaminated food and water may complicate control efforts. The public health risk varies by mammals, birds and reptile species, age group, husbandry practice and health status (Hoelzer *et al.*, 2011).

A study from Canada conducted between 1994 and 1996 illustrated the potential problem of reptile-associated salmonellosis for the first time. Investigations revealed that 3–5% of human *Salmonella* cases were associated with exposure to exotic pets with a great variety of *Salmonella* serovars involved, e.g. *S.* Paratyphi B var. Java, *S.* Stanley, *S.* Poona, *S.* Jangwani, *S.* Pomona, *S.* subsp. IV 48:g,z51:- (former *S.* Marina) and others (Woodward *et al.*, 1997). In 2011, a 13-month-old child from Austria passed away on the transport to the hospital with vomiting and diarrhoea. Local health authorities found that the infection was triggered by *S.* Kintambo and *S.* Poano found in the faeces of a monitor lizard kept in his family (Kornschober, Graz, pers. comm.). Several publications in the past decade (Cyriac and Wozniak, 2000; Ward, 2000; Willis *et al.*, 2002; Stam *et al.*, 2003; Wybo *et al.*, 2004; De Jong *et al.*, 2005; Bruins *et al.*, 2006; Corrente *et al.*, 2006; Berendes *et al.*, 2007; Brédart *et al.*, 2007; Hames *et al.*, 2008; O'Byrne and Mahon, 2008; Bertrand *et al.*, 2008) indicate that although infections attributed to exposure to reptiles and other exotic pets represent only a small proportion of all human salmonellosis cases, it is likely to be an underestimated and growing problem that deserves closer attention. In Spain *S.* Paratyphi B var. Java (d-tartrate positive, dT^+) and monophasic variants were associated with turtles (Hernández *et al.*, 2012). It is difficult to distinguish between pathovars of *S.* Paratyphi B.

The list of exotic *Salmonella* serovars transmitted by exotic pets becomes longer and longer, but *S.* Typhimurium has also been involved in outbreaks. A multi-state outbreak in the USA in 2008 was associated with pet turtle exposure. In nearly half of the 135 cases, children ≤5 years were affected. This outbreak was the third turtle-associated outbreak since 2006 (CDC, 2010). An increase of *S.* Typhimurium with the very rare phage type DT191a was recognized by the reference laboratory in England and Wales. A matched case–case study gave strong statistical evidence for a connection between illness and reptile keeping (mainly corn snakes). In this case, frozen feeder mice were suspected to be the source of infection and DT191a was found in three pools of sampled mice that could be traced back to a single supplier in the USA (Harker *et al.*, 2011). According to the ownership statistics gathered from APPA's (American Pet Products Association) 2011–2012 National Pet Owners Survey, 4.6 million US households own a pet reptile or 13 million reptiles live in US households, respectively (http://www.americanpetproducts.org/press_industrytrends.asp; AVMA, 2007).

The number of pet reptiles (bearded dragons, chameleons, geckos, snakes, skinks and turtles) is also steadily increasing in European countries, including Germany. In 2007 more than 500,000 reptiles were imported to Germany only via Frankfurt/Main airport (Hatt *et al.*, 2009). Reptile trade fairs are booming and a lot of exotic reptiles with CITES certificate are offered by Internet stores and swapping platforms. In the TESSy database the number of cases from children under 6 years old with REPAS-known serovars has increased in recent years (Table 18.4; Johanna Takkinen, ECDC, personal communication).

Table 18.4. Confirmed *Salmonella*-associated deaths in Germany.

2010	2009	2008	2007	2006	2005	2004
26	20	33	39	47	46[a]	52

[a]A 12-year-old boy died after eating Christmas cookie dough at a friendly family (Robert Koch-Institut, 2006).

Reptiles are known to release *Salmonella* frequently (Geue and Löschner, 2002) and reptile-associated salmonellosis has been recognized as an emerging zoonosis. Our own investigations of reptiles from households with confirmed salmonellosis in children demonstrated that the strains detected from the child can be regularly isolated from the choana, the cloaca and/or the ventral skin of the reptile. In the majority of the cases, multiple *Salmonella* serovars were isolated from the respective reptile (M. Pees, Clinic for birds and reptiles, Leipzig, unpublished data). Reptiles are frequently asymptomatic carriers of *Salmonella* and therefore an important reservoir for these bacteria. In fact, each reptile should be considered a *Salmonella* carrier until the contrary is proven (see Chapter 17, this volume).

Swedish import restrictions and information campaigns were shown to be effective public health measures against REPAS. When Sweden became a member of the European Union (EU) in January 1995 Sweden no longer required certificates stating that imported animals were free of *Salmonella* (De Jong *et al.*, 2005). In the USA, the Association of Reptilian and Amphibian Veterinarians (ARAV) published guidelines for reducing the risk of transmission of *Salmonella* from reptiles to humans, including a client hand-out distributed at the points of sale of these animals (Bradley *et al.*, 1998). Further, the US CDC published recommendations including hand washing after handling reptiles or their cages and keeping reptiles out of food preparation areas. The CDC also advises that pregnant women and young children should not keep reptiles as pets (CDC, 2008, 2010).

In Europe, recommendations related to the handling of reptiles and other exotic pets exist in the veterinarian sector but it appears that guidelines for prevention of *Salmonella* transmission from reptiles to humans should be extended to the field of local public health authorities, because at least one documented food-borne outbreak resulted from environmental contamination caused by a bearded dragon (Lowther *et al.*, 2011). The community needs to be cautioned about the risk of REPAS, and it is important that physicians and public health experts consider this way of transmission.

From the epidemiological point of view (Robert Koch Institute, 2013) and in addition to an earlier recommendation ('Reptile-Associated Salmonellosis', RAS, De Jong *et al.*, 2005), we propose to call this special type of epidemic 'Reptile-Exotic-Pet-Associated-Salmonellosis' (REPAS). The main argument for this proposal is that over recent years the method of trading reptiles has changed considerably and this will probably continue in the future. The main risk of *Salmonella* transmission from reptiles to humans is not due to European wild species but, as the results of this study also demonstrate, at present is mainly due to 'exotic' imported reptile species. Furthermore, following recent examinations *Salmonella* shedding is higher in reptiles kept in captivity in comparison to wild reptiles (Geue and Löschner, 2002; Scheelings *et al.*, 2011) and 'pet' reptiles are obviously in closer contact to humans. These arguments justify the inclusion of 'exotic pet' into the term describing the problem. The risk to human health connected with the reptile pet market has been highlighted recently (Arena *et al.*, 2012) and the accurate description of the problem using REPAS might be important to convey the problem in education and assist the European Commission to give recommendations to harmonize animal welfare and public health.

Clinical Manifestation of Salmonellosis

Although the vast majority of *Salmonella* infections show self-limiting characteristics and are restricted to gastrointestinal symptoms, salmonellosis is a potentially serious disease that results in several fatal cases each year (Table 18.5; Robert Koch Institut, 2011b).

Most cases were associated with *S.* Enteritidis, but in 2010 the number of *S.* Typhimurium-caused deaths was higher. As with most other enteric infections, infants, elderly and immunocompromised people or patients with underlying diseases are more likely to be infected and the outcome of the disease is likely to be more severe in these groups (Saphra and Winter, 1957; Gordon, 2008). Typical symptoms of patients during an

Table 18.5. Cases from children younger than 6 years reported to the European Surveillance System (TESSy, 29 May 2012).

Serovar or subspecies	2007	2008	2009	2010	Total
Apapa	5	5	4	10	24
Arizona (IIIa and IIIb)	28	9	55	54	146
Carmel	3	4	5	14	26
Ealing	6	8	7	10	31
Eastbourne	6	9	2	11	28
Mississippi	5	2	5	11	23
Monschaui	9	16	15	19	59
Oranienburg	32	57	45	73	207
Pomona	41	28	43	32	144
Poona	48	55	39	102	244
Subsp. II	5	4	13	14	36
Subsp. IIIa	4	0	9	7	20
Subsp. IIIb	5	15	10	23	53
Subsp. IV	8	11	8	29	56
Tennessee	32	30	41	51	154
Total cases (527 serovars)	34.059	28.787	24.133	23.791	110.770

egg-associated outbreak of *S.* Enteritidis had been diarrhoea (87%), abdominal pain (84%), feeling feverish (75%), nausea (65%), muscle pain (64%), vomiting (24%), headache (21%) and blood in stool (6%) (Stevens *et al.*, 1989).

The incubation period in cases of *Salmonella* food poisoning usually ranges between 6 and 72 h but occasionally it may extend to 1 week. In some outbreaks with probably very high numbers of ingested bacteria incubation times of 2.5 h have been reported (Stevens *et al.*, 1989). The consumption of alcoholic beverages as a protective factor for *Salmonella* infection during or immediately after uptake of contaminated food has been discussed in the past (Bellido-Blasco *et al.*, 2002). Further, an antacid therapy might be a risk factor for salmonellosis (Jansen *et al.*, 2008). Diarrhoea may vary in volume and frequency. In most cases, stools are loose and of moderate volume without blood or mucus. Occasionally, stools can be of large volume and watery. With the vast majority of *Salmonella* serovars isolated from humans, the symptoms are consistent with those described by Stevens *et al.* (1989). However, in a small proportion of cases (ca. 1%), *Salmonella* develops invasive characteristics potentially leading to bacteraemia and gram-negative sepsis. For certain serovars, especially *S.* Dublin, *S.* Choleraesuis and strains of *S.* Virchow, the incidence of extra-intestinal infections is higher. In up to 25% of *S.* Dublin, 75% of *S.* Choleraesuis and 4% of *S.* Virchow infections the bacteria can be isolated from blood cultures (Threlfall *et al.*, 1992).

Salmonella can also cause pseudoappendicitis similar to that produced by *Yersinia enterocolitica* and other enteric bacteria (Sullivan and Cunha, 1989) or cholangitis (Vogel *et al.*, 2007); soft tissue infections are described as well (Hames *et al.*, 2008). Endovascular and cardiovascular infections represent rare complications of non-typhoid salmonellosis (Fernández-Guerrero *et al.*, 2004; Hsu and Lin, 2005). To reduce the number of severe systemic infections it is important to identify high-risk patients and treat them as early as possible (Hibbert *et al.*, 2010).

Some patients with non-typhoid salmonellosis develop meningitis and this is more common in neonates and often associated with reptiles (Makin *et al.*, 1996; Cyriac and Wozniak, 2000; Wybo *et al.*, 2004; Milstone *et al.*, 2006). *Salmonella*-induced osteomyelitis most frequently occurs in children and is usually of haematogenous origin (Cohen *et al.*, 1987).

Most cases of septic arthritis occur in children, immunosuppressed people or patients with sickle cell disease (Cohen *et al.*, 1987). The latter almost always have associated osteomyelitis (Hernigou *et al.*, 2010).

A highly invasive form of non-typhoidal *Salmonella* (mainly *S.* Typhimurium) infection emerged as one of the major public health problems in sub-Saharan Africa (Gordon *et al.*, 2008). This disease is characterized by bacteraemia and/or meningitis, occasionally accompanied by septic arthritis. The clinical presentation is nonspecific, with fever often being the only clinical sign and a history of gastroenteritis present in less than 50% of the cases. Molecular investigations of these strains on genome level implicated host–pathogen interactions, suggesting that this lineage may represent a distinct pathotype of *S.* Typhimurium (Kingsley *et al.*, 2009). Other complications are indirect and include reactive arthritis and pancreatitis, of which the pathogenesis is not well understood (Lee *et al.*, 2005; Townes, 2010; Mertens *et al.*, 2012). Broncho-pulmonary salmonelloses are rare manifestations of extra-intestinal focal infections in adults caused by different subspecies of *Salmonella*. They may appear without previous gastroenteritic symptoms especially in patients older than 60 years, as well as in patients who are immunocompromised or suffer from chronic pulmonary diseases (Jüch *et al.*, 2013).

The volunteer studies conducted by McCullough and Eisele (1951) demonstrated that with *Salmonella* such as *S.* Bareilly and *S.* Newport, a dose of at least 100,000 cells was required to cause infection. This created the belief that infection was only possible if large numbers of cells were consumed. This view was supported by studies with other serovars, including *S.* Derby and *S.* Anatum, where it was necessary for volunteers to consume more than 10 million cells to elicit disease. Such numbers of *Salmonella* must be found relatively seldom in foods, apart from instances of gross mishandling. Epidemiological data suggest that infection can be initiated from a low infective dose, particularly where the bacteria are protected within a food matrix. Foods with a high fat content (D'Souza *et al.*, 2012) or a good buffering capacity may protect small numbers (Jasson *et al.*, 2011) of *Salmonella* during their passage through the acid regions of the stomach, thus permitting a lower dose of organisms to initiate infection. Examples of such foods and infectious doses associated with them are shown in Table 18.6. It has also been demonstrated that people on antacids, where gastric acidity has been lowered, or antimicrobials, which altered the gut flora, are more susceptible to infection. A food-borne outbreak caused by *S.* Enteritidis PT8/7 was characterized by prolonged duration and a low infection rate among

Table 18.6. Some examples of foods associated with low infective doses in outbreaks of salmonellosis (courtesy of P.J. Stephens).

Food vehicle	*Salmonella* serovar	Infective dose (cells per person)
Chocolate[1,2,3]	*S.* Eastbourne, *S.* Napoli, *S.* Typhimurium	10–100
Cheddar cheese[4,5]	*S.* Heidelberg, *S.* Typhimurium	1–100
Maize snack[6]	*S.* Agona	2–45
Hamburger[7]	*S.* Newport	10–100
Potato chips[8]	*S.* Saintpaul, *S.* Rubislaw, *S.* Javiana	4–45

[1]Craven *et al.*, 1975; [2]Greenwood and Hooper, 1983; [3]Kapperud *et al.*, 1990; [4]Fontaine *et al.*, 1980; [5]D'Aoust, 1985; [6]Killalea *et al.*, 1996; [7]Fontaine *et al.*, 1978; [8]Lehmacher *et al.*, 1995.

patients. The epidemiological investigation suggests that the kitchen staff, as carriers, had contributed to a low-level contamination of various foods for a long period. The intermittent occurrence of the cases is best explained by a low level of contaminated food that primarily led to clinical symptoms among especially vulnerable persons or older patients with antacids therapy (Jansen *et al.*, 2008).

The infective dose required in these people may also be lower. Minimal infective doses can also vary with age and state of health; in the young they are very low. Analysis of a large number of outbreaks demonstrated that, for non-typhoid salmonellosis, there was a relationship between infective dose and the severity of illness (Glynn and Bradley, 1992; Mintz *et al.*, 1994; Werber *et al.*, 2005).

The study of outbreaks can provide much interesting information concerning the pathogenicity of salmonellosis and human reaction to infection, as it permits observations on a population exposed to the same *Salmonella* within the same foods and at the same time. Such work has revealed that there can be marked variations in attack rates, although this may be explained in part by the uneven distribution of *Salmonella* in non-liquid foods. However, early studies by Hobbs (1971) on poultry-associated outbreaks of salmonellosis found attack rates varying from 8 to 86% (mean 20%). More recent investigations from 47 *Salmonella* outbreaks, involving a number of vehicles and five different serovars, calculated the attack rate as 56% (Glynn and Bradley, 1992).

Salmonellosis remains an internationally important human disease and presents many challenges to the food and agriculture industries and those charged with the protection of public health. Infection rates will only be reduced if there is the closest possible working relationship between all those involved with food production and the government agencies with responsibility for food safety.

Outlook

By the time the book *The World Problem of Salmonellosis* was released in 1964, NRCs for *Salmonella* had been established in several European countries and the Kauffmann–White scheme had already been proved to be a valuable tool for epidemiological investigations.

During that time the excessive import of feeding stuff and egg products from overseas introduced a lot of 'exotic' *Salmonella* serovars to Europe. However, there was no *S.* Enteritidis pandemic in Europe until that time. This started in the mid-1980s and was picked out as a central theme in the book *Salmonella in Domestic Animals*. Today, it seems that the *S.* Enteritidis problem in laying hen and chicken flocks has been overcome in Europe by the applied control measurements and that the mass outbreaks of the 1990s belong to history. The above-mentioned book also referred to the rapid dissemination of the multidrug-resistant *S.* Typhimurium DT104. Meanwhile the number of isolates expressing this particular phage type is also declining and involved in outbreaks only sporadically. It has been replaced by a likewise multiresistant monophasic variant of *S.* Typhimurium DT193 that entered the human food chain and is now drawing attention throughout Europe. It was once speculated that *S.* Typhimurium DT104 originated from Asia and early infections with the monophasic *S.* Typhimurium DT193 variant seemed to be related to travelling to Asian countries as well. Following this hypothesis would lead to the assumption that the vast human and farm animal populations in close neighbourhood together with often deficient sanitation may provide optimal conditions for pathogen dynamics as well as microevolution. Brought to Europe, these novel strains would be able to provoke mass infections in humans and livestock for many years. Antibiotic selective pressure and exchange of virulence markers by horizontal gene transfer via plasmids and bacteriophages will always support the maintenance of the most virulent *Salmonella* isolates. Therefore we should bear in mind that the application of antibiotics in sub-inhibitory concentrations can promote horizontal gene transfer by phage induction (Santos *et al.*, 2009), since most of the *Salmonella* phages have generalized transduction capacities (Schicklmaier *et al.*, 1998).

Costerton wrote in 1995 that bacteria live only temporary as single organisms but spend most of their life cycle outside warm-blooded hosts in biofilms (Costerton *et al.*, 1995). The formation of this multicellular state was also described for *Salmonella*. Attached to each other and embedded into a self-produced extracellular matrix, bacteria are able to colonize abiotic materials, plant surfaces and epithelial cells (Römling *et al.*, 2007). This might be an explanation for the increase in *Salmonella* infections caused by vegetable foods. The bacteria persist on or within the plant leaves as cellulose-encased particles. In this indigestible state they are protected from gastric acid and reach the small intestine unaffected, where they then infect the epithelial cells. Since the reservoirs of underground water are limited, more and more potentially contaminated surface water is used for irrigation. Due to the expression of flagella, *Salmonella* is able to move through the plant's stomata. Special fimbriae or a colonic acid capsule allow the bacteria to attach and, subsequently, to form a biofilm. This biofilm seems to be effective for survival to such an extent that it might be comparable with *Bacillus* or *Clostridium* spores. Biofilm formation is also observed in sewage sludge. If the sewage sludge comes into contact with surface water (e.g. in occasions of flooding) or is directly brought on to the fields, vegetables will be contaminated and become the source of animal and human infections.

In cases of host-adapted salmonellosis, the eradication within the stock may succeed at times as shown for *S*. Gallinarum and *S*. Pullorum. The avian-adapted *S*. Gallinarum was endemic within European and US poultry flocks in the early 20th century. Since *S*. Gallinarum has no other reservoir than domestic and aquatic fowl, the test-and-slaughter method led to its eradication from commercial poultry flocks in the USA, England and Wales in the 1970s. However, infections caused by *S*. Gallinarum are still common in free-range or specialist flocks, where hygiene standards and management might be less effective than on intensive farms (Hinz *et al.*, 1989). Further, we have to understand that the host-bound life cycle is different from non-host survival. Since the *S*. Gallinarum genome contains the operons for cellulose, colonic acid and curli production the serovar should be able to form biofilms where the bacteria can reside in inter-epidemic phases. So it might be only a matter of time before *S*. Gallinarum will be brought back to the European poultry flocks by imported feed or other vehicles carrying the '*Salmonella* Gallinarum-cellulose-matrix-complex'. Therefore, a global eradication as achieved for pox viruses or other viral pathogens has no reasonable chance in the case of salmonellosis in general. Only long-term strategies to combat *Salmonella* biofilms can help to reduce the burden of salmonellosis in future.

Acknowledgements

We thank Angelika Fruth and Marita Wahnfried for continuous serotyping, Rita Prager and Gerlinde Bartel for PFGE and ribotyping as well as Dagmar Busse and Susanne Kulbe for technical assistance in phage typing. We are grateful to Linda R. Ward and Elizabeth de Pinna (Health Protection Agency Microbiology Services Colindale, London, UK) for supporting us with typing phages over decades. Furthermore, many thanks to Christian Kornschober (National Reference Laboratory for Salmonella, Graz, Austria) for the fruitful cooperation in the field of reptile-associated salmonellosis.

References

Anderson, E.S., Ward, L.R., Saxe, M.J. and de Sa, J.D. (1977) Bacteriophage-typing designations of *Salmonella* Typhimurium. *Journal of Hygiene* 78, 297–300.

Arena, P.C., Steedman, C. and Warwick, C. (2012) Amphibian and reptile pet markets in the EU: An investigation and Assessment. Available at: http://animal-public.de/2012/05/wissenschaftler-fordern-verbot-von-terraristikborse (accessed 15 December 2012).

Aserkoff, B., Schroeder, S.A. and Brachman, P.S. (1970) Salmonellosis in the United States – a five-year review. *American Journal of Epidemiology* 92, 13–24.
AVMA (2007) *American Veterinary Medical Association. US pet ownership and demographics sourcebook*. American Veterinary Medical Association, Schaumberg, Illinois.
Bean, B.N. and Griffin, P.H. (1990) Foodborne disease outbreaks in the United States, 1973-1987: pathogens, vehicles, and trends. *Journal of Food Protection* 38, 804–817.
Bellido-Blasco, J.B., Arnedo-Pena, A., Cordero-Cutillas, E., Canós-Cabedo, M., Herrero-Carot, C. and Safont-Adsuara, L. (2002) The Protective Effect of Alcoholic Beverages on the Occurrence of a *Salmonella* Food-Borne Outbreak. *Epidemiology* 13, 228–230.
Berendes, T.D., Keijman, J.M., te Velde, L.F. and Oostenbroek, R.J. (2007) Splenic abscesses caused by a reptile-associated *Salmonella* infection. *Digestive Surgery* 24, 397–399.
Bertrand, S., Rimhanen-Finne, R., Weill, F.X., Rabsch, W., Thornton, L., Perevoscikovs, J., van Pelt, W. and Heck, M. (2008) *Salmonella* infections associated with reptiles: The current situation in Europe. *Eurosurveillance* 13, 18902.
Biesold, I. and Behrend, L. (1970) The dissemination of *salmonella* through utilization of waste water in agriculture. *Zeitschrift Gesamte Hygiene,* 16, 609–613.
Boyen, F., Haesebrouck, F., Maes, D., Van Immerseel, F., Ducatelle, R. and Pasmans, F. (2008) Non-typhoidal *Salmonella* infections in pigs: a closer look at epidemiology, pathogenesis and control. *Veterinary Microbiology* 130, 1–19.
Brandl, M. and Mandrell, R.E. (2002) Fitness of *Salmonella enterica* serovar Thompson in the cilantro phyllosphere. *Applied Environmental Microbiology* 68, 3614–3621.
Bradley, T., Angulo, F.J. and Raiti, P. (1998) Association of Reptilian and Amphibian Veterinarians guidelines for reducing risk of transmission of *Salmonella* spp. from reptiles to humans. *Journal of the American Veterinary Medical Association* 213, 51–52.
Brédart, S., Wastelin, M., Collard, J.M., Coppée, M. and Bodart, E. (2007) Pet turtle and septicemia: what is the relationship? *Revue Medicale de Liege* 62, 496–497.
Brockmann, S.O., Piechotowski, I. and Kimmig, P. (2004) *Salmonella* in sesame seed products. *Journal of Food Protection* 67, 178–180.
Bruins, M.J., de Boer, A.M. and Ruijs, G.J. (2006) Gastroenteritis caused by *Salmonella* from pet snakes. *Nederlands Tijdschrift voor Geneeskunde* 150, 2266–2269.
Callow, B.R. (1959) A new phage-typing scheme for *Salmonella* Typhimurium. *Journal of Hygiene (Cambridge)* 57, 346–359.
CDC (1998) Reptile-associated Salmonellosis – Selected States, 1996–1998. *Morbidity and Mortality Weekly Report* 48, 1009–1013.
CDC (2008) Multistate outbreak of human *Salmonella* infections associated with exposure to turtles – United States, 2007–2008. *Morbidity and Mortality Weekly Report* 57, 69–72.
CDC (2010) Multistate outbreak of human *Salmonella* Typhimurium infections associated with pet turtle exposure – United States, 2008. *Morbidity and Mortality Weekly Report* 59, 191–196.
Cogan, T.A. and Humphrey, T.J. (2003) The rise and fall of *Salmonella* Enteritidis in the UK. *Journal of Applied Microbiology* 94, 114S–119S.
Cohen, J.I., Bartlett, J.A. and Corey, G.R. (1987) Extra-intestinal manifestations of *Salmonella* infections. *Medicine (Baltimore)* 66, 349–388.
Corrente, M., Totaro, M., Martella, V., Campolo, M., Lorusso, A., Ricci, M. *et al.* (2006) Reptile-associated salmonellosis in man, Italy. *Emerging Infectious Diseases* 12, 358–359.
Costerton, J.W., Lewandowski, Z., Caldwell, D.E., Korber, D.R. and Lappin-Scott, H.M. (1995) Microbial biofilms. *Annual Reviews of Microbiology* 49, 711–745.
Craven, P.C., Mackel, D.C., Baine, W.B., Barker, W.H., Gangarosa, E.J., Goldfield, M., Rosenfield, H., Altman, R., Lachapelle, G., Davies, J.W. and Swanson, R.C. (1975) International outbreak of *Salmonella* Eastborne infection traced to contaminated chocolate. *Lancet* I, 788–793.
Crook, P.D., Aguilera, J.F., Threlfall, E.J., O'Brien, S.J., Sigmundsdóttir, G., Wilson, D., Fisher, I.S., Ammon, A., Briem, H., Cowden, J.M., Locking, M.E., Tschäpe, H., van Pelt, W., Ward, L.R. and Widdowson, M.A. (2003) A European outbreak of *Salmonella enterica* serotype Typhimurium definitive phage type 204b in 2000. *Clinical Microbiology and Infection* 9, 839–845.
Cyriac, J. and Wozniak, E.R. (2000) Infantile *Salmonella* meningitis associated with gecko-keeping. *Communicable Disease and Public Health* 3, 66–67.

Daoust, P.Y., Busby, D.G., Ferns, L., Goltz J., McBurney S., Poppe C. and Whitney H. (2000) Salmonellosis in songbirds in the Canadian Atlantic provinces during winter-summer 1997-98. *The Canadian Veterinary Journal* 41, 54–59.

D'Aoust, J.Y. (1985) Infective dose of *Salmonella* typhimurium in cheese. American *Journal of Food Science and Technology* 24, 305–316.

De Jong, B., Andersson, Y. and Ekdahl, K. (2005) Effect of regulation and education on reptile-associated salmonellosis. *Emerging Infectious Diseases* 11, 398–403.

Denny, J., Threlfall, J., Takkinen, J., Löfdahl, S., Westrell, T., Varela, C., Adak, B., Boxall, N., Ethelberg, S., Torpdahl, M., Straetemans, M. and van Pelt, W. (2007) Multinational *Salmonella* Paratyphi B variant Java (*Salmonella* Java) outbreak, August – December 2007. *Eurosurveillance* 12, E071220.2.

Doyle, M.P. and Erickson, M.C. (2008) Summer meeting 2007 – the problems with fresh produce: an overview. *Journal of Applied Microbiology* 105, 317–330.

D'Souza, T., Karwe, M. and Schaffner, D.W. (2012) Effect of high hydrostatic pressure and pressure cycling on a pathogenic *Salmonella enterica* serovar cocktail inoculated into creamy peanut butter. *Journal of Food Protection* 75,169–73.

Eberth, C.J. (1880) Die Organismen in den Organen von Typhus abdominalis. *Virchows Archiv der patholischen Anatomie* 81, 58–73.

EFSA (2010) EFSA Panel on Biological Hazards (BIOHAZ); Scientific Opinion on monitoring and assessment of the public health risk of '*Salmonella* Typhimurium-like' strains. *EFSA Journal* 8(10), 1826.

EFSA/ECDC (2010) The Community Summary Report on Trends and Sources of Zoonoses, Zoonotic Agents and Food-borne Outbreaks in the European Union in 2008. *EFSA Journal* 8(1), 1496.

Fernández-Guerrero, M.L., Aguado, J.M., Arribas, A., Lumbreras, C. and de Gorgolas, M. (2004) The spectrum of cardiovascular infections due to *Salmonella enterica*: a review of clinical features and factors determining outcome. *Medicine (Baltimore)* 83(2), 123–138.

Fontaine, R.E., Arnon, S., Martin, W.T., Vernon, T.M., Gangarosa, E.J., Farmer, J.J., Moram, A.B., Silliliker, J.H. and Decker, D.L. (1978) Raw hamburger, an interstate common source of human salmonellosis. *American Journal of Epidemiology* 107, 36–45.

Fontaine, R.E., Cohen, M.L., Martin, W.T. and Vernon, T.M. (1980) Epidemic salmonellosis from cheddar cheese: surveillance and prevention. *American Journal of Epidemiology* 111, 247–253.

Geue, L. and Löschner, U. (2002) *Salmonella enterica* in reptiles of German and Austrian origin. *Veterinary Microbiology* 84, 79–91.

Gilsdorf, A., Jansen, A., Alpers, K., Dieckmann, H., van Treeck, U., Hauri, A.M., Fell, G., Littmann, M., Rautenberg, P., Prager, R., Rabsch, W., Roggentin, P., Schroeter, A., Miko, A., Bartelt, E., Braunig, J. and Ammon, A. (2005) A nationwide outbreak of *Salmonella* Bovismorbificans PT24, Germany, December 2004 - March 2005. *Eurosurveillance* 10, E050324.1.

Glynn, J.R. and Bradley, D.J. (1992) The relationship between dose and severity of disease in reported outbreaks of *Salmonella* infection. *Epidemiology and Infection* 109, 371–388.

Gordon, M.A. (2008) *Salmonella* infections in immunocompromised adults. *Journal of Infection* 56, 413–422.

Gordon, M.A., Graham, S.M., Walsh, A.L., Phiri, L.W., Molyneux, E., Zijlstra, E.E., Heyderman, R.S., Hart, C.A. and Molyneux, M.E. (2008) Epidemics of invasive *Salmonella enterica* serovar enteritidis and *S. enterica* serovar typhimurium infection associated with multidrug resistance among adults and children in Malawi. *Clinical Infectious* Diseases 46, 963–969.

Greenwood, M.H. and Hooper, W.L. (1983) Chocolate bars contaminated with *Salmonella* napoli an infective study. *British Medical Journal* 286, 1394.

Guibourdenche, M., Roggentin, P., Mikoleit, M., Fields, P.I., Bockemühl, J., Grimont, P.A. and Weill, F.X. (2010) Supplement 2003-2007 (No. 47) to the White-Kauffmann-Le Minor scheme. *Research in Microbiology* 161, 26–29.

Hames, A., Mumford, J., Hale, J. and Galloway, A. (2008) *Salmonella* Michigan soft tissue infection in an immunocompromised child. *Journal of Clinical Pathology* 61, 773–774.

Hanning, I.B., Nutt, J.D. and Ricke, S.C. (2009) Salmonellosis outbreaks in the United States due to fresh produce: sources and potential intervention measures. *Foodborne Pathogens and Disease* 6, 635–648.

Harker, K.S., Lane, C., De Pinna, E. and Adak, G.K. (2011) An outbreak of *Salmonella* Typhimurium DT191a associated with reptile feeder mice. *Epidemiology and Infection* 139, 1254–1261.

Hartwig, H., Schlösser, A., Rabsch, W. and Beckmann, G. (2006) Salmonellen in Kräutern und Gewürzen. *Fleischwirtschaft* 3, 150–154.

Hatt, J.-M., Fruth, A. and Rabsch, W. (2009) Reptilienassoziierte Salmonellosen – aktuelle Informationen für Tierärztinnen und Tierärzte. *Zeitschrift Tierärztliche Praxis* 37, 188–193.

Hauser, E., Hühn, S., Junker, E., Jaber, M., Schroeter, A., Helmuth, R., Rabsch, W., Winterhoff, N. and Malorny, B. (2009) Anstieg der Isolate einer Variante des *Salmonella enterica* subsp. *enterica* Serovars Typhimuriums aus verendeten Wildvögeln und deren mögliche Übertragung auf Kleinkinder durch Katzen. *Berliner und Münchner Tierärztliche Wochenschrift* 122, 169–177.

Hauser, E., Tietze, E., Helmuth, R., Junker, E., Blank, K., Prager, R., Rabsch, W., Appel, B., Fruth, A. and Malorny, B. (2010) Pork contaminated with *Salmonella enterica* serovar 4,[5],12:i:-, an emerging health risk for humans. *Applied and Environmental Microbiology* 76, 4601–4610.

Hauser, E., Hebner, F., Tietze, E., Helmuth, R., Junker, E., Prager, R., Schroeter, A., Rabsch, W., Fruth, A. and Malorny, B. (2011) Diversity of *Salmonella enterica* serovar Derby isolated from pig, pork and humans in Germany. *International Journal of Food Microbiology* 151(2), 141–149.

Henzler, D.J., Ebel, E., Sanders, J., Kradel, D. and Mason, J. (1994) *Salmonella* enteritidis in eggs from commercial chicken layer flocks implicated in human outbreaks. *Avian Diseases* 38, 37–43.

Hernández, E., Rodriguez, J.L., Herrera-León, S., García, I., de Castro, V. and Muniozguren, N. (2012) *Salmonella* Paratyphi B var Java infections associated with exposure to turtles in Bizkaia, Spain, September 2010 to October 2011. *Eurosurveillance* 17, Issue 25, 21 June.

Hernigou, P., Daltro, G., Flouzat-Lachaniette, C.H., Roussignol, X. and Poignard, A. (2010) Septic arthritis in adults with sickle cell disease often is associated with osteomyelitis or osteonecrosis. *Clinical Orthopaedics and Related Research* 468, 1676–1681.

Heuvelink, A.E., Valkenburgh, S.M., Tilburg, J.J., Van Heerwaarden, C., Zwartkruis-Nahuis, J.T. and De Boer, E. (2007) Public farms: hygiene and zoonotic agents. *Epidemiology and Infection* 135, 1174–1183.

Hibbert, B., Costiniuk, C., Hibbert, R., Joseph, P., Alanazi, H., Dennie, S.T.C., Angel, J.B. and O'Brien, E.R. (2010) Cardiovascular complications of *Salmonella* Enteritidis infection. *Canadian Journal of Cardiology* 26, e323–e325.

Hinz, K.H., Glonder, G., Rottmann, S. and Friedrichs, M. (1989) Über *Salmonella* Gallinarum-Feldisolate der Biovare Pullorum und Gallinarum. *Berliner und Münchener Tierärztliche Wochenschrift* 102, 205–208.

Hobbs, B.C. (1971) Poultry disease and world economy. In: Gordon, R.F. and Freeman, B.M. (eds) *Poultry Disease and World Economy*. British Poultry Science, Edinburgh, UK, p. 65.

Hoelzer, K., Moreno Switt, A.I. and Wiedmann, M. (2011) Animal contact as a source of human non-typhoidal salmonellosis. *Veterinary Research* 42, 34.

Hopkins, K.L., Kirchner, M., Guerra, B., Granier, S.A., Lucarelli, C., Porrero, M.C., Jakubczak, A., Threlfall, E.J. and Mevius, D.J. (2010) Multiresistant *Salmonella enterica* serovar 4,[5],12:i:- in Europe: a new pandemic strain? *Eurosurveillance* 15, 19580.

Hsu, R.B. and Lin, F.Y. (2005) Risk factors for bacteraemia and endovascular infection due to non-typhoid *Salmonella*: a reappraisal. *An International Journal of Medicine QJM* 98, 821–827.

Jansen, A., Frank, C. and Stark, K. (2007) Pork and pork products as a source for human salmonellosis in Germany. *Berliner und Münchner Tierärztliche Wochenschrift* 120, 340–346.

Jansen, A., Hiller, P., Desai, S., Feier, B., Habermann, F., Baumann, A., Dreesmann, J., Beyrer, K., Pulz, M., von Benten, K., Malorny, B., Rabsch, W. and Stark, K. (2008) Protrahiert verlaufender nosokomialer Ausbruch von *Salmonella* Enteritidis LT 8/7. *Z. Gastroenterology* 46, 1270–1274.

Jasson, V., Baert, L. and Uyttendaele, M. (2011) Detection of low numbers of healthy and sub-lethally injured *Salmonella enterica* in chocolate. *International Journal of Microbiology* 145, 488–491.

Jüch, M., Grabert, E., Rabsch, W. and Achenbach, H.J. (2013) Broncho-pulmonary Salmonellosis – A Case Series and Review of the Literature. *Pneumologie* 67, 1–5.

Kapperud, G., Gustavsen, S., Hellesnes, I., Hansen, A.H., Lassen, J., Hirn, J., Jahkola, M., Montenegro, M.A. and Helmuth, R. (1990) Outbreak of *Salmonella* typhimurium infection traced to contaminated chocolate and caused by a strain lacking the 60-megadalton virulence plasmid. *Journal of Clinical Microbiology* 28, 2597–2601.

Kelterborn, E. (1967) Salmonella *Species. First isolation, names and occurrence*. S. Hirzel-Verlag, Leipzig.

Keymer, I.F., Gibson, E.A. and Reynolds, D.J. (1991) Zoonoses and other findings in hedgehogs (*Erinaceus europaeus*): a survey of mortality and review of the literature. *Veterinary Record* 128, 245–249.

Killalea, D., Ward, L.R., Roberts, D., de Louvois, J., Sufi, F., Stuart, J.M., Wall, P.G., Susman, M., Schwieger, M., Sanderson, P.J., Fisher, I.S.T., Mead, P.S., Gill, O.N., Bartlett, C.L.R and Rowe, B. (1996) International epidemiological and microbiological study of outbreak of *Salmonella* agona infection from a ready to eat savoury snack in England and Wales and the United States. *British Medical Journal* 313, 1105–1107.

Kingsley, R.A., Msefula, C.L., Thomson, N.R., Kariuki, S., Holt, K.E., Gordon, M.A., Harris, D., Clarke, L., Whitehead, S., Sangal, V., Marsh, K., Achtman, M., Molyneux, M.E., Cormican, M., Parkhill, J., MacLennan, C.A., Heyderman, R.S. and Dougan, G. (2009) Epidemic multiple drug resistant *Salmonella* Typhimurium causing invasive disease in sub-Saharan Africa have a distinct genotype. *Genome Research* 19, 2279–2287.

Kirk, M.D., Little, C.L., Lem, M., Fyfe, M., Genobile, D., Tan, A., Threlfall, J., Paccagnella, A., Lightfoot, D., Lyi, H., McIntyre, L., Ward, L., Brown, D.J., Surnam, S. and Fisher, I.S. (2004) An outbreak due to peanuts in their shell caused by *Salmonella enterica* serotypes Stanley and Newport-sharing molecular information to solve international outbreaks. *Epidemiology and Infection* 132, 571–577.

Koch, J., Schrauder, A., Alpers, K., Werber, D., Frank, C., Prager, R., Rabsch, W., Broll, S., Feil, F., Roggentin, P., Bockemühl, J., Tschäpe, H., Ammon, A. and Stark, K. (2005) *Salmonella* agona outbreak from contaminated aniseed, Germany. *Emerging Infectious Diseases* 11, 1124–1127.

Kolpinghaus Berlin report (1984) Salmonellose-Bekämpfung Ergebnisse eines WHO-Sachverständigen-Gespräch; Kolpinghaus Berlin 11.-14. Dec. 1984, *Veterinär Medizin Hefte, Robert von Ostertag Institut* 2, 1–47.

Kroupitski, Y., Golberg, D., Belausov, E., Pinto, R., Swartzberg, D., Granot, D. and Sela, S. (2009) Internalization of *Salmonella enterica* in leaves is induced by light and involves chemotaxis and penetration through open stomata. *Applied Environmental Microbiology* 75, 6076–6086.

Laszlo, V.G., Csorian, E.S. and Paszti, J. (1985) Phage types and epidemiological significance of *Salmonella* enteritidis strains in Hungary between 1976 and 1983. *Acta Microbiologica et Immunologica Hungarica* 32, 321–340.

Lee, A.T., Hall, R.G. and Pile, K.D. (2005) Reactive joint symptoms following an outbreak of *Salmonella* typhimurium phage type 135a. *The Journal of Rheumatology* 32, 524–527.

Lehmacher, A., Bockemühl, J. and Aleksic, S. (1995) Nationwide outbreak of human salmonellosis in Germany due to contaminated paprika-powdered potato chips. *Epidemiology and Infection* 115, 501–511.

Lowther, S.A., Medus, C., Scheffel, J., Leano, F., Jawahir, S. and Smith, K. (2011) Foodborne Outbreak of *Salmonella* Subspecies IV Infections Associated with Contamination from Bearded Dragons. *Zoonoses Public Health* 58, 560–566.

Makin, G., Abu-Harb, M., Flinn, A. and Partridge, S. (1996) *Salmonella* durban in an infant. *Lancet* 348, 200.

Malorny, B., Bunge, C. and Helmuth, R. (2003) Discrimination of d-tartrate-fermenting and -nonfermenting *Salmonella enterica* subsp. *enterica* isolates by genotypic and phenotypic methods. *Journal of Clinical Microbiology* 41, 4292–4297.

McCullough, N.B. and Eisele, C.W. (1951) Experimental human salmonellosis; pathogenicity of strains of *Salmonella* meleagridis and *Salmonella* anatum obtained from spray-dried whole egg. *Journal of Infectious Diseases* 88, 278–289.

Mertens, E., Kreher, H., Rabsch, W., Bornhofen, B., Alpers, K. and Burckhardt, F. (2012) Severe infections caused by *Salmonella* Enteritidis PT 8/7 linked to a private barbeque in Rhineland-Palatinate, Germany. *Epidemiology and Infection*, [Epub ahead of print].

Miller, T. (2009) *Development of a phage typing system for* Salmonella *Infantis for epidemiological purposes*. Institute of Food Hygiene, Faculty of Veterinary Medicine, University of Leipzig.

Milstone, A.M., Agwu, A.G. and Angulo, F.J. (2006) Alerting pregnant women to the risk of reptile-associated salmonellosis. *Obstetrics & Gynecology* 107, 516–518.

Mintz, E.D., Carter, M.L., Hadler, J.L., Wassell, J.T., Zingeser, J.A. and Tauxe, R.V. (1994) Dose-response effects in an outbreak of *Salmonella enteritidis*. *Epidemiology and Infection* 112, 13–23.

Mishu, B., Koehler, J., Lee, L.A., Rodrigue, D., Brenner, F.H., Blake, P. and Tauxe, R.V. (1994) Outbreaks of *Salmonella* Enteritidis infections in the United States, 1985-1991, *Journal of Infectious Diseases* 169, 547–552.

Mossong, J., Marques, P., Ragimbeau, C., Huberty-Krau, P., Losch, S., Meyer, G., Moris, G., Strottner, C., Rabsch, W. and Schneider, F. (2007) Outbreaks of monophasic *Salmonella enterica* serovar 4,[5],12:i:- in Luxembourg, 2006. *Eurosurveillance* 12, 11–12.

Nauerby, B., Pedersen, K., Dietz, H.H. and Madsen, M. (2000) Comparison of Danish isolates of *Salmonella enterica* serovar enteritidis PT9a and PT11 from hedgehogs (*Erinaceus europaeus*) and humans by plasmid profiling and pulsed-field gel electrophoresis. *Journal of Clinical Microbiology* 38, 3631–3635.

Noble, D.J., Lane, C., Little, C.L., Davies, R., De Pinna, E., Larkin, L. and Morgan, D. (2012) Revival of an old problem: an increase in *Salmonella enterica* serovar Typhimurium definitive phage type 8 infections in 2010 in England and Northern Ireland linked to duck eggs. *Epidemiology & Infection* 140, 146–149.

Nygård, K., Lassen, J., Vold, L., Andersson, Y., Fisher, I., Löfdahl, S., Threlfall, J., Luzzi, I., Peters, T., Hampton, M., Torpdahl, M., Kapperud, G. and Aavitsland, P. (2008) Outbreak of *Salmonella* Thompson infections linked to imported rucola lettuce. *Foodborne Pathogens and Disease* 5, 165–173.

O'Byrne, A.M. and Mahon, M. (2008) Reptile-associated salmonellosis in residents in the south east of Ireland 2005-2007. *Eurosurveillance* 13, 18830.

Pakalniskiene, J., Falkenhorst, G., Lisby, M., Madsen, S.B., Olsen, K.E., Nielsen, E.M., Mygh, A., Boel, J. and Mølbak, K. (2009) A foodborne outbreak of enterotoxigenic *E. coli* and *Salmonella* Anatum infection after a high-school dinner in Denmark, November 2006. *Epidemiology and Infection* 137(3), 396–401.

Pennycott, T.W., Ross, H.M., McLaren, I.M., Park, A., Hopkins, G.F. and Foster, G. (1998) Causes of death of wild birds of the family *Fringillidae* in Britain. *Veterinary Record* 143, 155–158.

Pessoa-Silva, C.L., Toscano, C.M., Moreira, B.M., Santos, A.L., Frota, A.C., Solari, C.A., Amorim, E.L., Carvalho, M.G., Teixeira, L.M. and Jarvis, W.R. (2002) Infection due to extended-spectrum beta-lactamase-producing *Salmonella enterica* subsp. *enterica* serotype infantis in a neonatal unit. *Journal of Pediatrics* 141, 381–387.

Pezzoli, L., Elson, R., Little, C.L., Yip, H., Fisher, I., Yishai, R., Anis, E., Valinsky, L., Biggerstaff, M., Patel, N., Mather, H., Brown, D.J., Coia, J.E., van Pelt, W., Nielsen, E.M., Ethelberg, S., de Pinna, E., Hampton, M.D., Peters, T. and Threlfall, J. (2008) Packed with *Salmonella* investigation of an international outbreak of *Salmonella* Senftenberg infection linked to contamination of prepacked basil in 2007. *Foodborne Pathogens and Disease* 5, 661–668.

Plenary meeting (1976) Vollversammlung des Bundesgesundheitsrates, Votum des Bundesgesundheitsrates zur *Salmonella*-Bekämpfung. *Bundesgesundheitsblatt* 22, 353–357.

Prager, R., Rabsch, W., Streckel, W., Voigt, W., Tietze, E. and Tschäpe, H. (2003) Molecular properties of *Salmonella enterica* serotype paratyphi B distinguish between its systemic and its enteric pathovars. *Journal of Clinical Microbiology* 41, 4270–4278.

Rabsch, W. (2009) International emergence and trends of *S.* Typhimurium DT193. In: *Second Annual Meeting of Food and Waterborne Diseases and Zoonoses Surveillance Network in Europe*, 24–25 September 2009, Malta.

Rabsch, W., Hargis, B.M., Tsolis, R.M., Kingsley, R.A., Hinz, K.H., Tschäpe, H. and Bäumler, A.J. (2000) Did the avian-adapted serovar *Salmonella* Gallinarum exclude *Salmonella* Enteritidis from poultry. *Emerging Infectious Diseases* 6, 443–448.

Rabsch, W., Tschäpe, H. and Bäumler, A.J. (2001a) Non-typhoidal Salmonellosis: Emerging problems. *Microbes and Infections* 3, 237–247.

Rabsch, W., Liesegang, A. and Tschäpe, H. (2001b) Laboratory-based surveillance of salmonellosis of humans in Germany – safety of *Salmonella* Typhimurium and *Salmonella* Enteritidis live vaccines *Berliner Münchner Tierärztliche Wochenschrift* 114, 433–437.

Rabsch, W., Andrews, H.L., Kingsley, R.A., Prager, R., Tschäpe, H., Adams, L.G. and Bäumler, A.J. (2002) *Salmonella enterica* serotype Typhimurium and its host-adapted variants. *Infection and Immunology* 70, 2249–2255.

Rabsch, W., Prager, R., Koch, J., Stark, K., Roggentin, P., Bockemühl, J., Beckmann, G., Stark, R., Siegl, W., Ammon, A. and Tschäpe, H. (2005) Molecular epidemiology of *Salmonella enterica* serovar Agona: characterization of a diffuse outbreak caused by aniseed-fennel-caraway infusion. *Epidemiology and Infection* 133, 837–844.

Rabsch, W., Truepschuch, S., Windhorst, D. and Gerlach, R.G. (2011) Typing phages and prophages of *Salmonella*. In: Porwollik, S. (ed.) Salmonella*: From Genome to Function*. Caister Academic Press, Norwich, UK, pp. 25–48.

Raybaudi-Massilia, R.M., Mosqueda-Melgar, J., Soliva-Fortuny, R. and Martín-Belloso, O. (2009) Control of pathogenic and spoilage microorganisms in fresh-cut fruits and fruit juices by traditional and alternative natural antimicrobials. *Comprehensive Reviews in Food Science and Food Safety* 8, 157–180.

Robert Koch Institut (2006) Death of a 12 year old boy by salmonellosis. *Epidemiologisches Bulletin* 5, 41.

Robert Koch Institut (2011a) SurvStat. Available at: http://www3.rki.de/SurvStat (accessed on 16 September 2011).

Robert Koch Institut (2011b) *Infektionsepidemiologisches Jahrbuch 2004-2010*. Robert Koch-Institut, Berlin.

Robert Koch Institut (2013) *Salmonella* infection in infants and young children by contact to exotic reptiles. *Epidemiologishes Bulletin* 9, 71.

Rodrigue, D.C., Tauxe, R.V. and Rowe, B. (1990) International increase in *Salmonella enteritidis* – a new pandemic. *Epidemiology and Infection* 105, 21–27.
Römling, U., Pesen, D. and Yaron, S. (2007) Biofilm formation of *Salmonella enterica*. In: Rhen, M., Maskell, D., Mastroeni, P. and Threlfall, J. (eds) Salmonella*: Molecular Biology and Pathogenesis*. Horizon Press, Norfolk, UK, pp. 127–145.
Schicklmaier, P., Moser, E., Wieland, T., Rabsch, W. and Schmieger, H. (1998) A comparative study on the frequency of prophages among natural isolates of *Salmonella* and *Escherichia coli* with emphasis on generalized transducers. *Antonie van Leeuwenhoek* 73, 49–54.
Santos, S.B., Carvalho, C.M., Sillankorva, S., Nicolau, A., Ferreira, E.C. and Azeredo, J. (2009) The use of antibiotics to improve phage detection and enumeration by the double-layer agar technique. *BMC Microbiology* 9, 148.
Saphra, I. and Winter, J.W. (1957) Clinical manifestations of salmonellosis in man; an evaluation of 7779 human infections identified at the New York *Salmonella* Center. *The New England Journal of Medicine* 256, 1128–1134.
Scheelings, T.F., Lightfoot, D. and Holz, P. (2011) Prevalence of *Salmonella* in Australian reptiles. *Journal of Wildlife Disease* 47, 1–11.
Sivapalasingam, S., Friedman, C.R., Cohen, L. and Tauxe, R.V. (2004) Fresh produce: a growing cause of outbreaks of foodborne illness in the United States, 1973 through 1997. *Journal of Food Protection* 67, 2342–2353.
Stam, F., Römkens, T.E., Hekker, T.A. and Smulders, Y.M. (2003) Turtle-associated human salmonellosis. *Clinical Infectious Diseases* 37, 167–169.
Stevens, A., Joseph, C., Bruce, J., Fenton, D., O'Mahoney, M., Cunningham, D., O'Connor, B. and Rowe, B. (1989) A large outbreak of *Salmonella enteritidis* phage type 4 associated with eggs from overseas. *Epidemiology and Infection* 103, 425–433.
St Louis, M.E., Morse, D.L., Potter, M.E., DeMelfi, T.M., Guzewich, J.J., Tauxe, R.V. and Blake, P.A. (1988) The emergence of grade A eggs as a major source of *Salmonella enteritidis* infections. New implications for the control of salmonellosis. *Journal of the American Medical Association* 259, 2103–2107.
Sullivan, C.L. and Cunha, B.A. (1989) Pseudoappendicitis caused by *Salmonella* heidelberg. *Heart & Lung* 18, 310–313.
Switt, A.I., Soyer, Y., Warnick, L.D. and Wiedmann, M. (2009) Emergence, distribution, and molecular and phenotypic characteristics of *Salmonella enterica* serotype 4,5,12:i. *Foodborne Pathogens and Disease* 6, 407–415.
Threlfall, E.J., Hall, M.L.M. and Rowe, B. (1992) *Salmonella* bacteraemia in England and Wales, 1981-1990. *Journal of Clinical Pathology* 45, 34–36.
Torpdahl, M., Litrup, E. and Nielsen, E.M. (2009) Characterisation and prevalence of *Salmonella* 4,5,12:i:- in Denmark, the monophasic variant of *Salmonella* Typhimurium. *ASM Conference on* Salmonella*: Biology Pathogenesis and Prevention*, Aix-en-Provence, France.
Townes, J.M. (2010) Reactive arthritis after enteric infections in the United States: the problem of definition. *Clinical Infectious Diseases* 50, 247–254.
Tschäpe, H., Liesegang, A., Gericke, B., Prager, R., Rabsch, W. and Helmuth, R. (1999) The ups and downs of *Salmonella enterica* in Serovar Enteritidis in Germany. In: Saeed, A.M. (ed.) Salmonella enterica *serovar Enteritidis in Humans and Animals*. Iowa State University Press, Ames, Iowa, pp. 51–62.
Van Pelt, W., van der Zee, H., Wannet, W.J., van de Giessen, A.W., Mevius, D.J., Bolder, N.M., Komijn, R.E. and van Duynhoven, Y.T. (2003) Explosive increase of *Salmonella* Java in poultry in the Netherlands: consequences for public health. *Eurosurveillance* 8, 31–35.
Vogel, Y., Tannapfel, A., Rabsch, W. and Henning, B. (2007) Cholangitis with hepatic microabscesses caused by *Salmonella enterica* serovar choleraesuis. *Deutsche Medizinische Wochenschrift* 132, 1214–1218.
Votum of Bundesgesundheitsrat (1985) *Bundesgesundheitsblatt* 28, 244–246
Wall, P.G. and Ward, L.R. (1999) Epidemiology of *Salmonella enterica* serovar Enteritidis phage type 4 in England and Wales. In: Saeed, A.M. (ed.) Salmonella enterica *serovar Enteritidis in Humans and Animals*. Iowa State University Press, Ames, Iowa, pp. 19–25.
Ward, L. (2000) *Salmonella* perils of pet reptiles. *Communicable Disease and Public Health* 3, 2–3.
Ward, L.R., de Sa, J.D. and Rowe, B. (1987) A phage-typing scheme for *Salmonella* enteritidis. *Epidemiology and Infection* 99, 291–294.
Watanabe, T. and Lyang, K.W. (1962) Episome-mediated transfer of drug resistance in Enterobacteriaceae. V. Spontaneous segregation and recombination of resistance factors in *Salmonella* typhimurium. *Journal of Bacteriology* 84, 422–430.

Wegener, H.C. and Baggesen, D.L. (1996) Investigation of an outbreak of human salmonellosis caused by *Salmonella enterica* ssp. *enterica* serovar Infantis by use of pulsed field gel electrophoresis. *International Journal of Food Microbiology* 32, 125–131.

Werber, D., Dreesman, J., Feil, F., van Treeck, U., Fell, G., Ethelberg, S., Hauri, A.M., Roggentin, P., Prager, R., Fisher, I.S., Behnke, S.C., Bartelt, E., Weise, E., Ellis, A., Siitonen, A., Andersson, Y., Tschäpe, H., Kramer, M.H. and Ammon, A. (2005) International outbreak of *Salmonella* Oranienburg due to German chocolate. *BMC Infectious Diseases* 5, 7.

Willis, C., Wilson, T., Greenwood, M. and Ward, L. (2002) Pet reptiles associated with a case of salmonellosis in an infant were carrying multiple strains of *Salmonella*. *Journal of Clinical Microbiology* 40, 4802–4803.

Winkle, S. and Rohde, R. (1979) Twenty-five Year Experience in Epidemiology and Prophylaxis of Epidemics at the Centre for *Salmonella* of Hamburg. *Zentralblatt Bakteriologie and Hygiene I Abteilung Originale A* 243, 392–411 [in German].

Woodward, D.L., Khakhria, R. and Johnson, W.M. (1997) Human salmonellosis associated with exotic pets. *Journal of Clinical Microbiology* 35, 2786–2790.

Wybo, I., Potters, D., Plaskie, K., Covens, L., Collard, J.M. and Lauwers, S. (2004) *Salmonella enterica* subspecies *houtenae* serotype 44:z4, z23: as a rare cause of meningitis. *Acta Clinica Belgica Journal* 59, 232–234.

19 *Salmonella* in Feed

Martin Wierup*
Department of Biomedical Sciences and Veterinary Public Health, Swedish University of Agricultural Sciences, Sweden

Introduction

Animal feed is a recognized source of hazards, being a health risk for both livestock and consumers. Historically this is well known for different microbes and toxins. The events often referred to as the BSE crisis (Prusiner, 1997) and the dioxin scandal (Bernard *et al.*, 2002) demonstrated the great potential for hazardous substances to be spread by feed. Those events also demonstrated the need to ensure consumer protection through a food safety approach that covers the whole food chain, from farm to fork. The feed is the first link of the food animal chain and among its microbiological hazards *Salmonella* requires special attention. Worldwide, *Salmonella* is one of the most common food-borne zoonoses (Crump *et al.*, 2004) and the cause of substantial economic losses. It is estimated that *Salmonella* globally causes around 94 million human infections and 155,000 deaths annually (Majowicz *et al.*, 2010). In the USA *Salmonella* is the leading food-borne pathogen, causing the largest number of deaths and the highest cost burden (Batz *et al.*, 2011). The annual costs for 2010 were estimated to US$2.71bn for 1.4 million cases (USDA, 2013).

The potential of *Salmonella*-contaminated feed to act as a source of human infections is exemplified by *S.* Agona, which emerged as a public health problem in several countries due to the use of contaminated fish meal as a feed ingredient. In the USA a rapid increase of human infections with *S.* Agona occurred from 1968 to 1972. Since then, *S.* Agona has been amongst the most prevalent serovars in humans, and in 2002 it was estimated that the serovar had caused more than 1 million human illnesses in the USA alone since it was introduced into the food chain (Clark *et al.*, 1973; Crump *et al.*, 2002).

Efforts to reduce *Salmonella* need to include measures to prevent the introduction of *Salmonella* to the food chain through contaminated feed. This approach is logical because in the same way as *Salmonella*-contaminated food is the main route for transmission of *Salmonella* infections in humans, ingestion of *Salmonella*-contaminated feed is a key route of transmission in animals (Fedorka-Cray *et al.*, 1995). This review will assess the possibilities for *Salmonella* to infect food animals through contaminated feed, and possibilities for control.

Feed Materials and Feeding Stuffs

The prevention and control of *Salmonella* contamination of feed requires an informed insight not only of the feed production but

* Author, e-mail: martin.wierup@slu.se

© CAB International 2013. *Salmonella in Domestic Animals, 2nd Edition* (eds P.A. Barrow and U. Methner)

also of the origin, trade and subsequent logistics of different feed materials through the production chain.

Usage of major feed materials

Animal feed includes of a variety of different feed materials primarily of vegetable and, to a limited extent, also of animal origin. Cereals and forages are the major feed components. In addition, fast-growing animals such as broiler chickens and fattening pigs, as well as high-producing dairy cows, require more protein and energy-rich feed. The feed composition varies by animal species, type of production and geographic regions. Statistics are available from different sources and the following data are provided by the European Feed Manufacturers Federation (FEFAC, 2009). The global industrial compound feed production is estimated to 739 Mt, of which Asia including China and Japan (32.9%), the USA (20.1%) and EU-27 (20.0%) are the major producers. For Europe about 460 Mt of feeding stuffs were consumed by the major food animal species (cattle, pigs and poultry) within the EU-27 during 2009. Out of this quantity, 228 Mt mostly were roughages grown and used on the farm of origin. The balance, i.e. 232 Mt, included cereals grown and used on the farm of origin (53 Mt) and feed purchased by livestock producers to supplement their own feed resources, either feed materials (31 Mt) or compound feed (148 Mt). Thus about 61% of the feed was grown and used on the farm of origin. Compound feed accounted for 32% of all feedstuffs recorded as being used for the major food animal species and of the feed purchased by livestock producers, compound feed accounted for 83%.

A split by feed materials shows that, of the compounded feed in the EU-27, 48% are feed cereals, 28% cakes and meals, 12% co-products from food industry, 3% minerals and additives and vitamins, 1% oils and fats each, 1% pulses dried forage, 1% dairy products, tapioca 0.5% and all others are 4%.

A large amount of feed is also produced for fish, although specific data are not readily available. If the small ruminants and the minor species such as rabbits, farmed game and so on are added, more than 600 Mt of animal feed are used for the production of animal protein for human consumption in the EU (EFSA, 2008).

Sources of protein-rich feed

The supply of protein-rich feed materials is essential in the light of the estimated need to increase the global food animal production by >70% within the coming 40 years to feed the global population (FAO, 2009). The demand for protein-rich feed is primarily met by a variety of products derived from vegetable protein. These products, often called cakes and meals, are generally by- or co-products from the food industry, e.g. from mills crushing plants for oilseeds, sugar-producing plants, distilleries and starch factories. In the EU-27, soymeal (68%) and rapeseed meal (15%) are the major sources of protein-rich feed materials used during 2009 followed by sunflower meal (5%) and to a lesser extent by other categories including copra and palm kernel meal, dried forage, pulses, maize gluten feed and cottonseed meal. Fish meal accounted for 2%. Meat and bone meals from slaughter or rendering plants are currently banned in the EU and elsewhere since the BSE crisis in the 1990s.

Globalized feed supply

In the same way as for food, the supply of animal feed for most countries is no longer solely based on domestic production. In Sweden only 72% of the non-forage feed materials for both swine and poultry are of domestic origin and for cattle the proportion is even lower (62%).

For the EU as a whole, about 36 Mt (6%) of the estimated total use of animal feed (600 Mt) were imported during 2009 (EFSA, 2008). The major components were oil meals (26.2 Mt; 72.7%) and cereals (4.5 Mt; 12.5%). Due to the fact that soybeans are rarely grown in Europe in contrast to e.g. the USA, the EU as well as several countries elsewhere with an intensive food animal production industry is dependent on importing vegetable protein, with soybeans or soybean meals being the major products. These are imported mainly from South America where Argentina and Brazil are the major producers. According to FEFAC the self-sufficiency in EU-25 is 2% for soybean and 93% for rapeseed meal (FEFAC, 2009). The protein from soybeans can be replaced only to a limited extent by rapeseed meal because the latter contains higher levels of antinutritional factors.

Feed production

Oilcakes and oil meals

Special attention is given here to oilseed meals because they appear to be the main by-product from the human food production that is often found to be a risk for contaminating animal feed with *Salmonella*. The oilseed processing involves the disaggregation of seeds, like soybeans, palm kernels, rape and sunflower seeds, into crude vegetable oil, animal feed and fibre. The crude oil is refined into food-grade, or may be used as an industrial or fuel feedstock. This process aims to release the oil and involves different methods for pressing or crushing the oilseed, the reason why these industries often are called 'crushers'. The process generally follows either alone or as combination of cold crushing, warm/hot crushing and extraction. In contrast to warm crushing, no preheating with steam is applied in the cold crushing process. The crushing involves either the use of a screw/expeller or hydraulic press between plates. Due to friction in the screw the temperature is raised up to 130–140°C, higher than in a hydraulic press and generally the material in the crushing plants reach >100°C for 20 min (Himathongkham *et al.*, 1996). The product after crushing is called cakes, which usually are ground to a meal. Solvent extraction is also done, typically with hexane, resulting in extraction meal that is further toasted or heat treated. The meals obtained are used as feed ingredients, usually under different names that reflect the different production methods applied, and consequently affect their nutritional properties and often also the hygienic quality.

The crushing plants are either located in the seed production area or at the area of animal production or close to harbours. This is typically the case for soybeans and, for example, Brazil's export to Europe is either soybean meal, crushed in Brazil or soybeans to be crushed in Europe. These products are transported by ships to the larger harbours of Europe for further transportation by smaller vessels or trucks to crushers or feed mills. To a certain extent soybean meal is also directly transported to and mixed into compounded feed at farms.

According to FEFANA (http://www.fefana.org/home.aspx) approximately 150 crushers operate in the EU. Some plants are located in major seaports and concentrate on one type of seed. Other plants process several types of seeds (soybean and/or rapeseed and/or sunflower or linseed), some of which are imported and some produced locally. Other plants depend almost exclusively on raw materials produced locally, e.g. rapeseed. Their capacities vary from 300 to 6000 t day^{-1} (EFSA, 2008). From the point of risk management of *Salmonella* contamination of feed it is interesting to note that in the EU more than 75% of the European crushing capacity belongs to a small number of major international groups and the majority (80%) of the oilseed producers ('the crushers') are organized in the EU Oil and Protein meal Industry; FEDIOL (http://www.fediol.be/http://www.fediol.be). Another major player is COCERAL (http://www.coceral.com), composed of national feed trade organizations, indicating the international activity of the supply of feed materials to the food animal production industry.

Compound feed

Compound feed is produced in feed mills. In contrast to feed ingredients, trade and distribution of the finished rations are usually regional. The output in terms of annual production of individual feed mills varies approximately between 30,000 and 120,000 t and in Europe the largest centralized plants are often found in countries with a small food animal industry, such as Finland and Sweden. The feed is produced in large volumes and even a medium-sized plant can produce around 20 t compound feed h^{-1} and usually operates 24 h day^{-1} and 5–7 days $week^{-1}$ (Binter *et al.*, 2011). The feed ingredients used vary with nutritional requirements for the intended livestock and rations are normally formulated on a least-cost basis, so that specific ingredients are chosen or substituted according to availability, quality and price.

Although the size, age and technical construction may vary between feed mills they have similar functions in common that can be seen from Fig. 19.1. Their basic functions include handling and storage of incoming ingredients, the processing of the ingredients and the conditioning and heat treatment of feed. As summarized by EFSA (EFSA, 2008), these functions include the following steps.

Major ingredients with low moisture content are deposited in the feed mills in the intake pit, while minor ingredients are brought into the feed mill by pneumatic transport or in bags. Intake pits are fitted with a conveyer in the bottom part transporting the ingredients to elevators that bring the ingredients to the storage bins inside the feed mill. Cereal grains are usually received directly from grain silos associated with the feed mill via conveyers or pneumatic transport systems, and are only stored within the feed mill in smaller quantities. Liquid ingredients, such as fat, are pumped to containers or storage tanks associated with the feed mill. Dry ingredients are delivered by trucks, rail cars or by transport ships, liquid ingredients by oil tankers.

The next step in the feed processing is weighing, followed by grinding or mixing of the different ingredients according to the feed formula. In some mills the entire mixture of ingredients is ground for each lot of feed, in other mills the individual ingredients are ground separately. Grinding is performed at ambient temperature but there is usually a slight increase in the temperature of the product after the grinding. Mixing of the ingredients takes place in the mixer where also liquid ingredients e.g. fat may be added. Afterwards the mixture of feed ingredients is transported and stored as meal or mash feed in the finished-product bins, or for heat treatment in a conditioning and pelleting process. The size of the mixer will determine the size of the feed lots being produced, which is usually 3–5 t in larger mills.

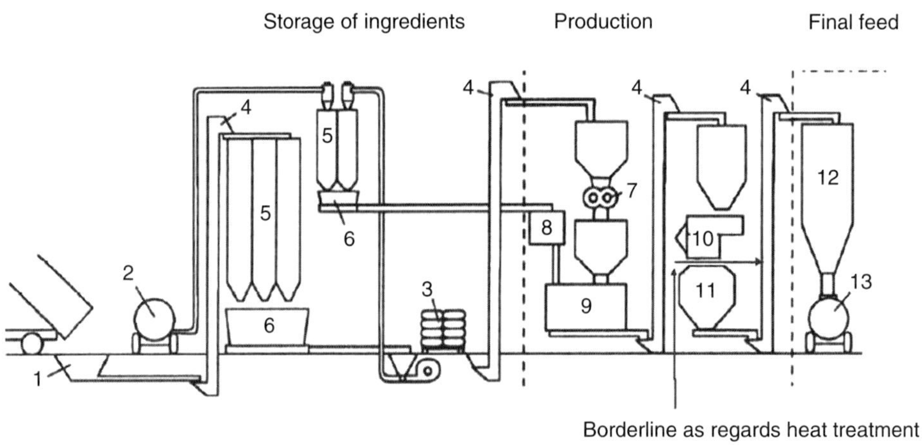

Fig. 19.1. Schematic diagram of a feed mill: 1, intake pit for trucks; 2, pneumatic intake for liquids; 3, intake hopper for bagged ingredients; 4, elevators; 5, storage bins for ingredients; 6, scales; 7, grinder; 8, pre-mix bins for pre-mixes, vitamins etc.; 9, mixer; 10, conditioner and pellet press; 11, pellet cooler; 12, storage bins for compound feeding stuffs; 13, feed truck being loaded at out-loading gantry. Arrows show the physical separation between 'clean' and 'non-clean' parts (Holmberg *et al.*, 1993).

Conditioning, followed by pelleting in a pellet press or expanding are the usual processing procedures performed in most feed mills when heat-treated feed is manufactured, although meals may also be heat treated, e.g. for poultry breeding flocks in some countries. Typically, the meal is introduced into the conditioner where steam is added to raise the temperature to a pre-set level. Conditioning and pelleting combined result in exposure of the feed to temperatures from around 50°C to 90°C. For ruminant and adult pig rations the temperature during pelleting is usually lower than for weaned pig or poultry feed. The moisture content of the feed after pelleting is approximately 15% and is cooled to ambient temperature and dried to approximately 12–13% as rapidly as possible to prevent condensation in the transport equipment and storage containers. Pelleted poultry feed is sometimes sprayed with liquid fat and other additives such as vitamins, enzymes and probiotics after cooling of the pellets. This is a risk and the use of imported brewer's yeast in this way has recently been the cause of several contamination incidents involving *S.* Virchow and *S.* Infantis in the UK (Rob Davies, Animal Health Veterinary Laboratories Agency, UK, pers. comm.). After processing, the feed is stored a short period of time in silos or out-loading bins for compound feeding stuffs before being transported to the farm. It is a feature of modern feed production that there is very limited storage capacity and most feed is dispatched within hours of production, so there is normally no opportunity for test and release programmes.

The design and construction of the feed plant will to varying degrees allow effective physical separation of the clean (post-processing) and non-clean (storage of ingredients and handling) parts of the production and likewise permit effective cleaning measures. The build-up of dust is a factor inherent in feed manufacturing. Therefore adequate dust aspiration systems and vacuum line cleaning equipment in the feed mill are important to keep the mill in a clean condition. It is also important that the aspiration of dust is not done with systems that contribute to circulation of potentially *Salmonella*-contaminated particles in the mill.

Farm-level production

Although a substantial proportion of animal feed is home-produced on farm, for certain sectors, and in particular for poultry, the majority of the feed is bought in as compound feed. For ruminants the predominant part of the feed ration is generally home-grown or local forage and cereals. For pigs around half of the feed is usually homemade, and in the UK the Meat and Livestock Commission has estimated that around 40% of feed produced for pigs is home-produced.

Traditionally the swine producers in the EU buy compound feed, or make their own feed based on home-produced cereals, which are ground in a hammer mill on the farm and mixed with purchased protein concentrate, minerals and vitamins. Home-mixed feed is rarely pelleted and never heat treated. Purchased feed is occasionally non-heat-treated meal, but is usually heat-treated pelleted feed. The meal feed, bought or homemade, is usually stored in 'closed' silos while the home produced grain often is stored on open flat stores. One reason for the producer to purchase compound feed is to obtain pelleted feed that improves feed intake, daily live weight gain and feed conversion. Pellets can also be fed on the floor without the need for expensive feeding equipment.

The specific ingredients finally chosen to feed the animals are largely based on availability, quality and price, although a more limited range of ingredients and sources are used for home-mixed feed, thus decreasing the risk of introduction of *Salmonella* organisms. The price is of significant importance and, for example in the USA and Canada, feed is estimated to represent 60% of the hog production cost and 40% of the total cost after slaughter (Lazaruk, 2009) and up to 70% of the cost of commercial broiler production (Anonymous, 2007). Consequently cost savings and efforts to find new feed ingredients is a continuously ongoing process. When available, by-products from the food industry such as whey, brewer's or distiller's grains and bakery waste is therefore included in non-poultry diets. This may involve the use of liquid feed systems.

Salmonella Contamination of Feed

The results from numerous studies on *Salmonella* in animal feed require careful evaluation. As an example, O'Connor *et al.* (2008) stated in a systematic review that only 277 out of 5071 publications in English were considered to be relevant for assessment of feeding management practice and *Salmonella* prevalence in live and market-weight finisher swine. The sampling procedures usually differ and typically have a low sensitivity for detecting *Salmonella* contamination, and may well lead to underestimate the level of contamination (Davies and Wales, 2010). In the absence of harmonized sampling procedures, results from testing of feed in different countries or in different studies are difficult to compare. The results of testing should be viewed as representing a minimum level of contamination. The same can be said for the data reported to EFSA from 19 EU member states during 2008, in which *Salmonella* positive findings ranged from 0% to 3.6% in cattle and pig feed and up to 8.3% in poultry feed (EFSA, 2010a).

Results of various studies also need to be related to the actual *Salmonella* situation. The EU harmonized studies have thus revealed significant difference between member states for the *Salmonella* status of poultry and swine and associated food products (EFSA, 2010a). Similarly, there is a wide variation between the control actions applied in feed and animal production – from non-acceptance of *Salmonella* contamination to no actions undertaken.

Data that document the importance of *Salmonella* in feed as well as of interventions are most easily achieved and performed in countries with a low level of *Salmonella* contamination as indicated in this review.

Detection and Sampling

Methods for detecting and subtyping

The authorized methods for isolation of *Salmonella* from feed and feed-associated samples follow standard bacteriological procedures, namely ISO 6579 and NMKL-71(Maciorowski *et al.*, 2006). The same methods are principally also applied in the food industry and on samples from different environmental as well as clinical sources. Modified Semisolid Rappaport Vassiliadis (MSRV)-based methods have been shown to be suitable for testing feed (Koyuncu and Häggblom, 2009). An official authorization also of their use for feed and feedstuffs as well as for samples from primary food animal production would offer significant benefits in terms of harmonization across the food chain. There may be strain variations and situations when some *Salmonella* organisms may be more difficult to isolate, but the above methods should in a reliable way detect *Salmonella* contamination in a sample as the level of competing flora is normally low.

Immunological (ELISA) and molecular PCR-based methods are available for an indirect detection of *Salmonella* contamination with the potential for faster detection of *Salmonella* contamination and identification of negative samples as a complement to the standard bacteriological procedures (Maciorowski *et al.*, 2005, 2006). These are sometimes used to screen ingredients before processing or by primary poultry breeding companies to test stored feed before placing on breeding farms.

Direct methods with isolation of the microbe are needed to identify the serovars, which is required for tracing and epidemiological studies. However, it should be highlighted that there is a risk that not all serovars present in a sample will be detected by these methods, if only one colony is selected for the final confirmation. A further subtyping of isolated serovars can be applied, e.g. by pulsed-field gel electrophoresis (PFGE) or variable number tandem repeat (VNTR), which can facilitate tracing and may be useful when different strains of the serovars or phage types occur (Xia *et al.*, 2009). A combination of antimicrobial resistance pattern and subtyping results in an often valuable additional discrimination of the *Salmonella* serovars.

Sampling methods

A major challenge is how to design a suitable sampling protocol to substantiate freedom from *Salmonella* contamination to a defined level of confidence, particular in large volumes of feed or feed ingredients, e.g. in a truck- or a shipload. In contrast to a herd of animals, which is made up of a defined number of discrete sampling units, i.e. the individual animals, no corresponding unit exists for feed. Instead a 25 g sample is often used as a sampling unit and 'freedom' from *Salmonella* defined as absence in the number of specified samples examined. The problem is that absence of *Salmonella* in the samples does not verify true absence of *Salmonella* in a feed batch.

Testing of a selected number of samples in these situations should give a representative measure of the *Salmonella* contamination in the whole lot. The sampling can be based on different methods such as simple random sampling, stratified random sampling and systemic random sampling according to principles described in different ISO documents and elsewhere. However, uncertainties exist, in particular relating to the uneven distribution of the low concentration of *Salmonella* contamination that is typically present in feed. Different statistically based models and methods have been worked out to address this challenge as described and reviewed by Biotracer. This is an integrated EU project established in 2007 with one of the objectives to suggest sampling for tracking and tracing contamination of *Salmonella* along the feed chain (http://www.biotracer.org). An EFSA opinion on microbial contamination of feed also highlighted the need for harmonized and validated methods (EFSA, 2008). Only a few countries are known to have implemented such sampling protocols, and in the absence of harmonized sampling or harmonized regulations for the control of *Salmonella* in feed or in feed production there seem to be no agreed standard methods available for ensuring freedom of *Salmonella*, e.g. in a feed ingredient before use in feed production or of a compounded feed as a guarantee for a farmer. When a control is applied, testing for 'freedom in a 25 g sample' is often used, but freedom in one 25 g sample of feed gives very unreliable information on the contamination in the situations described above (Andersson *et al.*, 2010). Foster (1971) and Dahms (2004) found that testing around 60 negative 25 g samples was required to conclude with 95% confidence that the contamination level is less than 1 cfu per 526 g feed, which indicates the level of sampling that would be required to provide a meaningful result for a large batch of feed.

Testing of the final product alone is usually not sufficient to ensure freedom of *Salmonella*. However, it is possible to ensure that a feed in practice is free from significant levels of *Salmonella* contamination if the whole production process is controlled. A *Salmonella*-free feed could thus be defined as coming from a '*Salmonella* safe feed production', since the possible contamination of *Salmonella* is so low that it is very unlikely that it would result in an infection in animals consuming the feed. The official approval of feed mills could be based on the existence of an appropriate HACCP-based control and associated strategies for interventions. This approach is successfully applied in Finland, Norway and Sweden and is also found to be effective when applied for crushing plants for rape seed and soybeans (Herland, 2006; EFSA, 2008).

If oilseed meal cannot be obtained from crushing plants under appropriate and effective HACCP programmes for control of *Salmonella* their products should be tested before introduction to the feed mill as applied in Sweden (Wierup and Häggblom, 2010). The surveillance of such high-risk feed ingredients is based on a sampling procedure that takes into consideration an uneven distribution of *Salmonella* and is designed to detect contamination in 5% of the batch with 95% probability (Ekbohm, 1993). The size of the analytical sample is 25 g and usually eight samples are analysed, each consisting of ten pooled sub-samples of 2.5 g.

A representative sampling meets large practical difficulties in particular from large volumes of feed or feed ingredients that seemingly are inaccessible. To overcome these problems it is advised to 'sample in a moving stream', meaning that samples are taken when the commodity is circulated. This can be done manually or by the use of an automated in-line statistical sampling device.

Salmonella in Different Feed Materials

Animal-derived protein

Animal-derived protein has historically been found to be contaminated by *Salmonella*. From the USA several studies describe a high rate of contamination in by-products of animal origin. For example, 43 serovars of *Salmonella* were isolated from 175 (18%) of 980 samples of such products from 22 states (Pomeroy and Grady, 1961), or 28 serovars from 37 (18.5%) out of 200 samples of poultry and other animal by-products used in poultry feeds (Watkins *et al.*, 1959). In a third study, 13% out of 5712 samples of bone meal, feather meal, fish meal and egg products were *Salmonella*-contaminated with 59 serovars (Morehouse and Wedman, 1961). Similar observations were made in Europe. The heavy contamination that could occur in these feed ingredients was demonstrated when up to 12 different serovars were isolated in a single contaminated batch, which in fact in Sweden in 1960 initiated an organized control programme for *Salmonella* in feed, in particular for high-risk products such as animal-derived protein (Rutqvist and Thal, 1958). The sources of the contamination appear to be *Salmonella*-infected animal carcasses that are subject to an ineffective rendering process. Before the BSE crisis, animals that might have died from different infections, so called fallen stock, were also generally rendered, resulting in the risk for feed-borne spread also of other infections (Rutqvist and Swahn, 1957). The treatment in the rendering process (133°C for at least 20 min at 3 bar pressure to inactivate BSE/TSE agents) should destroy all incoming *Salmonella* organisms. However, as for crushing plants and feed mills there is a significant high risk of recontamination from a *Salmonella*-contaminated environment in the absence of effective hygienic routines (EFSA, 2008) and leaking cooker seals can contaminate expellers with fluid from incompletely cooked material. The introduction of *Salmonella* through fish meal highlights a risk from proteins derived also from fish (Clark *et al.*, 1973; Crump *et al.*, 2002), although it is uncertain whether the fish themselves are the primary source of such contamination.

Vegetable proteins

Long-term experiences and data from several countries have highlighted and verified that vegetable protein, cakes and meal are frequently contaminated by *Salmonella*. In a comprehensive study based on an annual examination of up to 80,000 batches of feed, Kwiatek *et al.* (2008) reported that in Poland up to 15.0% of imported lots of soybean and rapeseed meal were found to be contaminated with *Salmonella* in 2005–2007. *Salmonella* is also frequently isolated from consignments of vegetable proteins, which are tested before being used as feed ingredients in Sweden. From 2004 to 2005, 5250 pooled samples were analysed from 795 consignments and 14.6% of the soybean meal and 10.0% of the rapeseed meal samples were contaminated (Wierup and Häggblom, 2010). When the majority of the imported soybean was from South America 20.1% of the consignments were contaminated and even higher levels, up to 30%, were regularly found in previous studies (Häggblom, 1993). The frequent isolation of *Salmonella* from vegetable proteins is in agreement with several observations from different countries (EFSA, 2008; Binter *et al.*, 2011).

Palm kernel and maize gluten are other feed sources of vegetable protein from which *Salmonella* are also frequently reported. Experiences indicate a lower prevalence and in a study by Wierup and Häggblom (2010) 9% out of 67 batches of maize meal and 1 out of 127 batches of palm kernel meal were *Salmonella*-contaminated during a 2-year period (2004–2005). The EFSA zoonoses report data also point out oilseeds, e.g. soybean products, as a risk factor for introducing *Salmonella* into the feed chain (EFSA, 2010a).

In summary, oilseed feed ingredients are often contaminated with *Salmonella* although it is difficult to compare the level of contamination between different studies due to variation in sampling and culture techniques applied. From an epidemiological point of view there is a need to raise awareness in the industry that raw oilseeds and pulses may already be frequently contaminated before entering the crushing plants. There is also a need to reflect why certain feed ingredients are frequently contaminated with *Salmonella* organisms, often with several serovars of *Salmonella*. Apart from in-house contamination in crushing plants and feed mills as well as contamination during transport and storage, studies indicate that e.g. soybeans are often heavily contaminated already when entering the crushing plant. In a Norwegian crushing plant, dust samples from imported soybeans were taken upon arrival as part of the HACCP control. During a 12-year period (1994–2005) *Salmonella* was on an annual average isolated from approximately 30% of the samples and in total 63 different serovars were identified (Wierup, 2006). Data on *Salmonella* contamination at the growing site seem to be lacking. However, it is logical to suggest that, as for vegetables, soybeans may be contaminated by *Salmonella*-contaminated water used for irrigation or through manure used as fertilizer (Greene *et al.*, 2008). This part of the *Salmonella* epidemiology requires further studies, but already indicates an infection cycle that includes links to faecal *Salmonella* contamination from both humans and animals.

Grain and forage

The other major feed ingredients, grain and forage, are not primarily considered as high-risk products for *Salmonella* contamination of feed. When these feed materials are found to be *Salmonella* contaminated it is considered as a result of contamination from wildlife and during storage as described below (Davies and Hinton, 2000). When present and if *Salmonella*-infected, wild birds and badgers have been reported to be the source of such a contamination. *Salmonella* Typhimurium from wild birds is a particular concern. When cereals are stored in open flat silos birds, rodents and cats may be additional sources for contamination of the feed material. However, *Salmonella* infection in rodents living close to animal holdings is usually a spill-over infection from the farm animals. Henzler and Opitz (1992) studied the role of mice in the epizootiology of *S.* Enteritidis in mice-infested poultry farms. *Salmonella* Enteritidis was only detected in mice on farms contaminated with that serovar but, when infected, *S.* Enteritidis persisted for at least 10 months in an infected mouse population. Rodents can thus maintain an infection on the farm, partly by contaminating the feed ingredients and the feed. Carrique-Mas *et al.* (2009) also found a longer persistence of *S.* Enteritidis infection in laying hens where rodents were present and clearance of the infection was related to elimination of rodents from the houses. Rodents may also acquire infection from contaminated feed and then amplify it, increasing the risk of infecting food-producing animals. Epidemiological experiences also suggest that birds, through faecal shedding, can infect animals via contaminated feed. The significance of this route was illustrated when virulent Newcastle Disease Virus, PPMV-1, caused 22 outbreaks in chickens in 1984. It is widely accepted that the source of the PPMV-1 was poultry feed contaminated with faeces from infected feral pigeons (Alexander *et al.*, 1984; Irvine *et al.*, 2009).

Methods of Prevention and Control

The prevention and control of *Salmonella* contamination of feed requires an integrated approach involving all links of the feed chain. Experiences have shown that there is no 'silver bullet' that can meet all the challenges involved. Instead, a combination of precautions and actions are needed and an overall strategic approach is required to avoid being lost in details. Jones (2011) has thus separated the control measures into three major strategies: prevention of contamination, reduction of multiplication and procedures to kill the pathogen. It is helpful to consider an overall flow chart of the possible sources of contamination throughout the process as presented by Sauli *et al.* (2005). Binter *et al.* (2011) described a conceptual model for the pig feed chain, which can be adapted and applied to formulate a control programme for the feed chain in question.

Feed mills and crushing plants

Although a lot of experiences on the control of *Salmonella* in feed mills have not been published in scientific literature the major risks for *Salmonella* contamination of compounded feed have been identified and also ways to minimize those risks (Häggblom, 1993; Davies and Wray, 1997; Davies and Hinton, 2000; EFSA, 2008; Davies and Wales, 2010; Binter *et al.*, 2011; Jones, 2011). The results of those studies are a good scientific basis for advice in individual situations.

The data and advice in this section, which mostly focus on feed mills, can also be used for crushing plants that work under similar hygienic conditions. This reflects that published data on hygienic routines for *Salmonella* control in crushing plants are surprisingly rare.

Major risks

Long-term experiences have demonstrated that the major primary source for *Salmonella* contamination of feed mills and the compounded feed are *Salmonella*-contaminated feed ingredients (Malmqvist *et al.*, 1995). Davies and Wray (1997) monitored nine feed mills and found that the intake pits were the most frequently contaminated sampling site and on average 24% of the samples were positive for *Salmonella*. This risk is rather similar for all feed production using vegetable proteins, which is a high-risk product for *Salmonella* contamination. In the EU this in particular concerns soybeans or soybean meal (98% imported from South America) and domestically produced rapeseed meal as well as some animal-derived proteins when used (FEFAC, 2009). In all countries there is thus a continuous risk for introducing *Salmonella* to the food chain via *Salmonella*-contaminated feed ingredients (EFSA, 2008).

To minimize the risk described above, the most logical approach would be to prevent or eliminate *Salmonella* contamination as early as possible in the feed chain. In the case of the high-risk feed materials (e.g. soybean meal, rapeseed meal, animal-derived protein) *Salmonella* should theoretically have been already eliminated at the crushing or rendering plants. As described above, the process in these industries normally includes heat treatment that should readily eliminate *Salmonella* contamination and if recontamination is avoided, would allow the production of *Salmonella*-free feed ingredients. However, available data indicate that that is generally not the case. Data on *Salmonella* contamination in crushing plants indicate the frequent occurrence of environmental contamination and cross-contamination, including recontamination of heat-treated products (Morita *et al.*, 2006; Jones, 2011). However, data from certain crushing plants also demonstrate that in spite of heavy *Salmonella* contamination of incoming soybeans (mean 30% of dust samples) it is possible to produce soybean meal that, based on testing and epidemiological experiences during several years, is found to be free from *Salmonella* (Wierup, 2006; EFSA, 2008). Similar experiences exist from a rapeseed crushing plant using the same control strategies as advised for feed mills (Herland, 2006).

The *Salmonella*-contaminated feed ingredients put an extra pressure on the feed mills to reduce the risk that incoming *Salmonella* is transmitted to the compounded feed. A strategy applied in Sweden to minimize this risk is to categorize the feed ingredients according to risk for *Salmonella* contamination. The high-risk feed categories have to be tested negative for *Salmonella* contamination before being used for feed production. They are not allowed to enter the feed mill before a negative test result is at hand. Consignments found to be *Salmonella* contaminated are decontaminated by organic acids followed by re-testing with negative result before use (Wierup and Häggblom, 2010).

As described below, heat treatment can be used to eliminate remaining *Salmonella* contamination. However, on an EU level only 30–40% of the industrial feed is estimated to be heat treated (Binter *et al.*, 2011), which emphasizes the importance of the *Salmonella* status of the feed ingredients. In the absence of heat treatment, *Salmonella* organisms from contaminated feed ingredients are easily transmitted to the compounded feed. In feed production lines without heat treatment the current methods for production of compounded feed do not include any specific processes aiming at reducing *Salmonella* contamination unless subsequent chemical antimicrobial treatment is applied. The observed decrease in the concentration of incoming *Salmonella* microbes in such production lines is primarily a result of dilution (Davies and Wales, 2010).

A second major source for *Salmonella* contamination at the feed mill is *Salmonella*-infected animal vectors, which can contaminate feed ingredients during storage, at the intake pit and as compounded feed. Davies and Wray (1997) frequently (10 out of 51 samples) isolated *Salmonella* from wild bird droppings from intake pit areas but also from warehouses and out loading gantries, and similar experiences are gained from other countries. Feed mills are thus attractive to birds as well as rodents if feed spillage and dust is not carefully and continuously removed from the environment. Such dust is thus often found to be *Salmonella* contaminated and wild birds, rodents as well as humans can serve as vectors for contamination of the feed production (Binter *et al.*, 2011). To minimize these risks the external environment of feed mills should be kept clean and, in addition to rodent control, wild birds should be prevented from nesting and perching in roof spaces and gantries to avoid risk for direct and indirect faecal contamination of the feed.

In addition to the previous risks of external contamination, the cooler area is identified as a most important risk due to its potential to multiply a *Salmonella* contamination from incoming organisms that either have survived the heat-treatment process or being introduced by the cooling air, if applied. The heat treatment associated with the pelleting process is thus also a potential hazard because steam is added to the feed. It is essential that this humidity as well as the heat is rapidly removed, which is done in the cooler by large volumes of air (Jones, 2011). If the feed is not properly cooled, the cooling area can act as an incubator, allowing for fast multiplication of existing *Salmonella* microbes. Such contamination can not only directly contaminate the compounded feed but also establish a contamination in moist and fatty aggregates that can persist and act as a source for recontamination of the feed (Israelsen *et al.*, 1996; Davies and Wray, 1997; Jones and Richardson, 2004). Experiences have shown that it is important to avoid the introduction of *Salmonella* by the cooling air. The air inlet to the cooling should be placed externally so that contamination by dust from e.g. potentially *Salmonella*-contaminated feed ingredients is minimized and that the air is passed through a filter that removes dust and particles.

In order to avoid bacterial growth, experiences have emphasized the need to avoid moisture in the whole feed production system as emphasized by Davies and Hinton (2000) and Jones (2011). Moisture can be caused by water cleaning, leakage and by condensation. In addition to the cooler area (see above), condensation of water may thus also occur in other places inside the feed transport systems as well as during storage (Binter *et al.*, 2011; Jones, 2011). Experiences from certain feed mills have also shown the existence of an in-house contamination indicated by the recurrent isolation of certain serovars of *Salmonella* during a period of many years in spite of various interventions (Wierup and Häggblom, 2010). This indicates that certain strains survive at unidentified spots or may be adapted to survive, e.g. by the help of biofilm formation (Vestby *et al.*, 2009).

There is also a need to develop methods for inspection and dry cleaning of the interior of the production line. Davies and Hinton (2000) have highlighted the problems associated with inspecting certain coolers and the removal of internal coatings. The mills, in particular those of older age, are not constructed to meet hygienic requirements for cleaning and disinfection and access to critical sites to allow inspection and cleaning of the inside of production lines (Davies and Hinton, 2000). When found necessary, new openings for inspections are required as well as in critical situations modifications of the basic building construction or equipment to overcome recurrent problems (Gabis, 1991). Decontamination of persistent contamination is demanding and requires special competence as described by Davies and Hinton (2000), and in difficult situations dismantling of the whole process line has been found necessary (Stig Widell, Swedish Board of Agriculture, pers. comm.).

Heat treatment

Various studies have verified the *Salmonella*-reducing effect of heat treatment (Himathongkham *et al.*, 1996). Jones and Richardson (2004) reported that heating between 80°C and 85°C for 1 min in most cases should eliminate *Salmonella*. However, the level of elimination is dependent on the level of initial contamination (Himathongkham *et al.*, 1996). Certain strains of *Salmonella* may also be more resistant to high temperatures, which might explain the occurrence of *Salmonella* in feed following heat treatment (Kirby and Davies, 1990; Habimana *et al.*, 2010). However, Davies and Wales (2010) reported that *Salmonella* contamination following heat treatment is most likely caused by internal contamination of the cooler.

The initial period after shut down of the production before the intended temperature is reached is identified as a risk. Destruction or manual recirculation of the first feed produced before the set temperature is reached or during temperature dips is applied to avoid that contaminating *Salmonella* may survive due to too low a temperature. Processes with automatic recirculation have been applied but were found to be a risk for residual *Salmonella* contaminations.

It is important to note that the purpose of pelleting and the associated heat treatment is primarily to improve the handling qualities and feed intake and not the hygienic feed quality, although its hygienic potential was recognized early (Swahn and Rutqvist, 1957). Temperature and time limits for the process are therefore guided to meet also nutritional requirements, and exposure of the feed to too high a temperature may have negative effects on certain feed ingredients such as amino acids and vitamins. As a complement to experimental data, empirical field data may give a more realistic result of the efficiency of heat treatment for eliminating *Salmonella*. Treatment at approximately 80–82°C for 30 s is generally applied by the feed industry in Sweden and found to result in *Salmonella*-free poultry feed as described above. In summary, it is not possible to specify a minimum temperature and time range that under all conditions would be sufficient to eliminate contaminations of *Salmonella* in industrial feed production (van Asselt and Zwietering, 2006). Instead, as applied in the food industry, monitoring of *Salmonella* and *Enterobacteriaceae* contamination is used to ensure the efficiency of the process.

Dry storage

In the same way as it is important to prevent and reduce contamination of *Salmonella* at all stages of the feed production, it is equally important to prevent multiplication of possibly contaminating *Salmonella* microbes that can survive for a considerable time in various materials (Jones, 2011). Keeping all feed ingredients and the compounded feed under dry conditions is, therefore, an essential requirement (Jones, 2011). In order to avoid microbial multiplication grains should be dried to approximately 13–14% and oilseeds to 7–9% moisture content corresponding to a water activity of around 0.4 to 0.7 (Eisenberg, 2007).

Chemical treatment

Chemical treatment, mostly by organic acids, has been used to control *Salmonella* in feed production (EFSA, 2008) as reviewed by Wales *et al.* (2010). Such treatment seems either to be used as a way to reduce or eliminate *Salmonella* contamination from a batch of feed ingredients or as a general treatment of the feed administered to animals. The former use is applied e.g. on feed ingredients found to be *Salmonella* contaminated before its use in feed production as described elsewhere in this chapter (Wierup and Häggblom, 2010). The latter use may have various purposes and in terms of *Salmonella* control it merely seems to be used in herds as a way to prevent intestinal colonization of *Salmonella* not only from feed but also from the environment. There is thus some evidence that some of the products may promote an unfavourable intestinal environment for colonization of animals by *Salmonella* originating from other sources, such as the environment. The use of such products can thus limit the within-flock prevalence of infection and the number of organisms excreted in faeces (EFSA, 2008). In addition, such feeding of pigs is found to improve feed conversion and growth rate (Partanen and Mroz, 1999).

Formaldehyde, which is found to be efficient for microbial decontamination of equipment and animal houses, is also effective with higher activity than acids for decontamination of feed (Smyser and Snoeyenbos, 1979; Moustafa *et al.*, 2002). Formaldehyde has been used in combination with organic acids in order to achieve a synergistic effect allowing lower levels of formaldehyde and acids that e.g. minimizes operator and possible food safety hazards. Carrique-Mas *et al.* (2007) found that such treatment can mask a subsequent isolation of *Salmonella*. Although many studies report that formaldehyde does not appear to cause adverse effects or tissue residues in animals given feed, the use of formaldehyde in the EU so far in the feed industry largely appears to be limited to equipment and feeding systems. According to the feed additive legislation, formaldehyde is only authorized at Community level as preservative for skimmed milk for pigs up to the age of 6 months and for all species or categories of animals as silage additive (EFSA, 2008).

Dust removal and cross-contamination

Dust and spillages are often found to be contaminated by *Salmonella* and therefore suitable for sampling (Davies and Wales, 2010). Programmes for avoiding and removing dust and spillage inside feed mill operations has been found to be another essential requirement for avoiding the build-up of a *Salmonella* contamination that easily can be spread by cross-contamination.

Jones (2011) has highlighted that the odds of contamination increase each time feed is handled and it is reported that some ingredients may be handled up to 15 times before transport to the user (Ratcliff, 2006). The logistics and management should thus be designed to avoid cross-contamination and separate storage of ingredients and the compounded feed and thus separating the so called clean and unclean parts of the mill. It should be ensured that equipment and tools for service and repair are kept separate clean and away from potentially contaminated areas. In some feed mills external service people are not allowed to bring in their own equipment, in order to avoid external contamination in critical places; accordingly, installation of second-hand processing equipment from other mills is a major risk.

HACCP including monitoring

The control of *Salmonella* in feed operation faces a continuously moving target. The risk for contamination varies over time but can never be excluded. An appropriate implementation of the control methods described above requires careful planning as well as the design of a monitoring system of *Salmonella* contamination. The monitoring for *Salmonella* should be based on the bacteriological examination of samples from dust and spillage (Davies and Wales, 2010; Binter *et al.*, 2011; Jones, 2011). As suggested by EFSA (2008), this process should follow the same principles as in food safety programmes and be based on hazard analysis and critical control point principles (HACCP). This should also include strategies for interventions when *Salmonella* contamination occurs. Due to the risk for contamination of the compounded feed and the build-up of in-house contamination it is important to endeavour to control *Salmonella* contamination whenever detected (Jones, 2011). The challenges to avoid *Salmonella* contamination in feed mills also apply for crushing plants; the outline of a HACCP programme for a crushing plant was described by Herland (2006). The HACCP programme has to be adapted to each feed operation.

For reasons described above, sampling only of the compounded feed is inappropriate. This was highlighted in Sweden in 1993 when sampling of the compounded feed was unable to detect a contamination by *S.* Livingstone in a feed mill in spite of the fact that this serovar was spread during a 7-month period by the feed from the mill and repeatedly infected flocks of broiler chickens at 15 producers (Wierup *et al.*, 1988). Based on this experience and following a poultry producer demand, the feed control was changed from sampling the end product to sampling at critical control points. The aim was to detect contamination of *Salmonella* as early as possible in the production process starting at the intake. The following control points were identified: top of bin for final feed (compound feed), room for pellet coolers, top of pellet cooler, dust from the production line and from the aspiration system (filter) and from intake pit/bottom part of elevator for feed materials (Malmqvist *et al.*, 1995). This event also demonstrates that trace-back investigations from *Salmonella*-infected herds can be used as part of monitoring to detect the spread of *Salmonella* by feed, as shown also by Österberg *et al.* (2006).

Usually most attention is paid to poultry feed because poultry are considered to be more sensitive to *Salmonella* exposure than e.g. ruminants. Accordingly, heat treatment of feed is in some countries a legal demand only for poultry feed. However, feed for poultry and for other food animal species is often produced in the same mill. Although separate production lines including the transport to farms should be applied, experiences have shown that cross-contamination easily occurs. In addition to experiences from cross-contamination with *Salmonella*, the risks for cross-contamination were typically visualized during the initial phase of the BSE crisis when feed intended for poultry and swine could end up in cattle feed. Other examples of cross-contamination occur when medicals are mixed into feed of one species and later on detected in another animal species. A way to avoid such problems is to apply the same standard for the control of *Salmonella* in feed for all animal species, which is in line with EFSA (2008) stating that an overall requirement should be the final feed to all food animals is free of *Salmonella*. When this is not the case, experience has shown that cross-contamination, e.g. between transports from feed mills to farms, may occur if cleaning and disinfection procedures are insufficient. Davies and Hinton (2000) emphasized the importance of letting transport wagons as well as other equipment dry after cleaning and disinfection.

Farm production

Contamination and multiplication during production and storage

There appears to be very little literature concerning the risk for introduction of *Salmonella* to livestock as a result of home-mixing of feed, although many studies were carried out in herds already infected with *Salmonella* organisms. The evaluation of the true importance of *Salmonella*-contaminated feed in such herds and in particular when they are contaminated by several serovars of *Salmonella* as described by Marin *et al.* (2011), requires comprehensive epidemiological studies. These need to be based on adequate monitoring for *Salmonella* and if possible the use of molecular typing methods to identify routes of *Salmonella* infection (Löfström *et al.*, 2006).

However, the same basic conditions and recommendations for minimizing the risks for contamination and multiplication of *Salmonella* during handling, storage and transport for feed mills also apply for farm feed production. In farms where the animals are already infected with *Salmonella* the environment and the animal stock are additional potential sources of *Salmonella* contamination. Outdoor feeding runs an additional risk. The feeding places are very attractive to wild birds as well as rodents. When such animals are infected, they can easily contaminate the feed with *Salmonella* and also maintain an infection as described above. The significance of this route of infection was shown in experimental studies in concentrated cattle-feeding operations in Texas, USA. Following an effective control of European starlings, the detection rate of *S. enterica* from feed bunks declined from 8% to 0% (Carlson *et al.*, 2011).

Due to the difficulties in detecting a *Salmonella* contamination, there are so far in practice no available simple methods for farmers to ensure that bought-in feed ingredients or compounded feed are free from *Salmonella.* Such a guarantee can only be obtained when the feed products are produced in mills or crushing plants operating with effective *Salmonella* control programmes. A quality control to ensure freedom of *Salmonella* contamination of feed ingredients and compounded feed on the market would enable farmers to use safe sourcing procedures to minimize the risk of introducing *Salmonella* through the feed.

Because heat treatment in practice cannot be implemented at farm level, there is no other specific measure with the potential to break the chain of *Salmonella* infections through the feed. As described above, instead different chemical treatments of the feed, in particular the use of organic acids, has been tried (Wingstrand *et al.*, 1997). When available, the inclusion of whey to the diet is shown to have a *Salmonella*-decreasing effect in pigs, perhaps due to the lowered pH (Lo Fo Wong *et al.*, 2004). Similar effects are also found in wet feed that is allowed to ferment at ambient temperature or where fermentation is controlled using a starter culture and controlled temperature conditions (EFSA, 2008). These treatments of feed can logically have a reducing effect on *Salmonella* even in already contaminated feed. However, the possible *Salmonella*-reducing effect is usually measured only through the prevalence of *Salmonella* infections of animals being fed. Such results are usually reported from countries with a medium or high prevalence of *Salmonella*. Possible sources of the *Salmonella* infection in animals under such conditions are thus not only the feed but most likely to a much larger extent the result of direct and indirect transmission from neighbouring animals. In addition to nutritional purposes, such treatments of the feed are thus used as a way to control *Salmonella* not primarily in the feed but at the farm level and are therefore out of the scope of this review. However, the use of pelleted feed merits a special focus.

Pelleted versus non-pelleted feed

Several studies, mostly from countries with a medium or high prevalence *Salmonella* status, have found that pigs fed pelleted feed often have a higher risk for becoming *Salmonella* infected than pigs fed non-pelleted diets (Lo Fo Wong *et al.*, 2004). The complex reasons behind these findings have been intensively studied and seem to be largely associated with the particle size of the feed, nutritional and fibre components of the diet and perhaps mostly due to a rapid passage of the pelleted feed through the stomach and upper small intestine (Hedemann *et al.*, 2005; Anguita *et al.*, 2006). Ingested *Salmonella* bacteria can thereby escape the *Salmonella*-reducing effect of the gastric acid. However, this also results in a dysbacteriosis in which protective lactobacilli and anaerobes are reduced and *Enterobacteriaceae,* including *Escherichia coli* and *Salmonella,* increase. Studies by Hedemann *et al.* (2005) also suggest that pigs fed pelleted diet secrete mucins that are capable of binding *Salmonella* and thereby facilitate colonization. These observations are in contrast to pigs fed coarsely ground meal feed, when the stomach acts as a barrier that decreases the occurrence of pathogenic bacteria (Mikkelsen *et al.*, 2004).

In fact, a concept for use of pelleted feed as a way to improve feed conversion is by decreasing the negative energy balance for the host of feed digestion in the upper digestive tract, in favour of the positive energy balance gained of the microbial fermentation in the lower digestive tract (Just *et al.*, 1983; Anguita *et al.*, 2006). The adverse effect, however, seems to be that the gastric barrier against incoming pathogens like *Salmonella* is compromised. This is a dilemma that can interfere with efforts to reduce the prevalence of *Salmonella*, particularly in herds where this prevalence is high. In such herds the major risk for exposure of the animals with

Salmonella is from other infected animals and their environment (EFSA, 2010b). To reduce the *Salmonella* problem in such herds, coarse-ground meal, barley or maize cob meal can be added to the diet (Jørgensen *et al.*, 1999). In a systemic review of the literature O'Connor *et al.* (2008) found a strong evidence of association that such an intervention reduces the *Salmonella* prevalence. The concept behind the *Salmonella*-reducing effect of such feeding seems to be partially associated with a slow-down of the passage in the stomach allowing for longer exposure to the gastric acid. Stomach contents from pigs fed a coarse-ground non-pelleted diet have been shown to increase the *in vitro* death rate of *S.* Typhimurium DT12 (Mikkelsen *et al.*, 2004). This may provide incentive to use non-pelleted feed with increased risk for introducing *Salmonella* through the feed if no additional measures are taken, although the use of non-pelleted feed reduces productivity and increases cost (Goldbach and Alban, 2006). A way to avoid that risk might be to crush the pelleted feed after the pelleting process if the particles of the feed then have a size of non-coarse-ground meal feed.

Significance of *Salmonella* in Feed

Epidemiological aspects

In older literature *Salmonella* was sometimes referred to as a ubiquitous bacterium, which, like *Escherichia coli*, normally exists in the intestinal flora of animals and in the environment. This is a gross simplification and is normally not the case, in particular not for the major food animal species, and the occurrence of *Salmonella* in their environment is usually a spill-over effect from *Salmonella*-infected animals (Quinn *et al.*, 2003). Its epidemiology is characterized by a great potential to survive in certain animal species and in the environment. Although *Salmonella* under certain conditions also may multiply in environmental niches such as in the feed, their reservoir and main localization for multiplication is infected animals (including wildlife) and humans following oral ingestion. *Salmonella* is then excreted in faeces during varying periods, often in large numbers in particular during the acute stage of the infection, e.g. 10^{6-7} cfu g^{-1} faeces (Gutzmann *et al.*, 1976).

As highlighted above one of the major risk products for *Salmonella* contamination of the feed, soybeans are often heavily contaminated with a variety of serovars already on entering the crushing plant, which indicates links to faecal contamination from both humans and animals. Irrespective of the primary source of this contamination, it is obvious that in the absence of effective *Salmonella* control of the feed probably for several decades, generations of food animals were continuously exposed to *Salmonella* through their feed. This is likely to be the primary source of most of the *Salmonella* infection that is now resident in food-animal breeding and production and in their environment in most countries.

Interestingly, the annual incidence of salmonellosis in humans in the industrialized world steadily increased from around the 1950s until it reached alarming proportions during the *S.* Enteritidis pandemic in the late 1980s and early 1990s, and annually for Germany alone it was estimated to have 2 million human food-borne infections (WHO, 1989). At that time WHO concluded that the industrialization of food-animal production had opened the door to the food chain for *Salmonella*. The meat inspection procedures that were designed to ensure food safety by detecting lesions due to tuberculosis and zoonotic parasites, such as *Trichinella*, could not detect and eliminate carcasses contaminated with *Salmonella*. There are still no effective means of ensuring *Salmonella*-safe food-animal products for humans at the slaughter stage, or in the marketing of shell eggs, without effective control in primary production, apart from heat treatment, decontamination and irradiation.

Following assessment of risk mitigation options of *Salmonella* in swine and pork production (EFSA, 2006) and in feed (EFSA, 2008), a quantitative risk assessment concluded that in both breeder and slaughter pigs, infected incoming pigs and *Salmonella*-contaminated feed are the major sources of

Salmonella (EFSA, 2010b). A similar situation is the case for poultry. The importance of feed is further emphasized in that *Salmonella*-free feed is required to maintain the breeding animals free from *Salmonella*.

Data that document the importance of *Salmonella* in feed as well as of interventions are most easy attained and performed in countries with a low level of *Salmonella* contamination. In other cases as described above, in-depth epidemiological studies are usually required. In such studies it is also essential to consider the time factor for accessing consequences of introduction of *Salmonella* as well as of interventions (EFSA, 2008). *Salmonella* Agona, introduced to USA and elsewhere by fishmeal in the late 1960s, is today not considered as being feed borne (Clark *et al.*, 1973; Crump *et al.*, 2002) even though this serovar is still regularly found in vegetable proteins and finished feed in many countries. The lack of targeted studies is probably a major reason why feed as a source of introduction of new serovars of *Salmonella* in animal herds is underestimated. The time factor also has to be considered when assessing interventions against *Salmonella* contamination in feed. In regions or farms with a high prevalence of *Salmonella* in animals, isolated interventions against *Salmonella* contamination on feed cannot directly be expected to result in a lower prevalence in animals or on carcasses after slaughter because other sources for the infection are much more important and need to be addressed simultaneously (Alban and Stärk, 2005; EFSA, 2010b; Carlson *et al.*, 2011).

Salmonella serovars involved

Salmonella organisms isolated from feed or feed ingredients include a wide range of serovars and to some extent also those serovars frequently causing disease in humans. In Sweden 38 serovars of *Salmonella* were isolated from feed-associated sources during a 2-year period. Four (10.5%) of the serovars isolated were among the ten most common isolates of human cases of salmonellosis in the EU, and 30 (78.9%) had also been isolated from human cases of salmonellosis diagnosed in Sweden during a 10-year period (Wierup and Häggblom, 2010). *Salmonella* serovars that frequently cause infections in both animals and humans, e.g. *S.* Enteritidis and *S.* Typhimurium, are regularly isolated also from feed (EFSA, 2008).

Only a limited number of the serovars normally cause disease in animals and the majority appears to be transient colonizers of the intestine. However, some of them can become adapted to certain animal species that facilitate their survival and spread. This was observed in Europe in the early 1980s, when a sharp increase in the prevalence of *S.* Derby in swine occurred in several countries (Wierup, 1994), probably because that serovar had become adapted to swine as suggested by Wray (1985). Another important example is *S.* Enteritidis phage type 4, which during the 1980s appears to have adapted to poultry and infection of their eggs, leading to a rapid spread throughout world poultry production and a pandemic spread in humans. *Salmonella* Enteritidis has since become the major *Salmonella* serovar causing food-borne illness in humans (Sobel *et al.*, 2000; EFSA, 2010a). Such events cannot be foreseen and because all serovars are considered to be potentially pathogenic for humans (EFSA, 2008) there is little scientific support for a *Salmonella* control policy in feed that is limited to only certain serovars.

The importance of control of *Salmonella* in the feed as well as of the breeding animals is also indicated by the fact that such control programmes prevented the spread of *S.* Enteritidis in the late 1980s in Swedish poultry production (Wierup *et al.*, 1995). However, the relatively low occurrence in animal feed of those serovars most frequently causing food-borne illness in humans has often been used as an argument against the potential importance of feed as a source of such infections. That argument is fallacious and seems to neglect that even an uncommon *Salmonella* following an oral ingestion in an animal causes an active infection, often with a rapid multiplication of the microbe in contrast to being a passive contamination in the environment, feed, and in the subsequent food chain (Jones, 2011). In fact the same message was already given in 1969 by a USDA Committee on *Salmonella*, which concluded that this discrepancy in the assessment probably has contributed more than anything else to the fact that effective action has not been taken to control contamination of feed (USDA, 1969).

Conclusions and Future Perspective

The initial strategy to prevent human food-borne salmonellosis at the consumer level by good hygiene and safe cooking was insufficient (Mosel and Kampelmacher, 1981). Instead, the annual increase in the incidence of human food-borne salmonellosis that was generally observed since around the 1950s and 1960s continued until the *S.* Enteritidis pandemic at the end of 1980s initiated more active control of *Salmonella* in poultry in the EU and elsewhere (WHO, 1989; Sobel *et al.*, 2000; EFSA, 2010a). In the EU, the control programmes that focus on actions at the pre-harvest level are considered as reason for the significant shift to a decreasing trend of human salmonellosis (EFSA, 2010a). However, due to less effective interventions in the USA, in 2011 food-borne salmonellosis is still one of the few food-borne pathogens for which illnesses have not significantly declined over the past 10 years (Batz *et al.*, 2011).

In the EU the control of *Salmonella* will not be restricted to poultry but will be extended to other food animals, starting with pigs. In addition the traditional meat inspection procedures are under review in the EU, guided by the need to improve food safety against today's major food-borne zoonotic agents.

Substantial efforts will be required to reduce the *Salmonella* prevalence in herds of pigs and cattle. It would therefore be logical and probably most cost-effective to start this process by efforts to prevent animals from becoming infected through their feed, as well as through the breeding pyramid, and so apply the top-down approach that has been a successful concept for the control of *Salmonella* in poultry (Sternberg Lewerin *et al.*, 2005). Because important feed ingredients are often contaminated, stringent efforts to control *Salmonella* have to be implemented at the crushing plants and feed mills. A HACCP-based quality control system to ensure freedom of *Salmonella* contamination of feed ingredients and compound feed on the market would enable farmers to minimize the risk of introducing *Salmonella* through the feed. That approach would also be necessary to avoid *Salmonella*-contaminated feed jeopardizing their efforts to eliminate *Salmonella* at the farms.

As described in this review, long-term experience has shown that it is possible to produce feed that is free from *Salmonella*. In many countries monitoring of *Salmonella* in feed and animals has also provided substantial experience on the epidemiology relating to the occurrence of *Salmonella* in feed. The missing point seems to be the lack of stringent regulatory or economic incentives needed to combine improved monitoring with appropriate interventions. A proactive policy would help to avoid urgent actions that might be imposed if new highly virulent serovars like *S.* Enteritidis should occur as an emerging threat to animal and public health in the future.

Acknowledgements

The kind support with reviewing and suggestions on the manuscript by Per Häggblom, Helene Wahlström, Ivar Vågsholm and in particular to Rob Davies is gratefully acknowledged.

References

Alban, L. and Stärk, K.D. (2005) Where should the effort be put to reduce the *Salmonella* prevalence in the slaughtered swine carcass effectively? *Preventive Veterinary Medicine* 68, 63–79.

Alexander, D.J., Parsons, G. and Marshall, R. (1984) Infections of fowls with Newcastle disease virus by food contamination with pigeon faeces. *Veterinary Record* 115, 601–602.

Andersson, G., Straver, J., Löfström, C., Lindqvist, P.-A. and Häggblom, P. (2010) Sampling for traceability and conformance testing of *Salmonella* in animal feedingstuffs. In: Colin, P. and Clement, G. (eds) *Proceedings of International Symposium of* Salmonella *and Salmonellosis*, 28–30 June 2010, Saint-Malo, France. ZOOPOLE développement-ISPAIA, Ploufragen, France, pp. 69–72.

Anguita, M., Canibe, N., Pérez, J.F. and Jensen, B.B. (2006) Influence of the amount of dietary fiber on the available energy from hindgut fermentation in growing pigs: use of cannulated pigs and *in vitro* fermentation1. *Journal of Animal Science* 84, 2766–2778.

Anonymous (2007) Economic approach to broiler production. Atlantic Poultry Research Institute. Available at: http://www.thepoultrysite.com/articles/894/economic-approach-to-broiler-production (accessed 13 March 2013).

Batz, M.B., Hoffmann, S. and Morris Jr, J.G. (2011) *Ranking the Risks; the 10 pathogen–food combinations with the greatest burden on public health*. Emerging Pathogen Institute, University of Florida, pp. 1–68.

Bernard, A., Broeckaert, F., De Poorter, G., De Cock, A., Hermans, C., Saegerman, C. and Houins, G. (2002) The Belgian PCB/dioxin incident: analysis of the food chain contamination and health risk evaluation. *Environmental Research* 88, 1–18.

Binter, C., Straver, J.M., Häggblom, P., Bruggeman, G., Lindqvist, P.A., Zentek, J. and Andersson, M.G. (2011) Transmission and control of *Salmonella* in the pig feed chain: a conceptual model. *International Journal of Food Microbiology* 145, 7–17.

Carlson, J.C., Engeman, R.M., Hyatt, D.R., Gilliland, R.L., Deliberto, T.J., Clark, L., Bodenchuk, M.J. and Linz, G.M. (2011) Efficacy of European starling control to reduce *Salmonella enterica* contamination in a concentrated animal feeding operation in the Texas panhandle. *BMC Veterinary Research* 7, 9.

Carrique-Mas, J.J., Bedford, S. and Davies, R.H. (2007) Organic acid and formaldehyde treatment of animal feeds to control *Salmonella*: efficacy and masking during culture. *Journal of Applied Microbiology* 103, 88–96.

Carrique-Mas, J.J., Breslin, M., Snow, L., McLaren, I., Sayers, A.R. and Davies, R.H. (2009) Persistence and clearance of different *Salmonella* serovars in buildings housing laying hens. *Epidemiology and Infection* 137, 837–846.

Clark, G.M., Kaufmann, A.F., Gangarosa, E.J. and Thompson, M.A. (1973) Epidemiology of an international outbreak of *Salmonella* Agona. *Lancet* 2(7827), 490–493.

Crump, J.A., Griffin, P.A. and Angulo, F.J. (2002) Bacterial contamination of animal feed and its relationship to human food borne illness. *Clinical Infectious Diseases* 35, 859–865.

Crump J.A., Luby, S.P. and Mintz, E.D. (2004) The global burden of typhoid fever. *Bulletin of the World Health Organization* 82, 346–353.

Dahms, S. (2004) Microbiological sampling plans – statistical aspects. Mitteilungen aus Lebensmitteluntersuchung und Hygiene 95, 32–44.

Davies, R.H. and Hinton, M. (2000) *Salmonella* in animal feed. In: Wray, C. (ed.) Salmonella *in Domestic Animals*. CAB International, Wallingford, UK, pp. 285–300.

Davies, R.H. and Wales, A.D. (2010) Investigations into *Salmonella* contamination in poultry feedmills in the United Kingdom. *Journal of Applied Microbiology* 109, 1430–1440.

Davies, R.H. and Wray, C. (1997) Distribution of *Salmonella* contamination in ten animal feedmills. *Veterinary Microbiology* 57, 159–169.

EFSA (2006) Opinion of the Scientific Panel on Biological Hazards on the request from the Commission related to 'Risk assessment and mitigation options of *Salmonella* in pig production'. *EFSA Journal* 341, 1–131.

EFSA (2008) Microbiological risk assessment in feedingstuffs for food-producing animals. *EFSA Journal* 720, 1–84.

EFSA (2010a) The community summary report on trends and sources of zoonoses, zoonotic agents, antimicrobial resistance and food-borne outbreaks in the European Union in 2008. *EFSA Journal* 8(1), 1496.

EFSA (2010b) Scientific Opinion on a Quantitative Microbiological Risk Assessment of *Salmonella* in slaughter and breeder pigs. *EFSA Journal* 8(4), 1547.

Eisenberg, S. (2007) Relative stability of selenites and selenates in feed premixes as a function of water activity. *Journal of AOAC International* 90, 349–353.

Ekbohm, G. (1993) On the determination of the number of samples required for control of *Salmonella* [In Swedish]. The Swedish Board of Agriculture.

FAO (2009) World summit on food security; Rome 16–18 November 2009. Available at: http://www.fao.org/wsfs/world-summit/en (accessed 13 March 2013).

Fedorka-Cray, P.J., Kelley, L.C., Stabel, T.J., Gray, J.T. and Laufer, J.A. (1995) Alternate routes of invasion may affect pathogenesis of *Salmonella* typhimurium in swine. *Infection and Immunity* 63, 2658–2664.

FEFAC (2009) Feed and food Statistical Yearbook 2009. Available at: http://www.fefac.eu/file.pdf?FileID=42596 (accessed 13 March 2013).

Foster, E.M. (1971) The control of *Salmonellae* in processed foods: a classification system and sampling plan. *Journal of the Association of Official Analytical Chemists* 54, 259–266.

Gabis, D.A. (1991) Environmental factors affecting enteropathogens in feed and feed mills. In: Blankenship, L.C. (ed.) *Colonisation Control of Human Bacterial Enteropathogens in Poultry*. Academic Press, London, pp. 22–27.

Goldbach, S.G. and Alban, L. (2006) A cost-benefit analysis of *Salmonella*-control strategies in Danish pork production. *Preventive Veterinary Medicine* 77, 1–14.

Greene, S.K., Daly, E.R., Talbot, E.A., Demma, L.J., Holzbauer, S., Patel, N.J., Hill, T.A., Walderhaug, M.O., Hoekstra, R.M., Lynch, M.F. and Painter, J.A. (2008) Recurrent multistate outbreak of *Salmonella* Newport associated with tomatoes from contaminated fields, 2005. *Epidemiology and Infection* 136, 157–165.

Gutzmann, F., Layton, H., Simkins, K. and Jarolmen, H. (1976) Influence of antibiotic- supplemented feed on occurrence and persistence of *Salmonella typhimurium* in experimentally infected swine. *American Journal of Veterinary Researches* 37, 649–655.

Habimana, O., Møretrø, T., Langsrud, S., Vestby, L.K., Nesse, L.L. and Heir, E. (2010) Micro ecosystems from feed industry surfaces: a survival and biofilm study of *Salmonella* versus host resident flora strains. *BMC Veterinary Research* 6, 48.

Häggblom, P. (1993) Monitoring and control of *Salmonella* in animal feed. In: *NVI/WHO International Course on Salmonella Control in Animal Production and Products*, 21–27 August 1993, Malmö, Sweden. National Veterinary Institute, Uppsala, Sweden, pp. 127–137.

Hedemann, M.S., Mikkelsen, L.L., Naughton, P.J. and Jensen, B.B. (2005) Effect of feed particle size and feed processing on morphological characteristics in the small and large intestine of pigs and on adhesion of *Salmonella enterica* serovar Typhimurium DT12 in the ileum *in vitro*. *Journal of Animal Science* 83, 1554–1562.

Henzler, D.J. and Opitz, H.M. (1992) The role of mice in the epizootiology of *Salmonella* enteritidis on chicken layer farms. *Avian Diseases* 36, 625–631.

Herland, P.J. (2006) *Salmonella* control of feed in the Swedish crushing industry. In: Wahlström, H. (coordinator) *Salmonella* Workshop: Control in Poultry from Feed to Farm, 13–17 March 2006, Uppsala, Sweden, pp. 26–27. Available at: http://s3.amazonaws.com/zanran_storage/www.agronavigator.cz/ContentPages/1852397210.pd (Accessed 13 March 2013).

Himathongkham, S., Pereira, M.G. and Riemann, H. (1996) Heat destruction of *Salmonella* in poultry feed: effect of time, temperature, and moisture. *Avian Diseases* 40, 72–77.

Holmberg, T., Häggblom, P., Jonsson, N. and Larsson, K. (1993) Swedish Board of Agriculture. In: *Technique and Hygiene During Feed Production*. Swedish Board of Agriculture, pp. 10–25.

Irvine, R.M., Aldous, E.W., Manvell, R.J., Cox, W.J., Ceeraz, V., Fuller, C.M., Wood, A.M., Milne, J.C., Wilson, M., Hepple, R.G., Hurst, A., Sharpe, C.E., Alexander, D.J. and Brown, I.H. (2009) Outbreak of Newcastle disease due to pigeon paramyxovirus type 1 in grey partridges (*Perdix perdix*) in Scotland in October 2006. *Veterinary Record* 165, 531–535.

Israelsen, M., Hansen, I.D. and Jacobsen, E. (1996) Don't grow *Salmonella* in the pellet cooler. *Feed International* 17, 34–38.

Jones, F.T. (2011) A review of practical *Salmonella* control measures in animal feed. *Journal of Applied Poultry Research* 20, 102–113.

Jones, F.T. and Richardson, K.E. (2004) *Salmonella* in commercially manufactured feeds. *Poultry Science* 83, 384–391.

Jørgensen, L., Dahl, J., Jensen, B.B. and Poulsen, H.D. (1999) Effects of expanding, pelleting, and grinding on *Salmonella* typhimurium infection, growth performance and gastrointestinal ecosystem in slaughter pigs. *Publication No. 426*. The Natl. Comm. for Pig Prod., Copenhagen, Denmark. [In Danish]

Just, A., Fernandez, J.A. and Jorgensen, H. (1983) The net energy value of diets for growth in pigs in relation to the fermentative processes in the digestive tract and the site of absorption of the nutrients. *Livestock Production Science* 10, 171–186.

Kirby, R.M. and Davies, R. (1990) Survival of dehydrated cells of *Salmonella* typhimurium LT2 at high temperatures. *Journal of Applied Bacteriology* 68, 241–246.

Koyuncu, S. and Häggblom, P.A. (2009) Comparative study of cultural methods for the detection of *Salmonella* in feed and feed ingredients. *BMC Veterinary Research* 5, 6.

Kwiatek, K., Kukier, E., Wasyl, D. and Hoszowski, A. (2008) Microbial quality of feed in Poland. *Medycyna Weterynaryjna* 64, 183–188. [In Polish with an English summary.]

Lazaruk, G. (2009) Cost of Production Forecast – US versus Canada Comparison. 38th Banff Pork Seminar 2009, Banff, Canada, January. Available at: http://www.thepigsite.com/articles/19/conferences-events/2614/banff-pork-seminar-2009 (accessed 13 March 2013).

Lo Fo Wong, D.M., Dahl, J., Stege, H., van der Wolf, P.J., Leontides, L., von Altrock, A. and Thorberg, B.M. (2004) Herd-level risk factors for subclinical *Salmonella* infection in European finishing-pig herds. *Preventive Veterinary Medicine* 62, 253–266.

Löfström, C., Eriksson, J., Aspán, A., Häggblom, P., Gunnarsson, A., Borch, E. and Rådström, P. (2006) Improvement and validation of RAPD in combination with PFGE analysis of *Salmonella enterica* ssp. *enterica* serovar Senftenberg strains isolated from feed mills. *Veterinary Microbiology* 114, 345–351Maciorowski, K.G., Pillai, S.D., Jones, F.T. and Ricke, S.C. (2005) Polymerase chain reaction detection of foodborne *Salmonella* spp. in animal feeds. *Critical Reviews in Microbiology* 31, 45–53.

Maciorowski, K.G., Herrera, P., Jones, F.T., Pillai, S.D. and Ricke, S.C. (2006) Cultural and Immunological Detection Methods for *Salmonella* spp. in Animal Feeds – A Review. *Veterinary Research Communications* 30, 127–137.

Majowicz, S.E., Musto, J. and Scallan, E. (2010) The global burden of nontyphoidal *Salmonella* 16 gastroenteritis. *Clinical Infectious Diseases* 50, 882–889.

Malmqvist, M., Jacobsson, K.G., Häggblom, P., Cerenius, F., Sjöland, L. and Gunnarsson, A. (1995) *Salmonella* isolated from animals and feedstuffs in Sweden during 1988-1992. *Acta Veterinaria Scandinavica* 36, 21–39.

Marin, C., Balasch, S., Vega, S. and Lainez, M. (2011) Sources of *Salmonella* contamination during broiler production in Eastern Spain. *Preventive Veterinary Medicine* 98, 39–45.

Mikkelsen, L.L., Naughton, P.J., Hedemann, M.S. and Jensen, B.B. (2004) Effects of physical properties of feed on microbial ecology and survival of *Salmonella enterica* serovar Typhimurium in the pig gastrointestinal tract. *Applied and Environmental Microbiology* 70, 3485–3492.

Morehouse, L.G. and Wedman, E.E. (1961) *Salmonella* and other disease producing organisms in animal by products – a survey. *Journal of the American Veterinary Medical Association* 139, 989.

Morita, T., Kitazawa, H., Iida, T. and Kamata, S. (2006) Prevention of *Salmonella* cross-contamination in an oilmeal manufacturing plant. *Journal of Applied Microbiology* 101, 464–473.

Mosel, D.A.A. and Kampelmacher, E.H. (1981) Prevention of salmonellosis. *The Lancet* 2, 208.

Moustafa, G.Z., Zaki, M.M. and Badawy, E.M. (2002) Hygienic control of *Salmonella* in artificially contaminated feed. *Veterinary Medical Journal Giza* 50, 239–246

O'Connor, A.M., Denagamage, T., Sargeant, J.M., Rajić, A. and McKean, J. (2008) Feeding management practices and feed characteristics associated with *Salmonella* prevalence in live and slaughtered market-weight finisher swine: a systematic review and summation of evidence from 1950 to 2005. *Preventive Veterinary Medicine* 87, 213–228.

Österberg, J., Vågsholm, I., Boqvist, S. and Lewerin, S.S. (2006) Feed-borne outbreak of *Salmonella* Cubana in Swedish pig farms: risk factors and factors affecting the restriction period in infected farms. *Acta Veterinaria Scandinavica* 47, 13–21.

Partanen, K.H. and Mroz, Z. (1999) Organic acids for performance enhancement in pig diets. *Nutrition Research Reviews* 12, 117–145.

Pomeroy, B.S. and Grady, M.K. (1961) *Salmonella* organisms isolated from feed ingredients. *Proc. US Livestock Sanit. Ass.* 65, 449.

Prusiner, S.B. (1997) Prion diseases and the BSE crisis. *Science* 278(5336), 245–251.

Quinn, P.J., Markey, B.K., Carter, M.E., Donnelly, W.J. and Leonard, F.C. (2003) *Veterinary Microbiology and Microbial Disease*. Blackwell Publishing Company, ISBN 0-632-05525-1.

Ratcliff, J. (2006) Pathogen control in feedmills. In: Feed Processing and Quality Control. Technical Report Series. American Soybean Association, Int. Marketing, Southeast Asia, Singapore, pp. 45–49. Available at: http://www.asaimsea. com/download_doc.php?file=ASA-TR-Processing.pdf (accessed November 2009).

Rutqvist, L. and Swahn, O. (1957) Epizootologiska och bakteriologiska undersökningar vid mjältbrandsepizootien i Sverige 1956-1957. *Nordisk Veterinaer Medicin* 9, 641–663.

Rutqvist, L. and Thal, E. (1958) *Salmonella* isolated from animals and animal products in Sweden during 1956-1967. *Nordisk Veterinaer Medicin* 10, 234–244.

Sauli, I., Danuser, J., Geeraerd, A.H., Van Impe, J.F., Rüfenacht, J., Bissig-Choisat, B., Wenk, C. and Stärk, K.D. (2005) Estimating the probability and level of contamination with *Salmonella* of feed for finishing pigs produced in Switzerland–the impact of the production pathway. *International Journal of Food Microbiology* 100, 289–310.

Smyser, C.F. and Snoeyenbos, G.H. (1979) Evaluation of organic acids and other compounds as *Salmonella* antagonists in meat and bone meal. *Poultry Science* 58, 50–54.

Sobel, J., Hirshfeld, A.B., McTigue, K., Burnett, C.L., Altekruse, S., Brenner, F., Malcolm, G., Mottice, S.L., Nichols, C.R. and Swerdlow, D.L. (2000) The pandemic of *Salmonella* enteritidis phage type 4 reaches Utah: a complex investigation confirms the need for continuing rigorous control measures. *Epidemiology and Infection* 125, 1–8.

Sternberg Lewerin, S., Boquist, B., Engström, P. and Häggblom, P. (2005) The effective control of *Salmonella* in Swedish poultry. In: Mead, G.C. (ed.) *Food Safety in the Poultry Industry*. Woodhouse Publishing in Food Science and Technology, CRC Press, Cambridge, UK.

Swahn, O. and Rutqvist, L. (1957) Pasteurisation of feed by heat pelleting. A way to reduce *Salmonella*? *Svenska Veterinärläkareföreningens medlemsblad* 9, 377–383. [English summary.]

USDA (1969) USDA Committee on *Salmonella*: An evaluation of the *Salmonella* problem. *Publication 1683*, National Academy of Science, Washington, DC, Library of Congress Catalog Card Number 76-600461.

USDA (2013) Foodborne Illness Cost Calculator: Salmonella. Available at: http://webarchives.cdlib.org/sw1rf5mh0k/http://www.ers.usda.gov/Data/FoodborneIllness/salm_Intro.asp (accessed 13 March 2013).

van Asselt, E.D. and Zwietering, M.H. (2006) A systematic approach to determine global thermal inactivation parameters for various food pathogens. *International Journal of Food Microbiology* 107, 73–82.

Vestby, L.K., Moretro, T., Langsrud, S., Heir, E. and Nesse, L.L. (2009) Biofilm forming abilities of *Salmonella* are correlated with persistence in fish meal- and feed factories. *BMC Veterinary Research* 5, 20–25.

Wales, A.D., Allen, V.M. and Davies, R.H. (2010) Chemical treatment of animal feed and water for the control of *Salmonella*. *Foodborne Pathogenesis and Disease* 7, 3–15.

Watkins, J.R., Flowers, A.I. and Grumbles, L.C. (1959) *Salmonella* organisms in animal products used in poultry feeds. *Avian Diseases* 3, 290.

WHO (1989) WHO-consultation on epidemiological emergency in poultry and egg salmonellosis. Geneva 20–23 March, 1989, *WHO/CDS/VPH* 89.92

Wierup, M. (1994) Control and prevention of salmonellosis in livestock farms. *16th Conference OIE Regional Commission for Europe*, Stockholm, Sweden, 28 June–1 July 1994, pp. 249–269.

Wierup, M. (2006) Contamination of Feed – an assessment on behalf of Swedish Board of Agriculture of risks in Sweden. Swedish Board of Agriculture, ISBN 91 88 264-32-7, pp. 1–132 [In Swedish – summary and key figures in English].

Wierup, M. and Häggblom, P. (2010) An assessment of soybeans and other vegetable proteins as source of *Salmonella* contamination in pig production. *Acta Veterinaria Scandinavica* 52, 15.

Wierup, M., Wold-Troell, M., Nurmi, E. and Häkkinen, M. (1988) Epidemiological evaluation of the *Salmonella*-controlling effect of a nationwide use of a competitive exclusion culture in poultry. *Poultry Science* 67, 1026–1033.

Wierup, M., Engström, B., Engvall, A. and Wahlström, H. (1995) Control of *Salmonella enteritidis* in Sweden. *International Journal of Food Microbiology* 25, 219–226.

Wingstrand, A., Dahl, J., Thomsen, L.K., Jørgensen, L. and Jensen, B.B. (1997) Influence of dietary administration of organic acids and increased feed structure on *Salmonella* Typhimurium infection in pigs. *Proceedings of the 2nd International Symposium on the Epidemiology and Control of* Salmonella *in Pork*, 20–22 August, Copenhagen, Denmark, pp. 170–172.

Wray, C. (1985) Is salmonellosis a serious problem in veterinary practice? *Veterinary Record* 485–489.

Xia, X., Zhao, S., Smith, A., McEvoy, J., Meng, J. and Bhagwat, A.A. (2009) Characterization of *Salmonella* isolates from retail foods based on serotyping, pulse field gel electrophoresis, antibiotic resistance and other phenotypic properties. *International Journal of Food Microbiology* 129, 93–98.

20 Environmental Aspects of *Salmonella*

Andrew Wales* and Robert H. Davies
Animal Health and Veterinary Laboratories Agency, Addlestone, UK

Introduction

Non-typhoidal *Salmonella* are zoonotic organisms that, depending on serovar and dose, may cause illness or asymptomatic carriage in exposed individuals. In the farmed species under modern husbandry, the latter appears to be most common outcome of infection. As a non-commensal pathogen *Salmonella* appears to be well adapted to cycle regularly through the environment, surviving external stresses en route to a new host (Winfield and Groisman, 2003). The source of contamination of processed foods and of animals can often be correlated with the *Salmonella* found in the local environment including contaminated housing and feed. However, as the environment is not normally a primary site of multiplication and contamination the organisms are likely to have been introduced previously into these sites by some agent such as wild or farmed animals, feedstuffs, or human or farm effluent. Having been introduced in this way contamination can multiply and persist, sometimes for decades, without further introductions in some special circumstances, e.g. feed industry cooling systems, hatcheries or abattoir equipment such as de-hairing or plucking equipment (Saide-Albornoz *et al.*, 1995; Heyndrickx *et al.*, 2002; Vestby *et al.*, 2009).

Various aspects of the behaviour and distribution of *Salmonella* in the environment have been reviewed previously (Murray, 1991; Wray, 1995). While some strains can be identified across host species, e.g. *Salmonella* (*S.*) Typhimurium definitive phage type 104, other strains have not moved out of one dominant species niche, despite ample opportunity to cross the species barrier, e.g. *S.* II Sofia in poultry in Australia. This host-species influence is also evident when reviewing serovars found in many animals, including wild animals. In particular, *Salmonella* species *bongori* and species *enterica*, subspecies other than *enterica* are more likely to be found in cold-blooded animals and their environment (Pignato *et al.*, 1998).

Trends in Farming, Biodiversity and *Salmonella* Isolation

In the developed world, there has been an emphasis on exclusion and eradication of infectious livestock diseases by various means including specific pathogen-free breeding, testing and removal, biosecurity and vaccination. Intensification and integration, particularly within the poultry and pig sectors, has allowed more control over breeding and biosecurity in particular. This has led

* Corresponding author, e-mail: andywales@fastmail.fm

© CAB International 2013. *Salmonella in Domestic Animals, 2nd Edition*
(eds P.A. Barrow and U. Methner)

to the virtual eradication in many regions of livestock salmonellosis caused by species-adapted variants such as *S.* Gallinarum biovars Gallinarum and Pullorum in poultry and *S.* Choleraesuis in pigs. In parallel with this process, breeding technologies and integrated, multinational breeding structures have led to increased genetic specialization and reduced genetic diversity among livestock, which might increase the *Salmonella* risk in situations where there is a breakdown in biosecurity (Hunter and Izsak, 1990).

One consequence of this has been the existence of large groups of animals that are free of clinical salmonellosis but which may have lowered immunological and genetic resistance to broad-host-range salmonellas. These may be introduced by stock, feed or other environmental carriers, and flourish in the absence of species-adapted competitor salmonellas. One example of this in recent years has been *S.* Enteritidis, a serovar that is genetically closely related to *S.* Gallinarum and which has proven recently to be a tenacious environmental pathogen of egg production (EFSA, 2010). It has been hypothesized that *S.* Enteritidis was not a major problem within the industry prior to the widespread eradication of *S.* Gallinarum owing to competitive exclusion of the former by the latter (Rabsch *et al.*, 2000). While this may be a simplistic view (*S.* Gallinarum and *S.* Enteritidis have been found to co-exist in some laying flocks; R.H. Davies, unpublished data), the result of eradicating a species-adapted *Salmonella*, with identifiable clinical signs and limited existence outside of the host, may be to reduce the immunological barrier to introduction of a broader host-range pathovar. Such strains can have an increased capacity for environmental persistence and spread, less tendency to cause identifiable disease, and greater potential to contaminate food of animal origin and infect humans.

Conversely, a non-species-adapted serovar that becomes established as an endemic *Salmonella* in an industry sector may be rather benign and act as a competitive excluder of potentially more problematic strains. It is hypothesized that this is what has happened with *S.* II Sofia in the Australian broiler industry (Murray, 2000; Chinivasagam *et al.*, 2010).

When *Salmonella* in livestock or food are investigated, the sources to which they may be traced (farms, hatchery, feed mill, transporters, wildlife, etc.) are diverse. Furthermore, when detailed studies are performed, certain persistent strains are often found in these locations. Such 'endemic' strains appear to be well adapted to the combination of environment and animals in a location. The scale of production and level of integration found in modern farming may elevate the risk of these non-species-adapted strains being propagated into the human food chain. Increased international trade in animals and standardization of farming practices may also promote the wide dissemination of such strains (Hunter and Izsak, 1990; Nakamura *et al.*, 1993).

By contrast, in remote areas such as the Kimberley region of Western Australia where food-animal contamination is less prominent and humans often rely on native fauna for food, serovars associated with wildlife (in this case reptiles) tend to predominate in humans and other mammals (Murray, 2000).

Salmonella Survival in the Environment

Salmonella may persist in a number of environments following excretion or the death of its host. The survival of *Salmonella* in diverse environments is documented in Table 20.1. The environmental conditions may change dramatically over time because of natural processes such as drying, decomposition or predation, or of human activities such as disinfection or sewage treatment. *Salmonella* can mount a range of more or less specific responses to physical, chemical and biological stressors and to starvation. Inevitably, responses to one stressor will affect susceptibility to others, and some may be considered general stress responses. These include the 'SOS' response of many bacteria in response to various internal and external triggers that include starvation and some metabolic and oxidative stresses (Erill *et al.*, 2007). The principal effect of SOS is to delay cell division

Table 20.1. Survival of *Salmonella* Typhimurium and other serovars in and on various matrices under differing environmental conditions.

Matrix	Serovar	Conditions	Initial count	Survival	Comments
Agar	Typhi	RT, sealed tubes		>40 years	
Broth, tryptose	Typhimurium	58°C	$1–3 \times 10^6$ ml^{-1}	D value 0.48–0.59 min (10 strains)	Stationary phase
Broth, heart infusion	Typhimurium	60°C	10^7 ml^{-1}	D value 0.2 – 0.9 min (14 strains)	Stationary phase, re-suspended
Chocolate	Typhimurium	20°C, a_w 0.37	1.1×10^5 100g^{-1}	83 days	
	Typhimurium	70°C and 90°C		D value (min) 70°C: 720; 90°C: 75	Median D values
Colostrum, bovine	Typhimurium	30°C (pH 6.4–4.4)	10^2 cfu ml^{-1}	>35 days	Rapid decline below pH 4.45
	Dublin	30°C (pH 6.4–4.3)		>5, <14 days	
Egg, fresh whole	Enteritidis	4°C and 25°C	approx 10^7 cfu	4°C: >270, <365 days; 25°C: >365 days	
	Typhimurium	4°C and 25°C	approx 10^7 cfu	4°C: >180, <270 days; 25°C: >365 days	
Faeces, poultry	Typhimurium	Fresh, 19°C (pH 8.9) and 5–8.9°C (pH 8.1–8.9)	10^8 cfu ml^{-1}	19°C: <6 days 5–8.9°C: >12, <25 days	*Salmonella*-impregnated silk immersed in faeces
Faeces, bovine	Typhimurium	18–20°C	Suspension of colony loop	Fresh: 166 days; autoclaved: 152 days	
Faeces, bovine[a]		Dried		≥1000 days	
Faeces, rodent[a]				148 days	
Feed, turkey mash[b]	Enteritidis	82°C, 15% moisture		3 log reduction in 47 s	Artificial contamination
Glass	Schottmulleri	4°C and 45°C, desiccated	Approx 5×10^7 cfu	4°C: 99 days; 45°C: 56 days	*S.* Typhi much shorter survival
Hatchery chick fluff	Senftenberg	RT	Natural contamination	≥1484 days	Stored in polythene bags
Ice cream	Typhimurium	–28°C	8.2×10^3 cfu g^{-1}	1.3 log unit reduction after 35 months	
Oil, paraffin	Typhimurium	25°C		2 years 6 months	Solid media overlain with oil
Pasture	Typhimurium	Summer, New Zealand	2×10^7 cfu 25cm^{-2}	>70, <84 days	Applied in faecal suspension
Semolina	Typhimurium	25°C, dried	23 cfu g^{-1}	≥360 days	Artificial contamination
Slurry, cow	Typhimurium	1–6°C and 18–20°C, pH 6.7	3×10^7 ml^{-1}	1–6°C: 70–84 days 18–20°C: 140–154 days	
Slurry, pig	Typhimurium	1–6°C and 18–20°C, pH 7.0	3×10^7 ml^{-1}	1–6°C: 150–364 days 18–20°C: 182–196 days	
Sweeper dust[a]				300 days	
Vegetables, various, surfaces	Typhimurium	Icebox and room temperatures	Approx 8×10^4 cfu cm^{-2}	Icebox: 35–77, median 49 days RT: 21–49, median 28 days	

Data abstracted from Mitscherlich and Marth (1984), except [a]Jones (2011) and [b]Himathongkham *et al.* (1996).
a_w, water activity; cfu, colony-forming units; min, minutes; RT, room temperature; s, seconds.

whilst promoting repair and replication of damaged DNA. One interesting aspect of the stress response in some substrates such as food is filamentation, in which *Salmonella* cells elongate rather than multiply and when more favourable conditions occur the filaments can septate and divide rapidly, resulting in a dramatic increase in the number of cells present (Humphrey, 2004).

Water activity, osmotic stress and desiccation

Protection against osmotic stress is provided initially by cellular accumulation of potassium ions, balanced by glutamate. If this is not adequate or possible with prevailing potassium concentrations, cells will take up or synthesize molecules such as trehalose, betaine and proline and effect alterations to outer membrane porins (Rychlik and Barrow, 2005). When water activity (a_w) is moderately depressed, down to around 0.92 to 0.95 (depending on solute) in nutrient broth or on agar, *Salmonella* will exhibit filamentation. Variations between strains and between solutes, plus heterogeneity within populations, have been observed in such responses (Mattick *et al.*, 2000; Kieboom *et al.*, 2006).

In *S.* Enteritidis, survival against the extreme water stress of desiccation appears to be greatly enhanced by the presence of an O-antigen capsule, chemically identical to the somatic antigen. Production of the capsule is co-regulated with biofilm elements, although the latter appear to be less significant in desiccation resistance (Gibson *et al.*, 2006). Interestingly, desiccation resistance *in vitro* was not correlated with persistence in feed factories or poultry production facilities (Broennum Pedersen *et al.*, 2008; Vestby *et al.*, 2009), suggesting that persistence may occur because of the processing equipment and its management rather than because the organisms have a dramatically increased environmental colonization potential.

Many interactions with other stressors have been observed. Reduced a_w protected *Salmonella* against heat (Palumbo *et al.*, 1995; Archer *et al.*, 1998) and oxidative (chlorine) stress (Kieboom *et al.*, 2006), whilst a dramatic increase in heat resistance was observed in *S.* Typhimurium following slow desiccation (Kirby and Davies, 1990). Osmotic stress with low nutrient availability in seawater is progressively lethal, but survival of *S.* Manhattan was enhanced by prior stress in waste water (Dupray *et al.*, 1995). In complex environments with other stressors, including microbiota, the effects of solutes and a_w may be difficult to predict: in one study soil moisture did not have a significant effect on *S.* Enteritidis survival (Danyluk *et al.*, 2008), and in another, *Salmonella* survival in poultry manure was minimal around 0.89 and significantly higher at lower a_w (Himathongkham *et al.*, 1999). In general however, *Salmonella* survives best in dry cool shady conditions and worst where there is moisture, heat and a predominant flora of environmental organisms.

Thermal stress

The acute thermal tolerance of environmental *Salmonella* will depend to a great extent on the moisture in the surroundings and the effects of other stressors. Growth occurs in media between about 7°C and 47°C (Mitscherlich and Marth, 1984). The effect of the immediate environment on thermotolerance can be gauged by the observation that the decimal reduction (D) value for *Salmonella* at 71°C is a few seconds in a liquid medium but varies between 4.5 and 6.6 min in feed (Bell, 2002). Survival in fatty or proteinaceous matrices such as egg and chocolate is also greater and this has resulted in various food-poisoning outbreaks following failure of what would normally be considered to be adequate levels of heat treatment or cooking (Krapf and Gantenbein-Demarchi, 2010). In the complex environment of soil, *Salmonella* appears to survive longest in the coolest temperatures, within the range 5–35°C (Danyluk *et al.*, 2008; García *et al.*, 2010), but temperature stability is also important for long survival (Semenov, 2008), since fluctuating temperatures, particularly freeze–thaw cycles, normally lead to rapid reduction in *Salmonella* counts. Although *Salmonella* can survive in frozen meat, there is normally some reduction in numbers and survival in faecal samples at −20°C is poorer than at −80°C (Turpin *et al.*, 1993a).

Chemical attack

There is a wide variety of potential chemical stresses, although most can be considered in broad categories such as pH, oxidation, membrane disruption, denaturation of critical macromolecules or metabolic poisons (Lambert, 2004; Wales *et al.*, 2010a). Experimentally, oxidative attack using chlorine is commonly used to assess resistance to chemical stress, and resistance to this correlates with resistance to other environmental phenomena including osmotic stress (Kieboom *et al.*, 2006) and starvation (Marsh *et al.*, 1998). It may be that *Salmonella* can mount particularly robust oxidative protection as a consequence of its adaptation to survive as an intracellular parasite of macrophages (Hebrard *et al.*, 2009). Biofilms are in general at least partially protective against chemical attack upon their residents (McDonnell and Russell, 1999), and *Salmonella* biofilms have been shown to protect against chlorine (Solano *et al.*, 2002; Lapidot *et al.*, 2006). Sublethal chemical stress can precondition *Salmonella* cells against more severe environmental challenges (Kwon *et al.*, 2000).

Radiation

Incident radiation in the environment is mostly in the form of visible and ultraviolet (UV) light. Experiments with *Salmonella* and other bacterial species have indicated that UV light, particularly of the shorter wavelengths (UV-B), appears to have a greater lethal effect than does visible light on organisms suspended in transparent media (Muela *et al.*, 2000; Oppezzo *et al.*, 2011). However, short wavelengths do not penetrate water as well as longer wavelengths, so in natural environments with deep water and suspended particulates, more lethal effect has been observed to be associated with visible than with UV light. A reduction in the lethal effect of visible light and of full-spectrum sunlight was observed following treatments to quench hydrogen peroxide and to reduce oxygen concentration, respectively (Arana *et al.*, 1992; Oppezzo *et al.*, 2011). This indicates a significant role for photodynamic generation of reactive oxygen in the killing of *Salmonella* and *Escherichia coli* by UV and visible light. UV irradiation is an established treatment in the wastewater industry (Hijnen *et al.*, 2006). Artificial UV and pulsed high intensity light have dramatic effects on exposed *Salmonella* and have been used as a decontamination method for clear liquids and the surfaces of eggs and meat (Lasagabaster *et al.*, 2011; Paskeviciute *et al.*, 2011).

Starvation

The details of starvation stress responses in *S.* Typhimurium have been reviewed (Foster and Spector, 1995). Nutrient limitation has been observed to prolong the tail of the survival graph for many Gram-negative organisms when subjected to a variety of disinfectants (Hoff and Akin, 1986), and this has been shown in the case of *Salmonella* for which the failure to detect persister cells (Jayaraman, 2008) may lead to later recrudescence of detectable contamination. The effects of nutrient limitation on bacterial resistance to antimicrobials are thought in Gram-negative organisms to be mediated largely by alterations in phospholipid, porin protein and cation components of the cell envelope (Brown *et al.*, 1990; McDonnell and Russell, 1999). Starvation in *Salmonella* is closely associated with development of the so-called viable but non-culturable (VBNC) state (discussed below), although how much this is a coordinated response to environmental stress is open to debate.

Predation and competition

Salmonella survival is significantly affected by the microbiota of its immediate environment. This may compete for oxygen and nutrients as well as producing antagonistic chemicals such as organic acids and bacteriocins. Lytic phage may also be involved in the decay of *Salmonella* in environmental samples (Joerger, 2003). Compared with untreated soil, *Salmonella* survived for longer in sterilized soil (Turpin *et al.*, 1993b) and for less long in manure-amended soil (García *et al.*, 2010). Sterilized environmental samples from a paper mill were more conducive to *Salmonella* survival than equivalent untreated samples (Degnan, 2008), and soil-associated cress plant contamination persisted for longer when *Salmonella* was added to sterilized growing soil (Cooley *et al.*, 2003).

Despite the evident negative effects of microbiological competition, *Salmonella* will survive and even grow following ingestion by grazing amoeboid and ciliate soil protozoa (Gaze *et al.*, 2003; Brandl *et al.*, 2005). Passage through protozoa may result in membrane-bound *Salmonella* aggregates or cells with altered morphology, and the former at least are relatively resistant to other environmental stresses (Brandl *et al.*, 2005). In addition to suppression and resistance, *Salmonella* interaction with other environmental microorganisms may extend to cooperation in biofilms.

Biofilms

The capacity to form biofilms varies between *Salmonella* strains (Solano *et al.*, 2002). There is some correlation with serovar, and the biofilming capacity on solid/air and liquid/air interfaces has been described as being correlated with observed persistence in feed and fish-meal factories (Vestby *et al.*, 2009), although other studies (R.H. Davies, unpublished) have failed to identify this phenomenon in persistent strains from feed mills and hatcheries. The principal elements of *Salmonella* biofilms are cellulose and thin aggregative (curli) fimbriae, although the exact components appear to vary with the investigative media (Solano *et al.*, 2002). Curli appear to be more important in resisting desiccation, whilst cellulose provides a matrix that inhibits oxidative chemical (chlorine) attack (White *et al.*, 2006). The loss of biofilm-forming capacity reduces *Salmonella* resistance to chlorine applied at a plant surface but it does not cripple the bacteria in this respect, implying that other protective mechanisms are likely, possibly involving incorporation into other biofilms (Lapidot *et al.*, 2006). Cooperative, synergistic biofilms have been observed experimentally between *Salmonella* and a variety of Gram-positive and Gram-negative bacteria, leading the authors to hypothesize that pre-existing biofilms of endemic bacteria may provide an environmental 'foothold' for *Salmonella* (Jones and Bradshaw, 1997; Habimana *et al.*, 2010).

Viable but non-culturable states

Viable but non-culturable (VBNC) states have been observed or inferred for many bacteria in hostile environments, where culture of cells is not possible using conventional methodology but there is evidence for active metabolism obtained by elongation in the presence of suitable nutrition (direct viable count), demonstration of respiration by fluorescent dyes, or other techniques (McDougald *et al.*, 1998). Such states have been reported for *Salmonella* under a wide variety of conditions and after widely varying experimental time intervals. A marked numerical divergence was observed between plate counts and green fluorescent protein-labelled cells of *S.* Typhi in groundwater over 25 days (Cho and Kim, 1999), and between plate and direct viable counts in phosphate buffer (but not saline) over 10 weeks at 21°C (Chmielewski and Frank, 1995). Salmonellas added to river water held at room temperature showed a marked drop in plate counts after 45 days, but a similar reduction in direct viable counts was not observed (Santo Domingo *et al.*, 2000). Loss of culturability of *S.* Typhimurium in buffered starvation medium over weeks to months, associated with a shift to coccoid forms, was seen at 5°C but not 20°C (Gupte *et al.*, 2003).

In more complex environments, *Salmonella* in non-sterile soil showed a progressive numerical divergence between respiring and culturable populations, associated with increased resistance to physical lysis (Marsh *et al.*, 1998). A similar divergence in respiring and culturable *S.* Typhimurium was observed in soil, with shrinkage of viable cells, compared with fragmentation of UV-killed cells (Turpin *et al.*, 1993b).

Resuscitation of *Salmonella* cells in a putative VBNC state has apparently been successful using a number of techniques, including: (i) broth culture either for hours at 37°C or with a brief temperature upshift to 56°C (Gupte *et al.*, 2003); and (ii) several day's broth culture at room temperature then addition of viable culture supernatant (Santo Domingo *et al.*, 2000). The last technique reflects experiences with *Micrococcus luteus*, where resuscitation using spent stationary phase culture supernatant suggests that a soluble cell signalling factor may be involved (Kaprelyants *et al.*, 1994). In some studies the VBNC state has been designated by failure to recover cells on inhibitory plating media, so the extent of non-culturability may have been over-estimated.

Evidence linking VBNC *Salmonella* to pathogenic potential is weak (Winfield and Groisman, 2003), and opinions differ on the significance of the VBNC state. Fractionation of stationary phase culture by density gradient centrifugation has shown VBNC-type cells to be present within 4 h of entering stationary phase, increasing over time and with associated increases in fractions of dying and dead cells (Passerat *et al.*, 2009). *Salmonella* Typhimurium in artificial seawater shows increasing population heterogeneity over time with respect to various dye uptakes (Barcina *et al.*, 1997). Evidence of this nature has led some to suggest that VBNC is not a programmed survival response to hostile environmental conditions, but part of a stepwise deterioration in cell state under conditions of sustained starvation and/or other stresses, that leads ultimately to loss of membrane integrity and death (McDougald *et al.*, 1998). By this view, resuscitation may be possible by certain poorly understood means up to quite a late stage of deterioration, but the significance of the VBNC state, in terms of environmental persistence with potential for reinfection of hosts, is unclear.

Aspects of the Molecular Biology of *Salmonella* Survival

Many environmental stresses, such as temperature, pH and osmotic shifts, competition and predation, are also encountered during infection of a host via the alimentary tract, so regulation and competence in environmental survival is also seen to be related to virulence. There are a host of regulatory and effector mechanisms allowing *Salmonella* to sense and adapt to environmental stress, but fundamental to many of these is regulation by sigma factors. These RNA polymerase subunits alter gene expression at the transcriptional level by affecting binding of the polymerase to promoter sequences. In *Salmonella*, three so-called 'alternative' sigma factors (RpoS, RpoH and RpoE) have significant stress response roles. Of these, RpoS has the most wide-ranging effects with in excess of 50 regulated genes identified in various bacteria, involving tolerance to heat and cold, oxidation, osmotic stress, starvation, pH, UV and sunlight radiation, amongst others (Munro *et al.*, 1995; Zaafrane *et al.*, 2004; Rychlik and Barrow, 2005; McMeechan *et al.*, 2007; Rangel, 2011). As might be expected for such a pivotal molecule, the control of RpoS itself is complex, involving regulation of transcription, translation and degradation (Moreno *et al.*, 2000; Rychlik and Barrow, 2005).

RpoH is associated with expression of heat shock proteins, produced in response to thermal stress, but also to other stresses including starvation, DNA damage and oxidative attack. It has less wide-ranging regulatory effects, with up-regulated products being concerned principally with repairing and removing heat-damaged proteins (Rychlik and Barrow, 2005; Rangel, 2011). RpoE similarly has a more restricted regulon than RpoS, principally associated with protection of proteins, and is induced by extracytoplasmic (envelope) stresses including cold and osmotic shock. Its effects appear to be additive or synergistic with RpoS, and under certain conditions and time frames its protective effects can be more marked (Rychlik and Barrow, 2005; McMeechan *et al.*, 2007).

In addition to sigma factors there are other regulatory and effector mechanisms (both within and separate from alternative sigma factor regulons), which integrate more than one stress response. The product of the *fur* gene acts as an iron-responsive DNA-binding transcriptional suppressor for iron uptake and transport genes, but also is a promoter for a short-term acid-tolerance response (Rychlik and Barrow, 2005). The OmpR/EnvZ signal transduction system is active both in osmo- and pH resistance (Rychlik and Barrow, 2005). Integration of curli fimbriae and cellulose production occurs via control by *agfD* (part of the *agfDEFG* and *agfBAC* curli operons) (White *et al.*, 2006), providing genetic regulation of biofilms and the associated rdar colony morphology. However, *agfD* also appears to regulate production of the O-antigen capsule (Gibson *et al.*, 2006).

Thus, in common with that observed at the cellular level, genetic stress responses are found to be a series of overlapping and co-regulated changes. This reflects the fact that many stressors result in similar injuries at the fundamental level of membranes and macromolecules, and it may also be true that rapid and stereotypical responses can best ensure survival in sometimes changeable environments.

Water, as Environment and Carrier for *Salmonella*

Salmonella are disseminated into the aquatic environment from a diverse range of sources, including effluent discharges, agricultural runoff and excretion by wild animals. Studies in European rivers and associated coastal waters have shown that spikes in the number and diversity of *Salmonella* in these environments are associated with episodes of high rainfall and flooding (Polo *et al.*, 1999; Baudart *et al.*, 2000a; Martinez-Urtaza *et al.*, 2004b), irrespective of season. This may be because of agricultural runoff and/or the disturbance of sediments (Baudart *et al.*, 2000b) with increased suspended particulate matter, a feature noted with other water-borne bacteria (Jackson, 1996). The topography of the land also plays a part, and concentration of *Salmonella* serovars that are associated with local farmed animals or wildlife can often be found in streams that run through pasture or woodland valleys (R.H. Davies, unpublished data).

Sediments may protect enteric bacteria from some of the stresses associated with aquatic environments and may provide nutrients that support bacterial growth. Experimental and observational studies indicate that *Salmonella* survives better in mineral sediments than in overlying fresh water (Fish and Pettibone, 1995; Moore *et al.*, 2003), and better in clay-rich sediments (Burton *et al.*, 1987). The sediments that accumulate in slow-moving water where streams bend are good sampling points to detect *Salmonella* that has passed down the stream previously. In marine waters, similar effects are found, sediments being important as bacteria may attach to particles and then settle into sediments for increased survival. Human-associated serovars may be prominent amongst coastal and river isolates near to population centres (Polo *et al.*, 1999; Martinez-Urtaza *et al.*, 2004a), although the contribution of agriculture to levels of the same serovars (e.g. Typhimurium) may be significant (Baudart *et al.*, 2000a).

Open seas are important for eliminating organisms, including *Salmonella*, from human activities via discharges and rivers. *Salmonella* multiply in sterile sea water and elimination of *Salmonella* in the North Sea has been demonstrated to be predominantly due to protozoa (Glaus and Heinemeyer, 1994). In filtered fresh water and sea water, the numbers of *Salmonella* remain relatively stable, while, in unfiltered samples of the same waters, a reduction in numbers occurs (Moriñigo *et al.*, 1989). In very cold seas, adaptation to low temperature occurs. Sub-lethal injury was demonstrated in sea water in the Antarctic at −1.8°C in 54–56 days (Smith *et al.*, 1994), with *Salmonella* slowly forming colonies on solid media at −1.8°C but losing the ability to grow at 37°C.

The consequences of sewage discharges for *Salmonella* contamination in river and coastal marine environments depend upon local conditions and the treatment to which such discharges have been subjected. Wastewater monitoring may reveal a regular input of *Salmonella* organisms into surface waters but the *Salmonella* types in associated river and coastal waters may not reflect this, perhaps because *Salmonella* do not survive long when expelled in treated water that (by contrast to agricultural runoff) contains little protective particulate matter (Baudart *et al.*, 2000b). The situation may therefore be different with the discharge of waste water that has not been subjected to adequate removal of suspended solids.

The inactivation of *Salmonella* is greater than for other coliforms, faecal streptococci or *Clostridium perfringens* in sea water (Moriñigo *et al.*, 1989) and several studies have shown that the presence and levels of faecal indicator bacteria do not correlate well with *Salmonella* in coastal (Baudart *et al.*, 2000b; Catalao Dionisio *et al.*, 2000; Obiri-Danso and Jones, 2000) and river (Prokšová *et al.*, 2002) waters. However, indirect evidence of the impact of human waste was observed following analysis of estuarine water and mollusc samples from northern Spain (Martinez-Urtaza *et al.*, 2004a, b). This revealed that the temporal pattern of *S.* Typhimurium contamination was distinct from other serovars, with Typhimurium isolates being most frequent in summer months and around heavily touristed areas. Furthermore, the *S.* Typhimurium isolates that were associated with this spike in contamination were of distinct subtypes from those that were not. In estuarine environments, *Salmonella* were found to survive for extended periods and could multiply when temperatures were above 18°C (Rhodes and Kator, 1988).

Inland freshwater pools may be contaminated with *Salmonella* even when there are no identifiable foci of faecal contamination in the catchment area (Townsend, 1992). In drinking water, *S.* Enteritidis survival time was reduced as cell density decreased, as temperature rose from 4°C to 20°C, and as organic pollution (measured by chemical oxygen demand) increased (Pokorny, 1988). The effect on *Salmonella* of organic soil in water probably depends on the balance between particulates and nutrients on the one hand, and competitor/predator microbiota on the other. Isolation of *Salmonella* from nutrient-depleted samples such as natural water and soil can be enhanced by the addition of ferrioxamine E (Davies *et al.*, 2001a).

Salmonella in Waste

Salmonella may be present in any waste from human or animal activities. Meat waste from domestic sources in the UK included a variety of serovars (Durrant and Beatson, 1981), with the potential for proliferation with subsequent dissemination by birds, rodents, insects and other scavengers when conditions of temperature and moisture are favourable. The dumping of potentially *Salmonella*-contaminated waste in sites with access for scavengers is not uncommon (Murray, 2000), nor is access of birds to contaminated by-products of animal processing plants, such as fish-meal factories (Nesse *et al.*, 2005). Other studies have documented the incidence of serovars in sewage and abattoir effluents (Linklater *et al.*, 1985; Fransen *et al.*, 1996), and it is idealistic to expect that waste will be decontaminated before disposal and that disposals will be performed to the requirements of regulatory agencies at all times.

Waste treatment

Numerous authors have investigated the occurrence of *Salmonella* in waste and the effects of different treatment processes (see Strauch, 1991). The risks associated with sewage sludges and their disposal include: contamination of waters leading to human and animal infections, contamination of aquatic flora and shellfish, and contamination of foods such as vegetables via irrigation (Danielsson, 1977). Treatment of human waste in developed countries is generally well controlled but the discharge of untreated sewage into the sea is still practised, either routinely or when heavy rainfall overwhelms treatment systems.

The incidence of *Salmonella* and the effects of treatments were investigated in eight treatment plants in the UK (Jones *et al.*, 1980). *Salmonella* was found to be present in 85% of settled sewage, 87% of raw sewage and 96% of anaerobically digested sludge, at levels generally less than 200 cfu $100\,ml^{-1}$. Aerobic digestion was more effective at reducing *Salmonella* than anaerobic digestion. Lime and copperas conditioning, followed by dewatering, which raises pH to above 10, effectively eliminated *Salmonella*. Other authors give an average figure of 10^5 *Salmonella* g^{-1} of total solids for anaerobically digested and dewatered sewage sludge (Russ and Yanko, 1981), which is a much higher figure even allowing for the different units. Composting reduced this to below detectable levels, and a moisture content of at least 20% was found to be required for *Salmonella* to grow in composted sewage sludge. There is a risk of repopulation and regrowth should moisture increase during storage. Lowering pH to control *Salmonella* in composted sludge is undesirable for geochemical reasons (Hussong *et al.*, 1985). National regulations governing the application of sewage sludge to land generally employ pathogen density limits to determine whether sludge is deemed safe for application followed by immediate or, alternatively, delayed use of the land for crops and public access (Horswell *et al.*, 2010).

Animal waste from farms does not usually receive the same attention and treatment as human waste, and it is common practice to use slurry or farmyard manure (FYM) as a means of removal of animal wastes. FYM has been shown to be more bio-safe than slurry due to its composting effect so will not be considered further. Subsequent dispersal on to land and pasture provides a means of disposal and reuse of nutrients but introduces the risk of spreading contamination and cross-species infection, e.g. exposure of cattle to contaminated slurry from pigs (Jones, 1980). The virulence of *S.* Dublin did not appear to be affected by storage in slurry (Jones, 1975), although earlier experiments had found that *S.* Dublin levels of $10^5\,cfu\,ml^{-1}$ in slurry were necessary to infect cattle grazing pasture spread with the contaminated slurry. A delay of 10–30 days between application of pig manure to pasture and access to the land by cattle was associated with no detectable infection of the cattle by the *Salmonella* serovars Derby and Krefeld, which were detected both in the manure and on the forage (Holley *et al.*, 2008). There remains a risk of acquisition by wildlife and transfer of infection to a situation where it can multiply.

Although the levels of *Salmonella* in slurry are usually less than $100\,cfu\,ml^{-1}$, the survival of the organism varies with the physical conditions, e.g. the initial pH of slurry ranges from 6.2 to 8.0, which is not lethal for *Salmonella* and decay is largely a function of the activity of competing microorganisms, as the ecology of manure can shift over time to become markedly suppressive of *Salmonella* (You *et al.*, 2006). Addition of nutrients such as waste animal feed or milk to slurry stores, or even mixing to bring the organisms into contact with an as yet untapped source of nutrient, may stimulate growth of *Salmonella*. In addition, continual topping up of slurry stores with fresh material does not facilitate adequate decay of organisms before spreading and a two-store system that enables a longer holding period has been made compulsory in some countries. Addition of ammonia, urea or lime can also hasten the decline of undesirable bacteria in faecal waste (Ottoson *et al.*, 2008).

Anaerobic thermophilic digestion may be used to treat cattle waste, with collection of gas for energy use. The control of pathogens is regarded as an important part of the evaluation process (Plym-Forshell, 1995). The studies showed that *Salmonella* are eliminated during digestion at 55°C for 24h, or at much lower temperatures in longer cycles (Massé *et al.*, 2011), but subsequent release into a manure pit was associated with recontamination of the treated waste. Similar findings have been reported where regrowth of *Salmonella* occurred after digestion (Larsen *et al.*, 1994).

Historically, reuse of waste water has developed from a need to prevent pollution of waterways and to conserve water and nutrients, and this remains important today. Shuval (1991) considered that, although scientific and technical advances have occurred, problems associated with many pathogens still remain. World Health Organization (WHO) guidelines for reuse of waste water for localized irrigation to root crops likely to be eaten uncooked are for a 4-log reduction in pathogen levels, with a verification monitoring level of not more than 10^3 *E. coli* $100\,ml^{-1}$. For localized irrigation of low-growing crops, again a 4-log reduction in pathogens is recommended, by a suitable combination of pre- and postharvest treatments (WHO, 2006). Waste water reuse in intensive operations such as slaughterhouses requires advanced treatments to avoid the risk of perpetuating and amplifying contamination (de Nardi *et al.*, 2011).

Soil and Crops

The observed survival times of *Salmonella* in soil vary widely, from less than 25 to in excess of 200 days (Mitscherlich and Marth, 1984; Jones, 2011), in consequence of the many influencing factors such as soil type, temperature profiles, moisture, indigenous microbiota, method by which *Salmonella* is introduced and strain variations. *Salmonella* Typhimurium applied to the top of soil cores survived longer at all depths and leached out in larger numbers when introduced in sewage sludge rather than in soil (Horswell *et al.*, 2010). Arthurson *et al.* (2011) noted enhanced survival of *Salmonella* in soil in the presence of manure. Experimentally, *S.* Newport survived for nearly 1 year when introduced in manure to soil (You *et al.*, 2006), but natural contamination by pig manure applied to plots appeared to be more short-lived, with *Salmonella* persistence for up to 54 days albeit with some spread to adjacent plots (Cote and Quessy, 2005). In contrast, survival for at least 8 months was demonstrated in pig and poultry range areas and abattoir holding paddocks for sheep (Davies and Wray, 1996b; Davies *et al.*, 2001b; Davies and Breslin, 2003b; Purvis *et al.*, 2005).

Additional factors that appear to enhance survival times in soil include: injection versus surface application of slurry, the absence of indigenous microbiota, anaerobic conditions, thermal stability and cooler temperatures (Natvig *et al.*, 2002; You *et al.*, 2006; Semenov, 2008).

Salmonella may also be introduced into soil and the adjacent environment by burial and decomposition of infected carcasses. One study (Davies and Wray, 1996b) examined calf carcasses artificially contaminated with *S.* Typhimurium. *Salmonella* isolations lasted for up to 6 months in local soil, blowfly larvae and bird droppings. During cold winter weather, *Salmonella* reappeared, possibly due to changes in other flora within the environment.

The contamination of plants by soil-associated *Salmonella* has been the subject of numerous investigations, but the methodologies and plants investigated have varied widely. Root crops may be contaminated by *S.* Typhimurium for a whole growing cycle following a single application of contaminated manure before planting (Islam *et al.*, 2004). Direct contact between the edible parts of aerial crops and soil may also generate contamination of food; for example the exposure of tomato fruits to *Salmonella*-contaminated soil permitted surface colonization, with increasing invasion of peripheral tissues over 10 days (Guo *et al.*, 2002). *Salmonella* strain and serovar variations were observed.

The potential of *Salmonella* to invade and spread on and within the aerial parts of crops appears to be quite limited with some plant/strain combinations, but less so with others. The stems and leaves of tomato seedlings were contaminated for several weeks by *Salmonella* applied to the soil 6 weeks or more before germination (Barak and Liang, 2008). Contamination of cress seeds by surface adsorption of *S.* Newport, or by irrigation of seedlings with the same strain, resulted in seedlings positive for *Salmonella* for up to 30 days (Cooley *et al.*, 2003). Numbers of *Salmonella* were highest on roots, with clustering at root tips and branching buds, and aerial parts of the plants were colonized in a motility-dependent manner over external surfaces. By contrast, there was no contamination of the leaves of spinach seedlings germinated in soil heavily (10^4–10^6 cfu g^{-1}) contaminated by *S.* Weltevreden (Arthurson *et al.*, 2011).

Heavy and repeated contamination of tomato plant soil by *S.* Newport (Hintz *et al.*,

2010) or *S.* Enteritidis (Jablasone *et al.*, 2004) was associated with a low frequency of internal contamination of tomatoes in the former study but with none in the latter. *Salmonella* was not found in stem, leaf or fruit samples of tomatoes grown from seedlings with repeated applications of *S.* Montevideo by irrigation (Miles *et al.*, 2009). *Salmonella* Typhimurium survived for months on barley and rosemary seedlings following application by spray and irrigation, and was associated with the emergence of rugose colony types, suggesting an increased production of biofilm components (Amel and Amina, 2007). However, the contamination did not spread to new parts of the plants as they grew. Greater spread was seen when *S.* Typhimurium was applied by soil irrigation to mature parsley plants, as it appeared rapidly and persistently in leaves and stems (Lapidot and Yaron, 2009). Biofilm-deficient mutants still spread, but in lower numbers.

Therefore, there is evidence of the risk for *Salmonella* contamination of crops via soil contamination, although the risk clearly differs between crops and most of the fragmentary evidence is based on heavy, experimental applications of *Salmonella* to plants or soil. Features that are already known to affect environmental survival, such as biofilm capability and motility, are also significant in spread and survival on and in plants.

The particular vulnerability of bean sprouts to heavy *Salmonella* contamination has been recognized, along with the risk to consumers of this product that is frequently consumed raw (Taormina *et al.*, 1999). *Salmonella* contaminating the seeds or irrigation water appears to be well able to take advantage of the warm, wet environmental conditions and growth surfaces available during the sprouting process to grow to heavy densities (Charkowski *et al.*, 2002).

Farmed Species

Poultry

Chicks may acquire *Salmonella* via 'vertical' transmission in the egg from the parent breeder flock, but 'horizontal' transmission from environmental contamination on the farm or in the hatchery can be a significant problem. The endemic contamination of hatcheries may occur with multiple serovars simultaneously but often there are one or two predominant serovars, which may persist for years (Pennington *et al.*, 1968; Byrd *et al.*, 1999), and which may not have a discernible link to the supplying breeder flocks (Bailey *et al.*, 2002). Elimination of an endemic serovar from a hatchery was followed by its decline in broiler flocks (Christensen *et al.*, 1997). Similar problems have been encountered in turkey hatcheries (Davies and Bedford, 2001).

In the absence of widespread infection of chicks from breeders, the persistence of contamination on commercial laying farms is currently considered to be the predominant environmental *Salmonella* problem in poultry in developed countries (Garber *et al.*, 2003; Carrique-Mas *et al.*, 2009). Amongst commercial layers, contaminated eggs will typically result from flock infections acquired via persistent environmental and wildlife-associated *Salmonella* (van de Giessen *et al.*, 1994; Kinde *et al.*, 1996; Wales *et al.*, 2006b), although feed and replacement pullets are other possible routes. *Salmonella* Enteritidis of the phage types associated with 18 egg-associated outbreaks studied by Altekruse *et al.* (1993) were found in the internal organs of birds in 71% of source flocks and in 79% of environmental samples from the sheds.

Dust has been found to contain *Salmonella* in broiler and layer houses (Morgan-Jones, 1980; Wales *et al.*, 2007). Release of contaminated dust from wall or ceiling spaces during repairs is often associated with contamination incidents and spikes of infection in hatcheries, feed mills and poultry houses. Contaminated water may provide a significant source for the spread of *Salmonella* between birds, but this is dependent on the drinker system, with troughs, bell and cup drinkers providing a greater risk than nipple lines. Litter has been found to be a more effective monitor of environmental contamination in broiler and turkey units than drinking water, and the *Salmonella* isolations from litter correlate with those in the birds (Poppe *et al.*, 1991; Irwin *et al.*, 1994). Sampling the litter by means of boot swabs further enhances isolation by more thorough and representative sampling of the faecal material on litter (Carrique-Mas and Davies, 2008).

In well-ventilated rooms, *S.* Enteritidis phage type 4 could be found in the air with chicks becoming colonized as a result of the exposure (Lever and Williams, 1996). Airborne transmission using *Salmonella*-contaminated dust has been experimentally demonstrated in turkeys (Harbaugh *et al.*, 2006). With older birds, airborne spread within and between poultry houses is dependent on the housing systems and weight of infection, so in many cases where pens within a house have separate feed and water supplies there is no spread of infection and this clustering effect can make detection of an infected flock rather difficult.

Salmonella Enteritidis can survive for at least 1 year in empty poultry sheds and free-range accommodation, where naturally infected flocks have previously been housed (Davies and Wray, 1996a; Davies and Breslin, 2003b). In these studies, *S.* Enteritidis persisted in food troughs, nesting boxes, unbedded floor areas and dust on fans. Association with dust particles appears to aid persistence, the organisms being found in dust remaining after cleaning and disinfection. *Salmonella* was also found outside the units, in litter, wild-bird droppings and in insects. Survival was demonstrated in feeds for at least 2 years. Seasonal changes in the ability to isolate *Salmonella* from the environment were noted in an empty poultry house (Davies and Wray, 1996b).

Contamination of the range area of free-range flocks can persist for many months but this is not normally associated with infection of subsequent flocks due to the prolonged interval for cleaning houses and acclimatizing birds. Pooled water on range areas and accumulated manure close to the houses are the most highly contaminated and should be dealt with if there is a short interval between use of the range between flocks (Davies and Carrique-Mas, 2010). Application of lime is sometimes used to decontaminate range areas, but this technique is often ineffective as insufficient quantity is used to achieve the sustained elevation in pH required (Nyberg *et al.*, 2011).

Infection of turkey flocks may be acquired from the hatchery, from environmental carry-over between flocks (Hoover *et al.*, 1997; Nayak *et al.*, 2004) or from feed (Davies and Wales, 2010b). A further source of dissemination may be rearing or brooder farms, in which *Salmonella* may persist, often mediated by wildlife vectors such as mice or litter beetles.

Cleaning and disinfection of poultry units is frequently inadequate for the elimination of *Salmonella*, as discussed below. The intermittent detection of the same *Salmonella* serovar on poultry premises may suggest that it is continuously present despite cleaning and disinfection, but that sampling and detection is failing to show this. This is borne out by longitudinal studies involving detailed subtyping of isolates (Broennum Pedersen *et al.*, 2008).

Pigs

Like poultry, the dominant mode of *Salmonella* infection in pigs is asymptomatic, although the endemic serovars, for example Typhimurium and Derby, differ from those in poultry. Environmental sources for *Salmonella* infection of pig production may include feed, wild birds and rodents, visitors, vehicles and other fomites, but most *Salmonella* risk factor studies reflect existing endemic infections on premises or within the breeding pyramid (Berends *et al.*, 1996; Lo Fo Wong *et al.*, 2004). Endemic infection is associated with contamination of buildings and equipment and ineffective cleaning, disinfection and pest control (Berends *et al.*, 1996; Wales *et al.*, 2009). Ingestion of contaminated soil along with feed is likely to be one of the factors responsible for the high within-herd prevalence and persistence of *Salmonella* in outdoor pig herds (Davies and Cook, 2008).

Where it is possible to use effectively cleaned and biosecure accommodation to house selected weaned piglets, the cycle of *Salmonella* infection can be broken (Wales *et al.*, 2011). Apart from this, eliminating endemic *Salmonella* on premises can be arduous and expensive, at least partly owing to the lack of regular cycles of complete depopulation of accommodation that are inherent in, for example, poultry production. However, experience in Sweden with contaminated premises indicates that an empirical procedure of intensive cleaning and disinfection plus segregation, testing and removal of pigs can, over time, exert sufficient negative pressure to eliminate *Salmonella* (Österberg, 2010). This demonstrates the necessity to address *Salmonella* in both stock and the farm environment if the organism is to be eliminated, rather than suppressed, on a unit.

Cattle

A common theme in investigations of bovine *Salmonella* infections has been the potential for the recycling or acquisition of infection through the farm environment and/or via manure or effluent. Housing of cattle and exposure of calving cows to accommodation previously occupied by sick animals were risk factors in a UK study (Evans and Davies, 1996). Sick pens, calving pens and manure stores were frequently contaminated on US dairy farms (Fossler *et al.*, 2005), and another American study identified human and farm effluents as vehicles for the acquisition and dissemination of *Salmonella* around dairy farms (Anderson *et al.*, 2001). In Australia, manure fertilizer and effluent were identified as agents for the importation and persistence, respectively, of *S.* Typhimurium on a dairy farm (Vanselow *et al.*, 2007b). Imported manure was a risk factor for *S.* Typhimurium on Dutch dairy farms (Veling *et al.*, 2002). *Salmonella* Montevideo was found in environmental samples, effluent and recycled wash water in the dairy of a farm 2 years after resolution of a clinical outbreak of salmonellosis caused by the same serovar (Gay and Hunsaker, 1993).

Although feed has not previously often been incriminated as the source of bovine *Salmonella* infection, there is evidence that feed stores can become contaminated by the excreta of *Salmonella*-positive farm wildlife or by effluent, and this may lead to re-exposure of animals or further dissemination of infection on a site or group of farms (Evans and Davies, 1996; Davies, 1997). The advent of year-round feeding of total mixed rations and zero grazing of cattle has more recently led to increases in persistent *S.* Mbandaka and *S.* Montevideo acquired from contaminated soya. These practices, together with increased herd size and increased use of purchased replacement cattle have in some cases overwhelmed the natural tendency for spontaneous regression of *Salmonella* infection as herd immunity increases.

Aquaculture

Extensive and intensive aquaculture ponds in South-east Asia were frequently contaminated with *Salmonella* (Reilly and Twiddy, 1992). Coastal marine environments are used to cultivate and harvest filter-feeding bivalve molluscs such as mussels, oysters and clams. These will accumulate suspended pathogens and, although elimination is efficient, the risk posed to human consumers will depend on the level of challenge and the mode of consumption (Hernroth *et al.*, 2010). The presence of *Salmonella* in bivalves is well established (Heinitz *et al.*, 2000; Martinez-Urtaza *et al.*, 2004b), although the frequency of related human salmonellosis appears to be low (Rippey, 1994; Potasman *et al.*, 2002). It was suspected that *S.* Senftenberg was being recycled into the sea and mussel beds via mussel processing plant waste, as the same subtypes were repeatedly isolated from seawater, mussels and mussel-processing plants in Galicia (Martinez-Urtaza and Liebana, 2005).

Cleaning and Disinfection of Animal Accommodation

Cleaning and disinfection (CandD) is pivotal to the control of *Salmonella* on farms, particularly in enterprises such as pig, broiler poultry, turkey and egg production where animals are housed and usually batch-managed. However, CandD frequently is not fully effective owing to limitations of cleaning, access, technique and disinfectants used (Davies and

Wray, 1995b; Davies and Breslin, 2003a; Wales *et al.*, 2006b, 2009; Mueller-Doblies *et al.*, 2010). Salmonellas are also often poorly controlled by CandD of calf accommodation (Wray *et al.*, 1987; Jones *et al.*, 2004; Wray and Davies, 2004).

The existence of physical niches that are difficult to clean or disinfect, plus the protective effect of organic residues and various survival features of *Salmonella* including oxidative resistance, biofilm formation, etc., render disinfectants less effective than laboratory assessments may predict (McLaren *et al.*, 2011). This is often compounded by the use of inappropriate disinfectant dilutions, inadequate technique and the permissive effect of moisture for growth among surviving *Salmonella*. In any contaminated farm unit, the elimination of *Salmonella* is favoured by a multifactorial approach, often needing repeated and thorough CandD, excellent control of vectors (particularly rodents) and the control of stock carriers by some combination of depopulation, vaccination and testing (Carrique-Mas *et al.*, 2009; Österberg, 2010). Where an uncommon or 'exotic' *Salmonella* serovar is persistent on premises and in stock despite vigorous attempts to eliminate it, a continuing feed source may be responsible, which can be difficult to trace with routine monitoring (Davies and Wales, 2010a).

Feed-Processing Plants

Modern farming practices make extensive use of prepared compounded feeds with multiple ingredients, and the subject is dealt with in depth in Chapter 19, this volume. Most protein ingredients of animal or vegetable origin are processed in a manner that should eliminate any *Salmonella* present in the raw materials. However, recontamination within the factory environment may occur after processing. Recontamination of cooked products can occur via leakage of untreated material from faulty cooker seals or via bio-aerosols or contact with contaminated surfaces (Bensink and Boland, 1979). *Salmonella* strains may establish themselves as endemic residents of diverse processing plants, including fishmeal, shellfish and oilseed processors and animal-feed compounders. (Davies and Wray, 1997; Nesse *et al.*, 2003; Morita *et al.*, 2004; Martinez-Urtaza and Liebana, 2005). Endemic strains are probably well adapted for the environmental conditions they inhabit, and this includes a capacity to form or join biofilm communities within cooling systems (Vestby *et al.*, 2009; Habimana *et al.*, 2010).

Detection of *Salmonella* in the Environment

The survival of *Salmonella* in dust is likely to be longer than survival in faeces or litter, thus rendering dust a more sensitive sampling medium for detection of infected poultry flocks in many cases. This is a function of the differential survival rates of *Salmonella* and competing organisms in the face of desiccation in dust (Wray and Davies, 1998). In feed mills, dust is also a good sample, by virtue of this differential survival plus the large surface area available for adsorption of *Salmonella* and the fact that it provides a natural subsample of a lot of the material that passes through the mill, which in itself may only be intermittently *Salmonella* positive. Intensive sampling of a mixture of matrices, including dust, may reveal *Salmonella* contamination that has been overlooked by routine monitoring (Davies and Wales, 2010b). Sampling floors and litter by means of boot 'socks' enhances isolation by allowing thorough and representative sampling of floor faecal material and dust whilst leaving the operator free to perform other tasks (Carrique-Mas and Davies, 2008). Issues of sample size, pooling and culture techniques for environmental samples have recently been reviewed (Carrique-Mas and Davies, 2008).

Vectors and Reservoirs

Rodents

Rodents are regarded as a potential risk to public health and rats are seen as an indication of unsatisfactory sanitation, although Healing (1991) concluded that they pose little direct *Salmonella* risk to humans in the UK. A high proportion of mice have been found to carry *S.* Enteritidis on poultry units where the same serovar is present in the stock (Davies and Wray, 1995a; Guard-Petter *et al.*, 1997), and there is a strong association between *Salmonella* in the stock and environment of layer units and *Salmonella* in associated mice (Henzler and Opitz, 1992; USDA, 2000).

When fed 10^3 or 10^5 cfu *S.* Enteritidis, wild mice excreted *Salmonella* for 5 weeks and 8 months, respectively. Chickens became infected when exposed to the faeces of mice infected 2 months previously with 10^5 cfu *Salmonella* (Davies and Wray, 1995a). Survey data support the view that poultry-house mouse faeces occasionally contains high numbers of *Salmonella* cells (Davies and Wray, 1995a; Wales *et al.*, 2006a), and rodents can become colonized and systemically infected for many months (Rabie *et al.*, 2010).

Mice need to be controlled as part of an overall plan of management of poultry units, in addition to efficient cleaning and disinfection, and there is evidence that good rodent control is a very significant factor for the absence (USDA, 2000; Garber *et al.*, 2003) and elimination (Carrique-Mas *et al.*, 2009) of *S.* Enterica in laying hen houses. Laying houses have more equipment (cages, nest boxes, etc.) and longer occupation times than other poultry accommodation, which may make them more vulnerable to the spread and maintenance of *Salmonella* via rodent infestation.

An association has also been made between rodent control and persistent *Salmonella* infections on pig units (Berends *et al.*, 1996; Wales *et al.*, 2009), and a study of cattle and sheep feed stored on barn floors resulted in estimates of an annual individual consumption of hundreds to thousands of rodent faecal pellets (Daniels *et al.*, 2003).

Arthropods

Evidence for the carriage and spread of *Salmonella* by arthropods (principally insects and acarids) has recently been reviewed (Wales *et al.*, 2010b). In general, a short-term vector role for arthropods and their larvae is inferred from observations of internal and external contamination of flies, beetles and their larvae on and around farms, plus experiments feeding contaminated arthropods to chicks. Insects may play a vector role by direct transfer between production units, by transfer to insectivorous birds or, in the case of wider-ranging flies, by transfer to human environments. Litter beetles can be relevant carriers on broiler and turkey farms where there is a short interval between successive flocks (Skov *et al.*, 2004), and control of litter beetles is becoming more difficult as resistance to acaricides increases. Heavy fly populations have been identified as a risk factor for *Salmonella* excretion by feedlot cattle in Australia (Vanselow *et al.*, 2007a).

Red mite (*Dermanyssus gallinae*), almost alone amongst arthropods, has been identified as a reservoir host for *Salmonella*. Mites will harbour (and retransmit experimentally to hens) *S.* Enteritidis for up to 14 days (Valiente Moro *et al.*, 2007) and *S.* Gallinarum biovar Gallinarum for in excess of 4 months (Zeman *et al.*, 1982; Parmar and Davies, 2007). Whilst transmission of *S.* Enteritidis does not appear to be an issue in the field, transmission via the feeding activities of red mites is the main means of spread and perpetuation of *S.* Gallinarum. The only way to eliminate red mites from an infested laying house is by expensive, prolonged heat treatment of houses and in some cases it is necessary to close farms or accept the permanent presence of fowl typhoid and the need for specific vaccination to reduce clinical disease. Some ticks can carry culturable *S.* Typhimurium naturally (Buriro, 1983), and experimentally they will harbour the serovar for many months and retransmit it to ducks by biting or when eaten (Glukhov, 1972).

Cockroaches have been reported to carry *Salmonella* in poultry units in the Middle East (Fathpour *et al.*, 2003) and in a hatchery and poultry feed mill in the USA (Kopanic *et al.*, 1994). These reports showed the transmission of salmonellae, including *S.* Typhimurium, on to other cockroaches and to eggshells. However, as with other insects, animals and birds, *Salmonella* in cockroaches may be a reflection of their environment, carried transiently as part of their gut flora as a result of feeding on sites contaminated with *Salmonella*, rather than being a primary source of the organisms.

Birds

Wild birds, particularly insectivorous birds such as swallows, rooks and cattle egrets, have been linked with the spread of *Salmonella* on cattle farms and in feedlots. In particular, dissemination of newly-emerged strains of monophasic *S.* Typhimurium (*S.* 4,[5],12:i:-) to poultry and cattle farms often appears to be associated with spread from pig farms via wild birds (Davies, 1997; Davies *et al.*, 2011). Gulls have been implicated in the transmission of *Salmonella* into and between fish-meal factories (Berg and Anderson, 1972; Nesse *et al.*, 2005). The spread or recycling of *Salmonella* infection among livestock by wild birds may occur through the contamination of water or feed, or the direct contamination of the environment (Watts and Wall, 1952; Daniels *et al.*, 2003).

The carriage of *Salmonella* by healthy wild birds is typically low and transient, and appears to reflect the serovars found in identified local sources such as farms, feed mills, rubbish tips and isolated ecosystems (Hart *et al.*, 1987; Cizek *et al.*, 1994; Davies and Wray, 1997; Skov *et al.*, 2008). None the less, gulls in particular appear to have a capacity to carry *Salmonella* over larger distances (Cizek *et al.*, 1994; Nesse *et al.*, 2005).

Whereas only 0.4% of trapped wild birds yielded *Salmonella* from cloacal swabs, 2.9% of 382 dead wild birds representing a diversity of UK bird types had *Salmonella* (Goodchild and Tucker, 1968). A higher percentage (22.5%) of 698 dead British garden birds examined by Lawson *et al.* (2010) was diagnosed with salmonellosis. Currently, *S.* Typhimurium is associated with a relatively high proportion of deaths among certain species of British wild passerine birds, although the strains involved appear to be largely restricted to those wild bird populations (Hughes *et al.*, 2008, 2010). Contemporary studies in several countries show widely varying findings, particularly in terms of prevalence, and many factors (such as species differences in feeding preferences and inherent resistance, geographical variations and methodologies) remain to be clarified (Skov *et al.*, 2008).

Wild animals

Animals in the natural environment may be reservoirs of *Salmonella*, irrespective of the country or region. These include wild animals, such as opossums (Runkel *et al.*, 1991) and hedgehogs (Keymer *et al.*, 1991), and domesticated animals including dogs, whether strays (Sugiyama *et al.*, 1993), household pets or kennel dogs (Shimi *et al.*, 1976), cats and reptiles (Borland, 1975). The serovars associated with reptiles and reptilian-associated infections are similar and are often unusual compared with the serovars within a human community (Ackman *et al.*, 1995).

Certain serovars (e.g. Binza and Agama) are associated with badgers in the UK (Wray *et al.*, 1977; Wilson *et al.*, 2003), and these same serovars are often encountered in domestically produced cereal ingredients (Davies and Hinton, 2000). This illustrates one of the routes by which *Salmonella* from wildlife that co-exists with crops can get into the human and livestock food chain.

Many wild animals are scavengers, although it is extremely difficult to investigate their microbial flora in pristine environments that are unaffected, either directly or indirectly, by the activities of humans. Scavengers, including rodents and opossums, in Panama had higher carriage rates of *Salmonella* than non-scavengers, most infected animals being near areas associated with human activity (Kourany *et al.*, 1976). *Salmonella* was isolated frequently from feral pigs and kangaroos in Australia, and often the serovars found were associated with humans (Murray, 2000).

Conclusion

Salmonella is a common and diverse pathogen that proves to be a hardy environmental contaminant in consequence of its lifestyle, cycling through animal alimentary tracts. The development of modern agricultural systems and breeds provides opportunities for larger-scale environmental contamination and transfer of *Salmonella* than previously, but conversely advances in understanding provide scope for better strategic control of *Salmonella*. Human populations and their activities provide ever greater opportunities for the concentration, recycling and dissemination of *Salmonella*. Therefore it is unrealistic to anticipate the elimination of *Salmonella* risk from human and domestic animal environments, but monitoring and understanding the role of environmental *Salmonella* provides tools for managing that risk.

References

Ackman, D.M., Drabkin, P., Birkhead, G. and Cieslak, P. (1995) Reptile-associated salmonellosis in New York State. *Pediatric Infectious Disease Journal* 14, 955–959.

Altekruse, S., Koehler, J., Hickman-Brenner, F., Tauxe, R.V. and Ferris, K. (1993) A comparison of *Salmonella enteritidis* phage types from egg-associated outbreaks and implicated laying flocks. *Epidemiology and Infection* 110, 17–22.

Amel, D. and Amina, B. (2007) Fate of *Salmonella typhimurium* on rosemary and barley grown in fields treated with contaminated irrigation water. *African Journal of Microbiology Research* 1, 42–45.

Anderson, R.J., House, J.K., Smith, B.P., Kinde, H., Walker, R.L., Vande Steeg, B.J. *et al.* (2001) Epidemiologic and biological characteristics of salmonellosis in three dairy herds. *Journal of the American Veterinary Medical Association* 219, 310–322.

Arana, I., Muela, A., Iriberri, J., Egea, L. and Barcina, I. (1992) Role of hydrogen peroxide in loss of culturability mediated by visible light in *Escherichia coli* in a freshwater ecosystem. *Applied and Environmental Microbiology* 58, 3903–3907.

Archer, J., Jervis, E.T., Bird, J. and Gaze, J.E. (1998) Heat resistance of *Salmonella weltevreden* in low-moisture environments. *Journal of Food Protection* 61, 969–973.

Arthurson, V., Sessitsch, A. and Jäderlund, L. (2011) Persistence and spread of *Salmonella enterica* serovar Weltevreden in soil and on spinach plants. *FEMS Microbiology Letters* 314, 67–74.

Bailey, J.S., Cox, N.A., Craven, S.E. and Cosby, D.E. (2002) Serotype tracking of *Salmonella* through integrated broiler chicken operations. *Journal of Food Protection* 65, 742–745.

Barak, J.D. and Liang, A.S. (2008) Role of soil, crop debris, and a plant pathogen in *Salmonella enterica* contamination of tomato plants. *PLoS ONE* 3, e1657.

Barcina, I., Lebaron, P. and Vives-Rego, J. (1997) Survival of allochthonous bacteria in aquatic systems: a biological approach. *FEMS Microbiology Ecology* 23, 1–9.

Baudart, J., Lemarchand, K., Brisabois, A. and Lebaron, P. (2000a) Diversity of *Salmonella* strains isolated from the aquatic environment as determined by serotyping and amplification of the ribosomal DNA spacer regions. *Applied and Environmental Microbiology* 66, 1544–1552.

Baudart, J., Grabulos, J., Barusseau, J.P. and Lebaron, P. (2000b) *Salmonella* spp. and fecal coliform loads in coastal waters from a point vs. nonpoint source of pollution. *Journal of Environmental Quality* 29, 241–250.

Bell, C.A.K. (2002) *Foodborne Pathogens*. Wood Head Publishing, CRC Press, Cambridge, UK.

Bensink, J.C. and Boland, P.H. (1979) Possible pathways of contamination of meat and bone meal with *Salmonella*. *Australian Veterinary Journal* 55, 521–524.

Berends, B.R., Urlings, H.A.P., Snijders, J.M.A. and Knapen, F.V. (1996) Identification and quantification of risk factors in animal management and transport regarding *Salmonella* spp. in pigs. *International Journal of Food Microbiology* 30, 37–53.

Berg, R.W. and Anderson, A.W. (1972) Salmonellae and *Edwardsiella tarda* in gull feces: a source of contamination in fish processing plants. *Applied Microbiology* 24, 501–503.

Borland, E.D. (1975) *Salmonella* infection in dogs, cats, tortoises and terrapins. *Veterinary Record* 96, 401–402.

Brandl, M.T., Rosenthal, B.M., Haxo, A.F. and Berk, S.G. (2005) Enhanced survival of *Salmonella enterica* in vesicles released by a soilborne *Tetrahymena* species. *Applied and Environmental Microbiology* 71, 1562–1569.

Broennum Pedersen, T., Elmerdahl Olsen, J. and Bisgaard, M. (2008) Persistence of *Salmonella* Senftenberg in poultry production environments and investigation of its resistance to desiccation. *Avian Pathology* 37, 421–427.

Brown, M.R., Collier, P.J. and Gilbert, P. (1990) Influence of growth rate on susceptibility to antimicrobial agents: modification of the cell envelope and batch and continuous culture studies. *Antimicrobial Agents and Chemotherapy* 34, 1623–1628.

Buriro, S.N. (1983) Relative abundance of different species of bacteria isolated from *Argas (persicargas) persicus,* Oken. *Pakistan Veterinary Journal* 3, 126–128.

Burton, G.A., Jr, Gunnison, D. and Lanza, G.R. (1987) Survival of pathogenic bacteria in various freshwater sediments. *Applied and Environmental Microbiology* 53, 633–638.

Byrd, J.A., DeLoach, J.R., Corrier, D.E., Nisbet, D.J. and Stanker, L.H. (1999) Evaluation of *Salmonella* serotype distributions from commercial broiler hatcheries and grower houses. *Avian Diseases* 43, 39–47.

Carrique-Mas, J. and Davies, R.H. (2008) Sampling and bacteriological detection of *Salmonella* in poultry and poultry premises: a review. *Revue Scientifique et Technique (Office International des Épizooties)* 27, 665–677.

Carrique-Mas, J.J., Breslin, M., Snow, L., McLaren, I., Sayers, A.R. and Davies, R.H. (2009) Persistence and clearance of different *Salmonella* serovars in buildings housing laying hens. *Epidemiology and Infection* 137, 837–846.

Catalao Dionisio, L.P., Joao, M., Soares Ferreiro, V., Leonor Fidalgo, M., García Rosado, M.E. and Borrego, J.J. (2000) Occurrence of *Salmonella* spp in estuarine and coastal waters of Portugal. *Antonie Van Leeuwenhoek* 78, 99–106.

Charkowski, A.O., Barak, J.D., Sarreal, C.Z. and Mandrell, R.E. (2002) Differences in growth of *Salmonella enterica* and *Escherichia coli* O157:H7 on alfalfa sprouts. *Applied and Environmental Microbiology* 68, 3114–3120.

Chinivasagam, H.N., Redding, M., Runge, G. and Blackall, P.J. (2010) Presence and incidence of food-borne pathogens in Australian chicken litter. *British Poultry Science* 51, 311–318.

Chmielewski, R.A.N. and Frank, J.F. (1995) Formation of viable but nonculturable *Salmonella* during starvation in chemically defined solutions. *Letters in Applied Microbiology* 20, 380–384.

Cho, J.-C. and Kim, S.-J. (1999) Viable, but non-culturable, state of a green fluorescence protein-tagged environmental isolate of *Salmonella typhi* in groundwater and pond water. *FEMS Microbiology Letters* 170, 257–264.

Christensen, J.P., Brown, D.J., Madsen, M., Olsen, J.E. and Bisgaard, M. (1997) Hatchery-borne *Salmonella enterica* serovar Tennessee infections in broilers. *Avian Pathology* 26, 155–168.

Cizek, A., Literak, I., Hejlicek, K., Treml, F. and Smola, J. (1994) *Salmonella* contamination of the environment and its incidence in wild birds. *Journal of Veterinary Medicine Series B - Infectious Diseases and Veterinary Public Health* 41, 320–327.

Cooley, M.B., Miller, W.G. and Mandrell, R.E. (2003) Colonization of *Arabidopsis thaliana* with *Salmonella enterica* and Enterohemorrhagic *Escherichia coli* O157:H7 and competition by *Enterobacter asburiae. Applied and Environmental Microbiology* 69, 4915–4926.

Cote, C. and Quessy, S. (2005) Persistence of *Escherichia coli* and *Salmonella* in surface soil following application of liquid hog manure for production of pickling cucumbers. *Journal of Food Protection* 68, 900–905.

Daniels, M.J., Hutchings, M.R. and Greig, A. (2003) The risk of disease transmission to livestock posed by contamination of farm stored feed by wildlife excreta. *Epidemiology and Infection* 130, 561–568.

Danielsson, M.L. (1977) *Salmonella* in sewage and sludge serological profiles of isolates their removal and-or survival in relation to potential health hazards to man and animals. *Acta Veterinaria Scandinavica* 1, 126.

Danyluk, M.D., Nozawa-Inoue, M., Hristova, K.R., Scow, K.M., Lampinen, B. and Harris, L.J. (2008) Survival and growth of *Salmonella* Enteritidis PT 30 in almond orchard soils. *Journal of Applied Microbiology* 104, 1391–1399.

Davies, R.H. (1997) A two year study of *Salmonella typhimurium* DT 104 infection and contamination on cattle farms. *Cattle Practice* 5, 189–194.

Davies, R.H. and Bedford, S. (2001) Observations on *Salmonella* contamination in five turkey hatcheries. *Research in Veterinary Science* 70, 26.

Davies, R. and Breslin, M. (2003a) Observations on *Salmonella* contamination of commercial laying farms before and after cleaning and disinfection. *Veterinary Record* 152, 283–287.

Davies, R.H. and Breslin, M. (2003b) Persistence of *Salmonella* Enteritidis phage type 4 in the environment and arthropod vectors on an empty free-range chicken farm. *Environmental Microbiology* 5, 79–84.

Davies, R. and Carrique-Mas, J. (2010) Clearance of *Salmonella* from laying flocks after eradication of rodents from laying houses. *Proceedings of the I3S International Symposium 'Salmonella and Salmonellosis'*, St Malo, France, 28–30 June, pp. 435–437.

Davies, R.H. and Cook, A.J. (2008) Why has the UK pig industry more *Salmonella* than other European pig industries and how can we lift our position? *Proceedings of 'Pigs': Meeting of Society of Feed Technologists and Home Grown Cereals Authority*, Coventry, UK, 6 November.

Davies, R.H. and Hinton, M.H. (2000) *Salmonella* in animal feed. In: Wray, C. and Wray, A. (eds) *Salmonella in Domestic Animals*, 1st edn. CAB International, Oxford, England, pp. 285–300.

Davies, R. and Wales, A. (2010a) Investigations into *Salmonella* contamination in poultry feedmills in the United Kingdom. *Journal of Applied Microbiology* 109, 1430–1440.

Davies, R.H. and Wales, A.D. (2010b) Investigations into *Salmonella* contamination in poultry feedmills in the United Kingdom. *Journal of Applied Microbiology* 109, 1430–1440.

Davies, R.H. and Wray, C. (1995a) Mice as carriers of *Salmonella* Enteritidis on persistently infected poultry units. *Veterinary Record* 137, 337–341.

Davies, R.H. and Wray, C. (1995b) Observations on disinfection regimens used on *Salmonella* Enteritidis infected poultry units. *Poultry Science* 74, 638–647.

Davies, R.H. and Wray, C. (1996a) Persistence of *Salmonella enteritidis* in poultry units and poultry food. *British Poultry Science* 37, 589–596.

Davies, R.H. and Wray, C. (1996b) Seasonal variations in the isolation of *Salmonella typhimurium*, *Salmonella enteritidis*, *Bacillus cereus* and *Clostridium perfringens* from environmental samples. *Journal of Veterinary Medicine Series B* 43, 119–127.

Davies, R.H. and Wray, C. (1997) Distribution of salmonella contamination in ten animal feedmills. *Veterinary Microbiology* 57, 159–169.

Davies, R.H., Bedford, S. and Shankster, S. (2001a) Enhanced culture techniques for detection of *Salmonella*. *Veterinary Record* 148, 539–540.

Davies, R.H., Bedford, S. and McLaren, I.M. (2001b) A six year study of the persistence of *Salmonella* Typhimurium DT104 on a farrow to finish pig farm. *Proceedings of the 4th International Symposium on the Epidemiology and Control of Salmonella and other Foodborne Pathogens in Pork*, Leipzig, Germany, 2–5 September, pp. 265–273.

Davies, R., Mueller-Doblies, D., Martelli, F. and Breslin, M. (2011) Observations on the distribution of monophasic *Salmonella* Typhimurium on pig farms in Great Britain. *Proceedings of the 9th International Conference on the Epidemiology and Control of Biological, Chemical and Physical hazards in Pigs and Pork (SafePork 2011)*, Maastricht, the Netherlands, 19–22 June, pp. 110–113.

de Nardi, I.R., Del Nery, V., Amorim, A.K.B., dos Santos, N.G. and Chimenes, F. (2011) Performances of SBR, chemical-DAF and UV disinfection for poultry slaughterhouse wastewater reclamation. *Desalination* 269, 184–189.

Degnan, A.J. (2008) Examination of indigenous microbiota and survival of *Escherichia coli* O157 and *Salmonella* in a paper milling environment. *Journal of Applied Microbiology* 104, 534–540.

Dupray, E., Derrien, A. and Pichon, R. (1995) Osmoregulation by trehalose synthesis in *Salmonella manhattan* after exposure to waste waters. *Letters in Applied Microbiology* 20, 148–151.

Durrant, D.S. and Beatson, S.H. (1981) Salmonellae isolated from domestic meat waste. *Journal of Hygiene* 86, 259–264.

EFSA (2010) Scientific Opinion on a quantitative estimate of the public health impact of setting a new target for the reduction of *Salmonella* in laying hens. *EFSA Journal* 8, 1546.

Erill, I., Campoy, S. and Barbé, J. (2007) Aeons of distress: an evolutionary perspective on the bacterial SOS response. *FEMS Microbiology Reviews* 31, 637–656.

Evans, S. and Davies, R. (1996) Case control study of multiple-resistant *Salmonella* typhimurium DT104 infection of cattle in Great Britain. *Veterinary Record* 139, 557–558.

Fathpour, H., Emtiazi, G. and Ghasemi, E. (2003) Cockroaches as reservoirs and vectors of drug resistant *Salmonella* spp. *Fresenius Environmental Bulletin* 12, 724–727.

Fish, J.T. and Pettibone, G.W. (1995) Influence of freshwater sediment on the survival of *Escherichia coli* and *Salmonella* sp. as measured by three methods of enumeration. *Letters in Applied Microbiology* 20, 277–281.

Fossler, C.P., Wells, S.J., Kaneene, J.B., Ruegg, P.L., Warnick, L.D., Eberly, L.E. *et al.* (2005) Cattle and environmental sample-level factors associated with the presence of *Salmonella* in a multi-state study of conventional and organic dairy farms. *Preventive Veterinary Medicine* 67, 39–53.

Foster, J.W. and Spector, M.P. (1995) How *Salmonella* survive against the odds. *Annual Review of Microbiology* 49, 145–174.

Fransen, N.G., van den Elzen, A.M., Urlings, B.A. and Bijker, P.G. (1996) Pathogenic micro-organisms in slaughterhouse sludge – a survey. *International Journal of Food Microbiology* 33, 245–256.

Garber, L., Smeltzer, M., Fedorka-Cray, P., Ladely, S. and Ferris, K. (2003) *Salmonella enterica* serotype Enteritidis in table egg layer house environments and in mice in US layer houses and associated risk factors. *Avian Diseases* 47, 134–142.

García, R., Bælum, J., Fredslund, L., Santorum, P. and Jacobsen, C.S. (2010) Influence of temperature and predation on survival of *Salmonella enterica* serovar Typhimurium and expression of *invA* in soil and manure-amended soil. *Applied and Environmental Microbiology* 76, 5025–5031.

Gay, J.M. and Hunsaker, M.E. (1993) Isolation of multiple *Salmonella* serovars from a dairy two years after a clinical salmonellosis outbreak. *Journal of the American Veterinary Medical Association* 203, 1314–1320.

Gaze, W.H., Burroughs, N., Gallagher, M.P. and Wellington, E.M.H. (2003) Interactions between *Salmonella typhimurium* and *Andacanthamoeba polyphaga*, and observation of a new mode of intracellular growth within contractile vacuoles. *Microbial Ecology* 46, 358–369.

Gibson, D.L., White, A.P., Snyder, S.D., Martin, S., Heiss, C., Azadi, P. *et al.* (2006) *Salmonella* produces an O-antigen capsule regulated by AgfD and important for environmental persistence. *Journal of Bacteriology* 188, 7722–7730.

Glaus, H. and Heinemeyer, E.A. (1994) The elimination of *Salmonella typhimurium* in coastal waters with various levels of microbiologically hygienic contamination. *Zentralblatt fur Hygiene und Umweltmedizin* 196, 312–326.

Glukhov, V.F. (1972) The role of ticks in the dissemination of fowl paratyphoid. *Veterinariya (Moscow)* 4, 49–50.

Goodchild, W.M. and Tucker, J.F. (1968) Salmonellae in British wild birds and their transfer to domestic fowl. *British Veterinary Journal* 124, 95–101.

Guard-Petter, J., Henzler, D.J., Rahman, M.M. and Carlson, R.W. (1997) On-farm monitoring of mouse-invasive *Salmonella enterica* serovar enteritidis and a model for its association with the production of contaminated eggs. *Applied and Environmental Microbiology* 63, 1588–1593.

Guo, X., Chen, J., Brackett, R. and Beuchat, L. (2002) Survival of *Salmonella* on tomatoes stored at high relative humidity, in soil, and on tomatoes in contact with soil. *Journal of Food Protection* 65, 274–279.

Gupte, A.R., de Rezende, C.L.E. and Joseph, S.W. (2003) Induction and resuscitation of viable but nonculturable *Salmonella enterica* serovar Typhimurium DT104. *Applied and Environmental Microbiology* 69, 6669–6675.

Habimana, O., Moretro, T., Langsrud, S., Vestby, L., Nesse, L. and Heir, E. (2010) Micro ecosystems from feed industry surfaces: a survival and biofilm study of *Salmonella* versus host resident flora strains. *BMC Veterinary Research* 6, 48.

Harbaugh, E., Trampel, D., Wesley, I., Hoff, S., Griffith, R. and Hurd, H. S. (2006) Rapid aerosol transmission of salmonella among turkeys in a simulated holding-shed environment. *Poultry Science* 85, 1693–1699.

Hart, R.P., Iveson, J.B. and Bradshaw, S.D. (1987) The ecology of *Salmonella* serotypes in a wild marsupial (the quokka *Setonix brachyurus*) in a disturbed environment. *Australian Journal of Ecology* 12, 267–279.

Healing, T.D. (1991) *Salmonella* in rodents: a risk to man? *Communicable Diseases Review* 1, R114–116.

Hebrard, M., Viala, J.P.M., Meresse, P., Barras, F. and Aussel, L. (2009) Redundant hydrogen peroxide scavengers contribute to *Salmonella* virulence and oxidative stress resistance. *Journal of Bacteriology* 191, 4605–4614.

Heinitz, M.L., Ruble, R.D., Wagner, D.E. and Tatini, S.R. (2000) Incidence of *Salmonella* in fish and seafood. *Journal of Food Protection* 63, 579–592.

Henzler, D.J. and Opitz, H.M. (1992) The role of mice in the epizootiology of *Salmonella enteritidis* infection on chicken layer farms. *Avian Diseases* 36, 625–631.

Hernroth, B., Lothigius, Å. and Bölin, I. (2010) Factors influencing survival of enterotoxigenic *Escherichia coli*, *Salmonella enterica* (serovar Typhimurium) and *Vibrio parahaemolyticus* in marine environments. *FEMS Microbiology Ecology* 71, 272–280.

Heyndrickx, M., Vandekerchove, D., Herman, L., Rollier, I., Grijspeerdt, K. and De Zutter, L. (2002) Routes for salmonella contamination of poultry meat: epidemiological study from hatchery to slaughterhouse. *Epidemiology and Infection* 129, 253–265.

Hijnen, W.A.M., Beerendonk, E.F. and Medema, G.J. (2006) Inactivation credit of UV radiation for viruses, bacteria and protozoan (oo)cysts in water: A review. *Water Research* 40, 3–22.

Himathongkham, S., Pereira, M.G. and Riemann, H. (1996) Heat destruction of *Salmonella* in poultry feed: effect of time, temperature, and moisture. *Avian Diseases* 40, 72–77.

Himathongkham, S., Nuanualsuwan, S. and Riemann, H. (1999) Survival of *Salmonella enteritidis* and *Salmonella typhimurium* in chicken manure at different levels of water activity. *FEMS Microbiology Letters* 172, 159–163.

Hintz, L.D., Boyer, R.R., Ponder, M.A., Williams, R.C. and Rideout, S.L. (2010) Recovery of *Salmonella enterica* Newport introduced through irrigation water from tomato (*Lycopersicum esculentum*) fruit, roots, stems, and leaves. *HortScience* 45, 675–678.

Hoff, J.C. and Akin, E.W. (1986) Microbial resistance to disinfectants – mechanisms and significance. *Environmental Health Perspectives* 69, 7–13.

Holley, R., Walkty, J., Blank, G., Tenuta, M., Ominski, K., Krause, D. *et al.* (2008) Examination of *Salmonella* and *Escherichia coli* translocation from hog manure to forage, soil, and cattle grazed on the hog manure-treated pasture. *Journal of Environmental Quality* 37, 2083–2092.

Hoover, N.J., Kenney, P.B., Amick, J.D. and Hypes, W.A. (1997) Preharvest sources of *Salmonella* colonization in turkey production. *Poultry Science* 76, 1232–1238.

Horswell, J., Hewitt, J., Prosser, J., Van Schaik, A., Croucher, D., Macdonald, C. *et al.* (2010) Mobility and survival of *Salmonella* Typhimurium and human adenovirus from spiked sewage sludge applied to soil columns. *Journal of Applied Microbiology* 108, 104–114.

Hughes, L., Shopland, S., Wigley, P., Bradon, H., Leatherbarrow, A.H., Williams, N. *et al.* (2008) Characterisation of *Salmonella enterica* serotype Typhimurium isolates from wild birds in northern England from 2005 - 2006. *BMC Veterinary Research* 4, 4.

Hughes, L.A., Wigley, P., Bennett, M., Chantrey, J. and Williams, N. (2010) Multi-locus sequence typing of *Salmonella enterica* serovar Typhimurium isolates from wild birds in northern England suggests host-adapted strain. *Letters in Applied Microbiology* 51, 477–479.

Humphrey, T. (2004) *Salmonella*, stress responses and food safety. *Nature Reviews Microbiology* 2, 504–509.

Hunter, P.R. and Izsak, J. (1990) Diversity studies of *Salmonella* incidents in some domestic livestock and their potential relevance as indicators of niche width. *Epidemiology and Infection* 105, 501–510.

Hussong, D., Burge, W.D. and Enkiri, N.K. (1985) Occurrence, growth, and suppression of salmonellae in composted sewage sludge. *Applied and Environmental Microbiology* 50, 887–893.

Irwin, R.J., Poppe, C., Messier, S., Finley, G.G. and Oggel, J. (1994) A national survey to estimate the prevalence of *Salmonella* species among Canadian registered commercial turkey flocks. *Canadian Journal of Veterinary Research* 58, 263–267.

Islam, M., Morgan, J., Doyle, M.P., Phatak, S.C., Millner, P. and Jiang, X. (2004) Fate of *Salmonella enterica* serovar Typhimurium on carrots and radishes grown in fields treated with contaminated manure composts or irrigation water. *Applied and Environmental Microbiology* 70, 2497–2502.

Jablasone, J., Brovko, L.Y. and Griffiths, M.W. (2004) A research note: the potential for transfer of *Salmonella* from irrigation water to tomatoes. *Journal of the Science of Food and Agriculture* 84, 287–289.

Jackson, G.F. (1996) Delivery of microbial indicator organisms to coastal waters from catchment sources. *Water Science and Technology* 33(2), 37–50.

Jayaraman, R. (2008) Bacterial persistence: some new insights into an old phenomenon. *Journal of Biosciences* 33, 795–805.

Joerger, R.D. (2003) Alternatives to antibiotics: bacteriocins, antimicrobial peptides and bacteriophages. *Poultry Science* 82, 640–647.

Jones, F.T. (2011) A review of practical *Salmonella* control measures in animal feed. *Journal of Applied Poultry Research* 20, 102–113.

Jones, K. and Bradshaw, S.B. (1997) Synergism in biofilm formation between *Salmonella enteritidis* and a nitrogen-fixing strain of *Klebsiella pneumoniae*. *Journal of Applied Microbiology* 82, 663–668.

Jones, P.W. (1975) The effect of storage in slurry on the virulence of *Salmonella dublin*. *Journal of Hygiene* 74, 65–70.

Jones, P.W. (1980) Animal health today – problems of large livestock units. Disease hazards associated with slurry disposal. *British Veterinary Journal* 136, 529–542.

Jones, P.W., Rennison, L.M., Lewin, V.H. and Redhead, D.L. (1980) The occurrence and significance to animal health of salmonellas in sewage and sewage sludges. *Journal of Hygiene* 84, 47–62.

Jones, P.W., Watson, P.R. and Wallis, T.S. (2004) Salmonellosis. In: Andrews, A.H., Blowey, R.W., Boyd, H. and Eddy, R.G. (eds) *Bovine Medicine – Diseases and Husbandry of Cattle*, 2nd edn. Blackwell Science, Oxford, UK, pp. 215–230.

Kaprelyants, A.S., Mukamolova, G.V. and Kell, D.B. (1994) Estimation of dormant *Micrococcus luteus* cells by penicillin lysis and by resuscitation in cell-free spent culture medium at high dilution. *FEMS Microbiology Letters* 115, 347–352.

Keymer, I.F., Gibson, E.A. and Reynolds, D.J. (1991) Zoonoses and other findings in hedgehogs (*Erinaceus europaeus*): a survey of mortality and review of the literature. *Veterinary Record* 128, 245–249.

Kieboom, J., Kusumaningrum, H., Tempelaars, M., Hazeleger, W., Abee, T. and Beumer, R. (2006) Survival, elongation, and elevated tolerance of *Salmonella enterica* serovar Enteritidis at reduced water activity. *Journal of Food Protection* 69, 2681–2686.

Kinde, H., Read, D.H., Chin, R.P., Bickford, A.A., Walker, R.L., Ardans, A. *et al.* (1996) *Salmonella enteritidis*, phage type 4 infection in a commercial layer flock in southern California: bacteriologic and epidemiologic findings. *Avian Diseases* 40, 665–671.

Kirby, R.M. and Davies, R. (1990) Survival of dehydrated cells of *Salmonella typhimurium* LT2 at high temperatures. *Journal of Applied Bacteriology* 68, 241–246.

Kopanic, R.J., Jr, Sheldon, B.W. and Wright, C.G. (1994) Cockroaches as vectors of *Salmonella*: laboratory and field trials. *Journal of Food Protection* 57, 125–132.

Kourany, M., Bowdre, L. and Herrer, A. (1976) Panamanian forest mammals as carriers of *Salmonella*. *American Journal of Tropical Medicine and Hygiene* 25, 449–455.

Krapf, T. and Gantenbein-Demarchi, C. (2010) Thermal inactivation of *Salmonella* spp. during conching. *LWT - Food Science and Technology* 43, 720–723.

Kwon, Y.M., Park, S.Y., Birkhold, S.G. and Ricke, S.C. (2000) Induction of resistance of *Salmonella typhimurium* to environmental stresses by exposure to short-chain fatty acids. *Journal of Food Science* 65, 1037–1040.

Lambert, P.A. (2004) Mechanisms of action of biocides. In: Fraise, A.P., Lambert, P.A. and Maillard, J.-Y. (eds) *Russell, Hugo and Ayliffe's Principles and Practice of Disinfection, Preservation and Sterilization*. Blackwell, Oxford, UK, pp. 139–153.

Lapidot, A. and Yaron, S. (2009) Transfer of *Salmonella enterica* serovar Typhimurium from contaminated irrigation water to parsley is dependent on curli and cellulose, the biofilm matrix components. *Journal of Food Protection* 72, 618–623.

Lapidot, A., Romling, U. and Yaron, S. (2006) Biofilm formation and the survival of *Salmonella* Typhimurium on parsley. *International Journal of Food Microbiology* 109, 229–233.

Larsen, H.F., Munch, B. and Schlundt, J. (1994) Use of indicators for monitoring the reduction of pathogens in animal waste treated in biogas plants. *Zentralblatt fur Hygiene und Umweltmedizin* 195, 544–555.

Lasagabaster, A., Arboleya, J.C. and de Maranon, I.M. (2011) Pulsed light technology for surface decontamination of eggs: impact on *Salmonella* inactivation and egg quality. *Innovative Food Science and Emerging Technologies* 12, 124–128.

Lawson, B., Howard, T., Kirkwood, J., Macgregor, S., Perkins, M., Robinson, R. *et al.* (2010) Epidemiology of salmonellosis in garden birds in England and Wales, 1993 to 2003. *EcoHealth* 7, 294–306.

Lever, M.S. and Williams, A. (1996) Cross-infection of chicks by airborne transmission of *Salmonella enteritidis* PT4. *Letters in Applied Microbiology* 23, 347–349.

Linklater, K.A., Graham, M.M. and Sharp, J.C. (1985) Salmonellae in sewage sludge and abattoir effluent in south-east Scotland. *Journal of Hygiene* 94, 301–307.

Lo Fo Wong, D.M.A., Dahl, J., Stege, H., van der Wolf, P.J., Leontides, L., von Altrock, A. *et al.* (2004) Herd-level risk factors for subclinical *Salmonella* infection in European finishing-pig herds. *Preventive Veterinary Medicine* 62, 253–266.

Marsh, P., Morris, N.Z. and Wellington, E.M.H. (1998) Quantitative molecular detection of *Salmonella typhimurium* in soil and demonstration of persistence of an active but non-culturable population. *FEMS Microbiology Ecology* 27, 351–363.

Martinez-Urtaza, J. and Liebana, E. (2005) Investigation of clonal distribution and persistence of *Salmonella* Senftenberg in the marine environment and identification of potential sources of contamination. *FEMS Microbiology Ecology* 52, 255–263.

Martinez-Urtaza, J., Liebana, E., Garcia-Migura, L., Perez-Pineiro, P. and Saco, M. (2004a) Characterization of *Salmonella enterica* serovar Typhimurium from marine environments in coastal waters of Galicia (Spain). *Applied and Environmental Microbiology* 70, 4030–4034.

Martinez-Urtaza, J., Saco, M., de Novoa, J., Perez-Pineiro, P., Peiteado, J., Lozano-Leon, A. *et al.* (2004b) Influence of environmental factors and human activity on the presence of *Salmonella* serovars in a marine environment. *Applied and Environmental Microbiology* 70, 2089–2097.

Massé, D., Gilbert, Y. and Topp, E. (2011) Pathogen removal in farm-scale psychrophilic anaerobic digesters processing swine manure. *Bioresource Technology* 102, 641–646.

Mattick, K.L., Jorgensen, F., Legan, J.D., Cole, M.B., Porter, J., Lappin-Scott, H.M. *et al.* (2000) Survival and filamentation of *Salmonella enterica* serovar Enteritidis PT4 and *Salmonella enterica* serovar Typhimurium DT104 at low water activity. *Applied and Environmental Microbiology* 66, 1274–1279.

McDonnell, G. and Russell, A.D. (1999) Antiseptics and disinfectants: activity, action, and resistance. *Clinical Microbiology Reviews* 12, 147–179.

McDougald, D., Rice, S.A., Weichart, D. and Kjelleberg, S. (1998) Nonculturability: adaptation or debilitation? *FEMS Microbiology Ecology* 25, 1–9.

McLaren, I., Wales, A., Breslin, M. and Davies, R. (2011) Evaluation of commonly-used farm disinfectants in wet and dry models of *Salmonella* farm contamination. *Avian Pathology* 40, 33–42.

McMeechan, A., Roberts, M., Cogan, T.A., Jørgensen, F., Stevenson, A., Lewis, C. *et al.* (2007) Role of the alternative sigma factors σ^E and σ^S in survival of *Salmonella enterica* serovar Typhimurium during starvation, refrigeration and osmotic shock. *Microbiology* 153, 263–269.

Miles, J., Sumner, S., Boyer, R., Williams, R., Latimer, J. and McKinney, J. (2009) Internalization of *Salmonella enterica* serovar Montevideo into greenhouse tomato plants through contaminated irrigation water or seed stock. *Journal of Food Protection* 72, 849–852.

Mitscherlich, E. and Marth, E.H. (1984) *Microbial Survival in the Environment*. Springer-Verlag, Berlin.

Moore, B.C., Martinez, E., Gay, J.M. and Rice, D.H. (2003) Survival of *Salmonella enterica* in freshwater and sediments and transmission by the aquatic midge *Chironomus tentans* (Chironomidae: Diptera). *Applied and Environmental Microbiology* 69, 4556–4560.

Moreno, M., Audia, J.P., Bearson, S.M.D., Webb, C. and Foster, J.W. (2000) Regulation of sigma S degradation in *Salmonella enterica* var *typhimurium*: *in vivo* interactions between sigma S, the response regulator MviA(RssB) and ClpX. *Journal of Molecular Microbiology and Biotechnology* 2, 245–254.

Morgan-Jones, S.C. (1980) The occurrence of salmonellae during the rearing of broiler birds. *British Poultry Science* 21, 463–470.

Moriñigo, M.A., Cornax, R., Muñoz, M.A., Romero, P. and Borrego, J.J. (1989) Viability of *Salmonella* species in natural waters. *Current Microbiology* 18, 267–273.

Morita, T., Kitazawa, H., Iida, T. and Kamata, S. (2004) Examination about survival of *Salmonella* in the environment of an oil-meal manufacturing plant. *Japanese Journal of Animal Hygiene* 30, 75–83.

Muela, A., Garcia-Bringas, J.M., Arana, I. and Barcina, I. (2000) The effect of simulated solar radiation on *Escherichia coli*: The relative roles of UV-B, UV-A, and photosynthetically active radiation. *Microbial Ecology* 39, 65–71.

Mueller-Doblies, D., Carrique-Mas, J.J., Sayers, A.R. and Davies, R.H. (2010) A comparison of the efficacy of different disinfection methods in eliminating *Salmonella* contamination from turkey houses. *Journal of Applied Microbiology* 109, 471–479.

Munro, P.M., Flatau, G.N., Clement, R.L. and Gauthier, M.J. (1995) Influence of the RpoS (KatF) sigma factor on maintenance of viability and culturability of *Escherichia coli* and *Salmonella typhimurium* in seawater. *Applied and Environmental Microbiology* 61, 1853–1858.

Murray, C.J. (1991) Salmonellae in the environment. *Revue Scientifique et Technique (Office International des Épizooties)* 10, 765–785.

Murray, C.J. (2000) Environmental aspects of *Salmonella*. In: Wray, C. and Wray, A. (eds) *Salmonella in Domestic Animals*. CAB International, Wallingford, UK, pp. 265–284.

Nakamura, M., Nagamine, N., Norimatsu, M., Suzuki, S., Ohishi, K., Kijima, M. *et al.* (1993) The ability of *Salmonella enteritidis* isolated from chicks imported from England to cause transovarian infection. *Journal of Veterinary Medical Science* 55, 135–136.

Natvig, E.E., Ingham, S.C., Ingham, B.H., Cooperband, L.R. and Roper, T.R. (2002) *Salmonella enterica* serovar Typhimurium and *Escherichia coli* contamination of root and leaf vegetables grown in soils with incorporated bovine manure. *Applied and Environmental Microbiology* 68, 2737–2744.

Nayak, R., Stewart, T., Wang, R.F., Lin, J., Cerniglia, C.E. and Kenney, P.B. (2004) Genetic diversity and virulence gene determinants of antibiotic-resistant *Salmonella* isolated from preharvest turkey production sources. *International Journal of Food Microbiology* 91, 51–62.

Nesse, L.L., Nordby, K., Heir, E., Bergsjoe, B., Vardund, T., Nygaard, H. *et al.* (2003) Molecular analyses of *Salmonella enterica* isolates from fish feed factories and fish feed ingredients. *Applied and Environmental Microbiology* 69, 1075–1081.

Nesse, L.L., Refsum, T., Heir, E., Nordby, K., Vardund, T. and Holstad, G. (2005) Molecular epidemiology of *Salmonella* spp. isolates from gulls, fish-meal factories, feed factories, animals and humans in Norway based on pulsed-field gel electrophoresis. *Epidemiology and Infection* 133, 53–58.

Nyberg, K.A., Vinnerås, B., Lewerin, S.S., Kjellberg, E. and Albihn, A. (2011) Treatment with $Ca(OH)_2$ for inactivation of *Salmonella* Typhimurium and *Enterococcus faecalis* in soil contaminated with infected horse manure. *Journal of Applied Microbiology* 110, 1515–1523.

Obiri-Danso, K. and Jones, K. (2000) Intertidal sediments as reservoirs for hippurate negative campylobacters, salmonellae and faecal indicators in three EU recognised bathing waters in North West England. *Water Research* 34, 519–527.

Oppezzo, O.J., Costa, C.S. and Pizarro, R.A. (2011) Influence of *rpoS* mutations on the response of *Salmonella enterica* serovar Typhimurium to solar radiation. *Journal of Photochemistry and Photobiology B: Biology* 102, 20–25.

Österberg, J. (2010) *Salmonella* in pigs: infection dynamics of different serotypes. PhD Thesis, Department of Faculty of Veterinary Medicine and Animal Sciences, Swedish University of Agricultural Sciences, 73 pp.

Ottoson, J., Nordin, A., von Rosen, D. and Vinnerås, B. (2008) *Salmonella* reduction in manure by the addition of urea and ammonia. *Bioresource Technology* 99, 1610–1615.

Palumbo, M.S., Beers, S.M., Bhaduri, S. and Palumbo, S.A. (1995) Thermal resistance of *Salmonella* spp. and *Listeria monocytogenes* in liquid egg yolk and egg yolk products. *Journal of Food Protection* 58, 960–966.

Parmar, D. and Davies, R. (2007) Fowl typhoid in a small backyard laying flock. *Veterinary Record* 160, 348.

Paskeviciute, E., Buchovec, I. and Luksiene, Z. (2011) High-power pulsed light for decontamination of chicken from food pathogens: a study on antimicrobial efficiency and organoleptic properties. *Journal of Food Safety* 31, 61–68.

Passerat, J., Got, P., Dukan, S. and Monfort, P. (2009) Respective roles of culturable and viable-but-nonculturable cells in the heterogeneity of *Salmonella enterica* serovar Typhimurium invasiveness. *Applied and Environmental Microbiology* 75, 5179–5185.

Pennington, J.H., Brooksbank, N.H., Poole, P.M. and Seymour, F. (1968) *Salmonella virchow* in a chicken-packing station and associated rearing units. *British Medical Journal* 4, 804–806.

Pignato, S., Giammanco, G., Santangelo, C. and Giammanco, G.M. (1998) Endemic presence of *Salmonella bongori* 48:z35:-causing enteritis in children in Sicily. *Research in Microbiology* 149, 429–431.

Plym-Forshell, L. (1995) Survival of salmonellas and *Ascaris suum* eggs in a thermophilic biogas plant. *Acta Veterinaria Scandinavica* 36, 79–85.

Pokorny, J. (1988) Survival and virulence of salmonellae in water. *Journal of Hygiene, Epidemiology, Microbiology and Immunology* 32, 361–366.

Polo, F., Figueras, M.J., Inza, I., Sala, J., Fleisher, J.M. and Guarro, J. (1999) Prevalence of *Salmonella* serotypes in environmental waters and their relationships with indicator organisms. *Antonie Van Leeuwenhoek* 75, 285–292.

Poppe, C., Irwin, R.J., Messier, S., Finley, G.G. and Oggel, J. (1991) The prevalence of *Salmonella enteritidis* and other *Salmonella* sp. among Canadian registered commercial chicken broiler flocks. *Epidemiology and Infection* 107, 201–211.

Potasman, I., Paz, A. and Odeh, M. (2002) Infectious outbreaks associated with bivalve shellfish consumption: a worldwide perspective. *Clinical Infectious Diseases* 35, 921–928.

Prokšová, M., Mogoŭová, E., Ferianc, P. and Harichová, J. (2002) The occurrence of *Salmonella* spp. in natural environment confirmed by biochemical and molecular methods. *Biologia, Bratislava* 57, 797–803.

Purvis, G.M., Hullah, K., Pascoe, S.J.S., Evans, S.J. and Davies, R.H. (2005) Persistence of *Salmonella* Typhimurium DT120 in abattoir paddocks holding sheep. *Veterinary Record* 157, 165–167.

Rabie, A., Carrique-Mas, J. and Davies, R. (2010) Persistence of *Salmonella* in rodent populations from infected farms in Great Britain. *Proceedings of the I3S International Symposium 'Salmonella and Salmonellosis'*, St Malo, France, 28–30 June, pp. 219–222.

Rabsch, W., Hargis, B.M., Tsolis, R.M., Kingsley, R.A., Hinz, K.H., Tschape, H. *et al.* (2000) Competitive exclusion of *Salmonella* Enteritidis by *Salmonella* Gallinarum in poultry. *Emerging Infectious Diseases* 6, 443–448.

Rangel, D.E.N. (2011) Stress induced cross-protection against environmental challenges on prokaryotic and eukaryotic microbes. *World Journal of Microbiology and Biotechnology* 27, 1281–1296.

Reilly, P.J. and Twiddy, D.R. (1992) *Salmonella* and *Vibrio cholerae* in brackishwater cultured tropical prawns. *International Journal of Food Microbiology* 16, 293–301.

Rhodes, M.W. and Kator, H. (1988) Survival of *Escherichia coli* and *Salmonella* spp. in estuarine environments. *Applied and Environmental Microbiology* 54, 2902–2907.
Rippey, S.R. (1994) Infectious diseases associated with molluscan shellfish consumption. *Clinical Microbiology Reviews* 7, 419–425.
Runkel, N.S., Rodriguez, L.F., Moody, F.G., LaRocco, M.T. and Blasdel, T. (1991) *Salmonella* infection of the biliary and intestinal tract of wild opossums. *Laboratory Animal Science* 41, 54–56.
Russ, C.F. and Yanko, W.A. (1981) Factors affecting salmonellae repopulation in composted sludges. *Applied and Environmental Microbiology* 41, 597–602.
Rychlik, I. and Barrow, P.A. (2005) *Salmonella* stress management and its relevance to behaviour during intestinal colonisation and infection. *FEMS Microbiology Reviews* 29, 1021–1040.
Saide-Albornoz, J.J., Knipe, C.L., Murano, E.A. and Beran, G.W. (1995) Contamination of pork carcasses during slaughter, fabrication, and chilled storage. *Journal of Food Protection* 58, 993–997.
Santo Domingo, J.W., Harmon, S. and Bennett, J. (2000) Survival of *Salmonella* species in river water. *Current Microbiology* 40, 409–417.
Semenov, A.V. (2008) Ecology and modelling of *Escherichia coli* O157:H7 and *Salmonella enterica* serovar Typhimurium in cattle manure and soil. PhD Thesis, Department of Biological Farming Systems Group, Wageningen University, the Netherlands, 212 pp.
Shimi, A., Keyhani, M. and Bolurchi, M. (1976) Salmonellosis in apparently healthy dogs. *Veterinary Record* 98, 110–111.
Shuval, H.I. (1991) Effects of wastewater irrigation of pastures on the health of farm animals and humans. *Revue Scientifique et Technique (Office International des Épizooties)* 10, 847–866.
Skov, M.N., Spencer, A.G., Hald, B., Petersen, L., Nauerby, B., Carstensen, B. *et al.* (2004) The role of litter beetles as potential reservoir for *Salmonella enterica* and thermophilic *Campylobacter* spp. between broiler flocks. *Avian Diseases* 48, 9–18.
Skov, M.N., Madsen, J.J., Rahbek, C., Lodal, J., Jespersen, J.B., Jørgensen, J.C. *et al.* (2008) Transmission of *Salmonella* between wildlife and meat-production animals in Denmark. *Journal of Applied Microbiology* 105, 1558–1568.
Smith, J.J., Howington, J.P. and McFeters, G.A. (1994) Survival, physiological response and recovery of enteric bacteria exposed to a polar marine environment. *Applied and Environmental Microbiology* 60, 2977–2984.
Solano, C., García, B., Valle, J., Berasain, C., Ghigo, J.-M., Gamazo, C. *et al.* (2002) Genetic analysis of *Salmonella enteritidis* biofilm formation: critical role of cellulose. *Molecular Microbiology* 43, 793–808.
Strauch, D. (1991) Survival of pathogenic micro-organisms and parasites in excreta, manure and sewage sludge. *Revue Scientifique et Technique (Office International des Épizooties)* 10, 813–846.
Sugiyama, Y., Sugiyama, F. and Yagami, K. (1993) Isolation of *Salmonella* from impounded dogs introduced to a laboratory. *Experimental Animals* 42, 119–121.
Taormina, P.J., Beuchat, L.R. and Slutsker, L. (1999) Infections associated with eating seed sprouts: an international concern. *Emerging Infectious Diseases* 5, 626–634.
Townsend, S.A. (1992) The relationships between salmonellas and faecal indicator concentrations in two pools in the Australian wet/dry tropics. *Journal of Applied Bacteriology* 73, 182–188.
Turpin, P.E., Maycroft, K.A., Rowlands, C.L. and Wellington, E.M. (1993a) An ion-exchange based extraction method for the detection of salmonellas in soil. *Journal of Applied Bacteriology* 74, 181–190.
Turpin, P.E., Maycroft, K.A., Rowlands, C.L. and Wellington, E.M. (1993b) Viable but non-culturable salmonellas in soil. *Journal of Applied Bacteriology* 74, 421–427.
USDA (2000) *Salmonella enterica* serotype Enteritidis in table egg layers in the U.S. National Animal Health Monitoring System CEAH. Fort Collins, Colorado. Available at: http://www.aphis.usda.gov/animal_health/nahms/poultry/downloads/layers99/Layers99_dr_Salmonella.pdf (accessed 4 March 2013).
Valiente Moro, C., Chauve, C. and Zenner, L. (2007) Experimental infection of *Salmonella* Enteritidis by the poultry red mite, *Dermanyssus gallinae*. *Veterinary Parasitology* 146, 329–336.
van de Giessen, A.W., Ament, A.J. and Notermans, S.H. (1994) Intervention strategies for *Salmonella enteritidis* in poultry flocks: a basic approach. *International Journal of Food Microbiology* 21, 145–154.
Vanselow, B.A., Hornitzky, M.A., Walker, K.H., Eamens, G.J., Bailey, G.D., Gill, P.A. *et al.* (2007a) *Salmonella* and on-farm risk factors in healthy slaughter-age cattle and sheep in eastern Australia. *Australian Veterinary Journal* 85, 498–502.
Vanselow, B.A., Hum, S., Hornitzky, M.A., Eamens, G.J. and Quinn, K. (2007b) *Salmonella* Typhimurium persistence in a Hunter Valley dairy herd. *Australian Veterinary Journal* 85, 446–450.

Veling, J., Wilpshaar, H., Frankena, K., Bartels, C. and Barkema, H.W. (2002) Risk factors for clinical *Salmonella enterica* subsp *enterica* serovar Typhimurium infection on Dutch dairy farms. *Preventive Veterinary Medicine* 54, 157–168.

Vestby, L., Møretrø, T., Langsrud, S., Heir, E. and Nesse, L. (2009) Biofilm forming abilities of *Salmonella* are correlated with persistence in fish meal- and feed factories. *BMC Veterinary Research* 5, 20.

Wales, A., Breslin, M. and Davies, R. (2006a) Semiquantitative assessment of the distribution of *Salmonella* in the environment of caged layer flocks. *Journal of Applied Microbiology* 101, 309–318.

Wales, A.D., Davies, R.H. and Breslin, M. (2006b) Assessment of cleaning and disinfection in *Salmonella*-contaminated poultry houses using qualitative and semi-quantitative culture techniques. *Veterinary Microbiology* 116, 283–293.

Wales, A., Breslin, M., Carter, B., Sayers, A.R. and Davies, R. (2007) A longitudinal study of environmental *Salmonella* contamination in caged and free-range layer flocks. *Avian Pathology* 36, 187–197.

Wales, A.D., McLaren, I.M., Bedford, S., Carrique-Mas, J.J., Cook, A.J.C. and Davies, R.H. (2009) Longitudinal survey of the occurrence of *Salmonella* in pigs and the environment of nucleus breeder and multiplier pig herds in England. *Veterinary Record* 165, 648–657.

Wales, A.D., Allen, V.M. and Davies, R.H. (2010a) Chemical treatment of animal feed and water for the control of *Salmonella*. *Foodborne Pathogens and Disease* 7, 3–15.

Wales, A.D., Carrique-Mas, J.J., Rankin, M., Bell, B., Thind, B.B. and Davies, R.H. (2010b) Review of the carriage of zoonotic bacteria by arthropods, with special reference to *Salmonella* in mites, flies and litter beetles. *Zoonoses and Public Health* 57, 299–314.

Wales, A.D., Cook, A.J.C. and Davies, R.H. (2011) Producing *Salmonella*-free pigs: a review focusing on interventions at weaning. *Veterinary Record* 168, 267–276.

Watts, P.S. and Wall, M. (1952) The 1951 *Salmonella typhimurium* epidemic in sheep in South Australia. *Australian Veterinary Journal* 28, 165–168.

White, A.P., Gibson, D.L., Kim, W., Kay, W.W. and Surette, M.G. (2006) Thin Aggregative Fimbriae and cellulose enhance long-term survival and persistence of *Salmonella*. *Journal of Bacteriology* 188, 3219–3227.

WHO (2006) WHO guidelines for the safe use of wastewater, excreta and greywater. World Health Organization. Geneva, WHO Press. Available at: http://www.who.int/water_sanitation_health/wastewater/en (accessed 4 March 2013).

Wilson, J.S., Hazel, S.M., Williams, N.J., Phiri, A., French, N.P. and Hart, C.A. (2003) Nontyphoidal salmonellae in United Kingdom badgers: prevalence and spatial distribution. *Applied and Environmental Microbiology* 69, 4312–4315.

Winfield, M.D. and Groisman, E.A. (2003) Role of nonhost environments in the lifestyles of *Salmonella* and *Escherichia coli*. *Applied and Environmental Microbiology* 69, 3687–3694.

Wray, C. (1995) Salmonellosis: a hundred years old and still going strong. *British Veterinary Journal* 151, 339–341.

Wray, C. and Davies, R.H. (1998) Environmental problems in poultry production: dust and pests. *Proceedings of the International Symposium on Food-borne* Salmonella, Baltimore, USA, 25–26 July, pp. 93–104.

Wray, C. and Davies, R. (2004) *Salmonella* in cattle: update. *Cattle Practice* 12, 313–316.

Wray, C., Baker, K., Gallagher, J. and Naylor, P. (1977) *Salmonella* infection in badgers in the South West of England. *British Veterinary Journal* 133, 526–529.

Wray, C., Todd, J.N. and Hinton, M. (1987) Epidemiology of *Salmonella typhimurium* infection in calves: excretion of *S. typhimurium* in the faeces of calves in different management systems. *Veterinary Record* 121, 293–296.

You, Y., Rankin, S.C., Aceto, H.W., Benson, C.E., Toth, J.D. and Dou, Z. (2006) Survival of *Salmonella enterica* serovar Newport in manure and manure-amended soils. *Applied and Environmental Microbiology* 72, 5777–5783.

Zaafrane, S., Maatouk, K., Gauthier, J.M. and Bakhrouf, A. (2004) Influence of preliminary cultivation conditions and the presence of the *rpoS* gene on the survival of *Salmonella typhimurium* in sea water exposed to sunlight. *Canadian Journal of Microbiology* 50, 341–350.

Zeman, P., Stika, V., Skalka, B., Bartik, M., Dusbabek, F. and Lavickova, M. (1982) Potential role of *Dermanyssus gallinae* in the circulation of the agent of pullurosis typhus in hens. *Folia Parasitologica* 29, 371–374.

21 Competitive Exclusion

Roberto La Ragione[1]* and Geoffrey Mead[2]
[1]*Animal Health and Veterinary Laboratories Agency, and Department of Microbial and Cellular Sciences, Faculty of Health and Medical Sciences, University of Surrey, UK;* [2]*Consultant, UK*

Introduction

Throughout the world, foods of animal origin, especially poultry and poultry products, including eggs, continue to be implicated in many sporadic cases and outbreaks of human salmonellosis (FAO/WHO, 2002, 2009). In response to this situation, greater efforts are now being made in some countries to control non-typhoid serovars of *Salmonella* in the poultry industry. In the European Union (EU), for example, deadlines have been set for the establishment of *Salmonella* reduction targets in breeders, layers, broilers and turkeys, and regular testing of flocks has become mandatory (EC, 2003a, b). Thus, the requirements for national control plans have been laid down and, ultimately, such measures are expected to have a beneficial effect on public health. They also have implications for international trade in poultry products (McCartney, 2008).

For most countries, total eradication of all salmonellas from raw poultry is unlikely to be cost-effective or even feasible (van Immerseel *et al.*, 2005; Mead *et al.*, 2010). However, knowledge of the epidemiology of *Salmonella* in poultry production and of the biology of the organism has led to the development of effective mitigation strategies. One such approach is based on the work of Nurmi and Rantala (1973), which recognized that the high susceptibility of newly hatched chicks to *Salmonella* colonization is due primarily to the lack of a mature gastrointestinal (GI) microflora to compete with any invading pathogen. Chicks could be protected from *Salmonella* infection by oral administration of a suspension or anaerobic culture of material taken from the alimentary tract of adult, *Salmonella*-free chickens (Nurmi and Rantala, 1973; Rantala and Nurmi, 1973). This kind of treatment preparation does not have a defined composition and its action against *Salmonella* (and possibly other pathogens) is broadly described by the term 'competitive exclusion' (CE). Over the years, the CE concept has been widely studied, both in the laboratory and under field conditions, and the treatment has been adapted for optimal commercial application. Because of its undefined nature, however, there is ongoing interest in developing simpler, defined microbial preparations with similar activity against *Salmonella*, which are termed 'probiotics'. This chapter will consider the advantages, limitations and current status in *Salmonella* control of both kinds of treatment, when applied to poultry.

* Corresponding author, e-mail: r.laragione@ahvla.defra.gsi.gov.uk; r.laragione@surrey.ac.uk

© CAB International 2013. *Salmonella in Domestic Animals, 2nd Edition* (eds P.A. Barrow and U. Methner)

The Intestinal Microflora

Studies involving cultural analytical techniques have shown that the intestinal microflora of the chick changes markedly with age. Initially, the gut contains bacteria belonging to only a few genera and these appear rapidly, derived, apparently, from the hatchery environment. Thus, within only a few hours of hatching, genera of Enterobacteriaceae and species of *Enterococcus* and *Clostridium* may occur in the caeca and scattered throughout the remainder of the alimentary tract. Species of *Lactobacillus* become established by about the third day after the start of feeding. The native adult flora in the small intestine appears within the first 2 weeks of life, but the caecal flora can take more than 4 weeks to develop fully (Barnes *et al.*, 1972, 1979b; Mead and Adams, 1975).

The caecal microflora is ultimately dominated by obligate anaerobes, including species of *Bacteroides*, *Fusobacterium*, *Peptostreptococcus*, anaerobic *Streptococcus*, *Eubacterium* and *Bifidobacterium*, and budding bacteria, such as *Gemmiger*. More than 40 different types of anaerobic Gram-negative and Gram-positive non-sporing rods and cocci have been isolated and characterized. Also, at least 17 different species of *Clostridium* have been isolated from the caecal contents (Barnes and Impey, 1970; Salanitro *et al.*, 1974, 1976; Barnes, 1979; Barnes *et al.*, 1979b; Croucher and Barnes, 1983). Apart from fusiforms, typical members of *Bacteroides* and *Bifidobacterium* do not appear as major components of the flora until 4 weeks of age (Barnes, 1977). More recently, the increasing diversity of the flora with age was confirmed by molecular metagenomic analytical methods involving analysis of 16S rRNA sequences (Hume *et al.*, 2003; Lu *et al.*, 2003; Amit-Romach *et al.*, 2004). These methods allow the component organisms to be studied without the inevitable bias of cultivation techniques, which permit the recovery of some organisms, but not others. Whatever the ultimate composition of the microflora, however, it is evident that its relatively slow rate of development makes the young chick particularly susceptible to colonization by enteropathogens such as *Salmonella*.

The 'Competitive Exclusion' Concept

The CE concept may be defined as 'the early establishment of an adult intestinal microflora to prevent subsequent colonization by enteropathogens'. The term 'competitive exclusion' was first used by Greenberg (1969), who showed that the normal microbiota in the maggots of blowflies prevented colonization by *S.* Typhimurium and only when the microbiota was absent or simplified did the pathogen become established. 'Colonization resistance' is an analogous term that was introduced by van der Waaij *et al.* (1971) in studying intestinal bacterial populations in mice. In the present context, the term 'competitive inhibition', as used by Lloyd *et al.* (1974), would appear to be more appropriate and exclusion of *Salmonella* is rarely complete under practical conditions.

Microbial interactions and the mechanisms by which indigenous intestinal microorganisms inhibit colonization by invading pathogens are not yet fully understood (Donoghue *et al.*, 2006). There is also a lack of information on the precise nature of the bacteria involved, although some effective mixtures of pure cultures have been developed for oral administration (see below). Apparently, the only universally accepted fact concerning the mechanism of CE is that protection depends upon the use of viable bacteria. According to Rantala (1974), only anaerobic cultures are fully effective in this respect but, more recently, similar levels of protection have been obtained with cultures incubated aerobically (de Oliviera *et al.*, 2000; Andreatti Filho *et al.*, 2003). This may be due to low redox potentials produced by growth of facultative anaerobes, which then allow multiplication of obligate anaerobes.

Blanchfield *et al.* (1982) obtained good protection of chicks against *Salmonella* infection by oral administration of 10^{-5} g of faeces from a *Salmonella*-free adult bird and similar protection was obtained with anaerobic broth cultures derived from 10^{-7} g of caecal or faecal material (Blanchfield *et al.*, 1984). As the quantity of inoculum was reduced from 10^{-7} g to 5×10^{-10} g, there was a gradual loss of protective activity. Excellent protection was evident with inocula of 10^{-7} g and even inocula of 10^{-8}g resulted in cultures that completely protected more than 50% of challenged chicks. Treatment cultures prepared from 10^{-10}g did not confer any protection. This suggests that all the bacterial species needed for fully protective cultures were present only at a level of 10^{-7} to 10^{-8}g^{-1} of caecal or faecal material.

Different kinds of *in vivo* and *in vitro* models have been used to study the mechanism of CE. *In vivo* models include infant, antibiotic-treated and germ-free animals, while *in vitro* models, which are considered to be less relevant than experiments with animals, include batch, continuous-flow (CF) and agar cultures (Savage, 1977; Barnes *et al.*, 1979a; Freter *et al.*, 1983; Rolfe, 1991; Nisbet, 2002).

The GI tract is a highly complex ecosystem. It involves a range of conditions, from some that favour colonization by a wide diversity of microbes to others in which few organisms can flourish. Within these different habitats, there is a variety of host–microbe and microbe–microbe interactions, most of which are still incompletely understood. Among the mechanisms by which one or more bacterial species may inhibit pathogen proliferation or reduce the numbers of competing organisms are the following (Rolfe, 1991; Donoghue *et al.*, 2006):

- Creation of a restrictive physiological environment;
- Competition for enteric receptor sites;
- Competition with the host and other microbes for nutrients;
- Production of antimicrobial compounds or agents such as bacteriocins and bacteriophage;
- Stimulation of the immune system.

These are described briefly in the following sections.

Creation of a restrictive physiological environment

One of the more immediate ways in which bacterial populations in the GI tract can influence the establishment of invading pathogens is through the production of short-chain fatty acids (SCFA) as metabolic end-products. Those produced by caecal anaerobes include acetic, butyric and propionic acids, and such acids are known to be inhibitory to *Salmonella*, especially in the un-dissociated state below pH 6.0. In studying the inhibition of *S.* Typhimurium in the mouse gut, Meynell (1963) concluded that the *Salmonella* failed to multiply because of the combined inhibitory effect of a low redox potential (E_h) and SCFA, both of which result from the activities of the indigenous microflora. The study involved elimination of the flora with streptomycin, which abolished the mechanism responsible for *Salmonella* inhibition. At the same time there was a decrease in SCFA concentration and a rise in pH and E_h. The importance of SCFA in the mechanism of CE has also been reported by others (Barnes *et al.*, 1979a; Nisbet *et al.*, 1993; Corrier *et al.*, 1995a, b; van der Wielen *et al.*, 2000). In relation to broiler chickens, van der Wielen *et al.* (2000) showed that SCFA concentrations increased from undetectable levels at day-old to the highest concentrations at 15 days of age. Although not fully understood, the antibacterial properties include bacteriostatic and bactericidal effects, which depend upon the physiological states of the bacteria and the physico-chemical characteristics of the external environment (Ricke, 2003).

Competition for enteric receptor sites

It has been reported (Seuna, 1979; Soerjadi *et al.*, 1981a) that, following administration of CE treatment, protection against an oral *Salmonella* challenge starts to become apparent within only 1–2 h. A similar observation was made by Mead *et al.* (1989b) when studying the effect of CE treatment on the transmission of *S.* Enteritidis between chicks contained in delivery boxes. All these studies indicate that, initially, protection is predominantly a physical phenomenon rather than one involving any metabolic process.

The ability of a bacterium to adhere rapidly to a suitable receptor is important in either establishing or maintaining colonization of the GI tract (Savage, 1977). The bacterial glycocalyx, which is considered to be any polysaccharide-containing component outside the cell wall (Costerton *et al.*, 1981), is thought to mediate adherence of protective bacteria to each other and to the intestinal epithelium of the bird (Soerjadi *et al.*, 1982b). Thus, a layer of cells is formed, and this appears to block receptor sites for *Salmonella* attachment (Fuller and Turvey, 1971; Snoeyenbos *et al.*, 1979; Savage, 1983). The process by which bacteria bind to the mucosal epithelium appears to be influenced by a variety of adherence factors (Donoghue *et al.*, 2006), including type 1 fimbriae, which mediate mannose-sensitive haemagglutination and have been implicated in initiating and maintaining colonization by some Enterobacteriaceae (Duguid and Campbell, 1969). Also, *S.* Typhimurium produces an exopolysaccharide that leads to biofilm formation and facilitates attachment of the organism to chicken gut epithelium (Ledeboer and Jones, 2005). In selecting bacterial strains from adult chickens for use in CE treatment preparations, Stavric and D'Aoust (1993) found that strains obtained from washed caeca had hydrophobic properties that improved their protective potential against *Salmonella*. Hydrophobicity of the outer surface of the bacterial cell is another factor that is thought to play a part in attachment of the organism to host tissue (Kiely and Olson, 2000).

Competition for nutrients

The importance of competition for growth-limiting nutrients as a means of controlling microbial populations in the GI tract has been difficult to evaluate *in vivo* because of other potentially inhibitory factors (Rolfe, 1991). Nevertheless, nutrient competition between indigenous organisms and invading pathogens is an accepted fact (Lan *et al.*, 2005). An example of a key nutrient is iron, which is essential for all living organisms. However, it is the ability to acquire iron that is critical in bacterial colonization and may confer a competitive advantage (Ratledge and Dover, 2000; van Vliet *et al.*, 2002; Ho *et al.*, 2004). Since most of the iron is stored intracellularly in host tissues, little is available to intestinal microbes, but many gram-negative organisms, including *Salmonella*, produce small iron-chelating molecules called siderophores that have a high affinity for ferric iron (Kingsley *et al.*, 1995; Neilands, 1995).

Other nutrients that may become limiting in the GI tract are certain amino acids, such as serine. Under anaerobic batch-culture conditions, reducing the serine concentration to a critical level slowed the growth rate of *S.* Typhimurium, but not that of an enteric coliform (Ha *et al.*, 1995). In this case, the inhibitory effect on the *Salmonella* was influenced by the E_h of the culture medium.

Production of antimicrobial agents

Microbes present in the GI tract are capable of producing a variety of antimicrobial agents that may affect the prevailing microbial balance. These include bacteriocins and bacteriocin-like substances, enzymes, free acids from microbial deconjugation of bile, hydrogen peroxide, hydrogen sulfide and SCFA that are either bacteriostatic or bactericidal (van der Wielen *et al.*, 2000). Another type of agent that may be present is bacteriophage, a virus capable of infecting and killing susceptible bacteria that are invariably specific target organisms. On the other hand, both *Salmonella* and *Campylobacter* spp. are known to be susceptible to reuterin, a bacteriocin produced by *Lactobacillus reuteri* (Mulder *et al.*, 1997). In general, however, the role of bacteriocins in naturally-occurring bacterial populations remains unclear.

Stimulation of the immune system

In birds, the intestine is a major part of the immune system; however, the natural resistance of the host to infectious agents is not fully developed in the young chick. At this stage, microbes present in the GI tract are important in stimulating the cellular components of the intestinal immune system and promoting maturation of the system (Donoghue *et al.*, 2006; Revolledo *et al.*, 2006).

Indigenous microbes also act to modulate the immune response by increasing or decreasing the amounts of mediator substances secreted by immunocompetent cells. Because of its diversity, the gut microbiota provides a considerable amount of antigenic material for the mucosal immune system.

The best-defined part of the system is secretory IgA, which initially mediates defence of the intestinal mucosal surface against enteric pathogens (Muir *et al.*, 2000). Young chicks have very few Ig-producing cells in the intestine, but the number increases in response to microbial colonization (Parry *et al.*, 1977). This may help to explain the relationship between the slow rate of gut colonization by indigenous microbes and susceptibility to *Salmonella* infection. Thus, enhancement of the local immune system via administration of a CE preparation or probiotic may have a significant effect in providing resistance to *Salmonella* colonization (Revolledo *et al.*, 2006).

Development of CE Preparations

Preparations of native intestinal microorganisms

Undefined, mixed cultures

In the publication that first described the CE concept in poultry, as the term is now understood, Nurmi and Rantala (1973) used diluted contents from the crop and GI tract of adult chickens to protect day-old chicks against a challenge with *S.* Infantis. Later, a similar degree of protection was obtained with an anaerobic broth culture of intestinal contents after sub-culturing on 3 successive days (Rantala and Nurmi, 1973). This approach provided more convenient and manageable treatment material that ultimately led to the development of the first commercial product (Schneitz, 1993). The results obtained for *Salmonella* control have been confirmed subsequently on many occasions by different research groups around the world and have been reviewed most recently by Schneitz and Mead (2010).

Much of the work done on undefined treatment preparations has utilized cultures of caecal content, because material from other parts of the alimentary tract was found to be less protective against *S.* Typhimurium (Lloyd *et al.*, 1977). Investigators using anaerobic broth cultures have usually employed a modified version of the French viande-levure (VL) medium (Barnes and Impey, 1971). The advantages of these cultures are that they can be subcultured many times without losing their effectiveness (Snoeyenbos *et al.*, 1978; Mead and Impey, 1986) and non-bacterial pathogens, such as viruses and protozoa, which are unable to proliferate in bacteriological culture media, are diluted out on subculture. The treatment cultures can also be tested using cultural and molecular techniques to ensure the absence of any known bacterial pathogen.

To minimize the risk of transferring pathogens from donor birds to recipients, Snoeyenbos *et al.* (1979) used faeces from a specific-pathogen-free (SPF) flock as the inoculum material. Birds in this flock had acquired their gut microflora by oral inoculation from a group of conventional birds, specially selected as one offering particularly good protection. This approach is said to avoid the problem of insufficient protection due to the retarded development of the intestinal microflora in SPF birds (Coloe *et al.*, 1984; Impey *et al.*, 1984; Mead and Impey, 1986).

Defined cultures

The main reason for developing defined treatment preparations is to avoid the necessity of testing the product for human and animal pathogens. Also, regulatory bodies are becoming stricter in their requirements and the days of undefined CE products may be coming to an end. Therefore, numerous attempts have been made to develop preparations containing one or more pure strains for protective purposes, but, despite some success, the earlier results were generally disappointing (Stavric and D'Aoust, 1993). Sometimes, the preparations studied have contained large numbers of bacterial strains that were developed for experimental purposes rather than commercial exploitation.

Newly hatched chicks were protected to some extent against colonization by *S.* Typhimurium when given pure cultures of a *Clostridium* spp. (Rigby *et al.*, 1977) or *Enterococcus faecalis* (Soerjadi *et al.*, 1978). Protection was also obtained with a mixture of 23 bacterial strains, including species of *Lactobacillus* and other facultatively and strictly anaerobic bacterial strains originating from caecal material (Barnes *et al.*, 1980b). Subsequently, Impey *et al.* (1982, 1984) reported protective activity equivalent to that of undefined caecal cultures with mixtures of 48 and 65 strains, in which *Bacteroides* spp. were numerically dominant. Unlike undefined preparations, however, neither of the two defined-culture mixtures from chicken provided any protection against *Salmonella* colonization of turkey poults (Impey *et al.*, 1984). Similarly, Stavric *et al.* (1985) succeeded in protecting chicks with a mixture of 50 strains. Less protection was evident when the challenge dose was increased above 10^4 colony-forming units (cfu) per chick or when the number of strains in the mixture was reduced. In a different approach, Nisbet *et al.* (1993) inoculated newly hatched chicks with a mixture of 11 strains originating from a CF culture of caecal material and gave the birds feed supplemented with lactose. Thus, caecal colonization was reduced by $\log_{10}$ 3.6 units compared with an untreated control group. By contrast, Goren *et al.* (1984a) obtained no protection against *S.* Infantis with a mixture of 295 strains of obligate anaerobes from gut material. This finding may suggest an important role for facultative anaerobes in host protection. A mixture of only three strains of *Escherichia coli*, isolated from sewage and an abattoir, produced a substantial reduction in caecal populations of *S.* Typhimurium over a period of 7 weeks (Barrow and Tucker, 1986). However, the strains were not so effective against other *Salmonella* serovars. With *S.* Typhimurium, Barrow *et al.* (1990) and Berchieri and Barrow (1990) obtained a profound inhibition of strain F98 by using an avirulent rough mutant of the same organism. A similar degree of inhibition was reported between two homologous strains of a *Citrobacter* sp. and the same occurred with *E. coli* (Barrow *et al.*, 1987). More recently, large numbers of facultative anaerobes have been screened for their *in vitro* ability to inhibit *Salmonella*. In one such study (Bielke *et al.*, 2003), a treatment preparation comprising 14 separate strains was developed. This included species of *Bacillus*, *Citrobacter*, *Enterobacter*, *Enterococcus*, *Escherichia*, *Klebsiella* and *Staphylococcus*. The protection conferred on turkey poults challenged with *S.* Enteritidis ranged from 0% to 100%, the greatest effect being unexpectedly associated with the lowest treatment doses. When 636 strains were isolated from nine donor chickens and tested *in vitro* for the ability to inhibit growth of both *Salmonella* and *Campylobacter jejuni*, 194 strains were strongly inhibitory for *C. jejuni* and 41 of them inhibited both *C. jejuni* and five different *Salmonella* serovars (Zhang *et al.*, 2007a). In a follow-up study (Zhang *et al.*, 2007b), the efficacy of 56 of the strains was tested *in vivo* in different combinations. A preparation containing one strain each of *La. salivarius* and *St. crispatus* yielded the best result, with a reduction of $\log_{10}$ 3.0 units in caecal colonization by *S.* Typhimurium.

The antagonistic effects of *Lactobacillus* spp. on the ability of different *Salmonella* serovars to colonize the alimentary tract of young poultry has been studied extensively and is reviewed by Juven *et al.* (1991). Overall, conflicting evidence has been obtained. Some positive effects have been reported by Edens *et al.* (1991) and Dunham *et al.* (1994) for *La. reuteri*, and Soerjadi *et al.* (1981b) showed that lactobacilli reduced *Salmonella* colonization of chicken crop epithelium by $\log_{10}$ 1–2 units. On the other hand, lactobacilli given alone or together with a few other bacterial strains had little or no effect in reducing *Salmonella* colonization of the GI tract of the chicken (Barnes *et al.*, 1980a; Weinack *et al.*, 1985b; La Ragione *et al.*, 2004).

Defined bacterial preparations, whatever their composition, tend to have one feature in common (disregarding mutant strains of *Salmonella* and *E. coli*, which may be unacceptable from the public health viewpoint): they may provide good or relatively good protection at first but, when used over a long period of time, they are inclined to lose their effectiveness. There is no clear explanation for this, but the use of artificial laboratory media in isolating and cultivating the organisms may well change their physiology and/or surface structure. Growing the strains together instead of individually partly overcomes the problem (Stavric, 1992). Furthermore, Nisbet *et al.* (1996) have claimed that growing the organisms as a mixture under conditions of continuous culture is a way of stabilizing their protective activity.

Commercial CE products

Several commercially available treatment products have been developed, including AviFree, Aviguard, Broilact and Preempt. All are essentially undefined, despite Preempt being described as a defined preparation.

AviFree

Evidently, AviFree is a mixed culture of whole caecal content from an adult chicken. It was developed by Alltech Ltd and launched in 1996. There is very little information available concerning the composition or effectiveness of this product but, according to Newman and Spring (1996), it was moderately protective against a strain of *S.* Typhimurium.

Aviguard

Aviguard is sold as a lyophilized product and was developed in the UK by Life-Care Products Ltd. It was launched in 1993. The product is a mixed culture of caecal content from an adult chicken. In small-scale trials, Aviguard protected newly hatched chicks against *S.* Enteritidis (Guillot *et al.*, 1997) and turkey poults against *S.* Kedougou (Ghazikhanian *et al.*, 1997) and *S.* Typhimurium (Cameron *et al.*, 1977). A highly successful series of field trials was also carried out (Deruyttere *et al.*, 1997). In addition, Aviguard was successfully given to older birds after therapeutic doses of antibiotics in order to regenerate the intestinal microflora and prevent reinfection with *Salmonella* (Reynolds *et al.*, 1997).

Broilact

Broilact was the first commercial CE product and was developed by the Orion Corporation in Finland. It was launched as a liquid product in Finland and Sweden in 1987, but has been sold in lyophilized form since 1994. Because competition for receptor sites on the mucosa is one of the suggested mechanisms of CE, Broilact is based on this hypothesis, being composed of bacteria that remain adhering to the caecal wall after a standard washing procedure (Nurmi *et al.*, 1987). Spore-forming organisms appear to be absent from the product. Experimental studies showed that newly hatched chicks given Broilact were largely protected against both *S.* Enteritidis and *S.* Typhimurium (Mead *et al.*, 1989b; Bolder *et al.*, 1992; Cameron and Carter, 1992; Nuotio *et al.*, 1992; Schneitz, 1992; Methner *et al.*, 1997). The treatment also protected the chicks against subsequent invasion of the heart, liver and spleen. Field trials on Broilact have confirmed the effectiveness of treatment in a number of studies (Wierup *et al.*, 1988, 1992; Bolder *et al.*, 1995; Palmu and Camelin, 1997). With older birds, Broilact administered following antibiotic therapy regenerated the intestinal microflora to prevent or minimize any reintroduction of *Salmonella* (Johnson, 1992; Humbert *et al.*, 1997; Reynolds *et al.*, 1997).

Preempt

Preempt, formerly known as CF3 (Hume *et al.*, 1998) or DeLoach 29 in Japan, is a mixed-culture preparation developed by Corrier *et al.* (1995a). It is based on the use of a CF culture system and a culture medium of low pH to favour the growth of certain facultative and obligate anaerobes. The starting material was an homogenate of caecal tissue and contents obtained from 10-week-old broiler chickens (Corrier *et al.*, 1995b; Nisbet *et al.*, 1995, 1996). The material was shown to reduce *Salmonella* colonization in both laboratory trials and field conditions, and to improve bird performance (Corrier *et al.*, 1995a, 1998).

The commercial version of CF3 was developed by Milk Specialities Co. (Burns, 1995). In attempting to define its composition, 29 bacterial strains were isolated, including 14 strictly anaerobic rods and cocci, representing seven genera, and 15 facultatively anaerobic rods and cocci, again representing seven genera. However, only one non-selective medium was used to isolate the anaerobes from CF3 and one non-selective and one selective medium for the facultative anaerobes (Corrier *et al.*, 1995a). Therefore, it is unlikely that all the organisms present would have been recovered. This preparation appears to be no longer available commercially.

It is evident from the literature that the CE preparations described above may differ in efficacy (Schneitz and Hakkinen, 1998; Nakamura *et al.*, 2002; Ferreira *et al.*, 2003). However, those used most widely, notably Aviguard and Broilact, have given good protection under various test conditions.

Other CE preparations

Saccharomyces boulardii

This is a yeast that is also used as a human probiotic. It was reported to reduce *Salmonella* infection of chicks when administered *in ovo* or via the feed, and has been given to broilers just before transportation from the farm to the processing plant (Line, 1997). Enteropathogens appear to adhere to the yeast surface and are removed from the bird when the yeast is voided with the faeces.

Vermicompost

The preparation known as vermicompost was produced by feeding the earthworm *Eisenia foetida* on a mixture of fresh chicken faeces and vegetable matter, the faeces being obtained from an SPF adult bird (Spencer and Garcia, 1995). This approach was seen as a means of producing large quantities of protective material easily and inexpensively. The material effectively protected chicks against a *Salmonella* challenge.

Used litter

The attraction of used litter as a potential source of a protective microflora is that the organisms present, while derived mainly from the birds, will have been exposed to the air and therefore are likely to be less oxygen-sensitive than the predominant bacteria in the GI tract. The impact on *Salmonella* colonization of dosing chicks with used-litter preparations was first studied by Rigby and Pettit (1980). In three separate trials, newly hatched broiler chicks were treated, respectively, with a lyophilized extract of breeder-flock nest litter, an anaerobic culture of this extract and an anaerobic culture of chicken faeces from an adult bird. Both treated and control chicks were challenged with *S.* Typhimurium at 3 days of age and reared for 7–8 weeks. Tests on litter samples and gut contents from the chicks showed that the prevalence of *Salmonella* infection at market age was significantly reduced in all treatment groups.

Subsequently, Corrier *et al.* (1992) placed newly hatched chicks on fresh, unused litter or on used litter that had been collected and stored for 1, 4 or 50 days before the start of the study. All chicks were challenged with *S.* Typhimurium at 3 days of age. The proportion of *Salmonella*-positive chicks and levels of caecal carriage were significantly lower in the birds reared on used litter of any age than in those on new litter initially. The birds reared on used litter also showed higher concentrations of caecal SCFA than birds given new litter.

Probiotics

Commercially available probiotics deemed to be safe for use in poultry by the EU Scientific Committee for Animal Nutrition and poultry probiotics available for use in food-producing animals in the UK are shown in Tables 21.1 and 21.2, respectively.

The CE concept is also associated with probiotics, the use of which originates from the work of Elie Metchnikoff, a Russian biologist working at the Pasteur Institute at the turn of the 20th century (Metchnikoff, 1908). He became convinced that fermented milks containing so-called 'lactic acid bacteria' were responsible for the longevity of Bulgarian farming families. It was assumed that the resultant introduction of a benign non-toxigenic gut

Table 21.1. Commercially available probiotics deemed to be safe for use in poultry by the EU Scientific Committee for Animal Nutrition (Adapted from the SCAN Opinion on the use of certain microorganisms as additives in feeding stuffs 26 September 1997: http://ec.europa.eu/food/fs/sc/scan/out93_en.pdf accessed on 19 December 2009).

Product name	Probiotic organisms	Culture collection	Target animal species
Lactobacillus acidophilus D2/CSL1	*Lactobacillus acidophilus*	CECT 4529	Broilers and laying hens
Bactocell1	*Pediococcus acidilacti*	CNCM MA18/5M	Broilers
Bioplus 2B1	*Bacillus licheniformis*, *Bacillus subtilis*	DSMZ 5749 DSMZ 5750	Piglets, sows, piglets for fattening, broilers, turkeys and calves
Oralin1	*Enterococcus faecium*	NCIMB 10415	Pigs for fattening, calves and broilers
Probios PDFM Granular1	*Enterococcus faecium*	DSMZ 4788 ATCC 53519 DSMZ 4789 ATCC 55593	Broilers
Microferm1	*Enterococcus faecium*	DSMZ 5464	Piglets, calves and broilers
Cylactin LBC1	*Enterococcus faecium*	NCIMB 10415	Piglets, pigs for fattening, calves and broilers

ATCC, American Type Culture Collection; CECT, Colección Española de Cultivos Tipo; DSM, Deutsche Sammlung von Mikroorganismen und Zellkulturen; CNCM, Collection Nationale de Cultures de Micro-organismes; NCIMB, National Collection of Industrial, Food and Marine Bacteria.

Table 21.2. Poultry probiotics available for use in food-producing animals in the UK (Adapted from the SCAN Opinion on the use of certain microorganisms as additives in feeding stuffs 26 September 1997: http://ec.europa.eu/food/fs/sc/scan/out93_en.pdf accessed on 19 December 2009).

Producer	Product name	Probiotic organisms	Target animal species
Protexin	Protexin Pro-soluble1	*Enterococcus faecium* (NCIMB 10415)	Cattle, poultry, pigs, lambs
Chr.Hansen Group	Gallipro1	*Bacillus subtilis*	Poultry
Medipharm (Chr.Hansen Group)	Lactiferm Caps1	Unknown	Cattle, poultry, pigs
Medipharm (Chr.Hansen Group)	Lactiferm Basic1	Unknown	Cattle, poultry, pigs
Medipharm (Chr.Hansen Group)	Lactiferm Spray1	Unknown strain M74	Cattle, poultry, pigs
Medipharm (Chr.Hansen Group)	Lactiferm DW (Drinking water) 1	Unknown strain M74	Cattle, poultry, pigs
Provita Eurotech	Provita lacteal1	*Lactobacillus acidophilus*, *Enterococcus faecium*, *Bacillus* spp.	Poultry

flora created conditions that favoured good health.

Probiotics have been used extensively in poultry since the 1970s, particularly in newly hatched chicks. The seminal work of Nurmi and Rantala (1973) first demonstrated the potential of live bacteria to protect chicks from *Salmonella* colonization by CE. Subsequently, a number of studies have demonstrated that the CE effects of probiotics can protect livestock against pathogens such as *Salmonella*, *Campylobacter*, *Yersinia* and *E. coli* (Weinack *et al.*, 1981, 1982; Soerjadi-Liem *et al.*, 1984a, b; Schoeni and Wong, 1994; La Ragione *et al.*, 2001; La Ragione and Woodward, 2003; Casey *et al.*, 2007; Zhang *et al.*, 2007a, b).

Probiotics can be effective in controlling *Salmonella* in poultry, and their use was extensively reviewed by Fuller (1992), Revolledo *et al.* (2006) and Schneitz and Mead (2010). Fuller (1992) noted that many published studies reported that administration of a probiotic produced marked effects on a number of host parameters including levels of vitamins and serum triglycerides. However, Fuller also concluded that little significant evidence existed to support these claims, even when those made for a particular probiotic product were substantial. In the years since the Fuller review, there is still limited evidence regarding any beneficial effects of probiotics in poultry other than for control of food-borne pathogens. At present, several research groups are working to define the mechanisms by which probiotics, including single-strain preparations, can control *S.* Typhimurium and *S.* Enteritidis infections in broilers (Carter, 2008). To facilitate application, a spray system has been used to dose chicks with a *Lactobacillus*-based probiotic (FM-Probiotic) (Higgins *et al.*, 2008).

Lactobacillus

A number of *Lactobacillus* strains have been tested as probiotics in poultry and, as described earlier, some with considerable success. Although the exact mechanism of action is still to be elucidated, their efficacy is thought to be closely linked to the production of lactic acid and other antimicrobial compounds. Of all the *Lactobacillus* spp. studied to date, *La. reuteri* has received the most attention in relation to poultry. The protective effect of *La. reuteri* against enteropathogens is based on its ability to produce reuterin, a broad-spectrum antibiotic (Talarico *et al.*, 1988). The organism has been shown to reduce colonization of chicks and turkey poults by *Salmonella* and *E. coli* (Edens *et al.*, 1997). Furthermore, it has been reported that a commercial *Lactobacillus* preparation, FM-B11, inhibited *S.* Enteritidis in commercial broilers (Higgins *et al.*, 2007; Vicente *et al.*, 2008). Both studies showed an overall reduction in *Salmonella* recovery, when the probiotic was administered prophylactically. Whilst demonstrating considerable promise, neither probiotic completely eliminated the *Salmonella* challenge strain (Higgins *et al.*, 2007; Vicente *et al.*, 2008).

Bacillus subtilis

The spores of *Bacillus* species are being used commercially as probiotics in poultry, however, their exact mode of action remains unclear. Cartman *et al.* (2008) demonstrated that *B. subtilis* spores can germinate in the chicken gut and it is feasible that the resultant vegetative cells then produce antimicrobial compounds. Furthermore, studies on mice given *B. subtilis* spores have shown that the organism may modulate the immune response of the host (Huang *et al.*, 2008).

Unlike the more commonly used *Lactobacillus*-type probiotics, spores are dormant life forms and thus have significant practical advantages with regard to storage and incorporation into water/feed (Casula and Cutting, 2002). La Ragione and Woodward (2003) demonstrated that a single oral inoculum of 1×10^9 *B. subtilis* spores administered 24 h prior to challenge with *S.*. Enteritidis was sufficient to suppress colonization and persistence of the *Salmonella*. In particular, faecal shedding of *S.* Enteritidis, as measured by a semi-quantitative, cloacal-swabbing technique, was reduced significantly for the 36 days of the experiment. *Bacillus subtilis* persisted in the gut, although with decreasing numbers, over the same period. More recently, Vilà *et al.* (2009) demonstrated that the administration of *B. cereus* var. *toyoi* to chickens reduced *S.* Enteritidis colonization and invasion. These data add further evidence that *Bacillus* spores may be effective in controlling avian diseases and food-borne pathogens (La Ragione *et al.*, 2001; La Ragione and Woodward, 2003).

Enterococcus faecium

As with lactobacilli the exact mechanisms of probiotic action are still to be fully elucidated for enterococci. However, the production of lactic acid and other antimicrobial compounds is thought to be a key part of their probiotic activity. In experimental studies, Audisio *et al.* (2000) showed that *Enterococcus faecium* J96 inhibited *S.* Pullorum infection in chickens. This organism was administered orally, either as a prophylactic or a therapeutic treatment. In the first case, the enterococcus was given to the chicks twice a day for 3 consecutive days. In the second, it was administered in the same way after a challenge at 24h with *S.* Pullorum. Caecal contents, livers and spleens were analysed. The chickens that were given the prophylactic treatment survived the *S.* Pullorum challenge, whereas those that were infected on the first day and then given the *Enterococcus* died 4 days later. The *Salmonella* was isolated from their livers and spleens. These studies indicate that *Ent. faecium* J96 can protect newly-hatched chicks from *S.* Pullorum infection, but only when used prophylactically and not as a therapeutic agent.

Levkut *et al.* (2009) studied the protective effect of *Ent. faecium* EF 55 against *S.* Enteritidis phage type 4 in day-old chicks. The enterococcus was administered daily for 7 days prior to challenge with *S.* Enteritidis. *Salmonella* levels in the faeces of *Enterococcus*-treated birds were significantly reduced on days 2 and 14 post-inoculation ($P<0.01$), in comparison with untreated controls. Furthermore, the numbers of *S.* Enteritidis in the caeca were significantly lower ($P<0.01$) at the end of the experiment (day 14) for the *Enterococcus*-treated group. At day 4, *Salmonella* levels in the livers were significantly lower for the treated group ($P<0.001$). Interestingly, the mean values for lymphocyte subpopulations in the blood and the relative percentages of caecal intraepithelial lymphocyte subpopulations (CD4, CD8, CD44, TCR, MHC II and IgM) were not significantly influenced by pretreatment with the enterococcus.

Prebiotics

Most prebiotic efficacy studies in livestock have involved poultry, for which compounds such as mannan- or fructo-oligosaccharides (MOS or FOS) have been used to modulate the resident gut flora of the host and subsequently reduce pathogen colonization (Fernandez *et al.*, 2002; Donalson *et al.*, 2008).

The application of MOS (Bio-MOS1) in broiler chickens has been associated with significant reductions in caecal colonization by *S.* Typhimurium ($P<0.05$) (Spring *et al.*, 2000). Additionally, β1–4 mannobiose reduced liver colonization by *S.* Enteritidis in broiler chickens at 7, 14 and 23 days post-infection ($P<0.05$) and also faecal shedding ($P<0.05$) (Agunos *et al.*, 2007).

Although prebiotics, such as MOS, have been shown to reduce *Salmonella* colonization in poultry, their precise mode of action is still uncertain. It has been demonstrated that prebiotics may increase populations of beneficial resident microflora, such as *Bifidobacterium* spp. Therefore, it is possible that increasing the abundance of bifidobacteria in the intestine reduces the availability of host receptors that are required for pathogen adherence. Alternatively, the reduction in pathogen colonization may be due to receptor mimicry or depletion of nutrients available to the pathogen as a consequence of stimulating the resident microbiota.

Stimulating proliferation of the microbiota can have a range of downstream effects on the host, such as an influence on the health and immune status of the host, SCFA production, the pH of the colon and suppression of pathogens by out-competing them. Thus, bifidobacteria are associated with increased host resistance to infection and diarrhoeal diseases, possibly through the ability to out-compete pathogens or by producing compounds such as organic acids, hydrogen peroxide and bacteriocins that have antagonistic effects on other microorganisms (Bernet-Camard *et al.*, 1997; Alakomi *et al.*, 2000; Mikolajczyk and Radowski, 2002; Skrivanova *et al.*, 2004; Fayol-Messaoudi *et al.*, 2005; Makras *et al.*, 2006; Skrivanova and Marounek, 2007).

Applicability of CE

Pathogen specificity

Studies carried out in several countries have shown that the CE concept appears to apply to all serovars of *Salmonella* that are capable of intestinal colonization in the chick (Pivnick and Nurmi, 1982; Schleifer, 1985; Mead and Impey, 1987; Schneitz, 1993; Stavric and D'Aoust, 1993).

Although aimed originally at the control of *Salmonella* infections, it has been shown experimentally that CE treatment also protects chicks against pathogenic *E. coli* (Soerjadi *et al.*, 1981a; Weinack *et al.*, 1981, 1982, 1984; Stavric *et al.*, 1992; Hakkinen and Schneitz, 1996), *Yersinia enterocolitica* (Soerjadi-Liem *et al.*, 1984b) and *Campylobacter jejuni* (Soerjadi *et al.*, 1982a; Soerjadi-Liem *et al.*, 1984a; Stern, 1994; Mead *et al.*, 1996). With *Campylobacter*, however, anaerobic preparations of adult caecal material, such as mucus, were clearly effective in protecting treated chicks, but less so when attempts were made to culture the material (Stern, 1994; Mead *et al.*, 1996).

In another potential application of CE treatment, there was a reduction in chicken mortality due to necrotic enteritis and hepatitis, and reduced levels of *Cl. perfringens*, which is one of the causative factors in necrotic enteritis (Barnes *et al.*, 1980b; Snoeyenbos *et al.*, 1983; Elwinger *et al.*, 1992; Kaldhusdal *et al.*, 1998). The use of CE treatment also reduced caecal colonization by *Listeria monocytogenes* in young chicks (Hume *et al.*, 1998). However, this organism appears to be a poor colonizer of the chicken and, in one study (Husu *et al.*, 1990), most chicks eliminated the bacterium from the gut within 9 days of per oral inoculation, and without any treatment.

Host specificity

Protection of newly hatched chicks against *Salmonella* colonization, using material from adult birds of the same species, seems to be independent of the breed, strain or sex of the bird, even though individual donors may show differences with respect to protective capability. Chickens can be protected to some extent by the microflora of a few other bird species (Snoeyenbos *et al.*, 1979; Weinack *et al.*, 1982; Impey *et al.*, 1984) but material from other animals, e.g. horse and cow, has proved to be ineffective (Rantala and Nurmi, 1973). Thus, mature chicken and turkey microfloras provide reciprocal protection for chicks and turkey poults (Weinack *et al.*, 1982; Impey *et al.*, 1984; Schneitz and Nuotio, 1992). However, defined mixtures of multiple strains used experimentally appear to be completely specific for the avian species from which the organisms were obtained (Impey *et al.*, 1984).

Laboratory experience

The effectiveness of CE treatment has been confirmed many times in laboratory-scale trials involving small groups of birds (reviewed by Pivnick and Nurmi, 1982; Schleifer, 1985; Mead, 2000; Schneitz and Mead, 2010). In these trials, the chicks were housed in cardboard boxes, cages or isolators with wire-mesh floors, or in wire-walled or solid-walled pens on concrete floors, with litter as a bedding. Three different methods of administering the treatment material have been used: dosing of individual birds, treatment via drinking water or by spraying. The most frequent method of challenge has been dosing of individual birds, although the seeder-bird technique and challenge via feed or water also have been used (Weinack *et al.*, 1979; Linton *et al.*, 1985; Mead *et al.*, 1989b; Hinton, M. *et al.*, 1991; Schneitz *et al.*, 1991; Schneitz, 1992; Bailey *et al.*, 1998; Corrier *et al.*, 1998). Usually, the trials last for 1 week. Both the rearing conditions and the method of administering the treatment may affect the results obtained. Chickens kept in cages with wire floors may be less prone to secondary challenge from their environment when any bird in the group starts to shed *Salmonella*. Dosing of individual birds is the most effective way of administering the treatment material, whereas spraying small groups of chicks effectively is difficult. The interval between treatment and challenge, and the length of the rearing period also may affect the results. Experience has shown that the results are improved if the interval between treatment and challenge is prolonged. A longer rearing period has the effect of reducing *Salmonella* levels in the caeca, since *Salmonella* infections tend to be self-limiting in older birds.

In an attempt to standardize the method used to evaluate different CE preparations, Mead *et al.* (1989a) developed an assay involving box-reared chicks. Newly hatched chicks were treated orally on day 1, challenged orally with *Salmonella* 24 h later and examined 5 days after challenge to determine both the proportion of positive birds in treated and control groups and the levels of *Salmonella* in any infected individuals. The efficacy of the treatment was determined by calculating an infection factor (IF) value, which is the geometric mean of the number of *Salmonella* per gram of caecal content for all chicks in a particular group, and a protection factor, which is obtained by dividing the IF value for the control group by that for the treated group (Pivnick *et al.*, 1985).

A different kind of assay was described by Wagner *et al.* (2002). This is carried out *in vitro* and avoids the need to use live chicks. Instead, the assay measures the ability of putative CE preparations to protect Caco-2 and CRL-2117 epithelial cells from invasion by *S.* Typhimurium and determines the effective concentration of the treatment preparation for each cell line. The test was not seen as an alternative to *in vivo* testing, but a convenient, rapid method for screening candidate bacterial strains and mixtures.

Field experience

It is difficult to carry out reliable field trials because artificial challenge cannot be used for birds intended for human consumption. Also, some of the chicks arriving at the farm may have been infected with *Salmonella* at the hatchery. Although there is evidence that levels of *Salmonella* infection in commercial broiler flocks can be significantly reduced by the use of CE treatment (Blankenship *et al.*, 1993; Bolder *et al.*, 1995; Deruyttere *et al.*, 1997; Palmu and Camelin, 1997), treatment must precede infection for maximum benefit (Seuna, 1979; Corrier *et al.*, 1998).

Some undefined CE preparations have been used widely throughout the world, but not in all countries. For example, their use is prohibited in the USA. In Sweden, where *Salmonella* has been virtually eliminated from the poultry supply chain, CE treatment was used routinely between 1981 and 1990, and played a major role in reducing the number of recurrent *Salmonella* infections in broilers (Wierup *et al.*, 1992). The treatment was part of an overall control programme for *Salmonella* that also included comprehensive biosecurity measures, and the benefit from CE in this situation may well have been cumulative because of its long-term application. Currently, CE products are not licensed for use in Swedish poultry. This is due to their undefined nature and the claim that their effectiveness has not been fully validated under commercial conditions (Sternberg Lewerin *et al.*, 2005). By international standards, Sweden has a very small poultry industry in comparison with, for example, Brazil. In the latter, CE treatment is used mainly in breeding stock along with other control measures, such as flock vaccination (Mead *et al.*, 2010). In the UK, CE products are recognized as valuable aids in the control of *Salmonella* and other pathogens (Davies, 2005), but tend to be used only on farms with recurrent problems from *Salmonella* (Mead, 2000). It is acknowledged that *Salmonella* is rarely excluded completely by this means, but usually there is a significant reduction in the prevalence of positive birds and in levels of intestinal carriage. However, it is questionable whether the benefits obtained are sufficient to be maintained throughout the poultry supply chain and up to the point of consumption. As indicated above, there is a lack of any definitive evidence for a clear reduction in the public health risk. When field trials on CE treatment were carried out in the Netherlands (Goren *et al.*, 1988), a statistically significant reduction in *Salmonella*-infected flocks was obtained, but, once the birds had been slaughtered and processed, there was no significant effect on carcass contamination. This was attributed to initial contamination of the birds from dirty transport crates and cross-contamination of carcasses during the various stages of processing. In contrast with the Dutch study, Palmu and Camelin (1997) carried out field trials in France and found a statistically significant reduction in *Salmonella* prevalence, both on the farm and in the processing plant from CE treatment. The carcasses were either processed first in the day or during a day when only CE-treated flocks were slaughtered, to prevent cross-contamination from untreated flocks. The only study in which all CE-treated broiler flocks were *Salmonella*-negative prior to slaughter was that of Deruyttere *et al.* (1997), but these were not followed through the processing plant.

Usually, CE preparations are given to newly hatched chicks or turkey poults as soon as possible after hatching, either at the hatchery or on the farm. Because the treatment is prophylactic rather than therapeutic, the birds should be *Salmonella*-free prior to treatment. Nevertheless, a reduction in *Salmonella* infection has been found in flocks that were *Salmonella*-positive in the hatchery before they were treated (Blankenship *et al.*, 1993; Bolder *et al.*, 1995; Palmu and Camelin, 1997). As mentioned above, the treatment is also given sometimes to older birds, following antibiotic therapy to eliminate an existing *Salmonella* infection (e.g. Johnson, 1992; Reynolds *et al.*, 1997). The two-stage treatment may thus avoid the necessity of slaughtering breeding stock that are infected with particular *Salmonella* serovars, such as *S.* Enteritidis and *S.* Typhimurium.

Both drinking-water administration and spraying at the hatchery are suitable for dosing birds under field conditions. Administering the treatment to birds individually is restricted to valuable elite stock, where the number of birds to be treated is low.

Initially, the only way of administering CE preparations in the field was via the first drinking water. This method was used successfully in Sweden (Wierup *et al.*, 1988, 1992). However, the method has its disadvantages. Sometimes, some of the chicks fail to drink prior to feeding and protection spreads unevenly among the flock (Schneitz *et al.*, 1991). Also, the viability of anaerobic organisms in the treatment preparation shows a rapid decline, especially in chlorinated water, and the product becomes ineffective before all the chicks have received an adequate dose (Seuna *et al.*, 1978). In addition, chicks may be exposed to *Salmonella* in the hatchery or during transportation to the farm, and even earlier if there is vertical transmission from infected breeders. In the first two cases, treatment on the farm via drinking water could be too late (Seuna, 1979). With respect to vertical transmission, CE treatment of chicks is likely to have little effect, although it may restrict the subsequent spread of *Salmonella* (Mead *et al.*, 1989b; Bailey *et al.*, 1998; Corrier *et al.*, 1998).

The use of aerosols as a method of administering CE preparations was suggested by Pivnick and Nurmi (1982). Subsequently, Goren *et al.* (1984b, 1988) developed a method of spray application to treat chicks at the hatchery, either in the hatchers themselves or when the chicks had been transferred to delivery boxes. Spraying in the hatcher followed by drinking-water administration on the farm was used by Blankenship *et al.* (1993) and shown to be effective in controlling *Salmonella* infection, but there is no evidence that a double treatment is necessary to obtain optimum protection and cost would be an important factor.

Spray application, either manual (Schneitz *et al.*, 1990) or automated (Schneitz, 1992), enables chicks to be treated at the earliest opportunity and ensures an even spread of the treatment material. It has no adverse effects on the health or performance of the birds during grow-out (Corrier *et al.*, 1995b; Palmu and Camelin, 1997). However, spray application may have to be carried out in a separate part of the hatchery to avoid contaminating a 'clean' area with microbes from the treatment material.

The possibility of chicks becoming infected with *Salmonella* in the hatchers has encouraged researchers to look for a method of administration that would enable the birds to be treated prior to hatching (Cox *et al.*, 1990, 1991). Therefore, an *in ovo* method was developed in which the CE preparation was introduced into either the air cell or the amnion of the egg a few days before hatching (Cox and Bailey, 1993). However, the use of a caecal culture containing highly proteolytic organisms and abundant gas-formers resulted in depressed hatchability when the material was introduced into the air cell (Cox *et al.*, 1992; Cox and Bailey, 1993). Inoculating the amnion prevented any of the chicks from hatching. Adverse effects on hatchability could be avoided by excluding strongly proteolytic and gas-forming organisms. Thus, instead of using an undefined CE preparation for this purpose, Edens *et al.* (1997) showed that *La. reuteri* could be administered *in ovo* without any loss of hatchability. Moreover, the lactobacillus was readily isolated from the hatched chicks. Unfortunately, the organism had little effect on colonization with *S.* Typhimurium.

Other Potential Beneficial Effects of CE

Although the normal microflora of the GI tract is known to have a negative impact on bird performance (Gabriel *et al.*, 2006), claims have been made that CE treatment enhances growth and reduces mortality in poultry. According to Goren *et al.* (1984b), an improvement in growth rate was observed in commercial broiler flocks spray-treated with a protective intestinal homogenate. When broiler chicks were given CE treatment on the day of hatch, Corrier *et al.* (1995b) found an improvement in the efficiency of feed utilization. Improvements in bird performance, in terms of higher body weight, better feed conversion and lower mortality, were reported by Abu-Ruwaida *et al.* (1995) and Palmu and Camelin (1997), although the effects were not always statistically significant. Higher body weight and lower mortality were also noted by Bolder *et al.* (1995).

In an attempt to explore further the nutritional effects of CE treatment, Schneitz *et al.* (1998) used Broilact as the treatment material and found a decrease in the viscosity of the ileal contents and an increase in faecal dry matter. There was also a 1.6% improvement in the metabolizable energy value of the feed, an increase in caecal propionic acid and a decrease in butyric acid in the ileal contents.

Factors Affecting the Efficacy of CE

In addition to certain antimicrobials that are used to treat infectious diseases in the birds, factors that can reduce the efficacy of CE treatment include stress and disease. Starving chicks for the first 24 h of life also has a negative effect (Goren *et al.*, 1984a), whereas, in older birds, the protective flora is more difficult to disrupt (Snoeyenbos *et al.*, 1985). With the day-old chick, physiological stress induced by high or low environmental temperatures, or removal of feed and water, either interfered with the colonization of protective organisms or reduced the protection they provided, however, there was no obvious effect at 2 weeks of age (Weinack *et al.*, 1985a).

Lafont *et al.* (1983) studied CE-treated chicks that were carrying low numbers of *Salmonella* in their intestines and administered oocysts of *Eimeria tenella* at a level known to produce caecal coccidiosis. The birds then shed large numbers of *Salmonella* for more than 2 weeks. Exposure of CE-treated chicks to aerosols of *Mycoplasma gallisepticum* and/or infectious bronchitis virus increased the number of birds shedding pathogenic *E. coli* or *S.* Typhimurium, following a challenge 2 days after protective treatment (Weinack *et al.*, 1984).

Induced moulting of white leghorn layers and subjecting market-age broilers to feed withdrawal also have been shown to increase both the numbers of *Salmonella* in the GI tract and the proportion of infected individuals (Holt and Porter, 1993; Holt *et al.*, 1995; Macri *et al.*, 1997; Raminez *et al.*, 1997).

As discussed earlier, vertical transmission of *Salmonella* via the egg or any *Salmonella* infection acquired before CE treatment can be administered will either reduce treatment efficacy in chicks or render it ineffective.

Potential for Combining CE with Other Treatments

CE treatments tend to reduce *Salmonella* colonization of poultry rather than completely eliminating the organisms. However, one of the advantages of CE treatment is that it can be combined with certain other anti-*Salmonella* measures to extend the protective capability. From the practical viewpoint, these treatment combinations are likely to be used only for breeding stock, because of cost, and some examples are described below.

One approach to enhancing the protective effects of undefined CE preparations is the incorporation of lactose in feed or drinking water. For example, lactose at a concentration of 2.5% in drinking water was shown to reduce subsequent colonization of chicks with *S.* Typhimurium (Hinton, A. *et al.*, 1991). The most effective protection, however, involving a $\log_{10}$ 5.5 reduction in caecal carriage resulted from the combined use of lactose and a protective caecal culture. Lactose reduced the pH of caecal contents in recipient chicks and increased concentrations of acetic, lactic and propionic acids. With turkey poults, Corrier *et al.* (1991) showed that protection against *Salmonella* colonization was similar for birds given anaerobic caecal cultures and those receiving dietary lactose, and a combined treatment resulted in a level of protection equal to or higher than that observed when either of the two treatments was given separately. Nisbet *et al.* (1993) reported that dietary lactose and a CF culture of chicken caecal bacteria controlled *Salmonella* colonization in newly-hatched broiler chicks. However, no beneficial effect of lactose against *Salmonella* was observed by Waldroup *et al.* (1992). The use of lactose tends to cause slight scouring in the birds and therefore wet litter, which may lead to skin lesions.

Treatment of poultry feed with organic acids, such as formic and propionic acids, is sometimes used to prevent the birds acquiring *Salmonella* from the feed itself, but the treatment has no effect on caecal carriage of the organism following challenge (Hinton, M. *et al.*, 1991). Acid usage is compatible with the application of CE preparations and the two may be combined to increase the overall protective capability. When chicks were treated with a probiotic containing 11 strains of lactic acid bacteria, a commercial water acidifier or both together, the combined treatment consistently and significantly reduced the prevalence of chicks colonized with *S.* Enteritidis in both crop and caecal tonsils, and was more effective in this respect than either individual treatment (Wolfenden *et al.*, 2007). By contrast, Jarquin *et al.* (2007) used a different, nine-strain probiotic and an organic-acid mixture containing tannic, lactic, butyric and acetic acids to study their effects on horizontal transmission of *S.* Enteritidis. *Salmonella* transmission was reduced with the acids alone or in combination with the probiotic, but there was no synergistic effect from combining the two treatments.

There is a potential benefit in using a CE preparation after antimicrobial therapy to regenerate the gut microflora of the bird and prevent reinfection (e.g. Reynolds *et al.*, 1997). However, according to Humbert *et al.* (1997), antimicrobial therapy, followed by transfer of the birds to a clean house and CE treatment, whether combined or not, had an effect in reducing *Salmonella* prevalence, but did not guarantee that the organism would be eliminated from all the birds. Nevertheless, in the study of Reynolds *et al.* (1997) no further isolates of *S.* Enteritidis were found during regular monitoring of hatchery samples and a long-term reduction in environmental *Salmonella* contamination was observed, following the combined treatment. Another antimicrobial combination treatment involved *in ovo* administration of gentamycin prior to a *Salmonella* challenge immediately after the chicks had hatched, and then a CE preparation 1 day later (Bailey and Line, 2001). In this case, there was a statistically significant cumulative effect and almost complete elimination of the *Salmonella* in all three replicate trials. It was suggested that the combined treatment could help to reduce cross-contamination of chicks in the hatcher.

CE treatment can also be combined successfully with vaccination. In a study carried out by Methner *et al.* (1999), young chicks were either given CE treatment, vaccinated with a live *S.* Typhimurium strain or given both together. The birds were then challenged on several occasions with the antibiotic-resistant but otherwise isogenic mutant of the vaccine strain. The commercial CE product used (Aviguard) gave considerable protection for at least 40 days, as did the vaccine strain alone, but there was a marked additive effect from the combined treatment, especially when the vaccine strain was administered prior to CE treatment or at the same time. This ensured adequate persistence of the vaccine strain as a prerequisite for colonization inhibition and a strong immune response. One advantage of the combined treatment was the degree of protection afforded to both young and older birds, although, for experimental purposes, only a non-attenuated vaccine strain was used in this study.

A different combination was studied by Toro *et al.* (2005) and involved the use of a 'cocktail' of *Salmonella*-specific bacteriophages and a CE product that was a poultry-specific probiotic comprising seven different bacterial strains. The CE product was given to chicks at hatch, while the phage preparation was administered several days before and after challenge with *S.* Typhimurium. The phages were readily isolated from the faeces of treated birds ca. 48 h after administration. Both treatments, whether separately or combined, reduced levels of *Salmonella* carriage in the ileum and caecum, although the extent of the reductions varied with the age of the birds and between trials. In this case, there was no obvious benefit from combining the two treatments, other than one treatment providing a 'back-up' for the other.

Safety Requirements for CE Preparations and Product Regulation

Undefined CE preparations have been used by poultry producers worldwide for more than 20 years, with no apparent harmful effects and with approval, in principle, from the World Health Organization (WHO, 1994). However, the WHO has suggested that these preparations should be distinguished from live probiotics that contain only one or a few microbial strains. Such products are not acceptable for use in all countries, due mainly to concerns about the possible presence of unknown or undetected pathogens and the potential for transmitting antimicrobial-resistant bacteria and resistance determinants, ultimately to humans via the food chain (Kruse, 1999).

The key to minimizing both concerns lies in the selection of one or more appropriate, adult donor birds and the use of suitable control measures in product manufacture. The donors should originate from a geographical area with a low risk of avian disease and from a farm in which flocks are kept under veterinary supervision, with regular health checks, avoiding antimicrobial therapy wherever possible. The microflora obtained from these birds can be administered to SPF chicks, which are then monitored for all the relevant antibodies associated with disease agents (Snoeyenbos *et al.*, 1979). Intestinal material from the SPF birds forms the basis of the CE treatment product and the organisms present will retain the protective capability of the original microflora. Even from this starting point, however, the gut material must be screened comprehensively for all relevant pathogens by standard laboratory tests. Other safety measures are described by Nurmi and Nuotio (1994) and include the use of good laboratory and manufacturing practices, and a series of dilution steps in the manufacturing process, so that the starting material is diluted to at least 1 in 100 million. The media and methods employed for propagation of the protective organisms do not support the proliferation of either mycoplasmas, viruses or protozoan parasites.

A study of prototype mixed cultures for CE purposes, using both cultural methods and culture-independent molecular techniques (Waters *et al.*, 2006), showed that many of the bacterial strains present could not be cultured on their own and, even among those isolated, a significant proportion could not be identified with known species. Of course, the same uncertainties are associated with the gut microflora of live poultry, where the component organisms are acquired naturally but by ways and means that are uncontrolled and not fully understood. By artificially establishing the flora from a carefully selected and fully-screened donor bird, any risk to public health from undetected pathogens should be substantially reduced.

With respect to antimicrobial-resistant bacteria, these organisms have been isolated frequently from commercial poultry reared intensively and they were found among various bacterial genera and species in an unidentified CE product by Wagner and Cerniglia (2005). Although the publication gives no information on the provenance of the CE product, it seems unlikely that the production process had followed all the precautions described above. Nevertheless, there is a need to clarify this aspect of product safety for CE preparations in general.

Animal feed additives (including yeasts and bacteria) are strictly regulated within the EU legislative framework. Since the decision was made to phase out antimicrobial feed supplements, there has been a great deal of interest in finding suitable alternatives and, consequently, the legislation and procedures governing this area have been undergoing significant change in recent years. Until May 2003, the risk assessment of animal feed additives for use in Europe was the responsibility of the Scientific Committee of Animal Nutrition (SCAN) (von Wright, 2005; Anadon *et al.*, 2006). After this date, the European Food Safety Authority (EFSA) took over the functions of SCAN. While EFSA provide expert scientific advice to the European Commission (EC), ultimately, the approval and risk management of a probiotic product is the responsibility of the EC and its constituent member states. In the USA a microorganism that is used as a feed additive is subject to approval by the Food and Drug Administration.

In order for a novel probiotic product to fulfil the current EU regulations on animal feed additives, the component(s) of the product must be clearly characterized and identified to species level, efficacy data must be provided in support of any claims made for the product, the product must be well tolerated by the target animal species (i.e. have no adverse effects on health or performance), it must be safe for the operator (i.e. have no adverse effects upon exposure) and it must not pose a risk to the safety of the end-consumer (SCAN, 2001). In addition, a novel probiotic product must not harbour any acquired antimicrobial resistance determinants that may be transferred to other bacteria (SCAN, 2001, 2003; EFSA, 2005).

Conclusions

There is continuing interest in developing better measures to reduce the symptomless carriage of human enteropathogens in food animals and thereby minimize the risk of consumer illness from contaminated products. The prospects for developing successful control programmes appear to be best for intensively-reared animals that are kept in controlled-environment housing, and poultry is a prime example. In this situation, the newly hatched chick should be regarded as a critical control point, because of its extreme susceptibility to colonization with pathogens such as *Salmonella*, a fact that can be attributed to the slow rate of development of a competing gut microflora under modern commercial conditions. Both the reason for chick susceptibility and a possible solution to the problem were highlighted in the seminal publication of Nurmi and Rantala (1973).

The use of an undefined CE preparation in *Salmonella* control has a number of advantages. The treatment is relatively cheap and easy to apply, and it appears to be effective against all non-host-specific *Salmonella* serovars that can colonize the GI tract of the bird. Treatment efficacy is unaffected by the breed, strain or sex of the bird and there are indications that other hazardous organisms, such as *Cl. perfringens* and pathogenic *E. coli*, may be controlled in the same way, should the need arise. Control of *C. jejuni* also appears to be possible by this means, but may involve different protective bacteria, perhaps reflecting the specific niche in the caecum occupied by campylobacters.

Treatment of chicks to establish a protective microflora is essentially a preventive measure that must be supported by an effective biosecurity programme on the farm. It also requires the use of good husbandry practice to minimize bird stress, otherwise the effectiveness of CE treatment is reduced (Weinack *et al.*, 1985a). Because of its preventive nature, a consistent supply of *Salmonella*-free chicks is needed and failure to meet one or other of these requirements may explain why some field trials have yielded poor results. Thus, CE treatment can only be a part of any programme aimed at controlling *Salmonella* infections in poultry. However, it can be readily combined with other measures, including, where appropriate, antimicrobial therapy, vaccination or the use of acid-treated feed. In some countries, there is an important application to adult breeder birds that are infected with certain *Salmonella* serovars and otherwise may have to be slaughtered.

The CE concept simply exploits a natural phenomenon relating to microbial competition in the GI tract, and the effect on any *Salmonella* ingested by the chick is to prevent multiplication (Impey and Mead, 1989). Thus, an invading *Salmonella* is unable to colonize and eventually would be flushed out of the gut. Most of the currently available treatment products are undefined and complex in composition, although at least two of them have been analysed and many of the component organisms identified and/or characterized. No preparation that completely excludes *Salmonella* from poultry has yet been developed and further work is needed to optimize the efficacy of CE treatment. Defined treatment preparations tend to be less effective than their undefined counterparts and progress in this area is hampered by a lack of knowledge of the precise mechanism(s) of protection and of the key properties of the organisms involved. Although commercial application of undefined preparations has a long history and no adverse effects on bird health or performance have been reported, the benefits claimed under some conditions in relation to bird growth, feed utilization and chick mortality require clarification.

Despite the long usage of undefined CE preparations in parts of Scandinavia and elsewhere, there is still reluctance on the part of regulatory authorities in some other countries to allow commercial application of these products. With appropriate precautions in the selection of donor birds and control of product manufacture to include comprehensive testing of donor material for all relevant pathogens, it can be argued that the resultant treatment preparation would offer a lower risk to human health than some of the microbes that are acquired naturally during poultry production. However, there is a need to determine whether this hypothesis can be supported by scientific evidence, especially in relation to antimicrobial resistance. It is probably less important that the treatment material is undefined and the WHO has suggested a special product category ('normal gut flora'), which distinguishes such products from conventional probiotics. Now that particular attention is being given to the development of improved defined-treatment preparations, to satisfy regulatory requirements, it will be interesting to see whether their protective capabilities will eventually match those of the undefined products currently available.

References

Abu-Ruwaida, A.S., Husseini, M. and Banat, I.M. (1995) Salmonella exclusion in broiler chicks by the competitive action of adult gut microflora. *Microbios* 83, 59–69.

Agunos, A., Ibuki, M., Yokomizo, F. and Mine, Y. (2007) Effect of dietary beta1–4 mannobiose in the prevention of *Salmonella* Enteritidis infection in broilers. *British Poultry Science* 48, 331–341.

Alakomi, H.L., Skytta, E., Saarela, M., Mattila-Sandholm, T., Latva-Kala, K. *et al.* (2000) Lactic acid permeabilizes Gram-negative bacteria by disrupting the outer membrane. *Applied and Environmental Microbiology* 66, 2001–2005.

Amit-Romach, E., Sklan, D. and Uni, Z. (2004) Microflora ecology of the chicken intestine using 16S ribosomal DNA primers. *Poultry Science* 83, 1093–1098.

Anadon, A., Martinez-Larranaga, M.R. and Aranzazu Martinez, M. (2006) Probiotics for animal nutrition in the European Union. Regulation and Safety assessment. *Regulatory Toxicology and Pharmacology* 45, 91–95.

Andreatti Filho, R.L., Sampaio, H.M., Barros, M.R., Gratao, P.R. and Cataneo, A. (2003) Use of caecal microflora cultured under aerobic or anaerobic conditions in the control of experimental infection of chicks with *Salmonella* Enteritidis. *Veterinary Microbiology* 92, 237–244.

Audisio, A.M., Oliver, G. and Apella, M.C. (2000) Protective effect of *Enterococcus faecium* J96, a potential probiotic strain, on chicks infected with *Salmonella* Pullorum. *Journal of Food Protection* 63, 1333–1337.

Bailey, J.S. and Line, E. (2001) In ovo gentamycin and mucosal starter culture to control *Salmonella* in broiler production. *Journal of Applied Poultry Research* 10, 1376–1379.

Bailey, J.S., Cason, J.A. and Cox, N.A. (1998) Effect of *Salmonella* in young chicks on competitive exclusion treatment. *Poultry Science* 77, 394–399.

Barnes, E.M. (1977) Ecological concepts of the anaerobic flora in the avian intestine. *American Journal of Clinical Nutrition* 30, 1793–1798.

Barnes, E.M. (1979) The intestinal microflora of poultry and game birds during life and after storage. *Journal of Applied Bacteriology* 46, 407–419.

Barnes, E.M. and Impey, C.S. (1970) The isolation and properties of the predominant anaerobic bacteria in the caeca of chickens and turkeys. *British Poultry Science* 11, 467–481.

Barnes, E..M. and Impey, C.S. (1971) The isolation of anaerobic bacteria from chicken caeca with particular reference to members of the family Bacteroidaceae. In: Shapton, D.A. and Board, R.G. (eds) *Isolation of Anaerobes*. Academic Press, London, pp. 115–123.

Barnes, E.M., Mead, G.C., Barnum, D.A. and Harry, E.G. (1972) The intestinal flora of the chicken in the period 2 to 6 weeks of age, with particular reference to the anaerobic bacteria. *British Poultry Science* 13, 311–326.

Barnes, E.M., Impey, C.S. and Stevens, J.H. (1979a) Factors affecting the incidence and anti-*Salmonella* activity of the anaerobic caecal flora of the young chick. *Journal of Hygiene* 82, 263–283.

Barnes, E.M., Mead, G.C., Impey, C.S. and Adams, B.W. (1979b) Analysis of the avian intestinal flora. In: Lovelock, D.W. and Davies, R. (eds) *Techniques for the Study of Mixed Populations*. Technical Series 11, Society for Applied Bacteriology, Academic Press, London, pp. 89–105.

Barnes, E.M., Impey, C.S. and Cooper, D.M. (1980a) Competitive exclusion of salmonellas from the newly hatched chick. *Veterinary Record* 106, 61.

Barnes, E.M., Impey, C.S. and Cooper, D.M. (1980b) Manipulation of the crop and intestinal flora of the newly hatched chick. *American Journal of Clinical Nutrition* 33, 2426–2433.

Barrow, P.A. and Tucker, J.F. (1986) Inhibition of colonization of the chicken caecum with *Salmonella* typhimurium by pre-treatment with strains of *Escherichia coli*. *Journal of Hygiene* 96, 161–169.

Barrow, P.A., Tucker, J.F. and Simpson, J.M. (1987) Inhibition of colonization of the chicken alimentary tract with *Salmonella* typhimurium by Gram-negative facultatively anaerobic bacteria. *Epidemiology and Infection* 98, 311–322.

Barrow, P.A., Hassan, J.O. and Berchieri, A., Jr (1990) Reduction in faecal excretion of *Salmonella* typhimurium strain F98 by chickens by vaccination with live and killed *S* typhimurium organisms. *Epidemiology and Infection* 104, 413–426.

Berchieri, A., Jr and Barrow, P.A. (1990) Further studies on the inhibition of colonization of the chicken alimentary tract with *Salmonella* typhimurium by pre-colonization with an avirulent mutant. *Epidemiology and Infection* 104, 427–441.

Bernet-Camard, M.F., Lievin, V., Brassart, D., Neeser, J.R., Servin, A.L. *et al.* (1997) The human *Lactobacillus acidophilus* strain LA1 secretes a nonbacteriocin antibacterial substance(s) active *in vitro* and *in vivo*. *Applied and Environmental Microbiology* 63, 2747–2753.

Bielke, L.R., Elwood, A.L., Donoghue, D.J., Donoghue, A.M., Newberry, L.A., Neighbor, N.K. and Hargis, B.M. (2003) Approach for selection of individual enteric bacteria for competitive exclusion in turkey poults. *Poultry Science* 82, 1378–1382.

Blanchfield, B., Gardiner, M.A. and Pivnick, H. (1982) Nurmi concept for preventing infection of chicks by *Salmonella*: comparison of fecal suspensions and fecal cultures administered into the crop and in drinking water. *Journal of Food Protection* 45, 345–347.

Blanchfield, B., Stavric, S., Gleeson, T. and Pivnick, H. (1984) Minimum intestinal inoculum for Nurmi cultures and a new method for determining competitive exclusion of *Salmonella* from chicks. *Journal of Food Protection* 47, 542–545.

Blankenship, L.C., Bailey, J.S., Cox, N.A., Stern, N.J., Brewer, R. and Williams, O. (1993) Two-step mucosal competitive exclusion flora to diminish salmonellae in commercial broiler chickens. *Poultry Science* 72, 1667–1672.

Bolder, N.M., van Lith, L.A.J.T., Putirulan, F.F., Jacobs-Reitsma, W.F. and Mulder, R.W.A.W. (1992) Prevention of colonization by *Salmonella enteritidis* PT4 in broiler chickens. *International Journal of Food Microbiology* 15, 313–317.

Bolder, N.M., Vereijken, P.F.G., Putirulan, F.F. and Mulder, R.W.A.W (1995) The effect of competitive exclusion on the *Salmonella* contamination of broilers (a field study). In: Briz, R.C. (ed.) *Proceedings of the 2nd Annual Meeting of EC COST Working Group No. 2*. Graficas Imprinter, Zaragoza, Spain, pp. 89–97.

Burns, R. (1995) Commercial competitive exclusion bacterial mix ready soon. *Feedstuffs*, 13 March, 27.

Cameron, D.M. and Carter, J.N. (1992) Evaluation of the efficacy of BROILACT in preventing infection of broiler chicks with *S.* enteritidis PT4. *International Journal of Food Microbiology* 15, 319–326.

Cameron, D.M., Carter, J.N., Mansell, P. and Redgrave, V.A. (1997) Floor-pen efficacy study with Aviguard against *Salmonella* typhimurium DT 104 colonization in turkeys. In: *Proceedings of the Salmonella and Salmonellosis Symposium Zoopôle Developpement,* Ploufragen, France, pp. 481–485.

Carter, A. (2008) An evaluation of the efficacy and safety of probiotic lactic acid bacteria. PhD thesis, University of Surrey, Guildford, UK.

Cartman, S.T., La Ragione, R.M. and Woodward, M.J. (2008) *Bacillus subtilis* spores germinate in the chicken gastrointestinal tract. *Applied and Environmental Microbiology* 74, 5254–5258.

Casey, P.G., Gardiner, G.E., Casey, G., Bradshaw, B., Lawlor, P.G. *et al.* (2007) A five-strain probiotic combination reduces pathogen shedding and alleviates disease signs in pigs challenged with *Salmonella enterica* Serovar Typhimurium. *Applied and Environmental Microbiology* 73, 1858–1863.

Casula, G. and Cutting, S.M. (2002) Bacillus probiotics: spore germination in the gastrointestinal tract. *Applied and Environmental Microbiology* 68, 2344–2352.

Coloe, P.J., Bagust, T.J. and Ireland, L. (1984) Development of the normal gastrointestinal microflora of specific pathogen-free chickens. *Journal of Hygiene, Cambridge* 92, 79–87.

Corrier, D.E., Hinton, A., Jr, Kubena, L.F., Ziprin, R.L. and DeLoach, J.R. (1991) Decreased *Salmonella* colonization in turkey poults inoculated with anaerobic cecal microflora and provided dietary lactose. *Poultry Science* 70, 1345–1350.

Corrier, D.E., Hinton, A., Jr, Hargis, B. and DeLoach, J.R. (1992) Effect of used litter from floor pens of adult broilers on *Salmonella* colonization of broiler chicks. *Avian Diseases* 36, 897–902.

Corrier, D.E., Nisbet, D.J., Scanlan, C.M., Hollister, A.G. and Deloach, J.R. (1995a) Control of *Salmonella* typhimurium colonization in broiler chicks with continuous-flow characterized mixed culture of cecal bacteria. *Poultry Science* 74, 916–924.

Corrier, D.E., Nisbet, D.J., Scanlan, C.M., Hollister, A.G., Caldwell, D.J., Thomas, L.A., Hargis, B.M., Tomkins, T. and Deloach, J.R. (1995b) Treatment of commercial broiler chickens with a characterized culture of cecal bacteria to reduce salmonellae colonization. *Poultry Science* 74, 1093–1101.

Corrier, D.E., Byrd, J.A., II, Hume, M.E., Nisbet, D.J. and Stanker, L.H. (1998) Effect of simultaneous or delayed competitive exclusion treatment on the spread of *Salmonella* in chicks. *Journal of Applied Poultry Research* 7, 132–137.

Costerton, J.W., Irvin, R.T. and Cheng, K.-J. (1981) The bacterial glycocalyx in nature and disease. *Annual Review of Microbiology* 35, 299–324.

Cox, N.A. and Bailey, J.S. (1993) Introduction of bacteria *in ovo*. United States Patent no. 5,206,015.

Cox, N.A., Bailey, J.S., Mauldin, J.M. and Blankenship, L.C. (1990) Presence and impact of salmonellae contamination in commercial broiler hatcheries. *Poultry Science* 69, 1606–1609.

Cox, N.A., Bailey, J.S., Mauldin, J.M. and Blankenship, L.C. (1991) Extent of salmonellae contamination in breeder hatcheries. *Poultry Science* 70, 416–418.

Cox, N.A., Bailey, J.S., Mauldin, J.M. and Blankenship, L.C. (1992) *In ovo* administration of a competitive exclusion treatment to broiler embryos. *Poultry Science* 71, 1781–1784.

Croucher, S.C. and Barnes, E.M. (1983) The occurrence and properties of *Gemmiger* formicilis and related budding bacteria in the avian caecum. *Journal of Applied Bacteriology* 54, 7–22.

Davies, R.H. (2005) Pathogen populations on poultry farms. In: Mead, G.C. (ed.) *Food Safety Control in the Poultry Industry.* Woodhead Publishing, Cambridge, UK, pp. 101–152.

de Oliviera, G.H., Berchieri, A. Jr and Barrow, P.A. (2000) Prevention of *Salmonella* infection by contact using intestinal flora of adult birds and/or a mixture of organic acids. *Brazilian Journal of Microbiology* 31, 116–120.

Deruyttere, L., Klaasen, J., Froyman, R. and Day, C.A. (1997) Field study to demonstrate the efficacy of Aviguard against intestinal *Salmonella* colonization in broilers. In: *Proceedings of the* Salmonella *and Salmonellosis Symposium,* Zoopôle Developpement, Ploufragan, France, pp. 523–525.

Donalson, L.M., McReynolds, J.L., Kim, W.K., Chalova, V.I., Woodward, C.L., Kubena, L.F., Nisbet, D.J. and Ricke, S.C. (2008) The influence of a fructooligosaccharide prebiotic combined with alfalfa molt diets on the gastrointestinal tract fermentation, *Salmonella* Enteritidis infection, and intestinal shedding in laying hens. *Poultry Science* 87, 1253–1262.

Donoghue, A.M., Farnell, M.B., Cole, K. and Donoghue, D.J. (2006) Mechanisms of pathogen control in the avian gastrointestinal tract. In: Perry, G.C. (ed.) *Avian Gut Function in Health and Disease.* Poultry Science Symposium Series, Vol. 28. CAB International, Wallingford, UK, pp. 138–155.

Duguid, J.P. and Campbell, I. (1969) Antigens of the type-1 fimbriae of *Salmonella* and other enterobacteria. *Journal of Medical Microbiology* 2, 535–553.

Dunham, H.J., Edens, F.W., Casas, I.A. and Dobrogosz, W.J. (1994) Efficacy of *Lactobacillus reuteri* as a probiotic for chickens and turkeys. *Microbial Ecology in Health and Disease* 7, 52–53.

EC (2003a) Regulation (EC) No. 2160/2003 of the European Parliament and of the Council of 17 November 2003 on the control of *Salmonella* and other specified food-borne zoonotic agents. *Official Journal of the European Union* L325, 1–15.

EC (2003b) Directive 2003/99/EC of the European Parliament and of the Council of 17 November 2003 on the monitoring of zoonoses and zoonotic agents. *Official Journal of the European Union* L325, 31.

Edens, F.W., Parkhurst, C.R. and Casas, I.A. (1991) *Lactobacillus reuteri* and whey reduce *Salmonella* colonization in the ceca of turkey poults. *Poultry Science* 70(Suppl. 1), 158.

Edens, F.W., Parkhurst, C.R., Casas, I.A. and Dobrogosz, W.J. (1997) Principles of *ex ovo* competitive exclusion and *in ovo* administration of *Lactobacillus reuteri*. *Poultry Science* 76, 179–196.

EFSA (2005) Opinion of the scientific panel on additives and products or substances used in animal feed on the updating of the criteria used in the assessment of bacteria for resistance to antibiotics of human and animal importance. *The EFSA Journal* 223, 1–12.

Elwinger, K., Schneitz, C., Berndtson, E., Fossum, O., Teglof, B. and Engstrom, B. (1992) Factors affecting the incidence of necrotic enteritis, caecal carriage of *Clostridium perfringens* and bird performance in broiler chicks. *Acta Veterinaria Scandinavica* 33, 369–378.

FAO/WHO (2002) *Risk Assessments of* Salmonella *in Eggs and Broiler Chickens.* Microbiological Risk Assessment Series No. 2. Food and Agriculture Organization of the United Nations, Rome and World Health Organization, Geneva.

FAO/WHO (2009) Salmonella *and* Campylobacter *in Chicken Meat.* Microbiological Risk Assessment Series No. 19. Food and Agriculture Organization of the United Nations, Rome and World Health Organization, Geneva.

Fayol-Messaoudi, D., Berger, C.N., Coconnier-Polter, M.H., Lievin-Le, Moal, V. and Servin, A.L. (2005) pH-, Lactic acid-, and non-lactic acid-dependent activities of probiotic Lactobacilli against *Salmonella enterica* Serovar Typhimurium. *Applied and Environmental Microbiology* 71, 6008–6013.

Fernandez, F., Hinton, M. and Van Gils, B. (2002) Dietary mannan-oligosaccharides and their effect on chicken caecal microflora in relation to *Salmonella* Enteritidis colonization. *Avian Pathology* 31, 49–58.

Ferreira, A.J.P., Ferreira, C.S.A., Knobl, T., Moreno, A.M., Bacarro, M.R., Chen, M., Robach, M. and Mead G.C. (2003) Comparison of three commercial competitive-exclusion products for controlling *Salmonella* colonization of broilers in Brazil. *Journal of Food Protection* 66, 490–492.

Freter, R., Stauffer, E., Cleven, D., Holdeman, L.V. and Moore, W.E.C. (1983) Continuous-flow cultures as *in vitro* models of the ecology of large intestinal flora. *Infection and Immunity* 39, 666–675.

Fuller, R. (1992) *Probiotics: The Scientific Basis.* Chapman & Hall, London.

Fuller, R. and Turvey, A. (1971) Bacteria associated with the intestinal wall of the fowl (*Gallus domesticus*). *Journal of Applied Bacteriology* 34, 617–622.

Gabriel, I., Lessire, M., Mallet, S. and Guillot, J.F. (2006) Microflora of the digestive tract: critical factors and consequences for poultry. *World's Poultry Science Journal* 62, 499–511.

Ghazikhanian, G.Y., Bland, M.C., Hofacre, C.L. and Froyman, R. (1997) Floor-pen study to determine the effect of Aviguard application to day-old turkey poults in reduction of clinical disease and intestinal colonization caused by *S.* kedougou infection. In: *Proceedings of the* Salmonella *and Salmonellosis Symposium*. Zoopôle Developpement, Ploufragan, France, pp. 531–533.

Goren, E., de Jong, W.A., Doornenbal, P., Koopman, J.P. and Kennis, H.M. (1984a) Protection of chicks against *Salmonella* infantis infection induced by strict anaerobically cultured intestinal microflora. *Veterinary Quarterly* 6, 22–26.

Goren, E., de Jong, W.A., Doornenbal, P., Koopman, J.P. and Kennis, H.M. (1984b) Protection of chicks against *Salmonella* infection induced by spray application of intestinal microflora in the hatchery. *Veterinary Quarterly* 6, 73–79.

Goren, E., de Jong, W.A., Doornenbal, P., Bolder, N.M., Mulder, R.W.A.W. and Jansen, A. (1988) Reduction of *Salmonella* infection of broilers by spray application of intestinal microflora: a longitudinal study. *Veterinary Quarterly* 10, 249–255.

Greenberg, B. (1969) *Salmonella* suppression by known populations of bacteria in flies. *Journal of Bacteriology* 99, 629–635.

Guillot, J.F., Salmon, A., Mouline, C., Delaporte, J. and Magnin, M. (1997) Effect of a gut microflora (Aviguard) against controlled *Salmonella* enteritidis contamination in chickens. In: *Proceedings of the* Salmonella *and Salmonellosis Symposium*. Zoopôle Developpement, Ploufragan, France, p. 521.

Ha, S.A., Ricke, S.C., Nisbet, D.J., Corrier, D.E. and DeLoach, J.R. (1995) Serine utilization as a potential competition mechanism between *Salmonella* Typhimurium and a chicken cecal bacterium. *Journal of Food Protection* 57, 1074–1079.

Hakkinen, M. and Schneitz, C. (1996) Efficacy of a commercial competitive exclusion product against chicken pathogenic *Escherichia coli* and *E coli* 0157:H7. *Veterinary Record* 139, 139–141.

Higgins, S.E., Erf, G.F., Higgins, J.P., Henderson, S.N., Wolfenden, A.D. *et al.* (2007) Effect of probiotic treatment in broiler chicks on intestinal macrophage numbers and phagocytosis of *Salmonella* Enteritidis by abdominal exudate cells. *Poultry Science* 86, 2315–2321.

Higgins, S.E., Higgins, J.P., Wolfenden, A.D., Henderson, S.N., Torres-Rodriguez, A. *et al.* (2008) Evaluation of a *Lactobacillus*-based probiotic culture for the reduction of *Salmonella* Enteritidis in neonatal broiler chicks. *Poultry Science* 87, 27–31.

Hinton, A., Jr, Corrier, D.E., Ziprin, R.L., Spates, G.E. and DeLoach, J.R. (1991) Comparison of the efficacy of cultures of cecal anaerobes as inocula to reduce *Salmonella* typhimurium colonization in chicks with or without dietary lactose. *Poultry Science* 70, 67–73.

Hinton, M., Mead, G.C. and Impey, C.S. (1991) Protection of chicks against environmental challenge with *Salmonella enteritidis* by 'competitive exclusion' and acid-treated feed. *Letters in Applied Microbiology* 12, 69–71.

Ho, W.L., Yu, R.C. and Chou, C.C. (2004) Effect of iron limitation on the growth and cytotoxin production of *Salmonella choleraesuis* SC-5. *International Journal of Food Microbiology* 90, 295–302.

Holt, P.S. and Porter, R.E., Jr (1993) Effect of induced molting on the recurrence of a previous *Salmonella enteritidis* infection. *Poultry Science* 72, 2069–2078.

Holt, P.S., Macri, P. and Porter, R.E., Jr (1995) Microbial analysis of the early *Salmonella enteritidis* infection in molted and unmolted hens. *Avian Diseases* 39, 55–63.

Huang, J.M., La Ragione, R.M., Cooley, W.A., Todryk, S. and Cutting, S.M. (2008) Cytoplasmic delivery of antigens, by *Bacillus subtilis* enhances Th1 responses. *Vaccine* 26, 6043–6052.

Humbert, F., Carraminana, F., Lalande, F. and Salvat, G. (1997) Bacteriological monitoring of *Salmonella enteritidis* carrier birds after decontamination using enrofloxacin, competitive exclusion and movement of birds. *Veterinary Record* 141, 297–299.

Hume, M.E., Byrd, J.A., Stanker, L.H. and Ziprin, R.L. (1998) Reduction of caecal *Listeria monocytogenes* in Leghorn chicks following treatment with a competitive exclusion culture (PREEMPT™). *Letters in Applied Microbiology* 26, 432–436.

Hume, M.E., Kubena, L.F., Edrington, T.S., Donskey, C.J., Moore, R.W., Ricke, S.C. and Nisbet, D.J. (2003) Poultry digestive microflora biodiversity as indicated by denaturing gradient gel electrophoresis. *Poultry Science* 82, 1100–1107.

Husu, J.R., Beery, J.T., Nurmi, E. and Doyle, M.P. (1990) Fate of Listeria monocytogenes in orally dosed chicks. *International Journal of Food Microbiology* 11, 259–269.

Impey, C.S. and Mead, G.C. (1989) Fate of salmonellas in the alimentary tract of chicks pretreated with a mature caecal microflora to increase colonization resistance. *Journal of Applied Bacteriology* 66, 469–475.

Impey, C.S., Mead, G.C. and George, S.M. (1982) Competitive exclusion of salmonellas from the chick caecum using a defined mixture of bacterial isolates from the caecal microflora of an adult bird. *Journal of Hygiene, Cambridge* 89, 479–490.

Impey, C.S., Mead, G.C. and George, S.M. (1984) Evaluation of treatment with defined and undefined mixtures of gut microorganisms for preventing *Salmonella* colonization in chicks and turkey poults. *Food Microbiology* 1, 143–147.

Jarquin, R.L., Nava, G.M., Wolfenden, A.D., Donoghue, A.M., Hanning, I., Higgins, S.E. and Hargis, B.M. (2007) The evaluation of organic acids and probiotic cultures to reduce *Salmonella enteritidis* horizontal transmission and crop infection in broiler chickens. *International Journal of Poultry Science* 6, 182–186.

Johnson, C.T. (1992) The use of an antimicrobial and competitive exclusion combination in *Salmonella*-infected pullet flocks. *International Journal of Food Microbiology* 15, 293–298.

Juven, B.J., Meinersman, R.J. and Stern, N.J. (1991) Antagonistic effects of lactobacilli and pediococci to control intestinal colonization by human enteropathogens in live poultry. *Journal of Applied Bacteriology* 70, 95–103.

Kaldhusdal, M., Schneitz, C., Hofshagen, M. and Skjerve, E. (1998) Broilact® reduces the incidence of necrotic enteritis in broiler chickens. In: Hakkinen, M., Nuotio, L., Nurmi, E. and Mead, G.C. (eds)

Proceedings of Cost Action 97, Working Group I, Helsinki, Finland. Office for Official Publications of the European Communities, Luxembourg, pp. 85–90.

Kiely, L.J. and Olson, N.F. (2000) The physicochemical surface characteristics of *Lactobacillus casei*. *Food Microbiology* 17, 277–291.

Kingsley, R., Rabsch, W., Stephens, P., Roberts, M., Reissbrodt, R. and Williams, P.H. (1995) Iron-supplying systems of *Salmonella* in diagnostics, epidemiology and infection. *FEMS Immunology and Medical Microbiology* 11, 257–267.

Kruse, H. (1999) Indirect transfer of antibiotic resistance genes to man. *Acta Veterinaria Scandinavica* 92 (Suppl.), 59–65.

La Ragione, R.M. and Woodward, M.J. (2003) Competitive exclusion by *Bacillus subtilis* spores of *Salmonella enterica* serotype Enteritidis and *Clostridium perfringens* in young chickens. *Veterinary Microbiology* 94, 245–256.

La Ragione, R.M., Casula, G., Cutting, S.M. and Woodward, M.J. (2001) *Bacillus subtilis* spores competitively exclude *Escherichia coli* O78:K80 in poultry. *Veterinary Microbiology* 79, 133–142.

La Ragione, R.M., Narbad, A., Gasson, M.J. and Woodward, M.J. (2004) *In vivo* characterization of *Lactobacillus johnsonii* FI9785 for use as a defined competitive exclusion agent against bacterial pathogens in poultry. *Letters in Applied Microbiology* 38, 197–205.

Lafont, J.P., Bree, A., Naciri, M., Yvoré, P., Guillot, J.F. and Chaslus-Dancla, E. (1983) Experimental study of some factors limiting 'competitive exclusion' of *Salmonella* in chickens. *Research in Veterinary Science* 34, 16–20.

Lan, Y., Verstegen, M.W.A., Tamminga, S. and Williams, B.A. (2005) The role of the commensal gut microbial community in broiler chickens. *World's Poultry Science Journal* 61, 95–104.

Ledeboer, N.A. and Jones, B.D. (2005) Exopolysaccharide sugars contribute to biofilm formation by *Salmonella enterica* serovar Typhimurium on HEp-2 and chicken intestinal epithelium. *Journal of Bacteriology* 187, 3214–3226.

Levkut, M., Pistl, J., Lauková, A., Revajová, V., Herich, R., Sevcíková, Z., Strompfová, V., Szabóová, R. and Kokincáková, T. (2009) Antimicrobial activity of *Enterococcus faecium* ef 55 against *Salmonella* Enteritidis in chicks. *Acta Veterinaria Hungarica* 57, 13–24.

Line, J.E. (1997) Administration of *Saccharomyces boulardii* to reduce salmonellae colonization in poultry. In: *Proceedings of the* Salmonella *and Salmonellosis Symposium*. Zoopôle Developpement, Ploufragan, France, pp. 475–479.

Linton, A.H., Al-Chalaby, Z.A.M. and Hinton, M.H. (1985) Natural subclinical *Salmonella* infection in chickens: a potential model for testing the effects of various procedures on *Salmonella* shedding. *Veterinary Record* 116, 361–364.

Lloyd, A.B., Cumming, R.B. and Kent, R.D. (1974) Competitive exclusion as exemplified by *Salmonella* typhimurium. In: *Proceedings of the Australian Poultry Science Convention*, Hobart, Tasmania, pp. 185–186.

Lloyd, A.B., Cumming, R.B. and Kent, R.D. (1977) Prevention of *Salmonella* typhimurium infection in poultry by pretreatment of chickens and poults with intestinal extracts. *Australian Veterinary Journal* 53, 82–87.

Lu, J., Idris, U., Harmon, B., Hofacre, C., Maurer, J.J. and Lee, M.D. (2003) Diversity and succession of the intestinal bacterial community of the maturing broiler chicken. *Applied and Environmental Microbiology* 69, 6816–6824.

Macri, N.P., Porter, R.E., Jr and Holt, P.S. (1997) The effects of induced molting on the severity of acute intestinal inflammation caused by *Salmonella enteritidis*. *Avian Diseases* 41, 117–124.

Makras, L., Triantafyllou, V., Fayol-Messaoudi, D., Adriany, T., Zoumpopoulou, G. *et al.* (2006) Kinetic analysis of the antibacterial activity of probiotic lactobacilli towards *Salmonella enterica* serovar Typhimurium reveals a role for lactic acid and other inhibitory compounds. *Research in Microbiology* 157, 241–247.

McCartney, E. (2008) Zapping salmonella – facing tougher limits. *World Poultry* 24(7), 34–36.

Mead, G.C. (2000) Prospects for 'competitive exclusion' treatment to control salmonellas and other foodborne pathogens in poultry. *Veterinary Journal* 159, 111–123.

Mead, G.C. and Adams, B.W. (1975) Some observations on the caecal microflora of the chick during the first two weeks of life. *British Poultry Science* 16, 169–176.

Mead, G.C. and Impey, C.S. (1986) Current progress in reducing salmonella colonization of poultry by 'competitive exclusion'. *Journal of Applied Bacteriology Symposium* Suppl. 61, 65S–75S.

Mead, G.C. and Impey, C.S. (1987) The present status of the Nurmi concept for reducing carriage of food-poisoning salmonellae and other pathogens in live poultry. In: Smulders, F.J.M. (ed.) *Elimination of*

Pathogenic Organisms from Meat and Poultry. Elsevier Science Publishers, Amsterdam, the Netherlands, pp. 57–77.

Mead, G.C., Barrow, P.A., Hinton, M.H., Humbert, F., Impey, C.S., Lahellec, C., Mulder, R.W.A.W., Stavric, S. and Stern, N.J. (1989a) Recommended assay for treatment of chicks to prevent *Salmonella* colonization by competitive exclusion. *Journal of Food Protection* 52, 500–502.

Mead, G.C., Schneitz, C.E., Nuotio, L.O. and Nurmi, E.V. (1989b) Treatment of chicks using competitive exclusion to prevent transmission of *Salmonella enteritidis* in delivery boxes. In: *IXth International Congress of the World Veterinary Poultry Association*, Brighton, UK, p. 115 (abstract).

Mead, G.C., Scott, M.J., Humphrey, T.J. and McAlpine, K. (1996) Observations on the control of *Campylobacter jejuni* infection of poultry by 'competitive exclusion'. *Avian Pathology* 25, 69–79.

Mead, G., Lammerding, A., Cox, N., Doyle, M.P., Humbert, F., Kulikovskiy, A., Panin, A., Pinheiro do Nascimento, V., Wierup, M. *et al.* (2010) Scientific and technical factors affecting the setting of *Salmonella* criteria for raw poultry: a global perspective. *Journal of Food Protection* 73, 1566–1590.

Metchnikoff, E. (1908) *Prolongation of Life*. G.P. Putnam and Sons, New York.

Methner, U., Barrow, P.A., Berndt, A. and Steinbach, G. (1999) Combination of vaccination and competitive exclusion to prevent *Salmonella* colonization in chickens: experimental studies. *International Journal of Food Microbiology* 49, 35–42.

Methner, U., Barrow, P.A., Martin, G. and Meyer, H. (1997) Comparative study of the protective effect against *Salmonella* colonization in newly-hatched SPF chickens using live, attenuated *Salmonella* vaccine strains, wild-type *Salmonella* strains or a competitive-exclusion product. *International Journal of Food Microbiology* 35, 223–230.

Meynell, G.G. (1963) Antibacterial mechanisms of the mouse gut. II The role of E_h and volatile fatty acids in the normal gut. *British Journal of Experimental Pathology* 44, 209–219.

Mikolajczyk, A. and Radowski, M. (2002) Elimination of *Salmonella* spp. by lactic acid. *Polish Journal of Veterinary Science* 5, 139–143.

Muir, W.L., Bryden, W.L. and Husband, A.J. (2000) Immunity, vaccination and the avian intestinal tract. *Developments in Comparative Immunology* 24, 325–342.

Mulder, R.W.A.W., Havenaar, R. and Huis in't Veldt, J.H.J. (1997) Intervention strategies: the use of probiotics and competitive exclusion microfloras against contamination with pathogens in pigs and poultry. In: Fuller, R. (ed.) *Probiotics 2: Applications and Practical Aspects*. Chapman & Hall, London, pp. 187–207.

Nakamura, A., Ota, Y., Mizukami, A., Ito, T., Ngwai, Y.B. and Adachi, Y. (2002) Evaluation of Aviguard, a commercial competitive exclusion product, for efficacy and after-effect on the antibody response of chicks to *Salmonella*. *Poultry Science* 81, 1653–1660.

Newman, K.E. and Spring, P. (1996) Effect of a commercial competitive exclusion culture (AviFree) on *Salmonella* typhimurium concentration in broiler chicks. In: *12th Annual Symposium on Biotechnology in the Feed Industry*. Enclosure Code AVI 2.1 (poster).

Neilands, J.B. (1995) Siderophores: structure and function of microbial iron transport compounds. *Journal of Biological Chemistry* 270, 26723–26726.

Nisbet, D. (2002) Defined competitive exclusion cultures in the prevention of enteropathogen colonization in poultry and swine. *Antonie van Leeuwenhoek* 81, 481–486.

Nisbet, D.J., Corrier, D.E., Scanlan, C.M., Hollister, A.G., Beier, R.C. and DeLoach, J.R. (1993) Effect of a defined continuous-flow derived bacterial culture and dietary lactose on *Salmonella* typhimurium colonization in broiler chickens. *Avian Diseases* 37, 1017–1025.

Nisbet, D.J., Corrier, D.E. and DeLoach, J.R. (1995) Probiotic for control of *Salmonella*. United States Patent 5,478,557.

Nisbet, D.J., Corrier, D.E., Ricke, S.C., Hume, M.E., Byrd, J.A., II and DeLoach, J.R. (1996) Maintenance of the biological efficacy in chicks of a cecal competitive-exclusion culture against *Salmonella* by continuous-flow fermentation. *Journal of Food Protection* 59, 1279–1283.

Nuotio, L., Schneitz, C., Halonen, U. and Nurmi, E. (1992) Use of competitive exclusion to protect newly-hatched chicks against intestinal colonization and invasion by *Salmonella enteritidis* PT4. *British Poultry Science* 33, 775–779.

Nurmi, E. and Nuotio, L. (1994) Safety requirements for commercial competitive exclusion products. In: *Proceedings of the 9th European Poultry Conference*, Vol. II. The World's Poultry Science Association, Glasgow, UK, pp. 90–93.

Nurmi, E.V. and Rantala, M. (1973) New aspects of *Salmonella* infection in broiler production. *Nature* 241, 210.

Nurmi, E.V., Schneitz, C.E. and Makela, P.H. (1987) Process for the production of a bacterial preparation for the prophylaxis of intestinal disturbances in poultry. US Patent 4,689,226.

Palmu, L. and Camelin, I. (1997) The use of competitive exclusion in broilers to reduce the level of *Salmonella* contamination on the farm and at the processing plant. *Poultry Science* 76, 1501–1505.
Parry, S.M., Allen, W.D. and Porter, P. (1977) Intestinal immune response to *E. coli* antigens in germ-free chickens. *Immunology* 32, 731–741.
Pivnick, H. and Nurmi, E. (1982) The Nurmi concept and its role in the control of *Salmonella* in poultry. In: Davies, R. (ed.) *Developments in Food Microbiology* – I. Applied Science Publishers, Barking, UK, pp. 41–70.
Pivnick, H., Barnum, D., Stavric, S., Gleeson, T. and Blanchfield, B. (1985) Investigations on the use of competitive exclusion to control *Salmonella* in poultry. In: Barnum, D.A. (ed.) *Proceedings of International Symposium on* Salmonella *and Prospects for Control*, University of Guelph, Ontario, 263 pp.
Raminez, G.A., Sarlin, L.L., Caldwell, D.J., Yezak, C.R., Hume, D.E., Corrier, D.E., DeLoach, J.R. and Hargis, B.M. (1997) Effect of feed withdrawal on the incidence of *Salmonella* in the crops and ceca of market age broiler-chickens. *Poultry Science* 76, 654–656.
Rantala, M. (1974) Cultivation of a bacterial flora able to prevent the colonization of *Salmonella infantis* in the intestines of broiler chickens, and its use. *Acta Pathologica Microbiologica Scandinavica* Section B 82, 75–80.
Rantala, M. and Nurmi, E. (1973) Prevention of the growth of *Salmonella* infantis in chicks by the flora of the alimentary tract of chickens. *British Poultry Science* 14, 627–630.
Ratledge, C. and Dover, L.G. (2000) Iron metabolism in pathogenic bacteria. *Annual Review of Microbiology* 54, 881–941.
Revolledo, L., Ferreira, A.J.P. and Mead, G.C. (2006) Prospects in *Salmonella* control: competitive exclusion, probiotics, and enhancement of avian intestinal immunity. *Journal of Applied Poultry Research* 15, 341–351.
Reynolds, D.J., Davies, R.H., Richards, M. and Wray, C. (1997) Evaluation of combined antibiotic and competitive exclusion treatment in broiler breeder flocks infected with *Salmonella enterica* serovar Enteritidis. *Avian Pathology* 26, 83–95.
Ricke, S.C. (2003) Perspectives on the use of organic acids and short chain fatty acids as antimicrobials. *Poultry Science* 82, 632–639.
Rigby, C.E. and Pettit, J.R. (1980) Observations on competitive exclusion for preventing *Salmonella* typhimurium infection of broiler chickens. *Avian Diseases* 24, 604–615.
Rigby, C.E., Pettit, J. and Robertson, A. (1977) The effects of normal intestinal flora on the *Salmonella* carrier state in poultry with special reference to *S.* thompson and *S.* typhimurium. In: Barnum, D.A. (ed.) *Proceedings of the International Symposium on* Salmonella *and Prospects for Control*. University of Guelph, Ontario, 263 pp.
Rolfe, R.D. (1991) Population dynamics of the intestinal tract. In: Blankenship, L.C. (ed.) *Colonization Control of Human Bacterial Enteropathogens in Poultry*. Academic Press, San Diego, pp. 59–75.
Salanitro, J.P., Fairchilds, I.G. and Zornicki, Y.D. (1974) Isolation, culture characteristics, and identification of anaerobic bacteria from the chicken caecum. *Applied Microbiology* 27, 678–687.
Salanitro, J.P., Muirhead, P.A. and Goodman, J.R. (1976) Morphological and physiological characteristics of *Gemmiger formicilis* isolates from chicken ceca. *Applied and Environmental Microbiology* 32, 623–632.
Savage, D.C. (1977) Microbial ecology of the gastrointestinal tract. *Annual Review of Microbiology* 31, 107–133.
Savage, D.C. (1983) Mechanisms by which indigenous microorganisms colonize gastrointestinal epithelial surfaces. *Progress in Food and Nutrition Science* 7, 65–74.
SCAN (2001) Guidelines for the assessment of additives in feedstuffs. Part II: Enzymes and micro-organisms. European Commission, health and consumer protection directorate-general. (SCAN) Scientific Committee on Animal Nutrition.
SCAN (2003) Opinion of the scientific committee on animal nutrition on the criteria for assessing the safety of micro-organisms resistant to antibiotics of human and veterinary importance. European commission, health and consumer protection directorate-general. (SCAN) Scientific Committee on Animal Nutrition.
Schleifer, J.H. (1985) A review of the efficacy and mechanism of competitive exclusion for the control of *Salmonella* in poultry. *World's Poultry Science Journal* 41, 72–83.
Schneitz, C. (1992) Automated droplet application of a competitive exclusion preparation. *Poultry Science* 71, 2125–2128.
Schneitz, C. (1993) Development and evaluation of a competitive exclusion product for poultry. PhD thesis, Department of Veterinary Medicine, University of Helsinki, Helsinki, Finland.

Schneitz, C. and Hakkinen, M. (1998) Comparison of two different types of competitive exclusion products. *Letters in Applied Microbiology* 26, 338–341.

Schneitz, C. and Mead, G. (2010) Competitive exclusion treatment in poultry management. In: Guerrero-Legarreta, I. and Hui, Y.H. (eds) *Handbook of Poultry Science and Technology*, Vol 1. John Wiley and Sons, Hoboken, New Jersey, pp. 19–44.

Schneitz, C. and Nuotio, L. (1992) Efficacy of different microbial preparations for controlling salmonella colonization in chicks and turkey poults by competitive exclusion. *British Poultry Science* 33, 207–211.

Schneitz, C., Hakkinen, M., Nuotio, L., Nurmi, E. and Mead, G. (1990) Droplet application for protecting chicks against *Salmonella* colonization by competitive exclusion. *Veterinary Record* 126, 510.

Schneitz, C., Nuotio, L., Kiiskinen, T. and Nurmi, E. (1991) Pilot-scale testing of the competitive exclusion method in chickens. *British Poultry Science* 32, 877–880.

Schneitz, C., Kiiskinen, T., Toivonen, V. and Näsi, M. (1998) Effect of Broilact® on the physicochemical conditions and nutrient digestibility in the gastrointestinal tract of broilers. *Poultry Science* 77, 426-432.

Schoeni, J.L. and Wong, A.C. (1994) Inhibition of *Campylobacter jejuni* colonization in chicks by defined competitive exclusion bacteria. *Applied and Environmental Microbiology* 60, 1191–1197.

Seuna, E. (1979) Sensitivity of young chickens to *Salmonella typhimurium* var Copenhagen and *S.* infantis infection and the preventive effect of cultured intestinal microflora. *Avian Diseases* 23, 392–400.

Seuna, E., Raevuori, M. and Nurmi, E. (1978) An epizootic of *Salmonella typhimurium* var. copenhagen in broilers and the use of cultured chicken intestinal flora for its control. *British Poultry Science* 19, 309–314.

Skrivanova, E. and Marounek, M. (2007) Influence of pH on antimicrobial activity of organic acids against rabbit enteropathogenic strain of *Escherichia coli. Folia Microbiologica (Praha)* 52, 70–72.

Skrivanova, E., Savka, O.G. and Marounek, M. (2004) *In vitro* effect of C2-C18 fatty acids on salmonellas. *Folia Microbiologica (Praha)* 49, 99–202.

Snoeyenbos, G.H., Weinack, O.M. and Smyser, C.F. (1978) Protecting chicks and poults from salmonellae by oral administration of 'normal' gut microflora. *Avian Diseases* 22, 273–286.

Snoeyenbos, G.H., Weinack, O.M. and Smyser, C.F. (1979) Further studies on competitive exclusion for controlling salmonellas in chickens. *Avian Diseases* 24, 904–914.

Snoeyenbos, G.H., Weinack, O.M. and Soerjadi, A.S. (1983) Our current understanding of the role of native microflora in limiting some bacterial pathogens of chickens and turkeys. In: *Australian Veterinary Poultry Association and International Union of Immunological Societies, Proceedings No 66, Disease Prevention and Control in Poultry Production*, Sydney, Australia, pp. 45–51.

Snoeyenbos, G.H., Weinack, O.M., Soerjadi-Liem, A.S., Miller, B.M., Woodward, D.E. and Weston, C.R. (1985) Large-scale trials to study competitive exclusion of *Salmonella* in chickens. *Avian Diseases* 29, 1004–1011.

Soerjadi, A.S., Lloyd, A.B. and Cumming, R.B. (1978) *Streptococcus faecalis*, a bacterial isolate which protects young chickens from enteric invasion by salmonellae. *Australian Veterinary Journal* 54, 549–550.

Soerjadi, A.S., Stehman, S.M., Snoeyenbos, G.H., Weinack, O.M. and Smyser, C.F. (1981a) Some measurements of protection against paratyphoid *Salmonella* and *Escherichia coli* by competitive exclusion in chickens. *Avian Diseases* 24, 706–712.

Soerjadi, A.S., Stehman, S.M., Snoeyenbos, G.H., Weinack, O.M. and Smyser, C.F. (1981b) The influence of lactobacilli on the competitive exclusion of paratyphoid salmonellae in chickens. *Avian Diseases* 25, 1027–1033.

Soerjadi, A.S., Snoeyenbos, G.H. and Weinack, O.M. (1982a) Intestinal colonization and competitive exclusion of *Campylobacter fetus* subsp. *jejuni* in young chicks. *Avian Diseases* 26, 520–524.

Soerjadi, A.S., Rufner, R., Snoeyenbos, G.H. and Weinack, O.M. (1982b) Adherence of salmonellae and native gut microflora to the gastrointestinal mucosa of chicks. *Avian Diseases* 26, 576–584.

Soerjadi-Liem, A.S., Snoeyenbos, G.H. and Weinack, O.M. (1984a) Comparative studies on competitive exclusion of three isolates of *Campylobacter fetus* subsp. *jejuni* in chickens by native gut microflora. *Avian Diseases* 28, 139–146.

Soerjadi-Liem, A.S., Snoeyenbos, G.H. and Weinack, O.M. (1984b) Establishment and competitive exclusion of *Yersinia enterocolitica* in the gut of monoxenic and holoxenic chicks. *Avian Diseases* 28, 256–260.

Spencer, J.L. and Garcia, M.M. (1995) Resistance of chicks and poults fed vermicompost to caecal colonization by *Salmonella. Avian Pathology* 24, 157–170.

Spring, P., Wenk, C., Dawson, K.A. and Newman, K.E. (2000) The effects of dietary mannanoligosaccharides on cecal parameters and the concentrations of enteric bacteria in the ceca of *Salmonella*-challenged broiler chicks. *Poultry Science* 79, 205–211.

Stavric, S. (1992) Defined cultures and prospects. *International Journal of Food Microbiology* 15, 245–263.

Stavric, S. and D'Aoust, J.-Y. (1993) Undefined and defined bacterial preparations for the competitive exclusion of *Salmonella* in poultry – a review. *Journal of Food Protection* 56, 173–180.

Stavric, S., Gleeson, T.M., Blanchfield, B. and Pivnick, H. (1985) Competitive exclusion of *Salmonella* from newly hatched chicks by mixtures of pure bacterial cultures isolated from fecal and cecal contents of adult birds. *Journal of Food Protection* 48, 778–782.

Stavric, S., Buchanan, B. and Gleeson, T.M. (1992) Competitive exclusion of *Escherichia coli* 0157:H7 from chicks with anaerobic cultures of faecal microflora. *Letters in Applied Microbiology* 14, 191–193.

Stern, N.J. (1994) Mucosal competitive exclusion to diminish colonization of chickens by *Campylobacter jejuni*. *Poultry Science* 73, 402–407.

Sternberg Lewerin, S., Boqvist, S., Engström, B. and Haggblöm, P. (2005) The effective control of *Salmonella* in Swedish poultry. In: Mead, G.C. (ed.) *Food Safety Control in the Poultry Industry.* Woodhead Publishing, Cambridge, UK, pp. 195–215.

Talarico, T.L., Casas, I.A., Cheng, T.C. and Dobrogosz, W.J. (1988) Production and isolation of reuterin, a growth inhibitor produced by *Lactobacillus reuteri*. *Antimicrobial Agents and Chemotherapy* 32, 1854–1858.

Toro, H., Price, S.B., McKee, S., Hoerr, F.J., Krehling, J., Perdue, M. and Bauermeister, L. (2005) Use of bacteriophages in combination with competitive exclusion to reduce *Salmonella* from infected chickens. *Avian Diseases* 49, 118–124.

van der Waaij, D., Berghuis-de Vries, J.M. and Lekkerkerk-van der Wees, J.E.C. (1971) Colonization resistance of the digestive tract in conventional and antibiotic-treated mice. *Journal of Hygiene, Cambridge* 69, 405–511.

van der Wielen, P.W.J.J., Biesterveld, S., Notermans, S., Hofstra, H., Urlings, B.A.P. and van Knapen, F. (2000) Role of volatile fatty acids in development of the cecal microflora in broiler chickens during growth. *Applied and Environmental Microbiology* 66, 2536–2540.

Van Immerseel, F., Methner, U., Rychlik, I., Nagy, B., Velge, P., Martin, G., Foster, N., Ducatelle, R. and Barrow, P.A. (2005) Vaccination and early protection against non-host-specific *Salmonella* serotypes in poultry: exploitation of innate immunity and microbial activity. *Epidemiology and Infection* 133, 959–978.

van Vliet, A.H.M., Ketley, J.M., Park, S.F. and Penn, C.W. (2002) The role of iron in *Campylobacter* gene regulation, metabolism and oxidative stress defense. *FEMS Microbiology Reviews* 26, 173–186.

Vicente, J.L., Torres-Rodriguez, A., Higgins, S.E., Pixley, C., Tellez, G. *et al.* (2008) Effect of a selected *Lactobacillus* spp.-based probiotic on *Salmonella enterica* serovar Enteritidis-infected broiler chicks. *Avian Diseases* 52, 143–146.

Vilà, B., Fontgibell, A., Badiola, I., Esteve-Garcia, E., Jiménez, G., Castillo, M. and Brufau, J. (2009) Reduction of *Salmonella enterica* var. Enteritidis colonization and invasion by *Bacillus cereus* var. *toyoi* inclusion in poultry feeds. *Poultry Science* 88, 975–979.

von Wright, A. (2005) Regulating the safety of probiotics – the European approach. *Current Pharmaceutical Design* 11, 17–23.

Wagner, R.D. and Cerniglia, C.E. (2005) Antimicrobial susceptibility patterns of competitive exclusion bacteria applied to newly hatched chickens. *International Journal of Food Microbiology* 102, 349–353.

Wagner, R.D., Holland, M. and Cerniglia, C.E. (2002) An *in vitro* assay to evaluate competitive exclusion products for poultry. *Journal of Food Protection* 65, 746–751.

Waldroup, A.L., Yamaguchi, W., Skinner, J.T. and Waldroup, P.W. (1992) Effects of dietary lactose on incidence and levels of salmonellae on carcasses of broiler chickens grown to market age. *Poultry Science* 71, 288–295.

Waters, S.M., Murphy, R.A. and Power, R.F.G. (2006) Characterisation of prototype Nurmi cultures using culture-based microbiological techniques and PCR-DGGE. *International Journal of Food Microbiology* 110, 268–277.

Weinack, O.M., Snoeyenbos, G.H. and Smyser, C.F. (1979) A supplemental test system to measure competitive exclusion of salmonellae by native microflora in the chicken gut. *Avian Diseases* 23, 1019–1030.

Weinack, O.M., Snoeyenbos, G.H., Smyser, C.F. and Soerjadi, A.S. (1981) Competitive exclusion of intestinal colonization of *Escherichia coli* in chicks. *Avian Diseases* 25, 696–705.

Weinack, O.M., Snoeyenbos, G.H., Smyser, C.F. and Soerjadi, A.S. (1982) Reciprocal competitive exclusion of *Salmonella* and *Escherichia coli* by native intestinal microflora of the chicken and turkey. *Avian Diseases* 26, 585–595.

Weinack, O.M., Snoeyenbos, G.H., Smyser, C.F. and Soerjadi-Liem, A.S. (1984) Influence of *Mycoplasma gallisepticum*, infectious bronchitis, and cyclophosphamide on chickens protected by native intestinal microflora against *Salmonella* typhimurium or *Escherichia coli*. *Avian Diseases* 28, 416–425.

Weinack, O.M., Snoeyenbos, G.H., Soerjadi-Liem, A.S. and Smyser, C.F. (1985a) Influence of temperature, social and dietary stress on development and stability of protective microflora in chickens against *S.* typhimurium. *Avian Diseases* 29, 1177-1183.

Weinack, O.M., Snoeyenbos, G.H. and Soerjadi-Liem, A.S. (1985b) Further studies on competitive exclusion of *Salmonella* typhimurium by lactobacilli in chickens. *Avian Diseases* 29, 1273–1277.

WHO (1994) Unpublished report of the WHO-FEDESA-FEP workshop on competitive exclusion, vaccination and antimicrobials in *Salmonella* control in poultry WHO/CDS/VPH/94. 134 WHO, Geneva.

Wierup, M., Wold-Troell, M., Nurmi, E. and Hakkinen, M. (1988) Epidemiological evaluation of the *Salmonella*-controlling effect of a nationwide use of a competitive exclusion culture in poultry. *Poultry Science* 67, 1026–1033.

Wierup, M., Wahlström, H. and Engström, B. (1992) Experience of a 10-year use of competitive exclusion treatment as part of the *Salmonella* control programme in Sweden. *International Journal of Food Microbiology* 5, 287–291.

Wolfenden, A.D., Vicente, J.L., Higgins, J.P., Andreatti Filho, R.L., Higgins, S.E., Hargis, B.M. and Tellez, G. (2007) Effect of organic acids on *Salmonella enteritidis* infection in broiler chickens. *International Journal of Poultry Science* 6, 403–405.

Zhang, G., Ma, L. and Doyle, M.P. (2007a) Potential competitive exclusion bacteria from poultry inhibitory to *Campylobacter jejuni* and *Salmonella*. *Journal of Food Protection* 70, 867–873.

Zhang, G., Ma, L. and Doyle, M.P. (2007b) Salmonellae reduction in poultry by competitive exclusion bacteria *Lactobacillus salivarius* and *Streptococcus crispatus*. *Journal of Food Protection* 70, 874–878.

22 Vaccination against *Salmonella* Infections in Food Animals: Rationale, Theoretical Basis and Practical Application

Paul A. Barrow[1]* and Ulrich Methner[2]
[1]*School of Veterinary Medicine and Science, University of Nottingham, UK;*
[2]*Institute of Bacterial Infections and Zoonoses at the Friedrich-Loeffler-Institute, Germany*

Introduction

During the early years of the last three decades, the animal and public health problems associated with *Salmonella* in poultry increased to such an extent to become major political issues, of which the general public become very aware. *Salmonella* Enteritidis, in particular, became a worldwide problem, arising mainly from poultry (Rodrigue *et al.*, 1990). In many countries, individual phage types of this serovar replaced *S.* Typhimurium as the most dominant type in poultry and humans. Control in poultry has become a major issue and immunity, whether acquired or, more speculatively, innate, is seen as one of the possible means of containing the problem. As a result, Commission Regulation (EC) No 1177/2006 (EC, 2006) prescribes the application of vaccination programmes against *S.* Enteritidis, at least during rearing, for all laying hens providing they did not demonstrate a prevalence of less than 10% (EC, 2006). In the UK cattle industry, clinical salmonellosis in its acute and chronic forms, together with subclinical infection, remains a major economic, welfare and health problem. While the incidence of acute clinical salmonellosis in pigs is less of a problem compared with that of cattle, subclinical *Salmonella* infections that result in carcass contamination lead to the introduction of the organism into the food chain (EFSA, 2008). Widespread use of antibiotics has led to the emergence of multiple antibiotic-resistant bacteria, especially *S.* Typhimurium. These problems have indicated to the industry and government agencies an increasing requirement for effective vaccines to control this important zoonotic infection.

This review discusses the reasons for the relatively poor success in immunizing food animals against those non-host-specific *Salmonella* serovars that usually produce food poisoning, compared with the success obtained with the small number of serovars that more typically produce systemic 'typhoid-like' diseases in a restricted range of host species. Most of our understanding of immunity to salmonellosis arises from experimental work with typhoid-like diseases, mainly *S.* Typhimurium infection in mice.

* Corresponding author, e-mail: paul.barrow@nottingham.ac.uk

© CAB International 2013. *Salmonella in Domestic Animals, 2nd Edition* (eds P.A. Barrow and U. Methner)

Such work may not be entirely relevant to the, often disease-free, colonization by most *Salmonella* serovars. However, during the last decade our knowledge, especially on the immune response of poultry after exposure to non-host-adapted serovars, has increased considerably. Whereas live, attenuated vaccines against host-specific serovars are highly protective, similarly developed vaccine strains have traditionally been less effective in protecting chickens, calves and pigs against intestinal colonization. Newer methods of attenuation are being developed, but their exploitation and success will depend on appropriate attenuation, delivery, their use for the types of infection that have been shown to be amenable to immune control and their effectiveness under field conditions. One of the key questions is to find the balance between an accepted level of attenuation and an unaffected ability to induce protection involving innate as well as adaptive immunity. This will be possible realistically only through the use of molecular genetics to generate precisely defined *Salmonella* mutants.

From the point of view of consumer safety there is a school of thought that considers inactivated or subunit vaccines to be the safest. The benefits of developing effective killed or subunit vaccines over the use of live vaccines are enormous. Recently, there have been significant advances in the development of adjuvants, for example microspheres or cytokines, which are capable of potent immunostimulation and modulating the immune response in a more controlled and specific manner (Morein *et al.*, 1996; Schmidt *et al.*, 2007; Dey and Srivastava, 2011). The exploitation of such technology in conjunction with the ongoing developments in identifying key *Salmonella* virulence determinants should form the next generation of *Salmonella* subunit vaccines for the control of this group of pathogens.

Pathogenesis of Salmonellosis

The development of an effective vaccine is dependent on an understanding of how *Salmonella* organisms infect their hosts and the host response to infection. A major problem with this goal is that *Salmonella* pathogenicity and virulence are both serovar- and host-dependent and that the factors influencing serovar–host specificity are not known (see Chapter 5, this volume).

From the point of view of the pathogenesis of *Salmonella* infections, *S. enterica* can be divided into two major groups. One group typically produces systemic disease and is rarely involved in human food poisoning, while the other typically produces food poisoning and only produces systemic disease under particular circumstances, such as immediately after parturition, at the onset of lay, in very young or old animals or after some viral or parasite infections. A comparison of the biological aspects of the two groups might explain our success in immunological control of the former group and our limited success in the control of the latter. It might also contribute to our understanding of the immune responses to infection and it is obviously central to any appraisal of experimental work on pathogenesis and immunity.

Our current understanding of *Salmonella* pathogenesis and immunity is largely derived from experimental infection studies, usually with *S.* Typhimurium, in inbred laboratory strains of mice. This type of infection is characteristic of a small number of serovars that produce severe systemic disease in adult animals, initially involving the reticuloendothelial system and the monocyte-macrophage series in a restricted number of host species. This type of infection is characteristic of *S.* Typhi in humans, *S.* Dublin in cattle and mice, *S.* Enteritidis in mice, *S.* Gallinarum in birds and *S.* Choleraesuis in a range of mammalian species including pigs. Following inoculation of mice with an infective dose, a systemic infection occurs without enteritis and with little intestinal colonization as a result of which they rarely enter the human food chain. Thus mice are only a useful model for studying the systemic form of disease. The severity of the infection is dependent on the virulence of the *Salmonella* strain, the route of infection, the innate resistance of the mouse strain used and its immune status. Similar information on *S.* Dublin in cattle or *S.* Gallinarum in poultry is much less complete. The second group comprises the remaining 2400 or more serovars. They are not restricted to particular host species and their epidemiology can therefore be complex. Most are able to colonize the alimentary tract of animals without production of disease. As a result of the intestinal colonization they contaminate the carcass and enter the human food chain resulting in food poisoning. Some strains of particular serovars, most notably *S.* Typhimurium and *S.* Enteritidis, are capable of producing systemic disease in addition to faecal excretion. This is particularly the case for young animals or during or after a period of physiological stress. The extent of disease and mortality varies according to the strain but there is always some invasion of the intestinal mucosa and reticuloendothelial system.

Vaccines for Poultry

Infection of poultry with its host-species-specific serovar *S.* Gallinarum-Pullorum induces a strong immunity against reinfection. Live, attenuated vaccines have been developed that can be administered parenterally and which are protective, because the disease is primarily systemic. The 9R *S.* Gallinarum vaccine (Smith, 1956) is an undefined rough strain produced by culture in defined media and, as a consequence of its roughness, it does not stimulate the production of antibodies to the somatic antigen. This is advantageous, since the vaccine's use will not interfere with serological tests to detect natural infection. A second vaccine, 9S, a smooth strain, is more protective but slightly more virulent (Smith, 1956). The 9R vaccine has been assessed and used extensively (Gordon and Luke, 1959; Gordon *et al.*, 1959; Silva *et al.*, 1981; Feberwee *et al*, 2001a; Lee *et al.*, 2005, 2007; Okamato *et al.*, 2010) and proved both safety and efficacious, although some residual virulence exists for highly susceptible breeds.

More recently, a number of other methods of attenuation for *S.* Gallinarum have been used. *Salmonella* Gallinarum strain 9, cured of its virulence plasmid is greatly attenuated for chickens of more than a few weeks old (Barrow *et al.*, 1987). Chickens that had received a parenteral inoculation with such a strain or an *aroA*-serC (aromatic-dependent) mutant were very resistant to reinfection with the parent strain (Barrow, 1990; Barrow *et al.*, 2001a). However, the resistance to oral challenge obtained by immunization with either this strain or a rough, phage-resistant derivative was not as great as that induced by the 9R strain, given either parenterally or orally (Barrow, 1990). An *aroA* mutant of strain 9 was generated by genetic deletion and, since the growth of these mutants requires *p*-aminobenzoic acid, which is not freely available in mammalian and avian tissues, such mutants are attenuated. The mutant was completely avirulent for 2-week-old chickens (increase in LD_{50} of 10^6). This strain was an effective vaccine, but, as with the virulence-plasmid-cured derivative, the degree of protection produced was not as great as that produced by 9R. However, it was suggested that such more attenuated, less protective vaccine strains might be used in more susceptible breeds, followed by a second vaccination with the 9R mutant (Griffin and Barrow, 1993).

The 9R vaccine of *S.* Gallinarum has been registered not only for use against *S.* Gallinarum but also against *S.* Enteritidis where it may be used by vaccinating 6-week-old laying hen chickens orally via drinking water followed by subcutaneous booster at 15 weeks of age as well as before the start of the laying period (Feberwee *et al.*, 2001b). However, this vaccine is no longer registered in many countries in Europe because of problems in differentiating between the 9R vaccine strain and *S.* Gallinarum wild-type strains. A *S.* Gallinarum strain with deletions in genes *cobS* and *cbiA*, involved in the biosynthesis of cobalmin, was used to immunize young chicks and tested for efficacy against *S.* Gallinarum and *S.* Enteritidis challenge. This attenuated vaccine candidate induced protective effects against both serovars (Penha Filho *et al.*, 2010)

There has also been increasing interest in vaccinating poultry against the serovars of major public health relevance, *S.* Enteritidis and *S.* Typhimurium. Vaccination of birds results in an additional increase in resistance against *Salmonella* infection above that observed in birds with a developed intestinal flora. The aim of vaccination is: (i) to reduce or prevent intestinal colonization, resulting in reduced faecal shedding and eggshell contamination; and (ii) to prevent systemic infection resulting in a diminished localization in the reproductive tissues. Vaccination is not a panacea but should always be used as a part of a comprehensive control programme. Although knowledge relating to the course of the innate and adaptive response to various *Salmonella* infection types is beginning to increase (Van Immerseel *et al.*, 2005; Smith and Beal, 2008), the development of vaccines for use with poultry has been almost exclusively empirical,.

A variety of live and inactivated (non-living) vaccine preparations have been developed and tested for their protective efficacy in poultry experimentally and in the field. Killed vaccines may be inactivated with formalin, acetone, glutaraldehyde or heat treatment. Oil adjuvants, aluminium hydroxide and other immune-stimulating compounds have been used to better stimulate the immune system. The inactivated vaccine preparations usually generate a detectable humoral immune response but they produce a poor or inconsistent protective effect. Some of this work is described below. In several experiments, Truscott (1981) immunized chickens with heated bacterial sonicates, prepared from different combinations of serovars and incorporated into the feed. This was followed some weeks later by oral challenge. The extent of protection in the different studies measured by isolation of the challenge strain from cloacal swabs varied from very good to poor. Other groups (Bisping *et al.*, 1971; Thain *et al.*, 1984) have found that heated, whole-cell bacterins have little effect on faecal shedding, either in vaccinated birds or when their newly hatched progeny were challenged. Some reductions in mortality have, however, been demonstrated (McCapes *et al.*, 1967; Truscott and Friars, 1972), but the biological significance of these findings in relation to faecal shedding and subsequent carcass contamination is unknown. *Salmonella* Enteritidis, grown under conditions of iron restriction, has been used to prepare an inactivated vaccine against *S.* Enteritidis infection in breeders and laying type chickens, which has been licensed in a number of European countries and shown efficacy in both experimental studies and large field trails (Feberwee *et al.*, 2000; Woodward *et al.*, 2002). One commercial inactivated bivalent *S.* Enteritidis and *S.* Typhimurium dual vaccine against both *S.* Enteritidis and *S.* Typhimurium has also been authorized (Clifton-Hadley *et al.*, 2002). Both killed vaccine types are based on bacterial cells cultured under conditions of iron depletion, despite the belief that iron depletion is necessarily the major environmental factor in the *Salmonella*-containing vacuole in the macrophage. Therefore, a more rational approach might be to culture cells under the conditions found inside the macrophage or other antigen-presenting cells, as currently understood (Eriksson *et al.*, 2003). A novel trivalent inactivated *Salmonella* vaccine consisting of *S.* Typhimurium, *S.* Enteritidis and *S.* Infantis was evaluated for safety and efficacy in chickens against exposure with the homologous serovars and *S.* Heidelberg. Compared to unvaccinated birds shedding of all challenge organisms was reduced in immunized chickens indicating protective effects against different serovars having O-antigens to those of the inactivated vaccine preparation (Deguchi *et al.*, 2009).

Parenteral administration of inactivated *Salmonella* vaccines to breeder birds will induce a strong production of antibodies, which will be transferred to the progeny. The maternally transferred antibodies persist for a few weeks and, although there seems to be some protective effect against systemic disease in the early post-hatch period, there is little effect on intestinal colonization by homologous challenge strains (Methner *et al.*, 1994; Methner and Steinbach, 1997; Young *et al.*, 2007) and it is therefore possible to immunize day-old chicks from vaccinated breeder birds effectively with live *Salmonella* vaccines (Methner *et al.*, 2002; Bailey *et al.*, 2007).

Although a number of different live *Salmonella* vaccine strains have been tested for their efficacy in experimental or semi-field studies only a few are authorized and commercially available for use in poultry in Europe (EFSA, 2004). A mutant of a mammalian *S.* Typhimurium defective in the enzyme UDP-galactose epimerase (*galE*), which persists for only a short time *in vivo*, was originally developed in mice for use with humans (Tagliabue *et al.*, 1986) and cattle (Wray *et al.*, 1977), but it has also been tested in poultry. Pritchard *et al.* (1978) vaccinated day-old chicks with this strain and challenged 2 weeks later with an avian *S.* Typhimurium strain. Small reductions were obtained in faecal excretion and in the number of isolations from the viscera and also when chickens were vaccinated twice, at 4 or 6 weeks of age, followed by challenge 2 weeks later. Surprisingly, protection was better when chickens were inoculated intramuscularly rather than orally (Subhabphant *et al.*, 1983). One drawback of the use of any *galE* mutant is the question of attenuation, because some mutants are known to retain some virulence for the host (Nnalue and Stocker, 1986; Hone *et al.*, 1988).

Some vaccine strains are excreted in the faeces for longer periods than are others. A general inverse correlation between virulence for chickens and the duration of faecal excretion can be found. More invasive strains may therefore stimulate a systemic as well as a local immune response, which should combine to clear such strains from the gut more quickly than might occur following colonization by less invasive strains. However, it might also follow that after immunization using an invasive strain, clearance of both invasive and less invasive challenge organisms might occur to the same extent (Smith and Tucker, 1980; Barrow *et al.*, 1988). Oral inoculation of 4-day-old chickens with a virulent avian *S.* Typhimurium strain, F98, resulted in faecal shedding for several weeks. When these birds were re-challenged orally after they had virtually ceased to shed the organism, the challenge strain was excreted in smaller numbers and for a shorter period of time than in a previously uninfected control group, demonstrating the induction of protective immunity controlling intestinal colonization and faecal shedding (Barrow *et al.*, 1990a). The use of a non-attenuated *Salmonella* wild-type strain as live vaccine strain was shown to be a valuable tool to evaluate the efficacy of any attenuated vaccine candidate as it can be assumed that a *Salmonella* wild-type strain induces the highest degree of protection against a subsequent *Salmonella* challenge (Methner *et al.*, 1995, 2011b).

An *aroA* mutant from *S.* Typhimurium F98 was produced and in addition a rough strain was selected by its resistance to virulent bacteriophage. When vaccinated intramuscularly, both mutants produced initially good reductions in faecal excretion of the challenge strain. By oral inoculation, the *aroA* mutant produced little protection, while the rough mutant was still very protective (Barrow *et al.*, 1990a). Oral ingestion of the mutants by human volunteers did not result in illness and the strains did not persist in their faeces for longer than 3 days.

An *aroA* mutant of *S.* Enteritidis has been tested in chickens. This also produces a good initial reduction in faecal excretion of a challenge *S.* Enteritidis strain, which, however, was of limited duration (Cooper *et al.*, 1990). However, when challenge was carried out by contact with orally infected birds, considerably better protection was obtained (Cooper *et al.*, 1992). Cross-protection against challenge with *S.* Typhimurium was not obtained.

Other auxotrophic mutants, including *pur* and *thy* mutations, have been produced, though some have not yet been tested thoroughly (O'Callaghan *et al.*, 1988; Sigwart *et al.*, 1989). In Germany and numerous other countries, registered live purine and histidine auxotrophic vaccines of *S.* Typhimurium and *S.* Enteritidis produced by chemical mutagenesis are being used extensively. The efficacy of these vaccines has been studied in experimental and field studies (Springer *et al.*, 2000, 2011). Although the precise nature of the attenuating mutations in these particular vaccine strains is unclear, most probably because of the two auxotrophic markers in these live vaccines, reversion to virulence has not been detected after their extensive use for more than 20 years (Rabsch *et al.*, 2001). Other *S.* Typhimurium and *S.* Enteritidis vaccines first authorized in Germany were developed on the basis of the principle of metabolic drift mutations (Vielitz *et al.*, 1992; Linde *et al.*, 1997; Hahn, 2000). These are negative mutations in essential enzymes and metabolic control centres of the bacterium resulting to prolonged generation times and reductions in virulence (Linde *et al.*, 1997). Apart from reducing intestinal colonization and systemic transmission of homologous challenge organisms after immunization of chickens (Hahn, 2000), reduction in internal egg contamination with *S.* Enteritidis wild-type strains was also found (Gantois *et al.*, 2006). In general, these vaccines are administered twice orally via drinking water in the first days after hatching and some weeks later as a booster vaccination. These attenuated vaccine strains are most effective against homologous challenge but also partly protective against heterologous exposure. Some of these *Salmonella* live vaccines have been characterized further by molecular methods (Schwarz and Liebisch, 1994).

Salmonella mutants lacking DNA adenine methylase (Dam) are highly attenuated and conferred considerable protection against challenge with homologous and moderate protection against infection with heterologous *Salmonella* serovars in chickens (Dueger *et al.*, 2003b).

Transposon and deletion mutants have also been produced, which are defective in adenylate cyclase activity (*cya*) or cyclic AMP receptor protein (*crp*) and which have been tested for their protective value in chickens (Hassan and Curtiss, 1994). A double-deletion mutant (*cya crp*) of *S.* Typhimurium was an effective vaccine when birds were challenged with homologous or heterologous serovars 2 weeks after the last vaccination. These strains remained virulent for germ-free pigs (Barrow *et al.*, 2001b).

A few studies were carried out to evaluate the potential and limitations on the combined use of vaccination and gut flora preparations (competitive exclusion cultures) in order to exploit the serovar non-specific competitive exclusion effects and the more serovar-specific vaccination effects (Methner *et al.*, 1999). Any efficacy of inactivated vaccines will not interfere with competitive exclusion effects after combined administration. However, it was clearly shown that live *Salmonella* vaccines need to be administered either before or simultaneously with the competitive exclusion cultures to ensure an adequate intestinal colonization of the vaccine strain and the development of a strong immune response. This combination has the potential to result in very young and older birds obtaining a degree of protection considerably beyond that afforded by single use of the two methods (Methner *et al.*, 1999, 2001).

Following vaccination, a protective adaptive immunity takes from several days to weeks to develop. This delay could be overcome by using a live strain, which, in newly hatched birds, shows a colonization-inhibition effect, a form of competitive exclusion that occurs between closely related enteric bacteria (Barrow *et al.*, 1987; Berchieri and Barrow, 1990; Methner *et al.*, 1999, 2001; Nogrady *et al.*, 2003). This might mean that an appropriate live, attenuated strain could protect against *Salmonella* infection acquired during the first few days of life, followed by the development of true immunity. A prerequisite is that attenuations in wild-type strains do not affect the potential to inhibit the intestinal colonization of *Salmonella* strains. It was found that vaccine strains produced by chemical mutagenesis or the principle of metabolic drift mutation were not able to express colonization-inhibition effects against closely related *Salmonella* strains (Methner *et al.*, 2001). Mutants with deletions in *phoP*, either alone or in combination with *rpoS*, resulted in a high level of attenuation, unimpaired ability to colonize the gut and a nearly unaffected potential to inhibit the challenge strain from caecal colonization (Methner *et al.*, 2004). Deletions in *hilA* but not in *sipA* or *ssrA* were also shown to be sufficiently attenuated and to induce a strong homologous colonization-inhibition effect against *S.* Enteritidis (Bohez *et al.*, 2007, 2008).

For the exploitation of this phenomenon information on colonization-inhibition between wild-type strains of different serovars is needed to ideally identify a *Salmonella* strain with a broad spectrum of inhibitory activity (Barrow *et al.*, 1987; Methner *et al.*, 2001, 2004; Nogrady *et al.*, 2003). It was shown in comprehensive experimental studies that the degree of colonization-inhibition between different serovars was not sufficiently high to identify a single strain that might inhibit a wide range of other *Salmonella* organisms (Methner *et al.*, 2011a). However, as *S.* Enteritidis is the dominant serovar in poultry in many countries and because of the profound colonization-inhibition within this serovar there is a considerable potential to exploit this phenomenon in the development of novel live *S.* Enteritidis vaccines. Moreover, treatment of young chicks with mixtures of different *Salmonella* serovars resulted not only in a very strong growth inhibition of the isogenic strains but also substantial inhibition of heterologous serovars (Methner *et al.*, 2011a).

The above studies indicated that in addition to intestinal-colonization inhibition between *Salmonella* organisms a rapid early invasion-inhibition effect might also occur after administration of live *Salmonella* strains. Invasive *Salmonella* strains induce a strong influx of heterophils in the caecal mucosa (Kogut *et al.*, 1993, 1994) followed by a substantial invasion-inhibition of both homologous and heterologous *Salmonella* challenge organisms administered 24 h later. Therefore, this invasion-inhibition effect should be considered in the development of future live vaccines (Methner *et al.*, 2010).

To further improve efficacy and acceptance of immunization against *Salmonella* infection in poultry vaccines should be generated that enable the serological differentiation between vaccinated and infected animals. It has been shown that deletions in *fliC* in *S.* Enteritidis, the most important serovar in the laying hen population in Europe, do not affect the immunogenic characteristics of the vaccine strain but enable the effective differentiation between vaccinated and infected chickens using an commercially available ELISA kit (Adriaensen *et al.*, 2007; Methner *et al.*, 2011b). Since it has been postulated that the innate response to *Salmonella* as a result of stimulation of TLR-5 via flagellin results in confinement of *S.* Enteritidis infection largely to the intestine, a *fliC* mutant might be expected to be more invasive, as occurs with *S.* Typhimurium, and highly immunogenic (Iqbal *et al.*, 2005).

Results from recent studies clearly indicate that there are many novel characteristics of live *Salmonella* vaccines that should be considered in the development of future vaccine candidates. One of the key questions is to find the balance between an accepted level of attenuation and an unaffected ability to induce protective effects of the innate as well as the adaptive immunity (Methner, 2007). This will be possible only by molecular genetics to generate defined *Salmonella* deletion mutants.

Vaccines for Cattle

Several studies show significant variation in the efficacy of vaccines based on dead *Salmonella* organisms, which might also be due to differences in the experimental designs used for potency testing of these preparations (Methner, 2001). A heat-inactivated *S.* Dublin vaccine administered intradermally was shown to be effective when the cattle were challenged by the intravenous route (Aitken *et al.*, 1982). Whether this type of vaccine would protect cattle against oral challenge was not determined. Acid-hydrolysed *S.* Typhimurium coated with alkali-hydrolysed LPS or LPS alone was ineffective in protecting cattle against challenge with this serovar (Anderson *et al.*, 1991). An inactivated commercial *S.* Typhimurium vaccine, registered for more than 20 years in Germany, has been proven to be effective against oral *S.* Typhimurium infection in both experimental as well as numerous field studies (Steinbach and Meyer, 1990). The efficacy of a *Salmonella* bacterin prepared from a *S.* Montevideo strain and a modified live *S.* Choleraesuis vaccine were compared after intramuscular injection of lactating cows. The herd was endemically infected with *S.* Montevideo (serogroup C1) as the dominating serovar but also with other different serovars. The live *S.* Choleraesuis vaccine resulted in a higher reduction of faecal shedding of serogroup C1 organisms by both cows and calves than did the bacterin-vaccinated animals indicating heterologous protective effects although the O-antigen was the same between these two serovars indicating the importance of this antigen (House *et al.*, 2001). It was shown more recently that subcutaneous injection of subclinically infected dairy cows with a commercial *S. enterica* subunit vaccine did not result in reduced shedding of *Salmonella* organisms by the animals (Heider *et al.*, 2008). An inactivated *S.* Newport vaccine preparation containing siderophore receptor and porin proteins was used to vaccinate cows and tested for effects on milk production and on shedding of *Salmonella* organisms (Hermesch *et al.*, 2008). The reason for the increase in milk production that was detected in cattle even in the absence of shedding of *S.* Newport or clinical signs of salmonellosis remained unclear.

Since calves may become infected with *Salmonella* within the first few days after birth (Jones *et al.*, 1983) and the peak of mortality occurs between 3 and 4 weeks of age, passive protection by vaccination of pregnant cows is one approach that can be adopted. Immunization of the dam 7 and 2 weeks prior to parturition, using formalin-killed, log-phase *S.* Typhimurium was shown to be safe and effective for preventing illness in the calf (Jones *et al.*, 1988a). However, the level of passive protection provided by immune colostrum reported in different studies varies considerably (House *et al.*, 2001).

Live, attenuated *Salmonella* vaccine strains have been assessed in cattle, with varying success rates. The most widely tested *Salmonella* vaccines in cattle are auxotrophic strains. Aromatic amino acid (*aro*) and purine (*pur*) auxotrophs are attenuated and stimulate protective immunity (Stocker, 1988). Many publications attest to the efficacy of live vaccines in experimental trials, but only few are available commercially. In Germany, however, the use of registered live auxotrophic (purine/histidine) mutants of *S.* Typhimurium and *S.* Dublin and a rough mutant of *S.* Choleraesuis has had a profound effect on the incidence of salmonellosis in calves and pigs after oral administration (Meyer *et al.*, 1992). Although the precise nature of the attenuating mutations in these particular vaccine strains is unclear, most probably because of the two auxotrophic markers in these live vaccines, reversion to virulence has not been detected after their extensive use for more than 20 years (Meyer *et al.*, 1992; Rabsch *et al.*, 2001). Clearly, live vaccines should ideally carry defined, multiple, attenuating mutations and specific genetic markers to distinguish them from wild-type strains. Much work has been spent on the development of auxotrophic aromatic-dependent *Salmonella* strains for use as vaccines in cattle. Three vaccine strains of *S.* Typhimurium carrying defined mutations in the *aroA* gene were tested for safety and efficacy in 2- to 3-week-old calves. All three strains were attenuated, although only one strain, SL1479, was protective after either oral or intramuscular administration (Smith *et al.*, 1984a). Of considerable concern, however, is that, when the same strain was assessed in 5-day-old calves, a lethal infection resulted (Mikula *et al.*, 1989). However, a double *S.* Typhimurium *aroA aroD* strain was shown to protect calves from challenge with virulent *S.* Typhimurium (Jones *et al.*, 1991; Villarreal *et al.*, 1998).

Live *S.* Dublin *aroA* vaccines have also been assessed in calves. Calves suffered a transient pyrexia and mild diarrhoea following intramuscular vaccination. When challenged orally with either wild-type *S.* Dublin or *S.* Typhimurium, some enteritis was seen, although all animals survived, demonstrating that cross-protection between serovars in large animals is possible (Smith *et al.*, 1984b), as had previously been reported with the live *S.* Dublin vaccine that was then commercially available (Rankin *et al.*, 1967). After oral administration of a live *S.* Dublin *aroA* vaccine strain and oral challenge with *S.* Dublin, protective effects could only be observed in case of very high vaccine doses, which makes the practical use in the field unlikely (Smith *et al.*, 1993). However, Segall and Lindberg (1991) concluded that *Salmonella* strains deleted in *aroA* are considerably attenuated, although high vaccine doses are recommended only in calves that are several weeks old or as booster vaccination.

The virulence plasmid of *S.* Dublin and *S.* Typhimurium was found not to be involved in either the enteric phase of infection or the systemic dissemination (Wallis *et al.*, 1995). However, plasmid-cured strains of *S.* Typhimurium were found to be attenuated and effective as vaccine strains after parenteral but not after oral administration (Van der Walt *et al.*, 2001).

The efficacy of an avirulent live *S.* Choleraesuis vaccine was tested in calves after intranasal administration against oral infection with *S.* Dublin. Although the attenuated *S.* Choleraesuis was not recovered from faecal samples after vaccination, immunization reduced clinical signs and bacterial shedding after oral infection with heterologous *S.* Dublin (Fox *et al.*, 1997). Mutations in the *dam* gene of *Salmonella*, which prevent expression of the DNA adenine methylase, result in highly attenuated organisms, which were used to study safety and efficacy against *Salmonella* challenge. Vaccination of calves with an attenuated *S.* Typhimurium *dam* strain conferred protection against *S.* Typhimurium infections in calves via both adaptive immunity and competitive exclusion mechanisms (Dueger *et al.*, 2003a). Moreover, immunization of young calves using a *S.* Typhimurium *dam* strain exhibited reduced clinical disease and a concomitant reduction in faecal shedding and lymph node colonization by the heterologous *S.* Dublin and *S.* Newport challenge organisms compared to non-vaccinated animals (Mohler *et al.*, 2006, 2008). Most of the commercial *Salmonella* vaccines licensed around the world are killed bacterins, which are usually administered parenterally in calves that are several weeks old and adult animals. The consensus of most reports on efficacy is that vaccination of calves with *Salmonella* bacterins provides partial protection against *Salmonella* infection. Live *Salmonella* vaccines are usually recommended to be administered orally to calves during the first weeks of life to reduce neonatal mortality and faecal shedding by *Salmonella* wild-type strains.

Vaccines for Pigs

Live, attenuated vaccine strains against the dominant *Salmonella* serovars Typhimurium and Choleraesuis have been assessed in pigs. In the USA, where there is a continuing problem with *S.* Choleraesuis, significant progress has been made with a live, attenuated vaccine strain of *S.* Choleraesuis (Roof and Doitchinoff, 1995). The strain was generated by repeated passage of a virulent strain through porcine neutrophils *in vitro* and was cured of the 50 kb virulence plasmid. Following oral administration, the vaccine was well tolerated and it provided significant protection for up to 20 weeks after vaccination. One slight concern with a vaccine of this type is the re-acquisition by the vaccine strain of the virulence plasmid from other *Salmonella* that may be present within the herd as a result of mobilization by other plasmids. This could possibly result in reversion of the vaccine strain to a virulent phenotype. Although this vaccine has been used in cattle it is not as effective as it is in pigs and can induce a significant pyrexia. This latter observation is not altogether surprising, as plasmid-free strains of *S.* Dublin and *S.* Typhimurium can induce a fatal enteritis in calves (Jones *et al.*, 1988b; Wallis *et al.*, 1995). Another plasmid-cured but also *crp*-gene deleted *S.* Choleraesuis strain was shown to be safe after immunization using high doses, not reverting to virulence and protective against heterologous challenge in piglets by simultaneously triggering humoral and cellular immune responses (Chu *et al.*, 2007). A *S.* Choleraesuis *cya crp* mutant with or without the virulence plasmid was evaluated for virulence and ability to elicit a protective immune response in weaned pigs. It did not provoke any adverse effects in the vaccinated animals and reduced clinical signs of morbidity significantly compared with non-vaccinated pigs after challenge with a highly virulent wild-type strain of *S.* Choleraesuis (Kennedy *et al.*, 1999). An auxotrophic double-attenuated *S.* Choleraesuis (pur$^-$/rough) vaccine, derived by chemical mutagenesis and registered in Germany as well as other countries, has been shown to be effective in control of *S.* Choleraesuis infection in both piglets and adult animals after oral and/or parenteral administration (Meyer *et al.*, 1993).

Numerous vaccine candidates have been developed to better control *S.* Typhimurium, the most important serovar in pigs in numerous countries. An *aroA* vaccine strain of *S.* Typhimurium was shown to be attenuated and it significantly reduced faecal shedding of a virulent strain following challenge, although in this study challenge was performed only 1 week after vaccination; thus the duration of protection is not clear and the protection obtained may have been the result of stimulation innate responses (Lumsden *et al.*, 1991). An *S.* Typhimurium *cya crp* vaccine strain was also shown to be protective in pigs; however, this strain caused significant pyrexia for 4 days post-vaccination (Coe and Wood, 1992). A *gyrA-cpxA-rpoB* mutant of *S.* Typhimurium was shown to be safe after oral immunization of 4-week-old piglets, preventing vaccinated pigs from clinical symptoms of salmonellosis and resulting in a significantly decreased colonization of inner organs compared with non-vaccinated controls (Roesler *et al.*, 2004). An auxotrophic double-attenuated *S.* Typhimurium vaccine strain has been evaluated for safety and potency in very young suckling piglets and animals that are several weeks old and is commercially available in Germany and other countries. Immunization of pigs either by the oral or the oral/parenteral route did not induce any adverse clinical signs but resulted in a significantly reduced colonization by *S.* Typhimurium challenge organisms in caecal and ileal mucosa as well as ileocaecal lymph nodes compared with unvaccinated animals (Springer *et al.*, 2001; Eddicks *et al.*, 2009). To enable the differentiation between vaccinated and infected pigs an *ompD* deletion mutant of this auxotrophic *S.* Typhimurium vaccine strain was produced. Safety and efficacy against infection with a virulent DT 104 strain of *S.* Typhimurium of this mutant in mice and pigs were confirmed. The problems with the use of vaccination in pigs and concurrent of serological differentiation between vaccinated and naturally infected pigs might be overcome using this approach (Selke *et al.*, 2007).

Besides live vaccines, inactivated *S.* Typhimurium vaccines have also been tested in pigs, mainly for their efficacy in protecting suckling pigs via maternal antibodies after parenteral administration of pregnant sows. *Salmonella* were not detected in piglets from sows vaccinated using a herd-specific *S.* Typhimurium strain whereas 47% of the piglets from non-vaccinated parent animals excreted the organisms (Roesler *et al.*, 2006), indicating the potential to decrease *Salmonella* prevalence in both sows and piglets.

Vaccines for Sheep

A number of vaccines have been developed to control *S.* Abortusovis and *S.* Typhimurium infection in sheep. A *S.* Abortusovis strain RV6, which represents a non-streptomycin-dependent reverse mutant selected from a streptomycin-dependent strain, has been evaluated in thousands of sheep in different parts of France (Pardon *et al.*, 1990). A metabolic-drift mutant of *S.* Typhimurium has been produced by Linde *et al.* (1992) and shown to protect against *S.* Abortusovis infection. Several studies evaluated the potential of aromatic-dependent mutants to protect sheep from clinical disease and abortion. Three live vaccine candidates of *S.* Abortusovis (Δ*aroA*, Δ*cya* Δ*crp* Δ*cdt*, and plasmid-cured strains) have been tested for their efficacy to induce humoral antibodies and protection against abortion after subcutaneous administration of the vaccines and after challenge with wild-type *S.* Abortusovis in pregnant ewes. The plasmid-cured derivative was as safe as the other vaccines and resulted in a greater reduction of pregnancy failure compared to Δ*aroA* or Δ*cya* Δ*crp* Δ*cdt* vaccine candidates (Uzzau *et al.*, 2005). Sheep immunized with a live *S.* Typhimurium *aroA* mutant strain by either the intramuscular or oral route were protected against oral challenge with a virulent ovine isolate of *S.* Typhimurium, whereas non-immunized animals died of acute enteritis within 7 days. As the different routes of administration of the vaccine obviously induced different immune parameters, protection against salmonellosis in sheep may involve several mechanisms (Mukkur *et al.*, 1987). Another live *aroA* mutant of *S.* Typhimurium was used to immunize sheep by the oral route. Compared to mice, vaccinated sheep did not reveal a strong vaccine-specific immune response but both mice and sheep were protected against challenge with a lethal dose of the virulent *S.* Typhimurium wild-type strain (Brennan *et al.*, 1994). An *aroA* mutant of *S.* Typhimurium was also tested for the potential to protect neonatal lambs via maternal antibodies containing colostrum after immunization of pregnant ewes (Mukkur *et al.*, 1998). Lambs from immunized and non-immunized dams were challenged with

S. Typhimurium during the first week of age and none of them displayed signs of clinical salmonellosis, However, lambs from immunized animals excreted the challenge organisms in significantly lower numbers and for a reduced period compared with control animals.

Subcutaneous administration of an inactivated *S.* Abortusovis vaccine preparation to ewes induced both humoral and cellular-mediated immune response and prevented abortion after infection using fully virulent *S.* Abortusovis. The supposed association between an inability to produce IFN-γ and abortion might be overcome by the use of an inactivated *S.* Abortusovis vaccine (Cagiola *et al.*, 2007). Because of the epidemiological importance of the serovar *S.* Brandenburg, different vaccine preparations were evaluated for their potential to induce protective effects against challenge by this serovar. A live *S.* Typhimurium mutant, a subunit preparation from *S.* Brandenburg and a commercial multivalent inactivated vaccine were used to immunize ewes twice. Several weeks after booster vaccination animals were challenged with *S.* Brandenburg and monitored for clinical signs, abortion and excretion of *Salmonella* challenge organisms. The use of these vaccine preparations did not, however, significantly protect sheep against lethal challenge with *S.* Brandenburg (Li *et al.*, 2005).

Although *S.* Abortusovis infection is a serious problem in some countries, most sheep are kept under free-range conditions and *Salmonella* infection is only a problem when sheep are stressed, e.g. under adverse weather conditions or when transported. Following an outbreak of salmonellosis, sheep are generally more resistant the following year and this should be borne in mind when evaluating vaccines (Pardon *et al.*, 1990).

Problems Associated with Killed Vaccines

Vaccines based on dead *Salmonella* bacteria have long been known to protect experimental animals and those in the field against salmonellosis, but, as indicated earlier, there are many contradictions in the scientific literature relating to their actual efficacy. In part, this is due to the huge variety of specific formulations, adjuvants, methods of bacterial inactivation and animal models, which make the different studies very difficult to compare. Parenteral administration of dead vaccines generally results in a potent serum antibody response, though often in the absence of secretory antibody and CMI responses. Widespread laboratory studies with genetically susceptible mouse strains have demonstrated that, in such animals, dead vaccines are not very effective. However, several studies, using outbred mice or genetically more resistant inbred mouse strains, have shown killed vaccines to be highly effective (Lindberg *et al.*, 1974; Kuusi et *al.*, 1981; Eisenstein *et al.*, 1984). Furthermore, a recent review was carried out comparing the efficacy of different types of *S.* Typhi vaccine in over 1.8 million humans. Whole-cell, killed vaccines were found to be more effective than a live, attenuated vaccine and a vaccine based on Vi capsular polysaccharide, although the killed vaccine was associated with more adverse side-effects (Engels *et al.*, 1998). Obviously, typhoid fever in humans represents a different form of infection from acute enteric salmonellosis in cattle and subclinical intestinal carriage in pigs and poultry, but killed vaccines should clearly not be dismissed on the basis of experimental laboratory studies using highly susceptible mouse strains.

There are three major potential problems with dead *Salmonella* vaccines. First, they only contain antigens induced by the environmental conditions *in vitro* in which they were grown, although this may be partially overcome by simulated *in vivo* conditions *in vitro* by, for example, growing organisms under appropriate nutritional or other environmental conditions. Second, they are generally believed to fail to elicit cell-mediated immune responses, which are considered important for long-term protection. This too may be overcome with the use of an appropriate adjuvant. Finally, they generally fail to elicit secretory IgA responses, which are potentially important in protecting mucosal surfaces although there is some evidence that immunoglobulin is not essential for controlling intestinal infections, at least in chickens

(Beal *et al.*, 2006). However, some dead vaccines have been shown to induce immune responses at mucosal surfaces. Baljer *et al.* (1986) protected calves by oral vaccination with repeated doses of heat-inactivated and disrupted cells, and found that anti-O antibody was produced in intestinal secretions. In the UK, at present only inactivated vaccines are licensed and therefore widely available for cattle, and these are claimed to be effective in combating outbreaks of disease in cattle. However, information relating to their actual efficacy is scarce.

Towards the Ideal Live Vaccine: Suggested Criteria for Effectiveness

A common problem with the use of live vaccine strains in calves is the mild enteritis and associated shedding of the vaccine strain that often follows oral vaccination. This is likely to be a reason for concern over their use in all food-producing animals. Not only is residual virulence for the host animal undesirable, but pathogenic effects on the human population are also possible, since the vaccine strains may conceivably enter the human food chain. Recent developments in our understanding of the virulence factors mediating *Salmonella*-induced enteritis are of potential value in further modifying the pre-existing live vaccine strains, in order to reduce these adverse side-effects. A virulence locus on the *Salmonella* chromosome, named *Salmonella* pathogenicity island 1 (SPI-1), encodes a protein secretory apparatus that translocates proteins into target eukaryotic cells (Galan, 1996; Hensel, 2004, 2007; Gerlach and Hensel, 2007). Mutation of genes in SPI-1 significantly reduces intestinal invasion of *S.* Typhimurium and *S.* Dublin in cattle (Watson *et al.*, 1995; Galyov *et al.*, 1997) as well as chickens (Rychlik *et al.*, 2009) and significantly attenuated *S.* Typhimurium in cattle, although mild pyrexia and scours still occurred (Watson *et al.*, 1998). The SopB and SopD effector proteins, which are secreted and translocated by SPI-1, are directly involved in the induction of enteritis (Galyov *et al.*, 1997; Norris *et al.*, 1998). Neither of these proteins is involved in mediating intestinal invasion and thus such mutants should be fully immunogenic. *SopB* maps to another pathogenicity island, called SPI-5, which encodes other proteins that influence enteropathogenesis in cattle but not systemic pathogenesis in mice (Wood *et al.*, 1998). The full potential of these new developments for vaccine design have not yet been investigated. The use of mutations that reduce enteritis, in conjunction with mutations that specifically prevent the systemic form of disease, has obvious potential benefits over the existing live, attenuated vaccine strains. However, the protective immune response operating in the gut, elicited in vaccinated and convalescent animals, is very serovar-specific (Villarreal *et al.*, 1997). This may be a consequence of these effector proteins being directly injected into cells by *Salmonella* and therefore avoiding immune defence mechanisms acting at the mucosal surface.

It should thus eventually be possible to delete from the *Salmonella* chromosome those genes responsible for fluid secretion (enterotoxigenicity), thereby producing a mutant that should behave like the parent strain in the alimentary tract of poultry but that would be avirulent for humans. The criteria in selecting an ideal vaccine have been discussed previously (Pritchard *et al.*, 1978; Barrow, 1991). These are outlined below.

Strong protection against intestinal and systemic infection is required. An additional requirement is stable avirulence for humans (see discussion above). In view of the current increased public awareness of *Salmonella* food poisoning, it is unclear whether the greatest fear will be of salmonellosis, thereby increasing the chance of acceptance of the use of live vaccines, or of the use of a live vaccine itself. There may always be some resistance to the use of a vaccine that is *Salmonella*-derived, unless it can be shown that the vaccine is no more virulent for humans than other microorganisms, which are also present on the carcass at slaughter. The virulence of some of these candidate vaccines for humans has been assessed (Barrow *et al.*, 1990b). Ideally, the vaccine strains should not enter the human food chain and, for this and reasons associated with the release of genetically modified organisms, the strain should not contaminate the environment.

Entry into the human food chain of live attenuated *Salmonella* strains is an issue although there is no evidence, from the widespread use of current live vaccines in poultry, that this is a problem. Since 1994 it has been obligatory in Germany to vaccinate all layer chickens during their rearing period using live *S.* Typhimurium or *S.* Enteritidis vaccines. Several hundred million doses of live vaccines from different producers have been administered since that time and there has been no evidence of reversion to virulence. Because of the broad use of live *Salmonella* vaccines in different animal species (poultry, calves, pigs, pigeons), in Germany the competent authority has established a lab-based surveillance system to monitor the occurrence of these live vaccine strains in the human population (Rabsch *et al.*, 2001). Since 2000 all strains of *S.* Typhimurium and *S.* Enteritidis from humans were examined in respect to their phage types and vaccine markers. From several thousands of isolates tested no live vaccine organism was detected from infections in humans.

There are additional potential concerns over the use of genetically modified strains as vaccines although there is clear logic in the use of deletion mutants that have defined genotypes and phenotypes, are antibiotic sensitive and can be easily differentiated from wild-type strains. Again the fact that extensive use of existing live vaccines in poultry in Europe suggests that this is a perceived rather than a real problem.

In Europe, the administration of live *Salmonella* vaccines in breeder birds and in chickens for table egg production has to guarantee by determining the appropriate withdrawal period, that *Salmonella* vaccine organisms do not enter the food chain via contaminated eggs (Directive 2001/82/EC; EC, 2001). As a result of this the use of live *Salmonella* vaccines in layer chickens is restricted to the rearing period. The period between the last application of the live vaccine strain and the beginning of the laying period must be long enough to ensure that no live *Salmonella* organism is excreted by the animals.

All *Salmonella* vaccines are immunological veterinary medicinal products in the EU and as such they are required to meet the requirements of national regulations in the member states of the EU and other countries in the world. International guidelines exist on the requirements for registration, including: (i) Directive 2001/82/EC of the European Parliament on the Community code relating to veterinary medicinal products; (ii) the European Pharmacopoeia; and (iii) the EP Monograph 62 on vaccines for veterinary use.

The ideal route of administration to poultry would be orally via the drinking water or food or by spray. For cattle and pigs, this should be achieved with a single dose. However, parenteral administration may be an additional requirement for maximum protection. Although the ideal vaccine should be avirulent for chickens, oral vaccination may require the use of an invasive strain to stimulate maximum immunity, because immunogenicity may be correlated with invasiveness. It seems likely that a strong secretory IgA response will be required for this. The vaccine must not affect animal productivity.

Protection should obviously last as long as possible. Protection of broilers is required for a matter of weeks. However, control in breeders and layers is an integral part of the European control programme, and here protection is needed for many months. Protection against *S.* Gallinarum induced either by the 9R vaccine (Smith, 1956) or by an *aroA* vaccine (Barrow *et al.*, 2001a) lasts for between 3 and 6 months. Immunity induced by an auxotrophic live *S.* Enteritidis vaccine and an inactivated *S.* Typhimurium/Enteritidis vaccine in chickens was detected for the whole laying period (Springer *et al.*, 2011).

Legislation in many countries requires that all isolations of *Salmonella* from poultry must be reported. Thus wild-type strains must be easily differentiated from vaccine strains. This can be achieved positively or negatively by antigenic markers for their absence, by auxotrophy or by molecular differentiation, many of which techniques would be beyond the competence of many laboratories. The use of antibiotic resistance is unlikely to be adopted, because it is so widespread, but resistance to heavy metals might be used. If monitoring is carried out serologically, the vaccine must not express the antigens responsible for stimulating antibodies detected in the test used.

Vaccination against salmonellosis can produce a degree of protection over and above that possessed by non-immunized chickens with a fully mature intestinal flora. Vaccination should therefore be compatible with the use of competitive exclusion (early application or replacement of gut flora). No problems should arise that are similar to those resulting from overuse of antibiotics. Vaccination should also be compatible with the use of growth-promoting antibiotics.

Cross-Protection Between Serovars

It is known that different serovars of *Salmonella*, either as virulent parent strains or when attenuated, induce different degrees of protection in the mouse typhoid model (Collins, 1974; Hormaeche *et al.*, 1991). The role of O-antigen in eliciting protective responses is unclear. Hybrid vaccine strains expressing O-antigen common to both *S.* Typhimurium and *S.* Dublin induced protection against both serovars in mice (Lindberg *et al.*, 1993), but not in cattle (Segall and Lindberg, 1993), suggesting that O-antigen is important in conferring protection in systemic salmonellosis in mice but not in enteritis in larger animals. In contrast, Hormaeche *et al.* (1991) found no key role for O-antigen in protection in mice, and proposed a role for other undefined antigens. Studies in poultry have been confusing. Cooper and his group (1993) have suggested that there is no cross-protection between *S.* Typhimurium and *S.* Enteritidis. However, more recently, Hassan and Curtiss (1994) indicated a considerable degree of cross-protection between a variety of serovars. It is assumed, however, that cross-protection between serovars does not generally occur and that protection lasts no longer than 6 months.

There is little evidence for any significant cross-protection between serogroups in mice (Hormaeche *et al.*, 1991; Lindberg *et al.*, 1993; Segall and Lindberg, 1993), cattle (Meyer *et al.*, 1992; Villarreal *et al.*, 1997) or chickens (Hassan and Curtiss, 1994; Curtiss and Hassan, 1996; Springer *et al.*, 2000), although the reason for this remains unclear. Some experimental evidence exists indicating little mutual protection between groups B and D in chickens. No published information exists for group C.

The problem of protecting animal herds against a broad spectrum of different *Salmonella* serovars remains unsolved. Whether or not it will ever be achievable is uncertain. No study to date has demonstrated good cross-protection between different *Salmonella* serovars for any significant duration after vaccination. Cross-protection was assessed in calves immunized with a live *S.* Typhimurium *aroA* or *S.* Dublin *aroA* and challenged with the homologous serovar to check (and boost) the protective immune response. When wild-type *S.* Typhimurium and *S.* Dublin strains were used to infect ligated ileal loops constructed in these immune animals 3 weeks after challenge with the virulent organism, serovar-specific protection was found. In animals vaccinated with *S.* Typhimurium, only *S.* Dublin strains invaded intestinal mucosa and elicited enteropathogenic responses and vice versa in *S.* Dublin-immunized cattle (Wallis *et al.*, 1995), despite these two serovars sharing common enteropathogenic virulence mechanisms (Wood *et al.*, 1998). This being the case, it is difficult to see how effective cross-protection between different serovars can be achieved in the future. One approach is to include different serovars in the vaccine preparation, be it live or dead. However, preliminary observations with dual, live *S.* Typhimurium *aroA* and *S.* Enteritidis *aroA* vaccination regimens in poultry suggest that the vaccine strains interfere with one another, reducing their efficacy compared with a monovalent regimen (M. Woodward, pers. comm.). It would appear that, at present, the only really effective means of controlling outbreaks of uncommon serovars is through the use of herd-specific killed vaccines, which have been shown to be protective in acute outbreaks (Bauer, 1986) and very effective in reducing faecal shedding (Aitken *et al.*, 1982; Weber *et al.*, 1993).

References

Adriaensen, C., DeGreve, H., Tian, J.Q., DeCraeye, S., Gubbels, E., Eeckhaut, V., Van Immerseel, F., Ducatelle, R., Kumar, M. and Hernalsteens J.-P. (2007) A live *Salmonella enterica* serovar Enteritidis vaccine allows serological differentiation between vaccinated and infected animals. *Infection and Immunity* 75, 2461–2468.

Aitken, M.M., Jones, P.W. and Brown, G.T. (1982) Protection of cattle against experimentally induced salmonellosis by intradermal injection of heat-killed *Salmonella dublin*. *Research in Veterinary Science* 32, 368–373.

Anderson, J., Smith, B.P. and Ulrich, J.T. (1991) Vaccination of calves with a modified bacterin or oil-in-water emulsion containing alkali-detoxified *Salmonella typhimurium* lipopolysaccharide. *American Journal of Veterinary Research* 52, 596–601.

Bailey, J.S., Rolon, A., Hofacre, C.L., Holt, P.S., Wilson, J.L., Cosby, D.E., Richardson, L.J. and Cox, N.A. (2007) Intestinal humoral immune response and resistance to *Salmonella* challenge of progeny from breeders vaccinated with killed antigen. *International Journal of Poultry Science* 6, 417–423.

Baljer, G., Hoerstke, M., Dirksen, G., Sailer, J. and Mayr, A. (1986) Efficacy of local and/or parenteral vaccination against calf salmonellosis with inactivated vaccines. *Journal of Veterinary Medicine* 33, 206–212.

Barrow, P.A. (1990) Immunity to experimental fowl typhoid in chickens induced by a virulence plasmid-cured derivative of *Salmonella gallinarum*. *Infection and Immunity* 58, 2283–2288

Barrow, P.A. (1991) Immunological control of *Salmonella* in poultry. In: Blankenship, L.C. (ed.) *Colonization Control of Human Bacterial Enteropathogens in Poultry*. Academic Press, San Diego, California, pp. 199–217.

Barrow, P.A., Simpson, J.M., Lovell, M.A. and Binns, M.M. (1987) Contribution of *Salmonella gallinarum* large plasmid towards virulence in fowl typhoid. *Infection and Immunity* 35, 388–392.

Barrow, P.A., Simpson, J.M. and Lovell, M.A. (1988) Intestinal colonization in the chicken by food-poisoning *Salmonella* serovars microbial characteristics associated with faecal excretion. *Avian Pathology* 17, 571–588.

Barrow, P.A., Hassan, J.O. and Berchieri, A. (1990a) Reduction in faecal excretion of *Salmonella typhimurium* strain F98 in chickens vaccinated with live and killed *S. typhimurium* organisms. *Epidemiology and Infection* 104, 413–426.

Barrow, P.A., Hassan, J.O. and Berchieri, A. (1990b) Immunisation of laying hens against *Salmonella enteritidis* phage type 4 with live, attenuated vaccines. *Veterinary Record* 126, 241–242.

Barrow, P.A., Lovell, M.A. and Stocker, B.A.D. (2001a) Protection against experimental fowl typhoid by parenteral administration of live SL5928, an *aroA-serC* (aromatic dependent) mutant of a wild-type *Salmonella* Gallinarum strain made lysogenic for P22*sie*. *Avian Pathology* 29, 423–431.

Barrow, P.A., Page, K. and Lovell, M.A. (2001b) The virulence for gnotobiotic pigs of live attenuated vaccine strains of *Salmonella enterica* serovar Typhimurium and Enteritidis. *Vaccine* 19, 3432–3436Bauer, K. (1986) Experiences with local administration of herd-specific vaccines *Tierärztliche Praxis* 14, 51–54.

Beal, R.K., Powers, C., Davison, T.F., Barrow, P.A. and Smith, A.L. (2006) Clearance of *Salmonella enterica* serovar Typhimurium in chickens is independent of B-cell function. *Infection and Immunity* 74, 1442–1444.

Berchieri, A. and Barrow, P.A. (1990) Further studies on the inhibition of colonization of the chicken alimentary tract with *Salmonella typhimurium* by pre-colonization with an avirulent mutant. *Epidemiology and Infection* 104, 427–441.

Bisping, W., Dimitriadis, I. and Seippel, M. (1971) Versuche zur oralen Immunisierung von Hühnern mit hitzeinaktivierter *Salmonella*-Vakzine 1. Mitteilung; Impf-und Infektionsversuche an Hühnerküken. *Zentralblatt für Veterinärmedizin B* 18, 337–346.

Bohez, L., Ducatelle, R., Pasmans, F., Haesebrouck, F. and Van Immerseel, F. (2007) Long-term colonization-inhibition studies to protect broilers against colonization with *Salmonella* Enteritidis, using *Salmonella* Pathogenicity Island 1and 2 mutants. *Vaccine* 25, 4235–4243.

Bohez, L., Dewulf, B., Ducatelle, R., Pasmans, F., Haesebrouck, F. and Van Immerseel, F. (2008) The effect of oral administration of a homologous *hilA* mutant strain on the long term colonization and transmission of *Salmonella* Enteritidis in broiler chickens. *Vaccine* 26, 372–378.

Brennan, F.R., Oliver, J.J. and Baird, G.D. (1994) Differences in the immune response of mice and sheep to an aromatic-dependent mutant of *Salmonella typhimurium*. *Journal of Medical Microbiology* 41, 20–28.

Cagiola, M., Severi, G., Forti, K., Menichelli, M., Papa, P., De Giuseppe, A. and Pasquali, P. (2007) Abortion due to *Salmonella enterica* serovar Abortusovis in ewes is associated to a lack of production of IFN-γ and can be prevented by immunization with inactivated *S.* Abortusovis vaccine. *Veterinary Microbiology* 121, 330–337.

Chu, C.-E., Wang, S.Y., Chen, Z.-W., Chien, M.-S., Huang, J.P., Chen, J.-J., Hoing, L.S., Shiau, A.L., Tsai, J.L. and Wu, C.L. (2007) Heterologous protection in pigs induced by a plasmid-cured and *crp* gene-deleted *Salmonella choleraesuis* live vaccine. *Vaccine* 25, 7031–7040.

Clifton-Hadley, F.A., Breslin, M., Venables, L.M., Sprigings, K.A., Cooles, S.W., Houghton, S. and Woodward, M.J. (2002) A laboratory study of an inactivated bivalent iron restricted *Salmonella enterica* serovar Enteritidis and Typhimurium dual vaccine against Typhimurium challenge in chickens. *Veterinary Microbiology* 89, 167–179.

Coe, N.E. and Wood, R.L. (1992) The effect of exposure to a Δcya Δcrp mutant *of Salmonella typhimurium* on the subsequent colonization of swine by the wild-type parent strain. *Veterinary Microbiology* 31, 207–220.

Collins, F.M. (1974) Vaccines and cell-mediated immunity. *Bacteriological Reviews* 38, 371–402.

Cooper, G.L., Nicholas, R.A.J., Cullen, G.A. and Hormaeche, C.E. (1990) Vaccination of chickens with a *Salmonella enteritidis aroA* live oral *Salmonella* vaccine. *Microbial Pathogenesis* 9, 255–265.

Cooper, G.L., Venables, L.M., Nicholas, R.A.J., Cullen, G.A. and Hormaeche, C.E. (1992) Vaccination of chickens with chicken-derived *Salmonella enteritidis* phage type 4 aroA live oral *Salmonella* vaccines. *Vaccine* 10, 247–254.

Cooper, G.L., Venables, L.M., Nicholas, R.A.J. and Cullen, G.A. (1993) Further studies of the application of live *Salmonella enteritidis* aroA vaccines *in* chickens. *Veterinary Record* 133, 31–36.

Curtiss, R. and Hassan, J.O. (1996) Nonrecombinant and recombinant avirulent *Salmonella* vaccines for poultry. *Veterinary Immunology and Immunopathology* 54, 365–372.

Deguchi, K., Yokoyama, E., Honda, T. and Mizuno, K. (2009) Efficacy of a novel trivalent inactivated vaccine against the shedding of *Salmonella* in a chicken challenge model. *Avian Diseases* 53, 281–286.

Dey, A.K. and Srivastava, I.K. (2011) Novel adjuvants and delivery systems for enhancing immune responses induced by immunogens. *Expert Review Vaccines* 10, 227–251.

Dueger, E.L., House, J.K., Heithoff, D.M. and Mahan, M.J. (2003a) *Salmonella* DNA adenine methylase mutants elicit early and late onset protective immune response in calves. *Vaccine* 21, 3249–3258.

Dueger, E.L., House, J.K., Heithoff, D.M. and Mahan, M.J. (2003b) *Salmonella* DNA adenine methylase mutants prevent colonization of newly hatched chickens by homologous and heterologous serovars. *International Journal of Food Microbiology* 80, 153–159.

EC (2001)Directive 2001/82/EC of the European Parliament and the council of 6 November 2001 on the Community code relating to veterinary medicinal products, 1–66.

EC (2006) Commission Regulation (EC) 1177/2006 of 1 August 2006 implementing Regulation (EC) No 2160/2003 of the European Parliament and of the Council as regards requirements for the use of specific control methods in the framework of the national programmes for the control of *Salmonella* in poultry.

Eddicks, M., Palzer, A., Hörmansdorfer, S., Ritzmann, M. and Heinritzi, K. (2009) Examination of the compatibility of a *Salmonella* Typhimurium live vaccine Salmoporc® for three days-old suckling piglets. *Deutsche Tierärztliche Wochenschrift* 116, 249–254.

EFSA (2004) Use of vaccines for the control of *Salmonella* in poultry. *The EFSA Journal* 114, 1–74.

EFSA (2008) Report of the task force on zoonoses data collection on the analysis of the baseline survey on the prevalence of *Salmonella* in slaughter pigs in the EU, 2006-2007. Part A: *Salmonella* prevalence estimates. *The EFSA Journal* 135, 1–111.

Eisenstein, T.K., Killar, L.M. and Sultzer, B.M. (1984) Immunity to infection with *Salmonella typhimurium*: mousestrain differences in vaccine- and serum-mediated protection. *Journal of Infectious Diseases* 150, 425–435.

Engels, E.A., Falagas, M.E., Lau, J. and Bennish, M.L. (1998) Typhoid fever vaccines: a meta-analysis of studies on efficacy and toxicity. *British Medical Journal* 316, 110–116.

Eriksson, S., Lucchini, S., Thompson, A., Rhen, M. and Hinton, J.C. (2003) Unravelling the biology of macrophage infection by gene expression profiling of intracellular *Salmonella enterica*. *Molecular Microbiology* 47, 103–118.

Feberwee, A., de Vries, T.S., Elbers, A.R. and de Jong, W.A. (2000) Results of a *Salmonella enteritidis* vaccination field trial in broiler-breeder flocks in The Netherlands. *Avian Disease* 44, 249–255.

Feberwee, A., Hartman, E.G., de Wit, J.J. and de Vries, T.S. (2001a) The spread of *Salmonella gallinarum* 9R vaccine strain under field conditions. *Avian Diseases* 45, 1024–1029.

Feberwee, A., de Vries, T.S., Hartman, E.G., de Wit, J.J., Elbers, A.R.W. and de Jong, W.A. (2001b) Vaccination against *Salmonella enteritidis* in Dutch commercial layer flocks with a vaccine based on a live

Salmonella gallinarum 9R strain: Evaluation of efficacy, safety, and performance of serologic *Salmonella* tests. *Avian Diseases* 45, 83–91.

Fox, B.C., Roof, M.B., Carter, D.P., Kesl, L.D. and Roth, J.A. (1997) Safety and efficacy of an avirulent live *Salmonella choleraesuis* vaccine for protection of calves against *Salmonella* dublin infection. *American Journal of Veterinary Research* 58, 265–271.

Galan, J.E. (1996) Molecular genetic bases of *Salmonella* entry into host cells. *Molecular Microbiology* 20, 263–271.

Galyov, E.E., Wood, M.W., Rosqvist, R., Mullen, P.B., Watson, P.R., Hedges, S. and Wallis, T.S. (1997) A secreted effector protein of *Salmonella* dublin is translocated into eukaryotic cells and mediates inflammation and fluid secretion in infected ileal mucosa. *Molecular Microbiology* 25, 903–912.

Gantois, I., Ducatelle, R., Timbermont, L., Bohez, L., Haesebrouck, F., Pasmans, F. and Van Immerseel, F. (2006) Oral immunisation of laying hens with live vaccine strains of TAD Salmonella vac® E and TAD Salmonella vac® T reduces internal egg contamination with *Salmonella* Enteritidis. *Vaccine* 24, 6250–6255.

Gerlach, R.G. and Hensel, M. (2007) *Salmonella* Pathogenicity islands in host specificity, host pathogen-interactions and antibiotics resistance of *Salmonella enterica*. *Berliner und Münchener Tierärztliche Wochenschrift* 120, 317–327.

Gordon, R.F. and Luke, D. (1959) A note on the use of the 9R fowl typhoid vaccine in poultry breeding flocks. *Veterinary Record* 71, 926–927.

Gordon, R.F., Garside, J.S. and Tucker, J.F. (1959) The use of living attenuated vaccines in the control of fowl typhoid. *Veterinary Record* 71, 300–305.

Griffin, H.G. and Barrow, P.A. (1993) Construction of an aroA mutant of *Salmonella* serovar Gallinarum – its effectiveness against experimental fowl typhoid. *Vaccine* 11, 457–462.

Hahn, I. (2000) A contribution to consumer protection: TAD *Salmonella* vac® E – a new live vaccine for chickens against *Salmonella* Enteritidis. *Lohmann Information* 23, 29–32.

Hassan, J.O. and Curtiss, R. (1994) Development and evaluation of an experimental vaccination program using a live-avirulent *Salmonella typhimurium* strain to protect immunized chickens against challenge with homologous and heterologous *Salmonella* serovars. *Infection and Immunity* 62, 5519–5527.

Heider, L.C., Meiring, R.W., Hoet, A.E., Gebreyes, W.A., Funk, J.A. and Wittum, T.E. (2008) Evaluation of vaccination with a commercial subunit vaccine on shedding of *Salmonella enterica* in subclinically infected dairy cows. *Journal of the American Veterinary Medical Association*. 233, 466–469.

Hensel, M. (2004) Evolution of pathogenicity islands of *Salmonella enterica*. *International Journal of Medical Microbiology* 294, 95–102.

Hensel, M. (2007) Genome-based identification and molecular analyses of pathogenicity islands and genomic islands in *Salmonella enterica*. *Methods in Molecular Biology* 394, 77–88.

Hermesch, D.R., Thomson, D.U., Loneragan, G.H., Renter, D.R. and White, B.J. (2008) Effects of a commercially available vaccine against *Salmonella enterica* serotype Newport on milk production, somatic cell count, and shedding of *Salmonella* organisms in female dairy cattle with no clinical signs of salmonellosis. *American Journal of Veterinary Research* 69, 1229–1234.

Hone, D.M., Attridge, S.R., Forrest, B., Morona, R., Daniels, D., La Brooy, J.L., Bartholomeusz, R.C.A., Shearman, D.J.C. and Hackett, J. (1988) A *galE Via* (Vi-antigen negative) mutant of *Salmonella* typhi Ty2 retains virulence in humans. *Infection and Immunity* 56, 1326–1333.

Hormaeche, C.E., Joysey, H.S., DeSilva, L., Izhar, M. and Stocker, B.A.D. (1991) Immunity conferred by aro-*Salmonella* live vaccines. *Microbial Pathogenesis* 10, 149–158.

House, J.K., Ontiveros, M.M., Blackmer, N.M., Dueger, E.L., Fitchhorn, J.B., McArthur, G.R. and Smith, B.P. (2001) Evaluation of an autogenous *Salmonella* bacterin and a modified live *Salmonella* serotype Choleraesuis vaccine on a commercial dairy farm. *American Journal of Veterinary Research* 62, 1897–1902.

Iqbal, M., Philbin, V.J., Withanage, G.S.K., Wigley, P., Beal, R.K., Goodchild, M.J., Barrow, P.A., McConnell, I., Maskell, D.J., Young, J.R., Bumstead, N., Boyd, Y. and Smith, A.L. (2005) Identification and functional characterization of chicken TLR5 reveals a fundamental role in the biology of infection with *Salmonella enterica* serovar Typhimurium. *Infection and Immunity* 73, 2344–2350.

Jones, P.W., Collins, P., Brown, G.T. and Aitken, M.M. (1983) *Salmonella* saint-paul infection in two dairy herds. *Journal of Hygiene, Cambridge* 91, 243–257.

Jones, P.W., Collins, P. and Aitken, M.M. (1988a) Passive protection of calves against experimental infection with *Salmonella typhimurium*. *Veterinary Record* 123, 536–541.

Jones, P.W., Collins, P. and Lax, A. (1988b) The role of large plasmids in the pathogenesis of salmonellosis in cattle [abstract]. *Journal of Medical Microbiology* 27, x.

Jones, P.W., Dougan, G., Hayward, C., Mackenzie, N., Collins, P. and Chatfield, S.N. (1991) Oral vaccination of calves against experimental salmonellosis using a double *aro* mutant of *Salmonella typhimurium*. *Vaccine* 9, 29–34.

Kennedy, M.J., Yancey, R.J., Sanchez, M.S., Rzepkowski, R.A., Kelly, S.M. and Curtiss III, R. (1999) Attenuation and immunogenicity of Δ*cya* Δ*crp* derivatives of *Salmonella choleraesuis* in pigs. *Infection and Immunity* 67, 4628–4636.

Kogut, M.H., Tellez, G., Hargis, B.M., Corrier, D.E. and Deloach, J.R. (1993) The effect of 5-fluorouracil treatment of chicks a cell depletion model for the study of avian polymorphonuclear leucocytes and natural host defences. *Poultry Science* 72, 1873–1880.

Kogut, M.H., Tellez, G.I., McGruder, E.D., Hargis, B.M., Williams, J.D., Corrier, D.E. and Deloach, J.R. (1994) Heterophils are decisive components in the early responses of chickens to *Salmonella enteritidis* infections. *Microbial Pathogenesis* 16, 141–151.

Kuusi, N., Nurminen, N., Saxen, H. and Makela, P.H. (1981) Immunization with outer membrane protein (Porin) preparations in experimental murine salmonellosis: effect of lipopolysaccharide. *Infection and Immunity* 34, 328–332.

Lee, Y.L., Mo, I.P. and Kang, M.S. (2005) Safety and efficacy of *Salmonella gallinarum* 9R vaccine in young laying chickens. *Avian Pathology* 34, 362–366.

Lee, Y.L., Mo, I.P. and Kang, M.S. (2007) Protective efficacy of live *Salmonella gallinarum* 9R vaccine in commercial layer flocks. *Avian Pathology* 36, 495–498.

Li, H., McFarlane, R.G. and Wagner, J. (2005) Vaccination of pregnant ewes against infection with *Salmonella* Brandenburg. *New Zealand Veterinary Journal* 53, 416–422.

Lindberg, A.A., Rosenberg, L.T., Ljunggren, A., Ganegg, P.J., Svensson, S. and Wallin, N.H. (1974) Effect of synthetic disaccharide-protein conjugate as immunogen in *Salmonella* infection in mice. *Infection and Immunity* 10, 541–545.

Lindberg, A.A., Segall, T., Weintraub, A. and Stocker, B.A.D. (1993) Antibody response and protection against challenge in mice vaccinated intraperitoneally with a live aroA 04-09 hybrid *Salmonella dublin* strain. *Infection and Immunity* 61, 1211–1221.

Linde, K., Bondarenko, V. and Sviridenko, V. (1992) Prophylaxis of *Salmonella abortus* ovis-induced abortion of sheep by a *Salmonella typhimurium* live vaccine. *Vaccine* 10, 337–340.

Linde, K., Hahn, I. and Vielitz, E. (1997) Development of live *Salmonella* vaccines optimally attenuated for chickens. *Lohmann Information* 20, 23–31.

Lumsden, J.S., Wilkie, B.N. and Clarke, R.C. (1991) Resistance to fecal shedding of salmonellae in pigs and chickens vaccinated with an aromatic-dependent mutant of *Salmonella typhimurium*. *American Journal of Veterinary Research* 52, 1784–1787.

McCapes, R.H., Coffland, R.T and Christie, L.E. (1967) Challenge of turkey poults originating from hens vaccinated with *Salmonella typhimurium* bacterins. *Avian Diseases* 11, 15–24.

Methner, U. (2001) The use of animal models in the development of classical vaccines. In: Schmidt, A. and Weber, O.F. (eds) *Animal Testing in Infectiology*. Karger Verlag, Basel, pp. 58–70.

Methner, U. (2007) Vaccination of poultry against *Salmonella:* What is the ideal vaccine strain? *XVIII European Symposium on the quality of poultry meat, eggs and egg products*, Prague, Czech Republic, 2–5 September 2007, pp. 56–59.

Methner, U. and Steinbach, G. (1997) Efficacy of maternal *Salmonella* antibodies against oral infection of chicks with *Salmonella* Enteritidis. *Berliner und Münchener Tierärztliche Wochenschrift* 110, 373–377.

Methner, U., Steinbach, G. and Meyer, H. (1994) Investigations on the efficacy of *Salmonella* immunization of broiler breeder birds to *Salmonella* colonization of these birds and their progeny following experimental oral infection. *Berliner und Münchener Tierärztliche Wochenschrift* 107, 192–198.

Methner, U., Koch, H. and Meyer, H. (1995) Model for experimental efficacy testing of control measures against *Salmonella* infections in poultry. *Deutsche Tierärztliche Wochenschrift* 102, 225–228.

Methner, U., Barrow, P.A., Berndt, A. and Steinbach, G. (1999) Combination of vaccination and competitive exclusion to prevent *Salmonella* colonization in chickens – Experimental studies. *International Journal of Food Microbiology* 49, 35–42.

Methner, U., Berndt, A. and Steinbach, G. (2001) Combination of competitive exclusion and immunization using an attenuated live *Salmonella* vaccine strain in chickens. *Avian Diseases* 45, 631–638.

Methner, U., Keiling, S., Kreutzer, B. and Schweinitz, P. (2002) Impact of maternal antibodies on the efficacy of immunisation of chicks with live *Salmonella* vaccines. *Deutsche Tierärztliche Wochenschrift* 109, 149–153.

Methner, U., Barrow, P.A., Gregorova, D. and Rychlik, I. (2004) Intestinal colonisation-inhibition and virulence of *Salmonella phoP, rpoS* and *ompC* deletion mutants in chickens. *Veterinary Microbiology* 98, 37–43.

Methner, U., Barrow, P.A. and Berndt, A. (2010) Induction of a homologous and heterologous invasion-inhibition effect after administration of *Salmonella* strains to newly hatched chicks. *Vaccine* 28, 6958–6963.

Methner, U., Haase, A., Berndt, A., Martin, G., Nagy, B. and Barrow, P.A. (2011a) Exploitation of intestinal colonisation-inhibition between *Salmonella* organisms for live vaccines in poultry: potential and limitations. *Zoonoses and Public Health* 58, 540–548.

Methner, U., Barrow, P.A., Berndt, A. and Rychlik, I. (2011b) *Salmonella* Enteritidis with double deletion in *phoP fliC* – a potential live *Salmonella* vaccine candidate with novel characteristics for use in chickens. *Vaccine* 29, 3248–3253.

Meyer, H., Barrow, P. and Pardon, P. (1992) *Salmonella* immunization in animals. In: *Proceedings of the International Symposium on Salmonella and Salmonellosis.* Ploufragan/St Brieuc, France, pp. 345–374.

Meyer, H., Koch, H., Methner, U. and Steinbach, G. (1993) Vaccines in salmonellosis control in animals. *Zentralblatt für Bakteriologie* 278, 407–415.

Mikula, I., Rosocha, J. and Pilipcinec, E. (1989) Immunization of calves with live and inactivated whole-cell vaccines against *Salmonella typhimurium* infection. *Acta Veterinaria Hungary* 37, 219–226.

Mohler, V.L., Heithoff, D.M., Mahan, M.J., Walker, K.H., Hornitzky, M.A., McConell, C.S., Shum, L.W.C. and House, J.K. (2006) Cross-protective immunity in calves conferred by a DNA adenine methylase deficient *Salmonella enterica* serovar Typhimurium vaccine. *Vaccine* 24, 1339–1345.

Mohler, V.L., Heithoff, D.M., Mahan, M.J., Walker, K.H., Hornitzky, M.A., Shum, L.W.C., Makin, K.J. and House, J.K. (2008) Cross-protective immunity conferred by a DNA adenine methylase deficient *Salmonella enterica* serovar Typhimurium vaccine in calves challenged with *Salmonella* serovar Newport. *Vaccine* 26, 1751–1758.

Morein, B., Villacres-Eriksson, M., Sjolander, A. and Bengtsson, K.L. (1996) Novel adjuvants and vaccine delivery systems. *Veterinary Immunology and Immunopathology* 54, 373–384.

Mukkur, T.K.S., McDowell, G.H., Stocker, B.A.D. and Lascelles, A.K. (1987) Protection against experimental salmonellosis in mice and sheep by immunisation with aromatic-dependent *Salmonella typhimurium*. *Journal of Medical Microbiology* 24, 11–19.

Mukkur, T.K.S., Walker, K.H. and McDowell, G.H. (1998) Passive immunisation of neonatal lambs via colostrum and milk of ewes previously immunised with live attenuated *Salmonella typhimurium* protects neonatal lambs from experimental salmonellosis. *Comparative Immunology, Microbiology and Infectious Diseases* 21, 327–336.

Nnalue, N.A. and Stocker, B.A.D. (1986) Some *galE* mutants of *Salmonella cholerae-suis* retain virulence. *Infection and Immunity* 54, 635–640.

Nogrady, N., Imre, A., Rychlik, I., Barrow, P.A. and Nagy, B. (2003) Growth and colonisation suppression of *Salmonella enterica* serovar Hadar *in vitro* and *in vivo*. *FEMS Microbiology Letters* 218, 127–133.

Norris, F.A., Wilson, M.P., Walks, T.S., Galyov, E.E. and Majerus, P. (1998) SopB, a protein required for virulence of *Salmonella* Dublin, is an inositol phosphate phosphatise. *Proceedings of the National Academy of Sciences USA* 95, 14057–14059.

O'Callaghan, D., Maskell, D., Liew, F.Y., Easmon, C.S.F. and Dougan, G. (1988) Characterization of aromatic-aro purine dependent *Salmonella typhimurium* attenuation, persistence and ability to induce protective immunity in Balb/C mice. *Infection and Immunity* 56, 419–423.

Okamato, A.S., Menconi, A., Goncalves G.A.M., Rocha, T.S., Andreatti, R.F., Savano, E.N. and Sesti, L. (2010) Reversion to virulence evaluation of a9R vaccine strain of *Salmonella enterica* serovar Gallonarum in commercial brown layers. *Brazilian Journal of Poultry Science* 12, 47–52.

Pardon, P., Sanchis, R., Marly, J., Lantier, F., Guilloteau, L., Buzoni-Gatei, D., Oswald, I.P., Pepin, M., Kaeffer, B. and Berthon, P. (1990) Experimental ovine salmonellosis (*Salmonella abortusovis*): pathogenesis and vaccination. *Research in Microbiology* 141, 945–953.

Penha Filho, R.A.C., de Paiva, J.B., da Silva, M.D., de Almeida, A.M. and Berchieri, A. (2010) Control of *Salmonella* Enteritidis and *Salmonella* Gallinarum in birds by using live vaccine candidate containing attenuated *Salmonella* Gallinarum mutant strain. *Vaccine* 28, 2853–2859.

Pritchard, D.G., Nivas, S.C., York, M.D. and Pomeroy, B.S. (1978) Effect of Gal-E mutant of *Salmonella typhimurium* on experimental salmonellosis in chickens. *Avian Diseases* 22, 562–575.

Rabsch, W., Liesegang, A. and Tschäpe, H. (2001) Laboratory-based surveillance of salmonellosis of humans in Germany – safety of *Salmonella typhimurium and Salmonella enteritidis* live vaccines. *Berliner und Münchener Tierärztliche Wochenschrift* 114, 433–437.

Rankin, J.D., Taylor, R.J. and Neaman, G. (1967) The protection of calves against infection with *Salmonella typhimurium* by means of a vaccine prepared from *Salmonella dublin* (strain 51). *Veterinary Record* 80, 720–726.

Rodrigue, D.C., Tauxe, R.V. and Rowe, B. (1990) International increase in *Salmonella enteritidis*: a new pandemic? *Epidemiology and Infection* 105, 21–27.

Roesler, U., Marg, H., Schöder, I., Mauer S., Arnold, T., Lehmann, J., Truyen, U. and Hensel, A. (2004) Oral vaccination of pigs with an invasive *gyrA-cpxA-rpoB Salmonella* Typhimurium mutant. *Vaccine* 23, 595–603.

Roesler, U., Heller, P., Waldmann, K.-H., Truyen, U. and Hensel, A. (2006) Immunization of sows in an integrated pig-breeding herd using a homologous inactivated *Salmonella* vaccine decreases the prevalence of *Salmonella typhimurium* infection in the offspring. *Journal of Veterinary Medicine, Series B* 53, 224–228.

Roof, M.B. and Doitchinoff, D.D. (1995) Safety, efficacy and duration of immunity induced in swine by use of an avirulent live *Salmonella* choleraesuis-containing vaccine. *American Journal of Veterinary Research* 56, 39–44.

Rychlik, I., Karasova, D., Sebkova, A., Volf, J., Sisak, F., Havlickova, H., Kummer, V., Imre, A., Szmolka, A. and Nagy, B. (2009) Virulence potential of five major pathogenicity islands (SPI-1 to SPI-5) of *Salmonella enterica* serovar Enteritidis for chickens. *BMC Microbiology* 9, 268–275.

Schmidt, C.S., Morrow, W.J.W. and Sheikh, N.A. (2007) Smart adjuvants. *Expert Review of Vaccines* 6, 391–400.

Schwarz, S. and Liebisch, B. (1994) Use of ribotyping, IS200 typing and plasmid analysis for the identification of *Salmonella enterica* subsp. *enterica* serovar Typhimurium vaccine strain Zoosaloral H and its differentiation from wild-type strains of the same serovar. *Zentralblatt für Bakteriologie* 281, 442–450.

Segall, T. and Lindberg, A.A. (1991) *Salmonella dublin* experimental infection in calves: protection after oral immunization with an auxotrophic *aroA* live vaccine. *Journal of Veterinary Medicine, Series B* 38, 142–160.

Segall, T. and Lindberg, A.A. (1993) Oral vaccination of calves with an aromatic-dependent *Salmonella dublin* (09, 12) hybrid expressing 04, 12 protects against *S dublin* (09, 12) but not against *Salmonella typhimurium* (04, 5, 12). *Infection and Immunity* 61, 1222–1231.

Selke, M., Meens, J., Springer, S., Frank, R. and Gerlach, G.-F. (2007) Immunization of pigs to prevent disease in humans: Construction and protective efficacy of a *Salmonella enterica* serovar Typhimurium live-negative-marker vaccine. *Infection and Immunity* 75, 2476–2483.

Sigwart, D., Stocker, B.A.D. and Clements, J.D. (1989) Effect of a *purA* mutation on efficacy of *Salmonella* live vaccine vectors. *Infection and Immunity* 57, 1858–1861.

Silva, E.N., Snoeyenbos, G.H., Weinack, O.M. and Smyser, C.F. (1981) Studies on the use of 9R strain of *Salmonella gallinarum* as a vaccine in chickens. *Avian Diseases* 25, 38–52.

Smith, A.L. and Beal, R. (2008) The avian enteric immune system in health and disease – Bacterial infections of the gut – *Salmonella*. In: Davison, F., Kaspers, B. and Schat, K.A. (eds) *Avian Immunology*. Academic Press, London, pp. 243–271.

Smith, B.P., Reina-Guerra, M., Hosieth, S.K., Stocker, B.A., Habasha, F., Johnson, E. and Merritt, F. (1984a) Aromatic-dependent *Salmonella typhimurium* as modified live vaccine for calves. *American Journal of Veterinary Research* 45, 59–66.

Smith, B.P., Reina-Guerra, M., Stocker, B.A.D., Hosieth, S.R. and Johnson, E. (1984b) Aromatic-dependent *Salmonella dublin* as a parenteral modified live vaccine for calves. *American Journal of Veterinary Research* 45, 2231–2235.

Smith, B.P., Dilling, G.W., Da Roden, L. and Stocker, B.A. (1993) Vaccination of calves with orally administered aromatic-dependent *Salmonella dublin*. *American Journal of Veterinary* Research 54, 1249–1255.

Smith, H.W. (1956) The use of live vaccines in experimental *Salmonella gallinarum* infection in chickens with observations on their interference effect. *Journal of Hygiene, Cambridge* 54, 419–432.

Smith, H.W. and Tucker, J.F. (1980) The virulence of *Salmonella* strains for chickens, their excretion by infected chickens. *Journal of Hygiene, Cambridge* 84, 479–488.

Springer, S., Lehmann, J., Lindner, Th., Thielebein, J., Alber, G. and Selbitz, H.-J. (2000) A new live *Salmonella* Enteritidis vaccine for chickens – experimental evidence of its safety and efficacy. *Berliner und Münchener Tierärztliche Wochenschrift* 113, 246–252.

Springer, S., Lindner, Th., Steinbach, G. and Selbitz, H.-J. (2001) Investigations on the efficacy of a genetically-stable live *Salmonella* Typhimurium vaccine for use in swine. *Berliner und Münchener Tierärztliche Wochenschrift* 114, 342–345.

Springer, S., Lindner, Th., Ahrens, M., Woitow, G., Prandini, F. and Selbitz, H.-J. (2011) Duration of immunity induced in chickens by an attenuated live *Salmonella enteritidis* vaccine and an inactivated *Salmonella enteritidis/typhimurium* vaccine. *Berliner und Münchener Tierärztliche Wochenschrift* 124, 89–93.

Steinbach, G. and Meyer, H. (1990) Investigations on the efficacy of subcutaneous vaccination with the *Salmonella* vaccine Murivac in calves. *Tierärztliche Praxis* 22, 529–531.

Stocker, B.A. (1988) Auxotrophic *Salmonella typhi* as live vaccine. *Vaccine* 6, 141–145.

Subhabphant, W., York, M.D. and Pomeroy, B.S. (1983) Use of two vaccines (live G30D or killed RW16) in the prevention of *Salmonella typhimurium* infections in chickens. *Avian Diseases* 27, 602–615.

Tagliabue, A., Villa, L., De Magistris, M.T., Romano, M., Silvestri, S., Boraschi, D. and Nencioni, L. (1986) IgA-driven T cell-mediated anti-bacterial immunity in man after live oral Ty 21a vaccine. *Journal of Immunology* 137, 1504–1510.

Thain, J.A., Baxter-Jones, C., Wilding, G.P. and Cullen, G.A. (1984) Serological response of turkey hens to vaccination with *Salmonella hadar* and its effect on their subsequently challenged embryos and poults. *Research in Veterinary Science* 36, 320–325.

Truscott, R.B. (1981) Oral *Salmonella* antigens for the control of *Salmonella* in chickens. *Avian Diseases* 25, 810–820.

Truscott, R.B. and Friars, G.W. (1972) The transfer of endotoxin induced immunity from hens to poults. *Canadian Journal of Comparative Medical and Veterinary Science* 36, 64–68.

Uzzau, S., Marogna, G., Leori, G.S., Curtiss III, R., Schianchi, G., Stocker, B.A.D. and Rubino, S. (2005) Virulence attenuation and live vaccine potential of *aroA, crp cdt cyp,* and plasmid-cured mutants of *Salmonella enterica* serovar Abortusovis in mice and sheep. *Infection and Immunity* 73, 4302–4308.

Van der Walt, M.L., Vorster, J.H., Steyn, H.C. and Greef, A.S. (2001) Auxotrophic, plasmid-cured *Salmonella enterica* serovar typhimurium for use as alive vaccine in calves. *Veterinary Microbiology* 80, 373–381.

Van Immerseel, F., Methner, U., Rychlik, I., Nagy, B., Velge, P., Martin, G., Foster, N., Ducatelle, R. and Barrow, P.A. (2005) Vaccination and early protection against non-host-specific *Salmonella* serotypes in poultry: exploitation of innate immunity and microbial activity. *Epidemiology and Infection* 133, 959–978.

Vielitz, E., Conrad, C., Voss, M., Löhren, U., Bachmeier, J. and Hahn, I. (1992) Immunization against *Salmonella*-infections using live and inactivated vaccine preparations. *Deutsche Tierärztliche Wochenschrift* 99, 483–485.

Villarreal, B., Paulin, S.M., Watson, P.R., Manser, J.M., Jones, P.W. and Wallis, T.S. (1997) Analysis of the specificity of protection induced by *Salmonella* in cattle In: *Proceedings of the 2nd International Symposium on* Salmonella *and Salmonellosis*, Ploufragran, France, pp. 471–473.

Villarreal, B., Manser, J., Collins, R.A., Dougan, G., Chatfield, S.N. and Howard, C.J. (1998) Immune response in calves immunised orally or subcutaneously with a live *Salmonella typhimurium* aro vaccine. *Vaccine* 16, 45–54.

Wallis, T.S., Paulin, S.M., Plested, J.S., Watson, P.R. and Jones, P.W. (1995) The *Salmonella dublin* virulence plasmid mediates systemic but not enteric phases of salmonellosis in cattle. *Infection and Immunity* 63, 2755–2761.

Watson, P.R., Paulin, S.M., Jones, P.W and Walks, T.S. (1995) Characterisation of intestinal invasion by *Salmonella typhimurium* and *Salmonella dublin* and effect of a mutation in the *invH* gene. *Infection and Immunity* 63, 2743–2754.

Watson, P.R., Galyov, E.E., Paulin, S.M., Jones, P.W. and Walks, T.S. (1998) *invH*, but not *stn*, influences *Salmonella*-induced enteritis in cattle. *Infection and Immunity* 66, 1432–1438.

Weber, A., Bernt, C., Bauer, K. and Mayr, A. (1993) Control of bovine salmonellosis under field conditions using herd-specific vaccines. *Tierärztliche Praxis* 21, 511–516.

Wood, M.W., Jones, M.A., Watson, P.R., Hedges, S., Wallis, T.S. and Galyov, E.E. (1998) Identification of a pathogenicity island required for *Salmonella* enteropathogenicity. *Molecular Microbiology* 29, 883–891.

Woodward, M.J., Gettinby, G., Breslin, M.F., Corkish, J.D. and Houghton, S. (2002) The efficacy of Salenvac, a *Salmonella enterica* subsp. *enterica* serotype Enteritidis iron-restricted bacterine vaccine, in laying chickens. *Avian Pathology* 31, 383–392.

Wray, C., Sojka, W.J., Morris, J.A. and Brinley-Morgan, W.J. (1977) The immunization of mice and calves with *galE* mutants of *Salmonella typhimurium*. *Journal of Hygiene, Cambridge* 79, 17–24.

Young, S.D., Olusanya, K.H., Jones, K.H., Liu, T., Liljelbjelke, K.A. and Hofacre, C.L. (2007) *Salmonella* incidence in broilers from breeders vaccinated with live and killed *Salmonella*. *Journal of Applied Poultry Research* 16, 521–528.

23 EU Legislation on the Control of *Salmonella*, Monitoring and Reporting

Kris De Smet[1]* and Pia Mäkelä†
[1]SANCO, European Commission, Belgium; [2]European Food Safety Authority, Biological Monitoring Unit, Italy

International Standards for *Salmonella*

European Union (EU) legislation intends to implement international standards for control of *Salmonella* in view of health protection and facilitating international trade of food and animals. Before presenting the EU legislation, an overview of these standards is opportune. The Codex Alimentarius Commission (CAC) and the World Organization for Animal Health (OIE) are two international bodies that developed standards and guidelines for the control of *Salmonella* in food and animals.

CAC is the international body responsible for making proposals on all matters pertaining to the implementation of the Joint Food Standards Programme of the World Health Organization (WHO) and the Food and Agriculture Organization of the United Nations (FAO) (CAC, Procedural Manual). The aim of the programme is to protect the health of consumers and to ensure fair practices of trade by promoting coordination of food standards.

CAC has developed in general 'Principles and Guidelines for the Conduct of Microbiological Risk Management' (CAC/GL 63-2007). In addition, CAC adopted in 2011 specific 'Guidelines for the Control of *Campylobacter* and *Salmonella* spp. in Chicken Meat' (CAC/GL78-2011). *Salmonella* control is targeted in different codes of hygiene practices for specific foods (CAC/RCP 15-1976, 39-1993, 58-2005, 66-2008) and CAC recommends the development of regulatory standards or performance objectives for *Salmonella*. Microbiological criteria should be established as part of risk management options in accordance with the 'Principles for the Establishment and Application of Microbiological Criteria for Foods' (CAC/GL 21-97). Specific *Salmonella* microbiological criteria have so far only be proposed by CAC for powdered infant formulae, formulae for special medical purposes intended for infants, human milk fortifiers, powdered follow-up formulae and formulae for special purposes for young children (CAC/RCP 66-2008).

The OIE intends to provide a better guarantee on the safety of food of animal origin by creating greater synergy between the activities of the OIE and those of the CAC. The

* Corresponding author, e-mail: Kris.De-Smet@ec.europa.eu
† The views or positions expressed in this text correspond to the authors and are not, and cannot be regarded as representing the position, the views or the policy of the European Commission nor EFSA.

© CAB International 2013. *Salmonella in Domestic Animals, 2nd Edition* (eds P.A. Barrow and U. Methner)

OIE's standard-setting activities in this field focus on eliminating potential hazards existing prior to the slaughter of animals or the primary processing of their products (meat, milk, eggs, etc.) that could be a source of risk for consumers. Chapter 6.5 of the OIE 'Terrestrial Animal Health Code' (OIE, 2011) provides recommendations on the on-farm prevention, detection and control of *Salmonella* in poultry and must be read together with the preceding Chapter 6.4 on 'Biosecurity Procedures in Poultry Production'. The OIE recommends *Salmonella* surveillance programmes in different poultry flocks. At import, absence of *S.* Enteritidis and *S.* Typhimurium based on these surveillance programmes, should be required:

- In the flock of origin at trade of live poultry;
- In the breeding flock of origin and the hatchery at trade of day-old birds;
- In the breeding flock of origin at trade of hatching eggs.

OIE requires similar conditions on *S.* Pullorum and *S.* Gallinarum for international trade of poultry and hatching eggs (Chapter 10.7 of the OIE Terrestrial Animal Health Code) for animal health protection.

Most countries in the world have introduced *Salmonella* control and monitoring programmes based on these CAC and OIE international standards. Some of them focus on flocks of breeding hens and/or laying hens (FDA, 2009), others lay down microbiological criteria (Brazil, 2003; USDA FSIS, 2010; FSANZ, 2011). In the EU, a comprehensive *Salmonella* strategy has been elaborated based on a farm to fork approach. The results are monitored in a harmonized way and published annually. Therefore it provides very useful examples of legislative *Salmonella* control tools and their results.

EU Risk Analysis Approach

The EU approach for *Salmonella* follows the CAC Working Principles for Risk Analysis, in particular consistency, transparency, scientific soundness, submission to evaluation and review in the light of new data (CAC, Procedural Manual). EU food safety must be based on risk analysis (EU, 2002). The players responsible for the three components of the risk analysis (risk assessment, risk management and risk communication) are clearly defined. The European Food Safety Authority (EFSA, http://www.efsa.eu) is the independent EU risk assessment body ensuring scientific integrity. EFSA has elaborated a whole series of opinions on various aspects providing the scientific basis for *Salmonella* control measures in the EU. While applying the CAC 'Principles and Procedures for the Conduct of Microbiological Risk Assessment' (CAC/GL 30-1999) in its opinions, EFSA collaborates intensively with the European Centre for Disease Prevention and Control (ECDC, http://www.ecdc.eu) and the European Medicines agency, as well other national scientific bodies. EFSA addresses the hazards identification in food and animals and the exposure assessment through food or other pathways, e.g. contact with animals, and provides in collaboration with ECDC the description of the severity and duration of adverse effects in humans (hazard characterization). The collection of information on the prevalence of the hazard in the food or animal population, e.g. by harmonized baseline surveys, is a very important part of a given risk assessment as it provides harmonized data in all EU member states. The EFSA opinions integrate these elements into a risk assessment. Such risk assessments typically identify risk factors and recommend risk management options. Often the reduction of human exposure to *Salmonella* infection by applying these options is estimated.

The selection and proposal of *Salmonella* risk management options is the task of the European Commission (EC), European Parliament and Council. The European Parliament and the Council adopt the major policy lines; the EC manages and refines the policy lines by delegated and implementing acts. Verification of the implementation by the competent authority in the member states is the task of the EC's Food and Veterinary Office, while the national authority ensures the implementation at national level and the verification of the application by the food business operators on their territory.

Monitoring of trends in the prevalence of the hazard in humans, food and animals provides essential information for risk assessment and is one of the tools to evaluate the effectiveness of the measures. ECDC is responsible for the coordination of human monitoring of salmonellosis and reporting while the collection of data from *Salmonella* monitoring in food and animals at EU level has been delegated by the EC to EFSA. The outcome may initiate requests of the Commission for a review or new scientific opinions, possibly resulting in amendments of control measures.

Risk communication happens within the competence of each body involved. Typically, consultation of EU member states takes place within dedicated networks. Before implementing a given measure, the EU risk managers involve relevant private stakeholders when performing impact assessments or cost–benefit studies in view of possible new measures and when considered appropriate within the development of risk assessments. The risk assessments as well as new measures to be implemented are widely communicated to the consumers through press communications at the publication of new scientific opinion and reports, and at the adoption of new control measures.

Based on the *Salmonella* risk assessments, control options have been selected in the EU. The legislative measures in the EU, their implementation at national level, and the monitoring of the prevalence are described in the next sections as examples of how risk assessments are translated practically and in a harmonized way into EU rules.

EU Control Approach

The focus of this chapter is on zoonotic, mostly food-borne, *Salmonella*. Some *Salmonella* spp. only cause disease in animals and not in humans. When specific animal health provisions exist, reference is made to them in the section on control in animals. Several measures, e.g. biosecurity measures, will have an impact on both public (zoonotic *Salmonella*) and animal health.

Some member states of the EU introduced *Salmonella* control measures in their national legislation several decennia ago, including microbiological criteria and *Salmonella* control programmes at farm level. Harmonized *Salmonella* microbiological criteria were laid down at EU level from 1990 on for certain products considered at risk (egg products, fishery products, bivalve molluscs, (drinking) milk and milk powder, minced meat and meat preparations). In 1992 (EU, 1992) EU requirements were introduced for the control of *Salmonella* in flocks of breeding hens. The requirements were first voluntary but became mandatory from 1 January 1998. They included marketing restrictions in flocks contaminated with *S.* Enteritidis or *S.* Typhimurium.

With the launching of the White Paper on Food Safety (COM, 2000), the EC enforced its strategy on food safety. The new strategy was triggered by a number of crises during the preceding years (BSE crisis, Belgian dioxin crisis of 1999) and the application of a single market for goods including food. The single market, allowing all operators to place their food on the markets of all member states, required a harmonization of food safety standards. Differences existed between member states as regards the control and prevalence of *Salmonella* in food. Harmonization needed to provide the same high consumers' protection level. Although health protection took priority, social, economic and environmental impacts were taken into account in the development of the policy. The high standards provided the best guarantee for ensuring export of food. A comprehensive and integrated approach to food safety was demanded at EU level. At the same time, EU legislation had to be enforceable in an efficient way in the member states. Responsibility for enforcement remained primarily a national, regional and local responsibility.

EU legislation strongly focuses on a farm to fork approach, with measures taken at all stages of the production chain to protect the public health. *Salmonella* is managed by a set of general and specific hygiene measures and a number of rules specific for the control of *Salmonella*.

Hygiene rules

Good hygiene practices are laid down for feeding stuffs for animals (EU, 2005a), primary production (farms) and processing, storage, transport and retail activities in food (EU, 2004a, b). They include hygiene provisions on the construction, equipment, conduct (personal hygiene, management of the animals/food and waste, temperature conditions etc.), water supply, treatment (heat or other), training etc., throughout the production chain. Procedures based on the application of Hazards Analysis and Critical Control Points (HACCP) principles are also mandatory for food business operators at all stages except primary production.

The hygiene rules to be complied with by the food business operators are supplemented by rules on food safety requirements, traceability, transparency, responsibility and liability (EU, 2002) and rules on official controls (EU, 2004c, d).

Specific control in feeding stuffs

All feed business operators, except farmers, carrying out any activity on feeding stuffs, including feed materials, must have procedures in place based on the HACCP principles (EU, 2005a). In the *Microbiological risk assessment in feedingstuffs for food-producing animals - Scientific Opinion of the Panel on Biological Hazards* published by EFSA (EFSA, 2008e), the EFSA Panel recommended that *Salmonella* process hygiene criteria should be established in crushing plants, rendering plants and feed mills as an integrated part of specific HACCP-based control programmes to maximize the control of *Salmonella* contamination for all food-production animal species. Animal by-products intended as feed material (e.g. fishmeal) must be free of *Salmonella* ($c = 0$). Five samples ($n = 5$) of 25 g must be tested (EU, 2011a).

Specific control in animal populations

As a follow-up of the White Paper on Food Safety of the European Commission an EU-wide specific *Salmonella* control strategy was enforced (EU, 2003a). The strategy introduces step by step controls in poultry and pig populations starting at the top of the production chain and taking into account the importance of the population as source of human salmonellosis at that time. The strategy may be extended to other animal species.

For each animal population a similar approach is followed:

1. EU-wide baseline studies on the prevalence of *Salmonella* are carried out. In this way, comparable information is collected from member states, intended to be reference values at the start of the EU strategy in a certain animal population (see 'Harmonization of monitoring and reporting').
2. Cost/benefit analyses on possible targets for reduction in the animal populations based on the baseline survey results.
3. EU targets for reduction are set for each population based on the outcome of the baseline and cost/benefit analysis. Such targets include the maximum percentage of epidemiological units (e.g. flocks) remaining infected or the minimum percentage of reduction in the units remaining infected, the maximum time limit to achieve the target, the testing scheme necessary to verify the achievement of the target and the *Salmonella* serovars covered by the target.
4. Once targets are set, member states have to develop or adapt, and implement national control programmes. The programmes need to be submitted to the EC for approval. Also non-member states can only import eggs or live poultry if an equivalent national control programme has been approved by the EC.
5. Trade restrictions on food or animals from each population become applicable when sufficient progress is or should have been made in the reduction of the prevalence of *Salmonella* in these populations and when an impact assessment shows a favourable balance between costs and benefits of such measures.

The purpose of control programmes at national level is to allow adaptations of *Salmonella* control measures, taking into account national or regional differences such as prevalence and production systems. However, a number of minimum requirements for all national control programmes have been adopted (EU, 2003a). These minimum requirements include requirements on the content of the programmes (e.g. information on production systems, competences, approved laboratories, official controls, measures in case of non-compliance, additional national rules or guidelines for hygiene, biosecurity measures, vaccination, record-keeping etc.), and harmonized monitoring requirements for food business operators and for official controls. The use of antibiotics has been prohibited as a specific method to control *Salmonella* in poultry except under clearly defined exceptional circumstances (EU, 2006a) as such use may result in an increase of antimicrobial resistance (ECDC *et al.*, 2009).

Most of the targets and trade restrictions focus on *S.* Enteritidis and *S.* Typhimurium. These two serovars represent about 80% of all human salmonellosis in the EU and are the most frequently reported serovars in flocks of breeding and laying hens and breeding turkeys (EFSA and ECDC, 2011a), which justifies the focus on these two serovars. However, in flocks of broilers and fattening turkeys, these serovars only represent from 10 to 20% of all serovars detected. Nevertheless, biosecurity and other measures taken in these flocks in order to achieve the target or to avoid trade restrictions on these two serovars are expected to result also in a reduction of other *Salmonella* serovars. Apart from this argument, the limitation to these two serovars in the case of the trade restrictions for fresh poultry meat was the outcome of an impact assessment by the EC. The impact assessment illustrated the best balance of such an approach between the expected public health impact and the economic and social consequences of the measures.

The EU *Salmonella* strategy, in particular the targets, may be reviewed taking into account trends in the *Salmonella* prevalence in humans, food and animals, the gravidity of its effects for humans, economic consequences for animal and human health care, and for feed and food business, new scientific advice, technological developments and requirements and trends concerning production methods. In 2011, such a review or rather clarification was introduced considering the monophasic variants of *Salmonella* Typhimurium-like with formula 1,4,[5],12:i:- as variants deriving from *S.* Typhimurium, based on EFSA advice (EFSA, 2010f). Several other EFSA opinions have also been published on a quantitative assessment to evaluate the public health impact of the strategies in the different poultry populations after the first years of implementation (EFSA, 2009c, 2010d, 2011a). They are being used to update the EU *Salmonella* control strategies. An overview of *Salmonella* control programmes is provided in Table 23.1.

Breeding hens of Gallus gallus

Since breeding hens are at the top of the egg and broiler meat production chain a reduction target for *Salmonella* was first adopted for these flocks in 2005 (EU, 2005b). From the end of 2009, a maximum of 1% of adult breeding flocks may remain infected with *S.* Enteritidis, *S.* Typhimurium, *S.* Hadar, *S.* Infantis and/or *S.* Virchow, five serovars of high public health importance in humans in the EU. Rearing flocks are monitored at three occasions by the farmer and every second week during the laying period (EU, 2003a).

Detailed harmonized rules for sampling by the operator and competent authorities and for testing and reporting are laid down (EU, 2010). Sampling may take place in the hatchery or at the farm. If *S.* Enteritidis or *S.* Typhimurium is detected, eggs may no longer be used for hatching and the hens are culled or slaughtered safely.

Laying hens

Because of the importance of eggs and egg products as the source of human salmonellosis cases and food-borne outbreaks (EFSA and ECDC, 2011a), a second target was set in flocks of laying hens (EU, 2006b). The baseline study (EU, 2004e) highlighted the major differences in prevalence in flocks of laying hens

Table 23.1. Summary of EU measures on the control of food-borne *Salmonella* in poultry.

Population		Start control programme	Minimum monitoring requirements		Target for reduction	Trade restrictions
			Operator	Competent authority		
Breeding hens of *Gallus gallus*	Rearing flocks	1/1/1998, renewed	Day-old chicks + 4 week old birds + 2 weeks before moving to laying phase or unit	None	No specific target	If *S.* Enteritidis or *S.* Typhimurium is found: slaughter or destruction so as to reduce as much as possible the spread of *Salmonella*
	Adult breeding flocks	1/1/1998, renewed 1/1/2007	Every 2nd week	At least at three occasions during the production cycle. Reduction is possible if the target has been met in a member state for at least 2 consecutive years	1% or less remaining positive for *S.* Enteritidis, *S.* Typhimurium, *S.* Hadar, *S.* Virchow + *S.* Infantis from 31 December 2009	Birds: see rearing; destruction of the eggs if *S.* Enteritidis or *S.* Typhimurium is found
Laying hens of *Gallus gallus*	Rearing flocks	1/2/2008	Day-old chicks + pullets 2 weeks before moving to laying phase or unit	None	No specific target	If *S.* Enteritidis or *S.* Typhimurium is found: slaughter or destruction so as to reduce as much as possible the spread of *Salmonella*
	Laying flocks	1/2/2008	Every 15 weeks, first sampling at 24 ± 2 weeks	At least one flock per holding per year + additional sampling under certain conditions (e.g. preceding flock positive)	10 to 40% reduction compared to preceding year until the prevalence of *S.* Enteritidis + *S.* Typhimurium is below 2%	Birds: see rearing; marking and placing on the market as class B eggs (only for egg products) if *S.* Enteritidis or *S.* Typhimurium is found
Broilers		1/1/2009	Not earlier than 3 weeks before slaughter; result must be available at slaughter	At least one flock per year in 10% of the holdings with more than 5000 birds	1% or less remaining positive for *S.* Enteritidis and *S.* Typhimurium from 31 December 2011	Absence of *S.* Enteritidis and *S.* Typhimurium must be ensured in 25 g of fresh meat

(*Continued*)

Table 23.1. (Continued)

Population		Start control programme	Minimum monitoring requirements		Target for reduction	Trade restrictions
			Operator	Competent authority		
Turkeys	Rearing flocks	1/1/2010	Day-old chicks + 4 week old birds + pullets 2 weeks before moving to laying phase or unit	None	1% or less remaining positive for *S.* Enteritidis and *S.* Typhimurium from 31 December 2012	If *S.* Enteritidis or *S.* Typhimurium is found: slaughter or destruction so as to reduce as much as possible the spread of *Salmonella*; destruction of the eggs if *S.* Enteritidis or *S.* Typhimurium is found
	Adult breeding flocks	1/1/2010	Every 3rd week	At least one flock per year in 10% of the holdings	1% or less remaining positive for *S.* Enteritidis and *S.* Typhimurium from 31 December 2012	If *S.* Enteritidis or *S.* Typhimurium is found: slaughter or destruction so as to reduce as much as possible the spread of *Salmonella*; destruction of the eggs if *S.* Enteritidis or *S.* Typhimurium is found
	Fattening flocks	1/1/2010	Not earlier than 3 weeks before slaughter; result must be available at slaughter and remains valid for 6 weeks	At least one flock per year in 10% of the holdings with more than 500 birds	1% or less remaining positive for *S.* Enteritidis and *S.* Typhimurium from 31 December 2012	Absence of *S.* Enteritidis and *S.* Typhimurium must be ensured in 25 g of fresh meat

in the member states, varying from 0% to over 50% of *Salmonella*-positive flocks (EFSA, 2009b). Due to this variation and high prevalence in a number of member states, a reduction target depending on the preceding year was set (10–40% reduction in following year) until the prevalence of *S.* Enteritidis and *S.* Typhimurium drops below 2%.

The *Salmonella* control programme in flocks of laying hens started in all member states on 1 February 2008 at the latest, including harmonized monitoring by operators every 15 weeks and competent authorities once a year (EU, 2011b). If the absence of *S.* Enteritidis or *S.* Typhimurium is not demonstrated according to the harmonized monitoring, table eggs can no longer be placed on the market after 1 January 2009 (EU, 2007a). Vaccination of all flocks of laying hens against *S.* Enteritidis is mandatory if its prevalence is above 10% (EU, 2006a).

The European farmers and agri-cooperatives (Copa-Cogeca) and the European Union of wholesale with eggs, egg products, poultry and game (EUWEP) developed a Community Guide for good hygiene practices in pullet rearing and egg-laying flocks with the purpose of assisting their members in applying biosecurity and other measures focused on *Salmonella* control (Copa-Cogeca and EUWEP, 2009).

Broilers

A baseline study on broiler flocks was conducted in the member states between October 2005 and September 2006 (EU, 2005c). Consequently, a reduction target for *S.* Enteritidis and *S.* Typhimurium of 1% or less of flocks remaining infected by 31 December 2011 was set (EU, 2007b).

The *Salmonella* control programmes for flocks of broilers started in all member states on 1 January 2009 at the latest, and include monitoring and testing of each flock before broilers are sent for slaughter. Flocks infected with *Salmonella* may still be slaughtered, however, measures must be taken to avoid further (cross-) contamination (e.g. logistic slaughter). In addition, from 1 December 2011, it must be ensured that *S.* Enteritidis and *S.* Typhimurium are absent in fresh poultry meat (25 g, $n=5$, $c=0$). Contaminated meat may be used for industrial heat treatment or another treatment to eliminate *Salmonella* before it reaches the final consumer (EU, 2003a).

Copa-Cogeca and the Association of Poultry Producers and Poultry Trade in the EU (AVEC) developed a guide to good hygiene practice for the prevention and control of *Salmonella* in broilers on farms, and during catching, loading and transport (Copa-Cogeca and AVEC, 2010).

Turkeys

A baseline study on fattening and breeding turkeys was carried out in the EU between October 2006 and September 2007 (EU, 2006c).

Based on the results of the baseline study (EFSA, 2008a), a reduction target for *S.* Enteritidis and *S.* Typhimurium of 1% or less of flocks of breeding and fattening turkeys remaining infected was set (EU, 2008b), which has to be reached by 31 December 2012. Harmonized sampling schemes have been introduced for breeding and fattening turkeys.

The trade restrictions for hatching eggs are the same as for breeding hens of *Gallus gallus* and the *Salmonella* criterion on fresh poultry meat is also applicable to turkey meat.

Control of Salmonella *Pullorum,* Salmonella *Gallinarum and* Salmonella *Arizonae*

S. Pullorum and *S.* Gallinarum do not cause disease in humans but are of major health interest for fowls (*Gallus gallus*), turkeys, guinea fowls, quails, pheasants, partridges and ducks.

At trade between member states and at import, all these birds in the consignment shall have been found negative in serological tests for *S.* Pullorum and *S.* Gallinarum antibodies in the month preceding the consignment (EU, 2009). In the case of hatching eggs or day-old chicks, the flock of origin shall be tested serologically for *S.* Pullorum and *S.* Gallinarum in the 3 months preceding the consignment at a level which gives 95%

confidence of detecting infection at 5% prevalence. Similar rules exist for *Salmonella* Arizonae in turkeys.

Slaughter and breeding pigs

Baseline studies on slaughter (EU, 2006d) and breeding pigs were carried out between October 2006 and September 2007 and from January to December 2008, respectively, in all member states to obtain a comparable view on the prevalence of *Salmonella* in slaughter and breeding pigs.

The outcome of the baseline surveys (EFSA, 2008b, 2009b) was used in a quantitative microbiological risk assessment on *Salmonella* in breeding and slaughter pigs (EFSA, 2010e) and in a further cost–benefit analysis on setting a target for reduction (FCC Consortium, 2010, 2011). These studies demonstrate the difficulties to reduce *Salmonella* in herds of pigs in certain EU member states in a cost-efficient way. In particular, the application of control options in herds with breeding pigs where all an in/all out policy is not obvious. Further cost–benefit analyses on measures after slaughter and discussions on the possible authorization of such measures (e.g. use of recycled water or lactic acid for carcass decontamination) are ongoing at the moment of this publication.

Some member states have already introduced *Salmonella* control programmes at national level. Finland and Sweden have a very low prevalence and, therefore, control programmes focus on prevention at farm level and culling of contaminated herds. Denmark, having a higher (but still relatively low) prevalence in its pig population, applies slaughter of pigs from infected herds in a dedicated plant and postharvest steam or hot water decontamination of carcasses.

Specific controls in food

In view of harmonizing microbiological criteria at EU level, the former Scientific Committee on Veterinary Measures relating to Public Health of the EC evaluated in 2003 the appropriateness of setting *Salmonella* criteria for different pathogens in food (EC, 2003). As an outcome, a number of *Salmonella* microbiological criteria were laid down in EU legislation and have to be complied with by food business operators (EU, 2005d). The use of these microbiological criteria forms an integral part of the implementation of HACCP-based procedures and other hygiene control measures by the food business operators. Sampling frequencies must be integrated in the HACCP plan. For reasons of harmonization and fair trade, the sampling frequency for *Salmonella* in certain types of meat has been laid down in legal provisions (EU, 2005d). It includes the possibility to reduce the frequency if preceding results are favourable or in small establishments.

Reference method for analysis of *Salmonella* in food is EN/ISO standard 6579. The use of alternative analytical methods by the food business operators is acceptable when the methods are validated against this method and if a proprietary method, certified by a third party in accordance with the protocol set out in EN/ISO standard 16140 or other internationally accepted similar protocols, is used.

Harmonized food safety criteria have been established for *Salmonella* in 19 groups of foodstuffs, including fresh poultry meat, minced meat and meat preparations, mechanically separated meat, egg products, ice cream and dried infant formulae. These criteria define the acceptability of foodstuffs placed on the market. The harmonization ensures that the same food safety standards are used at trade between member states and at import. Additional national food safety criteria are very rare, need to be thoroughly justified and notified, and should not result in trade barriers (but they can only be applied to domestically produced food).

Process hygiene criteria for *Salmonella* exist on carcasses of broilers, turkeys, pigs, cattle, sheep, goats and horses. They set an indicative value above which corrective action is required in order to maintain hygiene during processing. Flexibility is given to the member states on the application of these or alternative criteria that are for establishments on their own territory.

Salmonella spp. or certain *Salmonella* serovars need to be absent ($c=0$) in the food safety criteria. Such standard does not have the intention to reflect a zero-tolerance (which may not be realistic). The whole sampling and testing scheme including the sampling frequency, the sample size (e.g. 25 g), the number of samples to be taken from a batch (e.g. $n=5$), the number of samples allowed to be positive (e.g. none: $c=0$) and the analytical method used (with its sensitivity) define the chance that a contaminated batch is placed on the market and therefore the level of protection posed to the consumer. The same chance of acceptance can be achieved with a food safety criteria (keeping other factors unchanged) when $n=5$ and $c=0$ (absence in five samples), as when $c=1$ (one positive sample accepted) if a higher number of samples is taken (EFSA, 2010c). Such a 'tolerance' approach would result in substantially higher sampling and testing costs without changing the level of protection.

The use of substances for carcass decontamination or the use of bacteriophages is subject to authorization in the EU after thorough assessment of the efficacy, safety and, when relevant, effects on antimicrobial resistance and the environment. If authorized, they are considered as supplementary tools for control of *Salmonella* and other pathogens, without replacing measures at previous or later stages of production.

Consumers' Information

Consumers' information campaigns are often presented as alternatives to strict measures at productions (e.g. food safety criteria). Such campaigns can focus on good kitchen practices or the need to thoroughly cook the meat. At the same time, reluctance exists in many countries to put messages on the labels in order to remind consumers to certain precautions that can be taken. Because of this reluctance, initiatives in this field have been left to the individual member states. In general, it can be stated that awareness of *Salmonella* risks associated with the consumption of eggs and meat from poultry are well known by the European consumer. Nevertheless, many consumers expect that the food they buy is safe and not contaminated with *Salmonella* or another pathogen.

Special Guarantees

When Finland and Sweden became member states of the EU in 1995, these countries had reduced *Salmonella* in their animal populations and in food to a level substantially below the level in other member states. Strict control programmes for all *Salmonella* spp. had been introduced decennia ago and resulted in a very high level of protection of consumers to salmonellosis. In order not to reduce the level of protection of consumers in these member states, special *Salmonella* guarantees were granted to these member states at their accession. The guarantees are applicable at trade of live poultry, eggs and certain meat of poultry, pigs and cattle towards Finland and Sweden (EU, 1995, 2003b, 2004f, 2005e). They include comprehensive testing of the flocks of origin or the batch of meat with a negative outcome for all *Salmonella*. Other member states or regions may also be granted these special guarantees if applying an equivalent *Salmonella* control programme (EU, 2004b).

Norway, a non-member state, obtained similar guarantees within the agreement for the European Economic Area (EEA).

International Monitoring

In 2010, the World Health Organization (WHO) launched the WHO Global Salm-Surv programme, now known as the WHO Global Foodborne Infections Network (GFN), a global effort to build capacity to detect, control and prevent food-borne and other enteric infections from farm to table. A key objective of GFN is to enhance laboratory-based surveillance worldwide by improving laboratory capacity for serotyping of *Salmonella*. Laboratories participating in the GFN programme are encouraged to annually report the 15 most frequently isolated *Salmonella* serovars via an Internet-based country databank. Hendriksen *et al.* (2011) has analysed this data from years 2001–2007. They found *S.* Enteritidis and *S.* Typhimurium to be the most frequently isolated serovars form humans worldwide. While *S.* Enteritidis and

S. Typhimurium decreased during the observational period, other serovars such as *S.* Typhi, *S.* Infantis and *S.* Virchow increased in relative importance. However, the study showed large differences in the top 20 most commonly isolated serovars between regions, but lesser differences between the top 15 most commonly isolated serovars between countries within the same regions.

EU Monitoring and Reporting

In the EU, *Salmonella* is being monitored both in human cases as well as in food, feed and animals. In recent years all the 27 member states have submitted annual data on *Salmonella* to the EU level, and these data are summarized in the following.

All the EU member states have in place surveillance and reporting systems for salmonellosis cases in humans. At EU level these surveillance data are collected via The European Surveillance System (TESSy) from the EU member states, as well as Norway, Iceland and Liechtenstein. This system, which covers the most important communicable diseases, is run by the European Centre for Disease Prevention and Control (ECDC). For some diseases under enhanced surveillance, such as salmonellosis, a more in-depth set of variables is captured. These include mainly detailed laboratory information (for some diseases also on antimicrobial resistance testing), or whether the disease was likely to be imported or domestic (Ammon and Makela, 2010). In most countries the data sources are the national systems of disease notification.

Data on *Salmonella* in food, feed and animals are reported annually from the EU member states and additionally from Norway and Switzerland in accordance with EU legislation (EU, 2003c), which establishes a reporting framework for zoonotic agents in animals and food. This piece of legislation also requires reporting of food-borne outbreaks and antimicrobial resistance in *Salmonella* isolates. The information is submitted to the European Commission and EFSA through a web-based reporting system run by EFSA.

The main part of the data on the occurrence of *Salmonella* in food and feed in the member states derives from sampling undertaken by the competent authorities in the framework of the official controls or related monitoring of food. The member states coordinate the sampling at the central level through annual control and monitoring plans that define with varying details what food items should be sampled and analysed and sometimes also the number of samples taken. These plans are part of the multi-annual plan for official controls of foodstuffs and feeding stuffs required by EU legislation (EU, 2004e). A number of member states carry out regularly or occasionally specific surveys to examine *Salmonella* in foodstuffs. These surveys are often well designed and limited in duration and provide data of better quality.

The monitoring and reporting of *Salmonella* in poultry populations, i.e. laying hens, turkeys and their breeding flocks, is mandatory and harmonized by EU legislation (EU, 2005b, 2006b, 2007b, 2008b, 2010, 2011b). This legislation lays down *Salmonella* reduction targets and obliges the member states to run *Salmonella* control programmes. The reporting and monitoring of *Salmonella* in other animal species is less harmonized but still substantial amounts of data are reported regarding these animal species each year by the EU member states. Apart from the annual reporting, a set of fully harmonized EU-wide *Salmonella* baseline surveys have been carried out in the years 2004–2008 (EU, 2004c, 2005c, 2006c, d, 2007d, 2008a) and these surveys covered laying hens, flocks of broilers and turkeys, breeding pigs, slaughter pigs and broiler carcasses.

Analysis of the Data

The data received from the member states are analysed by EFSA and ECDC both descriptively and using statistical methods. Whenever possible the data are examined for trends over the reporting years. It is of interest to compare the trends in the human cases to those in food and animals, i.e. to see if similar trends are observed. The trend analysis is specifically a good tool to evaluate whether the EU or national control programmes are effective in reducing the occurrence of *Salmonella*. The analyses of *Salmonella* serovar distribution in human cases, animal populations and food provides information to source attribution analyses. Also data on food-borne outbreaks are interesting and analyses of it provide for information on the food vehicles involved in the reported *Salmonella* outbreaks, the settings of the outbreaks and the contributing factors involved. The results from the annual data analyses are each year published in European Union Summary Reports issued by EFSA and ECDC. The most recent one is from 2009 data (EFSA and ECDC, 2011a). The baseline survey analyses are published in separate reports of EFSA (EFSA, 2007b, c, d, 2008a, b, c, d, 2009b, 2010b, 2011b).

The Occurrence of *Salmonella* in Humans, Food and Animals in the EU

The information received in the framework of the annual data collection on *Salmonella* gives a picture of the situation and its developments throughout the EU. The main results of the *Salmonella* monitoring are summarized in the Community and EU Summary Reports on trends and sources of zoonoses, zoonotic agents and food-borne outbreaks in EU 2004–2009 (EFSA, 2005, 2006b, 2007e, 2009a, 2010a; EFSA and ECDC, 2011a).

Humans

The number of notified salmonellosis cases in humans has been constantly declining at EU level in the past years, and the decreasing trend over the years 2005–2009 is statistically significant, representing an average reduction of 12.0% per year (Fig. 23.1). It is assumed that this observed reduction of salmonellosis cases in humans is mainly due to successful *Salmonella* control programmes in fowl (*Gallus gallus*) populations that are in place in EU member states and that have particularly resulted in a lower occurrence of *Salmonella* in eggs. However, other control measures taken all along the food production chain may also have contributed to the decline of salmonellosis in humans. For many years salmonellosis has been the second most often notified zoonotic disease in humans following campylobacteriosis.

In humans, a total of 108,614 confirmed cases of human salmonellosis (TESSy) were reported in the EU in 2009, while in 2008 the

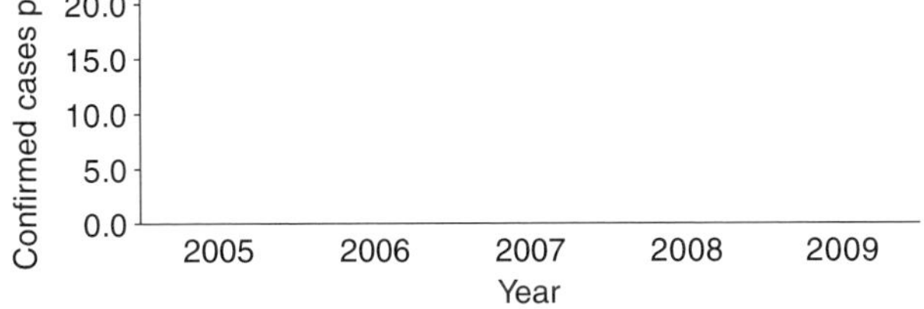

Fig. 23.1. Notification rate of reported confirmed cases of human salmonellosis in the EU (25 member states), 2005–2009 (EFSA and ECDC, 2011a; countries included: Austria, Belgium, Cyprus, Czech Republic, Denmark, Estonia, Finland, France, Germany, Greece, Hungary, Ireland, Italy, Latvia, Lithuania, Luxembourg, Malta, Netherlands, Poland, Portugal, Slovakia, Slovenia, Spain, Sweden and the UK).

number of confirmed cases was 131,468. EU notification rate for confirmed cases was 23.7 cases per 100,000 population, ranging from 2.1 to 100.1 per 100,000 population among the member states. *Salmonella* Enteritidis and *S.* Typhimurium have been the most frequently reported serovars (52.3% and 23.3%, respectively, of all known serovars in human cases in 2009).

Food-borne outbreaks

Salmonella has been the main cause of reported food-borne outbreaks in the EU in each of the years 2005–2009. The majority of the reported food-borne *Salmonella* outbreaks were related to eggs while different types of meats have been the second most common food vehicle in the outbreaks. The distribution of implicated food vehicles in the *Salmonella* outbreaks in 2009 is shown in Fig. 23.2. In 2009, 24 member states reported a total of 1722 food-borne outbreaks due to *Salmonella*, which constituted 31.0% of the total number of reported outbreaks in the EU.

The number of food-borne outbreaks caused by *Salmonella* within the EU has decreased markedly in recent years. From 2007 to 2009 the number of these outbreaks decreased by 23.6% and particularly the number of outbreaks caused by eggs has declined. This is in line with the general decline of notified human salmonellosis cases and the reduced prevalence of *Salmonella* in flocks of laying hens that have been observed within EU.

Food

Large numbers of food samples are each year tested by the member states for *Salmonella* and the results reported to the Commission and EFSA. According to these results *Salmonella* is most often detected in fresh (raw) poultry meat and raw products thereof. The EU baseline surveys also demonstrated that *Salmonella* was often isolated from broiler and pig carcasses.

In foodstuffs, the annual sampling and reporting on *Salmonella* is focused on food categories where EU legislation lays down *Salmonella* criteria (EU, 2005c). The food safety *Salmonella* criteria of absence in 25 g apply to products placed on the market during their shelf life. The highest levels of non-compliance with *Salmonella* criteria have

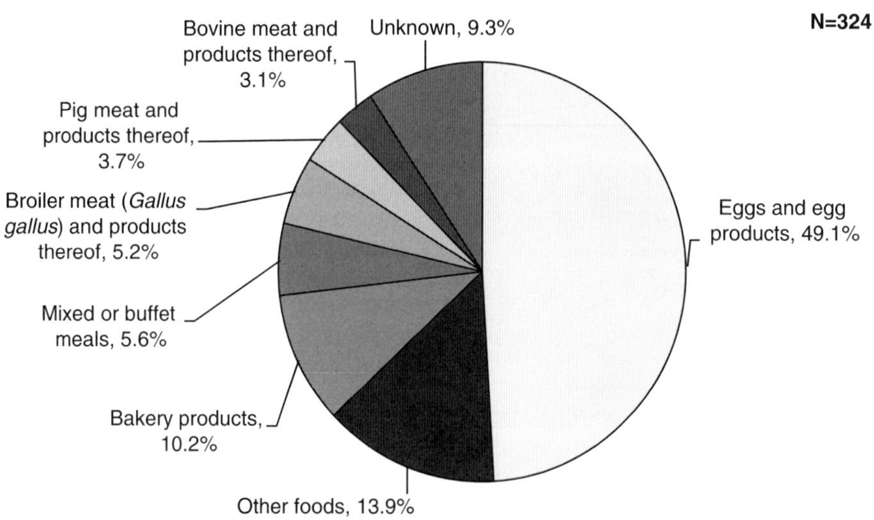

Fig. 23.2. Distribution of food vehicles in verified outbreaks caused by Salmonella in the EU, 2009 (EFSA and ECDC, 2011a).

generally occurred in foods of meat origin (Fig. 23.3). Minced meat and meat preparations from poultry had the highest proportion of samples containing *Salmonella* (6.7% and 8.7% in 2008 and 2009, respectively). These were followed by live bivalve molluscs and egg products where up to 3.4% and 2.8% of single samples, respectively, were *Salmonella* positive. Minced meat and meat preparations from animal species other than poultry intended to be eaten cooked, also had a relatively high proportion of positive samples (2.1% to 2.9% of single samples in 2008 and 2009). Of particular risk to human health are the *Salmonella* findings from the meat categories intended to be eaten raw, where from 1.0% to 1.7% of single sample units contained *Salmonella* in 2008–2009. In the other

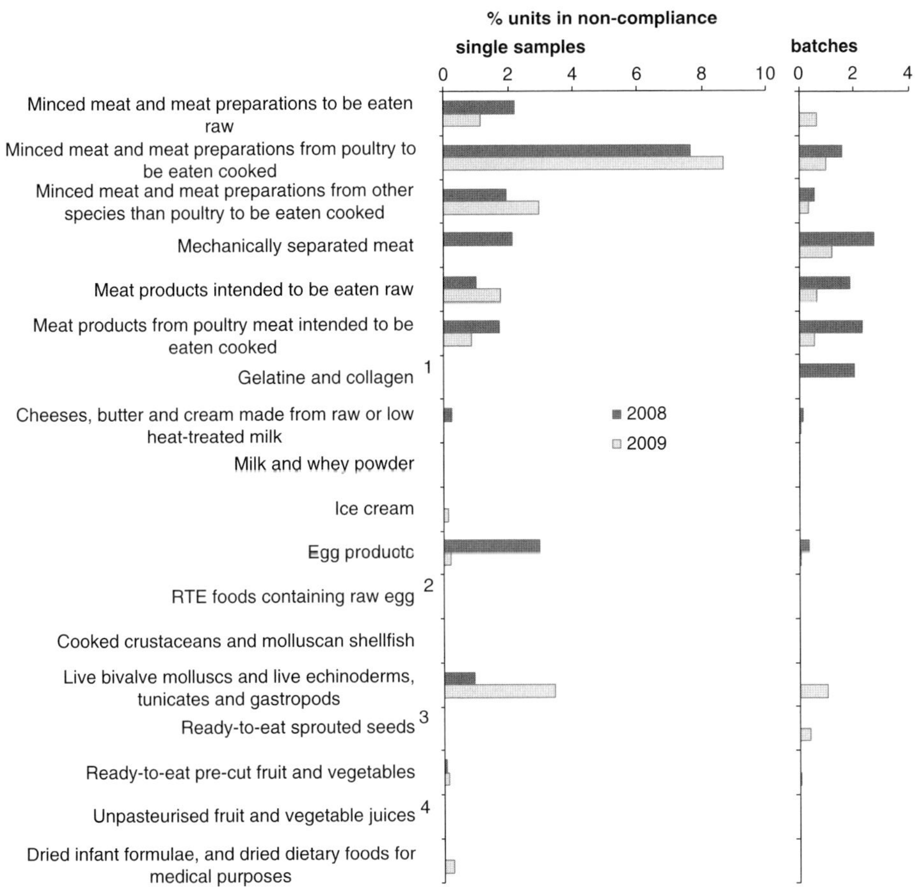

Note: only investigations covering 25 or more samples are included.

1. No investigations with more than 25 samples of gelatine and collagen in 2008 and batches in 2009.
2. No investigations with more than 25 samples of RTE foods containing raw egg in 2008 and 2009, or batches in 2009.
3. No investigations with more than 25 batches of RTE sprouted seeds in 2009.
4. No investigations with more than 25 samples of unpasteurised fruit and vegetable juices in 2008.

Fig. 23.3. Proportion of Salmonella-positive units in food categories for which EU *Salmonella* criteria (absence in 25 g) are applicable, 2008–2009 (EFSA and ECDC, 2011a).

food categories, the levels of non-compliance with the *Salmonella* criteria have been generally very low.

Member states also test great numbers of samples from different types of fresh meat, particularly of broiler, turkey, pig and bovine meat for *Salmonella*, and the reported annual results from the years 2008 and 2009 are summarized in Table 23.2. *Salmonella* was most often detected from fresh turkey meat followed by broiler meat, whereas in pig meat and bovine meat the prevalences at EU level were lower. However, the proportion of positive samples as well as the number of samples taken varied strongly between the member states. It is also good to note that the results from the EU-wide baseline surveys showed higher *Salmonella* prevalence in broiler and pig carcasses both in the EU and in many member states, most likely due to more sensitive sampling methods used in the surveys. The results from the baseline surveys are presented in Table 23.4.

Substantial numbers of other foodstuffs are also tested each year for *Salmonella* and the results regarding table eggs and fruits, vegetables and herbs are summarized in Table 23.2. In the category of fruits, vegetables and herbs the positive samples were most often reported from herbs. Member states also test large numbers of milk and dairy products each year for *Salmonella* with very few positive findings.

Animals

The EU member states report *Salmonella* findings in a wide range of animal species including both farm, pet and wildlife animal species. Most of the reports are from farm animals. According to the annual reporting and the EU-wide baseline surveys (Tables 23.3 and 23.4) prevalence of *Salmonella* is highest in domestic poultry and pig populations. The results also demonstrate that the EU *Salmonella* targets and related mandatory control programmes have reduced the *Salmonella* prevalence in the poultry population.

In animals, the reporting of the results from the national *Salmonella* control programmes for breeding flocks of *Gallus gallus*, laying hens, broilers and turkeys is mandatory according the EU legislation. Since the sampling in the control programmes is relatively well harmonized these results are comparable between the member states and the years. The prevalence of breeding flocks positive for *Salmonella* spp. and the five target serovars (*S*. Enteritidis, *S*. Typhimurium, *S*. Hadar, *S*. Infantis, *S*. Virchow) in the EU is low and has steadily declined from 2007 to 2009. *Salmonella* was more often detected from flocks of laying hens and broilers. Among laying hen flocks, where the mandatory control programmes have been implemented since 2008, the prevalence of two target serovars (*S*. Enteritidis and

Table 23.2. Occurrence of *Salmonella* in selected food categories in the EU in 2008–2009 (EFSA, 2010a; EFSA and ECDC, 2011a).

Food category	2008			2009			2008–2009
	No. MSs	*n*	Pos.	No MSs	*n*	Pos.	Range among MSs (%)
Poultry meat, fresh	19	15,355	5.1	19	26,591	5.4	0–75.5
Turkey meat, fresh	13	2,061	6.3	9	3,953	8.7	0–30.2
Pork, fresh	21	109,174	0.8	18	83,797	0.7	0–23.8
Beef, fresh	18	44,240	0.2	15	44,359	0.2	0–6.1
Table eggs	15	13,659	0.5	14	15,966	0.5	0–6.3
Fruits, vegetables and herbs	15	13,215	0.7	18	13,466	0.6	0–3.9

No. MSs: number of reporting member states; *n*, number of samples tested; Pos.,% of positive samples

Table 23.3. Prevalence of *Salmonella* in poultry flocks in the EU in 2008–2009 (EFSA, 2010a; EFSA and ECDC, 2011a).

Animal population	Year	No. of MSs	*n*	*S.* spp. Pos.	*S.* spp. Range in MSs (%)	5 target serovars Pos.	5 target range in MSs (%)
Breeding flocks of *Gallus gallus*	2007	25	15,949	2.9	0–26.3	1.4	0–15.4
	2008	25	12,499	2.7	0–9.1	1.3	0–5.7
	2009	25	13,983	2.7	0–10.3	1.2	0–7.0
						*S.*E./*S.*T. Pos.	*S.*E./*S.*T. range in MSs (%)
Flocks of laying hens	2008	25	27,826	5.9	0–34.9	3.5	0–15.6
	2009	27	28,050	6.7	0–41.7	3.2	0–10.9
Flock of broilers	2009	27	182,271	5.0	0–32.4	0.7	0–5.3

No. of MSs, number of reporting member states; *n*, number of samples tested; Pos.,% of positive flocks; *S.* spp., *Salmonella* spp.; 5 target serovars, *S.* Enteritidis, *S.* Typhimurium, *S.* Hadar, *S.* Infantis, *S.* Virchow; *S.*E./*S.*T. = *S.* Enteritidis and *S.* Typhimurium

Table 23.4. EU *Salmonella* prevalence observed in the EU-wide baseline surveys (EFSA, 2007b, c, 2008a, b, 2009b, 2010b).

Animal or food category	Year	No MSs	*n*	*S.* spp. Pos. (%)	*S.* spp. range among MSs (%)	*S.*E./*S.*T. Pos. (%)	*S.*E./*S.*T. range among MSs (%)
Holdings with laying hens	2004–2005	23	5,007	30.8	0–79.5	20.4	0–62.5
Flocks of broilers	2005–2006	23	7,120	23.7	0–68.2	11.0	0–39.3
Flocks of breeding turkeys	2006–2007	14	532	13.6	0–82.9	1.7	0–8.3
Flocks of fattening turkeys	2006–2007	22	3,702	30.7	0–78.5	3.8	0–18.4
Slaughter pigs – lymph node	2006–2007	25	18,663	10.3	0–29.0	4.7	0–16.1
Slaughter pigs – surface of carcass	2006–2007	13	5,736	8.3	0–20.0	3.9[a]	0–11.7[a]
Holdings with breeding pigs	2008	24	5,117	31.8	0–57.7	7.0[a]	0–17.5[a]
Broiler carcasses – skin sample	2008	26	9,249	15.6	0–85.6	3.6	0–9.6

No. MSs, number of reporting member states; *n*, number of samples tested; Pos.,% of positive units; *S.* spp., *Salmonella* spp.; *S.*E./*S.*T. = *S.* Enteritidis and *S.* Typhimurium
[a]Prevalence of *S.* Typhimurium only

S. Typhimurium) have reduced. In addition, member states have reported annually *Salmonella* findings in many other animal species, such as pigs, cattle, turkeys, ducks, geese, other domestic animals, pets and wildlife.

The results from the fully harmonized EU *Salmonella* baseline surveys in animals are summarized in Table 23.4. The observed *Salmonella* prevalence is higher than in the annual reporting by the member states, mainly due to more sensitive sampling methods applied in the surveys and also because the mandatory control programmes in the poultry populations have recently reduced the prevalence. The baseline survey results also demonstrated the large variation in the member states' specific *Salmonella* prevalence. In all the surveys some member states did not detect any positive samples whereas some other member states reported prevalence up to 83%.

Salmonella Enteritidis has been the most often isolated serovar in flocks of laying hens and broilers, whereas in pigs *S.* Typhimurium and *S.* Derby are the dominant serovars. In turkey flocks a number of different serovars are commonly detected. Resistance to antimicrobials is frequently detected among the *Salmonella* isolates from animals and food in the EU when using epidemiological cut-off values for defining the resistant isolates (EFSA and ECDC, 2011b).

Harmonization of Monitoring and Reporting

According to EU legislation (EU, 2003c) the monitoring of *Salmonella* in animals, feed and food is based on the systems in place in member states. However, harmonized monitoring and reporting schemes may be laid down by the Commission decision or technical specifications issued by EFSA. Indeed, substantial efforts have been made to harmonize the monitoring and reporting of *Salmonella* in the EU in order to make the data more comparable between the member states and reporting years.

The EU legislation laying down the *Salmonella* reduction targets and mandatory controls in poultry population (EU, 2005b, 2006b, 2007b, 2008b, 2010, 2011b) describes harmonized sampling and reporting schemes for each of the populations addressed: breeding flocks of fowl (*Gallus gallus*) and turkeys, flocks of laying hens, flocks of broilers and fattening turkeys. The breeding flocks are sampled either at hatchery or at farm whereas laying hen, broiler and fattening turkey flocks are always sampled at the farm. The detailed rules are described in Table 23.1. The sampling is carried out by using pooled faeces, boot/stock swabs or dust samples. The timing of sampling and the analyses methods are also described in the legislation.

The EU Regulations on microbiological criteria for foodstuffs (EU, 2005c) harmonize the testing against the *Salmonella* criteria by defining the reference analytical method, number of subsamples to be taken as well as in some cases also the type of specimen to be taken. At the slaughterhouse the sampling of carcasses takes place after dressing but before chilling. EFSA on its behalf has published an external report on development of harmonized survey methods for food-borne pathogens in foodstuffs in the EU (Käsbohrer *et al.*, 2010) that provides guidance on conducting surveys of *Salmonella* in various foodstuffs.

The monitoring of antimicrobial resistance in *Salmonella* isolates from animals is harmonized by EU legislation (EU, 2007c) and by EFSA's report on harmonized monitoring scheme of antimicrobial resistance in different animal populations (EFSA, 2007a).

Quality Assurance on Laboratory Analyses

Testing is an important part of *Salmonella* control and the outcome of testing may result in important consequences for the food business operators and for health protection. Therefore, guarantees must be provided on the quality of testing in the EU.

The EU reference laboratory (http://www.rivm.nl/crlsalmonella) and the national reference laboratories for *Salmonella* were introduced on 1 January 1994 (EU, 1992) to improve testing methodology and ensure high quality of laboratory analyses in all member states. The main tasks of the EU reference laboratory is to ensure and verify quality of testing in the national reference laboratories by providing details of analytic methods, coordinating application, in particular, by organizing comparative studies, coordination of practical arrangements to apply new methods and conducting training (EU, 2004d). It also provides scientific and technical assistance to the EC.

National reference laboratories have similar tasks towards laboratories carrying out official controls within member states. The network of the EU reference laboratory with the national reference laboratories ensures quick exchanges of information and experiences on testing throughout the EU.

Laboratories can carry out tests on samples taken by food business operators with the frame of control of *Salmonella* in animal population if these laboratories are designated by the competent authority and they apply quality assurance systems that conform to the requirements of the current EN/ ISO standard. In addition, these laboratories must regularly participate in collaborative testing, organized or coordinated by the national reference laboratory (EU, 2003a).

References

Ammon, A. and Makela, P. (2010) Integrated data collection on zoonoses in the European Union, from animals to humans, and the analyses of the data. *International Journal of Food Microbiology* 139, 43–47.

Brazil, Instrução Normativa SDA/MAA 70 (2003) (D.U.O. 10/10/2003) CAC, *Procedural Manual*.

CAC/GL 30 (1999) Principles and Guidelines for the Conduct of Microbiological Risk Assessment.

CAC/GL 21 (1997) Principles for the Establishment and Application of Microbiological Criteria in Foods.

CAC/GL 63 (2007) Principles and Guidelines for the Conduct of Microbiological Risk Management.

CAC Guidelines for the Control of *Campylobacter* and *Salmonella* spp. (2012) In: *Chicken Meat*.

CAC/RCP 15 (1976) Code of Hygienic Practice for Eggs and Egg products.

CAC/RCP 39 (1993) Code of Hygiene Practice for Precooked and Cooked Foods in Mass Catering.

CAC/RCP 58 (2005) Code of Hygiene Practice for Meat.

CAC/RCP 66 (2008) Code of Hygienic Practice for Powdered Formulae for Infants and Young Children.

Copa-Cogeca and EUWEP (2009) Community Guide for good hygiene practices in pullet rearing and egg laying flocks. Available at: http://ec.europa.eu/food/food/biosafety/salmonella/docs/community_guide_layers_hygiene_practice_pullet_egg_en.pdf (accessed 27 February 2013).

Copa-Cogeca and AVEC (2010) European poultrymeat industry guide [EPIG], Guide to Good Hygiene Practice for the Prevention and Control of Pathogenic Microorganisms with particular Reference to *Salmonella* in *Gallus gallus* (Broilers) reared for meat on farms, and during catching, loading and transport. Available at: http://ec.europa.eu/food/food/biosafety/salmonella/docs/community_guide_broilers_en.pdf (accessed 27 February 2013).

COM (2000) White Paper on Food Safety, COM (1999), 719 (final). Available at: http://eur-lex.europa.eu/LexUriServ/LexUriServ.do?uri=COM:1999:0719:FIN:EN:PDF (accessed 27 February 2013).

EC (European Commission) (2003) Opinion of the Scientific Committee on Veterinary Measures relating to Public Health on Salmonellae in Foodstuffs, adopted 14–15 April 2003. Available at: http://ec.europa.eu/food/fs/sc/scv/out66_en.pdf (accessed 27 February 2013).

ECDC, EFSA, EMA, SCENIHR (2009) Joint Opinion on antimicrobial resistance (AMR) focused on zoonotic infections, Question No. EFSA-Q-2008-781. doi:10.2903/j.efsa.2009.1372 European Medicines Agency Reference EMEA/CVMP/447259/2009. *The EFSA Journal* 7(11), 1372.

EFSA (2005) The Community Summary Report on Trends and Sources of Zoonoses, Zoonotic Agents, Antimicrobial resistance and Foodborne outbreaks in the European Union in 2004. *The EFSA Journal* 310, 280 pp.

EFSA (2006a) Preliminary Report on the Analysis of the Baseline Study on the Prevalence of *Salmonella* in Laying Hen Flocks of *Gallus gallus*. *The EFSA Journal* 81, 1–71.

EFSA (2006b) The Community Summary Report on Trends and Sources of Zoonoses, Zoonotic Agents, Antimicrobial Resistance and Foodborne Outbreaks in the European Union in 2005. *The EFSA Journal* 94, 288 pp.

EFSA (2007a) Report of the Task Force of Zoonoses Data Collection including a proposal for a harmonised monitoring scheme of antimicrobial resistance in *Salmonella* in fowl (*Gallus gallus*), turkeys, and pigs and *Campylobacter jejuni* and *C. coli* in broilers. *The EFSA Journal* 96, 1–46.

EFSA (2007b) Report of the Task Force on Zoonoses Data Collection on the Analysis of the baseline study on the prevalence of *Salmonella* in holdings of laying hen flocks of *Gallus gallus*. *The EFSA Journal* 97.

EFSA (2007c) Report of the Task Force on Zoonoses Data Collection on the Analysis of the baseline survey on the prevalence of *Salmonella* in broiler flocks of *Gallus gallus*, Part A. *The EFSA Journal* 98, 1–85.

EFSA (2007d) Report of the Task Force on Zoonoses Data Collection on the Analysis of the baseline survey on the prevalence of *Salmonella* in holdings of broiler flocks of *Gallus gallus*, Part B. *The EFSA Journal* 101, 1–86.

EFSA (2007e) The Community Summary Report on Trends and Sources of Zoonoses, Zoonotic Agents, Antimicrobial Resistance and Foodborne Outbreaks in the European Union in 2006. *The EFSA Journal* 130, 352 pp.

EFSA (2008a) Report of the Task Force on Zoonoses Data Collection on the Analysis of the baseline survey on the prevalence of *Salmonella* in turkey flocks, Part A. *The EFSA Journal* 134, 1–91.

EFSA (2008b) Report of the Task Force on Zoonoses Data Collection on the analysis of the baseline survey on the prevalence of *Salmonella* in slaughter pigs, in the EU, 2006-2007 – Part A: *Salmonella* prevalence estimates. *The EFSA Journal* 135, 1–111.

EFSA (2008c) Report of the Task Force on Zoonoses Data Collection on the Analysis of the baseline survey on the prevalence of *Salmonella* in turkey flocks, in the EU, 2006-2007: Part B: factors related to *Salmonella* flock prevalence and distribution of *Salmonella* serovars. *The EFSA Journal* 198, 1–224.

EFSA (2008d) Analysis of the baseline survey on the prevalence of *Salmonella* in slaughter pigs, in the EU, 2006-2007 – Part B: factors associated with *Salmonella* infection in lymph nodes, *Salmonella* surface contamination of carcasses, and the distribution of *Salmonella* serovars, *The EFSA Journal* 206, 1–111.

EFSA (2008e) Scientific Opinion of the Panel on Biological Hazards on a request from the Health and Consumer Protection, Directorate General, European Commission on Microbiological Risk Assessment in feedingstuffs for food producing animals. *The EFSA Journal* 720, 1–84.

EFSA (2009a) The Community Summary Report on Trends and Sources of Zoonoses and Zoonotic Agents in the European Union in 2007. *The EFSA Journal* 223, 320 pp.

EFSA (2009b) Scientific report on Analysis of the baseline survey on the prevalence of *Salmonella* in holdings with breeding pigs in the EU, 2008. Part A: *Salmonella* prevalence estimates. *EFSA Journal* 7(12), 93 pp.

EFSA (2009c) Scientific Opinion of the Panel on Biological Hazards on a request from European Commission on Quantitative estimation of the impact of setting a new target for the reduction of *Salmonella* in breeding hens of *Gallus gallus*. *The EFSA Journal* 1036, 1–68.

EFSA (2010a) The Community Summary Report on Trends and Sources of Zoonoses, Zoonotic Agents and Foodborne Outbreaks in the European Union in 2008. *The EFSA Journal* 8(1), 1496, 410 pp.

EFSA (2010b) Analysis of the baseline survey on the prevalence of *Campylobacter* in broiler batches and of *Campylobacter* and *Salmonella* on broiler carcasses in the EU, 2008 – Part A: *Campylobacter* and *Salmonella* prevalence estimates. *EFSA Journal* 8(03), 1503, 99 pp.

EFSA (2010c) EFSA Panel on Biological Hazards (BIOHAZ); Scientific Opinion on the link between *Salmonella* criteria at different stages of the poultry production chain. *EFSA Journal* 8(3), 1545, 66 pp.

EFSA (2010d) EFSA Panel on Biological Hazards (BIOHAZ); Scientific Opinion on a quantitative estimate of the public health impact of setting a new target for the reduction of *Salmonella* in laying hens. *EFSA Journal* 8(4), 1546, 86 pp.

EFSA (2010e) EFSA Panel on Biological Hazards; Scientific Opinion on a Quantitative Microbiological Risk Assessment of *Salmonella* in slaughter and breeder pigs. *EFSA Journal* 8(4), 1547, 90 pp.

EFSA (2010f) EFSA Panel on Biological Hazards (BIOHAZ); Scientific Opinion on monitoring and assessment of the public health risk of '*Salmonella* Typhimurium-like' strains. *EFSA Journal* 8(10), 1826, 48 pp. doi:10.2903/j.efsa.2010.1826.

EFSA (2011a) EFSA Panel on Biological Hazards (BIOHAZ); Scientific Opinion on a quantitative estimation of the public health impact of setting a new target for the reduction of *Salmonella* in broilers. *EFSA Journal* 9(7), 2106, 94pp.

EFSA (2011b) Analysis of the baseline survey on the prevalence of *Salmonella* in holdings with breeding pigs, in the EU, 2008 – Part B: factors associated with *Salmonella* pen positivity. *EFSA Journal* 9(7), 2329, 159 pp.

EFSA and ECDC (2011a) The European Union Summary Report on Trends and Sources of Zoonoses, Zoonotic Agents and Food-borne Outbreaks in 2009. *EFSA Journal* 9(3), 2090, 378 pp.

EFSA and ECDC (2011b) The European Union Summary Report on antimicrobial resistance in zoonotic and indicator bacteria from humans, animals and food in the European Union in 2009. *EFSA Journal* 9(6), 2154.

EU (1992) Council Directive 92/117/EEC of 17 December 1992 concerning measures for protection against specified zoonoses and specified zoonotic agents in animals and products of animal origin in order to prevent outbreaks of food-borne infections and intoxications. *Official Journal of the European Union L* 62, 15.3.1993, 38–48.

EU (1995) Council Decision 95/410/EC of 22 June 1995 laying down the rules for the microbiological testing by sampling in the establishment of origin of poultry for slaughter intended for Finland and Sweden. *Official Journal of the European Union L* 243, 11.10.1995, 25–28.

EU (2002) Regulation (EC) No 178/2002 of the European Parliament and of the Council of 28 January 2002 laying down the general principles and requirements of food law, establishing the European Food Safety Authority and laying down procedures in matters of food safety. *Official Journal of the European Union L* 31, 1.2.2002, 1–24.

EU (2003a) Regulation (EC) No 2160/2003 of the European Parliament and of the Council of 17 November 2003 on the control of *Salmonella* and other specified food-borne zoonotic agents. *Official Journal of the European Union L* 325, 12.12.2003, 1–15.

EU (2003b) Commission Decision 2003/644/EC of 8 September 2003 establishing additional guarantees regarding *Salmonella* for consignments to Finland and Sweden of breeding poultry and day-old chicks for introduction into flocks of breeding poultry or flocks of productive poultry. *Official Journal of the European Union L* 228, 12.9.2003, 29–34.

EU (2003c) Directive 2003/99/EC of the European Parliament and of the Council of 17 November 2003 on the monitoring of zoonoses and zoonotic agents. *Official Journal of the European Union L* 325, 12.12.2003, 31–40.

EU (2004a) Regulation (EC) No 852/2004 of the European Parliament and of the Council of 29 April 2004 on the hygiene of foodstuffs. *Official Journal of the European Union L* 139, 30.4.2004, 1; as corrected by *Official Journal of the European Union L* 226, 25.6.2004, 3–21.

EU (2004b) Regulation (EC) No 853/2004 of the European Parliament and of the Council of 29 April 2004 laying down specific hygiene rules for food of animal origin. *Official Journal of the European Union L* 139, 30.4.2004, 55; as corrected by *Official Journal of the European Union L* 226, 25.6.2004, 22–82.

EU (2004c) Regulation (EC) No 854/2004 of the European Parliament and of the Council of 29 April 2004 laying down specific rules for the organisation of official controls on products of animal origin intended for human consumption. *Official Journal of the European Union L* 139, 30.4.2004, 206; as corrected by *Official Journal of the European Union L* 226, 25.6.2004, 83–127.

EU (2004d) Regulation (EC) No 882/2004 of the European Parliament and of the Council of 29 April 2004 on official controls performed to ensure the verification of compliance with feed and food law, animal health and animal welfare rules. *Official Journal of the European Union L* 191, 30.4.2004, 1–65.

EU (2004e) Commission Decision 2004/665/EC of 22 September 2004 concerning a baseline study on the prevalence of *Salmonella* in laying flocks of *Gallus gallus*. *Official Journal of the European Union L* 303, 30.9.2004, 30–34.

EU (2004f) Commission Decision 2004/235/EC of 1 March 2004 establishing additional guarantees regarding *Salmonella* for consignments to Finland and Sweden of laying hens. *Official Journal of the European Union L* 72, 11.03.2004, 86–90.

EU (2005a) Regulation (EC) No 183/2005 of the European Parliament and of the Council of 12 January 2005 laying down requirements for feed hygiene. *Official Journal of the European Union L* 35, 8.2.2005, 1–22.

EU (2005b) Commission Regulation (EC) No 1003/2005 of 30 June 2005 implementing Regulation (EC) No 2160/2003 as regards a Community target for the reduction of the prevalence of certain *Salmonella* serovars in breeding flocks of *Gallus gallus* and amending Regulation (EC) No 2160/2003. *Official Journal of the European Union L* 170, 1.7.2005, 12–17.

EU (2005c) Commission Decision 2005/636/EC of 1 September 2005 concerning a financial contribution by the Community towards a baseline survey on the prevalence of *Salmonella* spp. in broiler flocks of *Gallus gallus* to be carried out in the Member States. *Official Journal of the European Union L* 228, 3.9.2005, 14–18.

EU (2005d) Commission Regulation (EC) No 2073/2005 of 15 November 2005 on microbiological criteria for foodstuffs. *Official Journal of the European Union L* 338, 22.12.2005, 1–26.

EU (2005e) Commission Regulation (EC) No 1688/2005 of 14 October 2005 implementing Regulation (EC) No 853/2004 of the European Parliament and of the Council as regards special guarantees concerning *Salmonella* for consignments to Finland and Sweden of certain meat and eggs. *Official Journal of the European Union L* 271, 15.10.2005, 17–28EU (2006a) Commission Regulation (EC) No 1177/2006 of 1

August 2006 Commission Regulation (EC) No 1177/2006 of 1 August 2006 implementing Regulation (EC) No 2160/2003 of the European Parliament and of the Council as regards requirements for the use of specific control methods in the framework of the national programmes for the control of *Salmonella* in poultry. *Official Journal of the European Union L* 212, 2.8.2006, 3–5.

EU (2006b) Commission Regulation (EC) No 1168/2006 of 31 July 2006 implementing Regulation (EC) No 2160/2003 as regards a Community target for the reduction of the prevalence of certain *Salmonella* serovars in laying hens of *Gallus gallus* and amending Regulation (EC) No 1003/2005. *Official Journal of the European Union L* 211, 1.8.2006, 4–8.

EU (2006c) Commission Decision 2006/662/EC of 29 September 2006 concerning a financial contribution from the Community towards a baseline survey on the prevalence of Salmonella in turkeys to be carried out in the Member States. *Official Journal of the European Union L* 272, 3.10.20006, 22–26.

EU (2006d) Commission Decision 2006/668/EC of 29 September 2006 concerning a financial contribution from the Community towards a baseline survey on the prevalence of *Salmonella* in slaughter pigs to be carried out in the Member States. *Official Journal of the European Union L* 275, 6.10.20006, 51–61.

EU (2007a) Commission Regulation (EC) No 1237/2007 of 23 October 2007 amending Regulation (EC) No 2160/2003 of the European Parliament and of the Council and Decision 2006/696/EC as regards the placing on the market of eggs from *Salmonella* infected flocks of laying hens. *Official Journal of the European Union L* 280, 24.10.2007, 5–9.

EU (2007b) Commission Regulation (EC) No 646/2007 of 12 June 2007 implementing Regulation (EC) No 2160/2003 of the European Parliament and of the Council as regards a Community target for the reduction of the prevalence of *Salmonella* Enteritidis and *Salmonella* Typhimurium in broilers and repealing Regulation (EC) No 1091/2005. *Official Journal of the European* Union *L* 151, 13.6.2007, 21–25.

EU (2007c) Commission Decision 2007/407/EC of 12 June 2007 on a harmonised monitoring of antimicrobial resistance in *Salmonella* in poultry and pigs. *Official Journal of the European Union L* 153, 14.6.2007, 26–29.

EU (2007d) Commission Decision (2007/516/EC) of 19 July 2007 concerning a financial contribution from the Community towards a survey on the prevalence and antimicrobial resistance of *Campylobacter* spp. in broiler flocks and on the prevalence of *Campylobacter* spp. and *Salmonella* spp. in broiler carcasses to be carried out in the Member States. *Official Journal of the European Union L* 190, 21.7.2007, 25–37.

EU (2008a) Commission Decision 2008/55/EC of 20 December 2007, concerning a financial contribution from the Community towards a survey on the prevalence of *Salmonella* spp. and Methicillin-resistant *Staphylococcus aureus* in herds of breeding pigs to be carried out in the Member States. *Official Journal of the European Union L* 14, 17.1.2008, 10–25.

EU (2008b) Commission Regulation (EC) No 584/2008 of 20 June 2008 implementing Regulation (EC) No 2160/2003 of the European Parliament and of the Council as regards a Community target for the reduction of the prevalence of *Salmonella* Enteritidis and *Salmonella* Typhimurium in turkeys. *Official Journal of the European Union L* 162, 21.6.2008, 3–8.

EU (2009) Council Directive 2009/158/EC of 30 November 2009 on animal health conditions governing intra-Community trade in, and imports from third countries of, poultry and hatching eggs. *Official Journal of the European Union L* 343, 22.12.2009, 74–113.

EU (2010) Commission Regulation (EU) No 200/2010 of 10 March 2010 implementing Regulation (EC) No 2160/2003 of the European Parliament and of the Council as regards a Union target for the reduction of the prevalence of *Salmonella* serovars in adult breeding flocks of *Gallus gallus*. *Official Journal of the European Union L* 61, 11.3.2010, 1–9.

EU (2011a) Commission Regulation (EU) No 142/2011 of 25 February 2011 implementing Regulation (EC) No 1069/2009 of the European Parliament and of the Council laying down health rules as regards animal by-products and derived products not intended for human consumption and implementing Council Directive 97/78/EC as regards certain samples and items exempt from veterinary checks at the border under that Directive Text with EEA relevance. *Official Journal of the European Union L* 54, 26.2.2011, 1–254.

EU (2011b) Commission Regulation (EU) No 517/2011 of 25 May 2011 implementing Regulation (EC) No 2160/2003 of the European Parliament and of the Council as regards a Union target for the reduction of the prevalence of certain *Salmonella* serovars in laying hens of *Gallus gallus* and amending Regulation (EC) No 2160/2003 and Commission Regulation (EU) No 200/2010. *Official Journal of the European Union L* 138, 26.5.2011, 45–51.

FCC Consortium (2010) Analysis of the costs and benefits of setting a target for the reduction of *Salmonella* in slaughter pigs for European Commission Health and Consumers Directorate-General, SANCO/2008/

E2/036 Final report, June 2010, Available at: http://ec.europa.eu/food/food/biosafety/salmonella/docs/fattening_pigs_analysis_costs.pdf (accessed 27 February 2013).

FCC Consortium (2011) Analysis of the costs and benefits of setting a target for the reduction of *Salmonella* in breeding pigs for European Commission Health and Consumers Directorate-General, SANCO/2008/E2/056 Final report, March 2011, Available at: http://ec.europa.eu/food/food/biosafety/salmonella/docs/br_pigs_repfor_submission_16032011_en.pdf (accessed 27 February 2013).

FDA (2009) Prevention of *Salmonella* Enteritidis in Shell Eggs During Production, Storage, and Transportation, 33030 Federal Register / Vol. 74, No. 130 / Thursday, 9 July 2009.

FSANZ (2011) Australia New Zealand Food Standards Code, Standard 1.6.1, Microbiological Limits for Food. Available at: http://www.foodstandards.gov.au/foodstandards/foodstandardscodeold (accessed 27 February 2013).

Hendriksen, R.S., Vieira, A.R., Karlsmose, S., Lo Fo Wong, D.M.A., Jensen, A.B., Wegener, H.C. and Aarestrup, F.M. (2011) Global monitoring of *Salmonella* serovar distribution from the World Health Organisation Global Foodborne Infections Network Country Data Bank: results of quality assured laboratories form 2001-2007. *Foodborne Pathogens and Disease* 8, 887–900.

Käsbohrer, A., Tenhagen, B.A., Appel, B. and Fetsch, A. (2010) Development of harmonised survey methods for food-borne pathogens in foodstuffs in the European Union. Scientific report submitted to EFSA, 9 December 2010.

OIE (2011) Terrestrial Animal Health Code. Available at: http://www.oie.int/international-standard-setting/terrestrial-code/access-online (accessed 27 February 2013).

USDA FSIS (2010) New Performance Standards for *Salmonella* and *Campylobacter* in Young Chicken and Turkey Slaughter Establishments; New Compliance Guides. *Federal Register Notice on 14 May 2010,* 75 FR 27288.

24 Current and New Approaches to Typing of *Salmonella*

John Wain[1]* and John E. Olsen[2]

[1]*The Norwich Medical School, University of East Anglia and The Laboratory of Gastrointestinal Pathogens, UK;* [2]*Department of Veterinary Disease Biology, University of Copenhagen, Denmark*

Introduction

As a group of organisms, *Salmonella* have been split more than most. There are two approved species within the genus, as described by DNA-DNA hybridization data: *Salmonella enterica* and *S. bongori*. Most human infections are caused by *S. enterica*, a species that has been further split into six subspecies as recognized by biochemical tests (Farmer, 2003). Using combinations of 46 O antigens and 114 H antigens, around ~2500 serovars are currently described within *S. enterica*. The most common subspecies in human infections is subspecies I (or *S. enterica* subsp. *enterica*), which is currently split into 1500 serotypes (Guibourdenche *et al.*, 2010). For some serotypes further subdivision into biotypes is used. The end result of all this typing is a magnificent classification known as the modified White–Kauffmann–Le Minor scheme (Grimont and Weill, 2007).

The main use for typing of *Salmonella* is to track changes in epidemiology and to trace sources of food-borne infections. A search of the NCBI database PubMed with the search words *Salmonella* AND typing or *Salmonella* AND PFGE revealed 566 and 334 hits between 2005 and 2010 to articles dealing with typing of *Salmonella*, often as part of an epidemiological investigation. On the one hand this shows that *Salmonella* is an important food-borne pathogen, on the other hand, it reflects that most typing investigations of this bacterial genus result in useful information. Good and validated typing methods are available and the genus has a suitable population structure for typing purposes. Originally it was described as strictly clonal with a low level of recombination based on analysis of multi-locus enzyme electrophoresis data (Smith *et al.*, 1993). However, more detailed analysis by multi-locus sequence typing (fragments of seven genes), SNP-detections (from 200 genes) (Rougmagnac *et al.*, 2006; Lan *et al.*, 2009) and sequence typing by genome sampling (approximately 10% of the core genome) (Didelot *et al.*, 2011) have revealed a good deal of recombination between lineages and even within some lineages of *S. enterica* subsp. *enterica*. It appears that the species has a good (for typing purposes) balance between stable lineages, created by genetic drift, that has resulted in an overall clonal framework and the more rapid variation

* Corresponding author, e-mail: john.wain@uea.ac.uk

© CAB International 2013. *Salmonella in Domestic Animals, 2nd Edition* (eds P.A. Barrow and U. Methner)

created by horizontal gene acquisition and diversifying selection that creates traceable differences between strains.

Recent reviews have detailed expertly the available typing techniques for *Salmonella* (Foley *et al.*, 2007; Malorny *et al.*, 2011; Wattiau *et al.*, 2011). In this chapter we therefore mainly address the question of why serotyping at the same time is such a 'good' typing scheme for *Salmonella*, but on the other hand is constantly under pressure to be replaced. The chapter also tries to predict which directions typing strategies for *Salmonella* will take in future. For the sake of overview, we first give a short introduction to the current typing strategies and methods in current use.

Current Strategies and Methods for Typing of *Salmonella*

Table 24.1 gives an overview of current typing schemes used for *Salmonella*. The sections below discuss the currently used definitive methods and how they are combined with molecular methods in current typing strategies.

Serotyping

Serotyping is based on the detection, by reaction with antibodies, of three types of antigens: O somatic antigens, H or flagella antigens and Vi or capsular antigens and discriminates between more than 2500 serotypes (Grimont and Weill, 2007). Antigenic formulae are written as follows: O:H1:H2.

The O antigens ($n=46$) are the sugar component of the lipopolysaccharide (LPS) exposed on the bacterial surface. The LPS is encoded by an array of genes, known as the *rfb* cluster, which provide enzymes for the biosynthesis and export of the molecule (Reeves *et al.*, 1996). Links between variation in LPS structure and immune selection are well described for other gram-negative organisms, such as *Pseudomonas* (Hajjar *et al.*, 2002), and one of the virulence factors in *Salmonella*, linked to invasive disease, is LPS (Fierer and Guiney, 2001). There is also a possible link between O type and host adaptation (Kingsley and Bäumler, 2000).

The H antigens are structural proteins on the surface of bacterial flagella ($n=114$). There is a one gene–one protein relationship for each of the two antigens: H1 is encoded by *fliC* and H2 by *fljB*. Expression is under the control of a phase switch mechanism and in any pure culture there is usually expression of one phase on the vast majority of cells – the other phase is expressed on a minority that is below the level of detection for antibody binding detected by agglutination. Therefore in order to serotype an isolate (for both H antigens) it is necessary to change the phase. This is achieved by incubating the test organism in the presence of an antibody to the expressed antigen; motility is impaired and only those expressing the minority antigen can swim. This characteristic is used in various formats to enrich for the minority antigen so that agglutination can be carried out. The whole process takes at least 2 days and more often longer than a working week.

For the capsular antigen there is only one, the Vi antigen of *S.* Typhi, Paratyphi C and rarely Dublin. The vast majority of fresh clinical isolates of *S.* Typhi express the Vi antigen (Wain *et al.*, 2005) but occasional geographic clusters of Vi-negative isolates are seen (Baker *et al.*, 2005). Thus the absence of Vi cannot rule out *S.* Typhi and neither can the presence be used as definitive identification. All isolates of *S.* Paratyphi C tested carry the genes and expressed the antigen, although in some cases at levels only detectable by ELISA (Wain, unpublished data). The genetics of the Vi antigen show clearly how selective advantage can create the same antigenic reaction in entirely different backgrounds. In *S.* Typhi and *S.* Paratyphi C the genes are within a large pathogenicity island, SPI-7, which is not unique even to the species *S. enterica* (Seth-Smith, 2008). There are significant differences between the islands found in different species and even between each serotype (Pickard *et al.*, 2003) but the expressed antigen reacts with the same antibody. This is a strong warning that any typing scheme dependent on the presence of a horizontally acquired, selectable island of genes is prone to the error of clustering entirely unrelated

Table 24.1. Current typing schemes for Salmonella

Technique	Brief description	Advantages	Currently available for	Disadvantages	Reference
Phenotypic					
Serotyping	Agglutination of somatic 'O' and flagella 'H' antigens. Requires phase change for full serotyping	Convenient; easy to perform. Represents a known method. Can be used to screen for *Salmonella* as well as serotyping	*Salmonella* subsp. I mainly	Is based on selectable markers and so does not reflect true classification. Need a very wide range of expensive antisera	Grimont and Weill, 2007
Phage type	Susceptibility of a bacterial isolate to a panel of bacteriophage	Well established and can be very quick. Provides useful, biologically relevant and epidemiological data	Serovars: Typhi Paratyphi A Paratyphi B Java Typhimurium Enteritidis Agona Virchow Hadar Pullorum Thompson	Is not widely available; is limited to reference labs because of need for phage maintenance. Molecular mechanism not defined for all serotypes	http://www.hpa.org/ then follow products and services/ infectious diseases/ Laboratories and Reference facilities/ LGP/SRU Kafatos *et al.*, 2009
Antibiotic resistance (R-type)	Susceptibility to different antibiotics	Easy and cheap to perform. Usefully discriminates between outbreak isolates of *S.* Enteritidis	All *Salmonella*	The same phenotypic resistance pattern may be due to different genetic mechanisms. Resistance may change very rapidly. Not a classification system	Threlfall and Frost, 1990
MALDI-Tof	Mass spectrometry of whole killed organisms	Quick and cheap	*S. enterica*	Current methods need an isolate and it is not discriminatory enough for subspecies typing	Personal experience
Genotypic					
RAPD – random amplification of polymorphic DNA	Amplification from random primers	Easy to perform. May be useful for outbreak investigation	All *Salmonella*	Not reproducible, not widely used	Dione *et al.*, 2012

PCR for specific genes, or islands	PCR for resistance genes, pathogenicity factors or metabolic markers	Straightforward to apply to isolates with known genetic difference(s)	Most serovars	To identify and validate candidate genes can be difficult – no standardization	Kim *et al.*, 2006
Plasmid profile	Analysis of plasmids harboured by isolate	Good in outbreak investigation	All *Salmonella*	Individual isolates may gain or lose plasmids readily. Not a true classification	Connerton *et al.*, 2000
Restriction digest of plasmids	Digestion of plasmid DNA with a restriction enzyme	Useful for describing the spread of resistance or virulence plasmids	All *Salmonella*	Can only be used for strains that contain similar plasmids. Tells you nothing about the bacterial host	Williamson *et al.*, 1988
PFGE – pulsed field gel electrophoresis	Restriction digestion of genomic DNA and separation on agarose gel used a pulsed electrical field	Has been standardized for comparison across different laboratories	All *Salmonella*	Expensive equipment and software needed for comparative results. Is limited to reference/research laboratories. Samples less than 1% of the sequence variation in *Salmonella* genomes	Baquar *et al.*, 1994; Olsen and Skov, 1994; Schwartz and Liebisch, 1994; Thong *et al.*, 1994; Baggesen *et al.*, 1996
Fragment length polymorphism (AFLP/ FALFP)	PCR-based modification of PFGE. Fluorescent markers included to improve discrimination of fragments	Is more robust than PFGE and provides a higher level of discrimination. Clustering matches serotype clusters	All *Salmonella*	Expensive equipment needed, only samples a small fraction of the genome; at the cut sites of the enzymes. Tried for *Salmonella* but not used currently	Arnold *et al.*, 1999
MLVA – multi-locus variable number tandem repeat (VNTR) analysis	Size of PCR products represents copy number of short repetitive sequences	Robust and reproducible, can be automated. Has been used for *S.* Typhi and Typhimurium. Attempts at standardization in progress for *E. coli* O157	Serovars: Typhimurium, Enteritidis	Needs to be defined for each of the current serotypes, may not discriminate as well as PFGE	Torpdal *et al.*, 2007

(*Continued*)

Table 24.1. (Continued)

Technique	Brief description	Advantages	Currently available for	Disadvantages	Reference
IS200 typing or ribotyping	Analysis of IS200 multi-copy elements or rRNA genes using either restriction digests or Southern blot	IS200 elements remain fairly constant in natural populations of bacteria. Has been used for several serotypes	All *Salmonella*	Discrimination between strains is not very high – database for identification not established	Baqar *et al.*, 1994
Multi-locus enzyme electrophoresis (MLEE)	Separate and detect activity and isoelectric point of enzymes	Very useful for global epidemiology	All *Salmonella*	Is a very difficult technique that cannot be automated	Smith *et al.*, 1990
Sequence-based					
MLST – multi-locus sequence typing	Compare the sequence of seven house-keeping genes	Redefines *Salmonella* into phylogenetic groups equivalent to serotypes. Is digital data and so very reproducible. Could be established as a SNP typing assay	All *Salmonella*	Does not differentiate within serotypes. Sequence analysis is currently expensive and so restricted to research or reference labs	Kidgell *et al.*, 2002

Microarrays, including Premi® test	DNA-DNA hybridization of the whole genome against an array of known sequences. Measures gene content	The presence or absence of genes can be defined across the whole genome of several isolates. Good for genetic diversity	All *Salmonella*	Detection of point mutations difficult. Can only detect features represented on array, cannot recognize novel insertions etc.	Porwollik *et al.*, 2002, 2004; Wattiau *et al.*, 2011
SNP typing	Platforms used vary	Reproducible, definitive and universally applicable	*S.* Typhi	Only as good as the strain collection originally sequenced	Roumagnac *et al.*, 2006
New generation genome sequencing	High coverage and depth – good for looking at conserved features of genomes. Read length not yet good enough to assemble the whole genome	Reproducible, definitive and universally applicable	All *Salmonella*	Interpretation currently at the research level – not yet established for *Salmonella* but has been used for investigation of *E. coli* outbreaks	Loman *et al.*, 2012

organisms. So why does serotyping work so well?

The population structure of *Salmonella* is probably the result of selection by diversity of niche (Butela and Lawrence, 2010). This has resulted in clusters of distinct strains, now spatially isolated, which represents an array of emerged variants. The rate of mutation in *Salmonella in vivo* is a matter of current research but is probably greater than 0.5 mutations per genome per year estimated for *Mycobacterium* (Ford *et al.*, 2011) and closer to the 1.1 mutations per genome per year estimated for *Escherichia coli* (Reeves *et al.*, 2011). Sequence variation, which encodes protein variation (non-synonymous base pair changes), is therefore slow to accumulate but expands if there is an advantage in a specific host. With selection helping to expand new variants, and niche adaptation allowing evolution in isolation, it is easy to see why there are so many different serotypes of *Salmonella* and why this traditional method of typing gives rise to such a robust classification scheme. The antigenic variants found in different hosts are actually indicators of different strains with associated chromosomal mutations fixed in the population. However, this may well break down in environments such as water where the spatial barriers to genetic exchange are relaxed.

Serotyping, as well as being a robust typing scheme, is a language by which interested parties (including basic scientists and government officials) can communicate with each other. In most cases it divides strains into biologically meaningful classes, for example we immediately associate serotype with biology when we mention the host-adapted serotypes (reviewed by Uzzau *et al.*, 2000); when an organism is described as *S.* Typhi, we have access to the antigenic formula and to the biology of a host-restricted and host-adapted pathogen for humans. However, serotyping is not perfect. When we describe an isolate as *S.* Newport or *S.* Choleraesuis it is less clear what we mean. Biotyping has been developed to split strains of the latter group into clinically relevant 'serotypes': *S.* Choleraesuis, *S.* Decatur and *S.* Paratyphi C. *Salmonella* Choleraesuis is associated with pigs and causes an invasive disease in immune-compromised human hosts, *Salmonella* Paratyphi C causes an invasive disease in humans, and *S.* Decatur causes gastroenteritis (Langridge *et al.*, 2008), and yet all have an identical antigenic formula: 6/7:c:1,5. Closer analysis of this group has shown that the LPS is identical but the flagella antigens H1:C and H2:1,5 show significant variation within the group. Within the population of strains known as *S.* Decatur there is a great deal of variation in both *fliC* and *fljB* but *S.* Choleraesuis and *S.* Paratyphi C have identical *fliC* and *fljB* genes. This is presumably because *S.* Choleraesuis and *S.* Paratyphi C have independently acquired mobile elements encoding *fliC* and *fljB* and that for serotype *S.* Decatur, which is rarely isolated, the antibodies used for their identification have not been purified as carefully as those antigens found in the more common serotypes. The situation for the very common serotype *S.* Enteritidis is very different. *Salmonella* Enteritidis expresses a G antigen. The capital letter G denotes a group of several closely related antigens, and the presence of a different G antigen is associated with a different serotype (e.g. *S.* Dublin is g,p and *S.* Enteritidis is g,m). As serotyping is based on LPS and flagella antigens, loss of either of these surface components leads to misclassification; for example, correct typing of the globally important *Salmonella* 4,[5],12:i:- monophasic variant of *S.* Typhimurium has been difficult (Hopkins *et al.*, 2010), and incorrect determination of second phase flagellar antigen, in general, account for most of the mistakes in serotyping (Hendriksen *et al.*, 2009).

The discriminatory power of serotyping is low in many outbreak situations because the majority of human non-Typhi isolates belong to one of the two serotypes *S.* Typhimurium and *S.* Enteritidis. In the European Union (EU), for example, 23.3% and 52.3% of all reported human cases in 2009 belonged to these serotypes (European Food Safety Authority, European Centre for Disease Prevention and Control, 2011) and a list of top ten serotypes in any country normally accounts for more than 95% of all isolates (for reference to USA and EU data see: Anon, 2008; European Food Safety Authority,

European Centre for Disease Prevention and Control, 2011). Nevertheless, results from serotyping are used to decide which additional typing methods are applied, in the case of rare serotypes no further typing needs to be carried out for outbreak detection.

Antibiogram typing

Antibiotic resistance is an acquired characteristic, which is then inherited under selective pressure. There is sometimes a cost associated with acquiring antibiotic resistance, especially plasmid-borne resistance, and so once the antibiotic producing the selective pressure is no longer in use and the pressure is lost the characteristic may disappear from the population. Furthermore, for resistance mediated by point mutations on the chromosome (such as resistance to nalidixic acid) mutations can occur in any organism at any time. If one believes therefore that typing schemes should allow the grouping of isolates by ancestry, then the antibiogram is a dreadful candidate for typing. Indeed the view expressed over 20 years ago was that 'because of the fluidity of resistance plasmids and transposons, antibiotic resistance patterns *per se* cannot be regarded as a satisfactory primary method for discrimination within serovars' (Threlfall and Frost, 1990). However, in public health microbiology it is sometimes the only characteristic that shows variation within circulating strains and antimicrobial resistance typing has been used successfully to define outbreaks of *S*.Typhimurium (Peters *et al*., 2010). The reason these 'unsatisfactory' methods are still in use is the lack of a viable alternative. One of the roles of public health microbiology is to confirm (or deny) the validity of links made by epidemiological investigation and sometimes the antibiogram is the best way to do this.

Phage typing

Phage typing for *Salmonella* is currently used by several European reference laboratories, and standardization has been largely achieved through the discontinuation of competing schemes related to the dwindling number of laboratories willing and able to propagate the phage. The utility of phage typing in public health investigations in the UK is not in doubt: 'Assuming no testing for phage-typing was undertaken it is likely that two out of five outbreaks would not have been detected' (Kafatos *et al*., 2009). Phage typing therefore remains a valuable tool in the detection of *Salmonella* outbreaks. However, the method is cumbersome, requiring propagation of viable virus particles and is very operator dependent. This makes it only suitable for reference laboratory use, which is not in keeping with the modern desire to get typing into the field using robust, easily accessible tests. For phage typing several weeks' training is required before even experienced microbiologists can be confirmed as competent to carry out the technique independently. The advantages of phage typing are, in the right hands: reproducibility; a high level of discrimination; and low cost in consumables and speed. During an outbreak the phage type can be produced from a purified culture in 24 h.

Phage typing is especially applied with the more commonly isolated serotypes. For example, most countries subject strains of *S*. Typhimurium to phage typing according to the scheme of Anderson *et al*. (1977) and strains of *S*. Enteritidis to phage typing according to Ward *et al*. (1987). The combined results of serotyping and phage typing define the current clonal framework, and further discrimination is considered a detailing of this framework. Like serotyping, phage typing carries with it a number of inherent weaknesses. Among other things, phage type reflects the presence or absence of the receptors for the lytic phage on the surface of the bacterium, and this may change by acquisition of mobile elements, such as plasmids (Brown *et al*., 1999; Cooke *et al*., 2007).

Molecular typing

A typing investigation of *Salmonella* always begins with serotyping according to the

Kauffmann-White scheme (Grimont and Weill, 2007) and if applicable, this is supplemented with phage typing. An additional level of typing is only performed if these results indicate so.

Serotyping and phage typing can easily demonstrate changes in the overall patterns of epidemiology, but outbreak investigations always rely on molecular typing. It is hard to believe that most of the techniques we now take for granted have only been around for a decade. Historically, molecular typing has benefitted from a series of method developments and currently investigations are carried out with a high degree of international standardization with regard to both the choice of methods and protocols used for each technique. Still, the fast development in DNA technology, especially in the fields of DNA sequencing and DNA-chip technology opens avenues of new approaches to typing, avenues that will be exploited to improve our current understanding of *Salmonella* population structure and epidemiology, and to improve typing strategies in relation to outbreak investigations.

No single method is suitable for all second-level typing of *Salmonella*. The choice of method depends on both the serotype/phage type combination and the typing situation. However, especially two methods have evolved as likely first choice methods for most situations.

PFGE

Pulsed field gel electrophoresis (PFGE) was developed by Schwartz *et al.* (1983) for the separation of eukaryotic chromosomes, and it quickly became a popular typing method for *Salmonella*. Early investigations were performed on an *ad hoc* basis with laboratory-specific protocols (see for example Baquar *et al.*, 1994; Olsen and Skov, 1994; Schwarz and Liebisch, 1994; Thong *et al.*, 1994; Baggesen *et al.*, 1996), but as the method grew in popularity, it became evident that a standardization of protocols between laboratories was needed to enable full use of the many typing investigations. SALM-NET (now Enter-Net; Fisher, 1995) was initiated in 1994 as a harmonization effort of phage typing schemes commonly used in *Salmonella* surveillance in Europe. From this network, SALM-Gene was developed to harmonize and communicate PFGE methods and molecular typing results between surveillance laboratories (Peters *et al.*, 2003) and most outbreak investigations carried out by authorized laboratories in Europe make use of this network. Through the database, members of the network have direct access to digitalized PFGE patterns of outbreak strains, enabling immediate recognition of trans-national outbreaks. A key component is a carefully standardized PFGE protocol (SALM-Gene-PFGE). A parallel network, Pulsenet-USA, was developed in the USA (reviewed by Gerner-Schmidt *et al.*, 2006). The standardized protocol used in this network has been published (Ribot *et al.*, 2006) and this method is now the most commonly applied PFGE protocol for typing of *Salmonella*.

MLVA

PFGE has been very successful to link isolates from even very large trans-national outbreaks (see for example a SALM-Gene study of *S.* Enteritidis major phage types; Peters *et al.*, 2007), but it fails to discriminate between highly related strains such as the penta-resistant *S.* Typhimurium DT104 (Murphy *et al.*, 2001), and it is a labour-intensive method. To overcome this problem and still maintain the possibility for sharing of data between laboratories, standardized protocols for PCR typing based on amplification of variable number of tandem repeats in the chromosome (VNTR typing) was developed, one method for *S.* Typhi (Liu *et al.*, 2003) and one for *S.* Typhimurium (Lindsted *et al.*, 2003). This method is now commonly referred to as MLVA-typing (multiple locus VNTR typing) with reference to the fact that several repeats, i.e. three with *S.* Typhi (Liu *et al.*, 2003; Hatta *et al.*, 2011) and five with *S.* Typhimurium (Lindsted *et al.*, 2004), are targeted. This method has become the first choice for second-line typing of *S.* Typhimurium in many countries, and large strain collections have been used to standardize the system and nomenclature, and to demonstrate that typing results are concurrent with PFGE typing but often gives higher discriminatory power (Best *et al.*, 2007; Torpdahl *et al.*, 2007; Larsson *et al.*, 2009). To aid in standardization, typing reference strains has been proposed (Torpdahl *et al.*, 2007). The method by now has proven its usefulness in even very large outbreak investigations (Ethelberg *et al.*, 2008). Based on the success with this method for typing of *S.* Typhimurium, it has been natural to investigate whether similar schemes can be developed for other serotypes with high public health importance, such as *S.* Enteritidis (first report by Boxrud *et al.*, 2007 and Malorny *et al.*, 2008) and *S.* Newport (Davis *et al.*, 2009).

Molecular Approaches to First-Line Typing of *Salmonella*

Efforts have been made to change the phenotypic characterization of serotypes to a DNA sequence-based method, and these will be discussed below, while method developments that are a streamlining of the use of the current typing-antibodies, such as protein arrays (Cai *et al.*, 2005), will not be covered. In essence, changing phenotypes to genotypes, but conserving the current grouping, does not improve the scheme, just replicates it. The genes responsible for the antigens tested by stereotyping, either the LPS cluster or those encoding flagella proteins, are under pressure from the host's immune defences and they may be horizontally exchangeable; this raises the possibility of the selection of certain genetic variants causing the emergence, and spread, of successful genes. This is turn would bias the typing scheme so that a single serotype could contain isolates from very different lineages, such as *S.* Paratyphi B and Newport (Sangal *et al.*, 2010) or different serotypes could actually represent the same lineage as with *S.* Sendai and Paratyphi A (Boyd *et al.*, 1993). As long as schemes, which reproduce serotyping, are sought, these inaccuracies will never be amended. Despite this the typing of *Salmonella* has been based on the Kauffmann-White scheme for longer than most of us can remember and the link between biological phenotype (for example the ability to cause enteric fever) and serotype is undeniable in most serotypes; the Kauffmann-White scheme works for the vast majority of serotypes, and it will therefore be very difficult to replace.

Serotyping by PCR and DNA array

Serotypes are recognized by the reaction of surface antigens with antibodies and so are dependent on the quality of the antibodies used. Good quality antibodies are not easily obtainable in all parts of the world. The effort to build genotype-based 'serotyping' of *Salmonella* is therefore a crucial step toward a broader access to this fundamental typing method. Since the genes encoding the O-antigens and the H-antigens are well described (Macnab, 1996; Raetz, 1996), a logical step towards molecular serotyping has been to PCR amplify the genes responsible for antigenicity, using primers that target regions that are responsible for the variation, or to produce DNA arrays with relevant gene and sequence combinations. As early as 1993, Luk *et al.* (1993) selected three sets of primers and used these in a multiplex PCR method targeting the *rfb* gene cluster to differentiate strains of serogroups A, B, C2 and D. This approach with division into the major serogroups has later been improved by including more serogroups and combining PCR with a bead-based suspension-array (Fitzgerald *et al.*, 2007), and by selecting serogroup-specific fragments from genomic sequence databases (Liu *et al.*, 2011), and while it is only the first step toward a molecular Kauffmann-White scheme, it serves to demonstrate the potential of PCR-based serotyping.

Similar to the methods targeting biosynthesis genes encoding the O-antigens, flagellin-specific PCR methods have been developed and used to differentiate between strains of *Salmonella*, both based on RFLP analysis of the PCR-amplified product (Hong *et al.*, 2003) and as classical PCR methods where positive reactions are scored on the basis of the number and size of the PCR products (Echeita *et al.*, 2002; Herrera-León *et al.*, 2004). It has been notoriously difficult to distinguish between some flagella antigenicities in the H:G complex., for example Herrera-León *et al.* (2004) failed to separate *S.* Enteritidis from other members of this group. The solution has been to include PCR methods for genes that are not involved in the traditional serotyping, for example *sdf* to identify *S.* Enteritidis. This is the case in most methods described below; however, the reader is referred to the original publications for details on which genes can be used for which serotypes. A complete H-antigen typing scheme based on multiplex PCR followed by hybridization to micro-bead-bound probes has recently been developed and extensively evaluated (McQuiston *et al.*, 2011). It takes advantage of the same bead system as used by Fitzgerald *et al.* (2007) for O-group identification. The two systems have not yet been combined. However, other studies have made this combination of O-antigen and H-antigen directed methods.

Cardona-Castro *et al.* (2009) combined two multiplex-methods; one PCR aimed at O-grouping and targeted LPS-synthesis genes with five primer sets and one PCR method primarily targeted *fliC* and *fljB* with 15 primer sets. The PCR reactions were performed individually, but when the results were combined, 96.5% of 386 strains were correctly identified and the rest (misclassified strains) could be explained by mistakes of the phenotypic method. To be attractive for routine use, the methods should be easy to perform and not dependent on visual scoring of PCR-bands. One direction has been to take advantage of the automatic reading features of real-time PCR. A two-step procedure based on three real-time multiplex PCRs was developed, all primarily targeting flagella genes, to detect the serotypes most commonly isolated in Europe (Rajtak *et al.*, 2011). In the final testing of 97 strains, all strains that belonged to the serotypes originally taken into account were correctly identified as were a number of additional strains, while strains of 18 serotypes were negative in the PCRs. Another technical solution to enhance the reliability of PCR serotyping has been to use automated PCR. Mertes *et al.* (2010) published a high-throughput PCR system, in which a universal TaqMan probe system (same probe for all PCR products) was combined with a nano-PCR chip, automated liquid-handling system and automated reading. This system was, however, based on a different approach as far as target genes are concerned, and it will be detailed below. The microarray format has also been used to detect different O-antigen and H-antigen combinations. Yoshida *et al.* (2007) constructed a prototype array with 117 sequences internal in LPS and flagella-associated genes and demonstrated the ability of such a platform to identify strains of 16 different serotypes. Based on the results, 31 antigenic-directed probes and three control probes were spotted on a final typing array. In *E. coli* the more flexible ArrayTube format has been used for serotyping (Ballmer *et al.*, 2007), and the final array of Yoshida *et al.* (2007) has been further developed in this format by combining O-antigen and H-antigen genes with serotype-specific SNPs to enable determination of a complete Kauffmann-White molecular serotype for subspecies I (*enterica*) strains. The array correctly identified all strains among serotypes used to design the array and 92% of strains in blind sample of 100 strains. Use of a PCR method directed against the gene *pepT* was shown to eliminate the most severe of the mistakes, since it allowed specific identification of strains of *S.* Enteritidis (Franklin *et al.*, 2011).

Salmonella strains of especially subspecies I have been compared by hybridization to DNA arrays consisting of all known genes in annotated genomes (Porwollik *et al.*, 2002, 2004). This enabled Kim *et al.* (2006) to design two multiplex PCR methods targeting six genetic loci from *S.* Typhimurium (STM1–6) and four from *S.* Typhi (STY1–4). The genes were selected to be able to distinguish the 30 clinically most relevant serotypes based on the presence and absence of the particular loci. By combining the results from the two methods, 22 serotypes were specifically identified, while eight serotypes fell in groups of two. With the addition of two more PCR methods, six of these were resolved, while *S. enterica* Java and *S. enterica* Paratyphi B remained un-separated. This system is fundamentally different from the PCR methods that target O-antigen and H-antigen encoding genes in the sense that it relies on determination of gene content in strains that have been typed by traditional phenotypic serotyping. It will therefore conserve inherent misclassifications of the current system. Nevertheless, it has formed the basis for two promising technological developments.

The high-throughput system of Mertes *et al.* (2010) mentioned above used these targets in the nanoPCR, while Peterson *et al.* (2010) validated multiplex PCR in a traditional set (capable of identifying 42 serovars) and constructed 70-mer oligonucleotides based on the sequence of the same loci and used these in a spotted microarray to obtain serotype-specific hybridization patterns. Included in this array were also genes supposed to give valuable prediction of pathogenicity (*sseL*, *invA* and *spvC*). Similar to this, Scaria *et al.* (2008) developed a typing array based on the core genome of *S. enterica*, and combined this with an identification program (Matlab based). It is likely that future setups will model this approach, i.e. a combination of probes that refers the strain to its Kauffmann White location, and additional probes that informs the typist of pathogenic potential and antimicrobial profile.

Several microarrays have been constructed in an attempt to perform a genotyping that predicts pathogenicity (Majtan *et al.*, 2007; Malorny *et al.*, 2007; Scaria *et al.*, 2008). However, the basic classification of strains into virulent/non-virulent is based on how often a serotype has been reported to be isolated from disease, and not on a virulence typing *per se*. Disappointingly, Littrup *et al.* (2010a) did not find any correlation between typing results on the array of Malorny *et al.* (2007) and the probability of *S.* Typhimurium causing severe systemic disease as opposed intestinal disease, nor could such a correlation be established when strains of *S.* Enteritidis, *S.* Derby, *S.* Dublin, *S.* Saintpaul, *S.* 4,5,12:i:-, *S.* Java, *S.* 4,5,12:b:- were compared, assuming that some serotypes were more virulent that others and also looking for associations between gene content and host adaptation (Littrup *et al.*, 2010b). In conclusion, the fundamentals for both PCR-based and microarray-based serotyping of *Salmonella* is in place, and commercially available systems must be foreseen soon. In addition to this, good information on antimicrobial patterns is easily included in such assays, while prediction of pathogenicity must await a better understanding of the bacterial factors that are responsible for virulence differences within *Salmonella*.

Phage typing by molecular methods

We currently lack a detailed understanding of the factors that determine the difference between strains with regard to phage-typing results. In this situation, the efforts to exchange phenotypic phage typing with molecular phage typing have concentrated on identification of associations between certain (important) phage types and variation in the genomic content. Microarray analysis and subtractive hybridization of epidemic strains of *S.* Typhimurium DT104 versus non-epidemic strains revealed that differences between epidemic and non-epidemic strains mostly concerned prophages and genomic island 1 (Kang *et al.*, 2006), and similar results were obtained when representative strains of a larger number of important phage types of this serotype were hybridized to a whole genome microarray (Cooke *et al.*, 2007). PCR methods directed against these variable elements can be used as a typing method to track strains and to identify new epidemic clones (Cooke *et al.*, 2007), but this is not a substitution for phage typing.

The first demonstration of a molecular phage typing scheme was published by Wang *et al.* (2008). They combined 26 PCRs directed against prophages, suggested as a good strategy from the investigations mentioned above, with 12 PCRs directed against phage type-specific AFLP fragments (amplified fragment length polymorphism, a PCR-based typing method; Hu *et al.*, 2002), into one multiplex PCR, and scored the PCR reactions using reverse line blot hybridization with streptavidin-labelled probes. A total of 168 strains of *S.* Typhimurium were typed into 102 unique patterns. This corresponded to a discriminatory power above that of PFGE and corresponding to MLVA, but more importantly, 99 strains were allocated to types, which were associated with particular phage types. Only 21 of the 46 phage types included in the study were reliably identified, but nevertheless it showed the potential for molecular phage typing, in particular since it provides (for the phage types where it worked) a likely phage type and a subtyping with a discriminatory power corresponding to MLVA typing.

A more recent approach is to utilize diversity array technology (DArT) to identify phage type-specific markers. The DArT array identifies DNA polymorphism using a DNA array without revealing sequence data (see Xia *et al*., 2005). DNA fragments representing all differences observed within 179 strains of nine *S*. Enteritidis and 14 *S*. Typhimurium phage types were spotted on two arrays, one for each serotype. Genomic DNA from each strain was prepared by a complexity reduction method for a proof of concept for this approach. Sets of four to five strains of each phage type were used to identify phage type-specific markers on the array. Eleven phage type-specific markers were finally utilized to obtain differentiation between strains of different phage types. The DArT array did not obtain complete differentiation between phage types of any of the serotypes, but the authors stated that this was most likely due to the use of the complexity reduction approach (Hackl *et al*., 2010).

In conclusion, the efforts to develop molecular phage typing so far have resulted in the proof of two concepts both based on the association between phage type and genomic content, but so far, none of the principles has been developed all the way to a full typing scheme for *S*. Enteritidis and *S*. Typhimurium.

New Approaches to Typing of *Salmonella*

Sample sequencing

Sample sequencing involves the sequencing of selected regions of the bacterial genome. If the regions selected are conserved then discrimination is low but the clustering is robust and related to ancestry. In this situation, it is straightforward to assess the relationship between isolates. This is, for example, the basis of 16S ribosomal sequence-based typing (see below). On the other hand, if the region selected is highly variable then a higher index of discrimination is possible but the relationship between isolates is not as clear. This is the basis of virulence typing, where the genotype may predict the clinical outcome but there is no phylogenetic context.

Multi locus sequence typing

Several schemes for MLST of *S. enterica* have been published. Most use the sequencing of fragments of genes, which encode housekeeping functions. The theory is that genes encoding products, which are essential for growth, are under selection to maintain the amino acid sequence of the active enzyme and are, as they are not exposed on the surface of the bacterial cell, very unlikely to be under any form of diversifying selection. Any genetic variation seen therefore is most likely to be the result of genetic drift giving rise to synonymous mutations, which will accumulate at a fixed rate. Therefore, the more variation seen in the population the older, in evolutionary terms, the population should be, and the more diverse two organisms are the longer ago it is since they shared a common ancestor and the further apart they will be in the typing scheme. This satisfies the need in public health microbiology to cluster isolates that are more likely to be from an outbreak because we assume that outbreak strains will share a more recent common ancestor than isolates from sporadic cases cultured at the same time. The technique also satisfies the need for a classification based on genetic relatedness to drive research into evolution, pathogenicity and the mapping of phenotype to genotype. It is therefore a very attractive method, but does it work?

The most widely used MLST scheme is that first described for exploring the genetic diversity in *S*. Typhi (Kidgell *et al*., 2002). Seven genes were chosen based on housekeeping function, lack of any trans-membrane domains, absence of proximity to likely horizontal acquisition sites such as tRNA genes or phage-related sequence and even distribution around the genome. An extensive and well-curated database of sequence types is available (http://www.mlst.net). Analysis of variation at the seven genes by clustering isolates, which share six identical alleles, gives a very good correlation with serotype (Achtman *et al.*, 2012). This holds very well for the common serotypes but the discrimination between the more rare serotypes, especially those towards the outer branches of the phylogeny, is less clear. The method seems robust and can be automated using robotic DNA isolation and SNP detection. Although well suited to clinical laboratories, the need to type to the level of serotype for clinical need is questionable, and a SNP test that recognizes only the most common and the most invasive serotypes may be more useful. To determine a full MLST using the Kidgell scheme requires sequencing of at least 14 DNA fragments. This is expensive and is challenged by the relentless reduction in cost of next-generation sequencing. Perhaps whole genome sequencing, as it becomes even cheaper, will replace MLST.

ISR analysis

A sequence-based ribo-typing method that uses sequence variation in the spaces between the DNA encoding the structural RNA subunits also shows promise, and when used in conjunction with *cyaA* sequencing, it is useful also for subtyping within the *S.* Enteritidis serotype (Morales *et al.*, 2006, 2007).

Mass spectrometry

Whole cell mass spectrometry by MALDI-TOF has proven a very useful tool in species identification of bacteria and has greatly reduced the manpower and time needed to handle large number of bacterial isolates in clinical laboratories (see review by Wieser *et al.*, 2012). Recently, Dieckmann and Malorny (2011) evaluated the potential of using serovar-specific biomarker ions for typing *Salmonella*. Strains of 89 different serovars were analysed, and based on this a classification algorithm was derived that allowed specific identification of the four most common serovars and for selected host-specific types with very good specificity. The authors concluded that MALDI-TOF can greatly reduce the number of strains that has to be submitted to traditional serotyping when used as a first screening tool, but presently it cannot substitute for serotyping.

Conclusion and Future Perspectives

Typing schemes and methods for *Salmonella* are highly developed, and the Kaufmann-White-Le Minor systems, combined with phage typing for the most common serotypes, constitute the current method for definition of the clonal framework. The optimal situation, however, is to have typing performed in a decentralized way, i.e. outside reference laboratories but with a central database of results. This is impractical with the current approach to serotyping and phage typing. Different molecular methods, both PCR and array-based, show promise to create a molecular mimic of the phenotypic methods; if this can be achieved, even if only for the most common serotypes, this must be considered an improvement. This is likely to happen in the near future.

It may be that sequence techniques improve so fast that soon all typing can be based on this technique. Clearly the use of DNA sequence data has moved forward massively our understanding of bacterial variation. The advent of next generation sequencing, short (but getting longer) reads with high depth, now promises the ability to detect SNPs for everyday use in diagnostic and public health laboratories. Initially DNA from isolates were pooled and sequenced as a whole, then tagging allowed multiplexing to be developed, and now new technologies – Illumina Miseq and Hi-seq, Ion Torrant, Pan Bio and most recently Oxford nanopore – all promise different things, but all have one thing in common, the rapid generation of cheap and accurate nucleic acid sequence data. This technology should be available to most scientists, both research and clinical in the very near future – the problem is – do they know what to do with the data that it generates? No doubt methods will be developed to reduce the waste information down to information that is useful for typing purposes. However, currently this remains the future.

References

Achtman, M., Wain, J., Weill, F.X., Nair, S., Zhou, Z., Sangal, V., Kranland, M.G., Hale, J.L., Harbottle, H., Usebeck, A., Dougan, G., Harrison, L.H., Brisse, S. and the *S. enterica* MLST Study Group (2012) Multilocus sequence typing as a replacement for serotyping in *Salmonella enterica*. PLoS Pathogens 8(6): e1002776 doi: 10.1371/journal.ppat.1002776

Anderson, E.S., Ward, L.R., de Saxe, M.J. and de Sa, J.D.H. (1977) Bacteriophage-typing designations of *Salmonella typhimurium*. *Journal of Hygiene, Cambridge* 78, 297–300.

Anon (2008) Preliminary FoodNet data on the incidence of infection with pathogens transmitted commonly through food – 10 States, 2007. MMWR 57, 366–370.

Arnold, C., Metherell, L., Willshaw, G., Maggs, A. and Stanley, J. (1999) Predictive fluorescent amplified-fragment length polymorphism analysis of Escherichia coli: high-resolution typing method with phylogenetic significance. *Journal of Clinical Microbiology* 37, 1274.

Baggesen, D.L., Wegener, H.C. and Christensen, J.P. (1996) Typing of *Salmonella enterica* serotype Saintpaul: an outbreak investigation. *APMIS* 104, 411–418.

Baker S., Sarwar Y., Aziz H., Haque, A., Ali, A., Dougan, G., Wain, J. and Haque, A. (2005) Detection of Vi-negative *Salmonella enterica* serovar typhi in the peripheral blood of patients with typhoid fever in the Faisalabad region of Pakistan. *Journal of Clincal Microbiology* 43, 4418–4425.

Ballmer, K., Kroczak, B.M., Kuhnert, P., Slickers, P., Ehricht, R. and Hächler, H. (2007) Fast DNA serotyping of *Escherichia coli* by use of an oligonucleotide microarray. *Journal of Clinical Microbiology* 45, 370–379.

Baquar, N., Burnens, A. and Stanley, J. (1994). Comparative evaluation of molecular typing of strains of a national epidemic due to *Salmonella brandenburg* by rRNA gene and IS*200* probes and pulsed-field gel electrophoresis. *Journal of Clinical Microbiology* 32, 1876–1880.

Best, E.L., Lindstedt, B.-A., Cook, A., Clifton Hadley, F.A., Threlfall, E.J. and Liebana, E. (2007) Multiple-locus variable-number tandem repeat analysis of *Salmonella enterica* subsp. *enterica* serovar Typhimurium: comparison of isolates from pigs, poultry and cases of human gastroenteritis. *Journal of Applied Microbiology* 103, 565–572.

Boxrud, D., Pederson-Gulrud, K., Wotton, J., Medus, C., Lyszkowicz, E., Besser, J. and Barkus, J.M. (2007) Comparison of multiple-locus variable-number tandem repeat analysis, pulsed field gel electrophoresis, and phage typing for subtyping analysis of *Salmonella enterica* serotype Enteritidis. *Journal of Clinical Microbiology* 45, 536–543.

Boyd, E.F., Wang, F.S., Beltran, P., Plock, S.A., Nelson, K. and Selander, R.K. (1993) *Salmonella* reference collection B (SARB): strains of 37 serovars of subspecies I. *Journal of General Microbiology* 139, 1125–1132.

Brown, D.J., Baggesen, D.L., Platt, D.J. and Olsen, J.E. (1999) Phage type conversion in *Salmonella enterica* serotype Enteritidis caused by the introduction of a resistant plasmid of incompatibility group X (incX). *Epidemiology and Infection* 122, 19–22.

Butela, K. and Lawrence, J. (2010) Population Genetics of *Salmonella*: Selection for Antigenic Diversity. In: Robinson, D., Falush, D. and Feil, E. (eds) *Bacterial Population Genetics in Infectious Disease*. John Wiley & Sons, Hoboken, New Jersey.

Cai, H.Y., Lu, L., Muckle, C.A., Prescott, J.F. and Chen, S. (2005) Development of a novel protein microarray method for serotyping of *Salmonella enterica* strains. *Journal of Clinical Microbiology* 43, 3427–3430.

Cardona-Castro, N., Sánchez-Jiméneza, M., Lavalettab, L., Múñozc, N. and Morenoc, J. (2009) Development and evaluation of a multiplex polymerase chain reaction assay to identify *Salmonella* serogroups and serotypes. *Diagnostic Microbiology and Infectious Diseases* 65, 327–330.

Connerton, P., Wain, J., Hien, T.T., Ali, T., Parry, C., Chinh, N.T., Vinh, H., Ho, V.A., Diep, T.S., Day, N.P.J., White, N.J., Dougan, G. and Farrar, J.J. (2000) Epidemic typhoid in Vietnam: molecular typing of multiple-antibiotic-resistant *Salmonella enterica* serotype Typhi from four outbreaks. *Journal of Clinical Microbiology* 38, 895–897.

Cooke, F.J., Wain, J., Fookes, M., Ivens, A., Thompson, N., Brown, D.J., Threlfall, E.J., Gunn, G., Foster, G. and Dougan, D. (2007) Prophage sequences defining hot spots of genome variation in *Salmonella enterica* serovar Typhimurium can be used to discriminate between field isolates. *Journal of Clinical Microbiology* 45, 2590–2598.

Davis, M.A., Baker, K.N., Call, D.R., Warnick, L.D., Soyer, Y., Wiedermann, M., Grohn, Y., Mcdonough, P.L., Hancock, D.D. and Besser, T.E. (2009) Multilocus variable-number tandem-repeat method for typing of *Salmonella enterica* serovar Newport. *Journal of Clinical Microbiology* 47, 1934–1938.

Didelot, X., Bowden, R., Street, T., Golubchik, T., Spencer, C., McVen, G., Sangal, V., Anjum, M.F., Actman, M., Falush, H.D. and Donelly, P. (2011) Recombination and population structure in *Salmonella enterica*. *PLOS Genetics* 7, e1002191.

Dieckmann, R. and Malorny, B. (2011) Rapid screening of epidemiologically important *Salmonella enterica* subsp. *enterica* serovars by whole-cell matrix-assisted laser desorption ionization-time mass spectrometry. *Applied and Environmental Microbiology* 77, 4136–3146.

Dione, M.M., Geerts, S. and Antonio, M. (2012) Characterisation of novel strains of multiply antibiotic-resistant *Salmonella* recovered from poultry in Southern Senegal. *Journal of Infection in Developing Countries* 6(5), 436–442.

Echeita, M.A., Herrera, S., Garaizar, J. and Usera, M.A. (2002) Multiplex PCR-based detection and identification of the most common *Salmonella* second-phase flagellar antigens. *Research in Microbiology* 153, 107–113.

Ethelberg, S., Wingstrand, A., Jensen, T., Sørensen, G., Müller, L., Lisby, M., Nielsen, E.M. and Mølbak, K. (2008) Large outbreaks of *Salmonella* Typhimurium infection in Denmark in 2008. *Euro Surveillance* 13, pii=19023.

European Food Safety Authority, European Centre for Disease Prevention and Control (2011) The European Union Summary Report on Trends and Sources of Zoonoses, Zoonotic Agents and Food-borne Outbreaks in 2009. *EFSA Journal* 9, 2090 doi:10.2903.

Fabre, L., Zhang, J., Guigon, G., Le Hello, S., Guibert, V., Accou-Demartin, M., de Romans, S., Lim, C., Roux, C., Passet, V., Diancourt, L., Guibourdench, M., Issenhuth-Jeanjean, S., Achtman, M., Brisse, S., Sola, C. and Francois-Xavier Weill (2012) CRISPR Typing and Subtyping for Improved Laboratory Surveillance of *Salmonella* Infections. *PLoS ONE* 7, e36995.

Farmer, I.J.J. (2003) *Enterobacteriaceae: Introduction and Identification. Manual of Clinical Microbiology*. ASM/MPR, Washington, DC, pp. 636–653.

Fierer, J. and Guiney, D.G. (2001) Diverse virulence traits underlying different clinical outcomes of *Salmonella* infection. *Journal of Clinical Investigations* 107, 775–780.

Fisher, I. (1995) Salm-Net: A network for human *Salmonella* surveillance in Europe. *Euro Surveillance* 0, pii=194.

Fitzgerald, C., Collins, M., van Duyne, S., Mikoleit, M., Brown, T. and Fields, P. (2007) Multiplex, bead-based suspension array for molecular determination of common *Salmonella* serogroups. *Journal of Clinical Microbiology* 45, 3323–3334.

Foley, S.L., Zhao, S. and Walker, R.D. (2007) Comparison of molecular typing methods for the differentiation of *Salmonella* foodborne pathogens. *Foodborne Pathogens and Disease* 4, 253–276.

Ford, C.B., Lin, P.L., Chase, M.R., Shah, R.R., Iartchouk, O., Galagan, J., Mohaideen, N., Ioerger, T.R., Sacchettini, J.C., Lipsitch, M., Flynn, J.A.L. and Forutne, S.M. (2011) Use of whole genome sequencing to estimate the mutation rate of Mycobacterium tuberculosis during latent infection. *Nature Genetics* 43, 482–487.

Franklin, K., Lingohr, E.J., Yoshida, C., Anjum, M., Bodrossy, L., Clark, C.G., Kropinski, A.M. and Karmali, M.A. (2011) Rapid genoserotyping tool for classification of *Salmonella* serotypes. *Journal of Clinical Microbiology* 49, 2954–2965.

Gerner-Schmidt, P., Hise, K., Kincaid, J., Hunter, S., Ronaldo, S., Hyyttä-Tress, E., Ribot, E.M., Swaminathan, B. and the Pulsenet taskforce (2006) Pulsenet-USA: a five year update. *Foodborne Pathogens and Disease* 3, 9–19.

Grimont, P.A. and Weill, F.-X. (2007) Antigenic formulas of the *Salmonella* serovars. WHO collaborating centre for reference and research on *Salmonella*, Institute Pasteur. Institut Pasteur, Paris, France. Available at: http://www.pasteur.fr/ip/portal/action/WebdriveActionEvent/oid/01s-000036-089 (accessed 1 March 2013).

Guibourdenche, M., Roggentin, P., Mikoleit, M., Fields, P.I., Bockemühl, J., Grimont, P.A.D. and Weill, F.X. (2010) Supplement 2003-2007 (No. 47) to the White-Kauffmann-Le Minor scheme. *Research in Microbiology* 161, 26–29.

Hackl, E., Konrad-Köszler, M., Kilian, A., Wenzl, P., Kornschober, C. and Sessitsch, A. (2010) Phage-type specific markers identified by diversity array technology (DArT) analysis of *Salmonella enterica* ssp. *enterica* serovars Enteritidis and Typhimurium. *Journal of Microbiological Methods* 80, 100–105.

Hajjar, A.M., Ernst, R.K., Tsai, J.H., Wilson, C.B. and Miller, S.I. (2002) Human Toll-like receptor 4 recognizes host-specific LPS modifications. *Nature Immunology* 3, 354–359.

Hatta, M., Pastoor, R., Scheelbeek, P.F.D., Sultan, A.R., Dwiyanti, R. *et al.* (2011) Multi-Locus variable-number tandem repeat profiling of *Salmonella enterica* serovar Typhi isolates from blood cultures and gallbladder specimens from Makassar, South-Sulawesi, Indonesia. *PLoS ONE* 6: e24983.

Hendriksen, R.S., Mikoleit, M., Carlson, V.P., Karlsmose, S., Viera, A.R., Jensen, A.B., Seyfarth, A.M., Delong, S.M., Weill, F.X., Lo Fo Wong, D.M.A., Anguola, F.J., Wegener, H.C. and Aarestrup, F.M. (2009) WHO global Salm-sruv external quality assurance system (EQAS) for serotyping of *Salmonella* isolates, 2000-2007. *Journal of Clinical Microbiology* 47, 2729–2736.

Herrera-León, S., McQuiston, J.R., Usera, M.A., Fields, P.I., Garaizar, J. and Echeita, M.A. (2004) Multiplex PCR for distinguishing the most common phase-1 flagellar antigens of *Salmonella* spp. *Journal of Clinical Microbiology* 42, 2581–2588.

Hong, Y., Liu, T., Hofacre, C., Maier, M., White, D.G., Ayers, S., Wang, L. and Maurer, J.J. (2003) A restriction fragment length polymorphism-based polymerase chain reaction as an alternative to serotyping for identification of *Salmonella* serotypes. *Avian Diseases* 47, 387–395.

Hopkins, K.L., Kirchner, M., Guerra, B., Granier, S.A., Lucarelli, C., Porrero, M.C., Jakubxzak, A., Threlfall, E.J. and Mevius, D.J. (2010) Multiresistant *Salmonella enterica* serovar 4, [5],12:i:- om Europe: a new pandemic strain? *Eurosurveillance* 15, pii:19580.

Hu, H., Lan, R. and Reeves, P.R. (2002) Fluorescent amplified fragment length polymorphism analysis of *Salmonella enterica* serovar Typhimurium reveals phage-type specific markers and potential for microarray typing. *Journal of Clinical Microbiology* 40, 3406–3415.

Kafatos, G., Andrews, N., Gillespie, I.A., Adak, G.K., De Pinna, E. and Threlfall, E.J. (2009) Impact of reduced numbers of isolates phage-typed on the detection of *Salmonella* outbreaks. *Epidemiology and Infection* 137, 821–827.

Kang, M.-S., Besser, T.E., Hancock, D.D., Porwollik, S., McClelland, M. and, Call, D.R. (2006) Identification of specific gene sequences conserved in contemporary epidemic strains of *Salmonella enterica*. *Applied and Environmental Microbiology* 72, 6938–6947.

Kidgell, C., Reichard, U., Wain, J., Linz, B., Torpdahl, M., Dougan, G. and Achtman, M. (2002) *Salmonella typhi*, the causative agent of typhoid fever, is approximately 50,000 years old. Infection, Genetics and Evolution 2, 39–45.

Kim, S., Frye, J.G., Hu, J., Fedorka-Cray, P.J., Gautom, R. and Boyle, D.S. (2006) Multiplex PCR-based method for identification of common clinical serotypes of *Salmonella enterica* subsp. *enterica*. *Journal of Clinical Microbiology* 44, 3608–3615.

Kingsley, R.A. and Bäumler, A.J. (2000) Host adaptation and the emergence of infectious disease: the *Salmonella* paradigm. *Molecular Microbiology* 36, 1006–1014.

Lan, R., Reeves, P.R. and Octavia, S. (2009) Population structure, origin and evolution of major *Salmonella enterica* clones. *Infection, Genetics and Evolution* 9, 996–1005.

Langridge, G.C., Wain, J. and Nair, S. (2008) Invasive salmonellosis in humans. Non-typhoidal *Salmonella* serovars cause different degrees of invasive disease globally. *Journal of Infectious Diseases* 199, 602.

Larsson, J.T., Torpdahl, M., Petersen, R.F., Sørensen, G., Lindstedt, B.A. and Nielsen, E.M. (2009) Development of a new nomenclature for *Salmonella* Typhimurium multilocus variable number of tandem repeats analysis (MLVA). *Euro Surveillance* 14, pii=19174.

Lindsted, B.A., Heir, E., Gjernes, E. and Kapperud, G. (2003) DNA fingerprinting of *Salmonella enterica* subspecies *enterica* serovar Typhimurium with emphasis on phage type DT104 based on variable number of tandem repeat loci. *Journal of Clinical Microbiology* 41, 1469–1479.

Lindsted, B.A., Vardund, T., Aas, L. and Kapperud, G. (2004) Multiple-locus variable number tandem repeats analysis of *Salmonella enterica* subspecies *enteria* serovar Typhimurium using PCR multiplexing and multicolor capillary electrophoresis. *Journal of Microbiological Methods* 59, 163–172.

Littrup, E., Torpdahl, M., Marlorny, B., Huehn, S., Helms, M., Christensen, H., Nielsen, E.M. (2010a) DNA microarray analysis of *Salmonella* serotype Typhimurium strains causing different symptoms of disease. *BMC Microbiology* 10, 96.

Littrup, E., Torpdahl, M., Marlorny, B., Huehn, S., Christensen, H. and Nielsen, E.M. (2010b) Association between phylogeny, virulence potential and serovars of *Salmonella enterica*. *Infection, Genetics and Evolution* 10, 1132–1139.

Liu, B., Zhang, L., Zhu, X., Shi, C., Chen, J., Jiu, W., He, X. and Shi, X. (2011) PCR identification of *Salmonella* serogroups based on specific targets obtained by comparative genomics. *International Journal of Food Microbiology* 144, 511–518.

Liu, Y., Lee, M.-A., Ooi, E.-E., Mavis, Y., Tan, A.-L. and Quek, H.-H. (2003) Molecular typing of *Salmonella enterica* serovar Typhi isolates from various countries in Asia by a multiplex PCR assay on variable-number tandem repeats. *Journal of Clinical Microbiology* 41, 4388–4394.

Loman, N.J., Misra, R., Dallman, T.J., Constantinidou, C., Gharbia, S.E., Wain, J. and Pallen, M.J. (2012) Performance comparison of benchtop high-throughput sequencing platforms. *Nature Biotechnology* 30, 434–439.

Luk, J.M., Kongmuang, U., Reeves, P.R. and Lindberg, A.A. (1993) Selective amplification of abequose and paratose synthase genes (*rfb*) by polymerase chain reaction for identification of *Salmonella* major serogroups (A, B, C2, and D). *Journal of Clinical Microbiology* 31, 2118–2123.

Macnab, R.M. (1996) Flagella and motility. In: Niedhardt, F.C. *et al.* (eds) *Escherichia coli and Salmonella: Cellular and Molecular Biology*, 2nd edn. AMS Press, Washington, DC, pp. 123–145.

Majtan, T., Majtanova, L., Timlo, J. and Majtan, V. (2007) Oligonucleotide microarray for molecular characterization and genotyping of *Salmonella* strains. *Journal of Antimicrobial Chemotherapy* 60, 937–946.

Malorny, B., Bunge, C., Guerra, B., Prietz, S. and Helmuth, R. (2007) Molecular characterization of *Salmonella* strains by an oligonucleotide multiprobe microarray. *Molecular and Cellular Probes* 21, 56–65.

Malorny, B., Junker, E. and Helmuth, R. (2008) Multi-locus variable-number tandem repeat analysis for outbreak studies of *Salmonella enterica* serotype Enteritidis. *BMC Microbiology* 8, 84.

Malorny, B., Hauser, E. and Diekerman, R. (2011) New Approaches in Subspecies-level *Salmonella* Classification. In: Porwollik, S. (ed.) *Salmonella, from Genome to Function*. Caister Academic Press, Norfolk, UK, pp. 1–24.

McQuiston, J.R., Waters, R.J., Dinsmore, B.A., Mikoleit, M.L. and Fields, P. (2011) Molecular determination of H antigens of *Salmonella* by use of a microsphere-based liquid array. *Journal of Clinical Microbiology* 49, 565–573.

Mertes, F., Biens, K., Lehrach, H., Wagner, M. and Dahl, A. (2010) High-throughput universal probe *Salmonella* serotyping (UPSS) by nanoPCR. *Journal of Microbiological Methods* 83, 217–223.

Morales, C.A., Gast, R. and Guard-Bouldin, J. (2006) Linkage of avian and reproductive tract tropism with sequence divergence adjacent to the 5S ribosomal subunit rrfH of *Salmonella enterica*. *FEMS Microbiology Letters* 264, 48–58.

Morales, C.A., Musgrove, M., Humphrey, J., Cates, C., Gast, R. and Guard-Bouldin, J. (2007) Pathotyping of *Salmonella enterica* by analysis of single-nucleotide polymorphisms in cyaA and flanking 23S ribosomal sequences. *Environmental Microbiology* 9, 1047–1059.

Murphy, T.M., McNamara, E., Hill, M., Rooney, N., Barry, J., Egan, J., O'Connell, A., O'Loughlin, J. and McFaddyen, S. (2001) Epidemiological studies on human and animal *Salmonella* Typhimurium DT104 and DT104b isolates in Ireland. *Epidemiology and Infection* 126, 3–9.

Olsen, J.E. and Skov, M.N. (1994) Genomic lineage of *Salmonella dublin*. *Veterinary Microbiology* 40, 271–282.

Peters, T.M., Maguire, C., Threlfall, E.J., Fisher, I.S., Gill, O.N. and Gatto, A.J. (2003) The Salm-gene project – a European collaboration for DNA fingerprinting for food-related salmonellosis. *Euro Surveillance* 8, pii=401.

Peters, T.M., Berghold, C., Brown, D., Coia, J., Dionisi, A.M., Echeita, A., Fisher, I.S.T., Gatto, A.J., Gill, N., Green, J., Gerner-Smidt, P., Heck, M., Lederer, I., Lukinmaa, S., Luzzi, I., Magurie, C., Prager, R., Usera, M., Siitinen, A., Threlfall, E.J., Torpdahl, M., Tschäpe, H., Wannet, W. and Van der Zwaluw, W.K. (2007) Relationship of pulsed-field profiles with key phage types of *Salmonella enterica* serotype Enteritidis in Europe: results of an international multi-centre study. *Epidemiology and Infection* 135, 1274–1281.

Peters, T., Hopkins, K.L., Lane, C., Nair, S., Wain, J. and De Pinna, E. (2010) Emergence and characterization of *Salmonella enterica* serovar Typhimurium phage type DT191a. *Journal of Clinical Microbiology* 48, 3375–3377.

Peterson, G., Gerdes, B., Berges, J., Nagaraja, T.G., Frey, J.G., Boyle, D.S., Narayanan, S. (2010) Development of microarray and multiplex polymerase chain reaction assays for identification of serovars and virulence genes in *Salmonella enterica* of human origin. *Journal of Veterinary Diagnostic Investigations* 22, 559–569.

Pickard, D., Wain, J., Baker, S., Line, A., Cohan, S., Fookes, M., Barron, A., Ogaora, P., Chbalgoity, A., Thanky, N., Scholes, C., Thomson, N., Parkhill, J. and Dougan, G. (2003) Composition, acquisition, and distribution of the Vi exopolysaccharide-encoding *Salmonella enterica* pathogenicity island SPI-7. *Journal of Bacteriology* 185, 5055–5065.

Porwollik, S., Wong, R.M. and McClelland, M. (2002) Evolutionary genomics of *Salmonella:* gene acquisitions revealed by microarray analysis. *Proceedings of the National Academy of Sciences, USA* 99, 8956–8961.

Porwollik, S., Boyed, S.F., Choy, C., Cheng, P., Florea, L., Proctor, E. and McClelland, M. (2004) Characterization of *Salmonella enterica* subspecies I genovars by use of microarrays. *Journal of Bacteriology* 186, 977–989.

Raetz, C.R.H. (1996) Bacterial lipopolysaccharides: a remarkable family of bioactive macroamphiphiles. In: Niedhardt, F.C *et al.* (eds) Escherichia coli *and* Salmonella*: Cellular and Molecular Biology*, 2nd edn. AMS Press, Washington, DC, pp. 1035–1063.

Rajtak, U., Leonard, N., Bolton, D. and Fanning, S. (2011) A real-time multiplex SYBR Green I polymerase chain reaction assay for rapid screening of *Salmonella* serotypes prevalent in the European Union. *Foodborne Pathogens and Disease* 8, 769–780.

Reeves, P.R., Hobbs, M., Miguel, A., Valvano, A.M., Skurnik, M., Whitfield, C., Coplin, D., Kido, N., Klena, K., Maskell, D., Raetz, R.H.C. and Rick P.D. (1996) Bacterial polysaccharide synthesis and gene nomenclature. *Trends in Microbiology* 4, 495–503.

Reeves, P.R., Liu, B., Zhou, Z., Li, D., Guo, D., Ren, Y., Clabots, C., Lan, R., Johnson, J.R. and Wang, L. (2011) Rates of Mutation and Host Transmission for an *Escherichia coli* Clone over 3 Years. *PLoS ONE* 6: e26907.

Ribot, E.M., Fair, M.A., Gautom, R., Cameron, D.N., Hunter, S.B., Swaminathan, B. and Barrett, T.J. (2006) Standardization of pulsed-field gel electrophoresis protocols for the subtyping of *Escherichia coli* O157:H7, *Salmonella*, and *Shigella* for PulseNet. *Foodborne Pathogens and Disease* 3, 59.

Roumagnac, P., Weill, F.X., Dolecek, C., Baker, S., Brisse, S., Chinh, N.T., Le, T.A., Acosta, C.J., Farrar, J., Dougan, G. and Achtman, M. (2006) Evolutionary history of *Salmonella* Typhi. *Science*, 1301–1304.

Sangal, V., Harbottle, H., Mazzoni, C.J., Helmuth, R., Guerra, B., Didelot, X., Paglietti, B., Rabsch, W., Brisse, S., Weill, F.-X., Roumagnac, P. and Achtman, M. (2010) Evolution and population structure of *Salmonella enterica* serovar Newport. *Journal of Bacteriology* 192, 6465-6476.

Scaria, J., Palaniappan, R.U.M., Chiu, D., Phan, J.A., Ponnala, L., McDonough, P., Grohn, Y., Prowollik, S., McClelland, M., Chiou, C.S., Chu, C. and Chang, Y.-F. (2008) Microarray for molecular typing of *Salmonella enterica* serovars. *Molecular and Cellular Probes* 22, 238–243.

Schwartz, D.C., Saffran, W., Welsh, J., Haas, R., Goldenberg, M. and Cantor, C.R. (1983) New techniques for purifying large DNAs and studying their properties and packaging. Cold Spring Harbor, *Symposia on Quantitative Biology* 47, 190–195.

Schwarz, S. and Liebisch, B. (1994) Pulsed field gel electrophoretic identification of *Salmonella enterica* serovar Typhimurium live vaccine strain Zoosaloral H. *Letters in Applied Microbiology* 19, 469–472.

Seth-Smith, H.M.B. (2008) SPI-7: *Salmonella's* Vi-Encoding Pathogenicity Island. *Journal of Infection in Developing Countries* 2, 267–271.

Smith, J.M., Smith, N.H., O'Rourke, M. and Spratt, B.G. (1993) How clonal are bacteria. *Proceedings of the National Academy of Sciences, USA* 90, 4384–4388.

Smith, N., Beltran, P. and Selander, R.K. (1990) Recombination of *Salmonella* Phase 1 Flagellin Genes Generates New Serovars. *Journal of Bacteriology* 172, 2209–2216.

Thong, K.L., Cheong, Y.M., Puthucheary, S., Koh, C.L. and Pang, T. (1994) Epidemiology analysis of sporadic *Salmonella typhi* isolates and those from outbreaks by pulsed-field gel electrophoresis. *Journal of Clinical Microbiology* 32, 1135–1141.

Threlfall, E.J. and Frost, J.A. (1990) The identification, typing and fingerprinting of *Salmonella*: laboratory aspects and epidemiological applications. *Journal of Applied Bacteriology* 68, 5–16.

Torpdahl, M., Sørensen, G., Lindstedt, B.-A. and Nielsen, E.M. (2007) Tandem repeat analysis for surveillance of human *Salmonella* Typhimurium infections. *Emerging Infectious Diseases* 13, 388–395.

Uzzau, S., Brown, D.J., Wallis, T.S., Rubino, S., Leori, G., Bernard, S., Casadesús, J., Platt, D.J. and Olsen, J.E. (2000) Host adapted serotypes of *Salmonella enterica*. *Epidemiology and Infection* 125, 229–255.

Wain, J., House, D., Zafa, A., Baker, S., Nair, S., Kidgell, C., Bhutta, Z., Dogan, G. and Hassan, R. (2005) Vi antigen expression in *Salmonella enterica* serovar Typhi clinical isolates from Pakistan. *Journal of Clinical Microbiology* 43, 1158–1165.

Wang, Q., Kong, F., Jelfs, P. and Gilbert, G.L. (2008) Extended phage locus typing of *Salmonella enterica* serovar Typhimurium using multiplex PCR-based revere line blot hybridization. *Journal of Medical Microbiology* 57, 827–838.

Ward, L.R., de Sa, J.D.H. and Rowe, B. (1987) A phage-typing scheme for *Salmonella enteritidis*. *Epidemiology and Infection* 99, 291–294.

Wattiau, P., Boland, C. and Bertrand, S. (2011) Methodologies for *Salmonella enterica* subsp. *enterica* subtyping: gold standards and alternatives. *Applied and Environmental Microbiology* 77, 7877–7885.

Wieser, A., Schneider, L., Jung, J. and Schubert, S. (2012) MALDI-TOF MS in microbiological diagnostics – identification and beyond. *Applied Microbiological Biotechnology* 93, 965–977.

Williamson, C., Bairdt, G.D. and Manning, E.J. (1988) A Common Virulence Region on Plasmids from Eleven Serotypes of *Salmonella*. *Journal of General Microbiology* 134, 975–982.

Xia, L., Peng, K., Yang, S., Wenzl, P., de Vicente, M.C., Fregen, M. and Kilian, A. (2005) DArT for high-throughput genotyping of Cassava (*Manihot esculenta*) and its wild relatives. *Theoretical and Applied Genetics* 100, 1092 1098.

Yoshida, C., Franklin, K.M., Konczy, P., Quiston, J.R., Fields, P., Nash, J.H., Taboada, E.N. and Rahn, K. (2007) Methodologies towards the development of an oligonucleotide microarray for determination of *Salmonella* serotypes. *Journal of Microbiological Methods* 70, 261–271.

25 Other Approaches to Infection Control

Filip van Immerseel[1]* and Robert J. Atterbury[2]
[1]Department of Pathology, Bacteriology and Avian Diseases, Ghent University, Belgium; [2]School of Veterinary Medicine and Science, University of Nottingham, UK

Introduction

The epidemiology of *Salmonella* infection in poultry is complex, but in summary, the major sources of infection for poultry are the birds themselves, feed and the environment (including housing). It is possible to rear poultry totally in the absence of *Salmonella*. Large breeding companies and research establishments do it at a high cost. This is done through the introduction of improved housing and diet, together with employment of skilled staff and efficient management structures. In addition, introduction of thorough hygiene and disinfection measures and other schemes to reduce the chances of cross-infection, such as 'all in-all out' rearing are required. In some cases these things will be possible and, as existing housing degenerates, requiring replacement, improvements can be made slowly. In countries with high ambient temperatures, open-sided housing may limit the extent to which improvements may contribute to reduce environmental sources of infection. However, the financial incentives to eliminate a food-poisoning pathogen from stock, which has very little direct impact on productivity and for which financial incentives are not available, poses considerable imponderable problems for poultry companies worldwide. It seems likely, therefore, for the foreseeable future, that biological control measures will be an increasingly attractive option. Some of the major options explored by poultry scientists over the years and used extensively include competitive exclusion (Chapter 21, this volume) and the use of vaccination (Chapter 22, this volume). In addition, antibiotic therapy or prophylaxis has been advocated at various times in the past but the general consensus of opinion is that it is less effective than would be expected and that it inevitably induces resistance either in the *Salmonella* themselves or in the normal flora (Chapter 7, this volume).

More recently other different approaches to infection control have been explored and this review summarizes the recent work in two of these areas, namely the use of volatile fatty acids as feed components and the use of lytic bacteriophages.

* Corresponding author, e-mail: filip.vanimmerseel@UGent.be

© CAB International 2013. *Salmonella in Domestic Animals, 2nd Edition* (eds P.A. Barrow and U. Methner)

The Use of Organic Acids as Feed or Drinking Water Additive to Control *Salmonella* in Pigs and Poultry

Antimicrobial activity of organic acids

Organic acids are a group of compounds characterized by a –COOH bond and with proton dissociation dependent on pH. Many different organic acids exist, from simple short-chain to medium- and long-chain fatty acids, to side-chained simple and complex acids, and aromatic acids. It is clear that the antibacterial activity of these acids differs between molecules, depending on the chemical structure. In addition, for certain acids there is a large difference in minimal inhibitory concentrations (MIC) when different bacterial species are exposed (Hsiao and Siebert, 1999). Not all acids are tested for their antibacterial properties against *Salmonella*, but for those that are potential feed additives (e.g. low toxicity, easy accessible, low price) some data on this exist.

Medium-chain fatty acids (C6 to C12; caproic, caprylic, capric and lauric acid) are much more antibacterial against *Salmonella* than the short-chain fatty acids (formic, acetic, propionic and butyric acid) (Van Immerseel *et al.*, 2003, 2004a; Thormar *et al.*, 2006; Boyen *et al.*, 2008). In an *in vitro* continuous culture system, simulating the porcine caecum, it was shown that caprylic acid reduced counts of *Salmonella* significantly, while the effect on the number of lactic acid bacteria and total anaerobes was much less pronounced (Messens *et al.*, 2010). Longer chain fatty acids are less or not at all bactericidal, depending on the specific compound (Sprong *et al.*, 2001).

The ability of organic acids to pass across the cell membrane and dissociate in the more alkaline cytoplasm resulting in acidification was years ago used to explain the antimicrobial properties of these acids (Kashket, 1987). Organic acids were compared to synthetic uncouplers that could remain membrane associated, and shuttle protons in a cyclic manner to dissipate the proton-motive force. This theory, however, did not explain the differences in susceptibility between bacterial species for acids and acidic compounds are charged and will not remain in the cell membrane as do synthetic uncouplers (Russell and Diez-Gonzalez, 1998). It became clear that anion accumulation is a major cytotoxic event for bacteria. Indeed, many bacteria have the potential to decrease their intracellular pH in an acidic extracellular environment, requiring a metabolism that is able to tolerate a low intracellular pH. When intracellular pH is required to remain high, the pH gradient across the cell membrane would become very large, resulting in pumping out protons from the cell. This would cause a logarithmic accumulation of the acid anions, which is thought to be toxic for the bacterial cell. If the bacterial mechanisms to withstand a decrease in intracellular pH function correctly, then the pH gradient across the cell membrane could be low and anion accumulation would not occur. Also the intracellular levels of ions that have a countering effect (such as K^+) are believed to be important in protection against anion accumulation resulting from exposure to acids (Diez-Gonzalez and Russell, 1997; Flythe and Russell, 2006, 2007; Van Immerseel *et al.*, 2006). The existence of stress response mechanisms that aid in protection against acid stresses has also been described, but the nature of these responses and the relative contribution is still not fully resolved.

Organic acids and their effects on virulence of *Salmonella*

Products for *Salmonella* aim to reduce shedding and colonization of the gut (and internal organs, e.g. to control egg contamination in layers). Thus one of the most important biological functions of *Salmonella* that must be controlled is invasion of intestinal epithelial cells, because this virulence attribute is directly linked to gut colonization in poultry and pigs (Boyen *et al.*, 2006; Bohez *et al.*, 2008). Invasion is dependent on invasion genes that are located on a pathogenicity island (SPI-1), and on the function encoded by other genes, indirectly linked to adhesion or invasion such as fimbriae and flagella. SPI-1 harbours genes encoding regulatory proteins, structural components of a needle complex and additional effector proteins that are injected in the cytoplasm of eukaryotic cells to induce actin rearrangements that promote uptake of the bacteria in the cells, defined as invasion. The most important regulatory gene of SPI-1 is the environmentally regulated gene *hilA*. Many triggers activate *hilA* expression, and organic acids have been shown to differentially regulate *hilA* expression, depending on the nature of the organic acid. *Salmonella* Enteritidis and Typhimurium were less invasive in human and porcine intestinal epithelial cell lines and primary chicken caecal epithelial cells *in vitro*, when pre-incubated with propionic and butyric acid, but more invasive when pre-incubated in medium supplemented with acetic acid (Durant *et al.*, 1999; Lawhon *et al.*, 2002; Van Immerseel *et al.*, 2004a, b; Boyen *et al.*, 2008). This was shown to be correlated with effects on *hilA* expression. Acetate, after its conversion to acetyl-phosphate, acts to phosphorylate BarA and subsequently SirA. The two-component system BarA/SirA is involved in sensing environmental triggers and *sirA* positively regulates *hilA*, hereby activating SPI-1 and stimulating invasion (Lawhon *et al.*, 2002). Propionate and butyrate decrease *hilA* expression (Lawhon *et al.*, 2002) explaining the decreased invasive phenotype. Interestingly, it was shown that very low concentrations of butyrate affect SPI-1 gene expression while not having effects on metabolic gene expression (Gantois *et al.*, 2006). Also *hilD*, a positive regulator of *hilA*, was shown to be down-regulated by butyrate. Although it is clear that butyrate is a specific inhibitor of SPI-1 gene expression, the actual mechanism of inhibition and the primary target of butyrate in *Salmonella* is still not clear. Short-chain fatty acids also activate acid-resistance phenotypes, which may be involved in survival in acidic environments, such as the stomach and the intracellular compartments in which they reside in macrophages (Kwon and Ricke, 1998). Whether this acid resistance is an important factor involved in pathogenesis is also not clear.

Efficacy of organic acids to decrease shedding and colonization of *Salmonella* inpigs andpoultry

The concept of using organic acids to control pathogens in food preservation has been understood for a long time. The use of organic acids to control *Salmonella* was initially based on decontamination of carcass meat and feed (Khan and Katamay, 1969). The original concept of incorporating acids into feed was based on the idea that the acids would decontaminate the feed itself and prevent *Salmonella* uptake by the animals, thereby preventing colonization and shedding. There are some studies showing significant decreases in the number of *Salmonella* bacteria in poultry feed when mixtures and formic and propionic acid were added to the feed with an associated lower caecal colonization when chickens were fed treated feed versus non-treated feed (Hinton and Linton, 1988; Iba and Berchieri, 1995). Humphrey and Lanning (1988) showed a decrease in the number of *Salmonella* positive feed samples from 4.1 to 1.1% after formic acid supplementation. Also the concept of drinking water decontamination was initially and still is meant to kill the bacteria in the drinking water, and not in the live animal. When the organic acid concentration in the drinking water is sufficiently high, the low pH in the drinking water will result in bacterial killing. Decontamination of both drinking water and feed will thus create a barrier to prevent uptake of *Salmonella* after contamination (feed) or recontamination (feed, drinking water from litter). As the antibacterial properties of organic acids are dependent on the temperature and water activity, there is a tendency to believe that, although some studies show good results, properly stored dry feed is not a good matrix for decontamination with organic acids. The observation that concentrations of organic acids also increased in the proximal gastrointestinal compartments, such as the crop in chickens, after uptake of acid-supplemented feed, steered the concept of administering acids to the feed and drinking water towards killing *Salmonella* in the live animal. The higher temperature and moistening of the feed would result in a much higher activity of the acids as compared to their within-feed activity. Short-chain fatty acid preparations that were on the market initially were powder-form, drinking water and feed additives. With powder-form products, the action is most likely limited to the upper gastrointestinal tract, such as the crop of chickens and the stomach. Indeed, it has been shown that short-chain fatty acids present in feed cannot be detected further down in the gastrointestinal tract, most likely due to absorption by the intestinal mucosa (Hume *et al.*, 1993; Thompson and Hinton, 1997). From the 1980s onwards, numerous studies have been published on the effects of supplementing powder-form organic acids in feed on colonization of *Salmonella*, mainly in chickens. These studies are summarized in a review of Van Immerseel *et al.* (2006) and show the efficacy of different acids, either or not in combination with each other, against colonization of different *Salmonella* serotypes. Studies using powder-form organic acids affecting shedding and intestinal colonization of pigs have also been published (Taube *et al.*, 2009; Martin-Pelaez *et al.*, 2010). Both short-chain and medium-chain fatty acids can have protective effects. To optimize the efficacy of the acid formulations, novel technologies have been developed to release the acids further down in the gastrointestinal tract. Systems to impregnate the acids into a carrier have been developed with different coatings, to prevent absorption of the acids in the upper gastrointestinal tract and ensure release further down in the gastrointestinal tract. There are few detailed studies showing dynamics of release of acids throughout the gastrointestinal tract using these delivery systems, and although many products are on the market, it is not clear what characteristics the coating material should have to ensure release of the acids at the site of action. Published studies either or do not show effects on *Salmonella* colonization depending on the acids and the formulation used, but the actual properties of the formulations are often not described in detail in such studies. Some studies using short-chain fatty acids encapsulated in micro-beads have been carried out in chickens and in pigs (Van Immerseel *et al.*, 2004c; Boyen *et al.*, 2008; Gebru *et al.*, 2010). In a study with chickens the effect on colonization of *S.* Enteritidis in caeca and internal organs of feed supplementation with micro-beads containing formic, acetic, propionic and butyric acid was studied (Van Immerseel *et al.*, 2004c). The nature of the acid was of crucial importance, as colonization of the caeca and internal organs was increased when acetic acid was used and decreased when propionic and butyric acid was used. Although these data look consistent with the differential ability of the acids to either or not increase invasiveness of the bacterium (see above), effects on the composition of the gut microbiota or on the intestinal architecture (epithelial integrity, inflammation, villus morphology) could also potentially have influenced *Salmonella* colonization. As an example, butyrate has been shown to serve as the direct energy source for colon epithelial cells, possess anti-inflammatory properties, stimulate production of mucins and host antimicrobial peptides and possibly as a consequence, it improves body weight gain in animals (reviewed by Guilloteau *et al.*, 2010). A comparative study of Van Immerseel *et al.* (2005) showed that a coated butyrate feed additive decreased shedding and caecal colonization of *Salmonella* in broiler chickens while a powder-form product had no effect. Coated butyrate also decreased shedding and intestinal colonization in pigs in contrast to uncoated butyric acid, supporting the data derived from chickens (Boyen *et al.*, 2008).

A novel strategy to increase gut health and control *Salmonella*: steering towards a butyrate-producing microbiota in the caeca

Feed and drinking water sanitation can prevent initial contamination and recontamination of animals with *Salmonella*. Powder-form applications in feed can decrease the bacterial load and the numbers of *Salmonella* bacteria in the upper gastrointestinal tract. New strategies are currently being explored to deliver acids further down in the gastrointestinal tract where the microbiota composition is such that short-chain fatty acid, such as butyrate, production is possible. This could theoretically be done using feed supplementation with compounds that are converted to butyrate by the resident microbiota, such as inulin and resistant starch, or by administration of bacteria, such as lactic acid bacteria, that are butyrogenic. The lactic acid produced is used by strictly anaerobic firmicute bacteria that belong to some specific clostridial clusters (IV, XIVa, XIVb, XVI) to produce butyric acid. This concept is called cross-feeding, and it could explain why the effect of administration of lactic acid bacteria is variable, i.e. the efficacy could depend on the quantity of butyrate-producing bacteria that are present in the caeca or the hindgut of poultry and pigs. Although these bacteria are well described for the human gut, the presence of these species in animals has only recently been described. In the broiler chicken caeca, the butyrate-producing *Clostridium* cluster XIVa and *Clostridium* cluster IV species were shown to be predominant (Gong *et al.*, 2002; Lan *et al.*, 2002; Zhu *et al.*, 2002; Dumonceaux *et al.*, 2006). In a recent study of Eeckhaut *etal.* (2011), 16 new butyrate-producing bacterial species of six novel genera were isolated from the chicken caecum, of which two have been described in detail (Eeckhaut *et al.*, 2008, 2010). Most of these species contain the butyryl-CoA:acetate CoA-transferase gene (Eeckhaut *et al.*, 2011), which can be used as a marker to quantify the potency of the chicken caecal microbiota to produce butyrate, and thus to evaluate the effect of prebiotic compounds to stimulate butyrate production. Whether the butyrate-producing species can be used in a probiotic approach is still not clear, because these species are not easy to culture and administration can be difficult as a result of their anaerobic nature. Stimulating colonization and butyrate production by these bacterial species could be an efficient alternative to the use of short-chain fatty acids in feed. Dietary composition might influence microbiota composition and stimulate the presence of these novel identified species, which could be a very cost-effective way to control *Salmonella*.

The success of organic acids: a dual function

As a result of the antimicrobial properties of organic acids they also improve nutrient digestibility, and thus enhance body weight gain and feed conversion. After the EU ban on the use of antimicrobial growth promoters (AGPs) in 2006, numerous novel compounds were used in the field that were claimed to restore performance parameters to normal levels. Based on the definition of AGPs these products should reduce the incidence and severity of subclinical infections, reduce the microbial use of nutrients, improve absorption of nutrients and reduce the amount of growth-depressing metabolites produced by gram-positive bacteria (reviewed by Huyghebaert *et al.*, 2011). A variety of compounds, under which prebiotics, probiotics, acids and, more recently, essential oils and herbicidal compounds have been suggested as alternatives for AGPs. Organic acids, including butyric acid, have been shown to be good candidates to, at least partially, replace AGPs. It is not surprising that, because of their growth-promoting and anti-*Salmonella* properties, organic acid products are currently widely used as feed and drinking water additives in different farm animal species, mainly pigs and poultry. They also seem to suppress novel disease entities that have emerged after the EU ban on AGPs, related to disturbances in the general homeostasis of the gut ecosystem, generally referred to as intestinal health problems. These multiple benefits, and mainly the economic advantage coupled to the use of organic acids, should give these compounds a long-lasting future as feed or drinking water additives in production animals.

Biological Approaches to Controlling *Salmonella*: Bacteriophage and *Bdellovibrio*

Introduction

Bacteriophage, often abbreviated to 'phage', are viruses that infect susceptible species of bacteria. As with all other viruses, phage are obligate intracellular parasites and are usually recovered from the same environments occupied by their hosts. They are thought to be the most abundant biological entity on the planet, with an estimated 10^{30} to 10^{32} virions in the biome (Boyd and Brussow, 2002; Rohwer and Edwards, 2002). Their discovery was credited separately to Twort (1915) and d'Herelle (1917), although observations by Hankin antedated both of these reports (Kutter, 2005). Bacteriophage can be ascribed to one of 12 families on the basis of morphological characteristics and nucleic acid content (Ackermann, 2001). The majority of bacteriophage isolated to date belong to the Caudovirales order (tailed phage, dsDNA genome), which comprises the *Myoviridae*, *Siphoviridae* and *Podoviridae* families (Ackermann, 2003).

The bacteriophage life cycle can be divided into two broad strategies, lysogenic or lytic. Both of these strategies begin in the same way, with attachment to and penetration of the host bacterium's cell wall and injection of the viral nucleic acid into the cytoplasm. From there onwards, the strategies diverge. The genome of a phage entering a lysogenic life cycle establishes a stable presence in its host (prophage) and is replicated, either autonomously or as an integrated region of the host chromosome, for an indefinite period of time until a change in the environment of the cell triggers entry into the lytic cycle. This trigger could result from any number of environmental changes. Induction of the lytic cycle in lambdoid phage can be achieved artificially by exposing lysogens to physical or chemical agents that damage DNA, such as UV light or mitomycin C (Smith *et al.*, 1983). Bacteriophages that enter a lytic life cycle without the capability of replicating in a lysogen are termed virulent. These phages sequester and redirect many of the host cell's metabolic pathways to produce a number of phage progeny. These daughter phages are released from the infected cell by enzymatic lysis of the cell wall after a relatively fixed interval.

One obvious potential application of bacteriophage is the treatment of bacterial diseases. Interest in the use of bacteriophage to control populations of pathogenic bacteria in animals, humans and the environment has grown considerably in the West over the past three decades. The main reason for this is the growing resistance of bacterial pathogens to antimicrobials, and the resulting limitations governments now place on the use of antibiotics, particularly in food animals. This section provides an overview and discussion of the main issues encountered when considering the use of phage therapy in the food chain, and how these apply specifically to *Salmonella*.

Bacteriophage therapy

The idea of using bacteriophage to reduce pathogen numbers is not new. In 1919, soon after his discovery of bacteriophage, d'Herelle used phage therapy to treat fowl cholera in chickens and bacterial dysentery in humans (Sulakvelidze and Barrow, 2005; Sulakvelidze and Kutter, 2005). Bacteriophage were soon recruited by other researchers to treat a range of diseases, including staphylococcal skin infections (Bruynoghe and Maisin, 1921) and bladder infections (Smith, 1978). However, not all of these early phage therapy trials were successful (Pyle, 1926; Clark and Clark, 1927). Interest in bacteriophage therapy declined in the West during the 1920s and 1930s, which was the result of a number of factors. In the first place, the poor efficacy of commercial bacteriophage products and the exaggerated claims made by their manufacturers badly damaged public confidence in these treatments (Sulakvelidze and Kutter, 2005). In the second place, influential reports by the American Medical Association (Eaton and Bayne-Jones, 1934; Krueger and Scribner, 1941), which both espoused a broadly negative assessment of phage treatments, reinforced the view that phage therapy was a pseudoscience. In the third place, the discovery of penicillin in the 1920s (Smith, 1953) eventually led to significant investment by governments and industry to search for new antimicrobial substances that could be exploited more easily than bacteriophage. The waning interest in phage therapy research as compared with antimicrobial chemotherapy in the West did not occur in

Eastern Europe and the Soviet Union, chiefly due to the paucity of antibiotics in these countries. A number of articles review the history and current development of phage-based treatments in Russia and Eastern Europe (Alisky *et al.*, 1998; Weber-Dabrowska *et al.*, 2000; Sulakvelidze *et al.*, 2001) and they will not be discussed further here.

Significant interest in phage therapy in the West began to grow again in the last two decades of the 20th century, at a time when antimicrobial resistance amongst human and animal pathogens was becoming a serious problem. In many countries the subsequent restrictions placed on the use of antimicrobials, particularly in food animals, served to increase the interest and demand for alternatives to chemotherapy. The potential of phage therapy to meet some of this demand was supported by the pioneering work of H. Williams Smith in the 1980s. His work focused chiefly on the treatment of *Escherichia coli* septicaemia and enteritis in a range of animals including mice, pigs, calves and lambs (Smith and Huggins, 1982, 1983; Smith *et al.*, 1987b). His key findings can be condensed into the following points:

- A single bacteriophage treatment was more effective at reducing mortality in mice with an *E. coli* infection than was eight doses of streptomycin (Smith, 1948).
- Prophylactic administration of bacteriophage 3–5 days before *E. coli* challenge protected mice against potentially lethal infection (Smith, 1948).
- Treating animals with bacteriophage after the onset of clinical symptoms may still result in a significant reduction in mortality compared with untreated control groups (Smith and Huggins, 1983).
- Phage could persist in the bloodstream for 24 h and for several days in the spleen (Smith, 1948).
- Bacteriophage-resistant *E. coli* mutants did develop, but were markedly less virulent than the parent strains (Smith and Huggins, 1983).

Bacteriophage therapy has many advantages when compared with antimicrobial chemotherapy. Phage are both self-replicating and self-limiting, replicating only when permissive hosts are available. Their host range tends to be restricted to one genus (or a cluster of closely related genera), so avoiding the potential disruption of commensal flora (dysbiosis) often seen during the use of broad spectrum antimicrobials. Phage therapy has been used to treat human diseases in countries formerly comprising the USSR, with minimal side effects (Sulakvelidze and Kutter, 2005). The seemingly innocuous nature of bacteriophage in humans was further supported by studies showing no detectable side effects after healthy volunteers were dosed with large numbers of bacteriophage (Ochs *et al.*, 1971; Bruttin and Brussow, 2005). Likewise, treating animals with bacteriophage does not appear to produce any abnormal histological changes, or increase morbidity or mortality (Merril *et al.*, 1996; Biswas *et al.*, 2002; Carlton *et al.*, 2005).

Bacteriophage therapy and *Salmonella*

Salmonella, along with *Campylobacter* and *Listeria*, has been one of main focuses of bacteriophage therapy trials. Most of these studies have used bacteriophage to control *Salmonella* in pigs and poultry rather than to treat human salmonellosis. This is due to several factors including the difficulty and cost of performing human trials, the relatively low financial rewards of developing a treatment for a human infection that can still be treated readily with antimicrobials, and the growing importance of food safety and security accompanied by increasingly stringent regulation of the food industry. Trials of phage-based treatments to reduce *Salmonella* in the food chain typically fall into two main areas, live animal models and surface sanitization.

Phage therapy in live animal models

Poultry

Bacteriophage have been used in various ways to reduce the carriage of *Salmonella* in food animals. The great majority of this work has focused on chickens, for obvious reasons. In fact, the first phage therapy trial was performed by Felix d'Herelle on chickens suffering from fowl typhoid (*S.* Gallinarum). Treatment of chickens with bacteriophage prevented disease in chickens, whereas all of the untreated birds became infected and died. Closer to the present day, Berchieri *et al.* (1991) performed a series of experiments to assess the ability of phage to control infections in 2-day-old chicks that had been challenged with *S.* Typhimurium F98. The results from this study were mixed, with treatment success seemingly dependent on two key factors: the choice and titre of phage. This study also found that the efficacy of some phage treatments was poor *in vivo*, despite the ability of these phage to infect *S.* Typhimurium F98 *in vitro*. Moreover, even phage that were effective *in vivo* needed to be administered in high titres ($>10^{11}$ PFU ml^{-1}) (PFU, plaque-forming units) if *Salmonella* numbers were to be reduced significantly (by 2 log_{10} colony-forming units (CFU) g^{-1} in the intestinal lumen), and even this effect was short-lived (<24h), notwithstanding a significant reduction in mortality. The contrast between the results obtained from this trial and those of d'Herelle serve to highlight the need to optimize phage therapy for different diseases and species, to a degree that may not be required for conventional treatments such as antimicrobial chemotherapy.

The study by Berchieri *et al.* (1991) outlined above studied the effect of administrating phage preparations by two routes, oral gavage and feed. However, as the two methods used different isolates and titres of phage, no robust comparison between these administration routes could be made. However, this aspect of phage therapy was further explored by Sklar and Joerger (2001). The aim of their study was to reduce the carriage of *S.* Enteritidis in the intestine of chicks by administration of phage either in water, feed or impregnated pieces of agar. In addition, the study compared *Salmonella* counts in birds given single and multiple phage treatments. Only two of the five trials performed resulted in statistically significant reductions in *Salmonella* numbers colonizing the chicken caeca compared with the control groups, and even then the reductions were small (0.3 to 1.3 log_{10} CFU g^{-1} caecal contents). The greatest reductions in *Salmonella* numbers were in birds given phage-treated feed. However, the authors noted that viability of phage in feed was poor, with a 1 log_{10} PFU reduction in recoverable phage after feed adsorption and a further 1 log_{10} PFU reduction over 14 days storage, presumably as a result of desiccation. This suggests either that chicken feed is not an ideal medium for phage delivery or that viability in feed matrices should be one of the criteria used to judge the suitability of phage for therapeutic applications. Similar experiments performed recently were successful in reducing *Campylobacter jejuni* colonization of chickens by administrating bacteriophage in feed (Carvalho *et al.*, 2010). However, in this study the feed was inoculated with a suspension of phage immediately before the experiment began, thereby avoiding issues of maintaining a high titre of phage in dry feed over a prolonged period.

Some studies searching for the best way to administer phage to animals have avoided feed altogether and instead focused on different ways of liquid suspension delivery. Borie *et al.* (2008) compared administration of phages by water and coarse spray to 10-day-old chickens 24h prior to challenge with *S.* Enteritidis. At 20 days of age the birds were euthanized and *Salmonella* numbers determined in the caecal contents. Both water and spray treatments resulted in a significant reduction in *Salmonella* colonization (1.42 and 1.63 log_{10} CFU g^{-1} caecal contents, respectively) compared with the control group. However, there was no appreciable difference between the two administration routes.

One of the challenges faced when using bacteriophage to reduce *Salmonella* carriage in animals is the wide range of serovars that may be encountered. One way of approaching this problem is to use cocktails of phage that are able to infect the predominant serovars present in particular animals. Atterbury and Allen (2007) used bacteriophage to reduce caecal colonization in chickens colonized with *Salmonella* serovars Enteritidis, Typhimurium or Hadar. Caecal colonization with the first two serovars was reduced by more than 2.19 log_{10} CFU g^{-1}, but birds colonized with *S.* Hadar remained unaffected. A repeat of the trial using a cocktail of phage with strong lytic activity against *S.* Hadar *in vitro* still did not lead to an appreciable reduction in *S.* Hadar colonization (unpublished data). Interestingly, colonies of *S.* Hadar recovered from phage-treated birds remained sensitive to phage infection, indicating that resistance was unlikely to be responsible for these results.

Another way of addressing the disadvantages of phage with relatively narrow serovar specificity is to complement phage therapy with treatments with a broad effect on *Salmonella* numbers, for example by using vaccination. However, the vaccine would have to be either a killed preparation or comprise live cells, which are not sensitive to phage infection which might otherwise reduce the efficacy of the vaccine. An alternative approach is to use competitive exclusion (CE) products. Toro *et al.* (2005) performed several trials that combined phage therapy with CE. In their first trial, SPF chicks (3 days of age) received a cocktail of three phage 3 days before and 3 days after challenge with *S.* Typhimurium. This resulted in a significant reduction of up to 1.1 $\log_{10}$ CFU g^{-1} in some intestinal compartments such as the ileum. In a second experiment, a phage cocktail was given to birds which had or had not received treatment with a CE product. Although significant reductions in *Salmonella* were achieved in this trial, the authors could find no evidence of synergy between CE and phage therapy. Different results were obtained from a similar study by Borie *et al.* (2009), which indicated that some synergy could be achieved between CE and phage therapy. In this study, groups of chicks were treated with a CE product at 1 day of age and then treated with a cocktail of bacteriophage at 6 days of age. This was followed by a *S.* Enteritidis challenge on day 7. The birds were euthanized 7 days after *Salmonella* challenge and quantitative bacteriology performed on the intestinal contents. Mean *Salmonella* colonization in the caeca of untreated control birds was 1.56×10^5 CFU g^{-1} compared with groups treated with phage only (9.48×10^3 CFU g^{-1}), CE only (4.23×10^3 CFU g^{-1}) or CE plus phage (1.6×10^2 CFU g^{-1}). It seems clear from this study that the combination of CE with phage therapy deserves further investigation.

The potential variability in the efficacy of phage therapy against different serovars highlighted by some of the above studies resulted in some groups developing alternatives to therapy with whole phage particles. In one such study, Waseh *et al.* (2010) used purified tail spike proteins from phage P22 (P22Tsp). These proteins do not kill *Salmonella*, rather they specifically agglutinate *Salmonella* cells even at very low concentrations (149 ng ml^{-1}). The authors demonstrated that P22Tsp are resistant to digestion by many intestinal proteases, and significantly reduce *Salmonella* motility, which is essential for efficient intestinal colonization and invasion by many serovars. Treatment of 2-day-old chicks colonized with *S.* Typhimurium with P22Tsp (30 μg × 3 treatments at 1 h, 18 h and 24 h) significantly reduced *Salmonella* colonization in the caeca, in some cases by greater than 2 $\log_{10}$ CFU g^{-1}. However, delaying treatment to 18 h post-infection did not lead to significant reductions in *Salmonella*. One possible explanation for this is that ingesta may remain in the chicken gizzard for several hours (Smith and Parsell, 1974) and the P22Tsp may have been mixed with *Salmonella* here rather than in the small intestine as was thought to be the case with complete phage in the study of Berchieri *et al.* (1991).

Pigs

Swine are a major source of *Salmonella* entering the food chain and a number of studies describe the use of bacteriophage to reduce *Salmonella* numbers in primary production. Wall *et al.* (2010) used a seeder model to investigate the ability of phage therapy to reduce *Salmonella* colonization and spread. Groups of adult pigs were challenged with *S.* Typhimurium, then after 48 h separate groups of pigs were treated either with a cocktail of 14 microencapsulated phage preparations or with the microencapsulation ingredients only (control). These pigs were then co-mingled with the pigs colonized with *S.* Typhimurium. Phage-treated pigs were re-administered phage every 2 h for 6 h, alongside equivalent treatments with microencapsulation ingredients for the control group. After 6 hours the pigs were euthanized and *Salmonella* enumerated in the intestinal contents. Phage treatment resulted in a significantly lower mean caecal colonization (1.5 $\log_{10}$ CFU ml^{-1}) than pigs given the control treatment (2.9 $\log_{10}$ CFU ml^{-1}). Phage therapy numerically reduced counts in other gut compartments but this was not statistically significant. Similar results were obtained by Smith *et al.* (1987a) who found that phage therapy could significantly reduce caecal populations of *S.* Typhimurium in growing swine by more than 1.4 $\log_{10}$ CFU g^{-1}. Similarly to Wall *et al.* (2010), this study found that *Salmonella* was reduced numerically in the rectum, but this was not statistically significant.

Phage treatments to sanitize surfaces

A range of studies have demonstrated the ability of some phage treatments to reduce *Salmonella* colonization in food animals with a view to this being used eventually on a farm. However, there are a number of potential problems with this approach such as the release and recycling of phage in the environment, which may lead to the development of resistance. Food animals may be reared in very different environments, be fed different diets and be given different vaccines and medications, all of which may affect the efficacy of phage therapy. As such, a number of studies have used phage to sanitize food postharvest where many of these factors can be more easily controlled. The direct application of phage to food surfaces may cause alarm to some members of the public, however it should be noted that phage have been recovered from a wide variety of foods and are regularly consumed by people without ill effects (Kennedy and Bitton, 1987).

Goode *et al.* (2003) experimentally contaminated sections of chicken skin with *S.* Enteritidis and then sprayed these sections with different titres of bacteriophage. The application of bacteriophage at a high multiplicity of infection (MOI) of 10^5 phage:bacteria led to a reduction in *Salmonella* numbers to below detectable limits as determined from *Salmonella* recovery 30 min after phage treatment. Hooton *et al.* (2011) performed similar experiments on the surface of pig skin contaminated with *S.* Typhimurium U288. The results of this study suggested *Salmonella* could be reduced by >1 $\log_{10}$ CFU cm^{-2} of pig skin provided that the MOI was greater than 10. Atterbury and Allen (2007) performed a number of phage surface sanitization trials using chicken skin sections from birds that had been experimentally colonized with different serovars of *Salmonella*, in an effort to produce a more representative distribution of *Salmonella* on the surface of the skin. Following the application of a high titre phage suspension (10^9 PFU), *Salmonella* numbers were reduced to below detectable levels in 73% of treated skin sections after 20 min incubation at room temperature. Although the above results are promising, it would be difficult to spray phage on to the surface of pig or poultry carcasses uniformly. This could result in untreated areas of skin containing high numbers of *Salmonella*.

This issue was addressed in part by Higgins *et al.* (2005), who took whole chicken carcasses from a commercial line, experimentally contaminated them with *S.* Enteritidis and then sprayed the carcass with different titres of bacteriophage (up to ~10^{10} PFU). After phage treatment, *Salmonella* was recovered using a whole carcass rinse, followed by selective culture. The number of carcasses testing positive for *Salmonella* following selective enrichment of the carcass rinses was reduced by up to 93% when compared with the untreated control group. However, this result was only achieved after spraying the carcass with 5.5 ml of a ≥10^8 PFU ml^{-1} phage suspension. In a similar study, Chighladze *et al.* (2001) found that a cocktail of phage could reduce *Salmonella* recovery on experimentally contaminated carcasses by >1000 fold compared with untreated controls.

The effect of temperature on the efficacy of bacteriophage treatment of food surfaces was investigated by Bigwood *et al.* (2008). In this study, cooked and raw beef surfaces were experimentally contaminated with *S.* Typhimurium or *C. jejuni* and then after 10 min, a phage suspension was pipetted on to the contaminated meat surface. Following incubation of the phage-treated and control meat slices at 5°C for 24 h, significant reductions in *Salmonella* numbers (>2 $\log_{10}$ CFU cm^{-2}) were recorded when the MOI was high (10^4). A smaller but significant reduction in *Salmonella* numbers was also seen in the contaminated cooked meat surface after phage treatment. The reduction in *Salmonella* numbers on phage-treated meat sections was maintained for up to 8 days when incubated at 5°C, despite no appreciable increase in phage numbers. Larger reductions in *Salmonella* (>5.9 $\log_{10}$ CFU cm^{-2}) were recorded for contaminated raw meat incubated at 24°C for 24 h. However, this does take into account the growth of *Salmonella* on control meat slices.

Advantages and disadvantages of phage therapy as a control for *Salmonella*

Salmonella is a genetically versatile and hardy organism capable of survival for prolonged periods in harsh environments. *Salmonella* is also able to colonize a wide range of warm- and cold-blooded vertebrate host species, many of which are food animals, with varying clinical consequences. Bacteriophage have some natural advantages over other types of treatment (e.g. antimicrobial chemotherapy) when used to reduce the numbers of *Salmonella* in the food chain. They are intrinsically more flexible and specific than antibiotics, so cocktails of phage can be targeted towards eliminating problem serovars, e.g. *S.* Enteritidis in chickens or *S.* Typhimurium in pigs. The careful selection of a cocktail of phage that adsorb to different surface receptors on *Salmonella* reduces the probability of resistance developing. Moreover, should phage resistance arise, the use of phage that adsorb to conserved receptors on *Salmonella*, preferably those that are involved in colonization or virulence, is more likely to result in mutants that have reduced virulence or colonization potential.

Notwithstanding these advantages, there are some potential pitfalls of phage therapy, some of which are more general problems with this approach and others that are more specific to *Salmonella*. Bacteriophage are capable of mediating the horizontal transfer of DNA between bacteria by specialized and generalized transduction. In some cases, this may result in the transfer of genes which may be associated with enhanced survival and virulence in an animal host. In addition, the phage themselves may carry genes that confer these properties on a bacterium. There are many examples of phage directly contributing to the pathogenicity of bacteria, e.g. *Corynebacterium diphtheriae, Vibrio cholerae, E. coli* O157:H7 (Waldor, 1998; Ho and Slauch, 2001). This is also the case for *Salmonella*, with phage-derived genes such as *sopE* (phage SopEφ), which enhances the uptake of *Salmonella* by eukaryotic cells, and *gipA* (phage Gifsy-1), which is necessary for optimal survival in the Peyer's patch (Wagner and Waldor, 2002). The genome of any one *Salmonella* strain may contain multiple prophages, for example *S.* Typhimurium typically contains between four and five whilst *S.* Typhi has been found to harbour up to seven (for a comprehensive review of *Salmonella* phage and prophage, see Kropinski, 2008). Regions of homology between different prophage, and the bacterial genome, may also lead to genome-wide recombination events and new strains of *Salmonella*. Prophage may also carry genes conferring immunity to super-infection by homologous phage. In the case of phage P22, this is achieved by either a prophage repressor, the prevention of DNA injection or serotype conversion (Kropinski, 2008). These factors make the outcome of any therapeutic application of whole, viable phage particles less certain.

The *in vivo* experimental models of phage therapy described earlier in this chapter have resulted in significant reductions in *Salmonella* colonization of chickens and pigs, but not elimination. Complete elimination of pathogens is not a realistic goal for phage therapy given the number of variables encountered in live animals such as phage resistance, access to and physiological state of the host bacterium, the consistency of gut contents and the presence of non-target 'decoy' bacteria. Even without these variables, mathematical models of phage therapy do not favour elimination, as a minimum density of bacteria is required to support an increase in phage numbers (proliferation threshold). If numbers of bacteria fall below this critical threshold bacteriophage numbers will decrease (O'Brien *et al.*, 1984). The resulting survival and recirculation of *Salmonella* in the animals' environment may reduce the efficacy of phage therapy in the medium to long term if the phage cocktail and method of administration do not change.

The efficacy of phage therapy is contingent upon a number of factors. Clearly, a robust system of selecting candidate therapeutic phage is an essential prerequisite to success. Only exclusively virulent phage should be selected as prospective therapeutic agents in order to minimize the risk of horizontal DNA transfer. In addition, the genomes of these phage should be screened for potentially harmful genes. Ideally, the phage should adsorb to a receptor on the bacterium that is abundant, present and un-obscured in all physiological states and highly conserved within the genus. A cocktail containing phage that separately adsorb to different receptors of this kind would greatly reduce the probability of resistance developing. Thorough characterization of viral replication dynamics is also important, although the results of *in vitro* experiments alone cannot be relied upon as accurate predictors of success *in vivo*. The modelling of phage–host interactions *in vitro* suggests that other characteristics such as the number of phage progeny per infected cell (burst size), the timing of the bacteriophage dose and the presence of decoy hosts are important (Wilkinson, 2001; Payne and Jansen, 2003). This is true, but these factors are necessarily affected by the environment of the animal or food surface to which the phage are being applied. As such, each phage cocktail needs to be optimized for use in a particular animal or food surface. For example, factors such as viability of phage in different parts of the gastrointestinal tract may have a significant impact on the efficacy of phage therapy. In one study, the viability of different *Salmonella* phage in porcine gastric juice could differ by >6 $\log_{10}$ PFU ml^{-1} within 30 min (O'Flynn *et al.*, 2006). The optimization required for treatments based on tail spike proteins or lytic enzymes may not be so onerous as the effects of the animal/food environment on efficacy are likely to be more predictable and reproducible when compared with a cocktail of viable bacteriophage.

The use of predatory bacteria to control *Salmonella* in animals

While bacteriophage therapy has received renewed and increasing interest over the last 30 years, it is by no means the only biological approach to controlling pathogenic bacteria. One relative newcomer to this area is *Bdellovibrio bacteriovorus*, a small, highly motile Gram-negative bacterium, which preys upon and kills other Gram-negative bacteria. *Bdellovibrio* has been shown to prey upon a number of pathogens, including *Salmonella*, and reduce their numbers under laboratory conditions (Dashiff and Kadouri, 2011; Dashiff *et al.*, 2011; Van Essche *et al.*, 2011). However, since the discovery of *B. bacteriovorus* in the early 1960s (Stolp and Starr, 1963), there has been relatively little interest in using this bacterium therapeutically. There are reports that *Bdellovibrio* has been isolated from the intestinal contents of live animals and humans (Schwudke *et al.*, 2001). In addition, some limited studies were undertaken to determine the effect of orally-delivered *Bdellovibrio* preparations on a number of animal species including fish, frogs, mice and rabbits (Westergaard and Kramer, 1977). The authors concluded that *Bdellovibrio* was non-pathogenic to these animal species when delivered orally. The same study also found that *Bdellovibrio* did not multiply inside rabbit ileal loops that were co-infected with enteropathogenic *E. coli*, implying that *Bdellovibrio* would be ineffective as a therapeutic agent in this model. In contrast, a study by Nakamura (1972) found that the injection of *Shigella flexneri* into 16 rabbit ileal loops resulted in fluid accumulation in all 16; whereas simultaneous injection of *S. flexneri* and *B. bacteriovorus* into 16 loops caused fluid accumulation in only one loop. This latter result suggested *Shigella* numbers were being reduced as a consequence of *Bdellovibrio* predation.

More recently, Atterbury *et al.* (2011) investigated the use *Bdellovibrio* to reduce *Salmonella* colonization in chickens. This study aimed to discover whether *Bdellovibrio* treatment was harmful to chickens, and whether *Bdellovibrio* therapy could reduce *Salmonella* numbers in chicken caeca. The first question was addressed by orally inoculating groups of birds with large numbers (1.9×10^6 PFU) of a genome-sequenced strain of *B. bacteriovorus* (HD100). No adverse effects on bird health or weight gain were recorded up to 28 days post-treatment with *Bdellovibrio*. In order to assess the therapeutic efficacy of *Bdellovibrio*, groups of birds were colonized with *S.* Enteritidis P125109 and then orally inoculated with either a wild-type predatory *Bdellovibrio* (HD100) or an isogenic non-predatory Δ*pilA* mutant or buffer (control). The number of *Salmonella* in the caecal contents of HD100-treated birds was significantly lower (by up to 1.09 $\log_{10}$ CFU g^{-1}) than in the buffer-treated control animals. *Salmonella* numbers were also lower in the caeca of HD100-treated birds than in birds treated with the non-predatory Δ*pilA* mutant (by up to 0.78 $\log_{10}$ CFU g^{-1}) which suggests that the reduction in *Salmonella* numbers was dependent upon the *Bdellovibrio* exhibiting a predatory phenotype. However, in concordance with the findings of previous studies, the survival of *Bdellovibrio* in the alimentary tract of chickens was found to be poor.

The therapeutic application of *Bdellovibrio* shares many of the features of bacteriophage therapy but has some important advantages. First, unlike bacteriophage, *Bdellovibrio* are highly motile and are not reliant on diffusion to locate new prey cells. Second, it appears that prey cannot become resistant to *Bdellovibrio* by simple mutation of receptors (as occurs with resistance to bacteriophage). In fact, only one mechanism of resistance to *Bdellovibrio* has ever been demonstrated, that being the production of an intact S-layer (Sockett, 2009). Notwithstanding these advantages, the production of *Bdellovibrio* progeny from a prey cell typically takes 3–4 h, which is generally much slower than bacteriophage replication. In addition, only three to six *Bdellovibrio* progeny are produced per prey cell (Sockett and Lambert, 2004), which is lower than the number of daughter phage produced from most lytic phage which have been characterized. *Bdellovibrio* therapy is still in its infancy and much remains to be discovered about the molecular mechanisms of predation, but this fascinating bacterium has significant potential as a novel therapeutic in the future.

Concluding Comments

Bacteriophage therapy is potentially an effective means by which *Salmonella* colonization can be reduced in food animals and associated products. However, there are a number of issues that need to be addressed before the widespread use of phage therapy could be considered as an alternative to antimicrobials. Among the most important of these are: (i) the development of resistance and recirculation of phage in the environment; (ii) the ability of phage to be used following the onset of clinical symptoms of disease, particularly with pathogens that are intracellular or where multiple bacteria are involved in the infection; (iii) the facilitation of DNA transfer between bacteria via transduction; and (iv) defensibility of intellectual property and regulatory approval. Notwithstanding these issues, phage-based biocontrol has a place in reducing *Salmonella* in the human food chain. The use of predatory bacteria such as *B. bacteriovorus* to control *Salmonella* in animals is a new approach, which warrants further investigation. *Bdellovibrio* shares many of the benefits of bacteriophage when applied therapeutically, whilst possessing unique advantages of its own, such as the ability to actively seek new prey cells and the limited ability of prey to become resistant to predation. Some recent studies have taken important first steps towards the use of *Bdellovibrio* to control bacterial pathogens, and with further optimization and development this bacterium has the potential to be a useful tool in the fight against antimicrobial-resistant pathogens.

References

Ackermann, H.W. (2001) Frequency of morphological phage descriptions in the year 2000. Brief review. *Archiv Virology* 146, 843–857.

Ackermann, H.W. (2003) Bacteriophage observations and evolution. *Research in Microbiology* 154, 245–251.

Alisky, J., Iczkowski, K., Rapaport, A. and Troitsky, N. (1998) Bacteriophages show promise as antimicrobial agents. *Journal of Infection* 36, 5–15.

Atterbury, R.J. and Allen, V.M. (2007) The use of bacteriophage to reduce the numbers of *Campylobacter* on the surface of chicken skin. *Zoonoses and Public Health* 54, 136–136.

Atterbury, R.J., Hobley, L., Till, R., Lambert, C., Capeness, M.J., Lerner, T.R., Fenton, A.K., Barrow, P. and Sockett, R.E. (2011) Effects of orally administered *Bdellovibrio bacteriovorus* on the well-being and *Salmonella* colonization of young chicks. *Applied and Environmental Microbiology* 77, 5794–5803.

Berchieri, A., Jr, Lovell, M.A. and Barrow, P.A. (1991) The activity in the chicken alimentary tract of bacteriophages lytic for *Salmonella typhimurium*. *Research in Microbiology* 142, 541–549.

Bigwood, T., Hudson, J.A., Billington, C., Carey-Smith, G.V. and Hememann, J.A. (2008) Phage inactivation of foodborne pathogens on cooked and raw meat. *Food Microbiology* 25, 400–406.

Biswas, B., Adhya, S., Washart, P., Paul, B., Trostel, A.N., Powell, B., Carlton, R. and Merril, C.R. (2002) Bacteriophage therapy rescues mice bacteremic from a clinical isolate of vancomycin-resistant *Enterococcus faecium*. *Infection and Immunity* 70, 204–210.

Bohez, L., Dewulf, J., Ducatelle, R., Pasmans, F., Haesebrouck, F. and Van Immerseel, F. (2008) The effect of oral administration of a homologous *hilA* mutant strain on the long-term colonization and transmission of *Salmonella* Enteritidis in broiler chickens. *Vaccine* 26, 372–378.

Borie, C., Albala, I., Sanchez, P., Sanchez, M.L., Ramirez, S., Navarro, C., Morales, M.A., Retamales, A.J. and Robeson, J. (2008) Bacteriophage treatment reduces *Salmonella* colonization of infected chickens. *Avian Diseases* 52, 64–67.

Borie, C., Sanchez, M.L., Navarro, C., Ramirez, S., Morales, M.A., Retamales, J. and Robeson, J. (2009) Aerosol spray treatment with bacteriophages and competitive exclusion reduces *Salmonella enteritidis* infection in chickens. *Avian Diseases* 53, 250–254.

Boyd, E.F. and Brussow, H. (2002) Common themes among bacteriophage-encoded virulence factors and diversity among the bacteriophages involved. *Trends in Microbiology* 10, 521–529.

Boyen, F., Pasmans, F., Van Immerseel, F., Morgan, E., Adriaensen, C., Hernalsteens, J.-P., Decostere, A., Ducatelle, R., and Haesebrouck, F. (2006) *Salmonella* Typhimurium SPI-1 genes promote intestinal but not tonsillar colonization in pigs. *Microbes and Infection* 8, 2899–2907.

Boyen, F., Haesebrouck, F., Vanparys, A., Volf, J., Mahu, M., Van Immerseel, F., Rychlick, I., Dewulf, J., Ducatelle, R. and Pasmans, F. (2008) Coated fatty acids alter virulence properties of *Salmonella* Typhimurium and decrease intestinal colonization of pigs. *Veterinary Microbiology* 132, 319–327.

Bruttin, A. and Brussow, H. (2005) Human volunteers receiving *Escherichia coli* phage T4 orally: a safety test of phage therapy. *Antimicrobial Agents and Chemotherapy* 49, 2874–2878.

Bruynoghe, R. and Maisin, J. (1921) Essais de therapeutique au moyem du bacteriophage. *Comptes Rendus des Séances et Mémoires de la Société de Biologie* 85, 1120–1121.

Carlton, R.M., Noordman, W.H., Biswas, B., De Meester, E.D. and Loessner, M.J. (2005) Bacteriophage P100 for control of *Listeria monocytogenes* in foods: Genome sequence, bioinformatic analyses, oral toxicity study, and application. *Regulatory Toxicology and Pharmacology* 43, 301–312.

Carvalho, C.M., Gannon, B.W., Halfhide, D.E., Santos, S.B., Hayes, C.M., Roe, J.M. and Azeredo, J. (2010) The *in vivo* efficacy of two administration routes of a phage cocktail to reduce numbers of *Campylobacter coli* and *Campylobacter jejuni* in chickens. *BMC Microbiology* 10, 232.

Chighladze, E., Alavidze, Z., Brown, T., Pasternack, G., Morris, J.G. and Sulakvelidze, A. (2001) Application of lytic phages for reducing contamination of poultry with selected *Salmonella* serotypes. *American Society for Microbiology General Meeting.* Available at: http://asmusa.org/memonly/abstracts/Abstractview.asp?AbstractID=4 9400 (accessed October 2002).

Clark, P.F. and Clark, A.S. (1927) A bacteriophage active against a virulent hemolytic streptococcus. *Proceedings of the Society for Experimental Biology and Medicine* 24, 635–639.

D'Herelle, F. (1917) Sur un microbe invisible antagoniste des bacilles dysenteriques. *Comptes rendus de l'Académie des sciences* 165, 373.

Dashiff, A. and Kadouri, D.E. (2011) Predation of oral pathogens by *Bdellovibrio bacteriovorus* 109J. *Molecular Oral Microbiology* 26, 19–34.

Dashiff, A., Junka, R.A., Libera, M. and Kadouri, D.E. (2011) Predation of human pathogens by the predatory bacteria *Micavibrio aeruginosavorus* and *Bdellovibrio bacteriovorus*. *Journal of Applied Microbiology* 110, 431–444.

Diez-Gonzalez, F. and Russell, J.B. (1997) The ability of *Escherichia coli* O157:H7 to decrease its intercellular pH and resist the toxicity of acetic acid. *Microbiology* 143, 1175–1180.

Dumonceaux, J.T., Hill, J.E., Hemmingsen, S.M. and Van Kessel, A.G. (2006) Characterisation of intestinal microbiota and response to dietary virginiamycin supplementation in the broiler chicken. *Applied and Environmental Microbiology* 72, 2815–2823.

Durant, J.A., Lowry, V.K., Nisbet, D.J., Stanker, L.H., Corrier, D.E. and Ricke, S.C. (1999) Short-chain fatty acids affect cell-association and invasion of Hep-2 cells by *Salmonella* Typhimurium. *Journal of Environmental Science and Health B* 34, 1083–1099.

Eaton, M.D. and Bayne-Jones, S. (1934) Bacteriophage therapy. *Journal of the American Medical Association* 103, 1769–1776.

Eeckhaut, V., Van Immerseel, F., Louis, P., Pasmans, F., Fievez, V., Haesebrouck, F., Ducatelle, R. and Vandamme, P. (2008) *Butyricicoccus pullicaecorum* gen. nov., sp. Nov., an anaerobic, butyrate producing bacterium isolated from the caecal content of a broiler chicken. *International Journal of Systematic and Evolutionary Microbiology* 58, 2799–2802.

Eeckhaut, V., Van Immerseel, F., Pasmans, F., De Brandt, E., Haesebrouck, F., Ducatelle, R. and Vandamme, P. (2010) *Anaerostipes butyraticus* sp. Nov., an anaerobic, butyrate-producing bacterium from Clotridium cluster XIVa, isolated from broiler chicken caecal content. *International Journal of Systematic and Evolutionary Microbiology* 60, 1108–1112.

Eeckhaut, V., Van Immerseel, F., Croubels, S., De Baere, S., Haesebrouck, F., Ducatelle, R., Louis, R. and Vandamme, P. (2011) Butyrate production in phylogenetically diverse firmicutes isolates from the chicken caecum. *Microbial Biotechnology* 4, 503–12

Flythe, M.D. and Russell, J.B. (2006) Fermentation acids inhibit amino acid deamination by Clostridium sporogenes MD1 via a mechanism involving a decline in intracellular glutamate rather than prootonmotive force. *Microbiology* 152, 2619–2624.

Flythe, M.D. and Russell, J.B. (2007) Effect of acidic pH on the ability of Clostridium sporogenes MD1 to take up and retain intracellular potassium. *FEMS Microbiology Letters* 267, 46–50.

Gantois, I., Ducatelle, R., Pasmans, F., Haesebrouck, F., Hautefort, I., Thompson, A., Hinton, J.C. and Van Immerseel, F. (2006) Butyrate specifically down-regulates *Salmonella* pathogenicity island I gene expression. *Applied and Environmental Microbiology 72*, 946–949.

Gebru, E., Lee, J.S., Son, J.C., Yang, S.Y., Shin, S.A., Kim, B., Kim, M.K. and Park, S.C. (2010) Effect of probiotic-, bacteriophage-, or organic acid-supplemented feeds or fermented soybean meal on the growth performance, acute-phase response, and bacterial shedding of grower pigs challenged with Salmonella enterica serotype Typhimurium. *Journal of Animal Science* 88(12), 3880–3886.

Gong, J., Forster, R.J., Yu, H., Chambers, J.R., Sabour, P.M., Wheatcroft, R. and Chen, S. (2002) Diversity and phylogenetic analysis of bacteria in the mucosa of chicken ceca and comparison with bacteria in the cecal lumen. *FEMS Microbiology Letters* 208, 1–7.

Goode, D., Allen, V.M. and Barrow, P.A. (2003) Reduction of experimental *Salmonella* and *Campylobacter* contamination of chicken skin by application of lytic bacteriophages. *Applied and Environmental Microbiology* 69, 5032–5036.

Guilloteau, P., Martin, L., Eeckhaut, V., Ducatelle, R., Zabielski, R. and Van Immerseel, F. (2010) From the gut to the peripheral tissues: the multiple effects of butyrate. *Nutrition Research Reviews* 23(2), 366–384.

Higgins, J.P., Higgins, S.E., Guenther, K.L., Huff, W., Donoghue, A.M., Donoghue, D.J. and Hargis, B.M. (2005) Use of a specific bacteriophage treatment to reduce *Salmonella* in poultry products. *Poultry Science* 84, 1141–1145.

Hinton, M. and Linton, A.H. (1988) Control of *Salmonella* infections in broiler chickens by the acid treatment of their feed. *The Veterinary Record* 123, 416-421.

Ho, T.D. and Slauch, J.M. (2001) OmpC is the receptor for Gifsy-1 and Gifsy-2 bacteriophages of *Salmonella*. *Journal of Bacteriology* 183, 1495–1498.

Hooton, S.P., Atterbury, R.J. and Connerton, I.F. (2011) Application of a bacteriophage cocktail to reduce *Salmonella* Typhimurium U288 contamination on pig skin. *International Journal of Food Microbiology* 151, 157–163.

Hsiao, C. and Siebert, K.J. (1999) Modelling the inhibitory effects of organic acids on bacteria. *International Journal of Food Microbiology* 47, 189–201.
Hume, M.E., Corrier, D.E., Ambrus, S., Hinton, A. and DeLoach, J.R. (1993) Effectiveness of dietary propionic acid in controlling *Salmonella* Typhimurium colonization in broiler chicks, *Avian Diseases* 37, 1051–1056.
Humphrey, T.J. and Lanning, D.G. (1988) The vertical transmission of *Salmonella* and formic acid treatment of chicken feed. *Epidemiology and Infection* 100, 43–49.
Huyghebaert, G., Ducatelle, R. and Van Immerseel, F. (2011) An update on alternatives to antimicrobial growth promoters for broilers. *Veterinary Journal* 187, 182–188.
Iba, A.M. and Berchieri, A. (1995) Studies on the use of a formic acid-propionic acid mixture (Bio-Add™) to control experimental *Salmonella* infection in broiler chickens. *Avian Pathology* 24, 303–311.
Kashket, E.R. (1987) Bioenergetics of lactic acid bacteria: cytoplasmic pH and osmotolerance. *FEMS Microbiology Reviews* 46, 233–244.
Kennedy J.E. and Bitton, G. (1987) Bacteriophages in foods. In: Goyal, S.M., Gerba, G.P. and Bitton, G. (eds) *Phage Ecology.* John Wiley & Sons, New York, pp. 289–316.
Khan, M. and Katamay, M. (1969) Antagonistic effects of fatty acids against *Salmonella* in meat and bone meal. *Applied Microbiology* 17, 402–404.
Kropinski, A.M. (2008) *Salmonella* phages and prophages – genomics and practical aspects. *Methods in Molecular Biology* 394, 133–175.
Krueger, A.P. and Scribner, E.J. (1941) The bacteriophage – its nature and its therapeutic use. *Journal of the American Medical Association* 116, 2160–2277.
Kutter, E. (2005) Phage therapy: Bacteriophages as natural, self-limiting antibiotics. In: Pizzorno, J.E. and Murray, M.T. (eds) *Textbook of Natural Medicine*, 3rd edn. Churchill Livingstone, London, pp. 1147–1161.
Kwon, Y.M. and Ricke, S.C. (1998) Induction of acid resistance of *Salmonella* Typhimurium by exposure to short-chain fatty acids. *Applied and Environmental Microbiology* 64, 3458–3463.
Lan, P.T., Hayashi, H., Sakamoto, M. and Benno, Y. (2002) Phylogenetic analysis of cecal microbiota in chicken by the use of 16S rDNA clone libraries. *Microbiology and Immunology* 46, 371–453.
Lawhon, S.D., Maurer, R., Suyemoto, M. and Altier, C. (2002) Intestinal short-chain fatty acids alter *Salmonella* Typhimurium invasion gene expression and virulence through BarA/SirA. *Molecular Microbiology* 46, 1451–1464.
Martin-Pelaez, S., Costabile, A., Hoyles, L., Rastall, R.A., Gibson, G.R., La Ragione, R.M., Woodward, M.J., Mateu, E. and Martin-Orue, S.M. (2010) Evaluation of the inclusion of a mixture of organic acids or lactulose into the feed of pigs experimentally challenged with Salmonella Typhimurium. *Veterinary Microbiology* 142, 337–345.
Merril, C.R., Biswas, B., Carlton, R., Jensen, N.C. and Creed, G.J. (1996) Long-circulating bacteriophage as antibacterial agents. *Proceedings of the National Academy of Sciences of the United States of America* 93, 3188–3192.
Messens, W., Goris, J., Dierick, N., Herman, L. and Heyndrickx, M. (2010) Inhibition of *Salmonella* Typhimurium by medium-chain fatty acids in an *in vitro* simulation of the porcine cecum. *Veterinary Microbiology* 141, 73–80.
Nakamura, M. (1972) Alteration of *Shigella* Pathogenicity by Other Bacteria. *American Journal of Clinical Nutrition* 25, 1441–1451.
O'Brien, A.D., Newland, J.W., Miller, S.F., Holmes, R.K., Smith, H.W. and Formal, S.B. (1984) Shiga-like toxin-converting phages from *Escherichia coli* strains that cause hemorrhagic colitis or infantile diarrhea. *Science* 226, 694–696.
O'Flynn, G., Coffey, A., Fitzgerald, G.F. and Ross, R.P. (2006) The newly isolated lytic bacteriophages st104a and st104b are highly virulent against *Salmonella enterica*. *Journal of Applied Microbiology* 101, 251–259.
Ochs, H.D., Davis, S.D. and Wedgwood, R.J. (1971) Immunologic responses to bacteriophage phi-X-174 in immunodeficiency diseases. *Journal of Clinical Investigation* 50, 2559–2568.
Payne, R.J. and Jansen, V.A. (2003) Pharmacokinetic principles of bacteriophage therapy. *Clinical Pharmacokinetics* 42, 315–325.
Pyle, N.J. (1926) The bacteriophage in relation to *Salmonella pullorum* infection in the domestic fowl. *Journal of Bacteriology* 12, 245–261.
Rohwer, F. and Edwards, R. (2002) The phage proteomic tree: a genome-based taxonomy for phage. *Journal of Bacteriology* 184, 4529–4535.

Russell, J.B. and Diez-Gonzalez, F. (1998) The effects of fermentation acids on bacterial growth. *Advances in Microbial Physiology* 39, 205–234.
Schwudke, D., Strauch, E., Krueger, M. and Appel, B. (2001) Taxonomic studies of predatory *Bdellovibrios* based on 16S rRNA analysis, ribotyping and the hit locus and characterization of isolates from the gut of animals. *Systematic and Applied Microbiology* 24, 385–394.
Sklar, I.B. and Joerger, R.D. (2001) Attempts to utilize bacteriophage to combat *Salmonella enterica* serovar Enteritidis infection in chickens. *Journal of Food Safety* 21, 15–30.
Smith, H.W. (1948) Calcium-deficient media; their effect on phage action. *Nature* 161, 397.
Smith, H.W. (1953) The effect of physical and chemical changes on the liberation of phage particles by lysogenic strains of *Salmonella*. *Journal of General Microbiology* 8, 116–134.
Smith, H.W. (1978) Arsenic resistance in *enterobacteria*: its transmission by conjugation and by phage. *Journal of General Microbiology* 109, 49–56.
Smith, H.W. and Huggins, M.B. (1982) Successful treatment of experimental *Escherichia coli* infections in mice using phage: its general superiority over antibiotics. *Journal of General Microbiology* 128, 307–318.
Smith, H.W. and Huggins, M.B. (1983). Effectiveness of phages in treating experimental *Escherichia coli* diarrhoea in calves, piglets and lambs. *Journal of General Microbiology* 129(8), 2659–2675.
Smith, H.W. and Parsell, Z. (1974) The effect of virulence of converting the O antigen of *Salmonella choleraesuis* from 627 to 617 by phage. *Journal of General Microbiology* 81, 217–224.
Smith, H.W., Green, P. and Parsell, Z. (1983) Vero cell toxins in *Escherichia coli* and related bacteria: transfer by phage and conjugation and toxic action in laboratory animals, chickens and pigs. *Journal of General Microbiology* 129, 3121–3137.
Smith, H.W., Hugins, M.B. and Shaw, K.M. (1987a) The control of experimental *Escherichia coli* diarrhoea in calves by means of bacteriophages. *Journal of General Microbiology* 133, 1111–1126.
Smith, H.W., Huggins, M.B. and Shaw, K.M. (1987b) Factors influencing the survival and multiplication of bacteriophages in calves and in their environment. *Journal of General Microbiology* 133 (5), 1127–1135.
Sockett, R.E. (2009) Predatory lifestyle of *Bdellovibrio bacteriovorus*. *Annual Review of Microbiology* 63, 523–539.
Sockett, R.E. and Lambert, C. (2004) *Bdellovibrio* as therapeutic agents: a predatory renaissance? *Nature Reviews Microbiology* 2, 669–675.
Sprong, R.C., Hulstein, M.F.E. and Van der Meer, R. (2001) Bactericidal activities of milk lipids. *Antimicrobial Agents and Chemotherapy* 45, 1298–1301.
Stolp, H. and Starr, M.P. (1963) *Bdellovibrio bacteriovorus* gen. et sp. n., a predatory, ectoparasitic, and bacteriolytic microorganism. *Antonie Van Leeuwenhoek* 29, 217–248.
Sulakvelidze, A. and Barrow, P. (2005) Phage therapy in animals and agribusiness. In: Kutter, E. and Sulakvelidze, A. (eds) *Bacteriophages: biology and applications*. CRC Press, Boca Raton, Florida.
Sulakvelidze, A. and Kutter, E. (2005) Bacteriophage therapy in humans. In: Kutter, E. and Sulakvelidze, A. (eds) *Bacteriophages: biology and applications*. CRC Press, Boca Raton, Florida.
Sulakvelidze, A., Alavidze, Z. and Morris, J.G., Jr (2001) Bacteriophage therapy. *Antimicrobial Agents and Chemotherapy* 45, 649–659.
Taube, V.A., Neu, M.E., Hassan, Y., Verspohl, J., Beyerbach, M. and Kamphues, J. (2009) Effects of dietary additives (potassium diformate/organic acids) as well as influences of grinding intensity (coarse/fine) of diets for weaned piglets experimentally infected with *Salmonella* Derby or *Escherichia coli*. *Journal of Animal Physiology and Animal Nutrition* 93, 350–358.
Thompson, J.L. and Hinton, M. (1997) Antibacterial activity of formic and propionic acids in the diet of hens on *Salmonella*s in the crop. *British Poultry Science* 38, 59–65.
Thormar, H., Hilmarsson, H. and Bersson, G. (2006) Stable concentrated emulsions of the 1-monoglyceride of capric acid (monocaprin) with microbicidal activities against the food-borne bacteria *Campylobacter jejuni*, *Salmonella* spp., and *Escherichia coli*. *Applied and Environmental Microbiology* 72, 522–526.
Toro, H., Price, S. B., McKee, S., Hoerr, F.J., Krehling, J., Perdue, M. and Bauermeister, L. (2005) Use of bacteriophages in combination with competitive exclusion to reduce *Salmonella* from infected chickens. *Avian Diseases* 49, 118–124.
Twort, F.W. (1915) An investigation on the nature of the ultra microscopic viruses. *Lancet* 2, 1241.
Van Essche, M., Quirynen, M., Sliepen, I., Loozen, G., Boon, N., Van Elderle, J. and Teughels, W. (2011) Killing of anaerobic pathogens by predatory bacteria. *Molecular Oral Microbiology* 26, 52–61.

Van Immerseel, F., De Buck, J., Meulemans, G., Pasmans, F., Velge, P., Bottreau, E., Haesebrouck, F. and Ducatelle, R. (2003) Invasion of *Salmonella* Enteritidis in avian intestinal epithelial cells *in vitro* is influenced by short-chain fatty acids. *International Journal of Food Microbiology* 85, 237–248.

Van Immerseel, F., De Buck, J., Boyen, F., Bohez, L., Pasmans, F., Volf, J., Sevcik, M., Rychlik, I., Haesebrouck, F. and Ducatelle, R. (2004a) Medium-chain fatty acids decrease colonization and invasion shortly after infection with *Salmonella* Enteritidis in chickens through *hilA* suppression. *Applied and Environmental Microbiology* 70, 3582–3587.

Van Immerseel, F., De Buck, J., De Smet, I., Pasmans, F., Haesebrouck, F. and Ducatelle, R. (2004b) Interactions of butyric acid and acetic acid-treated *Salmonella* with chicken primary cecal epithelial cells *in vitro*. *Avian Diseases* 48, 384–391.

Van Immerseel, F., Fievez, V., De Buck, J., Pasmans, F., Martel, A., Haesebrouck, F. and Ducatelle, R. (2004c) Microencapsulated short-chain fatty acids in feed modify colonization and invasion early after infection with *Salmonella* Enteritidis in young chickens. *Poultry Science* 83, 69–74.

Van Immerseel, F., Boyen, F., Gantois, I., Timbermont, L., Bohez, L., Pasmans, F., Haesebrouck, F. and Ducatelle, R. (2005) Supplementation of coated butyric acid in the feed reduces colonization and shedding of *Salmonella* in poultry. *Poultry Science* 84, 1851–1856.

Van Immerseel, F., Russell, J.B., Flythe, M.D., Gantois, I., Timbermont, L., Pasmans, F., Haesebrouck, F. and Ducatelle, R. (2006) The use of organic acids to combat *Salmonella* in poultry: a mechanistic explanation of the efficacy. *Avian Pathology* 35, 182–188.

Wagner, P.L. and Waldor, M.K. (2002) Bacteriophage control of bacterial virulence. *Infection and Immununity* 70, 3985–3993.

Waldor, M.K. (1998) Bacteriophage biology and bacterial virulence. *Trends in Microbiology* 6, 295–297.

Wall, S.K., Zhang, J., Rostagno, M.H. and Ebner, P.D. (2010) Phage therapy to reduce preprocessing *Salmonella* infections in market-weight swine. *Applied and Environmental Microbiology* 76, 48–53.

Waseh, S., Hanifi-Moghaddam, P., Coleman, R., Masotti, M., Ryan, S., Foss, M., Mackenzie, R., Henry, M., Szymanski, C.M. and Tanha, J. (2010) Orally administered P22 phage tailspike protein reduces *Salmonella* colonization in chickens: prospects of a novel therapy against bacterial infections. *PLoS One* 5, e13904.

Weber-Dabrowska, B., Mulczyk, M. and Gorski, A. (2000) Bacteriophage therapy of bacterial infections: an update of our institute's experience. *Archivum Immunologiae et Therapiae Experimentalis* 48, 547–551.

Westergaard, J.M. and Kramer, T.T. (1977) *Bdellovibrio* and intestinal flora of vertebrates. *Applied and Environmental Microbiology* 34, 506–511.

Wilkinson, M.H. (2001) Predation in the presence of decoys: an inhibitory factor on pathogen control by bacteriophages or bdellovibrios in dense and diverse ecosystems. *Journal of Theoretical Biology* 208, 27–36.

Zhu, X.Y., Zhong, Y., Pandya, Y. and Joerger, R.D. (2002) 16S rRNA-based analysis of microbiota from the cecum of broiler chickens. *Applied and Environmental Microbiology* 68, 124–137.

Index